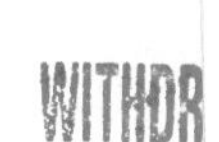

McGraw-Hill's
NAPLEX®
Review Guide

McGraw-Hill's NAPLEX® Review Guide

Editor

S. Scott Sutton, PharmD, BCPS (AQ ID)

Associate Clinical Professor
Department of Clinical Pharmacy & Outcomes Sciences
South Carolina College of Pharmacy
University of South Carolina
Columbia, South Carolina

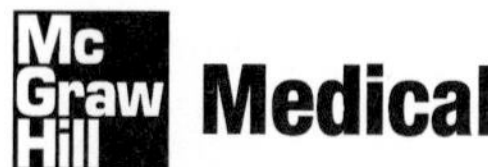

New York Chicago San Francisco Lisbon London Madrid Mexico City
Milan New Delhi San Juan Seoul Singapore Sydney Toronto

The McGraw-Hill Companies

McGraw-Hill's NAPLEX® Review Guide

1 2 3 4 5 6 7 8 9 0 QDB/QDB 14 13 12 11 10

Set ISBN 978-0-07-163012-2
Set MHID 0-07-163012-0
Book ISBN 978-0-07-175562-7
Book MHID 0-07-175562-4
CD-ROM ISBN 978-0-07-175496-5
CD-ROM MHID 0-07-175496-2

This book was set in Minion Pro by Glyph International.
The editors were Michael Weitz and Robert Pancotti.
The production supervisor was Catherine H. Saggese.
Project management was provided by Arushi Chawla, Glyph International.
The text designer was Elise Lansdon.
Quad/Graphics was printer and binder.

This book is printed on acid-free paper.

Library of Congress Cataloging-in-Publication Data

McGraw-Hill's NAPLEX review guide / by editor S. Scott Sutton.
p. ; cm.
Other title: NAPLEX review guide
Includes index.
ISBN-13: 978-0-07-163012-2 (pbk. : alk. paper)
ISBN-10: 0-07-163012-0 (pbk. : alk. paper)
1. Pharmacy—Outlines, syllabi, etc. 2. Pharmacy—Examinations, questions, etc. I. Sutton, S. Scott (Shawn Scott) II. Title: NAPLEX review guide.
[DNLM: 1. Pharmaceutical Preparations—Examination Questions. 2. Pharmaceutical Preparations—Outlines. 3. Drug Therapy—Examination Questions. 4. Drug Therapy—Outlines. QV 18.2]
RS98.M37 2010
615'.1—dc22

2010027272

To my students

You have inspired and challenged me for years; therefore, I have developed and dedicated this book for you. My desire is that this textbook will inspire and challenge you to be the best pharmacist you can be and to serve others; and I hope you ace the NAPLEX®.

About the Editor

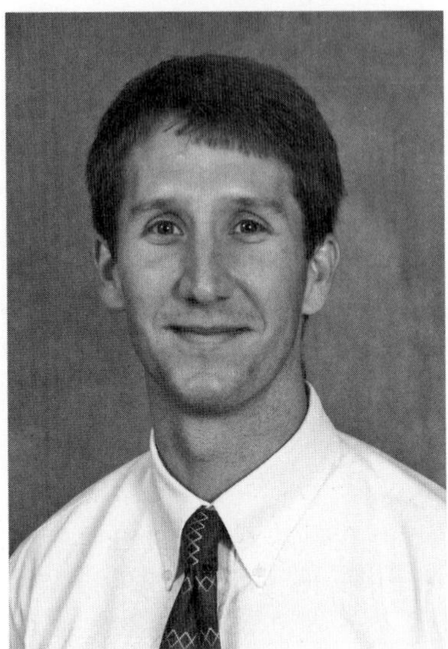

S. Scott Sutton, PharmD, BCPS (AQ ID), is an Associate Clinical Professor in the Department of Clinical Pharmacy and Outcomes Sciences at the South Carolina College of Pharmacy (SCCP). He received his Bachelor of Science and Doctor of Pharmacy degrees from the University of South Carolina and completed a clinical pharmacy residency in medicine and infectious diseases at the W.J.B. Dorn Veterans Affairs Medical Center in Columbia, South Carolina. He teaches in Pharmacotherapy, Pharmacokinetics, Clinical Applications, Infectious Diseases Pharmacotherapy, and Clinical Research. He also directs the clinical research program at the Dorn Research Institute for the postgraduate year-one pharmacy residents. His practice site is at the Veterans Affairs Medical Center in the areas of infectious diseases, internal medicine, and clinical research. He has received Teacher and Researcher of the Year awards from the University of South Carolina and has served as sports medicine pharmacist for the Department of Athletics. He is an educational consultant for Morris Cody and Associates, for which he teaches a national NAPLEX® Review course. He has taught thousands of students in this review course and continues teaching the course every spring. He is an avid Gamecock Fan, golfer, and guitarist. He enjoys spending time with his wife and they are expecting their first child in March 2011.

Contents

PART 11 Health and Wellness and Other Topics

Contributors

Jarrett R. Amsden, PharmD, BCPS
Assistant Professor, Department of Pharmacy Practice, Butler University College of Pharmacy and Health Sciences, Indianapolis, Indiana

Miranda R. Andrus, PharmD, BCPS, FCCP
Associate Clinical Professor of Pharmacy Practice, Auburn University Harrison School of Pharmacy, Huntsville, Alabama

Jennifer Baldock, PharmD
Oncology Pharmacy Specialty Resident, Department of Clinical Pharmacy, University of California, San Francisco, California

Charles L. Bennett, MD, PhD, MPP
COEE Endowed Chair in Mediation, Saftey and Efficacy, Frank P. and Josie M. Fletcher Professor of Pharmacy, South Carolina College of Pharmacy, University of South Carolina, Columbia, South Carolina

Elizabeth W. Blake, PharmD, BCPS
Clinical Associate Professor, Department of Clinical Pharmacy and Outcomes Sciences, South Carolina College of Pharmacy—University of South Carolina Campus, Columbia, South Carolina

Christopher M. Bland, PharmD, BCPS
Critical Care Pharmacist, Dwight D. Eisenhower Army Medical Center, Fort Gordon, Georgia

P. Brandon Bookstaver, PharmD, BCPS
Clinical Assistant Professor, Department of Clinical Pharmacy & Outcomes Sciences, University of South Carolina Campus, Columbia, South Carolina

Nancy Borja-Hart, PharmD, BCPS
Assistant Professor, Nova Southeastern University College of Pharmacy; Clinical Pharmacist, Sanford L. Ziff Health Care Center (Clinical Pharmacy), Fort Lauderdale, Florida

John A. Bosso, PharmD, FCCP, FIDSA
Professor and Chair, Department of Clinical Pharmacy & Outcome Sciences and Division of Infectious Diseases, Medical University of South Carolina, College of Medicine, Charleston, South Carolina

Michelle M. Bottenberg, PharmD, BCPS
Assistant Professor, Department of Clinical Sciences, College of Pharmacy and Health Sciences, Drake University, Des Moines, Iowa

Wendy Brown, PharmD, MPAS, PA-C, AE-C
Allergy and Asthma Care Center, North Dakota State University College of Pharmacy, Nursing, and Allied Sciences, Fargo, North Dakota

Reamer L. Bushardt, PharmD, PA-C
Associate Professor and Director, Division of Physician Assistant Studies, Medical University of South Carolina, Charleston, South Carolina

Joshua Caballero, PharmD, BCPP
Assistant Professor, Department of Pharmacy Practice, College of Pharmacy, Nova Southeastern University, Fort Lauderdale, Florida

Matthew A. Cantrell, PharmD, BCPS
Assistant Professor, University of Iowa College of Pharmacy; Clinical Pharmacy Specialist, Veterans Administration Medical Center, Iowa City, Iowa

Rachel S. Cathey, PharmD, CGP
Clinical Pharmacy Coordinator, W.J.B. Dorn Veterans Administration Medical Center, Columbia, South Carolina

Betty M. Chan, PharmD, BCOP
Assistant Professor of Clinical Pharmacy, University of Southern California School of Pharmacy; Clinical Pharmacist, University of Southern California/ Norris Comprehensive Cancer Center and Hospital, Los Angeles, California

Steven W. Chen, PharmD, FASHP
Associate Professor of Clinical Pharmacy and Pharmaceutical Economics & Policy, University of Southern California School of Pharmacy, Los Angeles, California

Vince Colucci, PharmD, BCPS
Associate Professor, Department of Pharmacy Practice, Skaggs School of Pharmacy, The University of Montana College of Health Professions and Biomedical Sciences, Missoula, Montana

Sheryl L. Compton, PharmD
Assistant Professor, Drake University; Clinical Pharmacist, Jordan Creek Internal Medicine, Des Moines, Iowa

Kristen Cook, PharmD, BCPS
Assistant Professor, Pharmacy Practice, University of Nebraska Medical Center College of Pharmacy, Omaha, Nebraska

Daniel G. Dauner, PharmD, MSPH, BCPS
Pharmacy Clinical Coordinator, St. Luke's Hospital, Duluth, Minnesota

David L. DeRemer, PharmD, BCOP
Clinical Assistant Professor, University of Georgia College of Pharmacy, Augusta, Georgia

Darla Klug Eastman, PharmD, BCPS
Assistant Professor of Pharmacy Practice, Drake University, College of Pharmacy and Health Sciences, Des Moines, Iowa

Rebecca F. Edwards, PharmD, BCPS, CDE, CPP
Instructor, General Internal Medicine, Wake Forest University School of Medicine; Clinical Assistant Professor, University of North Carolina Eshelman School of Pharmacy, Winston-Salem, North Carolina

Shareen Y. El-Ibiary, PharmD, BCPS
Associate Professor of Pharmacy Practice, Department of Pharmacy Practice, Midwestern University College of Pharmacy—Glendale, Glendale, Arizona

Benjamin J. Epstein, PharmD, BCPS
Assistant Professor of Pharmacy and Medicine, University of Florida, Gainesville, Florida; and President, East Coast Institute for Research, Jacksonville, Florida

Carmen M. Faulkner, PharmD, BCPS
Clinical Pharmacy Specialist in Infectious Diseases, Department of Pharmacy, Greenville Hospital System, University Medical Center, Greenville, South Carolina

Michele A. Faulkner, PharmD
Associate Professor of Pharmacy Practice and Medicine, School of Pharmacy and Health Professions, Creighton University, Omaha, Nebraska

Anisa Fornoff, PharmD
Assistant Professor, Clinical Sciences, Drake University, Des Moines, Iowa

Howell R. Foster, PharmD
Associate Professor, University of Arkansas for Medical Sciences, College of Pharmacy; Director, Arkansas Poison Control Center, Little Rock, Arkansas

L. Clifton Furman, PhD, RPh
Professor of Pharmaceutics, Presbyterian College School of Pharmacy, Clinton, South Carolina

Jennifer Ellis Girotto, PharmD, BCPS
Assistant Clinical Professor of Pharmacy Practice and Pediatrics, University of Connecticut Schools of Pharmacy and Medicine, Storrs, Connecticut

Amy D. Grant, PharmD
Director of Experimental Education, Clinical Assistant Professor, South Carolina College of Pharmacy—University of South Carolina Campus, Columbia, South Carolina

Joy B. Greene, PharmD
Assistant Professor of Pharmacy, Wingate University School of Pharmacy, Oakboro, North Carolina

William Joshua Guffey, PharmD
Clinical Assistant Professor, University of Georgia College of Pharmacy, Augusta, Georgia

Philip D. Hall, PharmD, FCCP, BCPS, BCOP
Professor, South Carolina College of Pharmacy, Hollings Cancer Center, Medical University of South Carolina, Charleston, South Carolina

Karly A. Hegge, PharmD, BCPS
Assistant Professor of Pharmacy Practice, South Dakota State University College of Pharmacy, Brookings, South Dakota

Brian A. Hemstreet, PharmD, BCPS
Department of Clinical Pharmacy, University of Colorado Denver School of Pharmacy, Aurora, Colorado

Mary L. Hewett, MS, PA-C
Assistant Professor, Medical University of South Carolina, College of Health Professions—Physician Assistant Program, Charleston, South Carolina

Ian B. Hollis, PharmD, BCPS
Clinical Specialist, Cardiothoracic Surgery, University of North Carolina Hospitals, Clinical Assistant Professor, University of North Carolina School of Pharmacy, Chapel Hill, North Carolina

Kristin K. Horning, PharmD, BCPS
Assistant Professor (Clinical), University of Iowa College of Pharmacy; Clinical Pharmacist, East Des Moines Family Care Center, Des Moines, Iowa

Kendrea M. Jones, PharmD, BCPS
Assistant Professor, University of Arkansas for Medical Sciences, College of Pharmacy; Clinical Pharmacist, Arkansas Children's Hospital, Little Rock, Arkansas

Margaret R. Jorgenson, PharmD, NCPS
Clinical Pharmacist, University of Wisconsin Hospital and Clinics Pharmacy—Inpatient Services, Madison, Wisconsin

Michael Kelly, PharmD, MS
Assistant Dean for Professional Education; Associate Professor, University of Iowa College of Pharmacy, Iowa City, Iowa

Jessica L. Kerr, PharmD, CDE
Assistant Professor, Southern Illinois University Edwardsville, School of Pharmacy, Edwardsville, Illinois

Carrie Foust Koenigsfeld, PharmD
Associate Professor, Department of Clinical Sciences, Drake College of Pharmacy and Health Sciences, Des Moines, Iowa

Peter J. S. Koo, PharmD
Clinical Professor of Pharmacy, University of California, San Francisco; Pharmacist Specialist, Pain Management, University of California Medical Center, San Francisco, California

Catherine H. Kuhn, PharmD
Pharmacist, Mansfield Patient Care Center, The Kroger Co., Mansfield, Ohio

Kelly C. Lee, PharmD, BCPP
Assistant Professor of Clinical Pharmacy, University of California, San Diego, California; Skaggs School of Pharmacy and Pharmaceutical Sciences, La Jolla, California

Donna Leverone, PharmD
Pharmacy Practice Resident, College of Medicine & Pharmacy, University of Florida—Shands Hospital, University of Florida, Gainesville, Florida

Daniel S. Longyhore, PharmD, BCPS
Department of Pharmacy Practice, Nesbitt College of Pharmacy & Nursing, Wilkes University, Wilkes-Barre, Pennsylvania

Bryan L. Love, PharmD, BCPS
Assistant Professor, South Carolina College of Pharmacy, University of South Carolina; Clinical Pharmacist, W.J.B. Dorn Veterans Administration Medical Center, Columbia, South Carolina

Tracy E. Macaulay, PharmD, BCPS
Assistant Professor (Adjunct), University of Kentucky College of Pharmacy and Clinical Pharmacy, Specialist—Cardiology, Department of Pharmacy Services, University of Kentucky Healthcare, Lexington, Kentucky

Jehan Marino, PharmD, BCPP
Assistant Professor, Department of Pharmacy Practice, College of Pharmacy, Nova Southeastern University, Fort Lauderdale, Florida

Keith R. McCain, PharmD, CSPI
Poison Control Specialist, Arkansas Poison Control Center; Assistant Professor, Department of Pharmacy Practice, University of Arkansas for Medical Sciences, College of Pharmacy, Little Rock, Arkansas

Karen H. McGee, PharmD, CDE
Certified Diabetes Educator (CDE) and Clinical Faculty, University of South Carolina College of Pharmacy, Columbia, South Carolina

Danny McNatty, PharmD, BCPS
Assistant Professor, Department of Pharmacy Practice, Midwestern University College of Pharmacy—Glendale, Glendale, Arizona

Lisa T. Meade, PharmD, CDE
Assistant Professor, Wingate University School of Pharmacy, Wingate, North Carolina

April D. Miller, PharmD, BCPS
Clinical Assistant Professor, South Carolina College of Pharmacy—University of South Carolina Campus; Clinical Pharmacy Specialist—Critical Care, Palmetto Health Richland, Columbia, South Carolina

Sarah J. Miller, PharmD, MS, BCNSP
Professor, University of Montana Skaggs School of Pharmacy; Pharmacy Clinical Coordinator, Saint Patrick Hospital and Health Sciences Center, Missoula, Montana

Michael P. Moranville, PharmD, BCPS
Clinical Pharmacy Specialist, Cardiology, University of Chicago Medical Center, Chicago, Illinois

Kathryn K. Neill, PharmD
Assistant Professor, University of Arkansas for Medical Sciences, College of Pharmacy; Clinical Pharmacist—Medical Intensive Care Unit, University Hospital of Arkansas, Little Rock, Arkansas

LeAnn B. Norris, PharmD, BCPS, BCOP
Assistant Professor, South Carolina College of Pharmacy—University of South Carolina Campus, Columbia, South Carolina

Kelly K. Nystrom, PharmD, BCOP
Associate Professor, Department of Pharmacy Practice, Creighton University School of Pharmacy and Health Professions, Omaha, Nebraska

Rory E. O'Callaghan, PharmD
Fellow in Ambulatory Care and Academia, University of Southern California, School of Pharmacy, Los Angeles, California

Thomas F. Oppelt, PharmD, BCPS
Regional Account Scientific Director, U.S. Medical Affairs and Regional Associate Scientific Director—Field Medical, Novartis Pharmaceutical Corporation, Wilmington, North Carolina

Kathleen Packard, PharmD, MS, BCPS
Assistant Professor, Department of Pharmacy Practice, Creighton University School of Pharmacy and Health Professions, Omaha, Nebraska

Jeong M. Park, MS, PharmD, BCPS
Clinical Associate Professor, Department of Clinical, Social and Administrative Sciences, College of Pharmacy; Clinical Transplant Pharmacist, Department of Pharmacy Services, University of Michigan, Ann Arbor, Michigan

Susie H. Park, PharmD, BCPP
Assistant Professor of Clinical Pharmacy, Titus Family Department of Clinical Pharmacy and Pharmaceutical Economics and Policy, University of Southern California, School of Pharmacy, Los Angeles, California

Krina H. Patel, PharmD
Assistant Professor, Department of Pharmacy Practice, Nesbitt College of Pharmacy and Nursing, Wilkes University, Wilkes-Barre, Pennsylvania

Beth Bryles Phillips, PharmD, FCCP, BCPS
Clinical Associate Professor, University of Georgia; Clinical Pharmacy Specialist, Charlie Norwood Veterans Administration Medical Center, Athens, Georgia

Cynthia M. Phillips, PharmD, CDE
Clinical Assistant Professor, South Carolina College of Pharmacy—University of South Carolina Campus, Columbia, South Carolina

Amy M. Pick, PharmD, BCOP
Assistant Professor, Department of Pharmacy Practice, Creighton University School of Pharmacy and Health Professions, Omaha, Nebraska

Patricia H. Powell, PharmD, BCPS
Clinical Assistant Professor, South Carolina College of Pharmacy—University of South Carolina Campus, Columbia, South Carolina

Alison M. Reta, PharmD
Fellow in Ambulatory Care and Academia, University of Southern California, School of Pharmacy, Los Angeles, California

Jo Ellen Rodgers, PharmD, FCCP, BCPS
Clinical Associate Professor, Eshelman School of Pharmacy, University of North Carolina—Chapel Hill, Chapel Hill, North Carolina

Brea O. Rowan, PharmD, BCPS
Clinical Pharmacy Specialist, Princeton Baptist Medical Center, Affiliate Clinical Faculty, Auburn University, Birmingham, Alabama

Randall C. Rowen, PharmD
Dean and Associate Professor, South Carolina College of Pharmacy—University of South Carolina Campus, Columbia, South Carolina

Laurajo Ryan, PharmD, MSc, BCPS, CDE
Clinical Assistant Professor, Pharmacotherapy Division, College of Pharmacy, The University of Texas—Austin; Department of Medicine & Pharmacotherapy Education Research Center, University of Texas Health Science Center, San Antonio, Texas

Julie M. Sease, PharmD, RPh, BCPS, CDE
Associate Professor of Pharmacy Practice, Presbyterian College School of Pharmacy, Clinton, South Carolina

Marintha R. Short, PharmD, BCPS
Clinical Pharmacy Specialist—Cardiology and Critical Care, Saint Joseph Hospital, Lexington, Kentucky

Douglas Slain, PharmD, BCPS, FCCP
Associate Professor, Infectious Diseases Specialist, West Virginia University, Morgantown, West Virginia

Lisa S. Smith, PharmD, BCPS
Assistant Professor, Wingate University School of Pharmacy, Wingate, North Carolina

Winter J. Smith, PharmD, BCPS
Assistant Professor, Department of Pharmacy, Clinical and Administrative Sciences, The University of Oklahoma Health Sciences Center College of Pharmacy; Clinical Pharmacist—Internal Medicine, Oklahoma University Medical Center, Oklahoma City, Oklahoma

Jessica Starr, PharmD, BCPS
Assistant Professor of Pharmacy Practice, Auburn University, Harrison School of Pharmacy, Birmingham, Alabama

Sharm Steadman, PharmD, BCPS CDE
Professor, Department of Family and Preventive Medicine, University of South Carolina School of Medicine, Columbia, South Carolina

S. Scott Sutton, PharmD, BCPS (AQ ID)
Associate Clinical Professor, Department of Clinical Pharmacy & Outcomes Sciences, South Carolina College of Pharmacy, University of South Carolina, Columbia, South Carolina

Robert K. Sylvester, PharmD
Associate Professor, Department of Pharmacy Practice, College of Pharmacy, Nursing and Allied Health, North Dakota State University; Clinical Specialist—Oncology, MeritCare Hospital, Fargo, North Dakota

Nancy Culberson Taylor, RPh, CDE
Instructor and Labs Coordinator, South Carolina College of Pharmacy, Columbia, South Carolina

Robyn Teply-Kondrack, PharmD, MBA
Assistant Professor, Department of Pharmacy Practice, Creighton University School of Pharmacy and Health Professions, Omaha, Nebraska

Sarah R. Tomasello, PharmD, BCPS
Clinical Associate Professor, Rutgers—The State University of New Jersey; Clinical Specialist, Nephrology, Robert Wood Johnson University Hospital, New Bruswick, New Jersey

John C. Voris, PharmD
Professor, South Carolina College of Pharmacy, University of South Carolina; Clinical Pharmacist, W.J.B. Dorn Veterans Administration Medical Center, Columbia, South Carolina

Scott M. Vouri, PharmD
PGY-1, Pharmacy Resident, Iowa City Veterans Administration Medical Center, Iowa City, Iowa

Kurt A. Wargo, PharmD, BCPS
Associate Clinical Professor, Department of Pharmacy Practice, Auburn University School of Pharmacy, Auburn, Alabama

T. Scott Warmack, PharmD, BCPS
Associate Professor, University of Arkansas for Medical Sciences, College of Pharmacy; Clinical Pharmacy Specialist, Central Arkansas Veterans Healthcare System, Little Rock, Arkansas

Holly J. Watson, RPh, PharmD
Clinical Assistant Professor, South Carolina College of Pharmacy, Columbia, South Carolina

Karen Whalen, PharmD, BCPS, CDE
Clinical Associate Professor, Department of Pharmacotherapy & Translational Research, University of Florida College of Pharmacy, Seminole, Florida

Patrick T. Wong, PharmD, BCPS, BCOP
Health Sciences Assistant Professor, Department of Clinical Pharmacy, School of Pharmacy, University of California, San Francisco, San Francisco, California

Assistant Editors

P. Brandon Bookstaver, PharmD, BCPS (AQ-ID), AAHIVE
South Carolina College of Pharmacy—University of South Carolina Campus, Columbia, South Carolina

Shareen Y. El-Ibiary, PharmD, BCPS
Midwestern University College of Pharmacy—Glendale, Glendale, Arizona

McKenzie C. Ferguson, PharmD, BCPS
Southern Illinois University Edwardsville, School of Pharmacy, Edwardsville, Illinois

Jessica L. Kerr, PharmD, CDE
Southern Illinois University Edwardsville, School of Pharmacy, Edwardsville, Illinois

April D. Miller, PharmD, BCPS
South Carolina College of Pharmacy—University of South Carolina Campus, Columbia, South Carolina

LeAnn B. Norris, PharmD, BCPS, BCOP
South Carolina College of Pharmacy—University of South Carolina Campus, Columbia, South Carolina

Julie M. Sease, PharmD, RPh, BCPS, CDE
Presbyterian College School of Pharmacy, Clinton, South Carolina

Peer Reviewers

Amanda M. Ball, PharmD, BCPS
The Hospital of the University of Pennsylvania, Philadelphia, Pennsylvania

Aida Rebecca Bickley, PharmD
Department of Pharmacy, Saint Joseph Hospital, Lexington, Kentucky

P. Brandon Bookstaver, PharmD, BCPS (AQ-ID), AAHIVE
South Carolina College of Pharmacy—University of South Carolina Campus, Columbia, South Carolina

Carole Bradley, PharmD, BCPS
Veterans Administration Medical Center, St. Louis, Missouri

Adrian Carlson, PharmD
Palmetto Health Richland, Columbia, South Carolina

Michael A. Dietrich, PharmD, BCPS
Midwestern University College of Pharmacy—Glendale, Glendale, Arizona

Emily A. Dill, PharmD
W.J.B. Dorn Veterans Administration Medical Center, Columbia, South Carolina

Cecily V. DiPiro, PharmD
Consultant Pharmacist, Charleston, South Carolina

Christian R. Dolder, PharmD, BCPS
Wingate University School of Pharmacy, Wingate, North Carolina

Brianne L. Dunn, PharmD
South Carolina College of Pharmacy, University of South Carolina, Columbia, South Carolina

Shareen Y. El-Ibiary, PharmD, BCPS
Midwestern University College of Pharmacy—Glendale, Glendale, Arizona

Ginger M. Eubank, PharmD
W.J.B. Dorn Veterans Administration Medical Center, Columbia, South Carolina

McKenzie C. Ferguson, PharmD, BCPS
Southern Illinois University Edwardsville, School of Pharmacy, Edwardsville, Illinois

Patrick R. Finley, PharmD, BCPP
University of California, San Francisco, California

Alicia B. Forinash, PharmD, BCPS, CCD
St. Louis College of Pharmacy, St. Louis, Missouri

L. Clifton Fuhrman, PhD, RPh
Presbyterian College School of Pharmacy, Clinton, South Carolina

Mandy L. Gatesman, PharmD, BCOP
Virginia Commonwealth University Health System, Richmond, Virginia

Douglas R. Geraets, PharmD, FCCP
Veterans Affairs Medical Center, Iowa City, Iowa

Lew Iacovelli, BS, PharmD, BCOP, CPP
The Moses Cone Regional Cancer Center, Greensboro, North Carolina

Tommy Johnson, PharmD, BC-ADM, CDE, FAADE
Presbyterian College School of Pharmacy, Clinton, South Carolina

Whitney A. Jones, PharmD
Wake Forest University Baptist Medical Center, Winston-Salem, North Carolina

Nicole M. Kase, PharmD
Veterans Administration Ann Arbor Healthcare System, Ann Arbor, Michigan

Kenneth Kennedy, PharmD
Saint Joseph Hospital, Lexington, Kentucky

Jessica L. Kerr, PharmD, CDE
Southern Illinois University Edwardsville, School of Pharmacy, Edwardsville, Illinois

Mary Lee, PharmD, BCPS, FCCP
Midwestern University, Downers Grove, Illinois

Laura Rickles Lehman, PharmD, BCPS, CACP
Carroll Hospital Center, Westminster, Maryland

Lisa M. Lundquist, PharmD, BCPS
Mercer University College of Pharmacy and Health Sciences, Atlanta, Georgia

J. Christopher Lynch, PharmD
Southern Illinois University Edwardsville, School of Pharmacy, Edwardsville, Illinois

Shalini S. Lynch, PharmD
University of California, School of Pharmacy, San Francisco, California

Heather Mandeville, PharmD, BCPS
SSM St. Mary's Health Center, St. Louis, Missouri

Karen H. McGee, PharmD, CDE
South Carolina College of Pharmacy—University of South Carolina and Palmetto SeniorCare, Columbia, South Carolina

Lewis N. McKelvey Jr., PharmD
Presbyterian College School of Pharmacy, Clinton, South Carolina

April D. Miller, PharmD, BCPS
South Carolina College of Pharmacy—University of South Carolina Campus, Columbia, South Carolina

Meredith T. Moorman, PharmD, BCOP
University of Oklahoma College of Pharmacy, Oklahoma City, Oklahoma

Khuong An Nguyen, PharmD
Saint Joseph Hospital, Lexington, Kentucky

LeAnn B. Norris, PharmD, BCPS, BCOP
South Carolina College of Pharmacy—University of South Carolina Campus, Columbia, South Carolina

Thomas F. Oppelt, PharmD, BCPS
U.S. Medical Affairs–Field Medical, Novartis Pharmaceutical Corporation, Wilmington, North Carolina

Adam B. Pesaturo, PharmD, BCPS
Baystate Medical Center, Springfield, Massachusetts

Kimberly A. Pesaturo, PharmD, BCPS
Massachusetts College of Pharmacy & Health Sciences—Worcester, Worcester, Massachusetts

Christina C. Piro, PharmD
Palmetto Health Children's Hospital, Columbia, South Carolina

Jamie M. Pitlick, PharmD
St. Louis College of Pharmacy, St. Louis, Missouri

David J. Quan, PharmD, BCPS
University of California, San Francisco, School of Pharmacy and UCSF Medical Center, San Francisco, California

Christie Robinson, PharmD, BCPS
University of California, San Francisco, School of Pharmacy, San Francisco, California

Celeste N. Rudisill, PharmD
South Carolina College of Pharmacy—University of South Carolina Campus, Columbia, South Carolina

J. Mark Ruscin, PharmD, BCPS
Southern Illinois University Edwardsville, School of Pharmacy, Edwardsville, Illinois

Julie M. Sease, PharmD, RPh, BCPS, CDE
Presbyterian College School of Pharmacy, Clinton, South Carolina

David W. Stewart, PharmD, BCPS
East Tennessee State University, Bill Gatton College of Pharmacy, Johnson City, Tennessee

Javad Tafreshi, PharmD, BCPS (AQ Cardiology)
Loma Linda University School of Pharmacy, Loma Linda, California

Erin M. Timpe, PharmD, BCPS
Southern Illinois University Edwardsville, School of Pharmacy, Edwardsville, Illinois

John C. Voris, PharmD
W.J.B. Dorn Veterans Administration Medical Center—Mental Health Service Line, Columbia, South Carolina

Abigail M. Yancey
St. Louis College of Pharmacy, St. Louis, Missouri

Preface

The North American Pharmacist Licensure Examination (NAPLEX®) measures a candidate's knowledge of pharmacy practice. The examination is used by Boards of Pharmacy as part of the assessment of a candidate's competency to practice pharmacy. The National Association of Boards of Pharmacy (NABP) publishes a competency statement that provides a blueprint of the topics covered in the examination. The blueprint offers important information about the knowledge and skills that are expected for an entry-level pharmacist. The NAPLEX® competency statement may be viewed at www.napb.net. The three areas of competency include:

- Assess pharmacotherapy to assure safe and effective therapeutic outcomes (56% of exam)
- Assess safe and accurate preparation and dispensing of medications (33% of exam)
- Assess, recommend, and provide health care information that promotes public health (11% of exam)

The *NAPLEX® Review Guide* published by McGraw-Hill has been organized around the NABP competencies and is designed to assist students in their preparation of the exam, stimulate critical thinking, consolidate key information, advance knowledge, and improve exam-taking ability.

The textbook was developed and reviewed by pharmacists, faculty, students, recent graduates, and education consultants with a priority focus on the NABP competency statements.

I have taught a NAPLEX® review course for Morris Cody and Associates since 2005 and have instructed thousands of students representing over 70 schools of pharmacy. I have been in a unique position to be able to talk with students and new graduates from across the country and discuss with them what they need to be successful when taking the exam and as a practicing pharmacist. The input given by the students and the faculty, pharmacists, and educational consultants was instrumental in the organization, development, and content of this textbook. As there are many ways to assess knowledge, there are equally as many ways to prepare for an exam. People are different and thrive in different preparatory methods. The development of this textbook was tailored to various learning and studying styles.

Each chapter within the textbook contains the following sections: Foundation Overview, Prevention or Treatment, Case Application questions, and Takeaway Points. The Foundation Overview consists of a general overview of the topic, pathophysiology, clinical presentation, and diagnosis. The Prevention or Treatment section provides a general overview and goals of prevention or treatment, followed by a focus on specific agents including indication, route of administration, rationale for use, and adverse reactions. Several chapters have incorporated and developed tables and figures for enhancement of the material in the chapter. The Case Application section is extremely unique and will provide students and graduates ample opportunity to apply their knowledge in each of the 70 chapters. Each chapter contains at least 20 case application questions (more than 1400 questions within the textbook). The case application questions are based on the material within the chapter with a focus on the NABP competency statements. Numerous students discussed with me their need and desire to have a lot of questions, especially questions that can serve as teaching points. Therefore, each case application question is provided with a detailed answer section at the end of the book. For each question, there is an explanation of why the correct answer is correct and why the other choices are incorrect. This is a valuable tool that you can tailor to your specific learning or studying style. At the end of each chapter, the Case Application questions are followed by the Takeaway Points section. The Takeaway Points summarize the key concepts within the text to bring together all the information you have studied and reviewed.

Finally, the textbook offers two complete practice exams on the accompanying CD-ROM. The 185-question practice exams (370 total questions) test the student's ability to measure pharmacotherapy and therapeutic outcomes, evaluate medications, and implement and recommend information for optimal patient care. The goal of the practice exams is to measure your knowledge and ability. The exams should be taken as you would take the NAPLEX®. Your goal during the practice exams should be to mimic the testing experience as closely as possible and identify areas that you need to continue reviewing.

The *NAPLEX® Review Guide* published by McGraw-Hill was developed for students and graduates to assist in their preparation of studying for the NAPLEX®. The textbook contains 70 chapters, more than 1400 case application questions with detailed explanations, and two practice exams. The textbook will assist in your preparation for the NAPLEX® and will also help you to improve your problem-solving skills and exam-taking ability, consolidate key information, and advance your knowledge base. In addition, the book can serve as a great resource for keeping up with pharmacy in the future after you have passed the NAPLEX®.

S. Scott Sutton
December 2010

Acknowledgments

I would like to acknowledge the commitment and dedication of the contributing authors and peer reviewers of the chapters contained within this text. I am very grateful to the staff of McGraw-Hill, especially Michael Weitz, Robert Pancotti, and Laura Libretti, for the opportunity to develop this textbook and for their dedication to this project. Finally, I would like to thank the students, graduates, faculty, pharmacists, and educational consultants who provided feedback for the development and design of this textbook.

PART

1 Cardiovascular Disorders

CHAPTER

1 Acute Decompensated Heart Failure

Ian B. Hollis and Jo Ellen Rodgers

FOUNDATION OVERVIEW

Acute decompensated heart failure (ADHF) is the leading cause of hospital admission in patients age 65 and older.[1] It is estimated that Americans are hospitalized for approximately 6.5 million patient-days per year due to this condition.[2] In 2009, the projected sum of direct and indirect costs from heart failure (HF) admissions is $36.2 billion with the majority of cost associated with hospitalization care.[3]

Unfortunately, patients who are hospitalized for ADHF have a high readmission rate in the 6 months following discharge.[2] Depending on the severity of disease, rates of in-hospital mortality range from 2% to 19%.[4] Despite the serious nature of the problem, relatively few prospective, randomized, clinical trials have been conducted to address the optimal treatment strategy for ADHF.

Pathophysiology

ADHF is commonly characterized by a relatively rapid (over days to weeks) decrease in cardiac output (CO) which triggers a variety of compensatory mechanisms in an attempt to maintain hemodynamic stability. Ultimately, activation of these compensatory neurohormonal pathways may result in fluid retention and vasoconstriction, both of which can further compromise cardiac function. Acute decompensation is frequently a consequence of disease progression in patients with chronic heart failure (HF).[5] It may also stem from medication or lifestyle noncompliance, such as failing to take evidence-based chronic heart failure medications as prescribed or indulging in excessive sodium or water intake (or both).

Key Definitions

ADHF = acute decompensated heart failure
BP = blood pressure
BNP = brain natriuretic peptide
CO = cardiac output
CI = cardiac index
EF = ejection fraction
HF = heart failure
HR = heart rate
PCWP = pulmonary capillary wedge pressure
RAAS = renin-angiotensin-aldosterone system
SNS = sympathetic nervous system
SVR = systemic vascular resistance
SV = stroke volume

Alternatively, ADHF may occur abruptly as a result of an acute insult such as the onset of atrial fibrillation, acute coronary syndrome, pneumonia, myocarditis, acute valvular dysfunction, acute kidney failure, or pulmonary embolism, among others.[6]

All of the above etiologies involve damage to or increased strain on cardiac tissue, triggering a series of neurohormonal responses. In response to a reduction in cardiac output and resultant hypoperfusion, activation of the sympathetic nervous system (SNS) and the renin-angiotensin-aldosterone system (RAAS) manifests as increased secretion of norepinephrine as well as angiotensin II and aldosterone, respectively. These effects are beneficial in maintaining cardiac output and vital organ perfusion in the short term; however, chronic activation of these systems worsens cardiac function in the long term. Chronic SNS activation can cause vasoconstriction, thereby increasing systemic vascular resistance (SVR, also known as afterload) and negative myocardial remodeling, and worsening pump dysfunction.[5] Activation of the RAAS also results in vasoconstriction as well as collagen deposition with fibrosis and further remodeling of myocardial tissue. In addition, RAAS activation causes renal sodium and water retention which increases intravascular fluid volume (also known as preload).[5]

Still another hormonal mechanism that occurs during ADHF is secretion of arginine vasopressin. Vasopressin acts as a vasoconstrictor and also causes free water retention, eventually leading to hyponatremia. The acute benefits of vasopressin are increased filling pressures (preload), which allow for preservation of stroke volume (SV) in the setting of declining cardiac function.

B-type natriuretic peptide (BNP) is secreted from ventricular tissue in response to the fluid overload and ventricular wall stretch. The physiologic effect of BNP is to induce natriuresis as well as venous and arterial vasodilation.[5] Unfortunately, an increased release of endogenous BNP only mildly attenuates the aforementioned negative compensatory neurohormonal cascade.[4]

Hemodynamic Equations

$BP = CO \times SVR$
$CO = SV \times HR$
$CI = CO/BSA$
$EF = (LVEDV - LVESV)/LVEDV$

The role of BNP in diagnosis and treatment of ADHF will be discussed in detail below.

Diagnosis

The presenting signs and symptoms of ADHF vary with degree of underlying disease. They are predominantly associated with fluid accumulation in a variety of locations throughout the body. Pulmonary symptoms such as dyspnea and orthopnea and signs such as rales, wheezing, and hypoxemia are often associated with an elevated pulmonary capillary wedge pressure (PCWP), a marker of fluid overload in the pulmonary vasculature. Peripheral edema, found in the lower extremities, abdomen (ascites), and liver (hepatomegaly, hepatojugular reflux) are systemic signs and symptoms of fluid overload. "Congested" patients may also present with some degree of systemic hypertension.[1,6]

Patients with "low output" cardiac failure are admitted with a different subset of clinical markers. Such patients may be fluid overloaded or congested as described above, presenting with a hypervolemic hyponatremia that is very characteristic of this type of HF. They may also present with signs and symptoms of end organ hypoperfusion. This may be evidenced by elevated serum creatinine (SCr), elevated hepatic transaminases, gut ischemia (manifesting as pain or vomiting with eating) or altered mental status. These patients may also present with hypotension, with systolic blood pressures (BP) of 90 to 100 mm Hg or lower.[1,6] It is important to confirm that such patients have adequate filling pressures, since a low volume state may contribute to or be the sole cause of low cardiac output.

A helpful biochemical marker in the diagnosis of ADHF is BNP. When used in conjunction with patient history and physical examination, the laboratory measurement of BNP can be especially helpful in distinguishing whether a patient who presents with acute dyspnea is suffering from ADHF or another condition altogether. It has been determined in clinical trials that a BNP level above 100 pg/mL is highly sensitive for ADHF and BNP levels below 50 pg/mL are likely due to an alternate, non-HF cause, such as pneumonia or a pulmonary embolism.[1,7]

Placement of a Swan-Ganz pulmonary artery catheter (PAC) may be helpful in distinguishing the precise cardiopulmonary hemodynamics of patients with ADHF. While such hemodynamic parameters may assist in determining an appropriate treatment course in select patients, the ESCAPE Trial demonstrated that routine PAC use did not improve outcomes but rather increased the number of adverse events experienced.[8] Subsequently, PAC use is not routinely recommended, and should only be employed in complex patients who do not respond to initial therapy, in patients whose volume status cannot be reliably assessed clinically, or in those who become hemodynamically unstable during treatment.[1]

Hemodynamic parameters acquired from PAC use can assist in providing some rough categorizations of patients presenting with ADHF, which may guide therapy. Patients with low cardiac index (CI < 2.2 L/min/m^2) are often referred to as "cold" due to the inability to perfuse, resulting in cold, clammy extremities. Patients with a CI > 2.2 L/min/m^2 who have reasonable perfusion to their extremities may be termed "warm." Another useful PAC measurement is the pulmonary capillary wedge pressure, a marker of intravascular fluid status and ventricular filling pressures. Normal, healthy persons have a PCWP approximately 10 mm Hg,[9] but those with chronic heart failure may require a PCWP of approximately 15 to 18 to optimize cardiac output in dilated ventricles. Patients with a PCWP >18 mm Hg are generally considered to be "wet," frequently presenting with signs and symptoms of fluid overload, with those with a PCWP of 15 to 18 mm Hg being termed "dry" (dry being a relative term for euvolemia). Using these measurements, patients may be classified as "warm and wet," "cold and wet," "warm and dry," or "cold and dry."[6] In addition to cardiac performance and fluid status values, a PAC also allows for the calculation of SVR. With a normal value of 800 to 1200 dyne/cm/s,[5] SVR represents the degree of arterial vasoconstriction with values >1200 representing a state of vasoconstriction and values <800 representing a state of vasodilation.[9]

TREATMENT

Goals of Therapy/Prognosis

The immediate goals of treatment for ADHF are return of the patient to hemodynamic stability and correction of pulmonary edema and other systemic fluid overload, which should reverse or remit the signs and symptoms that led to the hospital admission. Attempts should also be made to identify and manage any treatable underlying cause.[1,6] Hospital admissions also represent an important opportunity to educate patients about their disease, enact lifestyle modifications (such as sodium restriction or cardiovascular risk factor modification), and improve or optimize the patient's chronic oral HF medication regimen.[1]

Upon admission for ADHF, it is important to understand the severity of the patient's disease. Registry data has shown that on admission some key factors can be identified as predictors of poor prognosis: blood urea nitrogen (BUN) >43 mg/dL, systolic blood pressure <115 mm Hg, and serum creatinine >2.75 mg/dL. Risk increases incrementally as these factors are present alone or in combination, reaching approximately 20% in-hospital mortality during an ADHF admission if all three factors are present.[4] Hyponatremia as well as elevated serum troponin in the absence of acute coronary syndrome are also prognostic for poor outcomes.[6,10] Patients with these markers should be considered for mechanical assistance measures, or even transplant, as described in the section titled Nonpharmacologic Treatments below.

Pharmacologic Treatment

Initial Management of Chronic Heart Failure Medications

Well-managed patients with previously diagnosed HF will have a regimen of chronic, oral, home medications that may need to be temporarily modified upon admission for ADHF.

If patients present with hypotension (SBP <90 mm Hg), it may be necessary to decrease dose or even discontinue any evidence-based home medications that lower blood pressure such as angiotensin-converting enzyme inhibitors (ACE-inhibitors, such as enalapril, lisinopril, and ramipril), angiotensin receptor blockers (ARBs, such as valsartan, candesartan, and losartan), beta-blockers (such as carvedilol, metoprolol succinate, or bisoprolol), or the combination of hydralazine and isosorbide dinitrate. If beta-blocker initiation or uptitration is determined to be the cause of ADHF, a reduction in beta-blocker dose to the previously tolerated dose should occur. Discontinuation of beta-blocker therapy should only be considered in the setting of overt cardiogenic shock.[6]

Other chronic HF medications, such as spironolactone or digoxin, may need to be held during an ADHF admission if a patient presents with some degree of acute renal dysfunction. Spironolactone and ACE inhibitors can cause hyperkalemia, a condition that may be worsened in the setting of decreased urine output, and digoxin has a significant component of renal clearance, making accumulation and toxicity a concerning possibility. Measuring a serum digoxin level may be useful to determine whether it is safe to continue treatment. In the absence of the above situations, it is reasonable to continue these oral medications during inpatient ADHF treatment.

Intravenous Diuretics

The pharmacologic treatment of ADHF in patients who present with signs and symptoms of fluid overload should always begin with loop diuretics, given specifically by the intravenous (IV) route. When administered intravenously, loop diuretics can rapidly reduce elevated ventricular filling pressures and decrease PCWP by blocking sodium and chloride resorption in the Loop of Henle of the kidney, leading to osmotic fluid excretion.[1]

The type of loop diuretic used is unimportant; furosemide, bumetanide, and torsemide are all equally effective at equipotent doses. (Ethacrynic acid is a loop diuretic for patients with an allergic reaction to furosemide, bumetanide, and torsemide.) Administration is usually by intermittent boluses; doses of furosemide commonly range from 40 to 120 mg IV two to three times daily. The dose and frequency are often related to the patient's diuretic dose prior to admission and the perceived degree of fluid overload. To enhance diuresis in patients with inadequate urine output *after* initial intermittent bolus doses, it may be necessary to increase the dose size or to add a thiazide diuretic (such as oral hydrochlorothiazide or IV chlorothiazide) or a thiazide-like diuretic (such as metolazone) to the loop diuretic to reduce the reabsorption of sodium (and water) in the distal convoluted tubule.[1] Another viable alternative for diuretic resistance is the continuous infusion of loop diuretics.[1,11] Initial doses of furosemide infusions are commonly 5 to 15 mg/h, with titration to response. Table 1-1 lists IV diuretics used to treat heart failure related fluid retention.

Those who respond to loop diuretics should experience a net fluid loss of 1 to 2 L or more of urine every 24 hours, losing several kilograms of body weight each day in the process. At the initiation of treatment, it is useful to ascertain the "dry weight" or "goal weight" of a given patient which can serve as a goal for extent and duration of diuresis.[1]

It is very important to monitor for the adverse effects of loop diuretics during their administration. When rapid diuresis ensues, hypotension may be seen due to intravascular volume depletion, as mobilization of extravascular fluid into the intravascular space lags behind the rate of urinary fluid elimination. Monitoring of BP by arterial line or blood pressure cuff should occur at frequent intervals.[1] Decreased renal function and electrolyte abnormalities (hypokalemia, hypomagnesemia, and hyponatremia) are also common in patients exposed to high doses of loop diuretics, and thus, frequent laboratory monitoring should occur. When thiazide or thiazide-like diuretics are added to loop diuretics, the above hypotension and electrolyte abnormalities may be worsened, as well as potential for blood glucose variations and hyperuricemia leading to worsening of preexisting gout. Thiazides will also cause increased photosensitivity; patients should be counseled to take measures to avoid excessive sun exposure.

Intravenous Vasodilators

When patients present with hypertension and elevated SVR, in conjunction with congestive symptoms and an elevated PCWP (usually >20 mm Hg), IV vasodilator therapy is a reasonable concomitant therapy to IV loop diuretics. The three commonly used IV vasodilators for ADHF are nitroglycerin, nesiritide, and nitroprusside. ADHF guidelines indicate that these

TABLE 1-1 Intravenous Diuretics Used to Treat Heart Failure–Related Fluid Retention

	Onset of Action (min)	Duration of Action (h)	Relative Potency	Intermittent Bolus Dosing (mg)	Continuous Infusion Dosing (Bolus/Infusion)
Furosemide	2-5	6	40	20-200+	20-40/2.5-20
Torsemide	<10	6-12	20	10-100	20/2-10
Bumetanide	2-3	4-6	0.5	1-10	1-4/0.5-1
Ethacrynic acid	5-15	2-7		0.5-1 mg/kg/dose up to 100 mg/dose	

Adapted with permission from Vardeny O, Ng TMH. Heart failure. In: Chisholm-Burns MA, Wells BG, Schwinghammer TL, et al. *Pharmacotherapy Principles & Practice.* New York, NY: McGraw-Hill; 2008:33-61.

medications should be considered for rapid improvement in congestive symptoms in patients who do not present with low blood pressure (SBP <90 mm Hg).[1,6]

Nitroglycerin is a nitric oxide donor that leads to vascular smooth muscle relaxation and vasodilation. When given by IV infusion, nitroglycerin will reduce preload through the dilation of the venous blood vessels leading to a decrease in ventricular filling pressures and a reduction in pulmonary artery pressures.[12] This can serve to lessen wall strain on a failing ventricle that is occurring due to volume overload. Nitroglycerin will also dilate coronary arteries, lessening the effect of ADHF caused by acute or chronic ischemia. Nitroglycerin can be initiated at approximately 5 to 10 μg/min and titrated upward based on response, usually to dose of approximately 30 to 40 μg/min. At higher doses (>100 μg/min) nitroglycerin will also dilate the arterial vasculature, decreasing afterload and SVR and indirectly increasing cardiac output. Continuous BP monitoring is important with nitroglycerin, as hypotension is a common adverse effect. As with any nitrate, patients may also complain of headache.[6] If nitroglycerin is continuously infused for a period longer than 12 hours, nitrate tolerance may develop, necessitating increasing doses to maintain the pharmacologic effect.

Nesiritide is a recombinant BNP molecule that bears the same physiologic actions as the naturally occurring chemical, including natriuresis, venodilation, and arterial vasodilation. When administered as a continuous IV infusion, nesiritide has been shown to rapidly decrease PCWP,[13] indirectly increase cardiac output by decreasing SVR, and assist in diuresis when coadministered with loop diuretics. Nesiritide may be administered with or without a 2 μg/kg bolus dose, followed by a 0.01 μg/kg/min continuous infusion and titrated based on response. As with other vasodilators, frequent blood pressure monitoring is required, and the use of nesiritide in patients with low blood pressure on admission should be avoided. The impact of nesiritide on long-term outcomes such as renal function and mortality is currently being investigated.

Nitroprusside presents a third option for patients requiring vasodilation. It is a nitric oxide donor with potent effects on the smooth muscle of the vascular wall, which dilates venous and arterial vasculature equally and is also a potent pulmonary vasodilator. Nitroprusside will quickly decrease pulmonary artery pressures, while also decreasing preload and afterload, with a net increase in cardiac output. The ability to acutely dilate the pulmonary arteries has led to the use of nitroprusside in the assessment of a patient with pulmonary hypertension for heart transplant candidacy.[6] Response to nitroprusside as demonstrated by a decrease in pulmonary artery systolic pressures (PAS) indicates reversibility of pulmonary hypertension, which is a requirement for heart transplant listing.[1,6] Like the other vasodilators mentioned above, diligent blood pressure monitoring should be an expectation for patients receiving nitroprusside. Dosing begins approximately 0.1 to 0.2 μg/kg/min, with incremental titrations to effect (max dose: 10 μg/kg/min; doses >3 μg/kg/min are rarely necessary). Caution should be exercised in patients with hepatic and/or renal dysfunction, as nitroprusside is broken down to cyanide ion in the bloodstream, and the cyanide is conjugated to thiocyanate in the liver and excreted via the kidney. Hepatic or renal dysfunction can lead to accumulation of these toxic by-products; use in these patients should be very carefully monitored. This accumulation tends to be dose and time dependent; lower dose, shorter duration infusions are safer.[1,6]

Through acute vasodilatory effects, vasodilators are useful for quickly improving the subjective symptoms of pulmonary congestion in ADHF patients. They can assist in the mobilization of excess fluid volume by decreasing afterload, allowing the failing heart to successfully pump blood to the kidney for diuresis. Having a short half-life, they may also assist with transitioning patients to long-acting oral vasodilators used to manage chronic HF. It is important, however, to understand that the use of IV vasodilators, like other ADHF therapies, has not been shown to have a beneficial effect on mortality.[1]

Intravenous Inotropes

Some patients with low cardiac output present with low systolic blood pressure or low SVR, making them poor candidates for vasodilator therapy. In addition, diuretic refractory patients may require additional pharmacologic therapy to augment diuresis or experience worsening renal function with diuretic administration. In such situations, inotropic therapy is recommended.[1,6] Options include IV dobutamine and milrinone.

Dobutamine is an IV, nonselective beta-adrenergic receptor agonist, with some mild alpha-1-adrenergic effects. Clinically, dobutamine acts as a potent inotrope (increasing ventricular contractility) and chronotrope (increasing heart rate [HR]), with vasodilation due to the beta-2 effects and vasoconstriction due to the alpha-1 effects on peripheral vasculature. The net result is an increase in cardiac output with a very mild decrease in SVR. Initial doses frequently range from 2 to 5 μg/kg/min, with titration to effect (max dose: 20 μg/kg/min). Given the short half-life of dobutamine (~2 minutes), increases in cardiac output will often be seen within 10 minutes.[6,14]

Milrinone, an IV phosphodiesterase III (PDE_3) inhibitor, decreases the breakdown of cyclic adenosine monophosphate (cAMP) in cardiac tissue to result in an increase in cardiac contractility and output.[6,14] By increasing cAMP in vascular smooth muscle, systemic and pulmonary vascular resistance are also reduced, and thus, milrinone is often referred to as an "inodilator." Given its vasodilatory effects, milrinone should be used with caution in patients with hypotension.[6,14] Milrinone has a 30 to 60 minute half-life and is renally excreted. Accumulation can occur when used at normal doses in patients with renal dysfunction. Milrinone is administered at an initial dose of 0.1 to 0.375 μg/kg/min (max dose: 0.75 μg/kg/min). While a bolus dose may be considered, it is frequently avoided given the added risk of hypotension.

Both dobutamine and milrinone are useful agents for the acute management of ADHF, but they carry important cautions. Both drugs may cause sinus tachycardia and arrhythmias such as atrial fibrillation and ventricular tachycardia.[1,15] Dobutamine may induce hypokalemia due to robust stimulation of beta-receptors. There is also concern that administration of inotropes in the setting of ADHF may potentially worsen long-term prognosis.[1,14] In the OPTIME-CHF trial, patients with ADHF experienced sixfold more adverse events when treated with milrinone compared to placebo with no benefit in outcomes.[15] While still a very important option for the treatment of ADHF, inotropes should be reserved for managing patients being bridged to surgical devices or heart transplant or for palliative care of end-stage patients. See Tables 1-2 and 1-3 for hemodynamic effects, doses, and monitoring of commonly used IV agents for treatment of acute heart failure.

Nonpharmacologic Treatment

Pharmacologic treatment of episodes of ADHF can be augmented by mechanical support. Short-term options such as ultrafiltration and intra-aortic balloon pumps (IABPs) assist with the acute management of an exacerbation, and permanent options such as left ventricular assist devices (LVADs) and heart transplantation can be very helpful in prolonging survival and improving quality of life.

Ultrafiltration can be a safe and effective mechanism for removing excess fluid volume when diuretics and vasodilators prove unsuccessful or are undesirable. Much like continuous veno-venous hemofiltration (used for kidney failure), it removes water from the vasculature through cannulation of the venous system and filtration of excess water from the blood. Studies have shown this procedure to be a reasonable option for fluid removal (in lieu of IV diuretics) for patients admitted for ADHF.[16]

IABPs, consisting of a pneumatically inflated balloon at the end of a long catheter, can be inserted through a femoral artery and threaded up the aorta until the balloon rests just past the descending aortic arch. A mechanical pump deflates the balloon during systole, creating a small vacuum which decreases afterload, assisting with cardiac output. The balloon then inflates during diastole, forcing blood backward to the ascending aorta to aid in perfusion of the coronary arteries, which can improve cardiac oxygen supply and decrease ongoing ischemia.[6]

Heart transplantation remains the gold standard nonpharmacologic treatment for end-stage HF patients. Five- and 10-year year survival rates are approximately 70% and 50%, respectively.[17] Unfortunately, a limited number of organs (~4000) are available for transplantation each year, drastically less than the number of patients requiring them, leading to the development and improvement of the LVAD.

When acute and chronic medications prove unable to prolong life, and death seems imminent within 6 months, placement of an LVAD can prolong survival and markedly improve quality of life for several more years.[18,19] An LVAD is a small, mechanical pump (either pulsatile or axial continuous flow) that is permanently placed in the left ventricle, pumping blood into the aorta at a rate comparable to a normally functioning

TABLE 1-3 **Doses and Monitoring of Commonly Used Hemodynamic Medications**

Drug	Dose	Monitoring Variables[a]
Dobutamine	2.5-20 μg/kg/min	BP, HR urinary output and function, ECG
Milrinone	0.1-0.75 μg/kg/min	BP, HR, urinary output and function, ECG, changes in ischemic symptoms (eg, chest pain), electrolytes
Nitroprusside	0.25-3 μg/kg/min	BP, HR, liver and kidney function, blood cyanide and/or thiocyanate concentrations if toxicity suspected (nausea, vomiting, altered mental function)
Nitroglycerin	5-200+ μg/kg/min	BP, HR, ECG, changes in ischemic symptoms
Nesiritide	Bolus: 2 μg/kg Infusion: 0.01 μg/kg/min	BP, HR, urinary output and kidney function, blood BNP concentrations

[a]In addition to pulmonary capillary wedge pressure and cardiac output.

Abbreviations: BNP, B-type natriuretic peptide; BP, blood pressure; ECG, electrocardiogram; HR, heart rate.

Adapted with permission from Vardeny O, Ng TMH. Heart failure. In: Chisholm-Burns MA, Wells BG, Schwinghammer TL, et al. *Pharmacotherapy Principles & Practice.* New York, NY: McGraw-Hill; 2008:33-61.

TABLE 1-2 **Hemodynamic Effects of Commonly Used Intravenous Agents for Treatment of Acute or Severe Heart Failure**

Drug	CO	PCWP	SVR	BP	HR
Diuretics	↑/↓/0	↓		↓	0
Nitroglycerin	↑	↓↓	↓	↓↓	↑/0
Nitroprusside	↑	↓↓↓	↓↓↓	↓↓↓	↑
Nesiritide	↑	↓↓	↓↓	↓↓	0
Dobutamine	↑↑	↓/0	↓/0	↓/0	↑↑
Milrinone	↑↑	↓↓	↓	↓	↑

Abbreviations: BP, blood pressure; CO, cardiac output; HR, heart rate; PCWP, pulmonary capillary wedge pressure; SVR, systemic vascular resistance; ↑, increase; ↓, decrease; 0, no or little change.

Adapted with permission from Vardeny O, Ng TMH. Heart failure. In: Chisholm-Burns MA, Wells BG, Schwinghammer TL, et al. *Pharmacotherapy Principles & Practice.* New York, NY: McGraw-Hill; 2008:33-61.

heart. Patients' New York Heart Association HF functional class can significantly improve providing patients with a good medical option while they await heart transplantation.

Transition to Chronic Heart Failure Medications

Once patients have returned to a baseline fluid balance and have been successfully weaned from IV medications, attention turns to implementing the chronic, oral HF medications that will blunt disease progression, prolong life, and/or prevent readmission for further ADHF treatment.

The cornerstones of chronic heart failure treatment are ACE inhibitors and β-blockers. When titrated to the target doses, these agents have been demonstrated to reduce mortality, reduce hospitalizations, and improve quality of life. Other evidence-based medications that may improve long-term outcome in patients with ejection fraction (EF) < 35% to 40% are spironolactone, digoxin, and the combination of isosorbide dinitrate and hydralazine.

Also, when patients are admitted with ADHF, certain steps should be taken prior to their discharge to assure compliance with the American College of Cardiology/American Heart Association (ACC/AHA) Inpatient HF performance measures.[20] Measurement and documentation of LV systolic function before arrival, during the admission, or planning for measurement after discharge should be done. In the absence of contraindications, patients with HF should also be discharged with a prescription for an ACE-I or an ARB, and those with atrial fibrillation and HF should be prescribed an anticoagulant. Thorough discharge counseling and smoking cessation education should also be completed before a patient leaves the hospital. Adherence to these measures helps to ensure that HF care is optimized.

CASE Application

Questions 1 through 3 pertain to the following case.

JP is a 73-year-old man with nonischemic cardiomyopathy (EF 30%-35%) presenting to the emergency department (ED) with an acute HF exacerbation. His vital signs include BP 145/80 mm Hg, HR 92 beats per minute (bpm), respiratory rate (RR) 23 rpm, and O_2 sat 96% on 4 L/min of oxygen by nasal cannula (NC). Physical examination reveals 16 cm jugular venous distension (JVD), regular rate and rhythm (RRR), crackles bilaterally, and 3+ bilateral lower extremity edema. He admits to a 20-lb weight gain in the past 3 weeks since his carvedilol dose was increased and reports strict adherence to both dietary restrictions and medications. In the ED, he has already received a furosemide 40 mg IV × 1 dose with minimal response in urine output. Pertinent laboratory results include potassium 4.1 mmol/L, BNP 950 pg/mL, BUN 41 mg/dL, and creatinine 1.5 mg/dL (baseline). JP's home medications include enalapril 10 mg twice daily, carvedilol 12.5 mg twice daily, digoxin 0.125 mg/d, and furosemide 40 mg orally twice daily.

1. Based on the BNP result, JP is experiencing which one of the following?
   a. Active myocardial ischemia
   b. Shortness of breath due to a noncardiac etiology
   c. Significant volume overload and ventricular wall stretch
   d. Renal insufficiency

2. Which one of the following interventions is the best for JP on arrival to the intensive care unit (ICU)?
   a. Dobutamine 2.5 μg/kg/min infusion
   b. Milrinone 0.375 μg/kg/min infusion
   c. Furosemide 80 mg IV twice daily
   d. Metolazone 10 mg po now and then daily

3. Which of the following is appropriate management of JP's beta-blocker at this time?
   a. Continue carvedilol 12.5 mg twice daily.
   b. Increase carvedilol to 25 mg twice daily.
   c. Decrease carvedilol to 6.25 mg twice daily.
   d. Discontinue carvedilol.

4. Which of the following should be closely monitored during IV diuretic administration?
   a. Hypernatremia
   b. Hypertension
   c. Hypokalemia
   d. Hypouricemia

Questions 5 and 6 pertain to the following case.

AL is a 68-year-old woman complaining of "always tired these days." Her exercise tolerance is significantly less than it was 3 months ago; she now has to rest during daily activities. This has come on gradually. She has a history of hypertensive cardiomyopathy (LVEF 30% by ECHO 1 year ago). She is compliant with both diet restrictions and medications and her daughter confirms this as she prepares all meals for AL and fills her pillbox weekly. Vital signs include BP 92/57 mm Hg, HR 95 bpm (symptomatic orthostasis), and RR 16 rpm. AL has no complaints of dizziness or palpitations and her electrocardiogram (ECG) is normal. On physical examination, she has no jugular venous distention, clear lungs, and no ascites or lower extremity edema. Laboratory analysis reveals sodium 132 mmol/L, potassium 3.9 mmol/L, BUN 52 mg/dL, and serum creatinine (SCr) 1.8 mg/dL (baseline BUN/SCr 32/0.9). AL has been stable on the following oral regimen for several months: valsartan 80 mg twice daily, metoprolol XL 50 mg/d, furosemide 40 mg twice daily, amiodarone 200 mg/d, and digoxin 0.125 mg/d.

5. Which one of the following clinical categories best describes AL?
   a. Warm and dry
   b. Warm and wet
   c. Cold and dry
   d. Cold and wet

6. Which one of the following is the optimal initial intervention for AL?
   a. Change furosemide to 80 mg intravenously twice daily.
   b. Hold furosemide and begin cautious hydration with IV fluids.
   c. Hold metoprolol and begin dobutamine at 2 μg/kg/min.
   d. Increase metoprolol XL to 100 mg/d.

Question 7 pertains to the following case.

After your intervention, AL feels much better. Her vital signs today include BP 126/86 mm Hg, HR 83 bpm, and RR 21 rpm and orthostasis has resolved. An ECHO (done today) reveals an EF of 15% with increasing ventricular dilation. Her relevant laboratory values are sodium 125 mmol/L, potassium 4.9 mmol/L, BUN 38 mg/dL, and SCr 1.4 mg/dL.

7. Which one of the following most likely explains AL's decompensation?
   a. Acute arrhythmia
   b. Dietary nonadherence
   c. Renal insufficiency
   d. Progression of heart failure

Questions 8 through 12 pertain to the following case.

CJ is an 81-year-old woman who presents to the hospital with ADHF. Vital signs include BP 92/63 mm Hg, HR 72 bpm, and RR 19 rpm. Physical examination reveals JVP elevated to the jawline, +S3, bilateral rales on auscultation, 1+ abdominal ascites, and 3+ bilateral edema extending to her thighs. Chest radiograph reveals pulmonary edema and pleural effusions. Hemodynamic measurements obtained by pulmonary artery catheter (PAC) include PCWP 31 mm Hg, CI 1.9 L/min/m^2, and SVR 1400. Her laboratory values are all normal, except sodium 128 mmol/L, BUN 34 mg/dL, and SCr 1.5 mg/dL (baseline BUN/SCr 32 and 0.9). Her drugs on admission include lisinopril 20 mg/d, carvedilol 12.5 mg twice daily, bumetanide 2 mg twice daily, hydralazine 25 mg three times daily, isosorbide dinitrate 20 mg three times daily and aspirin 325 mg/d.

8. Which one of the following is a reasonable choice for diuretic therapy in CJ?
   a. CJ should not receive diuretic therapy because she is volume depleted.
   b. IV loop diuretic therapy should be given to provide a net fluid loss of 500 to 2000 mL/d.
   c. Metolazone should be considered a first-line option because of CJ's impaired renal function.
   d. Nesiritide therapy should be used as a replacement for diuretic therapy because CJ is volume overloaded.

9. Which of the following best describes what PCWP represents in CJ?
   a. Fluid status
   b. Inotropy
   c. Afterload
   d. Chronotropy

10. What is the desired PCWP for CJ?
    a. Less than 2.2 L/min/m^2
    b. Greater than 2.2 L/min/m^2
    c. Between 6 and 12 mm Hg
    d. Between 15 and 18 mm Hg

11. Once CJ has undergone successful diuresis, her CI and SVR do not change substantially and her vital signs and oral HF medications remain essentially unchanged with the exception of her diuretic dose. Which of the following therapies are now appropriate to manage CJ's ADHF?
    a. Nitroprusside
    b. Nesiritide
    c. Dobutamine
    d. Milrinone

12. Discharge for CJ is planned with outpatient inotropic therapy based on your recommendations. According to the American College of Cardiology/American Heart Association (ACC/AHA) Inpatient HF performance measures, which one of the following should be completed prior to CJ's discharge?
    a. Beta-blocker therapy in left ventricular systolic dysfunction (LVSD)
    b. Written documentation of her EF
    c. Care of her IV access site
    d. Advance directives

13. Which of the following should be assured prior to administering IV inotropes and vasodilators?
    a. Adequate filling pressures with a PCWP 6 to 12 mm Hg
    b. Adequate filling pressures with a PCWP >15 mm Hg
    c. Adequate filling pressure with an SVR >1200 dyne/s/cm^5
    d. Adequate filling pressure with an SVR >1500 dyne/s/cm^5

14. Which of the following would be a contraindication to IV vasodilators?
    a. Heart rate >90 bpm
    b. Heart rate >110 bpm
    c. Systolic blood pressure <90 mm Hg
    d. Systolic blood pressure <110 mm Hg

15. Which of the following are well-known adverse effects of dobutamine?
    a. Hyponatremia
    b. Renal dysfunction
    c. Hyperkalemia
    d. Arrhythmia

16. Which of the following is referred to as an "inodilator," having both inotropic and vasodilatory properties?
    a. Milrinone
    b. Dobutamine
    c. Nesiritide
    d. Nitroprusside

17. MJ is a 45-year old man (70 kg) admitted for ADHF refractory to aggressive outpatient titration of oral diuretics, including torsemide and metolazone. He is now receiving IV furosemide 30 mg/h and chlorothiazide 500 mg twice daily. While MJ's vital signs and renal function appear stable (BP 110/65 mm Hg, HR 85 bpm, SCr 1.3 mg/dL), his urine output is unchanged despite over 24 hours of the above regimen, and review of continuous telemetry demonstrates multiple 10-beat runs of ventricular tachycardia. Which of the following is an appropriate next step in therapy?
    a. Initiate milrinone 0.1 μg/kg/min
    b. Initiate dobutamine 2.5 μg/kg/min
    c. Initiate nesiritide 0.01 μg/kg/min
    d. Increase furosemide to 60 mg/h

18. AS is a 54-year old woman with NICM who is admitted to the critical care unit (CCU) for transplant work-up. A pulmonary artery catheter reveals elevated pulmonary pressures with a PAS 75 mm Hg despite normal fluid status. To best assess AS's appropriateness for transplant, her pulmonary pressures must be proven as reversible. Which of the following medications is commonly used for such purposes, given a short half-life and potent pulmonary vasodilator effects?
    a. Dobutamine
    b. Milrinone
    c. Hydralazine
    d. Nitroprusside

TAKEAWAY POINTS ››

- ADHF admissions are a common and costly occurrence, the result of medication or lifestyle noncompliance, an acute insult, or disease progression.
- Chronic up-regulation of the sympathetic nervous system and the renin-angiotensin-aldosterone system leads to ADHF.
- Measurement of a BNP level at admission can assist in the diagnosis of ADHF.
- Pulmonary artery catheter placement may assist in the management of complex AHDF patients, but should only be used in patients who do not respond to initial treatment, whose volume status is uncertain, or are hemodynamically unstable.
- Certain chronic HF medications such as β-blockers, ACE inhibitors, spironolactone, digoxin, or the combination of hydralazine and isosorbide dinitrate may need to have doses reduced or be stopped altogether at admission for ADHF, with attempt at reinitiation prior to discharge.
- Patients who present with fluid overload should be treated initially with IV loop diuretics.
- Patients with adequate filling pressure and blood pressure may benefit from the addition of either nitroglycerin or nitroprusside or nesiritide to their loop diuretic regimen.
- Patients who present with signs and symptoms of low cardiac output may require addition of dobutamine or milrinone to treat cardiogenic shock and to assist with systemic hypoperfusion.
- In patients with ADHF that is refractory to medical management, mechanical options such as ultrafiltration, intra-aortic balloon pumps, ventricular assist devices, and heart transplantation may prolong survival.
- Admission for ADHF presents an opportunity to improve care by measuring ejection fraction, optimizing medication regimens, and delivering smoking cessation and lifestyle counseling.

REFERENCES

1. Heart Failure Society of America. Evaluation and management of patients with acute decompensated heart failure. *J Card Fail.* 2006;12(1):e86-e103.
2. Fonarow GC, Corday E, ADHERE Scientific Advisory Committee. Overview of acutely decompensated congestive heart failure (ADHF): a report from the ADHERE Registry. *Heart Fail Rev.* 2004;9:179-85.
3. Lloyd-Jones D, Adams R, Carnethon M, et al. Heart Disease and Stroke Statistics—2009 Update: a report from the American Heart Association Statistics Committee and Stroke Statistics Subcommittee. *Circulation.* 2009;119:e21-e181.
4. Fonarow GC, Adams KF, Abraham WT. Risk stratification for in-hospital mortality in acutely decompensated heart failure: classification and decision tree analysis. *JAMA.* 2005;293(5):572-580.

5. Summers RL, Amsterdam E. Pathophysiology of acute decompensated heart failure. *Heart Fail Clin.* 2008;5:9-17.
6. Parker RB, Rodgers JE, Cavallari LH. Heart Failure. In: Dipiro JT, Talbert RL, Yee GC, et al, eds. *Pharmacotherapy: A Pathophysiologic Approach.* 7th ed. New York, NY: McGraw-Hill; 2008:173-216.
7. Maisel AS, Krishnaswamy P, Nowak RM, et al. Rapid measurement of B-type natriuretic peptide in the emergency diagnosis of heart failure. *N Engl J Med.* 2002;346(3):161-166.
8. The ESCAPE Investigators. Evaluation study of congestive heart failure and pulmonary artery catheterization effectiveness. *JAMA.* 2005;294:1625-1633.
9. Hoffman E. Basics of hemodynamic monitoring. *Drug Intell Clin Pharm.* 1982;16:657-664.
10. Peacock WF, De Marco T, Fonarow GC, et al. Cardiac troponin and outcome in heart failure. *N Engl J Med.* 2008;358:2017-2026.
11. Dormans TPJ, van Meyel JJM, Gerlag PGG, et al. Diuretic efficacy of high dose furosemide in severe heart failure: bolus injection versus continuous infusion. *J Am Coll Cardiol.* 1996;28:376-82.
12. Elkayam U, Bitar F, Akhter MW, et al. Intravenous nitroglycerin in the treatment of decompensated heart failure: potential benefits and limitations. *J Cardiovasc Pharmacol Ther.* 2004;9(4):227-241.
13. VMAC Investigators. Intravenous nesiritide vs. nitroglycerin for treatment of decompensated heart failure. *JAMA.* 2002;80:287:1531.
14. Bayram M, De Luca L, Massie MB et al. Reassessment of dobutamine, dopamine, and milrinone in the management of acute heart failure syndromes. *Am J Card.* 2005;96(suppl):47G-58G.
15. Cuffe MS, Califf RM, Adams KF, et al. Short-term intravenous milrinone for acute exacerbation of chronic heart failure. *JAMA.* 2002;287:1541.
16. Costanzo MR, Guglin ME, Saltzberg MT, et al. Ultrafiltration vs. intravenous diuretics for patients hospitalized for acute decompensated heart failure. *J Am Coll Cardiol.* 2007;49(6):675-683.
17. Taylor DO, Edwards LB, Bounce MM, et al. Registry of the international society for heart and lung transplantation: twenty-third official adult heart transplantation report—2006. *J Heart Lung Transplant.* 2006;25:869-879.
18. Rose EA, Gelijns AC, Moskowitz AJ, et al. Long-term use of a left ventricular assist device for end-stage heart failure. *N Engl J Med.* 2001;345(20):1435-1443.
19. Miller LW, Pagani FD, Russell SD, et al. Use of a continuous flow device in patients awaiting heart transplantation. *N Engl J Med.* 2005;357:885-896.
20. Bonow RO, Bennett S, Casey DE, et al. ACC/AHA Clinical Performance Measures for Adults With Chronic Heart Failure: A Report of the American College of Cardiology/American Heart Association Task Force on Performance Measures (Writing Committee to Develop Heart Failure Clinical Performance Measures): Endorsed by the Heart Failure Society of America. *Circulation.* 2005;112;1853-1887.

CHAPTER

2 Chronic Heart Failure

Michael P. Moranville and Jo Ellen Rodgers

FOUNDATION OVERVIEW

Heart failure (HF) is a syndrome of reduced cardiac output (CO) compromising the metabolic needs of bodily organs and tissues. Heart failure may result from dilation of the left ventricle and a subsequent reduction in left ventricular function (dilated cardiomyopathy or systolic dysfunction). Alternatively, HF may result from hypertrophy and subsequent underfilling of the left ventricle (hypertrophic cardiomyopathy, diastolic dysfunction, or HF with preserved ejection fraction). Progressive HF often severely limits exercise capacity, and mortality is most commonly associated with sudden cardiac death (SCD) or pump failure. Chronic HF may be managed with lifestyle modifications, medications, and implantable devices to delay progression and reduce mortality. Medical management aims at disrupting the neurohormonal pathways that are associated with the disease. Key targets include the sympathetic nervous system (SNS) and the renin angiotensin aldosterone (RAA) system.[1,2]

Approximately 5 million people in the United States are living with this disease and roughly 550,000 new diagnoses are made annually. After the age of 65, approximately 10 out of every 1000 people will be diagnosed and the numbers have steadily risen each year.[1] Although HF due to systolic dysfunction is the most well-recognized diagnosis, approximately 50% of cases are due to diastolic dysfunction. The majority of studies determining appropriate medical management of HF have been conducted in patients with systolic dysfunction, and thus, the discussion of drug therapy in this chapter will focus on that literature. Hospitalization rates for HF continue to rise and are its primary expense. In addition to hospital admissions and morbidity, HF causes significant mortality with an overall 50% 5-year mortality rate.

Disease severity is determined by evaluating functional capacity or structural heart changes. The New York Heart Association (NYHA) uses exercise tolerance and ability to perform activities of daily living. Patients may be classified as NYHA class I if there are no symptoms or restrictions in activity, class II or III if there are symptoms with moderate or mild physical activity, respectively, and class IV if symptoms are present at rest. The NYHA classification system allows a patient's current state of HF health to be assessed at a particular point in time. A patient may shift between classes as disease control improves or declines.[3] To classify patients in a sequential manner as the disease state progresses, the ACC/AHA developed a staging system based on risk factors for HF and structural determinants. Using this system, patients are categorized as being at risk of developing HF (stage A), having structural heart disease but no symptoms (stage B), developing HF signs and symptoms (stage C), and having end-stage disease despite maximal medical therapy (stage D).[1]

Key Definitions

ACC = American College of Cardiology
AHA = American Heart Association
CO = cardiac output
SV = stroke volume
HR = heart rate
BSA = body surface area
EF = ejection fraction
LVEDP = left ventricular end diastolic pressure
LVEDV = left ventricular end diastolic volume
LVESV = left ventricular end systolic volume

Diagnosis

Patients with HF commonly present with signs and symptoms associated with volume overload, low CO, or both. Patients with fluid overload may present with signs and symptoms of pulmonary congestion (eg, dyspnea, orthopnea, rales on auscultation) or peripheral congestion (eg, ascites, jugular venous distension, lower extremity edema). Signs and symptoms of low CO are less readily identified and may be very subjective. Vague symptoms of fatigue and nausea and vomiting are common. Worsening renal function is a common objective measure of low CO. Exercise intolerance and early satiety may be present with either fluid overload or low CO. Weight gain is the best predictor of fluid status since weight change often precedes overt HF signs and symptoms.[1,2]

A comprehensive patient history should be obtained to elucidate causes of HF. Both myocardial infarction (MI) and hypertension are common causes, and thus, cardiovascular risk factors should be addressed. Detailed medication histories should be completed to assure dietary and medication compliance and avoidance of substance abuse. Presence of medications known to exacerbate fluid retention (eg, nonsteroidal anti-inflammatory drugs), alter left ventricular function (eg, certain

Hemodynamic Equations

$CO = SV \times HR$
$CI = CO/BSA$
$EF = (LVEDV - LVESV)/LVEDV$

TABLE 2-1 **Drugs That May Precipitate or Exacerbate Heart Failure**

Negative Inotropic Effect
Antiarrhythmics (e g, disopyramide, flecainide, propafenone, and others)
Beta-blockers (e g, propranolol, metoprolol, atenolol, and others)
Calcium channel blockers (e g, verapamil, diltiazem)
Itraconazole
Terbinafine
Cardiotoxic
Doxorubicin
Daunomycin
Cyclophosphamide
Trastuzumab
Imatinib
Ethanol
Amphetamines (e g, cocaine, methamphetamine)
Sodium and Water Retention
Nonsteroidal anti-inflammatory drugs
Cyclooxygenase-2 inhibitors
Rosiglitazone and pioglitazone
Glucocorticoids
Androgens and estrogens
Salicylates (high dose)
Sodium-containing drugs (e g, piperacillin sodium)

Reproduced with permission from Parker RB, Rodgers JE, Cavallari LH. Heart failure. In: DiPiro JT, Talbert RL, Yee GC, Matzke GR, Wells BG, Posey LM. *Pharmacotherapy: A Pathophysiologic Approach*. 7th ed. New York, NY: McGraw-Hill; 2008:173-216.

antineoplastic agents), and those with negative inotropic effects (nondihydropyridine calcium channel blockers) should also be assessed (Table 2-1). Measurement of B-type natriuretic peptide (BNP) may be helpful in differentiating HF from other disease states that cause similar symptoms. An echocardiogram is necessary to evaluate left and right ventricular function to determine disease severity as well as valvular compliance to assess etiology.[1,2]

Pathophysiology

Heart failure is the result of any disorder that impairs the heart's ability to contract as it normally would. This syndrome may be of ischemic or nonischemic origin. Nonischemic etiologies include uncontrolled hypertension, viral diseases, sarcoidosis, peripartum cardiomyopathy, uncorrected valvular heart disease, or hyperthyroidism. In general, hypertension and ischemia are the most common causes.

In response to a decline in CO, numerous compensatory mechanisms are activated to maintain adequate CO and organ perfusion. Activation of the SNS and RAA system is primarily responsible for this compensatory response. Norepinephrine is released from the SNS in an effort to maintain CO by increasing contractility and heart rate (HR). Unfortunately, norepinephrine is a potent vasoconstrictor which only further worsens contractility by increasing afterload. Renal hypoperfusion results in RAA system activation with a resultant rise in serum angiotensin II and aldosterone levels. Like norepinephrine, angiotensin II is a potent vasoconstrictor, further compromising CO while aldosterone release causes sodium and fluid retention. Volume retention with elevated left ventricular end diastolic pressure (LVEDP) and increased preload as well as vasoconstriction with increased afterload initially improve organ perfusion; however, such neurohormonal activation ultimately result in further decline in CO. In addition, the SNS and the RAA system interrelate resulting in additional activation of one another. Finally, these neurohormones also contribute directly to ventricular remodeling and hypertrophy. This cycle of events propagates itself as further decline in CO results in additional release of these negative compensatory neurohormones. Finally, additional neurohormones are released including, but not limited to, vasopressin and nitric oxide.[4-7]

TREATMENT

General Considerations

The goals of managing HF are to maximize quality of life (QOL), minimize symptoms, prevent hospitalizations, slow disease progression, and prolong survival. Efforts should be made to prevent the development of HF in patients with risk factors (hypertension, diabetes mellitus, myocardial infarction). It is also important to identify and treat any reversible, underlying cause. All patients should be educated on fluid and sodium restrictions and encouraged to weigh themselves daily to assure early detection of changes in volume status. Drug therapy is focused on inhibiting the neurohormonal cascade described above and is the cornerstone of therapy (see Table 2-2 for dosing and monitoring of neurohormonal blocking agents).

Pharmacologic Therapy

Loop Diuretics

Sodium and fluid retention is common in HF and loop diuretics are the most frequently used medication to assist in fluid removal. Loop diuretics (furosemide, bumetanide, and torsemide) block sodium reabsorption in the ascending loop of Henle. This group of medications has not shown a mortality benefit, but provides symptomatic relief of fluid overload, improves exercise tolerance, and prevents hospitalization. Patients can develop resistance to loop diuretics requiring escalation in therapy or addition of thiazide diuretics. Common adverse effects include hypokalemia, hypomagnesemia, hypotension, and renal dysfunction. Weight should be monitored daily to prevent overdiuresis.[8,9]

Angiotensin-Converting Enzyme Inhibitors

Angiotensin-converting enzyme (ACE) inhibitors prevent the conversion of angiotensin I to angiotensin II. This medication class was the first and most widely studied in HF patients and has been proven effective at reducing mortality, slowing

TABLE 2-2 Dosing and Monitoring for Neurohormonal Blocking Agents

Drug	Initial Daily Dose	Target or Maximum Daily Dose	Monitoring
ACE Inhibitors			
Captopril Enalapril Fosinopril Lisinopril Perindopril Quinopril Ramipril Trandolapril	6.25 mg three times daily 2.5 mg twice daily 5-10 mg once daily 2.5-5 mg once daily 2 mg once daily 5 mg twice daily 1.25-2.5 mg once daily 1 mg once daily	50 mg three times daily 10-20 mg twice daily 40 mg once daily 20-40 mg once daily 8-16 mg once daily 20 mg twice daily 10 mg once daily 4 mg once daily	BP Electrolytes (K^+, BUN, SCr) at baseline, 2 wk, and after dose titration, CBC periodically Adverse effects: cough, angioedema
Angiotensin Receptor Blockers			
Candesartan Losartan Valsartan	4-8 mg once daily 25-50 mg once daily 20-40 mg twice daily	32 mg once daily 50-100 mg once daily 160 mg twice daily	BP Electrolytes (K^+, BUN, SCr) at baseline, 2 weeks, and after dose titration, CBC periodically Adverse effects: cough, angioedema
Aldosterone Antagonists			
Spironolactone Eplerenone	12.5-25 mg once daily 25 mg once daily	25 mg once daily or twice daily 50 mg once daily	BP Electrolytes (K^+) at baseline and within 1 wk of initiation and dose titration Adverse effects: gynecomastia or breast tenderness, menstrual changes, hirsutism
Beta-Blockers			
Bisoprolol Carvedilol Metoprolol succinate	1.25 mg once daily 3.125 mg twice daily 12.5-25 mg once daily	10 mg once daily 25 mg bid (50 mg twice daily for patients > 85 kg or 187 lb) 200 mg once daily	BP, HR baseline and after each dose titration, ECG Adverse effects: worsening HF symptoms (edema, SOB, fatigue), depression, sexual dysfunction

Abbreviations: BP, blood pressure; BUN, blood urea nitrate; CBC, complete blood cell count; ECG, electrocardiogram; HF, heart failure; HR, heart rate; K^+, potassium; SCr, serum creatinine; SOB, shortness of breath.

Adapted with permission from Vardeny O, Ng TMH. Heart failure. In: Chisholm-Burns MA, Wells BG, Schwinghammer TL, et al. *Pharmacotherapy Principles & Practice*. New York, NY: McGraw-Hill; 2008:33-61.

progression, preventing hospitalization, and providing symptomatic improvement.[10-12] Patients with risk factors for HF (hypertension, diabetes mellitus, myocardial infarction) and patients with a reduced EF, regardless of the absence of symptoms, are recommended to take an ACE inhibitor unless contraindicated. As tolerated, ACE inhibitors should be titrated to target doses as outlined in the ACC/AHA guidelines.[1] Patients should be monitored for hypotension, hyperkalemia, and renal dysfunction. Cough is the most common side effect while angioedema is rare but potentially life threatening. Absolute contraindications for this class include angioedema, bilateral renal artery stenosis, and pregnancy.[2]

Angiotensin Receptor Blockers

Angiotensin receptor blockers (ARB) competitively inhibit angiotensin II receptors. Unlike ACE inhibitors, bradykinin does not accumulate, and thus, cough and angioedema are less common. An ARB can be considered an alternative in patients who are intolerant of ACE inhibitors.[13,14] Patients who develop renal dysfunction, hyperkalemia, or hypotension associated with an ACE inhibitor are likely to experience similar adverse effects with an ARB. Studies evaluating the addition of an ARB to an ACE inhibitor have shown a decrease in cardiovascular mortality and hospitalizations but an increased risk of hypotension, hyperkalemia, and renal dysfunction.[15,16] ACE inhibitors remain first-line therapy for blocking angiotensin II since a significantly greater mortality benefit has not been demonstrated with an ARB.[14-17]

Beta-Adrenergic Blockers

Historically, beta-blockers were not used to manage HF due to the concern that negative inotropic effects associated with their use would worsen HF symptoms and outcomes. However, the long-term benefits of inhibiting the deleterious effects of the SNS with beta-receptor blockade outweigh short-term negative inotropic effects. Multiple large, randomized, placebo-controlled trials have demonstrated a significant mortality benefit when beta-blocker therapy is initiated in addition to background ACE inhibitor therapy. This benefit is present in patients of all HF severities.[18-20] As outlined in the ACC/AHA guidelines, titration to goal doses or to the highest tolerated dose is recommended.[21] Not all beta-blockers have proven effective in HF and only three agents are currently recommended: carvedilol, metoprolol succinate CR/XL, and bisoprolol. Beta-blockers should be started at low doses and up-titrated slowly when patients are euvolemic. Even when started or up-titrated under optimal conditions, a patient's symptoms may transiently worsen when these adjustments are made until a new equilibrium is established. Patients who require diuresis due to volume overload should have their doses held constant until excess fluid is removed. Patients should be monitored for hypotension, bradycardia, fluid retention, and fatigue. Comorbidities including diabetes mellitus, chronic obstructive pulmonary disease (COPD), asthma, and peripheral vascular disease (PVD) should not be considered absolute contraindications to beta-blocker. A beta-1-selective agent (metoprolol succinate, bisoprolol) is preferred in asthma patients.

Aldosterone Antagonists

Although ACE inhibitors reduce the amount of aldosterone release in the short term, additional suppression of aldosterone can be achieved with the aldosterone receptor antagonist (ARA), spironolactone. This agent has been shown to reduce all-cause mortality in patients with moderate to moderately severe (NYHA class III-IV) HF.[22] Eplerenone is an alternative ARA with mortality benefit demonstrated in patients with left ventricular dysfunction following MI.[23] It is recommended to avoid ARAs if serum potassium is >5 mmol/L or if creatinine clearance is <30 mL/min. Strict serum potassium and creatinine monitoring is necessary. Eplerenone is more mineralcorticoid specific and associated with less gynecomastia.[1]

Digoxin

While it was previously hypothesized that the benefits of digoxin were derived from its positive inotropic effects, more recent data has suggested that it has important neurohormonal modulating effects. Digoxin has not shown a mortality benefit in HF patients, but does significantly improve symptoms and reduce hospitalization.[24] And thus, digoxin is recommended in patients who remain symptomatic despite standard therapy with ACE inhibitors and beta-blockers. Serum digoxin concentrations should be maintained at a level between 0.5 to 1 ng/mL.[25] Digoxin discontinuation should be avoided since withdrawal of therapy has been shown to worsen HF symptoms in stable patients.[26,27] Digoxin dosing should be based upon renal function and lean body mass.

Isosorbide Dinitrate and Hydralazine

Several proposed mechanisms support the combined use of isosorbide dinitrate and hydralazine (ISDN-HYD) for HF. While ISDN is a venous vasodilator and HYD is an arterial vasodilator, ISDN also delivers nitric oxide which may be deficient in HF. In addition, hydralazine has antioxidant properties which eliminate the need for a nitrate free-interval with ISDN. The ISDN-HYD combination significantly reduces all-cause mortality and is recommended in African Americans with moderate to moderately severe (NYHA class III-IV) HF receiving standard HF therapy with ACE inhibitor and beta-blocker.[28-30] The combination may also be used in any patient who cannot tolerate an ACE inhibitor or ARB.[1] Dizziness and headache are the most common side effects with ISDN-HYD.

Nonpharmacologic Therapy

Ventricular arrhythmias and SCD are major causes of mortality in HF patients. Placement of an implantable cardioverter defibrillator (ICD) has been shown to significantly reduce mortality in patients with ischemic and nonischemic cardiomyopathies and an ejection fraction (EF) less than or equal to 30 percent despite standard HF therapy.[31-33] Ventricular dyssynchrony may further compromise CO in HF patients. Cardiac resynchronization therapy (CRT) with a biventricular pacemaker significantly reduces hospitalizations and improves QOL.[33,34] Patients with NYHA class III to IV HF despite standard HF therapy, a LVEF less than or equal to 35%, and a QRS interval greater than or equal to 120 ms are eligible for CRT.[1]

CASE Application

1. JB is a 45-year-old man with cardiomyopathy (LVEF 35%) following an acute MI. Immediately following his MI, he developed signs and symptoms of HF including shortness of breath (SOB) at rest. Which of the following best characterizes JB's current ACC/AHA HF stage and New York Heart Association (NYHA) class?
   a. Stage A, NYHA class not applicable
   b. Stage B, NYHA class I
   c. Stage C, NYHA class II
   d. Stage C, NYHA class IV

2. Which of the following is the best predictor of fluid status and should be monitored daily by all HF patients?
   a. Fatigue
   b. Shortness of breath
   c. Weight change
   d. Lower extremity edema

3. Which of the following laboratory values may be helpful in differentiating HF from other disease states that cause similar symptoms?
   a. Sodium
   b. Creatinine
   c. B-type natriuretic peptide (BNP)
   d. Hematocrit

4. AF is a 63-year-old woman with HF (NYHA class I) receiving furosemide 40 mg twice daily, lisinopril 10 mg daily, metoprolol XL 50 mg daily, digoxin 0.125 mg daily, and spironolactone 25 mg daily. During her routine clinic visit today, pertinent findings include: blood pressure (BP) 120/80 mm Hg, HR 70 bpm, RR 14 rpm, K^+ 5.1 mmol/L, BUN 35 mg/dL, creatinine 1.2 mg/dL (baseline), and SDC 0.7 ng/mL. Which of the following is the most appropriate change to optimize AF's medical regimen?

   a. Increase ACE inhibitor dose
   b. Increase beta-blocker dose
   c. Increase digoxin dose
   d. Increase spironolactone dose

Questions 5 through 8 pertain to the following case.

IH is a 54-year-old African American man with systolic heart failure presenting with a 2-week history of SOB which limits his normal daily activities and increases lower extremity edema. His weight has recently increased by 10 lb. His physical examination is notable for BP 148/72 mm Hg, HR 88 bpm, RR 24 rpm, rales, and 3+ lower extremity edema. Pertinent laboratory values include: sodium 138 mmol/L, potassium 5.4 mmol/L, BUN 35 mg/dL, creatinine 0.9 mg/dL, and digoxin 2.1 ng/mL. Past medical history is significant for hypertension (HTN), gout, COPD. Current medications include lisinopril 20 mg daily, diltiazem CD 120 mg daily, digoxin 0.250 mg daily salmeterol/fluticasone 250/50, two puffs bid. IH recently began taking naproxen 220 mg tid for gout pain.

5. In addition to counseling on salt and fluid restriction, which of the following pharmacologic options is most appropriate for managing IH's fluid overload?

   a. Initiate hydrochlorothiazide 50 mg daily.
   b. Initiate furosemide 40 mg twice daily.
   c. Initiate metolazone 2.5 mg daily.
   d. Initiate spironolactone 25 mg daily.

6. Within the following 24 hours, IH experiences a brisk diuresis with considerable improvement in HF signs and symptoms. What additional medication changes should be considered?

   a. Continue current regimen and initiate hydrochlorothiazide 50 mg daily.
   b. Continue current regimen and initiate spironolactone 25 mg daily.
   c. Discontinue lisinopril and initiate combination hydralazine 25 mg and isosorbide dinitrate 20 mg tid.
   d. Discontinue over-the-counter naproxen and initiate colchicine 0.6 mg tid until gout pain resolves.

7. Once optimal fluid status has been achieved, which of the following represents the best option to manage IH's hypertension?

   a. Discontinue diltiazem and initiate amlodipine 5 mg daily.
   b. Initiate carvedilol 3.125 mg twice daily.
   c. Discontinue diltiazem and initiate carvedilol 3.125 mg twice daily.
   d. Initiate prazosin 2 mg daily.

8. What additional medication change should be considered to decrease morbidity (ie, hospitalizations) outcomes for IH?

   a. Increase lisinopril to 40 mg daily.
   b. Reduce digoxin to 0.125 mg daily.
   c. Initiate spironolactone 25 mg daily.
   d. Initiate candesartan 4 mg daily.

Questions 9 and 10 pertain to the following case.

RJ is a 71-year-old woman with a history of ischemic cardiomyopathy who presents to clinic with symptoms consistent with NYHA class IV HF. Past medical history includes hyperlipidemia, diabetes mellitus, myocardial infarction, and hypothyroidism. RJ complains of progressive weight gain (~6 lb increase since her previous visit 3 months ago), SOB at rest, 2 pillow orthopnea, and occasional paroxysmal nocturnal dyspnea (PND). Her physical examination is positive for 1+ pitting edema in her ankles and minimal JVD. Vital signs include BP 105/70 mm Hg and HR 91 bpm. Laboratory results include potassium 3.6 mmol/L, BUN 39 mg/dL, and creatinine 1.4 mg/dL. RJ's current medications are levothyroxine 0.05 mg daily, furosemide 40 mg twice daily, lisinopril 20 mg daily, atorvastatin 40 mg daily, aspirin 81 mg daily, insulin glargine 46 units at bedtime, and insulin aspart 6 units before meals.

9. Which of the following is the best treatment option to manage RJ's hypokalemia and fluid overload?

   a. Continue furosemide 40 mg twice daily.
   b. Increase furosemide to 80 mg twice daily
   c. Initiate spironolactone 25 mg once daily.
   d. Increase furosemide to 80 mg twice daily and initiate spironolactone to 25 mg once daily.

10. RJ is approaching euvolemia and the medical team anticipates another 2 to 3 days of aggressive diuresis prior to achieving euvolemia. Which of the following represents the next best option to manage RJ's heart failure?

    a. Initiate metoprolol succinate 25 mg daily immediately.
    b. Initiate metoprolol succinate 25 mg daily once euvolemia is achieved.
    c. Initiate metoprolol tartrate 12.5 mg bid immediately.
    d. Initiate digoxin 0.25 mg daily.

11. Which of the following are absolute contraindications to the use of beta-blockers?

    a. Asthma with active bronchospasm
    b. Diabetes
    c. Chronic obstructive pulmonary disease
    d. Peripheral vascular disease

Questions 12 and 13 pertain to the following case.

BT is a 54-year-old African American man recently diagnosed with nonischemic cardiomyopathy. His past medical history is notable for moderate asthma since childhood and hypertension. Current medications include salmeterol one inhalation twice daily, fluticasone 88 μg inhaled twice daily, furosemide 80 mg twice daily, enalapril 20 mg twice daily, and spironolactone 25 mg daily.

12. Which of the following beta-blockers is the best option to treat BT's heart failure and minimize aggravating his asthma?
    a. Carvedilol
    b. Metoprolol succinate
    c. Propranolol
    d. Atenolol

13. Which of the following medication changes may provide further mortality benefit for BT?
    a. Digoxin 0.125 mg daily
    b. Combination hydralazine 25 mg and isosorbide dinitrate 10 mg three times daily
    c. Candesartan 8 mg daily
    d. Amlodipine 5 mg daily

14. Which of the following is an appropriate rationale to switch an ACE inhibitor to an ARB?
    a. Hypotension
    b. Renal dysfunction
    c. Hyperkalemia
    d. None of the above

15. TH is a 34-year-old man presenting with dizziness and orthostatic hypotension. His laboratory values reveal the following: potassium 5.8 mmol/L, BUN 60 mg/dL (baseline 18), creatinine 2.0 mg/dL (baseline 0.9). TH's medications include furosemide 80 mg twice daily, ramipril 5 mg twice daily, and metoprolol XL 50 mg daily. Which of the following immediate medication adjustments are appropriate?
    a. Temporarily hold furosemide.
    b. Temporarily hold metoprolol XL.
    c. Temporarily hold furosemide and ramipril.
    d. Continue current regimen with no changes.

16. Which of the following beta-blocker regimens would be a goal for most HF patients?
    a. Metoprolol succinate XL 150 mg once daily
    b. Carvedilol 25 mg twice daily
    c. Atenolol 100 mg once daily
    d. Bisoprolol 2.5 mg once daily

17. Which of the following are important to consider when initiating combination hydralazine and isosorbide dinitrate in an African American patient with HF?
    a. Initiate hydralazine 37.5 mg and isosorbide dinitrate 20 mg one tablet three times daily
    b. Discontinue background ACE inhibitor therapy
    c. Utilize a nitrate-free interval
    d. Therapy is commonly well tolerated

18. Which of the following is the primary cost driver in HF?
    a. Medication
    b. Physician visits
    c. Home health care
    d. Hospitalizations

19. Which of the following are important to monitor for when initiating beta-blocker therapy?
    a. Tachycardia
    b. Dehydration
    c. Fatigue
    d. Hyperkalemia

20. In which HF patients should aldosterone antagonists be avoided?
    a. Serum potassium <3.5 mmol/L
    b. Creatinine clearance is <30 mL/min
    c. Concomitant ARB therapy
    d. NYHA class III to IV despite standard HF therapy

TAKEAWAY POINTS ››

- Heart failure occurs most commonly due to myocardial infarction and uncontrolled hypertension.
- Heart failure may be categorized as having resulted from a reduction in left ventricular function (systolic dysfunction) or being associated with underfilling of the left ventricle (diastolic dysfunction or HF with preserved ejection fraction).
- Heart failure can be described by two classification systems. The NYHA classification system uses functional capacity to determine if patients are asymptomatic (class I), symptomatic with moderate or mild physical activity (class II or III), or symptomatic at rest (class IV), respectively, at a particular point in time. The ACC/AHA staging systems uses risk factors and structural changes to outline the progression of HF in a sequential manner as at risk for HF (Stage A), left ventricular dysfunction without symptoms (Stage B) or with symptoms (Stage C), or refractory end-stage HF (Stage D).
- Patients with HF commonly present with signs and symptoms of fluid overload such as dyspnea on exertion (DOE) and lower extremity edema. Less commonly, signs and symptoms of low cardiac output exist (ie, fatigue).

- Activation of neurohormonal pathways including the SNS and the RAA system occur in HF and result in vasoconstriction, sodium and fluid retention, and cardiac remodeling. Treatment strategies are aimed at blocking these neurohormonal systems.
- Lifestyle modifications such as fluid and sodium restriction are important in maintaining fluid balance. Achieving fluid balance commonly requires loop diuretic administration. Addition of thiazide diuretic may be considered in diuretic-refractory patients.
- The goals of HF drug therapy include reduction in mortality, prevention of progression, reduction in hospitalizations, and improvement in quality of life.
- Both ACE inhibitors and beta-blockers have been shown to reduce all-cause mortality in HF patients, and thus, standard HF therapy consists of both of these therapies. An ARB should be considered if a patient experiences intolerable cough or angioedema with an ACE inhibitor.
- The ARA, spironolactone, reduces mortality in moderate to moderately severe (NYHA class III-IV) HF despite standard HF therapy. Spironolactone should not be initiated in the setting of hyperkalemia or poor renal function and close monitoring is imperative.
- While digoxin does not reduce mortality, it does reduce hospitalizations and causes symptomatic improvement. It may be considered for patients who remain symptomatic despite standard HF therapy. Digoxin concentrations should generally be maintained at <1 ng/mL.
- The combination of ISDN-HYD has been shown to reduce mortality in African American patients who have moderate to moderately severe (NYHA class III-IV) HF despite standard HF therapy. In addition, any patient who is intolerant of ACE inhibitors and ARBs can also be considered for this drug combination.
- Implantation of an ICD significantly reduces SCD and should be considered in eligible patients. Biventricular pacing using CRT provides symptomatic improvement and reduces hospitalizations, but has not been shown to reduce mortality.

REFERENCES

1. Jessup M. ACC/AHA 2009 guideline update for the diagnosis and management of heart failure in the adults: a report of the American College of Cardiology Foundation/American Heart Association Task Force on Practice Guidelines: developed in collaboration with the International Society of Heart and Lung Transplantation (2009 writing group to review new evidence and update the 2005 Guideline for the Management Patients with Chronic Heart Failure). *Circulation* 2009;119:1977-2016.
2. Parker R, Rodgers J, Cavallari J. Heart failure. In: DiPiro J, Talbert R, Yee G, eds. *Pharmacotherapy: A Pathophysiologic Approach*. New York, NY: McGraw-Hill;2008:173-216.
3. Heart Failure Society of America. Evaluation and management of patients with acute decompensated heart failure. *J Card Fail.* 2006;12(1):e86-e103.
4. Colucci W, Braunwald E. Pathophysiology of heart failure. In: Braunwald E, Zipes DP, Libby P, eds. *Heart Disease: A Textbook of Cardiovascular Medicine*. 6th ed. Philadelphia, PA: Saunders, 2001:503-533.
5. Jessup M, Brozena S. Heart failure. *N Engl J Med.* 2003;348: 2007-2018.
6. Gheorghiade M, Bonow R. Chronic heart failure in the United States: a manifestation of coronary artery disease. *Circulation.* 1998;97:282-289.
7. Mann D. Mechanisms and models in heart failure: a combinatorial approach. *Circulation.* 1999;100:999-1008.
8. Brater DC. Diuretic therapy in congestive heart failure. *Congest Heart Fail.* 2000;6(4):197-201.
9. Shankar SS, Brater DC. Loop diuretics: from the Na-K-2Cl transporter to clinical use. *Am J Physiol Renal Physiol.* 2003;284(1):F11-F21.
10. The CONSENSUS Trial Study Group. The CTSG Effects of enalapril on mortality in severe congestive heart failure. Results of the Cooperative North Scandinavian Enalapril Survival Study (CONSENSUS). *N Engl J Med.* 1987;316(23):1429-1435.
11. The SOLVD Investigators. The SI effect of enalapril on mortality and the development of heart failure in asymptomatic patients with reduced left ventricular ejection fractions. *N Engl J Med.* 1992;327(10):685-691.
12. The SOLVD Investigators. The SI Effect of enalapril on survival in patients with reduced left ventricular ejection fractions and congestive heart failure. *N Engl J Med.* 1991;325(5):293-302.
13. Granger CB, McMurray JJ, Yusuf S, et al. Effects of candesartan in patients with chronic heart failure and reduced left-ventricular systolic function intolerant to angiotensin-converting-enzyme inhibitors: the CHARM-Alternative trial. *Lancet.* 2003;362(9386):772-776.
14. Cohn JN, Tognoni G. A randomized trial of the angiotensin-receptor blocker valsartan in chronic heart failure. *N Engl J Med.* 2001;345(23):1667-1675.
15. McMurray JJ, Ostergren J, Swedberg K, et al. Effects of candesartan in patients with chronic heart failure and reduced left-ventricular systolic function taking angiotensin-converting-enzyme inhibitors: the CHARM-added trial. *Lancet.* 2003;362(9386):767-771.
16. Pfeffer MA, McMurray JJ, Velazquez EJ, et al. Valsartan, captopril, or both in myocardial infarction complicated by heart failure, left ventricular dysfunction, or both. *N Engl J Med.* 2003;349(20):1893-1906.
17. Pfeffer MA, Swedberg K, Granger CB, et al. Effects of candesartan on mortality and morbidity in patients with chronic heart failure: the CHARM-Overall programme. *Lancet.* 2003;362(9386):759-766.
18. CIBIS-II. The Cardiac Insufficiency Bisoprolol Study II (CIBIS-II): a randomised trial. *Lancet.* 1999;353(9146):9-13.
19. MERIT-HF Study Group. Effect of metoprolol CR/XL in chronic heart failure: Metoprolol CR/XL Randomised Intervention Trial in Congestive Heart Failure (MERIT-HF). *Lancet.* 1999;353(9169):2001-2007.

20. Packer M, Bristow MR, Cohn JN, et al. The effect of carvedilol on morbidity and mortality in patients with chronic heart failure. U.S. Carvedilol Heart Failure Study Group. *N Engl J Med.* 1996;334(21):1349-1355.
21. Bristow MR, Gilbert EM, Abraham WT, et al. Carvedilol produces dose-related improvements in left ventricular function and survival in subjects with chronic heart failure. MOCHA Investigators. *Circulation.* 1996;94(11):2807-2816.
22. Pitt B, Zannad F, Remme WJ, et al. The effect of spironolactone on morbidity and mortality in patients with severe heart failure. Randomized Aldactone Evaluation Study Investigators. *N Engl J Med.* 1999;341(10):709-717.
23. Pitt B, Remme W, Zannad F, et al. Eplerenone, a selective aldosterone blocker, in patients with left ventricular dysfunction after myocardial infarction. *N Engl J Med.* 2003;348(14):1309-1321.
24. The DIG. The effect of digoxin on mortality and morbidity in patients with heart failure. The Digitalis Investigation Group. *N Engl J Med.* 1997;336(8):525-533.
25. Rathore SS, Curtis JP, Wang Y, Bristow MR, Krumholz HM. Association of serum digoxin concentration and outcomes in patients with heart failure. *JAMA.* 2003;289(7):871-878.
26. Packer M, Gheorghiade M, Young JB, et al. Withdrawal of digoxin from patients with chronic heart failure treated with angiotensin-converting-enzyme inhibitors. RADIANCE Study. *N Engl J Med.* 1993;329(1):1-7.
27. Uretsky BF, Young JB, Shahidi FE, Yellen LG, Harrison MC, Jolly MK. Randomized study assessing the effect of digoxin withdrawal in patients with mild to moderate chronic congestive heart failure: results of the PROVED trial. PROVED Investigative Group. *J Am Coll Cardiol.* 1993;22(4):955-962.
28. Cohn JN, Archibald DG, Ziesche S, et al. Effect of vasodilator therapy on mortality in chronic congestive heart failure. Results of a Veterans Administration Cooperative Study. *N Engl J Med.* 1986;314(24):1547-1552.
29. Cohn JN, Johnson G, Ziesche S, et al. A comparison of enalapril with hydralazine-isosorbide dinitrate in the treatment of chronic congestive heart failure. *N Engl J Med.* 1991;325(5):303-310.
30. Taylor AL, Ziesche S, Yancy C, et al. Combination of isosorbide dinitrate and hydralazine in blacks with heart failure. *N Engl J Med.* 2004;351(20):2049-2057.
31. Bardy GH, Lee KL, Mark DB, et al. Amiodarone or an implantable cardioverter-defibrillator for congestive heart failure. *N Engl J Med.* 2005;352(3):225-237.
32. Moss AJ, Zareba W, Hall WJ, et al. Prophylactic implantation of a defibrillator in patients with myocardial infarction and reduced ejection fraction. *N Engl J Med.* 2002;346(12):877-883.
33. Bristow MR, Saxon LA, Boehmer J, et al. Cardiac-resynchronization therapy with or without an implantable defibrillator in advanced chronic heart failure. *N Engl J Med.* 2004;350(21):2140-2150.
34. Young JB, Abraham WT, Smith AL, et al. Combined cardiac resynchronization and implantable cardioversion defibrillation in advanced chronic heart failure: the MIRACLE ICD Trial. *JAMA.* 2003;289(20):2685-2694.

CHAPTER

3 Hypertension

Benjamin J. Epstein and Donna Leverone

FOUNDATION OVERVIEW

It is estimated that hypertension affects one billion people globally.[1] In the United States, one in three Americans have elevated blood pressure (BP). Hypertension is responsible for 62% of cerebrovascular events and 49% of ischemic heart disease events. It is directly associated with 7.1 million deaths, making it the most common cause of death in the world. Despite these sobering statistics, 30% of adults in the United States are still unaware that they have hypertension, more than 40% are not being treated, and 65% have blood pressure levels that are above goal.[2] Blood pressure increases with age such that the lifetime risk of developing hypertension among normotensive persons older than 55 years is 90%.[3] The prevalence of hypertension in older women and men is 78% and 64%, respectively. The prevalence of hypertension will continue to grow due to a burgeoning population of senior citizens and an increase in factors that predispose patients to hypertension, such as obesity, diabetes, sedentary lifestyle, and dietary indiscretion.

Large observational studies demonstrate that the risk of death due to ischemic heart disease and stroke increases steeply beginning at blood pressure levels as low as 115/75 mm Hg.[4] Hypertension and blood pressure in the high-normal range (systolic BP [SBP] of 130 to 139 mm Hg and diastolic BP [DBP] of 85 to 89 mm Hg diastolic) are associated with a more than twofold increase in cardiovascular disease risk compared with BP <120/80 mm Hg. The importance of hypertension as a risk factor is illustrated by the high concordance between high blood pressure and first heart attack (69% have hypertension), first stroke (77% have hypertension), and heart failure (HF; 74% have hypertension). Correspondingly, lowering BP results in a cardiovascular risk reduction that is blood pressure dependent. A reduction in SBP as small as 2-mm Hg reduces the risk of death from ischemic heart disease or other vascular causes by 7% and from stroke by 10%.[4] These data highlight the importance of effective treatment of hypertension.

Pathophysiology

Blood pressure is the mathematical product of peripheral vascular resistance (PVR) and cardiac output (CO), the latter defined as the product of heart rate and stroke volume (Table 3-1). Hypertension is the result of increased CO and/or increased PVR. The same factors that normally regulate BP can be responsible for the development of hypertension. Aberrations in the normal function of neurohormonal systems such as the renin-angiotensin system (RAS) or sympathetic nervous system (SNS), abnormal neuronal mechanisms, defects in peripheral autoregulation, and disturbances in sodium, calcium, and natriuretic hormones have all been implicated in the pathophysiology of hypertension. Hypertension is usually multifactorial; consequently, multiple antihypertensive drugs targeting these mechanisms are often necessary to sufficiently control BP.[5]

The majority of patients with hypertension have essential hypertension because their BP is elevated for unknown reasons. Fewer than 10% of patients have secondary hypertension. Common causes of secondary hypertension, including medications, are listed in Table 3-2.

Diagnosis

Hypertension is diagnosed when the average of two or more BP measurements are elevated at two or more clinical encounters. This BP can also be used to classify the patient's hypertension. Table 3-3 lists the classifications of BP according to the Joint National Committee on Prevention, Detection, Evaluation, and Treatment of High Blood Pressure (JNC 7 Guidelines).[6] It is important that BP is properly measured with a brachial sphygmomanometer. The American Heart Association has published explicit criteria for the accurate measurement of BP.[7] Flawed assessment of BP can result in both undertreatment and overtreatment and is a common cause of pseudoresistant hypertension.

With increasing age the relative importance of systolic and diastolic BP varies. SBP increases progressively throughout life. On the other hand, DBP rises until approximately the age of 50 years and then plateaus; it may remain stable or fall after the age of 60 years.[8] Diastolic hypertension is common before the age of 50 years and may occur in isolation or coexist with systolic hypertension. After the age of 50 years, systolic hypertension prevails and SBP represents an important cardiovascular risk factor[9] (Figure 3-1). Systolic hypertension is more difficult to control than diastolic hypertension. Large outcome studies have demonstrated the benefit of treating isolated systolic hypertension.[10-12] These studies reported large reductions in the incidence of stroke, myocardial infarction, and cardiovascular death.

Evaluation

Because hypertension is asymptomatic, the evaluation of patients with elevated BP is an important part of the

TABLE 3-1 Pathophysiology of Hypertension

BP = PVR × CO CO = HR × SV	
Peripheral Vascular Resistance	**Increased Cardiac Output**
Excess stimulation of the RAS	Increased intravascular volume from excess sodium intake
SNS overactivity	Increased intravascular volume from renal sodium retention
Genetic alterations of cell membranes	Excess stimulation of the RAAS
Endothelial-derived factors	SNS overactivity
Hyperinsulinemia resulting from obesity or the metabolic syndrome	

Abbreviations: SNS, sympathetic nervous system; RAAS, renin-angiotensin aldosterone system.

management of hypertension. Assessment of the hypertensive patient should aim to identify cardiovascular risk factors and concomitant disorders that may affect prognosis and guide treatment, assess lifestyle factors that might contribute to hypertension, expose identifiable causes of high BP, and determine whether target organ damage and cardiovascular disease (CVD) are present. This can be accomplished by obtaining a thorough medical history, physical examination, routine laboratory tests, and other diagnostic procedures. It is recommended that the following tests are routinely performed before initiating therapy: a 12-lead electrocardiogram (ECG), urinalysis, blood glucose, hematocrit, serum potassium, creatinine, calcium, and a lipoprotein profile.

TREATMENT

Lifestyle Modification

Several lifestyle factors have been associated with the development of hypertension, including excess body weight; excess dietary sodium intake; reduced physical activity; inadequate intake of fruits, vegetables, and potassium; smoking; and excess alcohol intake.[13-20] Lifestyle modifications are critical for both the prevention and treatment of hypertension.[21] Not only do such modifications forestall the development and progression of hypertension, they also enhance antihypertensive drug efficacy and decrease overall cardiovascular risk. Implementing multiple lifestyle interventions simultaneously results in additive benefit.[22] Despite irrefutable evidence supporting the relationship between lifestyle choices and cardiovascular risk, there remains considerable resistance on the part of patients to implement these changes and nonadherence is high.

Goals

Table 3-4 lists the lifestyle modifications that have consistently been shown to lower BP. Clinicians should encourage patients to adopt a healthy lifestyle that incorporates these habits. Focus is centered on diet, exercise to maintain normal body weight, and moderation of alcohol. For overall cardiovascular risk reduction, patients should be strongly encouraged to quit smoking.

TABLE 3-2 Secondary Causes of Hypertension

Identifiable Causes
Chronic kidney disease
Coarctation of the aorta
Cushing syndrome and other glucocorticoid excess states including chronic steroid therapy
Drug induced or drug related
Obstructive uropathy
Pheochromocytoma
Primary aldosteronism and other mineralocorticoid excess states
Renovascular hypertension
Sleep apnea
Thyroid or parathyroid disease
Associated Conditions
Smoking
Obesity
Obstructive sleep apnea
Hyperinsulinemia
Excessive ethanol intake
Anxiety
Chronic pain
Raynaud arteritis
Medications
Nonsteroidal anti-inflammatory drugs (NSAIDs) and cyclooxygenase-2 inhibitors
Sympathomimetics
Oral contraceptives
Steroids
Cyclosporine
Erythropoietin
Antidepressants (SNRIs, MAO-Is, TCAs)
Licorice
Beta-blockers or centrally acting alpha-agonists
Illicit Drug Use
Anabolic steroids

Diet

A diet high in sodium as well as low in fruits and vegetables is believed to account for the rising prevalence of hypertension in developed countries. Average sodium intake in the United States is approximately 4100 mg/d for men and 2750 mg/d for women; 75% of sodium intake is derived from processed foods.[23,24] Additionally, <25% of patients consume five or more servings of fruits and vegetables daily.[25] The Dietary Approaches to Stop Hypertension (DASH) eating plan was devised to aid in the prevention and treatment of hypertension.[15] Recommendations include a high intake of fruits, vegetables, and low-fat dairy products along with a reduced content of dietary cholesterol, saturated fat, and total

TABLE 3-3 **Blood Pressure Classification**

BP Classification	SBP (mm Hg)	DBP (mm Hg)	Intervention	Threshold for Starting Combination Therapy
Normal	<120	and <80	Lifestyle modification	N/A
Prehypertension	120-139	or 80-89	Lifestyle modification	N/A
Stage 1 hypertension	140-159	or 90-99	Pharmacotherapy plus lifestyle modification	≥160 or ≥ 100 mm Hg
Stage 2 hypertension	≥160	or ≥100	Pharmacotherapy plus lifestyle modification	Already on combination therapy

fat. The diet is also rich in potassium and calcium and low in sodium.[16] The preferred intake of dietary sodium is no more than 100 mmol/d (2.4 g of sodium).[15-17]

Exercise

Less than 20% of Americans engage in regular physical activity.[26] Lack of physical activity is one of the most important cardiovascular risk factors because excess weight and obesity increase the risk for hypertension, hyperlipidemia, diabetes, and other forms of cardiovascular disease. Presently, at least 122 million Americans are overweight or obese, including one out of every three children.[27] Weight loss as little as 10 lb (4.5 kg) reduces BP and/or prevents hypertension in a large proportion of overweight persons. Patients should be encouraged to achieve normal body weight.[13-14] In the absence of contraindications or disability, all patients with hypertension should participate in regular, aerobic physical activity most days of the week, for example, brisk walking at least 30 min/d.[18,19]

Alcohol

Excessive consumption of alcohol can increase BP. Alcohol intake should be limited to 1 oz (30 mL) or less of ethanol, the equivalent of two drinks per day in most men and one drink (0.5 oz) per day in women and lighter weight persons.[20]

Pharmacotherapy

Control rates (SBP <140 mm Hg and DBP <90 mm Hg) in persons with hypertension have improved over the last several years; nevertheless, they are still far below the Healthy People goal of 50%.[28] This goal was originally set for the year 2000 and has since been extended to 2010. In most patients, lowering SBP has been considerably more difficult than reducing DBP. Low control rates are likely multifactorial and include lack of awareness, failure to act on elevated BP levels in timely fashion, improper selection of antihypertensive drugs, and nonadherence to medications and lifestyle modifications. The majority of patients with hypertension will require two or more antihypertensive medications to reach their BP goal.[29-31]

Goals

The ultimate goal of hypertension management is to reduce cardiovascular and renal morbidity and mortality. Most hypertensive patients, especially over the age of 50, will reach the DBP goal once the SBP goal is achieved. Therefore the primary focus should be on attaining the SBP goal. A target goal of <140/90 mm Hg is associated with a decrease in cardiovascular complications.[32] In patients with concomitant diabetes or renal disease, the BP goal is <130/80 mm Hg.[33,34] The American Heart Association recently extended this more stringent goal to the

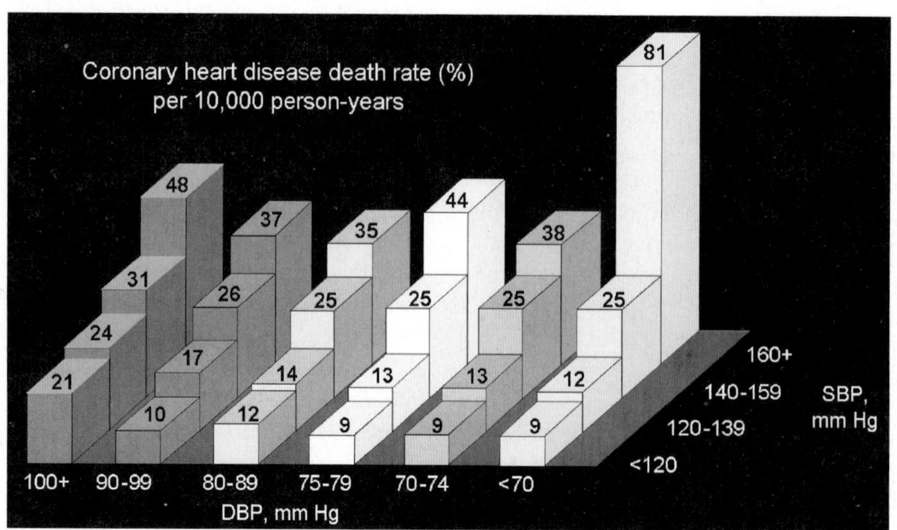

FIGURE 3-1 Systolic blood pressure is a more important cardiovascular risk factor than diastolic blood pressure.

TABLE 3-4 Lifestyle Modifications to Prevent and Manage Hypertension[a]

Modification	Recommendation	Approximate SBP Reduction (Range)[b]
Weight reduction	Maintain normal body weight (body mass index 18.5-24.9 kg/m^2)	5-20 mm Hg/10 kg[13,14]
Adopt DASH eating plan	Consume a diet rich in fruits, vegetables, and low-fat dairy products with a reduced content of saturated and total fat	8-14 mm Hg[15,16]
Dietary sodium reduction	Reduce dietary sodium intake to no more than 100 mmol/d (2.4 g sodium or 6 g sodium chloride)	2-8 mm Hg[15-17]
Physical activity	Engage in regular aerobic physical activity such as brisk walking (at least 30 min/d, most days of the week)	4-9 mm Hg[18,19]
Moderation of alcohol consumption	Limit consumption to no more than two drinks (eg, 24 oz beer, 10 oz wine, or 3 oz 80-proof whiskey) per day in most men, and to no more than one drink per day in women and lighter weight persons	2-4 mm Hg[20]

[a]For overall cardiovascular risk reduction, stop smoking.
[b]The effects of implementing these modifications are dose and time dependent, and could be greater for some individuals.
Abbreviations: DASH, dietary approaches to stop hypertension; SBP, systolic blood pressure.

following patient populations: high risk for coronary artery disease, stable angina, unstable angina, and ST elevation myocardial infarction.[35] In addition, the guidelines recommend a goal BP of <120/80 mm Hg in patients with left ventricular dysfunction. In clinical trials, antihypertensive therapy has been associated with reductions in (1) stroke incidence, averaging 35% to 40%; (2) myocardial infarction (MI), averaging 20% to 25%; and (3) HF, averaging >50%.[36] It is estimated that in patients with stage 1 hypertension (SBP 140-159 mm Hg and/or DBP 90-99 mm Hg) and additional cardiovascular risk factors, achieving a sustained 12 mm Hg reduction in SBP over 10 years will prevent 1 death for every 11 patients treated. In patients with established cardiovascular disease or target organ damage, only nine patients would require such BP reduction to prevent one death.[37]

Pharmacotherapy

Current targets for BP are listed in Table 3-5. Treatment of elevated blood pressure should begin immediately after the diagnosis of hypertension. A delay in pharmacotherapy in lieu of lifestyle changes is no longer recommended. A large selection of medications is currently available for the attainment of these goals. Tables 3-6 and 3-7 provide a list of the commonly used antihypertensive agents, their usual dose range, frequency of administration, available routes of administration, mechanism of action, adverse events, contraindications, and monitoring parameters. Table 3-8 lists the available combination products for the treatment of hypertension.

In order to achieve BP goals, over two-thirds of hypertensive patients will require two or more antihypertensive medications.[29,32,38-40] In the Antihypertensive and Lipid-Lowering Treatment to Prevent Heart Attack Trial (ALLHAT), one of the largest trials for hypertension, 60% of those whose BP was controlled to <140/90 mm Hg received two or more agents, and only 30% were controlled on one drug.[29] In hypertensive patients with tighter BP goals or with substantially elevated BP, three or more antihypertensive drugs may be required. As a result, guidelines recommend that treatment is started with combination therapy when the systolic BP is 20 mm Hg above goal or the diastolic BP is 10 mm Hg above goal.

In placebo-controlled trials, thiazide diuretics significantly reduced cardiovascular events, including stroke, coronary heart disease, and heart failure.[41-45] Hydrochlorothiazide (HCTZ) is the most commonly used thiazide diuretic in the United States, though most of the positive outcome data is with the thiazide diuretic chlorthalidone. ACEIs (angiotensin-converting enzyme inhibitors), ARBs (angiotensin receptor blockers), BBs (beta-blockers), and CCBs (calcium channel blockers) also reduce the complications of hypertension.[36,38,39,44,46-49] Several randomized, controlled trials have demonstrated reduction in CVD

TABLE 3-5 Recommended Blood Pressure Targets

Condition	SBP Goal (mm Hg)	DBP Goal (mm Hg)	Guideline
Uncomplicated hypertension	<140	<90	JNC 7, AHA
Diabetes	<130	<180	JNC 7
Renal disease	<130	<180	JNC 7
Proteinuria (>1 g/d)	<125	<75	JNC 7
Heart failure	<130	<80	JNC 7
	<120	<80	AHA
High CAD risk	<130	<80	AHA
UA, NSTEMI, STEMI	<130	<80	AHA

Abbreviations: SBP, systolic blood pressure; DBP, diastolic blood pressure; JNC 7, The Seventh Report of the Joint National Committee on Prevention, Detection, Evaluation, and Treatment of High Blood Pressure: the JNC 7 report; AHA, scientific statement from the American Heart Association Council for High Blood Pressure Research and the Councils on Clinical Cardiology and Epidemiology and Prevention; CAD, coronary artery disease; UA, unstable angina; NSTEMI, non-ST elevation myocardial infarction; STEMI, ST elevation myocardial infarction.

TABLE 3-6 **Oral Antihypertensive Drugs**[a]

Class	Drug (Trade Name)	Dose Range in mg/d[b]	Dose Frequency[b]	Most Common Routes of Administration
Thiazide diuretics	Chlorothiazide (Diuril)	125-500	1-2	po, IV
	Chlorthalidone (generic)	12.5-25	1	po
	Hydrochlorothiazide (Microzide, HydroDIURIL[c])	12.5-50	1	po
	Indapamide (Lozol[c])	1.25-2.5	1	po
	Metolazone (Mykrox)	0.5-1.0	1	po
	Metolazone (Zaroxolyn)	2.5-5	1	po
Loop diuretics	Bumetanide (Bumex[c]),	0.5-2	2	po, IV
	Furosemide (Lasix[c]),	20-80	2	po, IV
	Torsemide (Demadex[c])	2.5-10	1	po, IV
Potassium-sparing diuretics	Amiloride (Midamor[c])	5-10	1-2	po
	Triamterene (Dyrenium)	50-100	1-2	po
Aldosterone antagonists	Eplerenone (Inspra)	50-100	1	po
	Spironolactone (Aldactone[c])	25-50	1	po
BBs	Atenolol (Tenormin[c])	25-100	1	po, IV
	Betaxolol (Kerlone[c])	5-20	1	po
	Bisoprolol (Zebeta[c])	2.5-10	1	po
	Metoprolol (Lopressor[c])	50-100	1-2	po, IV
	Metoprolol extended release (Toprol XL)	50-100	1	po
	Nadolol (Corgard[c])	40-120	1	po
	Propranolol (Inderal[c])	40-160	2	po, IV
	Propranolol long acting (Inderal LA[c])	60-180	1	
	Timolol (Blocadren[c])	20-40	2	po
BBs with ISA	Acebutolol (Sectral[c])	200-800	2	po
	Penbutolol (Levatol)	10-40	1	po
	Pindolol (generic)	10-40	2	po
Combination alpha- and beta-blockers	Carvedilol (Coreg)	12.5-50	2	po
	Labetalol (Normodyne, Trandate[c])	200-800	2	po, IV
Beta-blocker with NO activity	Nebivolol (Bystolic)	5-40	1	po
ACE inhibitors	Benazepril (Lotensin[c])	10-40	1	po
	Captopril (Capoten[c])	25-100	2	po
	Enalapril (Vasotec[c])	5-40	1-2	po, IV
	Fosinopril (Monopril)	10-40	1	po
	Lisinopril (Prinivil, Zestril[c])	10-40	1	po
	Moexipril (Univasc)	7.5-30	1	po
	Perindopril (Aceon)	4-8	1	po
	Quinapril (Accupril)	10-80	1	po
	Ramipril (Altace)	2.5-20	1	po
	Trandolapril (Mavik)	1-4	1	po
Angiotensin II receptor blockers (ARB)	Candesartan (Atacand)	8-32	1	po
	Eprosartan (Teveten)	400-800	1-2	po
	Irbesartan (Avapro)	150-300	1	po
	Losartan (Cozaar)	25-100	1-2	po
	Olmesartan (Benicar)	20-40	1	po
	Telmisartan (Micardis)	20-80	1	po
	Valsartan (Diovan)	80-320	1-2	po
CCBs: non-dihydropyridines	Diltiazem extended release (Cardizem CD, Dilacor XR, Tiazac[c])	180-420	1	po, IV[d]
	Diltiazem extended release (Cardizem LA)	120-540	1	
	Verapamil immediate release (Calan, Isoptin[c])	80-320	2	
	Verapamil long acting (Calan SR, Isoptin SR[c])	120-480	1-2	
	Verapamil (Covera HS, Verelan PM)	120-360	1	
CCBs: dihydropyridines	Amlodipine (Norvasc)	2.5-10	1	po
	Felodipine (Plendil)	2.5-20	1	po
	Isradipine (Dynacirc CR)	2.5-10	2	
	Nicardipine sustained release (Cardene SR)	60-120	2	po, IV
	Nifedipine long-acting (Adalat CC, Procardia XL)	30-60	1	
	Nisoldipine (Sular)	10-40	1	po

(*Continued*)

TABLE 3-6 **Oral Antihypertensive Drugs[a] *(Continued)***

Class	Drug (Trade Name)	Dose Range in mg/d[b]	Dose Frequency[b]	Most Common Routes of Administration
Alpha-1 blockers	Doxazosin (Cardura)	1-16	1	po
	Prazosin (Minipress[c])	2-20	2-3	po
	Terazosin (Hytrin)	1-20	1-2	po
Central alpha-2 agonists	Clonidine (Catapres[c])	0.1-0.8	2	po, IV
	Clonidine patch (Catapres-TTS)	0.1-0.3	1/wk	Transdermal
	Methyldopa (Aldomet[c])	250-1000	2	po, IV
	Reserpine (generic)	0.1-0.25	1	
	Guanfacine (Tenex[c])	0.5-2	1	
Direct vasodilators	Hydralazine (Apresoline[c])	25-100	2	po, IV
	Minoxidil (Loniten[c])	2.5-80	1-2	po

[a]In some patients treated once daily, the antihypertensive effect may diminish toward the end of the dosing interval (trough effect).
[b]Dosage range and frequency are for oral dosage forms.
[c]Available now or becoming available soon in generic preparations.
[d]Diltiazem is also available as a powder for injection.
BP should be measured just prior to dosing to determine if satisfactory BP control is obtained. Accordingly, an increase in dosage or frequency may need to be considered. These dosages may vary from those listed in the *Physician's Desk Reference* (57th ed).
Abbreviations: ACEIs, angiotensin-converting enzyme inhibitors; BBs, beta blockers; CCBs, calcium channel blockers; ISA, intrinsic sympathomimetic activity; NO, nitric oxide.

with BBs, but the benefits are less consistent than with other antihypertensive agents (especially in older patients).[44,45] Table 3-7 lists commonly used antihypertensive agents and Table 3-8 lists agents that are available in fixed dose combinations.

Initial Therapy

Figure 3-2 depicts the treatment algorithm advocated by the JNC 7 guidelines. It is recommended that most patients be treated with a thiazide diuretic as initial therapy. The basis for this recommendation is the multiple clinical trials showing that thiazide diuretics lower BP and prevent cardiovascular events, along with the low cost of these agents and their acceptable side effect profile. An ACEI, ARB, CCB, or BB are acceptable alternatives to a thiazide diuretic as initial therapy if compelling indications are present or a thiazide is contraindicated.

Thiazide-Type Diuretic

Several large clinical trials have compared thiazide diuretics to other therapies, demonstrating that thiazides are equally effective in the prevention of cardiovascular complications secondary to hypertension. In the ALLHAT study, which enrolled more than 40,000 hypertensive patients, there were no differences in the primary CVD outcome or mortality among patients randomized to the thiazide-type diuretic chlorthalidone, the ACEI lisinopril, or the CCB amlodipine.[29] The incidence of stroke was greater with lisinopril than chlorthalidone, but these differences were primarily present in African Americans who also experienced less BP lowering with lisinopril than diuretics. The incidence of HF was greater in CCB-treated and ACEI-treated individuals as compared to those receiving the diuretic, in both African Americans and Caucasians.

Thiazide diuretics are especially effective in the elderly and in blacks where volume and heightened PVR are major contributors to elevated BP. In patients with renal insufficiency, thiazide diuretics are less effective. Thiazide diuretics become ineffective in the management of BP when creatinine clearance approaches 30 mL/min and below. At this point it becomes necessary to switch to (or add) a loop diuretic.

Diuretics are generally well tolerated at the doses currently employed in clinical practice, which are equivalent to 25 to 50 mg of hydrochlorothiazide or 12.5 to 25 mg of chlorthalidone.[29,40] Higher doses have demonstrated little additional antihypertensive efficacy, and are associated with more hypokalemia and other adverse effects.[50-53] Dysglycemia, dyslipidemia, hyperuricemia, sexual dysfunction, and nephrolithiasis may occur.[54] Unlike loop diuretics, thiazides increase renal tubular reabsorption of calcium.

Diuretics are capable of interfering with glucose homeostasis and can predispose patients to developing diabetes or make glucose control more challenging in patients with established disease. In ALLHAT, new-onset diabetes after 4 years of therapy occurred in 11.8% of patients on chlorthalidone, 9.6% on amlodipine, and 8.1% on lisinopril. However, those differences did not translate into fewer cardiovascular events for the ACEI or CCB groups.[29,46] In fact, those patients who were diabetic at baseline had fewer cardiovascular events following treatment with a diuretic compared to an ACEI. In general, trials of longer than 1 year using modest doses of diuretics have not shown an increase in serum cholesterol in diuretic-treated patients.[55,56] Routine laboratory monitoring is required with thiazide-type diuretics to ensure that electrolytes, uric acid, lipids, and blood glucose remain within the normal range.

Other Diuretics

In patients with significant renal impairment (creatinine clearance <30 mL/min), thiazide diuretics lose their effectiveness. In such patients, loop diuretics may be considered. Loop diuretics can also cause lipid and glucose disturbances in addition to

TABLE 3-7 Details of Oral Antihypertensive Agents

Class	Mechanism of Action	Adverse Reactions	Contraindications	Monitoring Parameters[a]
Thiazide diuretics	Increase the excretion of Na^+, Cl^+, and H_2O by inhibiting Na^+/Cl^- ion exchange in the early part of the distal tubule; lower blood pressure by decreasing extracellular fluid volume which decreases peripheral vascular resistance	Glucose disturbance Negative effects on lipids Electrolyte abnormalities ($\downarrow K^+$, Mg^{2+}, Cl^-, and HCO_3^-; $\uparrow$UA, Ca^{2+})	Anuria Thiazide or sulfonamide hypersensitivity	Blood glucose Lipids Electrolytes (Ca^{2+}, Mg^{2+}, K^+) BUN/SrCr UA
Loop diuretics	Inhibit the reabsorption of Na^+ and Cl^- in the ascending limb of the loop of Henle by interfering with the Cl^- binding of the $Na^+/K^+/2Cl^-$ cotransport system; renal vasodilation occurs, decreasing renal vascular resistance; reduce peripheral vascular resistance; the subsequent decrease in left ventricular filling pressure may contribute to the drug's beneficial effect in patients with congestive heart failure	Glucose disturbance Increase cholesterol and triglycerides Electrolyte abnormalities ($\downarrow$ Na^+, Cl^-, K^+, Ca^{2+}, Mg^{2+}, and HCO_3^-; $\uparrow$ UA)	Anuria	Audiometry Blood glucose BUN/SrCr Serum electrolytes UA Lipids
Potassium-sparing diuretics	Inhibit the Na^+/K^+ ion exchange in the distal renal tubule; inhibit sodium transport mechanisms directly, thereby setting up an electrical-potential difference across the membrane that blocks the passive distal tubular secretion of potassium; increase in urinary excretion of electrolytes and H_2O leads to a slight diuresis	Glucose disturbance Negative effects on lipids Electrolyte abnormalities ($\downarrow$ Na^+, HCO_3^+, Ca^{2+}, and Cl^-; $\uparrow$ K^+) Note: triamterene decreases Mg^{2+}, amiloride increases Mg^{2+}	Anuria Hepatic disease Renal failure Hyperkalemia	Blood glucose Lipids Serum electrolytes BUN/SrCr UA
Aldosterone antagonists	Inhibit effects of aldosterone on the distal renal tubules; enhance Na^+, Cl^-, and H_2O excretion; reduce the excretion of K^+, ammonium, and phosphate	Electrolyte abnormalities Gynecomastia and breast pain with spironolactone	Anuria Hyperkalemia Renal failure	BUN/SrCr Serum electrolytes
Beta-blockers	Reduce both resting and exercise heart rate, cardiac output, and both systolic and diastolic blood pressure; reduce sympathetic outflow from the CNS and suppress renin release from the kidneys; agents with ISA stimulate beta-receptors when sympathetic tone is low; agents that also block alpha-receptors or increase nitric oxide reduce peripheral vascular resistance	Exercise intolerance Fatigue Bradycardia Sexual dysfunction Depression Cold extremities Exacerbate reactive airway disease Exacerbate peripheral vascular disease Glucose disturbance $\uparrow$ Triglycerides $\downarrow$ HDL	AV block Cardiogenic shock Heart failure Hypotension	None
Angiotensin-converting enzyme inhibitors	Block the conversion of angiotensin I to angiotensin II by interfering with angiotensin-converting enzyme (ACE) activity; BP is also lowered through arterial dilation, lowering total peripheral vascular resistance; also inhibit kininase II (identical to ACE), an enzyme that degrades bradykinin, a potent vasodilator	Cough Angioedema Hyperkalemia Worsening renal function	Angioedema Hypersensitivity to ACE inhibitors Pregnancy	BUN/SrCr Electrolytes (K^+, Na^+)
Angiotensin II antagonists	Antagonize angiotensin II at the AT_1 receptor subtype, which decreases systemic vascular resistance	Angioedema Hyperkalemia Worsening renal function	Pregnancy	BUN/SrCr Electrolytes (K^+, Na^+)
Calcium channel blockers: non-dihydropyridines	Inhibit the influx of extracellular Ca^{2+} across the myocardial and vascular smooth muscle cell membranes; decrease in intracellular calcium inhibits the contractile processes of the myocardial smooth muscle cells, resulting in dilation of the coronary and systemic arteries	Bradycardia Constipation Gingival hyperplasia Worsening of heart failure due to negative inotropic effect	Acute myocardial infarction AV block Cardiogenic shock Heart failure Hypotension Lown-Ganong-Levine syndrome Sick sinus syndrome Ventricular dysfunction Ventricular tachycardia Wolff-Parkinson-White syndrome	ECG Echo LFTs

(Continued)

TABLE 3-7 Details of Oral Antihypertensive Agents (*Continued*)

Class	Mechanism of Action	Adverse Reactions	Contraindications	Monitoring Parameters[a]
Calcium channel blockers: dihydropyridines	Inhibit the influx of extracellular Ca^{2+} across the vascular smooth muscle cell membranes; decrease in intracellular calcium inhibits the contractile processes of smooth muscle cells, resulting primarily in dilation of arteries	Dose dependent peripheral edema Headache Flushing	Dihydropyridine sensitivity	None
Alpha-1 blockers	Cause peripheral vasodilation by selective, competitive inhibition of vascular postsynaptic alpha-1-adrenergic receptors, thereby reducing peripheral vascular resistance	Mild sexual dysfunction Nasal stuffiness Postural hypotension	None	None
Central alpha-2 agonists	Agonize presynaptic alpha-2-receptors in the medulla, inhibiting sympathetic outflow and tone; suppression of efferent sympathetic pathways decreases vascular tone in the heart, kidneys, and peripheral vasculature; lowers peripheral resistance	Bradycardia Dry mouth Orthostatic hypotension Rash (transdermal patch) Rebound hypertension	None	None
Direct vasodilators	Direct vasodilatory effect on arterial smooth muscle, reducing peripheral resistance; all direct vasodilators produce a compensatory sympathetic response including an increase in heart rate, stroke volume, and cardiac output, and a marked increase in plasma renin activity, which, in turn, leads to increased sodium and water retention	Orthostatic hypotension Reflex tachycardia (can abate with BB) Rebound Na^+ retention (abate with a loop diuretic) Minoxidil: hirsutism Hydralazine: drug-induced lupus	Minoxidil: pheochromocytoma Hydralazine: coronary heart disease, rheumatic heart disease	BUN/SrCr ANA with hydralazine

[a]With all antihypertensive medications, the response to therapy should be evaluated with careful monitoring of blood pressure and heart rate.

Abbreviations: ACEIs, angiotensin-converting enzyme inhibitors; BBs, beta-blockers; BUN, blood urea nitrogen; Ca^{2+}, calcium; CCBs, calcium channel blockers; Cl^-, chloride; ECG, electrocardiogram; ECHO, echocardiogram; HCO_3, bicarbonate; H_2O, water; ISA, intrinsic sympathomimetic activity; K^+, potassium; Mg^{2+}, magnesium; Na^+, sodium; SrCr, serum creatinine; UA, uric acid.

electrolyte imbalances, mandating the requirement of routine laboratory monitoring. At minimum, furosemide and bumetanide need to be administered in two or three divided doses to achieve 24-hour BP control. Like thiazide diuretics, loop diuretics increase the excretion of potassium and magnesium. An important distinction, however, is that loops increase calcium excretion while thiazides decrease calcium excretion.

Potassium-sparing diuretics, such as amiloride or triamterene, can be used in combination with other agents in order to offset hypokalemia. These agents are not used as monotherapy.

Aldosterone antagonists are reserved for treating patients with resistant hypertension, hyperaldosteronism, or compelling indications.[57] They can cause life-threatening hyperkalemia, especially when potassium is elevated at baseline, in patients with chronic kidney disease, or when concomitant medications (eg, NSAIDs) predispose patients to hyperkalemia.

ACE Inhibitors

The angiotensin-converting enzyme (ACE) converts angiotensin I to angiotensin II, a potent vasoconstrictor and negative-feedback mediator for renin activity. Angiotensin II is the primary vasoactive hormone of the RAS and plays an important role in the pathophysiology of hypertension and cardiovascular disease. ACEIs compete with angiotensin I for ACE and reduce the conversion of angiotensin I to angiotensin II. ACEIs also inhibit kininase II, an enzyme identical to ACE, which degrades the potent vasodilator bradykinin to inactive peptides. Bradykinin-induced vasodilation is thought to contribute to the blood-pressure lowering and cardiovascular protection afforded by ACEIs. Bradykinin has been implicated as the cause of ACEI-induced cough and angioneurotic edema.[58]

Compelling indications for the use of an ACEI as first-line therapy are listed in Table 3-9. In these clinical settings, ACEIs have been shown to reduce cardiovascular morbidity and mortality, and at least a fraction of the benefit cannot be explained by BP lowering. Results of the Heart Outcomes Prevention Evaluation (HOPE) trial, which studied the ACE-I ramipril versus placebo in high-risk patients without established CVD, demonstrated significant reductions in all primary cardiovascular endpoints in patients treated with ramipril (composite of MI, stroke, or death from CVD: 22% relative risk [RR], $P<0.001$; death from MI: 20% RR, $P<0.001$; death from stroke: 32% RR, $P<0.001$; death from CVD: 26% RR, $P<0.001$).[47] A subset of this study, Micro-HOPE, examined ramipril versus placebo in patients with established diabetes mellitus. The study was stopped 6 months early (after 4.5 years) by the independent data safety and monitoring board because of a consistent benefit of ramipril compared with placebo. Ramipril lowered the risk of the combined primary outcome by 25% (95% confidence interval [CI] 12-36, $P = 0.0004$), MI by 2% (6-36), stroke by 33% (10-50), cardiovascular death by 37% (21-51), total mortality by 24% (8-37), revascularization by 17% (2-30), and overt nephropathy by 24% (3-40, $P = 0.027$).[59] After adjustment for the changes in systolic (2.4 mm Hg) and

TABLE 3-8 Combination Drugs for Hypertension

Combination Type[a]	Fixed-Dose Combination (mg)[b]	Trade Name
ACEIs and CCBs	Amlodipine-benazepril hydrochloride (2.5/10, 5/10, 5/20, 10/20)	Lotrel
	Enalapril-felodipine (5/5)	Lexxel
	Trandolapril-verapamil (2/180, 1/240, 2/240, 4/240)	Tarka
ACEIs and diuretics	Benazepril-hydrochlorothiazide (5/6.25, 10/12.5, 20/12.5, 20/25)	Lotensin HCT
	Captopril-hydrochlorothiazide (25/15, 25/25, 50/15, 50/25)	Capozide
	Enalapril-hydrochlorothiazide (5/12.5, 10/25)	Vaseretic
	Fosinopril-hydrochlorothiazide (10/12.5, 20/12.5)	Monopril/HCT
	Lisinopril-hydrochlorothiazide (10/12.5, 20/12.5, 20/25)	Prinzide, Zestoretic
	Moexipril-hydrochlorothiazide (7.5/12.5, 15/25)	Uniretic
	Quinapril-hydrochlorothiazide (10/12.5, 20/12.5, 20/25)	Accuretic
ARBs and diuretics	Candesartan-hydrochlorothiazide (16/12.5, 32/12.5)	Atacand HCT
	Eprosartan-hydrochlorothiazide (600/12.5, 600/25)	Teveten-HCT
	Irbesartan-hydrochlorothiazide (150/12.5, 300/12.5)	Avalide
	Losartan-hydrochlorothiazide (50/12.5, 100/25)	Hyzaar
	Olmesartan medoxomil-hydrochlorothiazide (20/12.5, 40/12.5, 40/25)	Benicar HCT
	Telmisartan-hydrochlorothiazide (40/12.5, 80/12.5)	Micardis-HCT
	Valsartan-hydrochlorothiazide (80/12.5, 160/12.5, 160/25)	Diovan-HCT
ARBs, CCB, and diuretic	Valsartan-amlodipine-hydrochlorothiazide	Exforge
	Olmesartan-amlodipine-hydrochlorothiazide	Azor
BBs and diuretics	Atenolol-chlorthalidone (50/25, 100/25)	Tenoretic
	Bisoprolol-hydrochlorothiazide (2.5/6.25, 5/6.25, 10/6.25)	Ziac
	Metoprolol-hydrochlorothiazide (50/25, 100/25)	Lopressor HCT
	Nadolol-bendroflumethiazide (40/5, 80/5)	Corzide
	Propranolol LA-hydrochlorothiazide (40/25, 80/25)	Inderide LA
	Timolol-hydrochlorothiazide (10/25)	Timolide
Centrally acting drugs and diuretics	Methyldopa-hydrochlorothiazide (250/15, 250/25, 500/30, 500/50)	Aldoril
	Reserpine-chlorthalidone (0.125/25, 0.25/50)	Demi-Regroton, Regroton
	Reserpine-chlorothiazide (0.125/250, 0.25/500)	Diupres
	Reserpine-hydrochlorothiazide (0.125/25, 0.125/50)	Hydropres
Diuretic and diuretic	Amiloride-hydrochlorothiazide (5/50)	Moduretic
	Spironolactone-hydrochlorothiazide (25/25, 50/50)	Aldactazide
	Triamterene-hydrochlorothiazide (37.5/25, 75/50)	Dyazide, Maxzide

[a]ACEIs, angiotensin-converting enzyme inhibitors; ARBs, angiotensin receptor blockers; BBs, beta-blockers; CCBs, calcium channel blockers.
[b]Some drug combinations are available in multiple fixed doses. Each drug dose is reported in milligrams.

diastolic (1.0 mm Hg) BPs, ramipril still lowered the risk of the combined primary outcome by 25% (12-36, $P = 0.0004$).

Angiotensin II Antagonists

ARBs selectively block the effects of angiotensin II by binding to the AT_1 receptor subtype. Two angiotensin II receptors, AT_1 and AT_2, have been identified. By selectively blocking the AT_1 receptor in tissues such as vascular smooth muscle and the adrenal gland, ARBs block the vasoconstrictor, inflammatory, and aldosterone-secreting effects of angiotensin II. The Valsartan Antihypertensive Long-term Use Evaluation (VALUE) trial, which compared amlodipine and valsartan for the treatment of hypertension in high-risk patients, found no difference in the primary endpoint of CVD (hazard ratio 1.04, 95% CI 0.94-1.15, $P = 0.49$).[60] The recent Ongoing Telmisartan Alone and in combination with Ramipril Global Endpoint Trial (ONTARGET) illustrated the similar efficacy of ACEIs and ARBs in high-risk patients with hypertension.[61] ONTARGET randomized 8576 patients to ramipril and 8542 to telmisartan and reported that cardiovascular and renal events occurred in similar numbers of patients in both groups.

At a median follow-up of 56 months, the primary outcome had occurred in 1412 patients in the ramipril group (16.5%), as compared with 1423 patients in the telmisartan group (16.7%; RR, 1.01; 95% CI, 0.94-1.09). As compared with the ramipril group, the telmisartan group had lower rates of cough (1.1% vs 4.2%, $P < 0.001$) and angioedema (0.1% vs 0.3%, $P = 0.01$) as well as a higher rate of hypotensive symptoms (2.6% vs 1.7%, $P < 0.001$); the rate of syncope was the same in the two groups (0.2%). ARBs do not influence bradykinin metabolism and therefore do not cause cough. Rarely, they can cause angioneurotic edema but the incidence is less than for ACEIs. In patients who experience a cough during treatment with an ACEI, an ARB can safely be substituted.

While ACEIs initially suppress angiotensin II levels, other enzymes eventually restore angiotensin II production. These non-ACE pathways for angiotensin II formation have been deemed "ACE escape" and prompted the design of studies evaluating the benefit of combining an ACEI with an ARB. In the largest study conducted to date comparing the the combination of an ACEI plus ARB to monotherapy, mean BP

TABLE 3-9 **Compelling Indications for the Use of Select Antihypertensive Classes**

	Diuretic	BB	ACEI	ARB	CCB	AA
Heart failure	√	√	√	√		√
Post-MI		√	√	√[a]		√
CAD risk	√	√	√		√	
DM	√	√	√	√	√	
Renal disease			√	√		
Recurrent stroke prevention	√		√	√[a]		

[a]JNC 7 did not consider post-MI or recurrent stroke prevention compelling indications for ARB use; however, several subsequent studies have confirmed the efficacy of ARBs in these populations.

Abbreviations: AA, aldosterone antagonist; ACEI, angiotensin-converting enzyme inhibitor; ARB, angiotensin II receptor blocker; BB, beta-blocker; CCB, calcium channel blocker; DM, diabetes mellitus; post-MI, post-myocardial infarction.

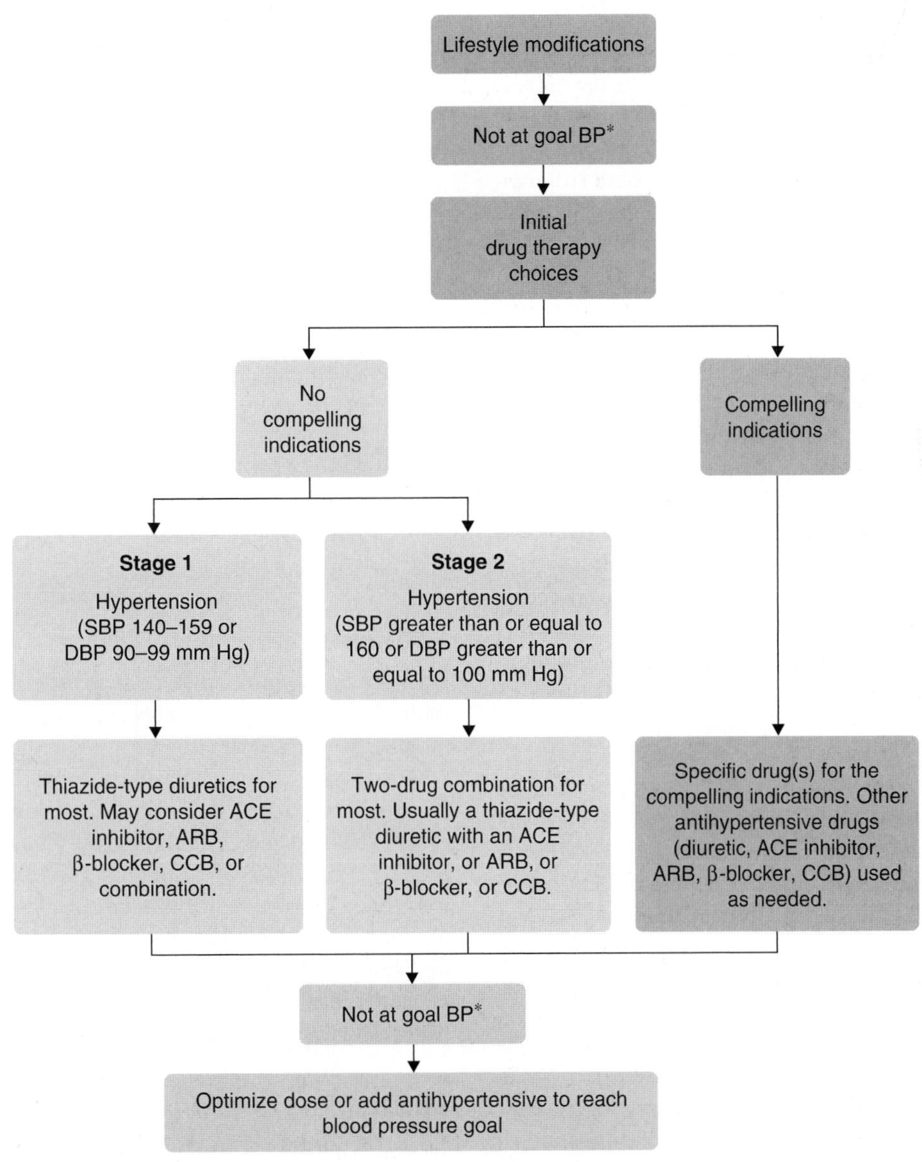

FIGURE 3-2 Treatment algorithm for the management of hypertension.
Reproduced with permission from Chisholm-Burns MA, Wells BG, Schwinghammer TL, et al, eds. *Pharmacotherapy Principles & Practice*. 2nd ed. New York, NY: McGraw-Hill; 2010:53.

was lower in the combination-therapy group (a 2.4/1.4 mm Hg greater reduction) than in the ramipril group;[62] however, there was an increased risk of hypotensive symptoms (4.8% vs 1.7%, P <0.001), syncope (0.3% vs 0.2%, P = 0.03), and renal dysfunction (13.5% vs 10.2%, P <0.001) with combination therapy. Based on these recent results, the combination of an ACEI and ARB is not recommended for the treatment of uncomplicated hypertension.

Calcium Channel Blockers

Both dihydropyridine (DHP) and nondihydropyridine (NDHP) CCBs have demonstrated efficacy in lowering BP and reducing cardiovascular events equal to that of other classes of blood-pressure medications.[30,32,46,63] As previously stated, the ALLHAT trial showed equal efficacy with the DHP CCB amlodipine compared to chlorthalidone and lisinopril for the primary composite endpoint of fatal and nonfatal coronary heart disease.[29] There was an increased risk of heart failure with amlodipine compared to chlorthalidone. In the Nordic Diltiazem (NORDIL) study, the NDHP CCB diltiazem was as effective as the diuretic, BB, or both in preventing the combined primary endpoint of all stroke, MI, and other cardiovascular death in hypertensive patients (BP reduction 20.3/18.7 vs 23.3/18.7 mm Hg; difference in systolic reduction P <0.001).[63] A primary endpoint occurred in 403 patients in the diltiazem group and in 400 in the diuretic and BB group (16.6 vs 16.2 events per 1000 patient-years; RR 1.00 [95% CI 0.87-1.15], P = 0.97). Fatal and nonfatal stroke occurred in 159 patients in the diltiazem group and in 196 patients in the diuretic and BB group (6.4 vs 7.9 events per 1000 patient-years; 0.80 [0.65-0.99], P = 0.04). Fatal and nonfatal MI occurred in 183 and 157 patients (7.4 vs 6.3 events per 1000 patient-years; 1.16 [0.94-1.44], P = 0.17). Based in these and other studies, CCBs should be considered an important part of the armamentarium. They are particularly useful in persons with angina. Short-acting CCBs, like immediate release formulations of nifedipine, should be avoided due to the potential for rapid and profound BP changes and the attendant risk of cardiovascular events.

Beta-Blockers

Originally, BBs were recommended as first-line therapy for the treatment of hypertension. Recent evidence has shown that in the absence of compelling indications, such as post-MI or HF, BBs are inferior to other classes of antihypertensive medications as first-line therapy.[63,64] In the Losartan Intervention for Endpoint Reduction in Hypertension (LIFE) study, high-risk patients with hypertension were randomized to treatment with either the BB, atenolol, or the ARB, losartan. Losartan reduced the incidence of CVD events by 13% relative to atenolol despite similar reductions in BP.[39] A recent meta-analysis showed the relative risk of stroke was 16% higher for BBs (95% CI 4%-30%) than for other drugs.[64] There was no difference in MI. When the effect of BBs was compared with that of placebo or no treatment, the relative risk of stroke was reduced by 19% for all BBs (7%-29%), about half of that expected from previous hypertension trials.

Notably, most of the studies included in the meta-analysis and the LIFE trial studied nonvasodilating, relatively short acting BBs, such as atenolol. At this time, it is not clear whether BBs are more effective if they are adequately dosed or if vasodilating BBs are superior. Newer BBs, such as those with alpha-blocking properties (carvedilol and labetalol) or the ability to increase the bioactivity of nitric oxide (nebivolol) might be more effective. Their vasodilating actions exert favorable effects on central aortic BP, are less likely to disturb glucose and lipid homeostasis, and may be better tolerated. Further studies are required to determine if these effects translate into meaningful differences in outcomes. In the meantime, BBs should be reserved for use in hypertension when compelling indications for beta-blockade are present.

Other Classes of Medications

Alpha-1 blockers, such as doxazosin, terazosin, and prazosin, should be reserved for patients with benign prostatic hypertrophy (BPH). In an earlier study by the ALLHAT collaborative research group, the doxazosin arm was discontinued prematurely due to an increased risk for stroke, combined CVD and HF.[65] Centrally-acting medications (ie, clonidine) and direct vasodilators (eg, minoxidil) should be reserved for resistant hypertension. When direct acting vasodilators are used for resistant hypertension, BBs and diuretics are often required to offset the reflex tachycardia and fluid retention that occurs with these agents. Recently, the first direct renin inhibitor, aliskiren, was approved for the treatment of hypertension.[66] Aliskiren blocks the enzymatic activity of renin thereby interrupting the conversion of angiotensinogen to angiotensin I. It is approximately as effective as other antihypertensives and like ACE inhibitors and ARBs it works well with diuretics and CCBs. Preliminary studies suggest that the addition of aliskiren to an ACE inhibitor or ARB is associated with favorable changes in surrogate markers in patients with heart failure, proteinuria, and left ventricular hypertrophy.

Follow-up and Monitoring

After the initiation of antihypertensive therapy, patients should return for follow-up at monthly intervals or until the BP goal is reached. More frequent visits are necessary for patients with stage 2 hypertension or complicating comorbid conditions. Once BP goal is reached, follow-up visits can be at 3- to 6-month intervals. Serum creatinine and electrolytes, most importantly potassium, should be monitored at least one to two times per year, perhaps more often in patients with chronic kidney disease. Comorbidities such as HF, associated diseases such as diabetes, and the need for laboratory testing all influence the frequency of visits. Other cardiovascular risk factors should be monitored and treated to their respective goals, especially the cessation of tobacco use.

Special Populations

Table 3-9 illustrates which classes of agents are listed for certain compelling indications.

Diabetes

Hypertension and diabetes frequently coexist and together they significantly increase the risk of CVD, stroke, progression of renal disease, and retinopathy.[67,68] Persons with diabetes manifest hypertension at a disproportionate rate and the converse is also true such that persons with elevated BP are 2.5 times more likely to develop diabetes within 5 years. Consequently, persons with hypertension and diabetes warrant a tailored approach to BP control.

Recommendations from the JNC 7 guidelines for the treatment of hypertension in patients with diabetes are consistent with those of the American Diabetes Association. Both recommend tight control of BP, aiming for levels <130/80 mm Hg, in order to mitigate the risk of cardiovascular events, end stage renal disease, and nephropathy. Several classes of medications including diuretics, ACEIs, BBs, ARBs, and CCBs have been proven effective for reducing risk in patients with type 1 and type 2 diabetes. Each of these medications can be considered to treat elevated BP in persons with diabetes; however, an ACEI, or ARB in ACEI intolerant patients, is considered first line based on results from several clinical trials suggesting a benefit beyond BP lowering and their favorable metabolic profile. The majority of patients with diabetes will need two or more medications to control their BP. The most rationale combinations include either an ACEI or ARB combined with a diuretic or CCB.

The ADA advocates for the use of ACEIs or ARBs in patients with diabetes over the age of 55 or at high risk for CVD. In the high-risk diabetic subpopulation of the HOPE study, the addition of an ACEI to conventional therapy reduced the composite endpoint of MI, stroke, and CVD death by 25% while stroke was reduced by 33%.[47] Furthermore, ACEIs and ARBs do not worsen glycemia and, compared with other antihypertensive medications, actually lower the risk of new-onset diabetes.[69]

Thiazide diuretics have been shown to be effective in patients with diabetic hypertension. In the ALLHAT trial, chlorthalidone was as effective as lisinopril and amlodipine in subjects with diabetes at baseline.[29] While thiazide-type diuretics do impair insulin sensitivity and increase the risk for new-onset diabetes, the effect on blood glucose is modest. Combining a thiazide-type diuretic with an ACEI or ARB as part of combination therapy neutralizes some of the thiazide's effect on glucose metabolism and improves BP control compared with a monotherapeutic approach.

BBs can be used in the management of hypertension in patients with diabetes, especially when used adjunctively with other medications. Their role as monotherapy is controversial except in the presence of another compelling indication, such as coronary artery disease. One disadvantage to using BBs in this population is the predilection for BBs to impair glucose homeostasis. BBs adversely affect insulin sensitivity and can mask signs and symptoms of hypoglycemia; however, this caution does not represent a contraindication to their use. When BBs are used, agents that are beta-1 selective or that have vasodilatory properties are preferred because they are less likely to increase blood glucose compared with nonselective, nonvasodilating agents.[70]

CCBs effectively lower BP in diabetic patients and recent studies have shown that they also reduce cardiovascular events. In recent studies, such as ALLHAT, VALUE, and comparison of amlodipine versus enalapril to limit occurrences of thrombosis (CAMELOT), amlodipine compared favorably with other antihypertensive medications in persons with hypertension and diabetes, though amlodipine might be less effective at protecting against the development of HF and nephropathy.[29,60,71] When nephropathy or HF is present, an ACEI or ARB should be used before a CCB.

Chronic Kidney Disease

More than 70% of patients with chronic kidney disease (CKD), defined as a glomerular filtration rate (GFR) <60 mL/min/1.73 m^2 or the presence of albuminuria (>300 mg/d or 200 mg/g creatinine), have comorbid hypertension. Age-related deterioration of renal function is closely linked to BP, making aggressive BP control an important consideration in the prevention of ESRD, dialysis, and renal transplant. Nevertheless, few patients with hypertension and CKD exhibit adequately controlled BP. Recommendations from the American Society of Nephrology and National Kidney Foundation recommend a goal BP of <130/80 mm Hg and state that the majority of patients will need multiple drugs to control their BP. Treatment should consist of either an ACEI or ARB and diuretic in most patients. A loop diuretic should be substituted for a thiazide agent when GFR is markedly reduced (<30 mL/min/1.73 m^2).

While ACEIs and ARBs are recommended to control BP in patients with CKD, it is not uncommon for the glomerular filtration rate (GFR) to decrease shortly after starting treatment. Angiotensin II is responsible for maintaining efferent arteriolar tone. Consequently, treatment with an ACE inhibitor or ARB will transiently reduce efferent arteriolar tone and lower GFR; this is a hemodynamic decline in GFR and does not represent kidney damage. In patients who experience a transient reduction in GFR, serum creatinine should not increase more than 30% and typically stabilizes or normalizes after 4 weeks. Treatment should continue in these patients. If creatinine increases by more than 30% or fails to stabilize after 4 weeks, other causes like NSAID use or volume depletion should be sought and corrected. Rarely, bilateral renal artery stenosis might be the culprit.

Heart Failure

Hypertension doubles the risk of developing HF and 90% of patients with HF have a history of hypertension. Both the sympathetic and renin-angiotensin systems are overactive in the setting of HF and they contribute to disease progression. For these reasons, ACEI, ARBs, and BBs are the cornerstone of treatment. These agents should be used routinely in patients with HF, in the absence of contraindications, because they reduce morbidity and mortality. Because volume retention is a hallmark of HF, loop diuretics are often necessary to control volume; however, these agents do not improve survival and thus should be used for symptomatic purposes. The aldosterone antagonists, spironolactone and eplerenone, reduce morbidity and mortality in advanced stages of HF, namely NYHA class III and IV disease. Spironolactone and eplerenone must be used cautiously in the setting of renal insufficiency because of the risk of hyperkalemia. While there are no authoritative recommendations for target BP in HF, there is irrefutable evidence to suggest that BP lowering is beneficial. In most clinical trials demonstrating benefit, systolic BP was lowered to the range of 110 to 130 mm Hg.

Ischemic Heart Disease

The presence of hypertension increases the risk of major coronary events and progression of atherosclerosis. Correspondingly, lowering BP reduces ischemic events and retards the progression of atherothrombotic disease in patients with ischemic heart disease. While lower BP generally improves outcomes, efforts should be made to maintain diastolic BP above 55 to 60 mm Hg. Levels below have been shown, in some studies, to increase the risk for CVD events presumably due to the impairment of coronary artery filling during diastole. This "J-shaped" phenomenon has not been detected with systolic BP.

In patients with angina, BBs should be used to lower heart rate and BP, alleviate angina symptoms, and improve survival. If a BB is not appropriate due to bradycardia, AV block or severe reactive airway or peripheral arterial disease, DHP or NDHP-type CCBs may be considered and are equally effective.[72]

Cerebrovascular Disease

The risk for ischemic stroke, hemorrhagic stroke, and dementia increases precipitously as a function of BP. BP control, rather than the selection of a specific agent is the most important factor in the prevention of cerebrovascular disease. No specific agent or class of agents has been identified as the preferred method for BP control though preference should be given to diuretics, ACEIs, and ARBs according to JNC 7 guidelines. In the LIFE study, losartan markedly reduced the risk of stroke compared to atenolol. Several studies have specifically evaluated the utility of antihypertensive medications for preventing recurrent stroke. The combination of an ACEI and diuretic reduced the risk of stroke by 43%.[48] Similarly, the ARBs have demonstrated efficacy in preventing recurrent stroke.[73] While not identified as a compelling indication for DHP, CCBs stroke was significantly reduced in several studies which employed long-acting DHP CCBs.[74,75]

In the setting of an acute stroke, the ideal strategy for BP control has not been elucidated. After an acute stroke, if systolic BP is above 220 mm Hg or diastolic BP is between 120 and 140 mm Hg, it should be lowered cautiously by 10% to 15%. Simultaneously, neurological function should be vigilantly monitored for deterioration.

Resistant Hypertension

When patients treated with full doses of an appropriate three-drug regimen that includes a diuretic fail to achieve BP goal they are said to have resistant hypertension. Implied within this definition is that patients are adherent to drug and lifestyle therapies and that a diuretic appropriate for renal function is being used. The causes of resistant hypertension are multifactorial and include both drug and nondrug factors (Table 3-10).

TABLE 3-10 **Causes of Resistant Hypertension**
Improper blood pressure measurement
Volume overload
Excess sodium intake
Volume retention from kidney disease
Inadequate diuretic therapy
Drug-induced or other causes
Nonadherence
Inadequate doses
Inappropriate combinations
Nonsteroidal anti-inflammatory drugs; cyclooxygenase 2 inhibitors
Cocaine, amphetamines, other illicit drugs
Sympathomimetics (decongestants, anorectics)
Oral contraceptive hormones
Adrenal steroid hormones
Cyclosporine and tacrolimus
Erythropoietin
Licorice (including some chewing tobacco)
Selected over-the-counter dietary supplements and medicines (eg, Ephedra, ma huang, bitter orange)
Associated conditions
Obesity
Excess alcohol intake

Improper measurement of BP is a common cause of falsely elevated BP. For example, use of a BP cuff that is too small in patients with obesity can result in an overestimation of BP. In patients with advanced atherosclerotic vascular disease, the brachial artery may not be easily compressible due to calcification and this may cause an overestimation of BP.

A transient rise in BP that occurs in the health-care setting, also known as white coat hypertension, can produce elevated BP readings in clinic settings but normal readings at home; this phenomenon can be documented with ambulatory BP monitoring or home BP measurements. Volume overload is a common cause of resistant hypertension. Fortunately, diuretic therapy can easily palliate this type of BP. While thiazides are recommended as initial therapy for most patients with hypertension, loop diuretics should be considered when GFR is reduced. Clinicians are sometimes reluctant to advance doses or add new medications in patients with uncontrolled BP and this can result in treatment resistance.

Drug interactions are frequent causes of resistant hypertension. NSAIDs, steroids, sympathomimetic agents in cold remedies, and some nontraditional remedies may increase BP or interfere with antihypertensive drugs. When remediable causes of secondary hypertension are unclear, secondary causes for hypertension should be explored. Of the secondary forms of hypertension, renal parenchymal disease is the most common secondary cause.

Other options in patients with resistant hypertension include the addition of spironolactone, direct acting vasodilators, or referral to a specialist.

Hypertensive Crises

A hypertensive emergency is defined by a BP above 180/120 mm Hg with evidence of impending or progressive target organ dysfunction. These patients are susceptible to developing hypertensive encephalopathy, intracerebral hemorrhage, acute MI, acute left ventricular failure with pulmonary edema, unstable angina pectoris, dissecting aortic aneurysm, or eclampsia. Immediate BP lowering is warranted but the extent and timing of BP lowering is not clearly defined. When target organ damage is absent but BP is severely elevated, the event is deemed a hypertensive urgency.

Hypertensive emergencies should be treated with a parenteral antihypertensive agent administered in an intensive care setting with continuous monitoring of BP. The goals of therapy are to avoid cardiovascular events and reduce mean arterial BP by up to 25% within the first hour, then, if stable, to 160/100 to 110 mm Hg within the next 2 to 6 hours. Gradual lowering of BP is necessary to avoid precipitating ischemic events. For this reason, short-acting formulations of nifedipine, which can profoundly lower BP and cannot be easily titrated, should be avoided. Normal BP should be achieved by 24 to 48 hours. In hypertensive urgency, immediate BP lowering is less urgent and rapid-acting oral agents such as captopril, labetalol, or clonidine can be considered; however, there is no evidence that these agents improve outcomes. When these therapies are used, it is important that patients have a follow-up visit within several days to ensure that BP has responded and that hypotension is not an issue. Alternatively, it is appropriate to adjust or titrate medications in treated patients and to encourage adherence.

Women

In women who are pregnant or are attempting to conceive, ACEIs and ARBs are contraindicated because of the risk of fetal developmental abnormalities. Lifestyle modification is the mainstay of treating hypertension in pregnant women. This includes restricting sodium intake and avoiding alcohol and smoking. When drug therapy is warranted, methyldopa is the drug of choice based on reports of stable uteroplacental blood flow and fetal hemodynamics and the absence of long-term (7.5-year follow-up) adverse effects on development of children exposed to methyldopa in utero. BBs, especially labetalol, are considered alternatives to methyldopa. These agents are better tolerated than methyldopa.

Diuretics are particularly useful in elderly individuals because of a decreased risk of hip fracture. Some antihypertensive drugs have gender-specific adverse effect profiles. For example, in the Treatment of Mild Hypertension Study (TOMHS study), women reported twice as many adverse effects as men.[76] Women are more likely to develop diuretic-induced hyponatremia, and men more likely to develop gout. Hypokalemia is more common in women taking a diuretic. ACEI-induced cough is twice as common in women as in men, and women are more likely to complain of CCB-related peripheral edema and minoxidil-induced hirsutism.

Minorities

Hypertension is more common, more severe, develops at an earlier age, and leads to more clinical sequelae in African Americans compared with persons of other descent. Mexican Americans and native Americans also exhibit poor BP control rates. Minorities may respond especially well to weight reduction and sodium restriction and these interventions should be encouraged. Drugs that block the RAS, such as ACEIs, ARBs, and BBs, lower BP slightly less in African Americans compared with whites. This disparity was apparent in the ALLHAT trial which enrolled more than 15,000 blacks.[29] The ACEI lisinopril were less effective in lowering BP than either the thiazide-type diuretic or the CCB and the BP disparity resulted in a 40% greater risk of stroke, 32% greater risk of HF, and 19% greater risk of CVD in those randomized to the ACEI versus the diuretic. When RAS-blocking agents are administered with either a diuretic or CCB, interracial differences are no longer present. African Americans and Asians are more susceptible to angioedema and cough is more prevalent with ACEI.

Other Special Considerations

In patients experiencing urinary outflow obstruction due to benign prostatic hypertrophy, alpha-1 receptor antagonists such should be used because they not only lower BP but also indirectly dilate prostatic and urinary sphincter smooth muscle.

CASE Application

1. What is the BP goal for a hypertensive patient without any comorbid conditions and who is at low risk for heart disease based on the Framingham risk score?

   a. <120/80 mm Hg
   b. <140/90 mm Hg
   c. <130/80 mm Hg
   d. <125/75 mm Hg
   e. <160/100 mm Hg

2. Which of the following recommendations for lifestyle modification is correct?

   a. Weight loss of at least 15 lb.
   b. Sodium restriction of 4 g or less per day.
   c. Moderation of alcohol to no more than two drinks a day for a woman, one for a man.
   d. Exercise for at least 30 minutes most days of the week.
   e. Adopt an eating plan low in potassium and carbohydrates.

3. JD is a 55-year-old African American woman with newly diagnosed hypertension. Her average BP is 167/92 mm Hg. Which of the following is the best recommendation for JD?

a. Begin hydrochlorothiazide and return to clinic in 3 months.
b. Begin metoprolol and prescribe monitoring blood pressure at home.
c. Begin two medications since most patients with stage 2 hypertension will not reach goal with one agent alone.
d. Prescribe lifestyle modifications first, and return to clinic in 1 month to determine if pharmacotherapy is warranted.
e. Begin clonidine patch since a once weekly patch increases patient compliance.

4. JD was started on a new medication for her blood pressure. About a week later she noticed a persistent cough. Which of the following medications could be the cause?

a. Maxzide
b. Bystolic
c. Vasotec
d. Diovan
e. Catapres

5. You have identified the cause of the cough. At the next visit, JD wants to change the medication as she cannot tolerate the cough. Unfortunately, she missed her follow-up and returns to you in 6 months. In between appointments, she was admitted to the hospital and diagnosed with type 2 diabetes. Which of the following recommendations is best for JD?

a. Switch to Lopressor.
b. Switch to Atacand.
c. Switch to Altace.
d. Switch to Cardizem.
e. Continue her current medication as this side effect usually resolves in a couple of months, and may take up to a year.

6. FS is a 50-year-old woman diagnosed with osteoporosis and hypertension. Which of the following antihypertensives is most likely to help the patient's osteoporosis in addition to lowering her BP?

a. Dyazide
b. Demadex
c. Microzide
d. Capoten
e. Toprol XL

7. Which of the following statements is true regarding lifestyle modifications?

a. They only decrease the risk for cardiovascular disease.
b. They decrease the risk for renal disease but not stroke.
c. Morbidity, not mortality, is decreased.
d. They are critical for the prevention of hypertension but not the treatment.
e. Risk for cardiovascular and renal disease and stroke are all decreased.

8. A patient presents to the emergency room (ER) with signs and symptoms of hyperkalemia. Electrolyte testing reveals serum potassium of 6.7 mmol/L. All of the following agents could cause or exacerbate the situation *except* for which one?

a. Bumex
b. Mavik
c. Dyrenium
d. Aldactone
e. Cozaar

9. Which of the following is true regarding the use of combination treatment with an ACE inhibitor and an ARB for the treatment of hypertension?

a. The combination significantly reduces the risk of cardiovascular events in this setting.
b. The combination increases the risk of hyperkalemia but is otherwise safe in this setting.
c. The combination improves renal function in this setting.
d. The combination is very effective for controlling blood pressure in this setting.
e. This combination is not currently recommended because it does not reduce cardiovascular events in this setting.

10. DL is a 35-year-old man recently diagnosed with diabetes, hypertension, hyperlipidemia, and sexual dysfunction induced by diabetic neuropathy. Which of the following two-drug regimens is most appropriate to initiate in DL for antihypertensive therapy?

a. Amlodipine + lisinopril
b. Short-acting nifedipine + trandolapril
c. Doxazosin + HCTZ
d. Pindolol + losartan
e. HCTZ + lisinopril

11. The risk for cardiovascular events increases sharply when blood pressure exceeds:

a. 100/60 mm Hg
b. 115/75 mm Hg
c. 130/80 mm Hg
d. 140/90 mm Hg
e. 160/100 mm Hg

12. Which of the following is most correct regarding the pathophysiology of hypertension?

a. Most patients with hypertension have an identifiable secondary cause such as hyperaldosteronism.
b. Peripheral vascular resistance is often increased because the activity of the renin-angiotensin system is decreased.
c. Cardiac output and peripheral vascular resistance are the two key factors that determine blood pressure.
d. Stroke volume and heart rate are the two key factors that determine blood pressure.
e. In the elderly, cardiac output rises, increasing the risk of hypertension, especially diastolic hypertension.

13. AC is a 46-year-old white man with a medical history significant for type 2 diabetes (4 years), obesity, and new-onset hypertension. He is treated for his diabetes and his current HA1c is 7.2%. He was started on lisinopril 10 mg 4 weeks ago and the dose was increased after 2 weeks to 20 mg. His BP is now 146/94 mm Hg and his heart rate is 67 beats per minute (bpm). Which of the following is the most appropriate recommendation for AC?
    a. Continue current regimen with no changes.
    b. Discontinue lisinopril and start diltiazem.
    c. Discontinue lisinopril and start HCTZ.
    d. Add atenolol.
    e. Add amlodipine.
14. TJ is a 64-year-old man with long-standing untreated hypertension. He has recently been diagnosed with chronic kidney disease and his estimated glomerular filtration rate (GFR) is 24 mL/min. He is currently taking ramipril 10 mg/d and verapamil ER 240 mg/d. His blood pressure is 138/86 mm Hg, heart rate (HR) is 58 bpm, and electrolytes notable for a potassium of 5.1 mEq/L. Which of the following would be the best recommendation?
    a. Continue current therapy and monitor BP regularly.
    b. Add HCTZ 12.5 mg daily.
    c. Add furosemide 20 mg twice daily.
    d. Increase verapamil ER to 360 mg daily.
    e. Add spironolactone 25 mg qd.
15. RE is a 47-year-old white woman who has been seen by her family physician twice in the last 2 weeks, and her BP (measured properly) was similar at both visits, averaging 138/98 mm Hg. RH has no significant medical history or risk factors for cardiovascular disease; she is relatively active and likes to exercise. Which of the following would be the most appropriate recommendation for RH?
    a. She should be seen again by her physician within 2 months to see if she has hypertension.
    b. She should be counseled to undertake an intensive weight reduction program, with follow-up in 2 months.
    c. Initiate treatment with ramipril.
    d. Initiate treatment with atenolol.
    e. Initiate treatment with clonidine.
16. In a patient with risk factors and history of hyperkalemia, which of the following agents would be the least likely to increase potassium?
    a. Amiloride
    b. Amlodipine
    c. Enalapril
    d. Spironolactone
    e. Valsartan
17. Which of the following agents is the least likely to increase blood glucose?
    a. Chlorthalidone
    b. Furosemide
    c. Hydrochlorothiazide
    d. Lisinopril
    e. Propranolol
18. FS is a 56-year-old man with diabetes mellitus and newly diagnosed hypertension. His mean blood pressure in clinic today after three proper measurements is 158/101 mm Hg. He is not currently on treatment. Which of the following drug regimens would be the most appropriate to treat FS?
    a. Chlorthalidone
    b. Quinapril
    c. Benazepril + amlodipine
    d. Benazepril + losartan
    e. Atenolol + HCTZ
19. How would you classify an average blood pressure of 158/104 mm Hg (it is taken properly and averaged over two clinical visits)?
    a. Normal
    b. Prehypertension
    c. Stage 1 hypertension
    d. Stage 2 hypertension
    e. None of the above
20. Which of the following does not require monitoring in a patient on HCTZ?
    a. Renal function
    b. Hepatic function
    c. Electrolytes
    d. Uric acid
    e. Blood glucose
21. Which of the following should be considered in patients with resistant hypertension?
    a. Volume overload is a common cause.
    b. Spironolactone might be effective.
    c. Minoxidil might be effective.
    d. A loop diuretic might be necessary.
    e. All of the above.

TAKEAWAY POINTS ››

- Hypertension is common, asymptomatic, and results in tremendous morbidity and mortality.
- Essential hypertension is the most common type of hypertension.
- Systolic blood pressure most closely reflects the true burden of hypertension in patients older than 50 years, whereas diastolic blood pressure is more predictive in younger patients.

- Medications such as NSAIDs, hormonal therapy, and corticosteroids can be a cause of secondary hypertension.
- Lifestyle modification is the cornerstone of effective treatment. Limiting sodium intake and increasing intake of calcium and potassium, increasing physical activity, and avoiding smoking and alcohol are important lifestyle changes.
- Diuretic therapy should be considered for most patients as the initial treatment.
- Combinations of agents should be considered as the initial treatment strategy in all patients unlikely to get to goal on a single drug, especially those whose systolic BP is ≥20 mm Hg above goal or diastolic BP is ≥10 mm Hg above goal.
- Certain comorbidities, such as chronic kidney disease, diabetes, and heart failure, should be considered in order to customize drug therapy.
- ACE inhibitors and ARBs are mainstays in the treatment of diabetes, heart failure, and post-MI.
- BBs are important in patients with ischemic heart disease, HF, post-MI, angina, and arrhythmias.
- Renal function and serum electrolytes should be monitored in patients treated with diuretics and antagonists of the renin-angiotensin system.
- Renin-angiotensin system blockers are contraindicated in pregnant women.
- Common side effects with antihypertensive medications include exercise intolerance and fatigue (beta-blockers), bradycardia (beta-blockers and nondihydropyridine calcium channel blockers), dose-dependent peripheral edema (dihydropyridine calcium channel blockers), electrolyte abnormalities (diuretics and RAS blockers), cough (ACEIs), and glucose and lipid disturbances (diuretics and beta-blockers).

REFERENCES

1. Lloyd-Jones D, Adams R, Carnethon M, et al. Heart Disease and Stroke Statistics—2009 Update A Report From the American Heart Association Statistics Committee and Stroke Statistics Subcommittee. *Circulation*. 2009;119:e21-e181.
2. Ong KL, Cheung BM, Man YB, et al. Prevalence, awareness, treatment, and control of hypertension among United States adults 1999-2004. *Hypertension*. 2007;1:69-75.
3. Vasan RS, Beiser A, Seshadri S, et al. Residual lifetime risk for developing hypertension in middle aged women and men: The Framingham Heart Study. *JAMA*. 2002;287:1003-1010.
4. Lewington S, Clarke R, Qizilbash N, et al. Age-specific relevance of usual blood pressure to vascular mortality: a meta-analysis of individual data for one million adults in 61 prospective studies. Prospective Studies Collaboration. *Lancet*. 2002;360:1903-1913.
5. Bernard W, Francois F, Luis M, et al. Fixed-Dose Combinations as Initial Therapy for Hypertension: a review of approved agents and a guide to patient selection. *Drugs*. 2009;69(13):1761-1776.
6. Chobanian AV, Bakris GL, Black HR, et al. The seventh report of the joint national committee on prevention, detection, evaluation, and treatment of high blood pressure: The JNC 7 report. *JAMA*. 2003;289(19):2560-2572.
7. Thomas G, Pickering MD, John EH, et al. Recommendations for Blood Pressure Measurement in Humans and Experimental Animals. Part 1: Blood Pressure Measurement in Humans. A Statement for professionals from the subcommittee of professional and public education of the American Heart Association Council on High Blood Pressure Research. *Hypertension*. 2005;45:142-161.
8. Franklin SS, Gustin W, Wong ND, et al. Hemodynamic patterns of age-related changes in blood pressure. The Framingham Heart Study. *Circulation*. 1997;96:308-315.
9. Neaton JD, Wentworth D. Serum cholesterol, blood pressure, cigarette smoking, and death from coronary heart disease. *Arch Intern Med* 1992;152:56-64.
10. Kostis JB, Davis BR, Cutler J, et al. Prevention of heart failure by antihypertensive drug treatment in older persons with isolated systolic hypertension. SHEP Cooperative Research Group. *JAMA*. 1997;278:212-216.
11. Staessen JA, Thijs L, Fagard R, et al. Predicting cardiovascular risk using conventional vs ambulatory blood pressure in older patients with systolic hypertension. Systolic Hypertension in Europe Trial Investigators. *JAMA*. 1999;282:539-546.
12. SHEP Cooperative Research Group. Prevention of stroke by antihypertensive drug treatment in older persons with isolated systolic hypertension. Final results of the Systolic Hypertension in the Elderly Program (SHEP). *JAMA*. 1991;265:3255-3264.
13. The Trials of Hypertension Prevention Collaborative Research Group. Effects of weight loss and sodium reduction intervention on blood pressure and hypertension incidence in overweight people with high-normal blood pressure. The Trials of Hypertension Prevention, phase II. *Arch Intern Med*. 1997;157:657-667.
14. He J, Whelton PK, Appel LJ, et al. Long-term effects of weight loss and dietary sodium reduction on incidence of hypertension. *Hypertension*. 2000;35:544-549.
15. Sacks FM, Svetkey LP, Vollmer WM, et al. Effects on blood pressure of reduced dietary sodium and the Dietary Approaches to Stop Hypertension (DASH) diet. DASH-Sodium Collaborative Research Group. *N Engl J Med*. 2001;344:3-10.
16. Vollmer WM, Sacks FM, Ard J, et al. Effects of diet and sodium intake on blood pressure: subgroup analysis of the DASH-sodium trial. *Ann Intern Med*. 2001;135:1019-1028.
17. Chobanian AV, Hill M. National Heart, Lung, and Blood Institute Workshop on Sodium and Blood Pressure: a critical review of current scientific evidence. *Hypertension*. 2000;35:858-863.
18. Kelley GA, Kelley KS. Progressive resistance exercise and resting blood pressure: a meta-analysis of randomized controlled trials. *Hypertension*. 2000;35:838-843.

19. Whelton SP, Chin A, Xin X, et al. Effect of aerobic exercise on blood pressure: a meta-analysis of randomized, controlled trials. *Ann Intern Med.* 2002;136:493-503.
20. Xin X, He J, Frontini MG, et al. Effects of alcohol reduction on blood pressure: a meta-analysis of randomized controlled trials. *Hypertension.* 2001;38:1112-1117.
21. Whelton PK, He J, Appel LJ, et al. Primary prevention of hypertension: clinical and public health advisory from The National High Blood Pressure Education Program. *JAMA.* 2002;288:1882-1888.
22. Appel LJ, Champagne CM, Harsha DW, et al. Effects of comprehensive lifestyle modification on blood pressure control: main results of the PREMIER clinical trial. Writing Group of the PREMIER Collaborative Research Group. *JAMA.* 2003;289:2083-2093.
23. Cleveland LE, Goldman JD, Borrud LG. Data Tables: results from USDA's 1994 Continuing Survey of Food Intakes by Individuals and 1994 Diet and Health Knowledge Survey. Riverdale, MD: Agricultural Research Service, U.S. Department of Agriculture; 1996.
24. James WP, Ralph A, Sanchez-Castillo CP. The dominance of salt in manufactured food in the sodium intake of affluent societies. *Lancet.* 1987;1:426-429.
25. Division of Adult and Community Health, National Center for Chronic Disease Prevention and Health Promotion, Centers for Disease Control and Prevention. A 5-day surveillance. Behavioral Risk Factor Surveillance System Online Prevalence Data, 1995-2000. Available at: http://apps.nccd.cdc.gov/5ADaySurveillance/. Accessed November, 2003.
26. U.S. Department of Health and Human Services. Physical activity and health: a report of the Surgeon General. Atlanta, GA: U.S. Department of Health and Human Services, Centers for Disease Control and Prevention, National Center for Chronic Disease Prevention and Health Promotion. 1996. http://www.cdc.gov/nccdphp/sgr/contents.htm.
27. Flegal KM, Carroll MD, Ogden CL, et al. Prevalence and trends in obesity among US adults, 1999-2000. *JAMA.* 2002;288:1723-1727.
28. Healthy People 2010. Available at: http://www.healthypeople.gov. Accessed September 2009.
29. The ALLHAT Officers and Coordinators for the ALLHAT Collaborative Research Group. Major outcomes in high-risk hypertensive patients randomized to angiotensin-converting enzyme inhibitor or calcium channel blocker vs diuretic: the Antihypertensive and Lipid-Lowering Treatment to Prevent Heart Attack Trial (ALLHAT). *JAMA.* 2002;288:2981-2997.
30. Black HR, Elliott WJ, Neaton JD, et al. Baseline characteristics and early blood pressure control in the CONVINCE trial. *Hypertension.* 2001;37:12-18.
31. Cooper-DeHoff RM, Bristol HA, Pepine CJ. Ethnic differences in systolic blood pressure control in hypertensive patients with coronary artery disease. *Am J Hyperten.* 2003;16:27A.
32. Hansson L, Zanchetti A, Carruthers SG, et al. Effects of intensive blood-pressure lowering and low-dose aspirin in patients with hypertension: principal results of the Hypertension Optimal Treatment (HOT) randomized trial. HOT Study Group. *Lancet.* 1998;351:1755-1762.
33. American Diabetes Association. Treatment of hypertension in adults with diabetes. *Diabetes Care.* 2003;26:S80-S82.
34. National Kidney Foundation Guideline. K/DOQI clinical practice guidelines for chronic kidney disease: evaluation, classification, and stratification. Kidney Disease Outcome Quality Initiative. *Am J Kidney Dis.* 2002;39:S1-S246.
35. Rosendorff C, Black HR, Cannon CP, et al. Treatment of hypertension in the prevention and management of ischemic heart disease: a scientific statement from the American Heart Association Council for High Blood Pressure Research and the Councils on Clinical Cardiology and Epidemiology and Prevention. *Circulation.* 2007;115:2761-2788.
36. Neal B, MacMahon S, Chapman N. Effects of ACE inhibitors, calcium antagonists, and other blood-pressure-lowering drugs: results of prospectively designed overviews of randomized trials. Blood Pressure Lowering Treatment Trialists' Collaboration. *Lancet.* 2000;356:1955-1964.
37. Ogden LG, He J, Lydick E, et al. Longterm absolute benefit of lowering blood pressure in hypertensive patients according to the JNC VI risk stratification. *Hypertension.* 2000;35:539-543.
38. Black HR, Elliott WJ, Grandits G, et al. Principal results of the Controlled Onset Verapamil Investigation of Cardiovascular End Points (CONVINCE) Trial. *JAMA.* 2003;289:2073-2082.
39. Dahlof B, Devereux RB, Kjeldsen SE, et al. Cardiovascular morbidity and mortality in the Losartan Intervention For Endpoint Reduction in Hypertension Study (LIFE): a randomized trial against atenolol. *Lancet.* 2002;359:995-1003.
40. Materson BJ, Reda DJ, Cushman WC, et al. Single-drug therapy for hypertension in men. A comparison of six antihypertensive agents with placebo. The Department of Veterans Affairs Cooperative Study Group on Antihypertensive Agents. *N Engl J Med.* 1993;328:914-921.
41. Cutler JA, MacMahon SW, Furberg CD. Controlled clinical trials of drug treatment for hypertension review. *Hypertension.* 1989;13:I36-I44.
42. Collins R, Peto R, Godwin J, et al. Blood pressure and coronary heart disease. *Lancet.* 1990;336:370-371.
43. Chalmers J, Zanchetti A. The 1996 report of a World Health Organization expert committee on hypertension control. *J Hypertension.* 1996;14:929-933.
44. Psaty BM, Smith NL, Siscovick DS, et al. Health outcomes associated with antihypertensive therapies used as first-line agents. A systematic review and meta-analysis. *JAMA.* 1997;277:739-745.
45. Psaty BM, Lumley T, Furberg CD, et al. Health outcomes associated with various antihypertensive therapies used as first-line agents: a network meta-analysis. *JAMA.* 2003;289:2534-2544.
46. Cushman WC, Ford CE, Cutler JA, et al. Success and predictors of blood pressure control in diverse North American settings: the Antihypertensive and Lipid-Lowering Treatment to Prevent Heart Attack Trial. *J Clin Hypertens.* 2002;4:393-404.
47. Heart Outcomes Prevention Evaluation Study Investigators. Effects of an angiotensin-converting enzyme inhibitor, ramipril, on cardiovascular events in high-risk patients. *N Engl J Med.* 2000;342:145-153.
48. PROGRESS Collaborative Group. Randomized trial of a perindopril-based blood-pressure-lowering regimen among 6,105 individuals with previous stroke or transient ischaemic attack. *Lancet.* 2001;358:1033-1041.
49. Wing LM, Reid CM, Ryan P, et al. A comparison of outcomes with angiotensin-converting enzyme inhibitors and diuretics for hypertension in the elderly. *N Engl J Med.* 2003;348:583-592.
50. Black HR. The evolution of low-dose diuretic therapy: the lessons from clinical trials. *Am J Med.* 1996;101:47S-52S.
51. Materson BJ, Cushman WC, Goldstein G, et al. Department of Veterans Affairs Cooperative Study Group on Antihypertensive Agents: treatment of hypertension in the elderly. I. Blood pressure and clinical changes. Results of a Department of Veterans Affairs Cooperative Study. *Hypertension.* 1990;15: 348-360.

52. Siscovick DS, Raghunathan TE, Psaty BM, et al. Diuretic therapy for hypertension and the risk of primary cardiac arrest. *N Engl J Med.* 1994;330:1852-1857.
53. Flack JM, Cushman WC. Evidence for the efficacy of low-dose diuretic monotherapy. *Am J Med.* 1996;101:53S-60S.
54. Grimm RH, Jr, Grandits GA, Prineas RJ, et al. Longterm effects on sexual function of five antihypertensive drugs and nutritional hygienic treatment in hypertensive men and women. Treatment of Mild Hypertension Study (TOMHS). *Hypertension.* 1997;29:8-14.
55. Moser M. Why are physicians not prescribing diuretics more frequently in the management of hypertension? *JAMA.* 1998;279:1813-1816.
56. Lakshman MR, Reda DJ, Materson BJ, et al. Diuretics and beta-blockers do not have adverse effects at 1 year on plasma lipid and lipoprotein profiles in men with hypertension. Department of Veterans Affairs Cooperative Study Group on Antihypertensive Agents. *Arch Intern Med.* 1999;159:551-558.
57. Jansen PM, Danser AH, Imholz BP, et al. Aldosterone-receptor antagonism in hypertension. *J Hypertension.* 2009;27:680-691.
58. Nussberger J, Cugno M, Amstutz C, et al. Plasma bradykinin in angioedema. *Lancet.* 1998;351:1693-1697.
59. Gerstein HC, Bosch J, Pogue J, et al. HOPE Study Investigators: rationale and design of a large study to evaluate the renal and cardiovascular effects of an ACE inhibitor and vitamin E in high-risk patients with diabetes: the MICRO-HOPE study. *Diabetes Care.* 1996;19:1225-1228.
60. Julius S, Kjeldsen SE, Weber M, et al. Outcomes in hypertensive patients at high cardiovascular risk treated with regimens based on valsartan or amlodipine: the VALUE randomised trial. *Lancet.* 2004;363:2022-2031.
61. Yusuf S, Teo KK, Pogue J. Telmisartan, ramipril, or both in patients at high risk for vascular events. *N Engl J Med.* 2008;358:1547-1559.
62. Unger T. The ongoing telmisartan alone and in combination with ramipril global endpoint trial program. 2003;91:28G-34G.
63. Hansson L, Hedner T, Lund-Johansen P, et al. Randomized trial of effects of calcium antagonists compared with diuretics and beta-blockers on cardiovascular morbidity and mortality in hypertension: the Nordic Diltiazem (NORDIL) study. *Lancet.* 2000;356:359-365.
64. Lindholm LH, Carlberg B, Samuelsson O. Should beta blockers remain first choice in the treatment of primary hypertension? A meta-analysis. *Lancet.* 2005;366:1545-1553.
65. ALLHAT Collaborative Research Group. Major cardiovascular events in hypertensive patients randomized to doxazosin vs chlorthalidone. *JAMA.* 2000;283:1967-1975.
66. Pinto R, Gradman AH. Direct renin inhibition: an update. *Curr Hypertens Rep.* 2009 Dec;11(6):456-462.
67. Fagan TC, Sowers J. Type 2 diabetes mellitus: greater cardiovascular risks and greater benefits of therapy. *Arch Intern Med.* 1999;159:1033-1034.
68. Davis TM, Millns H, Stratton IM, et al. Risk factors for stroke in type 2 diabetes mellitus: United Kingdom Prospective Diabetes Study (UKPDS) 29. *Arch Intern Med.* 1999;159:1097-1103.
69. Elliott WJ, Meyer PM. Incident diabetes in clinical trials of antihypertensive drugs: a network meta-analysis. *Lancet.* 2007;369:201-207.
70. Bakris GL, Fonseca V, Katholi RE, et al. Metabolic effects of carvedilol vs metoprolol in patients with type 2 diabetes mellitus and hypertension: a randomized controlled trial. *JAMA.* 2004;292:2227-2236.
71. Nissen SE, Tuzcu EM, Libby P, et al. Effect of antihypertenisve agents on cardiovascular events in patients with coronary disease and normal blood pressure: the CAMELOT study: a randomized controlled trial. *JAMA.* 2004;292:2217-2225.
72. Pepine CJ, Handberg EM, Cooper-DeHoff RM, et al. A calcium antagonist vs a non-calcium antagonist hypertension treatment strategy for patients with coronary artery disease. The International Verapamil-Trandolapril Study (INVEST): a randomized controlled trial. *JAMA.* 2003;290:2805-2816.
73. Epstein BJ, Gums JG. Can the renin-angiotensin system protect against stroke? A focus on angiotensin II receptor blockers. *Pharmacotherapy.* 2005;25:531-539.
74. Staessen JA, Fagard R, Thijs L, et al. Randomized double-blind comparison of placebo and active treatment for older patients with isolated systolic hypertension. The Systolic Hypertension in Europe (Syst-Eur) Trial Investigators. *Lancet.* 1997;350:757-764.
75. Wang JG, Staessen JA, Gong L, et al. Chinese trial on isolated systolic hypertension in the elderly. Systolic Hypertension in China (Syst-China) Collaborative Group. *Arch Intern Med.* 2000;160:211-220.
76. Lewis CE, Grandits A, Flack J, et al. Efficacy and tolerance of antihypertensive treatment in men and women with stage 1 diastolic hypertension: results of the Treatment of Mild Hypertension Study. *Arch Intern Med.* 1996;156:377-385.

CHAPTER

4 Dyslipidemia

Rebecca F. Edwards

FOUNDATION OVERVIEW

General Overview

Cardiovascular disease (CVD), which encompasses coronary heart disease, cerebrovascular disease, and peripheral arterial disease, is the leading cause of morbidity and mortality in the United States, resulting in 1 of every 2.9 deaths in 2006.[1-2] CVD is estimated to result in an average of one death in the United States every 37 seconds, nearly 2400 deaths every day.[1] The initial presentation in up to one-third of patients is sudden death.[3]

Hyperlipidemia is a major risk factor for coronary heart disease (CHD) and is found in approximately 16% of adults in the United States. CHD is a narrowing of the small blood vessels that lead to the heart, usually a result of atherosclerosis.[1,4-5] Low-density lipoprotein cholesterol (LDL-C) can provoke several components of the atherosclerotic inflammatory response, including promoting unstable lesions concentrated with lipid-laden macrophages.[6] For every 1 mg/dL change in LDL-C, the relative risk for CHD is changed in proportion by about 1%, although this link is weaker in women and in the elderly.[3-4,6] Elevated triglycerides (TG) can cause acute pancreatitis and may also predict CHD.[5-7] TG appear to have indirect atherosclerotic effects related to procoagulant properties, adverse impact on endothelial function, and correlation with low HDL-C and small, dense LDL-C particle formation.[6]

In contrast, high-density lipoprotein cholesterol (HDL-C) is a strong inverse predictor for CHD.[3,5] HDL-C is involved in reverse cholesterol transport, delivering cholesterol from the cell wall to the liver for disposal. HDL-C can prevent LDL-C oxidation and may also inhibit platelet aggregation and activation.[6,8] For every 1 mg/dL increase in HDL-C, the risk of future CVD is reduced by 2% in men and 3% in women; death from myocardial infarction or coronary disease is reduced by 6%.[7-8]

Diagnosis

A fasting lipoprotein profile is recommended once every 5 years in adults aged 20 years or older after a 9- to 12-hour fast.[4-5] If testing is nonfasting, only the HDL-C and total cholesterol (TC) will be accurate, and follow-up lipoprotein profile is required if total cholesterol is ≥200 or HDL-C is <40 mg/dL.[5] Most patients with diabetes should have a fasting lipid profile performed at least annually, although those with low-risk lipid values (LDL-C <100 mg/dL, HDL-C >50 mg/dL, and TG <150 mg/dL) may be repeated every 2 years.[9] Acutely ill patients or those with a recent stroke or myocardial infarction may have significant drops in LDL-C within 24 to 48 hours of the event and suppressed levels for many weeks. Therefore, clinicians should use lipid levels obtained within 24 hours of admission to guide initial choice of therapy, recognizing that medication requirements may increase over time.

The Adult Treatment Panel III (ATP III) of the National Cholesterol Education Program defines a total cholesterol <200 mg/dL as desirable, 200 to 239 as borderline high, and ≥240 as high. LDL-C <100 mg/dL is optimal, 100 to 129 near/above optimal, 130 to 159 borderline high, 160 to 189 high, and ≥190 very high. HDL-C <40 mg/dL is low and ≥60 is high. TG <150 mg/dL is normal, 150 to 199 borderline high, 200 to 499 high, and ≥500 very high.[4] The LDL-C can be measured directly or calculated using the Friedewald equation (LDL-C = TC – HDL-C – TG/5). This calculation is less accurate when TGs are >200 mg/dL and inaccurate when they are >400 mg/dL.[4,6]

PREVENTION

Many patients will develop abnormal lipid levels associated with obesity, sedentary lifestyle, poor dietary choices, and aging. Therapeutic lifestyle changes (TLC) are strongly encouraged for all persons with hyperlipidemia and may prevent hyperlipidemia development.[4] A minority of patients have genetic defects rendering lifestyle strategies less effective, including familial hypercholesterolemia (FH), which is an LDL-C receptor gene mutation, and other uncommon genetic disorders such as familial defective apolipoprotein (apo) B_{100}, familial combined hyperlipidemia, and familial hypertriglyceridemia.

TREATMENT

General Overview and Goals of Treatment

The primary goal of dyslipidemia management is to reduce cardiovascular morbidity and mortality. ATP III last issued evidence-based guidelines in 2001, with a 2004 update suggesting more aggressive LDL-C goals for high-risk patients.[4] LDL-C is considered the primary target for cholesterol-lowering therapy, and statins are first-line therapy.[2,4,10] There is currently no hard evidence that lowering LDL-C levels too far has intrinsic danger.[11] Multiple well-designed trials and meta-analyses have confirmed the beneficial effects of statins on cardiovascular endpoints, including a 12% to 13% reduction in all-cause

TABLE 4-1 Updated 2004 ATP III LDL-C Goals and Cutpoints for TLC and Drug Therapy

Risk Category	LDL-C Goal	Initiative TLC	Consider Drug Therapy
High risk: CHD or CHD risk equivalents (10-y risk >20%)[a]	<100 mg/dL (optional goal: <70 mg/dL if very high risk[b])	≥100 mg/dL	≥100 mg/dL (<100 mg/dL: consider drug options)
Moderately high risk: 2+ risk factors (10-y risk 10%-20%)	<130 mg/dL (optional goal: <100 mg/dL)	≥130 mg/dL	≥130 mg/dL (100-129 mg/dL: consider drug options)
Moderate risk: 2+ risk factors (10-y risk <10%)	<130 mg/dL	≥130 mg/dL	≥160 mg/dL
Lower risk: 0-1 risk factor	<160 mg/dL	≥160 mg/dL	≥190 mg/dL (160-189 mg/dL: LDL-lowering drug optional)

[a]Based on Framingham risk scoring available at www.nhlbi.nih.gov/guidelines/cholesterol.

[b]Very high risk defined as established CVD plus (1) multiple risk factors (especially diabetes), (2) severe and poorly controlled risk factors (especially continued cigarette smoking), (3) multiple risk factors of the metabolic syndrome (especially high TG ≥200 mg/dL plus non-HDL-C ≥130 mg/dL with low HDL-C [<40 mg/dL]), and (4) acute coronary syndromes.

Abbreviations: TLC, therapeutic lifestyle changes.

Data from Gluckman TJ, Baranowski B, Ashen MD, et al. A practical and evidence-based approach to cardiovascular disease risk reduction. *Arch Intern Med*. 2004;164:1490-1500.

mortality.[12-15] Recommended LDL-C goals and clinical strategies based on CHD risk are summarized in Tables 4-1 and 4-2. Framingham risk scoring is required in patients with two or more risk factors to triage them into three levels of 10-year risk for hard CHD events (CHD death, myocardial infarction).

The only exception to targeting LDL-C first is when TG ≥500 mg/dL, requiring immediate TG lowering to prevent pancreatitis. Fibrates, fish oil, or nicotinic acid may be used as initial drug therapy for these patients.[4,8-9,16] As benefits of lowering TG on CHD are unclear, non-HDL-C is the recommended secondary goal if the TG remain ≥200 mg/dL once LDL-C is at goal.[3] The non-HDL-C (total − HDL-C; sum of LDL-C + VLDL-C) goal is 30 mg/dL higher than the LDL-C goal. The non-HDL-C includes the atherogenic VLDL-C and LDL-C. Metabolic syndrome is also considered a potential secondary target.[5] If TG are <200 mg/dL but HDL-C is low, clinicians may consider a tertiary target of increasing HDL-C for patients with CHD and CHD risk equivalents.[4-5] However, controlled clinical trials do not provide evidence to warrant setting a specific goal for raising HDL-C.[3-5,8]

TABLE 4-2 ATP III Definitions

Major Risk Factors That Modify LDL Goals[a]	Cigarette smoking (within the past month) Hypertension (BP ≥140/90 mm Hg or on antihypertensive medication) Low HDL cholesterol (<40 mg/dL) Family history of premature CHD (CHD in male first-degree relative <55 y of age or in female first-degree relative <65 y of age) Age (men ≥45; women ≥55 years)
CHD Risk Equivalents	Peripheral arterial disease Abdominal aortic aneurysm Carotid artery disease (transient ischemic attacks or stroke of carotid origin or >50% obstruction of a carotid artery) Diabetes 2+ risk factors with 10-y risk for hard CHD >20%
CHD	Myocardial infarction Unstable angina Stable angina History of coronary artery procedures (angioplasty or bypass surgery) Evidence of clinically significant myocardial ischemia

[a]Note: HDL >60 mg/dL counts as "negative" risk factor, removing one risk factor from total count.

Data from Gluckman TJ, Baranowski B, Ashen MD, et al. A practical and evidence-based approach to cardiovascular disease risk reduction. *Arch Intern Med*. 2004;164:1490-1500.

A 2008 American Diabetes Association (ADA) and American College of Cardiology consensus panel recommends a greater focus on apo B and non-HDL-C, both clinical markers of small, dense LDL-C and better predictors of CVD risk than LDL-C.[3,7] They suggest an apo B goal of <80 mg/dL if the LDL-C goal is <70 mg/dL and apo B goal of <90 mg/dL if the LDL-C goal is <100 mg/dL.[3,9] The safety and benefit of combining statins with other agents to achieve lipid targets is inadequately studied, although pending trials should provide clarification.[3-5,9] The panel currently recommends niacin as the preferred agent to add to statins. Niacin has been shown to increase regression of atherosclerosis when combined with statins or bile acid sequestrants (BAS).[10,17-18] In one study, niacin resulted in a 26% decrease in myocardial infarction risk in men with hypercholesterolemia and CHD and also decreased mortality up to 11% after 15 years of follow up.[7,17]

Regarding outcomes with other classes of medications, a meta-analysis found a 32% reduction in cardiac mortality and a 23% reduction in overall mortality with use of omega-3 fatty acids.[12] BAS monotherapy reduced cardiac mortality by 30% with no apparent effect on overall mortality.[12] Fibrates increased risk of noncardiac mortality by 13% with no significant difference in overall and cardiac mortality, although there was a slight trend toward improvement in cardiac mortality.[12] Ezetimibe currently has no hard outcomes data.[7,18-20]

Response to therapy should be evaluated after 4 to 6 weeks of therapy. If the LDL-C goal is not achieved, therapy can be intensified with reassessment at 6-week intervals.[5-6] Once LDL-C is at target, clinicians can focus on other lipid and nonlipid risk factors.[5] Maintenance response is monitored every 6 to 12 months unless clinical changes require more frequent testing.[6]

Specific Agents

HMG-CoA Reductase Inhibitors (Statins)

Statins competitively inhibit 3-hydroxy-3-methylglutaryl coenzyme A (HMG-CoA) reductase, therefore reducing biosynthesis of mevalonate, a cholesterol precursor. LDL-C clearance is also increased by an increased expression of LDL receptors. Statins are the most effective class of drugs at reducing LDL-C (Table 4-3), and they also raise HDL-C 5% to 15% and lower TG 7% to 30%, with varying effects based on the statin and dose used.[4] In general, approximately a 6% decrease in LDL-C can be expected for every doubling of the statin dose.[4]

Statins also have pleiotropic effects beyond cholesterol lowering, including reduced inflammation, coronary plaque stabilization, improved endothelial cell function, reduced viscosity and fibrinogen levels, reduced uptake of aggregated LDL-C by vascular smooth muscle cells, suppressed release of tissue factor, and activation of endothelial nitric oxide synthase.

Statins are well tolerated, with side effects such as dyspepsia, headaches, insomnia, constipation, and diarrhea occurring in <5% of patients. Patients rarely report rash, arthralgia, peripheral neuropathy, tendon pain, and memory problems. Observational studies suggest myalgias, usually mild and tolerable, in up to 5% to 10% of patients.[21] Myalgia is usually symmetrical, impacting large proximal muscle groups. Myopathy, as defined by the National Lipid Association (NLA), describes all potential statin effects on muscle, including symptomatic myopathy (myalgias, weakness, and cramps), creatine kinase (CK) elevations with or without symptoms, and clinically important rhabdomyolysis, referring to any muscle cell destruction (regardless of CK level) thought to have caused changes in renal function.[22] Mild CK elevation is <10 times the upper limit of normal (ULN), moderate ≥10 but <50 times ULN, and marked ≥50 times ULN.[22] Moderate to marked CK elevations occurred in only 0.17% of statin-treated and 0.13% of placebo-treated patients in clinical trials, although higher risk populations were generally excluded.[23]

Although older guidelines recommended CK levels at baseline for all patients prior to starting statins, experts more recently recommend this practice only in high-risk individuals.[21-22] The CK should be checked in the event of unexplained muscle pain but not monitored on a routine basis.[22] Fatal rhabdomyolysis occurrence was not higher than placebo in trials of currently available statins.[18] Fatal rhabdomyolysis is estimated to occur in one per million person-years of statin use, with most cases involving a potential drug interaction with a fibrate or known CYP-3A4 inhibitor.[22-24]

Contraindications to statins include pregnancy and active liver disease.[18] Manufacturer recommendations vary, but liver function tests (LFTs) are generally checked before and 12 weeks after starting therapy, 12 weeks after any dose increase, and periodically thereafter. However, the NLA Statin Safety Assessment Task Force found no data to support routine monitoring of LFTs. Liver failure was not reported in clinical trials and is estimated to occur in only one per million person-years of statin use.[23] Although elevated LFTs occur in 0.5% to 2% of patients, they are generally transient and mild to moderate.[18,23,25]

TABLE 4-3 Percentage Reduction in Serum LDL-C Based on Statin and Daily Dose

	Daily Dose (mg)				
Statin	**5**	**10**	**20**	**40**	**80**
Atorvastatin	31%	37%	43%	49%	55%
Fluvastatin	10%	15%	21%	27%	33%
Lovastatin	—	21%	29%	37%	45%
Pravastatin	15%	20%	24%	29%	33%
Rosuvastatin	38%	43%	48%	53%	58%
Simvastatin	23%	27%	32%	37%	42%

Data from Neuvonen PJ, Niemi M, Backman JT. Drug interactions with lipid-lowering drugs: mechanisms and clinical relevance. *Clin Pharmacol Ther.* 2006;80:565-581 (estimated summary from 164 randomized, placebo-controlled trials).

Niacin/Nicotinic Acid

Niacin is a B-complex vitamin that inhibits hepatic production of VLDL-C by reducing mobilization of free fatty acids from adipose tissues. It also increases the rate of TG removal from plasma, resulting in a 20% to 50% decrease in TG.[4,10] Niacin reduces LDL-C 5% to 25% by reducing hepatic synthesis and causes a shift to larger, buoyant particles. Niacin is the most potent medication at increasing HDL-C (15%-35%) and the only lipid-lowering therapy that also reduces Lp(a).[4,6,26]

Prostaglandin-mediated flushing is a common side effect that usually mitigates over time. Patients may also experience paresthesias, headaches, pruritus, and syncope. Niacin can cause mild gastrointestinal (GI) effects such as dyspepsia, nausea, and diarrhea but may also more seriously activate peptic ulcers. Niacin can also cause hyperpigmentation, rash, maculopathy, and small decreases in phosphorus and platelet count. Niacin commonly increases LFTs and (unlike statins) is clearly linked to severe hepatic toxicity, especially with doses >2000 mg/d.[18]

LFTs should be checked at baseline, every 6 to 12 weeks for the first year, and then approximately every 6 months. Absolute contraindications include active liver disease or unexplained LFT elevations, active peptic ulcer disease, arterial bleeding, and known hypersensitivity. Precautious include unstable angina or acute phase of myocardial infarction, use of concomitant anticoagulants, concomitant vasodilators, renal disease, substantial alcohol consumption, and history of liver disease. Niacin should also be used with caution in patients with gout due to possible uric acid increases.[18] Although niacin can worsen glucose in patients with diabetes (a usually transient effect with an average 5% increase in fasting glucose and 0.3% increase in A_{1c}), it can be particularly beneficial for dyslipidemia in this patient population.[18]

Bile Acid Sequestrants

BAS bind to negatively charged, cholesterol-containing bile acids in the intestinal lumen, preventing their reabsorption. The liver then uses cholesterol to make more bile, which further lowers cholesterol.[10]

These agents lower LDL-C by 10% to 30%. They increase HDL-C by 3% to 5% and either have no effect or can increase TG.[4] Studies show a TG increase as much as 18% to 22% in patients taking insulin and sulfonylureas.[27] BAS can lower apo B, C-reactive protein, and in combination with a statin or niacin, reduce small, dense LDL-C particles.[3] Although all BAS can also lower fasting glucose and A_{1c} modestly, colesevelam is the only one approved for type 2 diabetes treatment.

BAS are nonsystemic drugs with primarily GI side effects such as constipation, nausea, vomiting, dyspepsia, bloating, flatulence, and aggravation of hemorrhoids. Side effects are less likely with colesevelam. BAS may interfere with absorption of fat and fat-soluble vitamins (A, D, E, K), and there are rare reports of increased bleeding tendency caused by vitamin K deficiency. Contraindications to BAS therapy include history of hypersensitivity, elevated TG >500 mg/dL (colesevelam) or hyperlipidemia types III, IV, or V (cholestyramine), history of bowel or biliary obstruction, and history of hypertriglyceridemia-induced pancreatitis. BAS are not generally recommended for patients at risk for bowel obstruction secondary to gastroparesis, GI motility disorders, and history of major GI surgery. Caution should be used for patients with TG >300 mg/dL, susceptibility to fat-soluble vitamin deficiencies, preexisting constipation, and dysphagia (colesevelam).

Omega-3-Acid Ethyl Esters

The active lipid-lowering components of fish oil are eicosapentaenoic acid (EPA) and docosahexaenoic acid (DHA), which both increase lipoprotein lipase activity, lower TG biosynthesis, and reduce hepatic lipogenesis.[18,28-29] EPA and DHA may also have direct cardioprotective effects, including reduced platelet aggregation, decreased inflammation, mildly decreased blood pressure, reduced arrhythmias, improved endothelial function, and enhanced nitric oxide production.[10,17,30] The American Heart Association (AHA) recommends all patients with CHD consume 1 g of EPA and DHA per day from fish and/or supplements. Higher doses of 3 to 4 g/d of EPA and DHA are usually needed for significant TG lowering.[30] These doses can lower TG by 25% to 52%, with an increase in LDL-C by 5% to 10% and HDL-C by 1% to 3%.[28-30] HDL-C and LDL-C can increase more impressively in patients with very high TG, as much as 5% to 14% and 49%, respectively.[28-29] However, increased LDL-C is caused primarily by a shift to larger, buoyant particles and does not appear to be atherogenic.

Fish oil supplements are well tolerated even at higher doses. Eructation, dyspepsia, taste perversion, flu-like syndrome, and infection are the most common adverse effects occurring in <5% of patients.[28] Patients may also report nausea, flatulence, bloating, and/or diarrhea. Fish oil has been shown to slightly prolong bleeding time and may theoretically increase bleeding risk at higher doses.[28-30] Fish oil may also increase risk of ventricular arrhythmias in patients with implantable defibrillators, although evidence is contradictory.[30] Alanine aminotransferase and LDL-C should be monitored periodically due to occasional increases.[28] Clinically significant drug interactions are unlikely, with the exception of orlistat which reduces absorption. A prescription omega-3-acid ethyl esters product, approved for treatment of very high (≥500 mg/dL) TG in adults, is contraindicated only in patients with past hypersensitivity (eg, anaphylaxis) to any product ingredient.[29]

Fibric Acid Derivatives (Fibrates)

Fibrates activate peroxisome proliferator–activated receptors to stimulate lipoprotein lipase, accelerating lipoprotein degradation. Fibrates also reduce hepatic apoprotein synthesis, resulting in lower TG and higher HDL-C.[10] Fibrates lower LDL-C by 5% to 20% (more with fenofibrate) and cause a beneficial shift in particle size. Generally, TGs are decreased by 20% to 50% and HDL-C increased by 10% to 20%.[4]

GI effects such as abdominal discomfort are generally transient but occur in approximately 10% of patients receiving gemfibrozil and clofibrate. Fenofibrate appears better tolerated. Fibrates can cause elevated creatinine, increased LFTs, gallstones, and myopathy.[18,22] Anemia and white blood cell decreases have been observed and usually stabilize with long-term use. Other adverse effects include urticaria, increased homocysteine, acute hypersensitivity reactions, and rarely, venous thromboembolism.[17-18] Patients on warfarin should be closely monitored since fibrates can increase prothrombin time.

Contraindications to fibrates include gallbladder disease, history of hypersensitivity reactions, hepatic dysfunction, and severe renal impairment (defined by manufacturer as CrCl <30 mL/min for fenofibrate and <10 mL/min for gemfibrozil). Fibrates require renal adjustment in patients with mild to moderate renal impairment. Fenofibrate is also contraindicated in nursing mothers, and gemfibrozil is contraindicated in patients taking repaglinide (due to increased risk of severe hypoglycemia). Monitor CBC periodically during the first year of therapy, CK in patients with muscle pain or on other myopathy-associated medications, LFTs every 3 months during first year of gemfibrozil and then periodically thereafter, and LFTs periodically throughout therapy with fenofibrate.

Cholesterol Absorption Inhibitors

Ezetimibe inhibits dietary cholesterol absorption at the brush border of the small intestine. Ezetimibe also increases cholesterol clearance from the plasma, reduces formation of LDL-C, lowers apo B, and decreases hepatic cholesterol stores.[10] LDL-C is reduced by 16% to 21%, TG reduced by 8% to 12% and HDL-C increased by 1% to 5% with therapy.[18] Ezetimibe is approved as monotherapy and in combination with a statin or fenofibrate, but it should not be combined with gemfibrozil because of increased risk of cholelithiasis. No dose adjustments are necessary in renal or hepatic impairment, although it should be avoided in patients with moderate to severe hepatic disease.

Ezetimibe is generally well tolerated. Adverse reactions occurring in <4% of patients include diarrhea, fatigue, upper respiratory infection, arthralgia, fatigue, and myagias.[6] There are rare case reports of myopathy and rhabdomyolysis, usually when combined with a statin or fibrate, but also with monotherapy.[25,31] There are rare reports of angioedema and allergic reactions, and ezetimibe is contraindicated in patients with past hypersensitivity reactions. Patients on ezetimibe with statins are more likely to have elevated LFTs compared to statin monotherapy, and LFTs should be monitored per statin recommendations. Increase in cancer observed in the SEAS trial was not replicated in larger studies but requires follow-up of longer duration.[7,20,32]

Special Populations

Elderly

Most new CHD events and coronary deaths occur in the elderly, and there are no clear age restrictions for drug therapy. Trials have demonstrated risk reduction with statin therapy in older persons with and without established CVD up to 82 years of age.[4] Older patients are at greater risk for adverse effects and may require lower doses. However, the safety and efficacy of statins, fish oil, ezetimibe, niacin (Niaspan), colesevelam, and fenofibrate did not appear different for elderly subjects in clinical trials. Although the PROSPER trial found a 25% increase in new cancer in elderly subjects randomized to pravastatin, subsequent meta-analyses have found no increase in cancer incidence.[4,12-13,33]

Children

Coronary atherosclerosis begins in childhood, and high cholesterol in children and young adults is associated with greater risk of premature CHD in middle age.[5-6,34] Therefore, cholesterol screening is recommended in children over 2 years of age and no later than 10 years of age if there is a positive family history of dyslipidemia or premature CVD.[34] Children should also be screened if the family history is unknown or if they have other CVD risk factors (overweight or obese, hypertension, smoking, or diabetes). High-risk children with values within the reference range are retested every 3 to 5 years.[34]

The 2008 American Academy of Pediatrics recommends consideration of drug therapy following ineffective diet changes in children 8 years of age with very high LDL-C (≥190 mg/dL), those with family history of early CHD or with two or more additional risk factors with LDL-C ≥160 mg/dL, and those with diabetes when LDL-C is ≥130 mg/dL.[5,34]

Pharmacologic intervention should be considered in children younger than 8 years old only for dramatic LDL-C elevations (>500 mg/dL).[34]

SPECIAL CONSIDERATIONS

Before starting lipid-lowering therapy, secondary causes of hyperlipidemia should be managed, such as obstructive liver disease, Cushing syndrome, alcohol overuse, hypothyroidism, nephrotic syndrome, and undiagnosed or uncontrolled diabetes. In patients with diabetes, TG levels can be lowered with optimal glucose control.[6] Many medications also increase cholesterol, for example, β-blockers, estrogens, androgens, rosiglitazone, thiazide diuretics, corticosteroids, isotretinoin, protease inhibitors, and cyclosporine.[5-6,17]

CASE Application

1. MM is a 74-year-old woman with a past medical history (PMH) of unstable angina, hypertension, and diabetes. She smokes two packs of cigarettes daily. Her LDL-C is 120 mg/dL, HDL-C 48 mg/dL, and TG 220 mg/dL. Which of the following is *not* an acceptable LDL-C goal for MM?
   a. <70 mg/dL
   b. <100 mg/dL
   c. A 20% to 30% decrease
   d. A 30% to 40% decrease

2. KW is a 53-year-old Asian woman with an LDL-C of 210 mg/dL, HDL-C 56 mg/dL, and TG 182 mg/dL. Her PMH is notable for hypertension with a recent BP of 118/70 mm Hg on lisinopril monotherapy. She is a nonsmoker. Her father died of a myocardial infarction at age 58. Which of the following are ATP III major risk factors for CHD that modify her LDL-C goal?
   a. Her age
   b. Family history of heart disease
   c. Hypertension
   d. Low HDL-C

3. KW's physician elects to use rosuvastatin to treat her hyperlipidemia and requests a dosing recommendation. Select the most appropriate starting dose for this patient, keeping in mind genetic factors.
   a. 5 mg daily
   b. 10 mg daily
   c. 20 mg daily
   d. 40 mg daily
   e. 80 mg daily

4. LE is a 33-year-old woman currently attempting to become pregnant. Her physician decides that benefits of hyperlipidemia treatment outweigh fetal risks. Her LDL-C is 240 mg/dL, HDL-C 64 mg/dL, and TG 132 mg/dL. Her PMH includes recent cholelithiasis. What is the most appropriate medication for LE?
   a. Rosuvastatin
   b. Niacin
   c. Colesevelam
   d. Gemfibrozil
   e. Omega-3-acid ethyl esters

5. MJ has a history of subtherapeutic anticoagulation on warfarin (due to poor adherence) until the administration time was changed from evening to morning. The patient also frequently skips meals and takes antacids for reflux. Which of the following statins is optimal for this patient?

   a. Pravastatin
   b. Atorvastatin
   c. Lovastatin
   d. Rosuvastatin
   e. Fluvastatin

6. CE is a 74-year-old man with a PMH of CHD, stroke, and hypothyroidism. He currently takes aspirin, levothyroxine, and simvastatin and has now been prescribed cholestyramine. What will you discuss with the patient?

   a. Take on an empty stomach once daily.
   b. Mix each dose with at least 12 oz of juice or soda.
   c. Sip slowly to reduce side effects.
   d. Take other medications at least 1 to 2 hours before or 4 to 6 after cholestyramine.

7. Select the brand name for fenofibrate.

   a. Fenoglide
   b. Tricor
   c. Triglide
   d. Lipofen
   e. All of the above

8. What medication for hyperlipidemia may be used in a patient with active hepatic disease?

   a. Colesevelam
   b. Simvastatin
   c. Ezetimibe
   d. Niacin
   e. Gemfibrozil

9. JM is a 64-year-old woman with a PMH of pancreatitis (when TGs were 2200 mg/dL), uncontrolled gout, severe psoriasis, recurrent infections requiring hospitalization, and lovastatin-associated myopathy. Her current medications include rosuvastatin, prednisone, and allopurinol. Colchicine was also added a few days ago for a gout exacerbation. She reports an anaphylactic reaction after eating seafood in college. Her LDL-C is 96 mg/dL, HDL-C 42 mg/dL, and TG 540 mg/dL. Which of the following is the safest addition to her therapy?

   a. Niacin
   b. Colesevelam
   c. Fish oil
   d. Gemfibrozil
   e. Fenofibrate

10. Select the brand name for lovastatin.

    a. Lescol
    b. Crestor
    c. Mevacor
    d. Pravachol
    e. Zocor

11. Which of the following statins should be temporarily discontinued for a patient starting a short course of clarithromycin?

    a. Simvastatin
    b. Pravastatin
    c. Lovastatin
    d. Atorvastatin
    e. a and c

12. Which of the following statin doses may be dispensed to a patient also taking gemfibrozil?

    a. Rosuvastatin 20 mg
    b. Simvastatin 20 mg
    c. Lovastatin 40 mg
    d. Fluvastatin 40 mg

13. LR is a 54-year-old woman with elevated TG who wants to substitute OTC fish oil instead of omega-3-acid ethyl esters (Lovaza) to save money. Her physician approves this change. She mentions past GI problems with dietary fish. What should you advise the patient regarding a product with 180 mg of EPA and 120 mg of DHA per capsule?

    a. Change to the more concentrated cod liver oil.
    b. Six capsules a day will equal the dose of the prescription product.
    c. Take on an empty stomach to improve tolerability.
    d. Eleven capsules a day will equal the dose of the prescription product.
    e. Have your mercury levels tested periodically.

14. RR is a 56-year-old Asian man with an LDL-C of 180 mg/dL, HDL-C 28 mg/dL, and TG 140 mg/dL. His fasting glucose is 96 mg/dL, waist circumference 41 in, and BP 128/82 mm Hg. His medications include hydrochlorothiazide and gemfibrozil. Which of the following does *not* potentially indicate metabolic syndrome in RR?

    a. HDL-C
    b. TG
    c. Fasting glucose
    d. Waist circumference
    e. BP

15. Which of the following key ATP III therapeutic lifestyle changes (TLC) should be recommended to patients with hyperlipidemia?

    a. Increase soluble fiber to at least 50 g/d.
    b. Limit cholesterol intake to <400 mg/d.
    c. Reduce trans fat and limit saturated fat to <15% of calories.
    d. Engage in regular physical activity.
    e. Eat one serving per week of fatty fish.

16. Select a patient risk factor for development of myopathy on statin therapy.
    a. Larger body size
    b. Hyperthyroidism
    c. Male sex
    d. Vitamin D deficiency
    e. Young age

17. CL is a 10-year-old boy with familial hyperlipidemia (FH). His physician wishes to use drug therapy since TLC has failed. His LDL-C is 320 mg/dL. Which of the following medications would you recommend?
    a. Atorvastatin
    b. Colesevelam
    c. Ezetimibe
    d. Niacin
    e. Fenofibrate

18. Select the lipid-lowering medication that requires adjustment in a patient with renal impairment.
    a. Atorvastatin
    b. Gemfibrozil
    c. Ezetimibe
    d. Cholestyramine
    e. Niacin

19. A patient on simvastatin complains of muscle pain, weakness, and cramps since running a marathon this past weekend. His CK is 1760 U/L today (normal range, 50-160) and 280 U/L when checked 3 months ago. His Cr is 1.0 mg/dL. How should you manage this patient?
    a. Continue therapy and closely monitor the CK.
    b. Stop simvastatin until symptoms and CK improve, then try another statin.
    c. Add coenzyme Q10.
    d. Change simvastatin to ezetimibe.

20. JT is a 62-year-old woman with low HDL-C who was prescribed niacin. She did not fill her prescription because of the expense and instead took five 100-mg immediate-release niacin tablets at bedtime. She complains of flushing and dizziness after the first dose that almost caused her to fall. What is the best recommendation to improve overall tolerability?
    a. Change to a "no flush" formulation.
    b. Take 81 mg of aspirin 30 to 60 minutes before each dose.
    c. Start with 100 mg tid.
    d. Take with food and a hot liquid.
    e. Change to sustained-release OTC formulation.

TAKEAWAY POINTS ››

- Hyperlipidemia, particularly elevated LDL-C, is strongly associated with CHD.
- Total cholesterol <200 mg/dL, LDL-C <100 mg/dL, HDL-C ≥60 mg/dL, and TG <150 mg/dL are considered optimal.
- Adults over 20 years of age should be screened for hyperlipidemia every 5 years.
- Children over 2 years of age with certain risk factors should be screened every 3 to 5 years.
- Therapeutic lifestyle changes are strongly indicated for all individuals with hyperlipidemia.
- LDL-C is the primary target of drug therapy unless TG ≥500 mg/dL.
- Secondary lipid goals include non-HDL-C, apo B, and metabolic syndrome.
- A more aggressive LDL-C goal <70 mg/dL can be considered in patients at very high risk.
- Statins are first-line for patients with hyperlipidemia, improving both cardiovascular and total mortality.
- Niacin is currently the preferred agent to add to statins in high-risk patients when lipid goals are not met.
- Niacin, fish oil, or gemfibrozil are preferred treatments for patients with TG>500 mg/dL.
- BAS and fish oil reduce cardiac mortality with no apparent difference in overall mortality.
- Fibrates appear to increase noncardiac mortality and may have no effect on overall and cardiac mortality.
- Widespread ezetimibe use cannot be supported due to lack of evidence of positive outcomes at this time.
- Fatal rhabdomyolysis with statins is rare. Myopathy is usually associated with preventable drug interactions (eg, gemfibrozil) or underlying patient risk factors.
- Elderly patients benefit from hyperlipidemia treatment but require closer monitoring.
- Statins and BAS are approved for treatment of hyperlipidemia in children.
- BAS are generally preferred agents for pregnant or breastfeeding women and patients with hepatic disease.
- Many medications can cause or worsen hyperlipidemia.

REFERENCES

1. Lloyd-Jones D, Adams R, Carnethon M, et al. Heart disease and stroke statistics—2009 update. A report from the American Heart Association Statistics Committee and Stroke Statistics Subcommittee. *Circulation*. 2009;119:480-486.
2. Gluckman TJ, Baranowski B, Ashen MD, et al. A practical and evidence-based approach to cardiovascular disease risk reduction. *Arch Intern Med*. 2004;164:1490-1500.
3. Brunzell JD, Davidson M, Furberg CD, et al. Lipoprotein management in patients with cardiometabolic risk: consensus conference report from the American Diabetes Association and the American College of Cardiology Foundation. *J Am Coll Cardiol*. 2008;51:1512-1524.
4. Grundy SM, Cleeman JI, Merz CN et al. Implications of the recent clinical trials for the National Cholesterol Education Program Adult Treatment Panel III Guidelines. *Circulation*. 2004;110:227-239.
5. Expert Panel on Detection, Evaluation, and Treatment of High Blood Cholesterol in Adults. Executive Summary of the Third Report of the National Cholesterol Education Program (NCEP) Expert Panel on Detection, Evaluation, and Treatment of High Blood Cholesterol in Adults (Adult Treatment Panel III). *JAMA*. 2001;285(19):2486-2497.
6. Jellinger PS, Dickey RA, Ganda OP, et al. The American Association of Clinical Endocrinologists Medical Guidelines for Clinical Practice for the Diagnosis and Treatment of Dyslipidemia and Prevention of Atherosclerosis. *Endocrin Pract*. 2000;6(2):162-203.
7. Preiss D, Sattar N. Lipids, lipid modifying agents and cardiovascular risk: a review of the evidence. *Clin Endocrin*. 2009;70:815-828.
8. Ashen MD, Blumenthal RS. Low HDL cholesterol levels. *N Engl J Med*. 2005;353:1252-1260.
9. American Diabetes Association. Standards of Medical Care in Diabetes—2009. *Diabetes Care*. 2009;32(suppl 1):S13-S61.
10. American Association of Clinical Endocrinologists (AACE) Clinical Practice Guidelines Task Force. AACE Medical Guidelines for Clinical Practice for the Management of Diabetes Mellitus. *Endocrin Pract*. 2007;13(suppl 1):S3-S68.
11. Steinberg D, Glass CK, Witztum JL. Evidence mandating earlier and more aggressive treatment of hypercholesterolemia. *Circulation*. 2008;118:672-677.
12. Studer M, Briel M, Leimenstoll B, et al. Effect of different antilipidemic agents and diets on mortality: a systematic review. *Arch Intern Med*. 2005;165:725-730.
13. Cholesterol Treatment Trialists' (CTT) Collaborators. Efficacy and safety of cholesterol-lowering treatment: prospective meta-analysis of data from 90,056 participants in 14 randomized trials of statins. *Lancet*. 2005;366:1267-1278.
14. Brugts JJ, Yetgin T, Hoeks SE, et al. The benefits of statins in people without established cardiovascular disease but with cardiovascular risk factors: a meta-analysis of randomized controlled trials. *BMJ*. 2009;338:b2376.
15. Delahoy PJ, Magliano DJ, Webb K, et al. The relationship between reduction in low-density lipoprotein cholesterol by statins and reduction in risk of cardiovascular outcomes: an updated meta-analysis. *Clin Ther*. 2009;31:236-244.
16. Grundy SM, Cleeman JI, Daniels SR, et al. Diagnosis and Management of the Metabolic Syndrome. An American Heart Association/National Heart, Lung, Blood Institute Scientific Statement. *Circulation*. 2005;112(17):2735-2752.
17. Brunzell JD. Hypertriglyceridemia. *N Engl J Med*. 2007;357:1009-1017.
18. Tannock LR. Advances in the management of hyperlipidemia-induced atherosclerosis. *Expert Rev Cardiovasc Ther*. 2008;6(3):369-383.
19. Toth PP, Davidson MH. High-dose statin therapy: benefits and safety in aggressive lipid lowering. *J Fam Pract*. 2008;57(suppl 5):S29-S36.
20. Rossebo AB, Pedersen TR, Boman K, et al. Intensive lipid lowering with simvastatin and ezetimibe in aortic stenosis. *N Engl J Med*. 2008;359:1343-1356.
21. Joy TR, Hegele RA. Narrative review: statin-related myopathy. *Ann Intern Med*. 2009;150:858-868.
22. Thompson PD, Clarkson PM, Rosenson RS. An assessment of statin safety by muscle experts. *Am J Cardiol*. 2006;97(suppl):69C-76C.
23. Law MR, Wald NJ, Rudnicka AR. Quantifying effect of statins on low density lipoprotein cholesterol, ischemic heart disease, and stroke: systematic review and meta-analysis. *BMJ*. 2003;326:1423.
24. Bottorff MB. Statin safety and drug interactions: clinical implications. *Am J Cardiol*. 2006;97(suppl):27C-31C.
25. Frishman WH, Horn J. Statin-drug interactions: not a class effect. *Cardiol Rev*. 2008;16:205-212.
26. Knopp RH. Drug treatment of lipid disorders. *N Engl J Med*. 1999;341:498-511.
27. Welchol (colesevelam) [package insert]. Parsippany, NJ: Daiichi Sankyo, Inc.; 2008.
28. McKenney JM, Sica D. Role of prescription omega-3 fatty acids in the treatment of hypertriglyceridemia. *Pharmacotherapy*. 2007;27(5):715-728.
29. Lovaza (omega-3-acid ethyl esters) [package insert]. Research Triangle Park, NC: GlaxoSmithKline; 2008.
30. Kris-Etherton PM, Harris WS, Appel LJ. American Heart Association Scientific Statement. Fish consumption, fish oil, omega-3 fatty acids, and cardiovascular disease. *Circulation*. 2002;106:2747-2757.
31. Neuvonen PJ, Niemi M, Backman JT. Drug interactions with lipid-lowering drugs: mechanisms and clinical relevance. *Clin Pharmacol Ther*. 2006;80:565-581.
32. Peto R, Emberson J, Landray M, et al. Analyses of cancer data from three ezetimibe trials. *N Engl J Med*. 2008;359:1357-1366.
33. Dale KM, Coleman CI, Henyan NN, et al. Statins and cancer risk: a meta-analysis. *JAMA*. 2006;295:74-80.
34. Daniels SR, Greer FR, and the Committee on Nutrition. American Academy of Pediatrics Clinical Report. Lipid screening and cardiovascular health in children. *Pediatrics*. 2008;122:198-208.

CHAPTER

5 Stroke

Jessica Starr and Brea O. Rowan

FOUNDATION OVERVIEW

Stroke is the third leading cause of death in the United States behind cardiovascular disease and cancer. Approximately 2.7% of men and 2.5% of women > 18 years of age have a history of stroke and there are nearly 800,000 stroke occurrences each year with a mortality rate approaching 150,000.[1] Of all strokes, 87% are ischemic in origin with the remainder hemorrhagic.[2] This chapter will focus on ischemic strokes.

Most cranial occlusions result from an embolus formed in either the carotid arteries or the ventricles of the heart. Atherosclerosis of the carotid arteries commonly leads to plaque formation. If plaque rupture occurs, collagen is exposed which results in platelet aggregation and thrombus formation. When a clot forms, it can break off and travel distally to the cranial vasculature. This causes cranial vessel occlusion which decreases blood flow to the brain region it supplies, ultimately resulting in ischemia. Strokes originating from a cardioembolic source are presumed to originate from thrombus formation in the left ventricle.

Ischemic stroke commonly presents as an acute onset of focal neurological deficit lasting greater than 24 hours.[3] Most patients present with weakness on one side of the body, visual impairment, and inability to speak. Diagnosis is confirmed with computed tomography (CT) scanning and magnetic resonance imaging (MRI). Patients at highest risk of developing an ischemic stroke are those with hypertension, diabetes, dyslipidemia, atrial fibrillation, cigarette smoking, and obesity (Table 5-1).[3,4]

The immediate goal of therapy in acute stroke is to reduce neurologic injury and long-term disability. Once the patient is through the hyperacute period, the goal of therapy is to prevent reoccurrence and ultimately decrease mortality.[3,4]

PREVENTION

Primary prevention against ischemic stroke focuses on the reduction of modifiable risk factors (see Table 5-1).

ACUTE TREATMENT

The treatment for acute ischemic stroke has a narrow therapeutic window making a timely evaluation and diagnosis essential.[5] Currently, only two pharmacologic agents have received a Class I, Level of Evidence A recommendation from the American Heart Association Stroke Council for use in treatment of acute stroke. These agents are intravenous (IV) recombinant tissue plasminogen activator (rtPA) and aspirin.[5]

rtPA is the only fibrinolytic agent used in the treatment of acute stroke. It is recommended due to its ability to achieve early reperfusion and improve neurological outcomes.[5] rtPA exerts its effects via the initiation of local fibrinolysis. It binds directly to fibrin thereby causing plasminogen to convert to plasmin.[5,6] Plasmin is the enzyme responsible for clot dissolution. Currently, it is recommended to administer rtPA intravenously at a dose of 0.9 mg/kg with 10% of the total dose given as an IV bolus over 1 minute and the remainder of the dose given over 1 hour. The maximum dose is 90 mg in patients weighing >100 kg.[7]

Timing is crucial when considering the use of rtPA in acute stroke. The 2007 guidelines set forth by the American Heart Association Stroke Council recommend that rtPA be administered within 3 hours of symptom onset.[5] If the time of onset is unknown, patients are ineligible to receive rtPA. Recently, the benefit of rtPA up to 4.5 hours after symptom onset was established in specific patients.[8] As a result, the American Heart Association Stroke Council amended its guidelines to extend the consideration for rtPA use in acute stroke out to 4.5 hours.[9] Patients who are excluded from consideration for the extended duration include: (1) age over 80 years, (2) oral anticoagulation regardless of the international normalized ratio (INR) value, (3) score >25 on National Institutes of Health Stroke Scale, and (4) history of both diabetes and stroke together. Patients falling into these four exclusion criteria may still be considered for rtPA use if they present within 3 hours of symptom onset.[9]

Due to its effects on fibrin, rtPA puts patients at risk for major bleeding. Therefore, there are multiple other exclusion criteria, in addition to timing, that must be considered when evaluating patients for its use. Some of these exclusion criteria are recent head trauma, major surgery, myocardial infarction, elevated aPTT or INR, gastrointestinal bleed, or blood pressure greater than 185/110 mm Hg (Table 5-2).[5]

The only other pharmacologic agent approved for use in acute stroke is aspirin. Aspirin generates a small decrease in morbidity and mortality when administered within 24 to 48 hours of stroke onset.[10,11] The recommended initial dose is 325 mg.[5] Unlike rtPA, aspirin does not appear to alter the neurological outcomes of stroke. Instead, its primary role is in the prevention of early recurrent events. If a patient receives rtPA, aspirin, along with all other antithrombotic agents, should be withheld for at least 24 hours after rtPA is administered.[5]

TABLE 5-1 Risk Factors for Ischemic Stroke[3,4]

Nonmodifiable	
Age	Risk doubles every 10 y after 55 y of age
Race	African Americans have a greater risk than Hispanics who have a greater risk than Caucasians
Gender	Men have a greater risk than women
Modifiable	
Hypertension	Risk is decreased by 50% if blood pressure is lowered to <120/80 mm Hg compared to patients with HTN
Dyslipidemia	25% reduction in risk with concomitant use of statin therapy
Diabetes	There is no correlation with glycemic control; however, risk is reduced when blood pressure is lowered to <130/80 mm Hg
Cigarette smoking	Risk is decreased by 50% within 1 y of quitting
Atrial fibrillation	Risk is decreased with concomitant use of warfarin therapy

In addition to evaluating patients for rtPA use in the acute setting, another important part of initial stroke treatment is blood pressure control. Neurological deterioration can be seen with both low and high blood pressures. Current consensus recommendations state that blood pressure treatment should be withheld unless systolic blood pressure is above 220 mm Hg or diastolic blood pressure is above 120 mm Hg.[5] However, if a patient meets all other criteria for rtPA, except elevated blood pressure, the recommendation is to decrease the blood pressure to <185/110 mm Hg. Frequent blood pressure monitoring should occur during rtPA administration and during the subsequent 24 hours. Several antihypertensive agents are recommended for use during acute stroke. These include labetalol, nicardipine, and sodium nitroprusside. Sodium nitroprusside is typically reserved for blood pressure not controlled by labetalol and nicardipine, and it should be used with caution in patients with renal insufficiency due to the risk of cyanide toxicity with prolonged use. If antihypertensive therapy is necessary, the blood pressure should be decreased by approximately 15% to 25% within the first day.[12]

TABLE 5-2 Exclusion Criteria for rt-PA[5,9]

- Subarachnoid hemorrhage
- Neurological signs that are minor, isolated, or that clear spontaneously
- Symptom onset >4.5 h
- Symptom onset >3 h if age is >80 y, if NIHSS score is > 25, if taking oral anticoagulants regardless of INR value, or if there is a history of both diabetes and previous stroke together
- Head trauma, myocardial infarction, or prior stroke within the previous 3 mo
- History of intracranial hemorrhage
- Active bleeding or trauma on exam
- Gastrointestinal or urinary tract hemorrhage within the previous 3 wk
- Major surgery within the previous 2 wk
- Arterial puncture at a noncompressible site within the previous 7 d
- Blood pressure >185/110 mm Hg
- Oral anticoagulation *and* INR >1.7
- Heparin therapy within previous 48 h *and* elevated aPTT
- Platelets <100,000 mm^3
- Blood glucose <50 mg/dL
- Seizure with postictal residual neurological impairments
- CT with multilobar infarction
- Patient and family are not informed of risks/benefits

SECONDARY PREVENTION

Patients with a history of an ischemic stroke are at significantly increased risk of having another stroke.[3] The American Heart Association Stroke Council recommends several different pharmacotherapy options for secondary prevention. The mainstay of therapy is long-term treatment with an antiplatelet agent; however, blood pressure and cholesterol lowering also play a role.[3,13] Currently, aspirin, clopidogrel, and extended-release dipyridamole plus aspirin are all acceptable antiplatelet options for initial therapy.[13] However, the American Heart Association Stroke Council gives preference to the use of extended-release dipyridamole plus aspirin over aspirin monotherapy (Table 5-3).[13,14,15] Currently, ticlopidine is not recommended for use. Patients with a cardioembolic source, most commonly due to atrial fibrillation, should be treated with warfarin therapy to achieve an INR goal of 2 to 3.[3]

Aspirin is the most well-studied antiplatelet agent used in the secondary prevention of stroke. Its antithrombotic effects occur by irreversible inhibition of platelet cyclooxygenase ultimately leading to a reduction in platelet aggregation.[16] The current dosing recommendation varies from 50 to 325 mg/d with doses as large as 1300 mg/d reported in the literature.[3,13] Most studies have shown that both high- and low-dose aspirin prevent the reoccurrence of stroke with higher doses associated with a greater risk of gastrointestinal hemorrhage. Common adverse reactions are gastrointestinal ulcerations and duodenal ulcers.

Clopidogrel works through selective, irreversible inhibition of adenosine diphosphate–induced platelet aggregation.[17] It is given as a 75-mg tablet once daily. The safety of clopidogrel is comparable to that of aspirin and the incidence of neutropenia and thrombotic thrombocytopenic purpura are low.[3,18] Clopidogrel is an excellent alternative to aspirin in those patients who are allergic to aspirin.[13] The combination of clopidogrel with aspirin is not recommended as there is an increased risk of hemorrhage.[19,20]

Platelet aggregation is inhibited to a greater extent with the combination of aspirin and dipyridamole than with either agent alone. Dipyridamole is an inhibitor of phosphodiesterase, which results in accumulation of adenosine and cyclic-3′,5′-adenosine monophosphate thereby inhibiting platelet aggregation.[21] This combination is given as a capsule that contains dipyridamole extended-release pellets in 200 mg and immediate-release aspirin in 25 mg.[21] The combination

TABLE 5-3 **Antiplatelet Therapy Recommendations for the Secondary Prevention of Ischemic Stroke**[13]

Antiplatelet Therapy	Recommendation	Evidence
Aspirin 50-325 mg po daily	Acceptable initial therapy	IA
Clopidogrel 75 mg po daily	Acceptable initial therapy Consider over aspirin alone Alternative to aspirin-allergic patients Do not use in combination with aspirin	IA IIb B IIa B III
Extended-release dipyridamole 200 mg plus aspirin 25 mg po twice daily	Acceptable initial therapy Recommended over aspirin alone	IA IB

capsule is taken twice daily. The most common adverse effects are headache, dyspepsia, and abdominal pain.

Ticlopidine is not currently recommended by the American Heart Association Stroke Council due to its significant side effect profile. It can cause severe gastrointestinal sides effects and there have been reports of neutropenia, agranulocytosis, aplastic anemia, and thrombotic thrombocytopenic purpura.[22]

Warfarin is the most effective treatment option for the prevention of stroke in patients with a cardioembolic source.[3,23,24] Warfarin is a vitamin K antagonist and inhibits the vitamin K-dependent coagulation factors II, VII, IX, and X in the liver thereby preventing the initial formation and propagation of thrombosis.[25] The most common adverse effects are bleeding, hemorrhage, and skin necrosis.

Antihypertensive treatment is recommended for all patients with a history of ischemic stroke regardless of whether or not the patient has a history of hypertension. Blood pressure lowering should be withheld in the acute setting.[3] The optimal medication regimen remains unknown; however, there is good data to support the use of a thiazide-type diuretic or an angiotensin-converting enzyme inhibitor plus a thiazide-type diuretic.[3]

All patients with atherosclerotic, ischemic stroke should receive HMG-CoA reductase inhibitors (statins) to reduce the risk of recurrent events.[13] Patients should be treated to a goal LDL cholesterol level of 100 mg/dL with an optional goal of <70 mg/dL.[13]

CASE Application

1. A 47-year-old white man with a PMH significant for hypertension, diabetes, and chronic alcoholism comes to your clinic for routine follow-up. His social history is significant for alcohol and tobacco abuse. He currently drinks one case of beer per night and smokes two packs per day. Pertinent laboratory findings are as follows: TC 182 mg/dL, TG 218 mg/dL, LDL 96 mg/dL, HDL 52 mg/dL, glucose 146 mg/dL. Current blood pressure is 158/94 mm Hg and HR is 92 beats per minute (bpm). He is 69 inches tall and weighs 232 lb.

   Which of the following is a risk factor for ischemic stroke in this patient?

   i. Hypertension
   ii. Obesity
   iii. Diabetes

   a. Only i is correct.
   b. Only iii is correct.
   c. Only i and ii are correct.
   d. Only ii and iii are correct.
   e. i, ii, and iii are all correct.

2. Which of the following statements most accurately describes the acute presentation of ischemic stroke?

   a. Focal neurological deficit lasting <24 hours, one-sided weakness, systolic blood pressure >200 mm Hg
   b. Focal neurological deficit lasting >24 hours, one-sided weakness, visual impairment
   c. Diffuse neurological deficit lasting <24 hours, one-sided weakness, visual impairment
   d. Diffuse neurological deficit lasting >24 hours, one-sided weakness, blood glucose >200 mm Hg

3. JS is a 78-year-old white woman with a PMH significant for atrial fibrillation, systolic heart failure with an ejection fraction of 35%, and hypertension. She presents to the emergency department with symptoms of right-sided paralysis. She is not able to communicate, but her family member states that the symptoms began approximately 5 hours ago. MRI of the brain confirms the patient has had an ischemic stroke. At home she takes metoprolol 100 mg po bid, lisinopril 40 mg po daily, and furosemide 20 mg po daily. Which of the following medications would be the most appropriate for secondary stroke prevention in JS?

   a. Aspirin
   b. Clopidogrel
   c. Warfarin
   d. Extended-release dipyridamole plus aspirin
   e. Ticlopidine

4. HB is a 54-year-old African American man who presents to the emergency department with symptoms of left-sided paralysis and visual impairment. He has a PMH significant for hypertension, dyslipidemia, and benign prostatic hyperplasia. MRI of the brain confirms the patient has had an ischemic stroke. Which of the following medications would be the most appropriate for secondary stroke prevention in HB?

   a. Ticlopidine
   b. Dipyridamole
   c. Aspirin

d. Clopidogrel plus aspirin
e. Warfarin

5. Which of the following is a common side effect of extended-release dipyridamole plus aspirin?

a. Agranulocytosis
b. Visual disturbances
c. Pancreatitis
d. Headache

6. A 63-year-old African American man with a PMH significant for dyslipidemia presented to the emergency department several days ago with symptoms of an acute stroke. The physician you are working with wants your recommendations on what to send this patient home on for blood pressure control. Current vitals are as follows: BP 138/88 mm Hg, HR 86 bpm. What do you recommend?

a. Beta-blocker.
b. Nondihydropyridine calcium channel blocker.
c. Angiotensin-converting enzyme inhibitor plus a diuretic.
d. Angiotensin-converting enzyme inhibitor.
e. No blood pressure medication. The patient's blood pressure is at goal.

7. What is the brand name of extended-release dipyridamole 200 mg plus aspirin 25 mg?

a. Angiomax
b. Aggrastat
c. Aggrenox
d. Abraxane
e. Anaprox

8. A 49-year-old white man with a PMH significant only for osteoarthritis was diagnosed with an ischemic stroke several days ago. The patient drinks one to two beers per day and denies smoking. Family history is unremarkable. His current lipid panel is as follows: TC 168 mg/dL, TG 88 mg/dL, HDL 44 mg/dL, LDL 116 mg/dL. Vitals: BP 136/84 mm Hg, HR 78 bpm. The physician you are working with wants to know if this patient needs to be placed on statin therapy. What do you recommend?

a. This patient's only major risk factor for coronary heart disease is his age. His goal LDL is <160 mg/dL. He does not need to be placed on statin therapy.
b. This patient's only major risk factors for coronary heart disease are his age and history of previous ischemic stroke. His goal LDL is <130 mg/dL. He does not need to be placed on statin therapy.
c. This patient's only major risk factors for coronary heart disease are his age and history of previous ischemic stroke. His goal LDL is <100 mg/dL. He does not need to be placed on statin therapy. Therapeutic lifestyle recommendation should be initiated.
d. Statin therapy is recommended for all patients with an ischemic stroke. His LDL goal is <100 mg/dL with a preference of <70 mg/dL. He should be put on statin therapy.

9. Which of the following medications inhibit platelet activity?

i. Clopidogrel
ii. Aspirin
iii. Dipyridamole

a. Only i is correct.
b. Only iii is correct.
c. Only i and ii are correct.
d. Only ii and iii are correct.
e. i, ii, and iii are all correct.

10. Which of the following is the most appropriate way for you to tell your patient to take extended-release dipyridamole plus aspirin therapy?

a. Extended-release dipyridamole 200 mg plus aspirin 25 mg po daily
b. Extended-release dipyridamole 25 mg plus aspirin 200 mg po daily
c. Extended-release dipyridamole 200 mg plus aspirin 25 mg po bid
d. Extended-release dipyridamole 25 mg plus aspirin 200 mg po bid
e. Extended-release dipyridamole 200 mg plus aspirin 25 mg two capsules po bid

11. CS is a 61-year-old white woman who has a PMH significant for hypertension and diabetes mellitus. She presents to the emergency department with signs and symptoms of an ischemic stroke. CT of the brain confirmed this diagnosis. Which of the following medications would be the most appropriate for secondary stroke prevention in CS?

a. Extended-release dipyridamole 200 mg plus aspirin 25 mg two capsules po bid
b. Aspirin 81 mg po daily
c. Clopidogrel 75 mg po bid
d. Clopidogrel 150 mg po daily
e. Warfarin 5 mg po daily

12. Which of the following best describes the mechanism of action of clopidogrel?

a. Irreversible inhibition of adenosine diphosphate–induced platelet aggregation
b. Irreversible inhibition of platelet cyclooxygenase
c. Reversible inhibition of adenosine diphosphate–induced platelet aggregation
d. Reversible inhibition of platelet cyclooxygenase

13. Which of the following medications works by binding to fibrin and subsequently converting plasminogen to plasmin?

a. Plavix
b. Aggrenox

c. Ticlid
d. Argatroban
e. Activase

14. Which of the following is the correct dose of aspirin for use during an acute stroke?

i. Aspirin 81 mg within 48 hours
ii. Aspirin 160 mg within 48 hours
iii. Aspirin 325 mg within 48 hours

a. Only i is correct.
b. Only ii is correct.
c. Only iii is correct.
d. ii and iii are correct.
e. i, ii, and iii are all correct.

15. A 68-year-old man with a PMH significant for diabetes mellitus, DVT 5 years ago, and GI bleed 2 weeks ago presents with right-sided weakness and right facial droop that began 2 hours ago. CT of the head confirms ischemic stroke. Home medications include: warfarin 5 mg po daily, pantoprazole 40 mg po daily, and metformin 1000 mg po bid. Pertinent laboratory values on admission include INR 1.4, hemoglobin 14, hematocrit 41, platelets 175,000, and glucose 200 mg/dL. Blood pressure on admission is 160/90 mm Hg. Which of the following is an exclusion criterion for this patient to receive rtPA?

a. Elevated INR
b. Low platelets
c. Recent GI bleed
d. Elevated blood pressure on admission
e. Time elapsed since onset of symptoms

16. A 72-year-old woman (68 in, 111 kg) is admitted for acute ischemic stroke confirmed by CT of the head. She presents within 1.5 hours of symptom onset and meets all criteria to receive rtPA. The physician asks you what the appropriate dose is for this patient and how to administer it. Your response is:

a. 100 mg IV over 1 hour
b. 90 mg IV over 1 hour
c. 10 mg IV bolus over 10 minutes and then 90 mg over an hour
d. 9 mg IV bolus over 1 minute and then 81 mg over an hour
e. 10 mg IV bolus over 1 minute and then 90 mg over an hour

17. In May 2009, the American Heart Association Stroke Council updated their guidelines to consider the use of rtPA up to 4.5 hours after symptom onset in certain patients. Patients who are not candidates for this extended window of rtPA use include:

a. Age >80 years
b. Patients taking oral anticoagulants regardless of INR
c. Score of >25 on the National Institutes of Health Stroke Scale
d. History of both stroke and diabetes together
e. All of the above

18. An 81-year-old man with a PMH significant for diabetes, hypertension, and ischemic stroke 3 years ago presents with slurred speech and left-sided weakness that began 3.5 hours ago. NIH stroke score is calculated to be 15. Home medications include lisinopril 40 mg po daily and glipizide 5 mg po bid. Laboratory values are within normal limits and blood pressure is 150/84 mm Hg. Patient weighs 80 kg. Which of the following may be used as initial treatment for ischemic stroke in this patient?

i. rtPA 72 mg (10% IV bolus over 1 minute and the remainder over 1 hour)
ii. Aspirin 325 mg po
iii. Aspirin 162 mg po
iv. Lovenox 1 mg/kg SQ q12h

a. Only i
b. Only ii
c. i and ii
d. ii and iv
e. iii and iv

19. Which of the following may be used to treat elevated blood pressure in acute stroke patients who have concomitant renal dysfunction?

i. Labetalol
ii. Nicardipine
iii. Sodium nitroprusside

a. Only i
b. Only ii
c. Only iii
d. i and ii
e. ii and iii

20. A 62-year-old woman is admitted 2 hours after onset of acute stroke symptoms including blurred vision, slurred speech, and right facial droop. CT of the head confirms ischemic stroke. Past medical history is nonsignificant, and the patient takes no medications at home. All laboratory values are within normal limits. Blood pressure is 200/110 mm Hg. Patient meets all other inclusion criteria for rtPA use. Which of the following is the best option for blood pressure control in this patient?

a. No treatment should be given since the systolic blood pressure is <220 mm Hg and the diastolic blood pressure is <120 mm Hg.
b. Since the patient meets all other inclusion criteria for rtPA, labetalol should be given to lower blood pressure to <185/110 mm Hg so that the patient can receive rtPA.
c. Since the patient meets all other inclusion criteria for rtPA, nicardipine infusion should be initiated to lower blood pressure to <140/90 mm Hg.
d. Since the patient meets all other inclusion criteria for rtPA, sodium nitroprusside should be initiated to lower the blood pressure by 15% to 25% within the first day.

TAKEAWAY POINTS ››

- Stroke is the third leading cause of death in the United States.
- Ischemic stroke commonly presents as an acute onset of focal neurological deficit lasting >24 hours.
- Patients at highest risk of developing an ischemic stroke are those with hypertension, diabetes, dyslipidemia, atrial fibrillation, cigarette smoking, and obesity.
- Intravenous rtPA and aspirin are the two pharmacologic agents recommended for use in the treatment of acute ischemic stroke.
- rtPA is recommended within 3 hours of symptom onset due to its ability to achieve early reperfusion and improve neurological outcomes. Some patients may be able to receive rtPA with 4.5 hours of symptom onset.
- Aspirin, clopidogrel, and extended-release dipyridamole plus aspirin are the cornerstone of antiplatelet options for the secondary prevention of ischemic stroke.
- Warfarin is the preferred antithrombotic agent for the secondary prevention of ischemic stroke in patients with a cardioembolic source.
- Antihypertensive treatment is recommended for all patients with a history of ischemic stroke regardless of whether or not the patient has a history of hypertension.
- All patients with atherosclerotic, ischemic stroke should receive HMG-CoA reductase inhibitors to reduce the risk of recurrent events.

REFERENCES

1. Lloyd-Jones D, Adams R, Carnethon M, et al. Heart disease and stroke statistics-2009 update: a report from the American Heart Association Statistics Committee and Stroke Statistics Subcommittee. *Circulation.* 2009;119:e21-e181.
2. *Incidence and Prevalence: 2006 Chart Book on Cardiovascular and Lung Diseases*. Bethesda, MD: National Heart, Lung, and Blood Institute; 2006.
3. Sacco RL, Adams R, Albers G, et al. Guidelines for prevention of stroke in patients with ischemic stroke or transient ischemic attack. A statement for health care professionals from the American Heart Association/American Stroke Association Council on Stroke. *Stroke.* 2006;37:577-617.
4. Goldstein L, Appel L, Brass L, et al. Primary Prevention of Ischemic Stroke: a Guideline from the American Heart Association/American Stroke Association Stroke Council. *Stroke.* 2006;37:1583-1633.
5. Adams HP Jr, del Zoppo G, Alberts MJ, et al. Guidelines for the early management of adults with ischemic stroke: a guideline from the American Heart Association. *Stroke.* 2007;38:1655-1711.
6. Activase [package insert]. San Fransisco, CA: Genentech; 2006.
7. The National Institute of Neurological Disorders and Stroke rt-PA Stroke Study Group. Tissue plasminogen activator for acute ischemic stroke. *N Engl J Med.* 1995;333:1581-1587.
8. Hacke W, Kaste M, Bluhmki E, et al. Thrombolysis with alteplase 3 to 4.5 hours after acute ischemic stroke. *N Engl J Med.* 2008;359:1317-1329.
9. del Zoppo GJ, Saver JL, Jauch EC, et al. Expansion of the time window for treatment of acute ischemic stroke with intravenous tissue plasminogen activator. *Stroke.* 2009;40:2945-2948.
10. International Stroke Trial Collaborative Group. The International Stroke Trial (IST): a randomized trial of aspirin, subcutaneous heparin, both, or neither among 19435 patients with acute ischemic stroke. *Lancet.* 1997;349:1569-1581.
11. CAST (Chinese Acute Stroke Trial) Collaborative Group. CAST: randomized placebo-controlled trial of early aspirin use in 20,000 patients with acute ischemic stroke. *Lancet.* 1997;349:1641-1649.
12. Grossman E, Ironi AN, Messerli FH. Comparative tolerability profile of hypertensive crisis treatments. *Drug Saf.* 1998;19:99-122.
13. Adams RJ, Albers G, Alberts MJ, et al. Update to the AHA/ASA recommendations for the prevention of stroke in patients with stroke and transient ischemic attack. *Stroke.* 2008;39:1647-1652.
14. Diener HC, Cunha L, Forbes C, et al. European Stroke Prevention Study, 2: dipyridamole and acetylsalicylic acid in the secondary prevention of stroke. *J Neurol Sci.* 1996;143:1-13.
15. ESPRIT Study Group. Aspirin plus dipyridamole versus aspirin alone after cerebral ischemia of arterial origin (ESPRIT): randomized controlled trial. *Lancet.* 2006;367:1665-1673.
16. Aspirin [package insert]. Morristown, NJ: Bayer Corportation; 2006.
17. Plavix [package insert]. Bridgewater, NJ: Bristol-Myers Squibb; 2009.
18. Bennett CL, Connors JM, Carwile JM, et al. Thrombotic thrombocytopenic purpura associated with clopidogrel. *N Engl J Med.* 2000;342:1773-1777.
19. Diener HC, Bogousslavsky J, Brass LM, et al. MATCH Investigators. Aspirin and clopidogrel compared with clopidogrel alone after recent ischemic stroke or transient ischemic attack in high-risk patients (MATCH): randomized, double-blind, placebo-controlled trial. *Lancet.* 2004;364:331-337.
20. Bhatt DL, Fox KA, Hacke W, et al. CHARISMA Investigators. Clopidogrel and aspirin versus aspirin alone for the prevention of atherothrombotic events. *N Engl J Med.* 2006;354:1706-1717.
21. Aggreonx [package insert]. Ridgefield, CT: Boehringer Ingelheim Pharmaceuticals, Inc; 2009.
22. Hass WK, Easton JD, Adams HP Jr, et al. A randomized trial comparing ticlopidine hydrochloride with aspirin for the prevention of stroke in high-risk patients: Ticlopidine Aspirin Stroke Study Group. *N Engl J Med.* 1989;321:501-507.
23. Hart RG, Benevente O, McBride R, et al. Antithrombotic therapy to prevent stroke in patients with atrial fibrillation: a meta-analysis. *Ann Intern Med.* 1999;131:492-501.
24. Hart RG, Halperin JL, Pearce LA, et al. Lessons from the stroke prevention in atrial fibrillation trials. *Ann Intern Med.* 2003;138:831-838.
25. Coumadin [package insert]. Princeton, NJ: Bristol-Myers Squibb; 2009.

CHAPTER

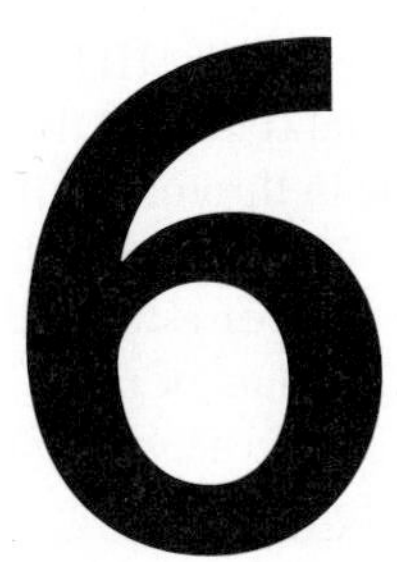

Anticoagulation/Venous Thromboembolism

William Joshua Guffey and Beth Bryles Phillips

FOUNDATION OVERVIEW

Venous thromboembolism (VTE) is a significant cause of morbidity and mortality in the United States. Each year approximately 2 million people develop VTE and 60,000 of these are fatal.[1] The economic burden to the health-care system is roughly $1.5 billion/year.[2] VTE encompasses both deep venous thrombosis (DVT) and pulmonary embolism (PE). The mainstay of treatment for VTE is anticoagulant agents. Anticoagulants are also used short and long term to prevent thromboembolic events, including those associated with cardiac valve replacement and myocardial infarction, thromboembolic stroke related to atrial fibrillation, high-risk hospitalized patients, and high-risk patients undergoing surgery.

Hemostasis, or termination of bleeding, is a fundamental bodily process. However, the balance between hemostasis and pathogenic thrombus formation is sensitive and depends on the stability and collaboration of three primary components known as Virchow's triad: venous stasis, vascular wall injury, or hypercoagulability.[3] A disruption in any of these components can result in thrombosis.

Patients presenting with VTE often have one or more risk factors for thromboembolism (Table 6-1).[4] Classic symptoms of a DVT include unilateral pain, swelling, erythema, and tenderness usually of the lower extremity; although some patients may be symptom free. Ultrasound (duplex ultrasonography) is typically used to diagnose a DVT. The symptoms of a PE are nonspecific and may include chest pain, shortness of breath, tachypnea, dyspnea, and hemoptysis. Most PEs originate from a DVT. The diagnosis of a PE is made by the presence of symptoms in conjunction with findings on ventilation-perfusion (V/Q) and computerized tomography scans. Medical work-up of patients presenting with VTE include determination of risk factors for VTE. Certain risk factors are reversible (eg, estrogen use, recent orthopedic surgery, prolonged immobility) and may be eliminated over time. The presence of irreversible or continuing risk factors (eg, cancer, thrombophilia, previous history of VTE) requires longer or indefinite duration of therapy. Short- and long-term sequelae of VTE include recurring thromboembolic events, death, and postphlebitic syndrome.

Key Definitions

Anticoagulation—the process of preventing blood clot formation

Deep venous thrombosis (DVT)—blood clot formation in a deep vein, usually in the leg (eg, iliac vein)

Postphlebitic syndrome—chronic condition occurring after DVT characterized by venous insufficiency, pain, edema, stasis dermatitis, varicose veins, and ulceration

Pulmonary embolism (PE)—blockage of a pulmonary artery, usually from a thrombus that has traveled from another site, such as the leg

Thromboembolism—occlusion of a blood vessel due to a blood clot that has broken away and traveled from its place of origin

Thrombophilia—genetic or acquired predisposition to thrombosis

Thrombosis—pathologic blood clot formation

TREATMENT OPTIONS

The goals of treatment in the management of VTE include the following: (1) prevention of thrombus extension, (2) prevention of development of PE, (3) prevention of recurrence of VTE, (4) decrease in mortality, and (5) prevention of postphlebitic syndrome. Anticoagulants are the primary drug therapy used to achieve these goals. These agents may be classified by basic mechanism of action into three groups: indirect thrombin inhibitors, direct thrombin inhibitors, and vitamin K antagonists. The parenteral indirect thrombin inhibitors are used for initial treatment of VTE. In most cases, oral anticoagulation with warfarin is initiated at the same time and the parenteral anticoagulants are discontinued once therapeutic anticoagulation with warfarin has been achieved. Anticoagulants are also used in the prevention of VTE and other thromboembolic disorders in high-risk patients.

Treatment

Indirect Thrombin Inhibitors

Heparin, low molecular weight heparins (LMWH), and fondaparinux comprise the commercially available indirect thrombin inhibitors (Table 6-2). These parenteral agents mediate their anticoagulant effect by activating antithrombin, an inhibitor of activated clotting factors.

Heparin and LMWH bind to antithrombin to exert their pharmacologic effects. The heparin–antithrombin complex inactivates factors IIa (thrombin), Xa, IXa, XIa, and XIIa. Both factor IIa and Xa, the main components responsible for the anticoagulant activity, are inactivated to an equal extent by heparin. The LMWH have a higher affinity for binding to factor Xa and inhibit its activity two to four times more than activity of factor IIa. Additionally, heparin binds to platelets, osteoblasts, macrophages, and a number of plasma proteins

TABLE 6-1 **Risk Factors for Venous Thromboembolism**[4]

Surgery
Major trauma
Prolonged immobility
Cancer
History of previous VTE
Estrogen-containing therapies
Selective estrogen receptor modulators (eg, Raloxifene)
Pregnancy
Advancing age
Inherited thrombophilia
Antithrombin deficiency
Factor V Leiden
Prothrombin gene mutation
Protein C deficiency
Protein S deficiency
Acquired thrombophilia
Antiphospholipid antibodies
Lupus anticoagulant
Anticardiolipin antibody

LMWH bind to these other targets to a lesser extent. Both heparin and LMWH have a short onset of anticoagulant effect, making them good choices for initial treatment of DVT.

Heparin may be administered by the intravenous (IV) or subcutaneous (SQ) route. In the treatment of VTE, an initial IV weight-based bolus dose is given followed by a weight-based continuous infusion. Heparin must be monitored closely by the activated partial thromboplastin time (aPTT) for efficacy and risk of bleeding. For the prevention of VTE, heparin is generally administered SQ at lower fixed doses.

The LMWH are administered SQ on a weight-based regimen once or twice daily for the treatment of VTE. Like heparin, lower fixed doses are used in the prevention of VTE, varying according to indication and patient characteristics. Unlike heparin, the LMWH exhibit a predictable dose–response relationship and routine monitoring is not needed. However, monitoring of anti-Xa activity is recommended for treatment in pregnant patients where variability in weight exists.[5]

Bleeding is the most common adverse effect associated with heparin and LMWH therapies, ranging from minor to severe and life threatening. The bleeding risk increases in heparin patients with advanced age and those receiving higher doses. In many cases, bleeding may be managed by suspending the continuous infusion for a few hours. For more severe cases, protamine sulfate may be administered to reverse the effects of heparin. Protamine may also be used to reverse the effects of LMWH administered within the previous 8 hours, but the reversal provided is incomplete.

One of the most serious complications associated with heparin is an antibody-mediated drop in platelets known as heparin-induced thrombocytopenia (HIT). This is a potentially critical and sometimes fatal condition that can be associated with a paradoxical increase in thrombosis. HIT is suspected if the platelet count decreases 50% or more within 5 to 14 days after initiation of therapy. In some cases, a rapid decline in platelet count may be seen after 24 hours of initiation of therapy if a patient was previously exposed to heparin within 100 days prior to therapy. This phenomenon is known as "rapid-onset HIT".[6] Heparin should be discontinued immediately in patients with HIT. When HIT develops in a patient receiving treatment with heparin or LMWH, alternative anticoagulation with a direct thrombin inhibitor must be administered to treat or prevent thrombosis until the platelet count has recovered (see Table 6-2). Fondaparinux may also be used but the dosing of this agent in HIT is less clear. LMWH have a much lower incidence of HIT due to the fact they have a much lower binding affinity to platelets. However, cross-reactivity can occur and LMWH should be avoided in suspected HIT. If indicated, the initiation of warfarin therapy should be delayed until the platelet count has recovered. For patients with a history of HIT in whom circulating antibodies are no longer present (usually 80-100 days after initial diagnosis), heparin and LMWH may theoretically be used with caution. However, many clinicians and patients are reluctant to do so due to the serious nature of HIT.

Other adverse effects associated with heparin therapy include osteoporosis, skin necrosis, hyperkalemia, hypersensitivity, and an elevation in hepatic transaminases.[5] The LMWH are associated with a lower risk of osteoporosis when compared to heparin. Contraindications to heparin and LMWH include active bleeding, hypersensitivity, and HIT. Heparin should be used over LMWH in renal insufficiency with creatinine clearance (CrCl) <30 mL/min in the treatment of VTE. In the prevention of VTE, lower doses are generally recommended when CrCl is <30 mL/min. Additionally, the LMWH carry a black box warning regarding the use of these agents in patients undergoing epidural anesthesia due to the potential for development of spinal hematoma and long-term or permanent paralysis. The use of platelet inhibitors, other anticoagulants, or nonsteroidal anti-inflammatory drugs concomitantly increases this risk.

Fondaparinux (Arixtra) is classified as a factor Xa inhibitor which exerts its anticoagulant effect by binding to antithrombin and inactivating factor Xa. It is administered SQ once daily and may be used in the treatment or prevention of VTE. It has a rapid onset of anticoagulation and a long half-life. Like LMWH, it has a predictable dose–response relationship and routine laboratory monitoring is not necessary. Bleeding is the most common adverse effect associated with fondaparinux. The anticoagulant effects may not be reversed with protamine. Fondaparinux does not bind to platelets and is not associated with HIT. It is contraindicated in patients with renal insufficiency and CrCl <30 mL/min.

Direct Thrombin Inhibitors

Direct thrombin inhibitors (DTIs) prevent clot formation by binding directly to thrombin and inactivating it. These drugs

TABLE 6-2 **Properties of Parenteral Anticoagulants**[5]

	Indirect Thrombin Inhibitors			
Properties	**Heparin**	**LMWH**	**Factor Xa inhibitor**	**Direct Thrombin Inhibitors**
Available agents	Heparin	Enoxaparin (Lovenox) Dalteparin (Fragmin) Tinzaparin (Innohep)	Fondaparinux (Arixtra)	Argatroban Bivalirudin (Angiomax) Lepirudin (Refludan)
Mechanism of action	Inhibits IIa, Xa, IXa, and XIIa through AT-III–binding complex	Inhibits Xa to greater extent through AT-III–binding complex	Selective Factor Xa inhibitor through AT-binding complex	Binds to and inactivates thrombin
Thrombin binding	N/A	N/A	N/A	Reversible: argatroban, bivalirudin Irreversible: lepirudin
Source	Porcine or bovine mucosa	Depolymerization of heparin	Synthetic	Synthetic: argatroban, bivalirudin Recombinant analog of hirudin: lepirudin
Avg MW (daltons)	15,000	4000-6000	1728	Argatroban: 526 Lepirudin: 6979 Bivalirudin: 2180
Anti-Xa/Anti-IIa ratio	1	Dalteparin 2.7 Enoxaparin 3.8 Tinzaparin 1.9	Anti-Xa only	Anti-IIa only
Plasma half-life	30-90 min	110-234 min	15-18 h	10-80 min
Elimination	Multifactorial	Renal	Renal	Hepatic: argatroban Renal: bivalirudin, lepirudin
Monitoring	aPTT; monitor closely	Not routinely done; anti-Xa activity in select patients	Not routinely done	aPTT; monitor closely
Protamine reversal	Yes	Yes; incomplete	No	No
Interaction with platelets	High	Low	No	No
May be used in HIT	No	No	Yes	Yes

are administered as continuous IV infusions and their effects are monitored by the aPTT. DTIs are the preferred agents to prevent and treat thrombosis associated with HIT. When used in this case, they should be continued until the platelet count has completely recovered. Bleeding is the most common adverse effect associated with DTIs. No specific agents exist that can reverse the anticoagulant effects. Hypersensitivity may occur in patients exposed to lepirudin. When used in combination with warfarin therapy, DTIs increase the international normalized ratio (INR). Argatroban has the most effect on the INR when compared to the other DTIs. Argatroban should be avoided in patients with hepatic dysfunction. Lepirudin should be avoided in patients with renal insufficiency and CrCl <30 mL/min. Bivalirudin is used primarily in patients undergoing cardiac procedures.

Vitamin K Antagonist

Warfarin sodium is the only oral anticoagulant available in the United States. It is consistently among the top 300 most commonly dispensed drugs in the United States each year.[7] When used for the treatment of VTE, the typical duration of therapy is 3 to 6 months if a reversible risk factor is present. Therapy may continue for several months or indefinitely if no specific risk factor for VTE was identified (ie, unprovoked), or if the patient has a continuing risk factor.

Warfarin reduces thrombus formation by inhibiting the activation of the vitamin K-dependent clotting factors, II, VII, IX, and X. The anticoagulant effect produced by warfarin is delayed and it takes several days to achieve a steady state anticoagulant effect due to its dependence on the depletion of these activated clotting factors. Warfarin is a racemic mixture of R and S enantiomers, each metabolized by a different cytochrome P (CYP)-450 pathway. S-warfarin, the more potent enantiomer, is metabolized by CYP-2C9, and R-warfarin is metabolized by CYP-3A4 and CYP-1A2.

In the treatment of VTE, warfarin therapy is used in combination with a parenteral anticoagulant until therapeutic levels are achieved. The recommended starting dose for most patients is 5 mg daily. Loading doses (generally >10 mg daily) are dangerous and no longer recommended for most patients. Lower starting doses of warfarin are recommended in certain situations, including elderly or malnourished patients, patients with moderate to severe heart failure or liver disease, or patients with a history of recent major surgery or medications that increase sensitivity to warfarin.[8] The maintenance dose required to maintain a therapeutic INR, the laboratory test used to monitor warfarin, must be individualized and adjusted as needed. The target INR is 2.5 (range 2.0-3.0) for most patients. A higher target INR of 3.0 (range 2.5-3.5) is recommended for patients with mitral and high-risk aortic mechanical cardiac valve replacements and patients who failed therapy with the lower target INR. Genetic variants may alter individual maintenance warfarin doses. For example, patients with CYP-2C9 polymorphisms often require lower warfarin doses, and patients with a vitamin K epoxide reductase complex 1 (VKORC1) mutation may be more sensitive or resistant to warfarin therapy.[8,9] Current guidelines do not support the use of genetic testing to determine initial warfarin dosing.[8]

Warfarin has a narrow therapeutic index, exhibits variability in individual dose requirements, and is subject to a number of drug–drug, drug–food, and drug–disease interactions, all of which necessitate close patient monitoring preferably by a specialized anticoagulation monitoring service. Warfarin therapy is adjusted to a target INR range. Patients with subtherapeutic INRs are at higher risk of thromboembolic complications and patients with supratherapeutic INRs are at higher risk of bleeding. Bleeding is the most significant adverse effect associated with warfarin and may range from minor epistaxis to life-threatening intracranial hemorrhage. One of the most important risk factors for bleeding is intensity of anticoagulation. Other risk factors include concomitant use of other drugs increasing bleeding risk (eg, antiplatelets or nonsteroidal anti-inflammatory drugs), advanced age, history of previous gastrointestinal bleed, and concomitant disease states. Patients with genetic polymorphisms in CYP-2C9 may also have a higher risk of bleeding.[10] The effects of warfarin may be reversed by administration of vitamin K. Oral vitamin K is preferred but IV vitamin K may be administered when urgent reversal is needed. Other uncommon adverse effects associated with warfarin include skin necrosis and purple toe syndrome.

Warfarin is perhaps one of the best known agents with many drug–drug interactions. Drugs may interact with warfarin based on a number of different mechanisms, including stereoselective interactions (eg, CYP-2C9/-3A4/-1A2), impaired absorption (eg, bile acid sequestrants), degradation of clotting factors (eg, levothyroxine), inhibition of cyclic conversion of vitamin K (eg, 2nd and 3rd generation cephalosporins), and potentiation of bleeding. Drugs that interact with warfarin by inhibiting or inducing CYP-2C9, which metabolizes S-warfarin, have the greatest and most consistent effect on the INR (Table 6-3). Drugs inhibiting or inducing CYP-3A4 or CYP-1A2, which metabolize the less potent R-warfarin, have a less consistent effect on the INR. Table 6-4 lists several drugs that increase the risk of bleeding when used in combination with warfarin.

TABLE 6-3 Stereoselective CYP-2C9 Warfarin Drug–Drug Interactions

Mechanism of Interaction	Effect on INR	Responsible Drugs
Inhibition of CYP-2C9 (S warfarin)	Increase	Amiodarone Azole antifungals Metronidazole Sulfamethoxazole/Trimethoprim
Induction of CYP-2C9 (S warfarin)	Decrease	Carbamazepine Rifampin Dicloxacillin Phenytoin Phenobarbital

TABLE 6-4 Select Drugs Increasing the Bleeding Risk with Warfarin[8]

Antiplatelets
Nonsteroidal anti-inflammatory drugs (NSAIDs)
Cyclooxygenase-2 (COX2) inhibitors
Aspirin
High-dose penicillins
Moxalactam

Another important interaction unique to warfarin is the drug–food interaction with vitamin-K–containing foods. Achieving a therapeutic warfarin dose is a fine balance with the vitamin K–dependent clotting factors. Introducing more or less vitamin K to the system upsets this balance and changes the INR. Common foods high in vitamin K content include dark green, leafy vegetables, green cabbage, and beef liver. Patients should be aware of this interaction and make an effort to keep their diet consistent in vitamin K. Patients and clinicians should also be aware of other sources of vitamin K, such as multivitamins and dietary supplements, which can alter the INR.

In addition to drug–drug and drug–food interactions, several other factors can affect the INR and therapeutic anticoagulation. An exacerbation of heart failure can increase the INR, while hypothyroidism can decrease warfarin sensitivity. Nonadherence to therapy can cause a decrease in the INR. Acute and chronic alcohol use can alter warfarin response as well. For these reasons, thorough and frequent patient education is essential for all patients receiving chronic warfarin therapy.

CASE Application

1. Which of the following agents would be the most appropriate reversal agent to be used in the case of warfarin overdose?
   a. Phenprocoumon
   b. Protamine sulfate
   c. Vitamin K
   d. Activated charcoal
   e. Ipecac syrup

2. Which of the following is not an adverse reaction associated with vitamin K antagonist use?
   a. Hematochezia
   b. Cardiac arrhythmias (QT prolongation)
   c. Bleeding
   d. Purple toe syndrome
   e. Anemia

3. Which of the following agents would result in a major drug interaction in conjunction with warfarin use?
   a. Lisinopril
   b. Metoprolol
   c. Darvon
   d. Lanoxin
   e. Fluconazole

4. Which of the following would be the best agent for treatment of DVT in a patient with heparin-induced thrombocytopenia?
   a. Enoxaparin
   b. Argatroban
   c. Aspirin
   d. Unfractionated heparin
   e. Fragmin

5. JC is a 36-year-old pregnant woman with an active DVT. She takes no other medications and has no significant past medical history. Which of the following agents would be the best choice for the initial treatment of her DVT?
   a. Enoxaparin
   b. Clopidogrel
   c. Aspirin
   d. Warfarin
   e. Apidra

6. Which of the following would be the most appropriate test for monitoring the efficacy of dalteparin in a pregnant female?
   a. International normalized ratio
   b. Liver enzymes
   c. Prothrombin time
   d. Anti-Xa activity
   e. Complete blood count

7. Which of the following choices below represents an appropriate initial regimen for a patient weighing 60 kg recently diagnosed with a PE?

   i. Coumadin 5 mg po daily
   ii. Lovenox 60 mg SQ bid
   iii. Plavix 75 mg po daily

   a. i only
   b. iii only
   c. i and ii only
   d. ii and iii only
   e. i, ii, and iii

8. Which of the following drugs can be used safely in an HIT patient with a creatinine clearance of 25 mL/min?
   a. Lepirudin
   b. Enoxaparin
   c. Dalteparin
   d. Fondaparinux
   e. Argatroban

9. Which of the following agents has a delayed onset of anticoagulant effect?
   a. Unfractionated heparin
   b. Lovenox
   c. Arixtra
   d. Warfarin
   e. Innohep

10. A 57-year-old woman (65 kg, BMI 28) was just admitted to the hospital for treatment of a PE. An order was written for heparin IV bolus 80 U/kg followed by a continuous infusion of 18 U/kg/h. What are respective heparin bolus dose and continuous infusion rate for this patient?
    a. 5000 U IV bolus; 1200 U/h infusion
    b. 4000 U IV bolus; 800 U/h infusion
    c. 6000 U IV bolus; 1150 U/h infusion
    d. 6000 U IV bolus; 1200 U/h infusion
    e. 4000 U IV bolus; 1150 U/h infusion

11. Which of the following over-the-counter products can be initiated safely in a patient on chronic warfarin therapy?
    a. Aspirin
    b. Naproxen
    c. Centrum Silver multivitamin
    d. Loratadine
    e. Micatin topical

12. From which of the following routes may unfractionated heparin be administered?

    i. Intravenously
    ii. Subcutaneously
    iii. Intramuscularly

    a. i and iii
    b. iii only
    c. i and ii only
    d. ii and iii only
    e. i, ii, and iii

13. Which of the following statements is appropriate for educating patients taking chronic warfarin therapy?
    a. Report any missed warfarin doses to your physician or clinic.
    b. Avoid foods high in vitamin K content.
    c. All herbal therapies are safe in combination with warfarin therapy.
    d. Over-the-counter analgesics are safe in combination with warfarin therapy.
    e. Alcohol consumption does not affect warfarin therapy.

14. JT is a 62-year-old man with a history of atrial fibrillation, coronary heart disease, hypertension, and benign prostatic hyperplasia. His current medications include warfarin 5 mg daily, amlodipine 5 mg daily, clopidogrel 75 mg daily, lisinopril 10 mg daily, finasteride 5 mg daily, and acetaminophen 500 mg prn. Which of the medications he is currently taking increases the risk of bleeding with warfarin?
   a. Clopidogrel
   b. Amlodipine
   c. Finasteride
   d. Acetaminophen
   e. Lisinopril

15. Which antibiotic would be expected to have the least effect on warfarin therapy in a 32-year-old woman with a urinary tract infection?
   a. Sulfamethoxazole-trimethoprim
   b. Nitrofurantoin
   c. Ciprofloxacin
   d. Dicloxacillin
   e. Metronidazole

16. A middle-aged woman presents a new prescription for her husband to your pharmacy for enoxaparin (Lovenox) 240 mg subcutaneously twice daily for 7 days for deep venous thrombosis. The patient's weight is 150 kg. Of the following choices, what is the most appropriate action for dispensing the medication?
   a. Dispense 21 80-mg syringes with instructions to inject three 80-mg syringes daily.
   b. Repackage the 240 mg dose in one syringe and dispense seven 220-mg syringes.
   c. Call the prescriber and recommend changing the dose to 150 mg twice daily.
   d. Call the prescriber and recommend changing the dose to 200 mg daily.
   e. Call the prescriber and recommend changing enoxaparin to warfarin 5 mg daily instead.

17. In which of the following patient types are lower initial doses of warfarin recommended?
   a. Pediatric
   b. Elderly
   c. Stroke
   d. Atrial fibrillation
   e. Hypothyroidism

18. A patient comes to your pharmacy requesting help in choosing a Boost dietary supplement. In your discussion, she tells you that she is also taking warfarin for recurrent DVT. Which of the following is a likely consequence of starting this dietary supplement in someone who is receiving chronic warfarin therapy?
   a. Increased risk of bleeding
   b. Increase in the INR
   c. Decrease in the INR
   d. Decrease in warfarin dose
   e. Warfarin-induced skin necrosis

19. Which of the following medications should be avoided in pregnant women (pregnancy category X)?
   a. Unfractionated heparin
   b. Enoxaparin
   c. Fondaparinux
   d. Argatroban
   e. Warfarin

20. Which of the following is *not* an appropriate counseling point when counseling a patient on Lovenox?
   a. Rotate injection site to minimize bruising and pain.
   b. Inject at least 2 inches from your belly button and out toward your sides.
   c. Prior to injection, gently press the plunger to remove the air bubble from the syringe.
   d. Dispose of used syringe in thick plastic container or biohazard container.
   e. Avoid rubbing site of injection after administration to minimize risk of bruising.

21. Which of the following agents would be the best pain management option in a patient with chronic warfarin therapy?
   a. Celebrex
   b. Ibuprofen
   c. Excedrin
   d. Aspirin
   e. Acetaminophen

22. In which of the following procedures should Lovenox use be avoided?
   a. Computed tomography (CT) scan
   b. Magnetic resonance imaging (MRI) scan
   c. Epidural anesthesia
   d. 24 hour urine collection
   e. Liver biopsy

TAKEAWAY POINTS ››

- Anticoagulants are frequently used drugs for the treatment of VTE and prevention of thromboembolic events associated with a variety of disorders, such as recurrent VTE, atrial fibrillation, mechanical cardiac valve placement, and myocardial infarction.
- VTE encompasses both DVT and PE. Complications of DVT include PE and development of the postphlebitic syndrome. PEs are potentially fatal and are often not preceded by a symptomatic DVT.

- The duration of VTE treatment is determined by the presence of a reversible risk factor, presence of a continuing risk factor, or absence of an identifiable risk factor.
- Bleeding is the most common adverse effect of oral and parenteral anticoagulants.
- Heparin therapy is monitored by the aPTT. Routine monitoring of LWMH by anti-factor Xa activity is not performed except in select patient populations (eg, pregnant women).
- Protamine sulfate may be used to reverse heparin therapy and may partially reverse LMWH. There is no reversal agent for fondaparinux.
- Heparin may cause an immune-mediated thrombocytopenia, known as HIT. This significant complication may also occur with LMWH but it is less common. Heparin and LMWH are contraindicated in patients who have developed HIT.
- Drugs inhibiting or inducing cytochrome P-450-2C9 are expected to have the greatest effect on INR values when used in combination with warfarin therapy.
- The anticoagulant effect of warfarin is delayed and steady state anticoagulation occurs only after several days of therapy.
- Warfarin has a significant drug–food interaction with vitamin K–containing foods and supplements. Foods with high vitamin K content typically include dark green, leafy vegetables. Patients should be educated to keep their diet consistent with respect to vitamin K–containing foods.
- Warfarin therapy should be avoided in pregnant women (pregnancy category X).

REFERENCES

1. Buller HR, Agnelli G, Hull RD, Hyers TM, Prins MH, Rasbkob GE. Antithrombotic therapy for venous thromboembolic disease: The Seventh ACCP Conference on Antithrombotic and Thrombolytic Therapy. *Chest*. 2004;126:401S-428S.
2. Spyropoulos AC, Hurley JS, Ciesla GN, de Lissovoy G. Management of acute proximal deep vein thrombosis: pharmacoeconomic evaluation of outpatient treatment with enoxaparin vs inpatient treatment with unfractionated heparin. *Chest*. 2002;122:108-114.
3. Haines ST, Bussey HI. Thrombosis and the pharmacology of antithrombotic agents. *Ann Pharmacother*. 1995;29:892-905.
4. Bates SM, Ginsberg JS. Treatment of deep-vein thrombosis. *N Engl J Med*. 2004;351:268-277.
5. Hirsh J, Bauer KA, Donati MB, Gould M, Samama MM, Weitz JI. Parenteral anticoagulants. *Chest*. 2008;133;141S-159S
6. Warkentin TE, Greinacher A, Koster A, Lincoff AM. Heparin-induced thrombocytopenia. *Chest*. 2008;133;340S-380S
7. The Internet Drug Index. Available at: http://www.rxlist.com/script/main/art.asp?articlekey=79509. Accessed July 28, 2009.
8. Ansell J, Hirsh J, Hylek E, Jacobson A, Crowther M, Palareti G. Pharmacology and management of the vitamin K antagonists. *Chest*. 2008;133:160S-198S
9. Rieder MJ, Reiner AP, Gage BF, et al. Effect of VKORC1 haplotypes on transcriptional regulation and warfarin dose. *N Engl J Med*. 2005;352:2285-2293.
10. Higashi MK, Veenstra DL, Kondo M, et al. Association between CYP2C9 genetic variants and anticoagulation-related outcomes during warfarin therapy. *JAMA*. 2002;287:1690-1698.

CHAPTER

7 Acute Coronary Syndromes

Tracy E. Macaulay and Marintha R. Short

FOUNDATION OVERVIEW

Acute Coronary Syndrome (ACS) is a set of cardiovascular diagnoses that have similar underlying pathophysiology, involving atherosclerosis and acute thrombosis. In the United States, cardiovascular disease, including ACS, is the single leading cause of death among males and females.[1] Over 900,000 patients present with ACS each year, with mortality ranging from 3% to 15% depending on the subtype of ACS.[1] The prevalence of ACS makes knowledge of appropriate treatment of great importance to both inpatient and community pharmacists.

Diagnosis as to the subtype of ACS is important to guide early and potentially life-saving interventions, such as percutaneous transluminal coronary angioplasty (PTCA) and other percutaneous coronary interventions (PCI). The first step in the recognition of ACS is to understand the classic clinical presentation. As the word "acute" implies, all subtypes of ACS have a sudden onset, differentiating them from stable angina. A patient presenting with ACS typically describes crushing chest pressure with radiation to the jaw, arm, and shoulder. They may also have a combination of nonspecific symptoms including diaphoresis, nausea, vomiting, and a sense of illness (Table 7-1). It is important to note that ACS presentation can also be clinically silent, particularly in women.[2] Beyond presenting symptoms, diagnosis is confirmed with electrocardiography (ECG), which should be immediately performed by emergency medical services (EMS) or upon arrival to the emergency department (ED). This important step is used to differentiate T-wave changes and/or ST-segment depressions seen with unstable angina (UA) and non-ST segment elevation myocardial infarctions (NSTEMI) from the ST-segment elevation observed with ST-segment elevation myocardial infarctions (STEMI). Because UA is not associated with heart muscle damage, while NSTEMI and STEMI result in cell death, cardiac biomarkers (troponin, creatine kinase-MB) are used to further stratify unstable angina from heart attacks.

PRIMARY PREVENTION

Due to the vast number of people afflicted with ACS each year, there is great interest in prevention of ACS. Large cohort studies have been performed to identify characteristics that put individuals at increased risk of developing coronary artery disease. About 90% of patients presenting with ACS have at least one of the following risk factors for atherosclerosis: high total cholesterol measurement (or treatment with cholesterol-lowering medications), hypertension (or current treatment), current cigarette smoking, or history of diabetes.[3] Other modifiable risk factors include abdominal obesity, low fruit and vegetable consumption, lack of physical activity, and some psychosocial situations.[4] If these risk factors are prevented or aggressively treated, the prevalence of ACS would likely decrease. Once ACS events occur, initial treatments, medical management, and secondary prevention become vitally important.

TREATMENT

Overview and Treatment Goals

In the treatment of ACS, a clear delineation must be made between the emergency of STEMI and the urgency of NSTEMI and UA. In patients experiencing STEMI, complete occlusion of a coronary artery results in elimination of blood flow to the distal heart muscle. It is vital that this vessel be opened in the shortest time possible from the onset of symptoms.[5] Therefore, patients with STEMI should proceed emergently to reperfusion therapy. Beyond 24 hours, it is likely that even if blood flow were restored, lack of oxygen would result in permanent muscle loss. Patients with NSTEMI and UA may undergo early PCI or be managed more conservatively with medical therapy alone.[6] For survivors of ACS, secondary prevention begins immediately and is similar in all subtypes.

Symptomatic Therapies

During the processes of diagnosing the patient with ACS and while early treatment strategies are being decided, several therapies can be administered that are potentially life-saving and improve symptoms. These include nitroglycerin (NTG), analgesia, oxygen, and antiplatelet therapies (Figure 7-1).

Because nitric oxide is an endogenous vasodilator that is decreased in patients with coronary artery disease, nitroglycerin can be given as an exogenous source of this vasodilator. In patients experiencing ACS, it is recommended to give nitroglycerin (NTG) as a sublingual tablet or spray to relieve symptoms associated with myocardial ischemia. For patients with home NTG prescriptions, they may take one sublingual tablet or spray, and if there is no chest pain relief, EMS should be notified.[7] The patient can continue taking NTG every

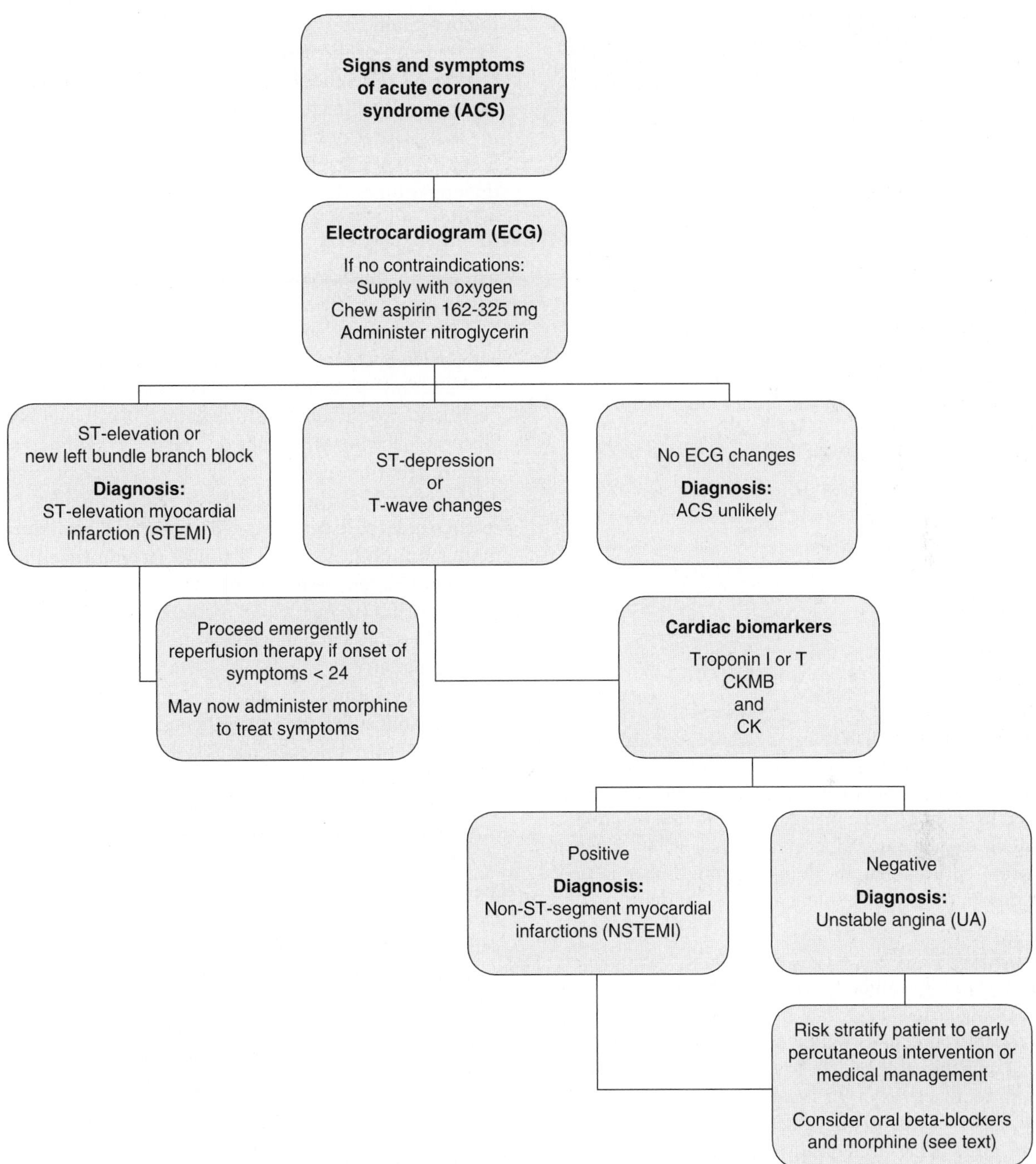

FIGURE 7-1 Diagnosis of acute coronary syndrome and treatment overview.

5 minutes (maximum of three doses in 15 minutes) until EMS arrives. Upon arrival to the hospital, intravenous nitroglycerin may be initiated and continued for the first 48 hours to treat ongoing ischemia, heart failure, or hypertension. Due to the risk of hypotension, NTG should be avoided in patients with evidence of right heart failure or low blood pressure.[7]

In patients with ongoing chest pain, despite treatment with NTG, morphine 2 to 4 mg intravenously every 5 to 15 minutes may be given to aid in pain control. In addition to opiate mediated analgesia, morphine causes vasodilation of both veins (preload) and arteries (afterload), which decreases myocardial oxygen demand. Although, morphine is the analgesic of choice in patients experiencing STEMI, studies have brought into question the safety of use in NSTEMI and UA. One observational analysis showed that morphine increased mortality in NSTEMI patients.[8] This resulted in a slight downgrading of guideline recommendations regarding morphine use, and a call for a randomized trial to evaluate morphine safety in this setting.[9] Morphine related vasodilation may also cause hypotension, limiting its usefulness in certain patients and requires blood pressure monitoring in all recipients.

TABLE 7-1 **Signs and Symptoms of Acute Coronary Syndrome**

Signs of Acute Coronary Syndrome
▪ Elevated cardiac biomarkers
▪ Troponin I or T
▪ CKMB
▪ Other potentially abnormal laboratory values
▪ Elevated white blood count
▪ Increased aspartate transaminase (AST)
▪ Elevated lactate dehydrogenase (LDH)
▪ ECG findings
▪ ST-segment elevations myocardial infarction (STEMI)
▪ New left bundle branch block
▪ ST-segment depressions
▪ T-wave changes
Symptoms of Acute Coronary Syndrome
▪ Chest pain
▪ Chest tightness / pressure
▪ Pain radiation to the left arm and/or jaw
▪ Diaphoresis (sweating)
▪ Nausea
▪ Vomiting
▪ Shortness of breath
▪ Palpitations
▪ Anxiety or sense of doom

In all patients experiencing ACS, supplemental oxygen (delivered by nasal cannula or face mask) should be provided to maintain oxygen saturation greater than 90%.[7] Adequate oxygenation ensures that all blood reaching ischemic tissue has the maximum oxygen content available for delivery.

Initial Treatment

Aspirin irreversibly inhibits formation of thromboxane A2, thus inhibiting platelet aggregation. At the onset of chest pain, patients should chew and swallow aspirin 162 to 325 mg (two to four 81 mg chewable tablets are preferred). If not taken at home (or unknown), aspirin should immediately be administered by EMS or upon arrival to ED. The benefit of aspirin in patients with ACS has been clearly established and is strongly recommended in American Heart Associations and the American College of Cardiology's (AHA/ACC) guidelines.[7,9,10]

In addition to aspirin, it is recommended that patients with ACS be loaded on a thienopyridine (ticlopidine, clopidogrel, or prasugrel). Thienopyridines inhibit platelet activation by irreversibly blocking the P2Y12 component of adenosine diphosphate receptors. Dual antiplatelet therapy with a thienopyridine plus aspirin, has demonstrated benefit over aspirin monotherapy both in medical management of ACS and following coronary stent placement.[11,12] The main thienopyridine utilized in the United States is clopidogrel, as severe toxicities associated with ticlopidine, including hematologic side effects, limit its use. Clopidogrel is typically administered as 300 to 600 mg oral loading dose followed by 75 mg daily. Prasugrel, the recently Food and Drug Administration approved thienopyridine, may infer increased antiplatelet benefits with the trade off of increased bleeding.[13] An important pharmacodynamic difference in clopidogrel and prasugrel may be the onset of full antiplatelet activity; following clopidogrel loading, antiplatelet onset takes 1 to 6 hours (depending on the dose), while prasugrel's antiplatelet onset is 30 minutes. Following thienopyridines discontinuation, it takes 5 to 7 days for restoration of normal platelet function. If surgery is performed in this platelet restoration window, increased bleeding is likely.[11,13] A thienopyridine alone may be given if the patient has an aspirin allergy.

Beta-blockers are a diverse class of medications that antagonize β_1-receptor with various other effects (Table 7-2). In the setting of ACS, beta-blockers decrease heart rate which decreases myocardial oxygen demand. Other benefits of beta-blockers following MI include decreasing arrhythmias and preventing recurrent events. It was previously recommended to give metoprolol 5 mg intravenously every 5 minutes; however, recent studies have demonstrated that early IV beta-blockers are more harmful than good.[14] It is now recommended that early oral beta-blockers are reasonable for patients that have high-risk characteristics (ie, high blood pressure), and who are hemodynamically stable without hypotension, evidence of heart failure, cardiogenic shock or bradycardia. The current goal is to initiate oral therapy within 24 to 48 hours post-MI. If there are contraindications at that time, the patient should be reevaluated at a later time for beta-blockers use as secondary prevention.[14]

Upon presentation to ED, while STEMI patients must receive reperfusion, patients with UA or NSTEMI may be treated in a variety of ways. Some may proceed to early invasive PCI while others will be managed conservatively with medical therapy alone or as a bridge to delayed PCI. Medical regimens involve several acceptable anticoagulant schemes, with a gold standard of unfractionated heparin (UFH), given as an IV loading dose and then a continuous maintenance infusion adjusted to maintain activated partial thromboplastin time (aPTT) 1.5 to 2 times baseline or 50 to 70 seconds (Table 7-3). Although aPTT is the gold standard for UFH monitoring, an increasing number of institutions are utilizing anti-factor Xa for adjusting heparin across a variety of clinical scenarios. Determination of most appropriate anti-factor Xa level in ACS requires further study.[15] Anticoagulation should be continued for 48 hours up to 7 days, or at least until PCI, along with aspirin and clopidogrel.[9,16] Additional anticoagulation options include low molecular weight heparin (LMWH), fondaparinux, or bivalirudin. Advantages of LMWH include ease of administration, lack of routine monitoring, and improved outcomes over heparinoids.[15] Fondaparinux is preferred if the patient is at an increased risk of bleeding, but only if PCI is not planned.[17] Finally, bivalirudin is recommended if PCI is planned, as a bridge to this ultimate therapy. When bivalirudin is initiated prior to PCI, a small bolus (0.1 mg/kg) and low infusion rate are utilized (0.25 mg/kg/h). If bivalirudin is chosen when the patient arrives in the cardiac path lab for PCI, they receive a second larger bolus and the infusion rate is increased.[18] Higher doses used during PCI are potent inhibitors of platelet activity.[19]

TABLE 7-2 **Beta-Blockers**

Agent/ Parameter	Brand Names	Pharmacology	Dose (po)	Dose (IV)	A	D	M	E	Role in Therapy
Propranolol	Inderal, Inderal LA	β_1 and β_2 blocker	80-320 mg divided 2-4 times daily	1 mg/dose over 5 min (MAX 10 mg)	Almost complete	Extensive	Hepatic	$t_{1/2}$ = 4 h LA: $t_{1/2}$ = 10 h	Angina, thyroid storm, migraine
Atenolol	Tenormin	β_1-selective	50-100 mg once twice daily	5 mg IV every 10 min	F = 0.5	6%-16% protein bound	None	> 50% renal, 50% unchanged $t_{1/2}$ = 6-7 h	Tachyarrhythmias, post-ACS/MI
Metoprolol	Lopressor Toprol XL	β_1-selective	100 to 400 mg daily (divided twice to three times daily)	5 mg IV every 5 min 3 times	Tartrate: rapid and complete Succinate: F = 0.77	12% protein bound	Hepatic, >50% first-pass	< 5% renal Tartrate: $t_{1/2}$ = 3-7 h Succinate: $t_{1/2}$ = 4-10 h	Consider metoprolol succinate in patients with decreased left ventricular ejection fraction (LVEF)
Carvedilol	Coreg Coreg CR	α, β_1, β_2 blocker	3.125-50 mg twice daily	n/a	F = 0.25 to 0.3	98% protein bound	Hepatic via CYP2D6	$t_{1/2}$ = 7-10 h	Consider using carvedilol in patients with decreased LVEF
Acebutolol	Sectral	β_1-selective mild ISMA	600-1600 mg	n/a	F = 0.4	26% protein bound	Extensive first-pass	Biliary and 30%-50% renal	Hypertension
Labetalol	Normodyne Trandate	α, β_1, β_2 blocker	200-400 mg bid or tid	0.25 mg/kg (20mg)every 10 min	F = 0.25	50% protein bound	Hepatic conjugation	Fecal, renal (55%-60%) $t_{1/2}$ = 6-8 h (po), 5.5 h IV	Treatment of emergent hypertension
Esmolol	Brevibloc	β_1	n/a	500 µg/kg IV bolus, 50 µg/kg/min	n/a	55% protein bound	Esterases, hydrolysis	73%-88% renal $t_{1/2}$ = 9 min	Aortic aneurysm, tachyarrhythmias
Nebivolol	Bystolic	β_1-selective vasodilatory properties	5-40 mg once daily	n/a	F = 0.12 to 0.96	98% protein bound	Hepatic, CYP2D6	Fecal 44%, renal 38%-67% $t_{1/2}$ = 12-19 h	Hypertension

Abbreviations: po, oral; IV, intravenous; A, absorption; D, distribution; M, metabolism; E, elimination; n/a, not available; ISMA, intrinsic sympathomimetic activity; F, bioavailability.

TABLE 7-3 **Anticoagulants for Treatment of Acute Coronary Syndrome**

Parameter	UFH	Enoxaparin[a]	Fondaparinux	Bivalirudin
Mechanism	Inactivates IIa, IX, X, XI, XII, and plasmin	Inactivates Xa, IIa	Xa inhibitor	Direct thrombin inhibitor
Excretion	Hepatic (reticuloendothelial system)	Hepatic and renal	Renal	< 20% renal
Half-life	1.5 h	4.5-7 h	17-21 h	25-57 min
Dose	60 units/kg IVP (maximum of 4000 units), then 12 units/kg/h (maximum 1000 units/h) to target aPTT 50-70 s (or 1.5-2 times control)	NSTEMI/UA: 1 mg/kg every 12 h STEMI with lytics: 0.3 mg/kg IV bolus, followed by 1 mg/kg every 12 h (0.75 mg/kg every 12 h in patients > 75 y)	2.5 mg subcutaneously daily (for medical management only, if given before PCI change to UFH for antithrombotic during procedure)	0.1 mg/kg IVP then 0.25 mg/kg/h with extra 0.5 mg/kg upon arrival to cath lab and increase infusion to 1.75 mg/kg/h
Contraindications	History of heparin-induced thrombocytopenia	SCr > 2.5 mg/dL	SCr > 3.0 mg/dL	Renal failure
Monitoring	aPTT and ACT during PCI	None required, anti-Xa possible	None	aPTT
Reversibility	Protamine	66% by protamine, FFP	FFP	None

[a]Dose during PCI dependent on the timing of the last subcutaneous dose and concomitant IIb/IIIa use.

Abbreviations: FFP, fresh frozen plasma; UFH, unfractionated heparin.

Glycoprotein IIb/IIIa inhibitors (GPI) block the final step of platelet aggregation. These medications have an established role during PCI, to prevent early in-stent thrombosis following stent deployment.[20] However, several of these medications have also demonstrated benefit when started before PCI and in the conservatively (medically) managed patient. Eptifibatide and tirofiban can be used in addition to anticoagulants and oral antiplatelets in patients who will be medically managed or if delayed-PCI is anticipated.[21] Abciximab, like bivalirudin, should be reserved for patients who are managed with PCI only. Utility of GPI for medical management and as adjunctive treatment with PCI should be balanced with an increased bleeding risk and contraindications should be strictly observed (Table 7-4).

TABLE 7-4 **Antiplatelet Therapies for Acute Coronary Syndrome**

Drug	Aspirin	Ticlopidine	Clopidogrel	Prasugrel	Eptifibitide[a]	Tirofiban[a]	Abciximab
MOA	Block production of thromboxane A2	Block production of adenosine diphosphate	Block production of adenosine diphosphate	Block production of adenosine diphosphate	Cyclic heptatide: blocks GPIIb/IIIa receptor	Nonpeptide inhibitor of GPIIb/IIIa	Antibody Fab fragment GPIIb/IIIa
Dose	162-325 mg	250 mg bid	LD: 300-600 mg MD: 75 mg daily	LD: 60 mg MD: 10 mg daily	180 µg/kg IV bolus followed by 1-2 µg/kg/min for 12-96 h	Rapid infusion of 0.4 µg/kg/min for 30 min, then 0.1 µg/kg/min for 12-24 h	Not recommended
PCI dose	Ideally, give at least 1 h before PCI	n/a	Load 2-6 h before PCI	Load 30 min before PCI	180 µg/kg IV bolus 2, times 10 min apart with an infusion of 1-2 µg/kg/min for 18 h	25 µg/kg over 3 min, then 0.15 µg/kg/min for 24-48 h	0.25 µg/kg IV bolus; 0.125 µg/kg/min (max 10 µg/kg/min) for 12 h
Metabolism	Hepatic esterases	CYP-450	Transformed to active metabolite by mainly CYP-450 2D6	Multiple CYP450 isoenzymes	Nonhepatic	Metabolism unknown 65% renal excreted	Unknown
Elimination half-life	15-20 min parent drug; 3 h for metabolites	12 h	7-8 h	7 h (range 2-15 h)	2.5 h	90-180 min	Phase 1 = 10 min Phase 2 = 30 min
Onset of antiplatelet effect	1-2 h	2-5 d	2-6 h	30 min	Within 20 min	Within 20 min	Within 20 min
Offset of antiplatelet effects	6 h	6 d	5-7 d	5-7 d	5-10 h	4-8 h	Usual 12 h, up to 24-48 h
CI	Severe thrombocytopenia (TTP/ITP), hematologic disorders, active bleeding, recent major surgery, hypersensitivity reactions	Active peptic ulcer disease (PUD) or intracranial hemorrhage (ICH); severe liver dysfunction; hematopoietic disorders	High risk for bleeding or severe HF, taking OAC, revascularization in previous 3 mo, received IIB/IIIa inhibitors within 3 d; PUD, ICH	Patients > 75 y, history of ischemic or hemorrhagic stroke, and weight < 60 kg (FDA blackbox warning)	Thrombocytopenia < 100, renal insufficiency, allergy, severe uncontrolled hypertension, pregnancy, history of hemorrhagic stroke, recent ischemic stroke/TIA (within 3 mo)	Hypersensitivity, active bleeding, history of intracranial hemorrhage, aneurysm, thrombocytopenia, ischemic stroke within 30 d, hypertension, pericarditis, thrombocytopenia < 150	Hypersensitivity, active bleeding, history of intracranial hemorrhage, pregnancy, ischemic stroke or TIA within 2 y, recent GI bleeding, major surgery, thrombocytopenia < 100
ADE	Bleeding, GI ulcers	Increased cholesterol and triglycerides, TTP, diarrhea, life-threatening hematologic reactions, liver injury	GI: abdominal pain, vomiting dyspepsia, bleeding	Bleeding	Severe bleeding, hypotension (6%), thrombocytopenia (rare)	Major bleeding (1.4%), minor bleeding (10.5%), thrombocytopenia	Bleeding, GI hemorrhage, severe thrombocytopenia, hypotension (14.4%), bradycardia, GI intolerance

[a]Require renal adjustment.

Abbreviations: MOA, mechanism of action; PCI, percutaneous coronary intervention; CI, contraindications; ADE, adverse drug effects.

TABLE 7-5 **Thrombolytics for Treatment of STEMI**

Drug[a]	Dose
Streptokinase (SK, Streptase)	1.5 million units IV over 60 min
Alteplase (tPA)	15 mg IV bolus followed by 0.75 mg/kg IV over 30 min (max 50 mg) followed by 0.5 mg/kg (max 35 mg) over 60 min
Reteplase (rPA, Retevase)	10 units IV bolus over 10 min 2 times, 30 min apart
Tenecteplase (TNK)	< 60 kg give 30 mg IV bolus over 5 s
	60-69.9 kg give 35 mg IV bolus
	70-79.9 kg give 40 mg IV bolus
	80-89.9 kg give 45 mg IV bolus
	> 90 kg give 50 mg IV bolus

[a]Administer with UFH or LMWH for at least 48 hours.

Reperfusion Therapy

If STEMI is diagnosed, the primary goal is to open the vessel in the shortest time possible with either fibrinolysis or percutaneous coronary intervention (PCI). Fibrinolytics (Table 7-5) catalyze the conversion of endogenous plasminogen to plasmin, which degrades fibrin and results in lysis of the thrombus. Although fibrinolysis may be administered up to 12 hours after the onset of chest pain, accrediting bodies have developed standards to guide how rapidly this emergency should be handled. The standard for fibrinolysis is a goal "door to needle time" of less than 30 minutes. Prior to administration of these potentially deleterious medications, it is always important to ensure that the patient does not have contraindications to fibrinolysis (Table 7-6). Because fibrinolytic therapy is unsuccessful in approximately 1/4th of patients, PCI with balloon angioplasty followed by coronary stenting is the preferred method of reperfusion. The standard goal "door to balloon time" with angioplasty (PCI) is less than 90 minutes. Unfortunately PCI is not always possible, making fibrinolytics a viable option for hospitals that do not have 24 hour cardiac catheterization laboratories. To prevent recurrent coronary thrombosis, anticoagulants (UFH, LMWH) should be used as adjunct with fibrinolytics for a minimum of 48 hours and recommended for the duration of the index visit up to 8 days.[7]

TABLE 7-6 **Thrombolytic Absolute and Relative Contraindications**

Absolute Contraindications
▪ Any history of intracranial hemorrhage (ICH)
▪ Known malignant intracranial neoplasm (primary or metastatic)
▪ Ischemic stroke within 3 mo
▪ Suspected aortic dissection
▪ Active bleeding or bleeding diathesis (excluding menses)
▪ Significant closed-head or facial trauma within 3 mo
▪ Major surgery within 14 d
Relative Contraindications
▪ Chronic, severe, poorly controlled hypertension
▪ Severe uncontrolled hypertension on presentation (SBP >180 mm Hg)
▪ Traumatic or prolonged (>10 min) cardiopulmonary resuscitation (CPR)
▪ Major surgery within 14-21 d
▪ Internal bleeding within 2-4 wk
▪ Noncompressible vascular punctures
▪ Pregnancy
▪ Active peptic ulcer
▪ Concurrent use with oral anticoagulant (correct INR first with fresh frozen plasma)

SECONDARY PREVENTION

The prevention of reinfarction and other complications from ACS begin immediately. Prevention of rethrombosis is aided by the previously mentioned antiplatelet therapies and short-term anticoagulation, but other medications have also been proven effective. These include HMG-CoA reductase inhibitors (statins), beta-blockers, and in certain patients, angiotensin converting enzyme inhibitors (ACE-I) or angiotensin receptor blockers (ARB).

Aspirin should be given initially and then continued indefinitely in all patients without contraindication. To minimize bleeding complications, it is recommended to give aspirin at the lowest effective dose in patients on dual antiplatelet therapy.[22] Continuation of a thienopyridine is indicated for 1 to 12 months following index event, and may be considered longer in patients who receive drug eluting stents.[11,23] While the current guidelines do not yet include the recently FDA approved thienopyridine, prasugrel, there appears to be improved antiplatelet effect with prasugrel compared to clopidogrel. However, this benefit comes with the distinct disadvantage of increased bleeding.[13]

Hydroxy-methylglutaryl (HMG) coenzyme A reductase is the rate-limiting step in synthesis of atherogenic low-density lipoproteins (LDL). The pharmacologic class of HMG-CoA reductase inhibitors (statin) that target this process have become an essential part of secondary prevention of ACS. Data supports early and ongoing treatment with high-dose statin therapy following ACS. Benefits of statin therapy seem to go beyond lipid lowering capabilities, which is why guidelines recommend use in patients whose cholesterol levels are unknown at the time of their event. The LDL goals have been a moving target over the past 5 years. Current guidelines recommend substantially below 100 mg/dL,[7] with less than 70 mg/dL as a reasonable target. In many patients this goal is difficult to achieve without using potent statins at high doses. The majority of evidence in this area supports the use of atorvastatin 80 mg initiated early after index event, and continued indefinitely.[24]

Use of long-term beta-blocker therapy is highly recommended in patients without absolute contraindications.[7] In the first 48 hours following MI, patients are at an increased risk of ventricular arrhythmias, sudden cardiac death, and are at the highest risk for recurrent ischemia. Long-term benefits of beta-blockers are well established, particularly in patients with impaired ventricular function (heart failure);[25] however, initiation should be with low doses and slow titration in these patients. Individual differences in the medications help guide which beta-blocker to choose (Table 7-2). For example, patients with asthma should receive a β_1-selective beta-blocker, while heart failure patients should receive metoprolol succinate, carvedilol, or bisoprolol.

Several studies have evaluated the use of ACE-I in patients post-ACS.[26-28] According to ACC/AHA guidelines, ACE-I therapy should be considered in all patients post-ACS. ACE-I therapy is particularly useful in patients with the highest risk of recurrent MI (smokers, diabetics, multiple vessel disease, hypertension) and in those with heart failure.[27] Contraindications include allergy (history of angioedema to ACE-I), acute renal failure, bilateral renal artery stenosis, and hyperkalemia. During initiation of ACE-I therapy, serum creatinine, potassium, and blood pressure should be monitored. In patients who experience bradykinin-mediated cough, angiotensin receptor blockers (ARBs) are a reasonable alternative. Finally, the aldosterone antagonist eplerenone showed mortality benefit when evaluated in patients post-ACS with an ejection fraction less than 40%, and either symptoms of heart failure or diabetes.[29]

Similar to primary prevention, aggressively treating modifiable risk factors for coronary artery disease is essential to secondary prevention as well. These goals include: blood pressure < 130/80 mm Hg, smoking cessation, exercise (30 minutes a day 5 to 7 days per week), weight reduction (body mass index to 18.5-24.9 kg/m^2), and treatment of diabetes (HbA$_{1C}$ < 7%). The therapeutic impact of reaching these goals has led to the development of many cardiac rehabilitation programs. All eligible patients should be offered cardiac rehabilitation, beginning in the hospital at many medical centers and continuing after hospital discharge.

CASE Application

Questions 1 to 3 refer to the following patient case.

TS is a 75-year-old woman who presents to the emergency department(ED) via EMS to a large academic medical center (with a coronary catheterization lab) complaining of sudden onset of diaphoresis and nausea. She states, "About 5 hours ago my chest started hurting and I just don't feel well." TS's weight is 65 kg.

Past medical history: Coronary artery disease and arthritis

Family history: Father died of acute myocardial infarction at 76 years of age and mother passed away at age 70 from pneumonia

Social history: Does not drink; smokes 1 pack of cigarettes per week

Medications: aspirin 81 mg orally once daily, atorvastatin 40 mg orally at bedtime, conjugated estrogens 0.625 mg, and celecoxib 200 mg orally daily

Laboratory data: SCr = 1.9 mg/dL, total cholesterol 250 mg/dL, triglycerides 150 mg/dL, high-density lipoprotein (HDL) = 40 mg/dL, LDL = 130 mg/dL, troponin I = 5.7 ng/mL

Electrocardiogram: ST-segment elevation

1. Which one of the following is the preferred approach to reperfuse this patient?
   a. Chew aspirin 81 mg, clopidogrel 75 mg, UFH for 48 hours
   b. Reteplase 10 units IV for two doses 30 minutes apart and UFH for 48 hours
   c. Chew aspirin 324 mg, administer clopidogrel 600 mg orally once, abciximab 16.25 μg IV bolus and percutaneous intervention with coronary stent placement
   d. Streptokinase 1,500,000 units IV over 30 minutes, aspirin 81 mg, clopidogrel 300 mg

2. The physicians are debating on whether TS should receive early oral beta-blockers after receiving aspirin, clopidogrel, oxygen, nitrates, and morphine. Which of the following vital signs for TS would be conducive for early beta-blocker use?
   a. Heart rate 110 beats per minutes (bpm); systolic blood pressure 85 mm Hg
   b. Heart rate 50 bpm; systolic blood pressure 120 mm Hg
   c. Heart rate 120 bpm; systolic blood pressure 120 mm Hg
   d. Heart rate 120 bpm; systolic blood pressure 120 mm Hg with rales and rhonchi on physical examination

3. Which one of the following statements would you *not* suggest to the attending physician prior to patient discharge regarding her home medication regimen?
   a. Discontinue conjugated estrogens
   b. Discontinue aspirin
   c. Discontinue celecoxib
   d. Start a beta-blocker
   e. All of the above should be suggested prior to discharge

4. A patient experiencing chest pain for a few hours decides to take a SL tablet of nitroglycerin (NTG). The first tablet provides no pain relief, so EMS is contacted. The patient continued to take the NTG every 5 minutes. The third tablet she took provided relief. How do nitrates decrease chest pain?
   a. Vasoconstriction of venous vasculature
   b. Vasodilation of arterial vasculature
   c. Vasodilation of venous vasculature
   d. Decreased cardiac output

5. What is the mechanism of clopidogrel's benefit in a STEMI patient that has already received aspirin, oxygen, nitrates, and morphine?
   a. Clopidogrel improves myocardial oxygen supply.
   b. Clopidogrel opens up the infarct-related artery.
   c. Clopidogrel reduces myocardial oxygen demand.
   d. Clopidogrel prevents myocardial reinfarction.

Questions 6 to 8 refer to the following patient case.

MS is a 68-year-old man who presents to his local physician's office after eating lunch at McDonald's. He complains of chest pain with radiation to his jaw. His physician has him chew aspirin 325 mg and calls 911. MS is transported to the local hospital where electrocardiogram shows ST-segment elevation.

Past medical history: Hypertension, coronary artery disease, chronic obstructive pulmonary disease (COPD), stage IV chronic kidney disease, cerebrovascular accident 2 months ago

Family history: Mother died of a stroke at 85 years and father passed away at 75 years in a car accident.

Social history: Smokes 1.5 pack of cigarettes per day for 50 years; no alcohol history

Medications: Hydrochlorothiazide 25 mg orally daily, metoprolol 25 mg orally bid, tiotropium 18 μg inhaled once daily, albuterol inhaler 1 puff every 6 hours PRN, fluticasone/salmeterol 250/50 μg inhaled bid

Vital signs: Blood pressure 150/90 mm Hg, heart rate (HR) 98 beats per minute (bpm), respiratory rate 22 rpm, O_2 sat 88%, weight 100 kg

Laboratory data: Unavailable

Allergies: Heparin

6. MS presents at a hospital that does not have a cardiac catheterization laboratory, therefore they have 30 minutes to verify his candidacy for fibrinolytic therapy. Which of the following is a contraindication to MS receiving a fibrinolytic?
   a. MS already received aspirin and clopidogrel.
   b. MS's blood pressure is 150/90 mm Hg.
   c. Ms had a recent cerebrovascular accident.
   d. MS has an allergy to heparin.

7. Given MS's contraindication to fibrinolytic therapy, he was life-flighted to a hospital with 24 hour cardiac catheterization capabilities. The plan is for emergent PCI on arrival. Which of the following statements about abciximab (glycoprotein IIb/IIIa inhibitor) is true?
   a. Abciximab needs to be renally adjusted.
   b. Abciximab can be reversed with platelet transfusion.
   c. Abciximab is administered as two subcutaneous boluses.
   d. Abciximab is the only glycoprotein IIb/IIIa inhibitor that is indicated as an adjunct to PCI.
   e. Abciximab is safe to give in this patient.

8. Which of the following beta-blockers would be most appropriate in MS?
   a. Propranolol ER
   b. Atenolol
   c. Carvedilol
   d. Acebutolol
   e. Esmolol

9. Which anticoagulant is treatment of choice in a STEMI patient who is also dialysis dependent?
   a. Enoxaparin
   b. Dalteparin
   c. Fondaparinux
   d. Heparin

10. What laboratory value is traditionally used to monitor the level of anticoagulation achieved with unfractionated heparin?
    a. International normalized ratio (INR)
    b. PT (Prothrombin time)
    c. Anti-Xa level
    d. Activated partial thromboplastin time (aPTT)

11. Which of the following antiplatelet/anticoagulant regimens would be recommended for treatment of a NSTEMI patient with a heparin allergy? The patient is going to receive PCI later in the day.
    a. Bivalirudin
    b. Eptifibatide and low molecular weight heparin
    c. Abciximab and unfractionated heparin
    d. Fondaparinux

12. Which of the following agents is *not* indicated in the setting of NSTEMI?
    a. Eptifibatide
    b. Unfractionated heparin (UFH)
    c. Aspirin
    d. Reteplase
    e. Clopidogrel

13. Once the acute phase of myocardial infarction has passed, which of the following therapies is most likely to slow the development of heart failure(HF)?
    a. Clopidogrel
    b. Atenolol
    c. Ramipril
    d. Amiodarone
    e. Isosorbide mononitrate

14. TL is an 82-year-old woman who is status post drug-eluting stent placement following presentations with a STEMI. She has a past medical history significant for

hypertension, dyslipidemia, and hypothyroidism. She has no known drug allergies. Which of the following is the best choice of long-term antiplatelet therapy?

a. Aspirin 325 mg orally daily
b. Aspirin 81 mg plus prasugrel 10 mg daily
c. Prasugrel 5 mg orally daily
d. Aspirin 81 mg plus clopidogrel 75 mg orally daily
e. Clopidogrel 75 mg orally daily

15. Which of the following is the most appropriate lipid lowering regimen to give a patient with recent NSTEMI with an LDL of 150 mg/dL, TC of 192 mg/dL, TG of 140 mg/dL, and HDL of 47 mg/dL? The patient has no allergies or intolerances.

a. Pravastatin 40 mg qhs
b. Simvastatin 20 mg daily
c. Atorvastatin 80 mg daily
d. Niacin 500 mg qhs
e. Rosuvastatin 10 mg qhs

16. Which of the following therapies requires monitoring of serum creatinine and potassium?

a. Carvedilol
b. Spironolactone
c. Atenolol
d. Pravastatin
e. Clopidogrel

17. Which of the following is an appropriate fibrinolytic dosing regimen for a 78-kg person with STEMI?

a. Streptase 1 million units IV over 20 minutes.
b. Reteplase or rPA 10 units IV bolus twice 30 minutes apart.
c. Tenecteplase or TNK 50 mg IV bolus once.
d. Alteplase 100 mg IV over 2 hours.

18. PK presents with chest pain, nausea, vomiting, and diaphoresis. He is diagnosed with a NSTEMI. Current blood pressure is 92/56 mm Hg and HR is 105 bpm. Which of the following should be given immediately?

a. ASA EC 325 mg orally once
b. ASA 81 mg two tablets chewed once
c. NTG IV drip at 20 μg/min
d. IV metoprolol 5 mg IV once
e. Morphine 2 to 4 mg IV every 2 hours

19. When completing a home medication evaluation for a patient admitted with unstable angina you notice he is on sildenafil. Which of the following statements is true regarding this medication?

a. He probably has not taken it in a while; so I can disregard the information.
b. Nitroglycerin IV does not interfere with sildenafil like sublingual tablets.
c. The patient does not need the medication restarted while he is in the hospital.
d. a and c
e. None of the above

20. DL is a 62-year-old woman who presents to the ED with NSTEMI. She has no significant past medical history. Pertinent data includes, blood pressure 125/79 mm Hg, heart rate 75 bpm, SCr 1.2 mg/dL, platelet count 142 k/uL, weight 94 kg. She has allergies to penicillin, sulfa, and aspirin. Which of the following regimens are okay to give DL while she waits for her PCI?

a. Aspirin 324 mg once, then 81 mg daily
b. Clopidogrel 300 mg once, then 75 mg daily
c. Aspirin 162 mg once, then 81 mg daily plus clopidogrel 600 mg once, then 75 mg daily
d. Prasugrel 60 mg once then 5 mg daily
e. None of the above.

21. Which of the following beta-blockers are available in both oral and IV formulations?

a. Atenolol
b. Esmolol
c. Metoprolol
d. Carvedilol
e. a and c

22. Secondary prevention of acute coronary syndrome should include which of the following therapies?

a. HMG-CoA reductase inhibitors
b. Aspirin
c. Calcium channel blockers
d. Fenofibrates
e. a and b

TAKEAWAY POINTS ››

- Acute coronary syndrome is associated with a high morbidity / mortality and hospitalization rates in male and female patients.
- Hyperlipidemia, hypertension, tobacco abuse, and diabetes are major risk factors for development of acute coronary syndrome.
- Reperfusion with fibrinolysis or percutaneous coronary intervention, in order to restore blood flow to the heart muscle, is the primary goal for treatment of ST-segment elevation myocardial infarction.
- Home medications that increase risk for coronary events should be discontinued at the time of acute

coronary syndrome event (ie, hormone replacement therapy and NSAIDS).

- Aspirin should be chewed at the onset of chest pain to prevent thrombosis extension and continued for life for prevention of future cardiovascular events.
- When added to aspirin, thienopyridines have been shown to decrease recurrent ischemic events. This benefit has to be balanced with the increased risk of bleeding.
- Morphine is the analgesic of choice for pain related to ACS; however, morphine should be used cautiously in patients who are hypotensive and those without planned PCI.
- Nitrates should be given at onset of chest pain as long as patient is not hypotensive or have used phosphodiesterase inhibitors (sildenafil) within the last 24 hours.
- Secondary prevention of ACS begins immediately with antiplatelet medications, HMG-CoA reductase inhibitors, beta-blockers, and angiotensin converting enzyme inhibitors.
- Secondary prevention includes aggressive treatment of modifiable risk factors (smoking, hypertension, dyslipidemia, diabetes, obesity, diet, physical inactivity)
- Glycoprotein IIb/IIIa inhibitors or direct thrombin inhibitors should be considered for management of patients with non-ST-segment elevation myocardial infarctions and unstable angina, reserving abciximab and bivalirudin for patients with planned (within 24 hours) PCI.

REFERENCES

1. Writing Group M, Lloyd-Jones D, Adams R, et al. Heart disease and stroke statistics–2009 update: a report from the American Heart Association Statistics Committee and Stroke Statistics Subcommittee. *Circulation.* January 27, 2009;119(3):e21-e181.
2. Hochman JS, Tamis JE, Thompson TD, et al. Sex, clinical presentation, and outcome in patients with acute coronary syndromes. Global use of strategies to open occluded coronary arteries in acute coronary syndromes IIb investigators. *N Engl J Med.* Jul 22 1999;341(4):226-232.
3. Greenland P, Knoll MD, Stamler J, et al. Major risk factors as antecedents of fatal and nonfatal coronary heart disease events. *JAMA.* Aug 20 2003;290(7):891-897.
4. Yusuf S, Hawken S, Ounpuu S, et al. Effect of potentially modifiable risk factors associated with myocardial infarction in 52 countries (the INTERHEART study): case-control study. *Lancet.* Sep 11-17 2004;364(9438):937-952.
5. Rokos IC, French WJ, Koenig WJ, et al. Integration of pre-hospital electrocardiograms and ST-elevation myocardial infarction receiving center (SRC) networks: impact on Door-to-Balloon times across 10 independent regions. *JACC Cardiovasc Interv.* Apr 2009;2(4):339-346.
6. Boden WE, O'Rourke RA, Teo KK, et al. Optimal medical therapy with or without PCI for stable coronary disease. *N Engl J Med.* Apr 12 2007;356(15):1503-1516.
7. Antman EM, Hand M, Armstrong PW, et al. 2007 focused update of the ACC/AHA 2004 guidelines for the management of patients with ST-elevation myocardial infarction: a report of the American College of Cardiology/American Heart Association Task Force on Practice Guidelines: developed in collaboration with the Canadian Cardiovascular Society endorsed by the American Academy of Family Physicians: 2007 writing group to review new evidence and update the ACC/AHA 2004 guidelines for the management of patients with ST-elevation myocardial infarction, writing on behalf of the 2004 Writing Committee. *Circulation.* Jan 15 2008;117(2):296-329.
8. Meine TJ, Roe MT, Chen AY, et al. Association of intravenous morphine use and outcomes in acute coronary syndromes: results from the CRUSADE quality improvement initiative. *Am Heart J.* Jun 2005;149(6):1043-1049.
9. Anderson JL, Adams CD, Antman EM, et al. ACC/AHA 2007 guidelines for the management of patients with unstable angina/non ST-elevation myocardial infarction: a report of the American College of Cardiology/American Heart Association Task Force on Practice Guidelines (Writing Committee to revise the 2002 guidelines for the management of patients with unstable angina/non ST-elevation myocardial infarction): developed in collaboration with the American College of Emergency Physicians, the Society for Cardiovascular Angiography and Interventions, and the Society of Thoracic Surgeons: endorsed by the American Association of Cardiovascular and Pulmonary Rehabilitation and the Society for Academic Emergency Medicine. *Circulation.* Aug 14 2007;116(7):e148-e304.
10. Randomized trial of intravenous streptokinase, oral aspirin, both, or neither among 17,187 cases of suspected acute myocardial infarction: ISIS-2.ISIS-2 (Second International Study of Infarct Survival) Collaborative Group. *J Am Coll Cardiol.* Dec 1988;12(suppl 6 A):3A-13A.
11. Yusuf S, Zhao F, Mehta SR, Chrolavicius S, Tognoni G, Fox KK. Effects of clopidogrel in addition to aspirin in patients with acute coronary syndromes without ST-segment elevation. *N Engl J Med.* Aug 16 2001;345(7):494-502.
12. Steinhubl SR, Berger PB, Mann JT, 3rd, et al. Early and sustained dual oral antiplatelet therapy following percutaneous coronary intervention: a randomized controlled trial. *JAMA.* Nov 20 2002;288(19):2411-2420.
13. Wiviott SD, Braunwald E, McCabe CH, et al. Prasugrel versus clopidogrel in patients with acute coronary syndromes. *N Engl J Med.* Nov 15 2007;357(20):2001-2015.
14. Chen ZM, Pan HC, Chen YP, et al. Early intravenous then oral metoprolol in 45,852 patients with acute myocardial infarction: randomised placebo-controlled trial. *Lancet.* Nov 5 2005;366(9497):1622-1632.
15. Lee MS, Menon V, Schappert J, Wilentz JR, Singh V, Hochman JS. Establishing a new target range for unfractionated heparin for acute coronary syndromes. *J Thromb Thrombolysis.* Apr 2004;17(2):121-126.
16. Cohen M, Demers C, Gurfinkel EP, et al. Low-molecular-weight heparins in non-ST-segment elevation ischemia: the ESSENCE

trial. Efficacy and Safety of Subcutaneous Enoxaparin versus intravenous unfractionated heparin, in non-Q-wave Coronary Events. *Am J Cardiol.* Sep 10 1998;82(5B):19L-24L.

17. Yusuf S, Mehta SR, Chrolavicius S, et al. Comparison of fondaparinux and enoxaparin in acute coronary syndromes. *N Engl J Med.* Apr 6 2006;354(14):1464-1476.
18. Stone GW, McLaurin BT, Cox DA, et al. Bivalirudin for patients with acute coronary syndromes. *N Engl J Med.* Nov 23 2006;355(21):2203-2216.
19. Lincoff AM, Bittl JA, Harrington RA, et al. Bivalirudin and provisional glycoprotein IIb/IIIa blockade compared with heparin and planned glycoprotein IIb/IIIa blockade during percutaneous coronary intervention: REPLACE-2 randomized trial. *JAMA.* Feb 19 2003;289(7):853-863.
20. Randomised placebo-controlled and balloon-angioplasty-controlled trial to assess safety of coronary stenting with use of platelet glycoprotein-IIb/IIIa blockade. *Lancet.* Jul 11 1998;352(9122):87-92.
21. Inhibition of platelet glycoprotein IIb/IIIa with eptifibatide in patients with acute coronary syndromes. The PURSUIT trial investigators. Platelet glycoprotein IIb/IIIa in unstable angina: receptor suppression using integrilin therapy. *N Engl J Med.* Aug 13 1998;339(7):436-443.
22. Campbell CL, Smyth S, Montalescot G, Steinhubl SR. Aspirin dose for the prevention of cardiovascular disease: a systematic review. *JAMA.* May 9, 2007;297(18):2018-2024.
23. Sabatine MS, Cannon CP, Gibson CM, et al. Addition of clopidogrel to aspirin and fibrinolytic therapy for myocardial infarction with ST-segment elevation. *N Engl J Med.* Mar 24 2005;352(12):1179-1189.
24. Ridker PM, Cannon CP, Morrow D, et al. C-reactive protein levels and outcomes after statin therapy. *N Engl J Med.* Jan 6 2005;352(1):20-28.
25. Dargie HJ. Effect of carvedilol on outcome after myocardial infarction in patients with left-ventricular dysfunction: the CAPRICORN randomised trial. *Lancet.* May 5 2001;357(9266):1385-1390.
26. Fourth International Study of Infarct Survival Collaborative Group. ISIS-4: a randomised factorial trial assessing early oral captopril, oral mononitrate, and intravenous magnesium sulphate in 58,050 patients with suspected acute myocardial infarction. ISIS-4 (Fourth International Study of Infarct Survival) collaborative group. *Lancet.* Mar 18 1995;345(8951): 669-685.
27. Yusuf S, Sleight P, Pogue J, Bosch J, Davies R, Dagenais G. Effects of an angiotensin-converting-enzyme inhibitor, ramipril, on cardiovascular events in high-risk patients. The Heart Outcomes Prevention Evaluation Study Investigators. *N Engl J Med.* Jan 20 2000;342(3):145-153.
28. Braunwald E, Domanski MJ, Fowler SE, et al. Angiotensin-converting-enzyme inhibition in stable coronary artery disease. *N Engl J Med.* Nov 11 2004;351(20):2058-2068.
29. Pitt B, Remme W, Zannad F, et al. Eplerenone, a selective aldosterone blocker, in patients with left-ventricular dysfunction after myocardial infarction. *N Engl J Med.* Apr 3 2003;348(14): 1309-1321.

CHAPTER

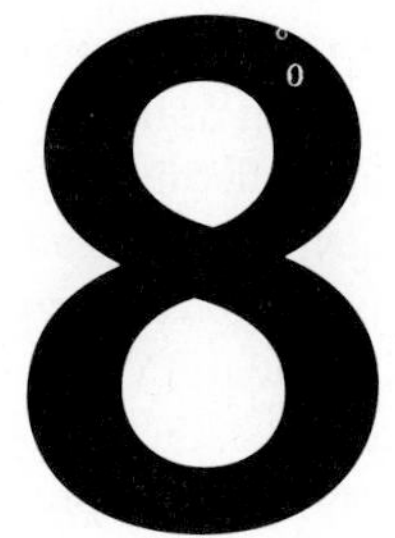

Arrhythmias

Robyn Teply-Kondrack and Kathleen Packard

FOUNDATION OVERVIEW

Normal conduction and cardiac rhythm is initiated by the sinoatrial (SA) node. The electrical current then travels through the conduction network and enters the ventricle via the atrioventricular (AV) node and bundle of His. From the bundle of His, the electrical activity moves into the branch-like system called the Purkinje system. As the current flows through the myocardium, the excitation coordinates the contraction of the atria and ventricles. After stimulation, each group of cells experiences a refractory period in which it cannot be excited. As the electrical current meets refractory tissue, the stimulation ceases allowing for the process to begin again.[1]

Conduction of electrical impulses through the myocardium is represented on an electrocardiogram (ECG) as waves of depolarization and repolarization. As depolarization occurs, the heart's myocytes become positive and contract. Recovery immediately follows as the myocytes return to their resting negative charge during repolarization. The initial p wave on an ECG represents depolarization and contraction of the atria, or top chambers of the heart. The QRS complex on an ECG represents depolarization of the ventricles and subsequent ventricular contraction. Finally, the T wave represents ventricular repolarization. One cardiac cycle consists of atrial systole, then ventricular systole, and finally a resting phase.[2]

Atrial Fibrillation

Atrial fibrillation (AF) can be described as disorganized atrial activation and subsequent uncoordinated atrial contraction.[3] AF can be symptomatic, lead to hemodynamic compromise and result in significant morbidity and mortality.[4,5] AF can be characterized as recurrent (having presented with two or more episodes), paroxysmal (if the recurrent AF terminates spontaneously), persistent (if it is sustained for at least 7 days), or permanent (in which attempts to convert to sinus rhythm have failed).[3] It is the most common cardiac arrhythmia and it is estimated that up to 5 million people living in the United States have been diagnosed with either paroxysmal or persistent AF.[5,6] The onset of AF is strongly associated with increasing age, male sex, and presence of cardiovascular disease.[4,6] AF can be asymptomatic in some patients and in others it can lead to complaints of palpitations, shortness of breath, and fatigue. The ECG reading of a patient with AF is described as an irregularly, irregular supraventricular rhythm, with no discernable p waves, and a variable ventricular rate between 120 and 180 bpm.[1]

Paroxysmal Supraventricular Tachycardia

Paroxysmal supraventricular tachycardia (PSVT) is a tachyarrhythmia with an abrupt onset and termination which results from an arrhythmia originating or involving supraventricular tissue. In an epidemiological study, an evaluation of medical records revealed that the prevalence of PSVT was 2.25 per 1000 and the incidence was 35 per 100,000 person-years.[7] Many patients with PSVT are asymptomatic while others have symptoms including palpitations, fatigue, light-headedness, chest discomfort, and dyspnea.[8]

Premature Ventricular Complexes

Premature ventricular complexes (PVCs) are a common, most often benign, arrhythmia originating from the ventricular tissue. In the general population, PVCs are present in people with and without structural heart disease.[9] For patients with a previous myocardial infarction or who have structural heart disease, PVCs have greater prognostic value and have been associated with an increased risk of sudden death.[9,10] Many patients are asymptomatic and the diagnosis of PVC is found incidentally on an ECG. If symptomatic, patients present with palpitations, dyspnea, chest pain, syncope, and presyncope.[11]

Ventricular Tachycardia and Ventricular Fibrillation

Ventricular tachycardia (VT) can be described as nonsustained VT (three or more beats in duration which terminate in less than 30 seconds) or sustained VT (VT lasting greater than 30 seconds in duration and/or involving hemodynamic compromise in less than 30 seconds).[11] Torsade de pointes is a rapid form of VT seen when the QTc interval is prolonged greater than 500 milliseconds and is diagnosed by an undulating, "party-streamer" appearance on the ECG. VT can result from the fibrous scar tissue formed after an acute myocardial infarction or from nonischemic cardiomyopathy.[12,13]

Ventricular Fibrillation (VF) is a rapid (300 bpm), irregular ventricular rhythm leading to asynchronous contraction of the left ventricle and rapid hemodynamic compromise. Sudden cardiac death can occur rapidly if medical intervention is not attempted.[11] Sudden cardiac death (SCD) accounts for approximately 300,000 deaths in the United States each year and most often are due to ventricular arrhythmias (VT or VF).[14] In hemodynamically stable patients with VT, symptoms include palpitations and in those that are unstable, patients can experience light-headedness, dizziness, loss of consciousness, and potentially sudden cardiac death.[11]

Sinus Bradycardia

Sinus bradycardia is described as having a heart rate of less than 60 bpm. It can be asymptomatic in young, active individuals or symptomatic in patients with etiologies such as sinus node dysfunction. The resulting decrease in cardiac output causes hypotension in which patients complain of dizziness, syncope, fatigue, and confusion.[1]

TREATMENT

Classification of the antiarrhythmic drugs including mechanism of action, side effects, and contraindications can be found in Table 8-1.

Atrial Fibrillation

Management of AF involves evaluating the need for immediate treatment, assessing the need for rate and/or rhythm control, and evaluating the need for anticoagulation for the prevention of thromboembolic complications. Acute treatment is warranted if the patient is hemodynamically unstable and direct current cardioversion (DCC) is indicated. If the patient has been in AF for less than 48 hours, DCC can proceed without anticoagulation if the patient has no risk factors for stroke. If the patient has risk factors for stroke, if the AF duration is unknown, or if the AF duration is greater than 48 hours, a transesophageal echocardiogram and intravenous (IV) unfractionated heparin (UFH) or low-molecular weight heparin (LMWH) are recommended prior to the DCC. If the patient is stable, the focus of their therapy should be rate control and anticoagulation leading up to DCC. With no comorbid conditions, initial therapy choices for rate control are β-blockers or nondihydropyridine calcium channel blockers (diltiazem, verapamil). In patients with decreased LV function (EF ≤ 40%), digoxin or amiodarone are recommended for rate control. If the patient has paroxysmal AF, digoxin should be avoided. Patients should be anticoagulated to an INR range of 2 to 3 prior to DCC (3-4 weeks) and 4 weeks post-DCC. Sinus rhythm can be restored through DCC or pharmacologic cardioversion. In patients without structural heart disease, flecainide, propafenone, or ibutilide can be used and in patients with structural heart disease amiodarone or dofetilide are the drugs of choice for pharmacologic cardioversion.[15]

For the chronic management of patients with AF, there is ongoing debate on whether therapy should be focused on controlling the patient's heart rate or maintaining sinus rhythm. The AFFIRM (Atrial Fibrillation Follow-up Investigation of Rhythm Management) study is the largest study to date evaluating this controversy and it concluded that there is no statistical difference in overall mortality between the two treatment strategies.[16] If patients are symptomatic despite rate control, chronic rhythm control can be attempted through antiarrhythmic agents chosen according to comorbid conditions. If no heart disease is present or if the patient has hypertension with no LV hypertrophy, flecainide, propafenone, and sotalol are the first-choice agents and amiodarone, dofetilide, and catheter ablation are second-choice therapies. If the patient has hypertension with substantial LV hypertrophy, amiodarone is the drug of choice and catheter ablation is second-line therapy. If coronary artery disease is present, dofetilide or sotalol are the first-choice agents and amiodarone or catheter ablation are second-choice therapies. If the patient has heart failure, amiodarone or dofetilide are the drugs of choice and catheter ablation is second line.[15]

To prevent thromboembolic complications in patients with AF, those who have had a prior ischemic stroke, transient ischemic attack (TIA), or systemic embolism, it is recommended that these patients receive long-term anticoagulation with an oral vitamin K antagonist such as warfarin with an INR goal of 2 to 3. For patients that have two or more risk factors for ischemic stroke (age > 75 years, history of hypertension, diabetes mellitus, moderately or severely impaired left ventricular systolic function, and/or heart failure) it is recommended that they receive long-term anticoagulation with warfarin with an INR goal of 2 to 3. If patients have only one risk factor for ischemic stroke, it is suggested that these patients receive long-term anticoagulation with warfarin with an INR goal of 2 to 3 (intermediate risk) or aspirin at a dose of 75 to 325 mg/d (low risk). In patients that are less than 75 years of age and have no risk factors for ischemic stroke, it is recommended that these patients receive long-term aspirin therapy with a dose of 75 to 325 mg/d.[17]

Paroxysmal Supraventricular Tachycardia

In the acute management of paroxysmal supraventricular tachycardia (PSVT), if the symptoms are severe (syncope, angina, severe HF), DCC is the treatment of choice. If the symptoms are mild, vasovagal maneuvers (ie, unilateral carotid sinus massage, Valsalva maneuver, ice water facial immersion, or induced retching) can be attempted first. If unsuccessful, acute treatment is based on the patient's ECG findings: (1) narrow QRS interval and regular rhythm, drugs of choice are adenosine, verapamil, or diltiazem; (2) wide QRS interval and regular rhythm, drugs of choice are adenosine or procainamide; (3) wide QRS interval and irregular rhythm, drugs of choice are procainamide or amiodarone. After a definitive diagnosis is made, the treatment of choice for those with severe and frequent symptoms is catheter ablation and if symptoms are mild and infrequent, antiarrhythmics can be used as needed.[8]

Premature Ventricular Complexes

Many patients with premature ventricular complexes (PVCs) do not require intervention. Treatment of symptomatic patients with PVCs should be limited to the use of β-blockers. Class Ic agents should be avoided due to the increased risk of mortality post-myocardial infarction[11].

TABLE 8-1 **Antiarrhythmic Drugs**

Type	Generic Name/ Route of Administration	Brand Name	Mechanism	Side Effects	Contraindications
Ia	Quinidine IV, IM, po	Quinidex, Quinaglute	Slow depolarization through Na^+ channel blockade	N/V/D, cinchonism, TdP	
	Procainamide IV, IM	Pronestyl, Procan, Procanbid		Lupus-like-syndrome, N/V/D, hypotension, TdP	LVEF < 40%
	Disopyramide po	Norpace		Anticholinergic symptoms, N, anorexia, TdP, HF	Glaucoma
Ib	Lidocaine IV, IO, ET	Xylocaine		CNS including slurred speech, blurry vision, tinnitus, seizures	Third-degree AV heart block
	Mexiletine po	Mexitil		CNS including tremors, dizziness, confusion	Third-degree AV heart block
Ic	Flecainide po	Tambocor		Blurry vision, dizziness, tremor, HF	HF, CAD, valvular disease, LVH
	Propafenone po	Rhythmol		Taste disturbances, dizziness, HF, bronchospasm, bradycardia	HF (NHYA III-IV), liver disease, valvular disease
II	Metoprolol IV, po Esmolol IV Atenolol po	Toprol XL, Lopressor Brevibloc Tenormin	Slow AV nodal conduction through β-blockade	Hypotension, bradycardia, dizziness	Severe COPD/asthma, severe bradycardia, heart block, severe hypotension, decompensated heart failure
III	Amiodarone IV, po	Cordarone	Slow repolarization through K^+ channel blockade	QT prolongation, pulmonary fibrosis, hypothyroidism, hyperthyroidism, CNS toxicity, photosensitivity, corneal deposits, macular degeneration, hepatitis, blue-gray skin, heart block	Iodine hypersensitivity, hyperthyroidism, third degree heart block
	Dofetilide po	Tikosyn		TdP, dizziness, diarrhea	Baseline QTc >440 ms, CrCl <20 mL/min
	Sotalol po	Betapace, Sorine		HF, bradycardia, TdP, bronchospasm, dizziness, fatigue, N/V/D	Baseline QTc >440 ms, CrCl <40 mL/min
	Ibutilide IV	Covert		TdP, heart block, hypotension	Baseline QTc >440 ms, concomitant antiarrhythmics, LVEF < 30%
	Dronedarone po	Multaq		QT prolongation, increased SCr	NYHA Class IV HF or recent decompensation, QTc ≥ 500
IV	Verapamil IV, po	Calan, Covera, Isoptin, Verelan	Slow AV nodal conduction through Ca^+ channel blockade	Gingival hyperplasia, constipation	LV dysfunction, SBP < 90 mm Hg, sick sinus syndrome, AV block
	Diltiazem IV, po	Cardizem, -CD, -LA, Cartia XT, Dilacor XR, Dilt-XR,-CD, Diltia XT, Diltzac, Taztia XT, Tiazac		Edema, headache	Sick sinus syndrome, AV block, SBP < 90 mm Hg, pulmonary congestion

Abbreviations: AV, atrioventricular; N, nausea; V, vomiting; D, diarrhea; TdP, torsade de pointes; LVEF, left ventricular ejection fraction; HF, heart failure; CAD, coronary artery disease; NYHA, New York Heart Association Classification; CrCl, creatinine clearance; IV, intravenous; IM, intramuscular; po, oral; IO, intraosseous; ET, endotracheal; SCr, serum creatinine; SBP, systolic blood pressure; QTc, corrected QT interval.

Ventricular Tachycardia

For stable patients with monomorphic ventricular tachycardia (VT), a loading dose of amiodarone (150 mg) over 10 minutes followed by an amiodarone drip is indicated. After the drip has been started, prepare for DCC. If the patient is unstable, perform immediate DCC. If the patient is experiencing polymorphic VT (torsades de pointes), the first step is to discontinue any potential offending agents (Class Ia or III antiarrhythmics, erythromycin, clarithromycin, levofloxacin, pentamide, fluconazole, haloperidol, phenothiazines, tricyclic antidepressants, diuretics, or other agents causing electrolyte disturbances). If the patient is unstable, DCC is indicated and magnesium 1 to 2 g IV is recommended regardless of serum electrolyte concentrations. If the patient is stable, administer 1 to 2 g IV of magnesium.

Ventricular Fibrillation or Pulseless Ventricular Tachycardia

If a patient is found to be in VF or pulseless VT, begin advanced cardiopulmonary life support. After the primary ABCDs (airway, breathing, circulation, defibrillation) have been enacted and a shockable rhythm has been detected, initiate DCC. Following cardiopulmonary resuscitation (CPR) and DCC, give epinephrine 1 mg IV every 3 to 5 minutes (no maximum) or vasopressin 40 IU as a single dose (replaces first or second epinephrine doses). Repeat DCC and resume CPR immediately. Antiarrhythmics can be considered at this time, amiodarone 300 mg IV one time and repeated at a dose of 150 mg IV or lidocaine 1 to 1.5 mg/kg IV and repeated at a dose of 0.5 to 0.75 mg/kg IV every 5 to 10 minutes (maximum dose of 3 mg/kg). If the rhythm is not shockable (pulseless electrical activity or asystole), begin CPR. Give epinephrine 1 mg IV every 3 to 5 minutes or vasopressin 40 IU as a single dose one time. If the heart rate is < 60 bpm, consider atropine 1 mg every 3 to 5 minutes and may be repeated up to 3 total doses.[11]

Sinus Bradycardia

If the patient is stable, observe and monitor the patient. If the patient is hemodynamically unstable, begin transcutaneous pacing and consider atropine 0.5 mg IV which can be repeated up to 3 mg total. If the patient does not respond, an infusion of epinephrine at 2 to 10 μg/min or dopamine at 2 to10 μg/kg/min can be initiated. The long-term therapy of choice in patients with symptomatic bradycardia is the implantation of a permanent pacemaker.

CASE Application

1. A patient with a HR of 53 bpm is complaining of shortness of breath (SOB), light-headedness, and has a BP of 80/58 mm Hg. Transcutaneous pacing is being prepared. What is the first drug and dose that should be administered?
   a. Epinephrine 1 mg IV
   b. Atropine 0.5 mg IV
   c. Atropine 1 mg IV
   d. Dopamine 1 to 5 μg/kg/min IV

2. You respond with the code team to a patient that is in cardiac arrest. High quality chest compressions are being given. The patient is intubated and an IV has been started. ECG reveals that patient is in asystole. The first IV drug and dose to administer is:
   a. Amiodarone 300 mg IV
   b. Epinephrine 1 mg IV
   c. Dopamine 1 to 5 μg/kg/min
   d. Lidocaine 1 to1.5 mg/kg IV

3. Which of the following antiarrhythmic drugs is *least likely* to cause torsade de pointes?
   a. Quinidine
   b. Sotalol
   c. Lidocaine
   d. Dofetilide

4. A 78-year-old woman with recurrent persistent atrial fibrillation is referred to your ambulatory care clinic for consideration of possible anticoagulation therapy. Her current medications include amiodarone 200 mg daily, simvastatin 10 mg HS for hyperlipidemia, lisinopril 10 mg daily for hypertension, and sitagliptin 50 mg daily for diabetes. Based on her risk of stroke, which of the following recommendations would be appropriate?
   a. Aspirin 325 mg daily
   b. Warfarin with a target INR 2.5
   c. Warfarin with a target INR 3.5
   d. None of the above

5. A nonresponsive patient in ventricular fibrillation has received multiple appropriate defibrillations, and epinephrine 1 mg IV twice. Which antiarrhythmic drug can be used next?
   a. Cordarone
   b. Isoptin
   c. Brevibloc
   d. Quinidex

6. A 79-year-old man presents to your hospital emergency room with newly discovered atrial fibrillation with rapid ventricular response and is very symptomatic despite some rate control with a diltiazem drip. It is decided by the attending physician to proceed with electrical cardioversion. The patient's wife reports that he underwent a cardiac workup the day before for routine knee replacement surgery. The ECG from that workup is retrieved and shows normal sinus rhythm. What is the next appropriate step in this patient's care?
   a. Proceed with synchronized direct cardioversion
   b. Anticoagulate with warfarin for 3 weeks, target INR 2.0 to 3.0, then cardioversion

c. Obtain transesophageal ECHO to rule out thrombus then cardioversion
d. None of the above

7. Which of the following drug(s) are considered safe and effective when utilized for pharmacologic cardioversion of atrial fibrillation in patients with structural heart disease?

i. Flecainide
ii. Sotalol
iii. Dofetilide

a. i only
b. iii only
c. i and ii
d. ii and iii
e. i, ii, and iii

8. Amiodarone requires substantial safety monitoring during long-term therapy due to its numerous side effects. Which of the following does not have to be routinely performed in a patient on long-term amiodarone therapy?

a. Hepatic function panel
b. Thyroid function tests
c. Ophthalmologic examination
d. B-type natriuretic peptide levels

9. Dofetilide is contraindicated in all of the following situations *except*:

a. A patient initiated in an outpatient setting
b. A patient with CrCl <20 mL/min
c. A baseline QT_c 510 millisecond
d. A patient with left ventricular hypertrophy

10. Which antiarrhythmic drug is safe to use for maintenance of sinus rhythm in a patient with atrial fibrillation, heart failure, and an ejection fraction of 15%.

a. Sotalol
b. Flecainide
c. Amiodarone
d. Procainamide

11. RT is a 65-year-old woman who presents with paroxysmal supraventricular tachycardia (PSVT) with a regular rhythm. RT is experiencing mild symptoms and was given unilateral carotid sinus massage with no success. What medication(s) are first-line agents to treat this patient?

i. Adenosine
ii. Verapamil
iii. Procainamide

a. i only
b. iii only
c. i and ii
d. ii and iii
e. i, ii, and iii

12. What antiarrhythmic drug has the potential for causing taste disturbances?

a. Norpace
b. Mexitil
c. Betapace
d. Rythmol

13. KG is a 55-year-old man who presents with complaints of shortness of breath and describes feeling like his heart is racing. An ECG is performed and it is determined that he is in atrial fibrillation with a ventricular rate of 160 bpm. An evaluation of his left ventricular function concluded that his ejection fraction is 35%. While the patient was still in the examination room, he reports that his symptoms had subsided and a repeat ECG was completed and it was found that the patient was in normal sinus rhythm. What medication should be prescribed to KG to control his rate?

a. Digoxin
b. Amiodarone
c. Diltiazem
d. Verapamil

14. Potential side effect(s) of dronedarone is (are):

i. Gingival hyperplasia
ii. Increased serum creatinine
iii. QT prolongation

a. i only
b. iii only
c. i and ii
d. ii and iii
e. i, ii, and iii

15. CB is a 56-year-old woman who presents with palpitations, dyspnea, and presyncope. An ECG is performed and premature ventricular complexes are found. CB has a past medical history of hypertension, hyperlipidemia, and post-myocardial infarction 2 years ago. What is the treatment of choice for CB?

a. Flecainide
b. Propafenone
c. Metoprolol succinate
d. Amiodarone

16. What is the initial step in therapy for a stable patient presenting with monomorphic VT?

a. Epinephrine
b. Amiodarone
c. Lidocaine
d. Immediate DCC

17. Which of the following medications given during the treatment of VF or pulseless VT has no dose maximum?
    i. Vasopressin
    ii. Epinephrine
    iii. Lidocaine
    a. i only
    b. ii only
    c. i and ii
    d. ii and iii
    e. i, ii, and iii
18. JL is a 58-year-old woman whose past medical history includes atrial fibrillation and seasonal allergies. What is the indicated treatment to prevent thromboembolic complications in JL?
    a. Aspirin 325 mg daily
    b. Warfarin with a target INR 2.5
    c. Warfarin with a target INR 3.5
    d. None of the above
19. Which of the following medications slows depolarization through sodium channel blockade?
    a. Brevibloc
    b. Tambocor
    c. Tiazac
    d. Covert
20. TG is an 85-year-old woman who is currently hospitalized for pneumonia. Her current medications include levofloxacin, albuterol via nebulization, zolpidem, and acetaminophen. On the second day of her hospitalization, her ECG reveals that she is experiencing polymorphic VT. If TG remains stable, what would the first step of treatment?
    a. Immediate DCC
    b. Epinephrine 1 mg IV
    c. Discontinue levofloxacin
    d. Amiodarone 150 mg over 10 minutes

TAKEAWAY POINTS ››

- Arrhythmias can occur in a variety of patient populations with atrial fibrillation being the most common type.
- Arrhythmias can be asymptomatic and incidentally discovered on an ECG.
- Potential symptoms associated with arrhythmias are palpitations, shortness of breath, fatigue, and in more serious situations loss of consciousness.
- Immediate cardioversion for atrial fibrillation is necessary if the patient is hemodynamically unstable with the need for concurrent anticoagulation based on the duration of AF and risk for stroke.
- The focus of AF therapy in stable patients is rate control and prevention of thromboembolic complications with rhythm control measures used if the patient continues to be symptomatic.
- If symptoms are severe, the acute management of a patient with PSVT is DCC.
- If symptoms are mild in a patient with PSVT, vasovagal maneuvers should initially be attempted. If unsuccessful, pharmacologic therapy should be based on the ECG findings.
- Treatment of symptomatic patients with PVCs should be limited to the use of β-blockers.
- In unstable patients with monomorphic VT, immediate DCC should be performed.
- In addition to pharmacologic measures used to treat a patient with VT, discontinue any agent that has the potential for inducing the arrhythmia.
- If a patient is found to be in VF or pulseless VT, initiate advanced cardiopulmonary life support and if the rhythm is shockable, proceed with DCC.
- If the patient has been shocked or if the rhythm is not shockable, proceed with pharmacologic measures in addition to CPR.
- If a patient presents with symptomatic bradycardia, begin transcutaneous pacing and start atropine.

REFERENCES

1. Sanoski CA, Schoen MD, Bauman JL. The arrhythmias. Section 2: Cardiovascular disorders. In: DiPiro JT, Talbert RL, Yee GC, Matzke GR, Wells BG, Posey LM, eds. *Pharmacotherapy: A Pathophysiologic Approach.* 7th ed. New York, NY : McGraw-Hill; 2008:279.
2. Dubin D. *Rapid Interpretation of EKG's.* 6th ed. Florida, FL: Cover: 2000.
3. Prystowsky Eric N, Waldo Albert L. Atrial fibrillation, atrial flutter, and atrial tachycardia. Fuster V, O'Rourke RA, Walsh RA, Poole-Wilson P, eds. King SB, Roberts R, Nash IS, Prystowsky EN, Assoc. eds.: *Hurst's the Heart,* 12e. http://www.accessmedicine. 772.com.cuhsl.creighton.edu/content.aspx?aID=3048. Accessed September 8, 2009.
4. Furberg CD, Psaty BM, Manolio TA, Gardin JM, Smith VE, Rautaharju PM. Prevalence of atrial fibrillation in elderly subjects (the Cardiovascular Health Study). *Am J Cardiol.* 1994;74(3):236-241.
5. Go AS, Hylek EM, Phillips KA, et al. Prevalence of diagnosed atrial fibrillation in adults: national implications for rhythm management and stroke prevention: the Anticoagulation and Risk Factors in Atrial Fibrillation (ATRIA) Study. *JAMA.* 2001;285(18):2370-2375.
6. Psaty BM, Manolio TA, Kuller LH, et al. Incidence of and risk factors for atrial fibrillation in older adults. *Circulation.* 1997;96(7):2455-2461.

7. Orejarena LA, Vidaillet H, Jr, DeStefano F, et al. Paroxysmal supraventricular tachycardia in the general population. *J Am Coll Cardiol.* 1998;31(1):150-157.
8. Blomstrom-Lundqvist C, Scheinman MM, Aliot EM, et al. ACC/AHA/ESC guidelines for the management of patients with supraventricular arrhythmias—executive summary: a report of the American College of Cardiology/American Heart Association Task Force on Practice Guidelines and the European Society of Cardiology Committee for Practice Guidelines (Writing Committee to Develop Guidelines for the Management of Patients With Supraventricular Arrhythmias) developed in collaboration with NASPE-Heart Rhythm Society. *J Am Coll Cardiol.* 2003;42(8):1493-1531.
9. Horan MJ, Kennedy HL. Ventricular ectopy: History, epidemiology, and clinical implications. *JAMA.* 1984;251(3):380-386.
10. Myerburg RJ, Mitrani R, Interian A, Jr, Castellanos A. Interpretation of outcomes of antiarrhythmic clinical trials: design features and population impact. *Circulation.* 1998;97(15):1514-1521.
11. Zipes DP, Camm AJ, Borggrefe M, et al. ACC/AHA/ESC 2006 guidelines for management of patients with ventricular arrhythmias and the prevention of sudden cardiac death: a report of the American College of Cardiology/American Heart Association Task Force and the European Society of Cardiology Committee for Practice Guidelines (Writing Committee to Develop Guidelines for Management of Patients With Ventricular Arrhythmias and the Prevention of Sudden Cardiac Death): developed in collaboration with the European Heart Rhythm Association and the Heart Rhythm Society. *Circulation.* 2006;114(10):e385-e484.
12. de Bakker JM, van Capelle FJ, Janse MJ, et al. Reentry as a cause of ventricular tachycardia in patients with chronic ischemic heart disease: electrophysiologic and anatomic correlation. *Circulation.* 1988;77(3):589-606.
13. Josephson ME, Horowitz LN, Farshidi A. Continuous local electrical activity. A mechanism of recurrent ventricular tachycardia. *Circulation.* 1978;57(4):659-665.
14. Myerburg RJ, Interian A, Jr, Mitrani RM, Kessler KM, Castellanos A. Frequency of sudden cardiac death and profiles of risk. *Am J Cardiol.* 1997;80(5B):10F-19F.
15. Estes NA,3rd, Halperin JL, Calkins H, et al. ACC/AHA/Physician Consortium 2008 Clinical Performance Measures for Adults with Nonvalvular Atrial Fibrillation or Atrial Flutter: a report of the American College of Cardiology/American Heart Association Task Force on Performance Measures and the Physician Consortium for Performance Improvement (Writing Committee to Develop Clinical Performance Measures for Atrial Fibrillation) Developed in Collaboration with the Heart Rhythm Society. *J Am Coll Cardiol.* 2008;51(8):865-884.
16. Wyse DG, Waldo AL, DiMarco JP, et al. A comparison of rate control and rhythm control in patients with atrial fibrillation. *N Engl J Med.* 2002;347(23):1825-1833.
17. Singer DE, Albers GW, Dalen JE, et al. Antithrombotic therapy in atrial fibrillation: American College of Chest Physicians Evidence-Based Clinical Practice Guidelines (8th ed.). *Chest.* 2008;133(suppl 6):546S-592S.

CHAPTER

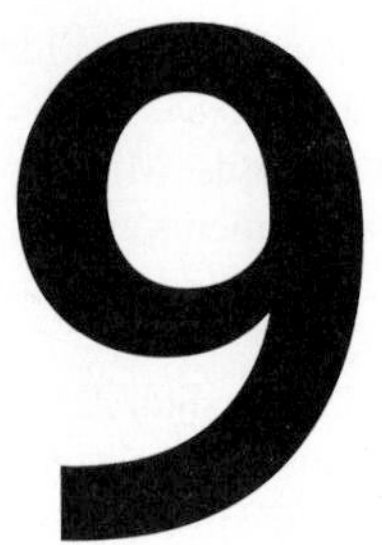

Peripheral Arterial Disease

Reamer L. Bushardt, Mary L. Hewett, and Julie M. Sease

FOUNDATION OVERVIEW

The term peripheral arterial disease (PAD) encompasses a number of disorders that affect the arterial beds of the body aside from the coronary arteries.[1] The arteries of the lower extremities are one of the main areas affected by PAD. PAD is defined by an ankle-brachial index (ABI) of ≤ 0.90.[2] PAD is a manifestation of atherosclerosis in the body and shares risk factors with coronary atherosclerosis. Data from the Framingham Heart Study determined the risk for developing PAD was increased when several common conditions were present including diabetes, hypercholesterolemia, cigarette smoking, and hypertension.[3]

PAD patients are often asymptomatic, but may present with symptoms of impaired lower extremity arterial circulation including aching, pain, discomfort, and fatigue in leg muscles upon exertion.[2] Symptoms are relieved with rest. This type of leg ischemia is also referred to as intermittent claudication, or simply claudication.[1] PAD is stratified in clinical practice guidelines based on presentation with the following classifications being used: asymptomatic, atypical leg pain, classic claudication, and critical limb ischemia.

The prevalence of PAD increases with age beginning after 40 years and affects 10% to 15% of the US population.[2] Unfortunately, most patients with PAD do not know that they have the disease even though awareness is necessary for successful treatment. The presence of PAD is indicative of advanced atherosclerotic disease. Sixty percent of patients with PAD have polyvascular disease or manifestations of atherosclerosis in the cardiovascular or cerebrovascular systems as well.[4] Therefore, PAD is considered a surrogate marker for coronary atherosclerosis.

Clinical history and physical examination findings are not reliable for detecting PAD; therefore diagnostic tests are critical.[2] Diagnostic tests for PAD commonly are ABI and exercise treadmill testing. Segmental limb pressure and volume plethysmography can be used to verify and gauge the extent of disease. Duplex ultrasonography is used to evaluate anatomy and avoid unnecessary angiography. Computed tomographic angiography, magnetic resonance angiography, and contrast angiography may also play a role in the diagnosis and evaluation of PAD. Table 9-1 lists key factors associated with the clinical presentation of PAD.

TREATMENT

The first steps in the treatment of PAD include exercise training and risk factor modification. Specific goals for the first steps of PAD treatment include:

1. Exercise rehabilitation through 30 to 45 minute sessions three times per week for 12 weeks with exercise to the point of symptom-limiting claudication[1,2]
2. Control of comorbid conditions and risk factors:
   a. Smoking cessation[5]
   b. Diabetes control with hemoglobin A_{1c} goal of less than 7%[5]
   c. Hypertension control with a blood pressure goal of less than 140/90 mm Hg[5]
      i. Beta blockers are no longer considered contraindicated in PAD though they were once thought to cause worsening of claudication symptoms[6,7]
   d. Hyperlipidemia control with a low density lipoprotein cholesterol goal of less than 100 mg/dL or less than 70 mg/dL if the patient also has other atherosclerotic disease[5]

Nonpharmacologic Treatment

Surgical treatment is reserved for patients in the following situations:[1,5]

a. Limb-threatening ischemia manifested as rest pain, ischemic ulcers, or gangrene
b. Inadequate response or predicted inadequate response to exercise rehabilitation and pharmacologic therapy
c. Significant disability due to intermittent claudication manifested by inability to perform normal work or other activities

Patients may require palliative analgesic medications while awaiting surgical intervention.

Pharmacologic Treatment

Pharmacologic interventions for PAD involve antiplatelet drug therapies and medications to combat intermittent claudication symptoms.[1] As per the American College of Cardiology/American Heart Association (ACC/AHA) guidelines, antiplatelet therapy is indicated to reduce the risk of myocardial infarction, stroke, or vascular death in individuals with atherosclerotic lower extremity PAD. Antiplatelet medications recommended in the ACC/AHA guidelines with the purpose of decreasing cardiovascular risk include aspirin and clopidogrel. Claudication therapies recommended include cilostazol and pentoxifylline. Table 9-2 lists key medication properties.

TABLE 9-1 Clinical Presentation of Peripheral Arterial Disease

General
▪ Patients with PAD are likely to be 40 y of age and older with hypertension, hypercholesterolemia, diabetes, and/or a history of smoking.
Signs and Symptoms
▪ The clinical presentation of PAD is variable and includes symptoms ranging from no symptoms at all (typically early in the disease) to pain and discomfort.
▪ The two most common characteristics of PAD are intermittent claudication and pain at rest in the lower extremities.
▪ Intermittent claudication is regarded as the primary indicator of PAD. It is described as fatigue, discomfort, cramping, pain, or numbness in the affected extremities (typically the buttocks, thigh, or calf) during exercise and resolves within a few minutes at rest.
▪ Physical examination may reveal nonspecific signs of decreased blood flow to the extremities (eg, cool skin temperature, shiny skin, thickened toenails, and/or lack of hair on the calf).
Laboratory Tests
▪ None specific to PAD
Other Diagnostic Tests
▪ An ABI is a simple, noninvasive, quantitative test that has been proven to be highly sensitive and specific in the diagnosis of PAD.

Aspirin

Aspirin, at doses of 75 to 325 mg per day, is recommended by the ACC/AHA for patients with PAD and is the drug of choice because of its lower cost and the high concomitant incidence of coronary atherosclerosis among PAD patients.[1,2] Aspirin is administered orally and should be taken with a full glass of water, 8 oz or more. Enteric coated products should be swallowed intact and not be chewed or crushed. Aspirin is a more potent inhibitor of both prostaglandin synthesis and platelet aggregation compared to other salicylic derivatives due to the acetyl group on the aspirin molecule. The acetyl group inactivates cyclooxygenase via acetylation. Aspirin inhibits platelet aggregation by irreversibly inhibiting platelet cyclooxygenase; therefore, it prevents the production of thromboxane A2, a powerful inducer of platelet aggregation and vasoconstriction.

Contraindications to the use of aspirin include:

- Hypersensitivity to nonsteroidal anti-inflammatory drugs or salicylates
- Use in children and teenagers (less than 16 years of age) with chickenpox or flu symptoms because of the risk of Reye syndrome
- Use in individuals with asthma, rhinitis, and nasal polyps

Precautions for the utilization of aspirin include alcohol use (three or more standard servings per day), pregnancy (especially third trimester; FDA Category D), gastrointestinal symptoms, peptic ulcer disease, renal failure, and severe hepatic insufficiency. The recommendation regarding the use of aspirin in women who are breast feeding is as follows: aspirin has been associated with significant effects on some nursing infants and should be given to nursing mothers with caution.

Common adverse effects with aspirin use are gastrointestinal (indigestion, nausea, and vomiting). Serious adverse effects are gastrointestinal (peptic ulcer disease, bleeding), hematologic (thrombocytopenia, anemia), otic (tinnitus), and respiratory (bronchospasm). Angioedema and Reye syndrome are also potential serious adverse effects associated with aspirin use. The range of toxicity for salicylates is as follows: acute ingestions greater than 150 mg/kg are toxic and should be referred to a health care facility; chronic ingestions of greater than 100 mg/kg/d for 2 days may cause toxicity.

Clopidogrel

Clopidogrel (Plavix), at a dose of 75 mg per day, is recommended as an alternative antiplatelet therapy for patients who do not tolerate aspirin.[1] In the Clopidogrel versus Aspirin in Patients at Risk of Ischemic Events trial, clopidogrel reduced the risk of heart attack, stroke, or vascular death among patients with PAD by 23.8% as compared with aspirin.[8] Clopidogrel carries an FDA labeled indication for the treatment of PAD.[9] Clopidogrel requires in vivo biotransformation to an active metabolite. The clopidogrel active metabolite inhibits platelet aggregation by selectively and irreversibly inhibiting the binding of adenosine diphosphate (ADP) to its platelet receptor and the subsequent activation of ADP-mediated glycoprotein GPIIb/IIIa complex. Since this action is irreversible, the remainder of the platelet life span is affected.

Contraindications for the use of clopidogrel are active bleeding (such as peptic ulcer or intracranial hemorrhage) and/or hypersensitivity to clopidogrel or any component of the product. Precautions for the use of clopidogrel are:

- Concomitant use with proton pump inhibitors (may reduce clopidogrel efficacy)
- Patients scheduled for elective surgery (clopidogrel should be discontinued 5 days prior)
- Patients with severe liver disease
- Patients at risk of increased bleeding from trauma or surgery
- Patients with severe renal impairment
- Patients undergoing transbronchial lung biopsy are at an increased risk of bleeding
- Thrombotic thrombocytopenic purpura (TTP), sometimes life-threatening, may occur with clopidogrel use

The FDA assigns clopidogrel to a Category B in pregnancy, but reports state that the use of clopidogrel in breast-feeding women may pose infant risk. Common adverse effects of clopidogrel include chest pain, hypertension, rash, constipation, diarrhea, gastritis, bleeding, and headache. Serious adverse effects include gastrointestinal hemorrhage, gastrointestinal ulcer, agranulocytosis, thrombotic thrombocytopenic purpura (rare), and abnormal liver function tests (rare).

TABLE 9-2 Pharmacotherapy Options for Patients with Peripheral Arterial Disease

Medication	Typical Dose	Side Effects	Contraindications	Mechanism of Action	Miscellaneous
Aspirin (Bayer, Bufferin, numerous others)	75 mg to 325 mg daily	Common: Indigestion/gastritis Serious: Stomach ulcer, bleeding, tinnitus, bronchospasm, Reye syndrome, angioedema	Hypersensitivity to NSAIDs; children <16 y with chickenpox or flu-like symptoms; syndrome of asthma, rhinitis, nasal polyps; active bleeding, thrombocytopenia	Irreversibly inhibits prostaglandin cyclooxygenase in platelets, preventing formation of thromboxane A2, which inhibits platelet aggregation	Take with food or large volume of water to minimize GI upset; do not crush sustained release or enteric coated
Clopidogrel (Plavix)	75 mg daily	Common: Headache, hypertension, purpura, rash, gastrointestinal Serious: Gastrointestinal bleeding, thrombotic thrombocytopenia purpura Chest pain	Hypersensitivity to clopidogrel or any component of the formulation, active bleeding, intracranial hemorrhage	Selectively and irreversibly inhibits ADP binding to its platelet receptor and subsequently activates the ADP-mediated glycoprotein GPIIb/IIIa complex	CYP 450 substrate: CYP 2C19 (minor), 3A4 (minor); 1A2 (minor); CYP 450 inhibitor: 2C9 (weak)
Ticlopidine (Ticlid)	250 mg bid	Common: Rash, dizziness, diarrhea, nausea Serious: Bleeding, bone marrow suppression	Active bleeding, severe hepatic impairment, neutropenia, thrombocytopenia	Irreversibly alters platelet membrane function resulting in platelet aggregation inhibition	Take with food; a complete blood count should be obtained every 2 wk starting the second week through the third month of treatment; more frequent monitoring is recommended for patients whose neutrophils have been decreasing or are less than 30% of baseline; ticlopidine is a substrate of CYP 3A4 (major) and inhibits 1A2 (weak), 2C9 (weak), 2C19 (strong), 2D6 (moderate), 2E1 (weak), 3A4 (weak)
Cilostazol (Pletal)	100 mg bid	Common: Palpitations, tachycardia, edema, headache, diarrhea, dizziness, infection, cough, rhinitis Serious: Heart failure, leukopenia, aplastic anemia, thrombocytopenia, fever from infection	All degrees of HF, active bleeding	Inhibit phosphodiesterase and suppresses cAMP degradation resulting in increased cAMP in platelets and blood vessels Reversible inhibitor of platelet aggregation Produces vasodilation, but not in renal arteries	High-fat food increases absorption; take 30 min before or 2 h after a meal; substrate of CYP 1A2 (minor), 2C19 (minor), 2D6 (minor), 3A4 (major)
Pentoxifylline (Trental)	400 mg tid	Common: Nausea, vomiting, dizziness, headache Serious: Angioedema, anemia, blurred vision, bone marrow suppression, and purpura	Recent cerebral or retinal hemorrhage, active bleeding	Reduces blood viscosity and improves erythrocyte flexibility, inhibits platelet aggregation, decreases fibrinogen concentrations	Take with food; inhibits CYP 450 1A2 (weak); tablets should be swallowed whole

Ticlopidine

Ticlopidine (Ticlid) is a thienopyridine antiplatelet drug structurally similar to clopidogrel.[10] Hematologic effects of ticlopidine limit its utilization in patients with PAD. Ticlopidine has a black box warning—may cause life-threatening hematologic reactions, including neutropenia, agranulocytosis, thrombotic thrombocytopenic purpura, and aplastic anemia.

Cilostazol

Cilostazol (Pletal) is indicated for patients with intermittent claudication based on significant improvement in maximal walking distances found with this agent.[1] The dosing of cilostazol for intermittent claudication is 100 mg orally bid. Cilostazol dosing adjustments are required for concomitant use with diltiazem, ketoconazole, erythromycin, omeprazole, and other cytochrome P450 3A4 or 2C19 inhibitors (decrease dose to 50 mg orally bid).[11] Cilostazol and its metabolites are inhibitors of phosphodiesterase III. As a result, cyclic adenosine monophosphate is increased leading to reversible inhibition of platelet aggregation, vasodilation, and inhibition of vascular smooth muscle cell proliferation.

Contraindications to the use of cilostazol include heart failure of any severity (black box warning), hemostatic disorders or active pathological bleeding (bleeding peptic ulcer or intracranial bleeding), and hypersensitivity to cilostazol or any of its components. Precautions associated with the use of cilostazol include concomitant therapy with platelet-aggregation inhibitors, or in patients with thrombocytopenia, renal impairment (creatinine clearance less than 25 mL/min) or hepatic impairment. Hematologic events, such as thrombocytopenia or leukopenia progressing to agranulocytosis, have been reported with the use of this drug. The FDA assigns cilostazol to the Category C in pregnancy.

Common side effects associated with cilostazol include: headache, abnormal stools, diarrhea, rhinitis, and infection. Other side effects include: edema, nausea, and abdominal pain. Rare life-threatening reactions include agranulocytosis, anemia, heart failure, and hemorrhage.

Pentoxifylline

Pentoxifylline (Trental) is a second line alternative therapy after cilostazol to improve walking distance in patients with PAD.[1] Pentoxifylline does not increase the ABI.[12] Pentoxifylline reduces blood viscosity via increased leukocyte and erythrocyte deformability and decreased neutrophil activation.[13] It improves tissue oxygenation presumably through enhanced blood flow. Pentoxifylline is dosed 400 mg tid with meals (may reduce dose to 400 mg bid if gastrointestinal or central nervous system side effects occur). Tablets should be swallowed whole; not chewed, broken, or crushed. Maximal therapeutic benefit may take 2 to 4 weeks to develop.

Contraindications for pentoxifylline include hypersensitivity to pentoxifylline, xanthenes (eg, caffeine, theophylline), and recent cerebral and/or retinal hemorrhage. Side effects associated with pentoxifylline include gastrointestinal problems (nausea and vomiting). Rare life-threatening reactions include angioedema, anemia, blurred vision, bone marrow suppression, and purpura.

CASE Application

1. Risk factors for the development and progression of PAD include which of the following?
   a. Tobacco abuse
   b. Hypertension
   c. Diabetes mellitus
   d. All of the above

2. A 40-year-old smoker with hypertension, diabetes, hypercholesterolemia, and PAD complains of pain in his calves when he walks two to three blocks. What therapy might offer him the greatest benefit in symptom reduction and in overall mortality?
   a. Limb revascularization procedure
   b. Cilostazol
   c. Smoking cessation
   d. Pravastatin

3. The gold standard diagnostic test for PAD is arteriography. Another test which is useful in the diagnosis is which of the following?
   a. Systolic blood pressure
   b. Diastolic blood pressure
   c. Cardiac angiography
   d. Resting ankle-brachial index (ABI)

4. Aspirin carries non-FDA labeled indications (Class IIb, Category B) for PAD, thrombosis, and prophylaxis. Which of the following are contraindications to the use of aspirin in this patient population?
   a. Asthma
   b. Hypersensitivity to NSAIDS
   c. Nasal polyps
   d. All of the above

5. Which of the following is recommended as an effective alternative antiplatelet therapy for patients who do not tolerate aspirin?
   a. Dipyridamole
   b. Clopidogrel, 150 mg a day
   c. Clopidogrel, 75 mg a day
   d. Pentoxifylline

6. Which of the following pharmacologic interventions is least appropriate for achieving a reduction in serious vascular events for a patient with established peripheral artery disease?
   a. Aspirin
   b. Clopidogrel
   c. Aspirin plus extended release dipyridamole
   d. Pentoxifylline

7. A 58-year-old man with peripheral artery disease, hypertension, hyperlipidemia, and New York Heart Association class III heart failure is noted to have significant functional impairment due to intermittent claudication. Which of the following pharmacologic interventions should be avoided due to safety issues which led to a black box warning from the FDA?
   a. Aspirin
   b. Clopidogrel
   c. Simvastatin
   d. Cilostazol

8. Which of the following antiplatelet agents should be monitored with periodic complete blood count testing related to potential hematologic complications that include agranulocytosis and aplastic anemia?
   a. Aspirin
   b. Simvastatin
   c. Ticlopidine
   d. Dipyridamole plus aspirin

9. Which of the following patients should not be given cilostazol as treatment for peripheral artery disease?

a. A 49-year-old woman with hypertension
b. A 60-year-old man with a history of benign prostatic hypertrophy
c. A 48-year-old man with congestive heart failure
d. A 52-year-old woman with hypothyroidism

10. Which medication(s) should be avoided in a 53-year-old patient with peripheral artery disease, asthma, and allergic rhinitis (with nasal polyps) who is currently taking albuterol as needed and flunisolide for his asthma and loratadine for allergic rhinitis?

a. Aspirin
b. Trental
c. Plavix
d. a and c

11. Which of the following mechanisms of action is associated with pentoxifylline?

a. Reduces blood viscosity
b. Improves erythrocyte flexibility
c. Inhibits platelet aggregation
d. All of the above

12. A patient is prescribed cilostazol for diagnosis of peripheral artery disease. What would be appropriate monitoring or evaluation points for patients receiving a prescription for cilostazol?

a. Evaluation of medications that inhibit the CYP 450 3A4
b. Evaluation of medications that inhibit the CYP 450 2C19
c. Evaluation of comorbidities (eg, heart failure)
d. All of the above

13. Select the treatment goal(s) for PAD in patient with intermittent claudication.

a. Increase maximal walking distance
b. Increase duration of walking
c. Increase amount of pain-free walking
d. All of the above

14. A 48-year-old cancer patient presents to the clinic and states to feel terrible (weakness, fatigue) after his last chemotherapy session. His medication list includes the antiplatelet ticlopidine (Ticlid) for peripheral arterial disease. Select the condition that may be caused by ticlopidine that may contribute to the patient's symptoms.

a. Anemia
b. Reye syndrome
c. Headache
d. Rash

15. Select the risk factors (comorbidities) that should be controlled in a patient with PAD.

a. Hypertension
b. Hyperlipdemia
c. Diabetes
d. All of the above

16. Select the primary pharmacologic management for PAD.

a. Anticoagulant
b. Antiplatelet
c. Antihypertensive
d. Antisympathomimetic

17. A 28-year-old mother with no significant medical history states her doctor wants her to start taking low-dose aspirin and thinks it is a good idea to keep a bottle in the house in case anyone in her family gets a headache or has some mild pain. Which of the following would be *inappropriate* counseling points?

a. Low-dose aspirin is perfectly fine to have around the house. Many people find it works well for mild pains and headache and it is safe for anyone over the age of 12.
b. Since you will be taking aspirin daily, you should know that some of the common side effects include indigestion and nausea and some of the serious side effects include bleeding, ringing in the ears, and peptic ulcer disease.
c. Should you decide to become pregnant while you are taking aspirin, let your doctor know right away because aspirin may not be safe while pregnant, especially during the third trimester.
d. Do not give aspirin to anyone in your home who has asthma or breathing problems because aspirin can cause bronchospasm.

18. Select the dose(s) of aspirin utilized in the management of PAD.

a. 81 mg
b. 162 mg
c. 325 mg
d. All of the above

19. Clopidogrel works by which of the following mechanisms ?

a. Selectively and irreversibly inhibits ADP-induced platelet aggregation.
b. Reversibly inhibits platelet aggregation.
c. Reduces blood viscosity by inhibiting phosphodiesterase.
d. Suppresses cyclic adenosine monophosphate (cAMP) degradation, which produces vasodilation.

20. Which of the following medications is contraindicated in patients with hypersensitivity to xanthenes?

a. Aspirin
b. Plavix
c. Trental
d. Pletal

TAKEAWAY POINTS ››

- Peripheral arterial disease (PAD) involves atherosclerotic occlusion of the lower extremities and is one of many potential manifestations of systemic atherosclerosis.
- A higher prevalence of PAD is associated with increased age, tobacco abuse, diabetes mellitus, hypertension, and hyperlipidemia.
- Patients with PAD have approximately the same relative risk of death from cardiovascular disease as patients with a history of coronary or cerebrovascular disease, and PAD should be considered a surrogate marker of subclinical coronary artery disease.
- PAD is caused by atherosclerotic plaque formation in the arteries that results in decreased blood flow to the legs.
- Specific goals should include:
  - Increasing maximal walking distance, duration of walking, and amount of pain-free walking
  - Improving control of comorbid conditions that contribute to morbidity (eg, hypertension, hyperlipidemia, and diabetes). Improving control of comorbid conditions can result in improvement in overall quality of life and reduction in cardiovascular complications and death.
- Risk factor reduction and controlling underlying causes such as diabetes mellitus, hypertension, and hyperlipidemia should be included in the treatment strategy as well as smoking cessation and exercise rehabilitation.
- Primary pharmacologic interventions for PAD involve antiplatelet drug therapies.
- Antiplatelet therapy is indicated to reduce the risk of myocardial infarction, stroke, or vascular death in individuals with atherosclerotic lower extremity PAD.
- Aspirin, clopidogrel, cilostazol, and pentoxifylline are commonly prescribed antiplatelet agents for the treatment of PAD.

REFERENCES

1. Hirsch AT, Haskal ZJ, Hertzer NR, et al. ACC/AHA guidelines for the management of patients with peripheral arterial disease (lower extremity, renal, mesenteric, and abdominal aortic): executive summary: a collaborative report from the American Association for Vascular Surgery/Society for Vascular Surgery, Society for Vascular Medicine and Biology, Society of Interventional Radiology, and the ACC/AHA Task Force on Practice Guidelines. *J Am Coll.* 2006;46:1239-1312. Available at: http://www.acc.org/clinical/guidelines/pad/summary.pdf. Accessed January 5, 2010.
2. Aslam F, Haque A, Foody J, et al. Peripheral arterial disease: current perspectives and new trends in management. *South Med J.* 2009;102:1141-1149.
3. Murabito JM, D'Agostino RB, Silbershatz H, Wilson WF. Intermittent claudication: a risk profile from the Framingham Heart Study. *Circulation.* 1997;96:44-49.
4. Aronow H, Hiatt WR. The burden of peripheral artery disease and the role of anti-platelet therapy. *Postgrad Med.* 2009;121:123-135.
5. Norgren L, Hiatt WR, Dormandy JA, et al. TASC II Working Group. Inter-society consensus for the management of peripheral arterial disease (TASC II). *J Vasc Surg.* 2007;45(suppl S): S5-S67.
6. Radack K, Deck C. Beta-adrenergic blocker therapy does not worsen intermittent claudication in subjects with peripheral arterial disease: a meta-analysis of randomized controlled trials. *AMA Arch.* 1991;151:1769-1776.
7. Thandani U, Whitsett TL. Beta-adrenergic blockers and intermittent claudication: time for reappraisal. *AMA Arch.* 1991;151:1705-1707.
8. CAPRIE Steering Committee. A randomised, blinded, trial of clopidogrel versus aspirin in patients at risk of ischaemic events (CAPRIE). *Lancet.* 1996;348:1329-1339.
9. Plavix [package insert]. Bridgewater, NJ: Bristol-Myers Squibb/Sanofi Pharmaceuticals Partnership; 2009.
10. Ticlid [package insert]. Nutley, NJ: Roche Pharmaceuticals; 2001.
11. Pletal [package insert]. Rockville, MD: Otsuka America Pharma; 2000.
12. Girolami B, Bernardi E, Prins MH, et al. Treatment of intermittent claudication with physical training, smoking cessation, pentoxifylline, or nafornyl: a meta-analysis. *AMA Arch.* 1999;159:337-345.
13. Trental [package insert]. Bridgewater, NJ: Sanofi-Aventis; 2007.

PART

2 Immunologic, Hematologic, and Oncologic Disorders

CHAPTER

10 Anemia

S. Scott Sutton and LeAnn B. Norris

FOUNDATION OVERVIEW

Anemia is a decline in the concentration of hemoglobin resulting in a reduction of the oxygen-carrying capacity of the blood.[1] The prevalence of anemia varies based upon age, gender, race/ethnicity, and comorbid conditions (Table 10-1).[2-7] Patients with anemia may be asymptomatic initially, but the lack of oxygen eventually results in fatigue, lethargy, shortness of breath, headache, edema, and tachycardia. Complications of anemia arise when the hemoglobin concentration is below 7 to 7.9 g/dL (70-79 g/L or 4.34-4.9 mmol/L). Anemia complications include cardiovascular sequelae and hypoxia. Common causes of anemia include blood loss, decreased production of red blood cells (RBCs), increased destruction of RBCs, or a combination of these factors. Comorbid conditions increase the risk of anemia, particularly in cancer patients receiving chemotherapy and chronic kidney disease (CKD) patients. Factors leading to hypo-productive anemia are: nutritional (such as iron, vitamin B_{12}, and folic acid), cancer, and CKD. Patients with immune-related diseases (such as rheumatoid arthritis and systemic lupus erythematosus) can develop anemia as a complication of their disease. Anemia related to these chronic inflammatory conditions is termed anemia of chronic disease. Management of the anemia is determined by the underlying cause. Drug therapy is a key component to decreased production and will be the focus of this chapter.

Erythropoiesis is a process that starts with a pluripotent stem cell in the bone marrow that eventually differentiates into an erythroid colony-forming unit (CFU-E). The development of these cells depends on stimulation from appropriate growth factors, primarily erythropoietin.[8-10] Other cytokines involved include granulocyte-monocyte colony-stimulating factor (GM-CSF) and interleukin-3. Eventually, the CFU-Es differentiate into reticulocytes and cross from the bone marrow in the peripheral blood. Finally, these reticulocytes mature into erythrocytes after 1 to 2 days in the bloodstream. Throughout this process, the cells gradually accumulate more hemoglobin and lose their nuclei.[8-12] The following are areas that disrupt this process:

- Deficiencies in nutrients such as folic acid and vitamin B_{12} hinder the process of erythrocyte maturation. Folic acid and vitamin B_{12} are required for the formation of DNA. Poor diet can be a contributor to the vitamin deficiencies. Patients with pernicious anemia are not able to absorb vitamin B_{12} from the gastrointestinal tract.
- Iron is another vital nutrient in the development of erythrocytes. Iron deficiency decreases hemoglobin synthesis and ultimately red blood cells.
- Patients with cancer may suffer from anemia because of chemotherapy or tumor effects. Chemotherapy may cause destruction of proliferating stem cells, thereby decreasing erythrocyte production and decreasing the life span of RBCs. Tumors cause anemia via hemorrhage, replacing normal bone marrow with malignant cells, and releasing cytokines that decrease erythropoietin production.
- CKD patients develop anemia because erythropoietin is produced in the kidneys.
- Anemia of chronic disease patients has a diminished production of erythropoietin and also has a blunted response to the limited supply that is made. Anemia of chronic disease also affects iron homeostasis via iron sequestration, thereby decreasing the amount available to the rest of the body.

Anemia is classified on the basis of the RBC morphology, etiology, or pathophysiology (Table 10-2). Characteristic changes in the size of RBCs seen in erythrocyte indices can be the first step in the morphologic classification and understanding of anemia. Anemias are classified by RBC size as macrocytic, normocytic, or microcytic. Vitamin B_{12} and folic acid deficiency are macrocytic anemias, iron deficiency is a microcytic anemia, and normocytic anemia is associated with recent blood loss or chronic disease. Multiple anemias and etiologies can occur concurrently. Laboratory evaluation of anemia includes a complete blood count, reticulocyte count, and examination of stool for occult blood. Table 10-3 lists and defines normal hematologic values, although these values may differ in certain populations, such as individuals living at high altitudes or endurance athletes. Figure 10-1 is an algorithm for the diagnosis of anemias based upon laboratory data. The algorithm is less useful in the presence of more than one cause of anemia.

TREATMENT

The goal of anemia therapy is to increase the hemoglobin level, which will improve the red cell oxygen-carrying capacity, alleviate symptoms, and prevent anemia complications. The underlying cause of anemia must be determined to guide therapy.

TABLE 10-1 Prevalence of Anemia[2-7]

Children (1-16 y)	6%-9%
Adults (> 65 y)	11%
Adults (> 85 y)	20%
Women (reproductive years 17-49 y)	12%
Men (17-49 y)	2%
Non-Hispanic whites	9%
Non-Hispanic blacks	28%

Nonpharmacologic Therapy

Nonpharmacologic therapy plays a limited role in the management of anemia. Diets lacking key nutrients are rarely the sole cause of anemia in the United States. Therefore, ingesting a diet rich in iron, folic acid, or vitamin B_{12} should not be the only modality of treatment. Symptomatic anemia patients with a hemoglobin concentration less than 7 g/dL (70 g/L or 4.34 mmol/L) are candidates for transfusion of red blood cells.[12,13] Because of the risk of infection, immunosuppression, and microcirculatory complications, the threshold for transfusion has been debated. Generally, only patients requiring immediate correction receive blood transfusions.

Pharmacologic Therapy

Iron Deficiency Anemia

Treatment of iron-deficiency anemia is oral iron therapy with 200 mg of elemental iron daily. There are different iron products and salt forms available (Table 10-4), with different amounts of elemental iron in each product. Iron supplementation resolves anemia by replacing iron stores in the body that are necessary for red blood cell production and maturation.[12-15] A response (presence of reticulocytosis) should be seen in 7 to 10 days and the hemoglobin values should rise by approximately 1 g/dL

TABLE 10-2 Classification System for Anemias

- I. Morphology
  - Macrocytic anemias
    - Megaloblastic anemias
      - Vitamin B_{12} deficiency
      - Folic acid deficiency anemia
  - Microcytic hypochromic anemias
    - Iron-deficiency anemia
    - Genetic anomaly
      - Sickle cell anemia
      - Thalassemia
      - Other hemoglobinopathies (abnormal hemoglobins)
  - Normocytic anemias
    - Recent blood loss
    - Hemolysis
    - Bone marrow failure
    - Anemia of chronic disease
  - Renal failure
  - Endocrine disorders
  - Myelodysplastic anemias
- II. Etiology
  - Deficiency
    - Iron
    - Vitamin B_{12}
    - Folic acid
    - Pyridoxine
  - Central, caused by impaired bone marrow function
    - Anemia of chronic disease
    - Anemia of the elderly
    - Malignant bone marrow disorders
  - Peripheral
    - Bleeding (hemorrhage)
    - Hemolysis (hemolytic anemias)
- III. Pathophysiology
  - Excessive blood loss
    - Recent hemorrhage
    - Trauma
    - Peptic ulcer
    - Gastritis
    - Hemorrhoids
  - Chronic hemorrhage
    - Vaginal bleeding
    - Peptic ulcer
    - Intestinal parasites
    - Aspirin and other nonsteroidal anti-inflammatory agents
  - Excessive RBC destruction
    - Extracorpuscular (outside the cell) factors
      - RBC antibodies
      - Drugs
      - Physical trauma to RBC (artificial valves)
      - Excessive sequestration in the spleen
    - Intracorpuscular factors
      - Heredity
      - Disorders of hemoglobin synthesis
  - Inadequate production of mature RBCs
    - Deficiency of nutrients (B_{12}, folic acid, iron, protein)
    - Deficiency of erythroblasts
      - Aplastic anemia
      - Isolated (often transient) erythroblastopenia
      - Folic acid antagonists
      - Antibodies
  - Conditions with infiltration of bone marrow
    - Lymphoma
    - Leukemia
    - Myelofibrosis
    - Carcinoma
  - Endocrine abnormalities
    - Hypothyroidism
    - Adrenal insufficiency
    - Pituitary insufficiency
  - Chronic renal disease
  - Chronic inflammatory disease
    - Granulomatous diseases
    - Collagen vascular diseases
  - Hepatic disease

RBC, red blood cell.

Reproduced with permission from Ineck B, Mason BJ, Lyons W. Anemias. In: DiPiro JT, Talbert RL, Yee GC, Matzke GR, Wells BG, Posey LM, eds. *Pharmacotherapy: A Pathophysiologic Approach*. 7th ed. New York, NY: McGraw-Hill; 2008:1639-1663.

TABLE 10-3 **Laboratory Tests in the Evaluation of Anemia**

Test Name	Normal Range	Description/Significance
Complete Blood Count		
Hemoglobin (Hgb)	Males: 14-17.5 g/dL (140-175 g/L or 8.69-10.9 mmol/L) Females: 12.3-15.3 g/dL (123-153 g/L or 7.63-9.5 mmol/L)	Amount of hemoglobin in the blood; signifies oxygen-carrying capacity of the blood and determines if a patient is anemic.
Hematocrit (Hct)	Males: 42%-50% (0.42-0.50) Females: 36%-45% (0.36-0.45)	The percent of blood that the erythrocytes encompass; also indicates anemia; the hemoglobin is measured, and the hematocrit is calculated.
Red blood cell count (RBC)	Males: 4.5-5.9 × 10^6 cells/mL (4.5-5.9 × 10^{12} cells/L) Females: 4.1-5.1 × 10^6 cells/mL (4.1-5.1 × 10^{12} cells/L)	The number of erythrocytes in a volume of blood; also indicates anemia, but seldom used.
Red Blood Cell Indices		
Mean cell volume (MCV)	80-96 fL/cell	A widely used laboratory value to measure RBC "size"; higher values indicate macrocytosis and lower values indicate microcytosis.
Mean cell hemoglobin (MCH)	27-33 pg/cell	Amount of Hgb per RBC; may be decreased in iron deficiency anemia.
Mean cell hemoglobin concentration (MCHC)	33.4-35.5 g/dL (334-355 g/L)	Hemoglobin divided by the hematocrit; also low in iron-deficiency anemia.
Iron Studies		
Serum iron Males Females	 45-160 μg/dL (8.1-31.3 μmol/L) 30-160 μg/dL (5.4-31.3 μmol/L)	Measures amount of iron bound to transferrin; low in iron-deficiency anemia.
Serum ferritin	Less than 10-20 μg/L (22-44 pmol/L)	Ferritin is the protein-iron complex found in macrophages used for iron storage; low in iron-deficiency anemia.
Total iron-binding capacity (TIBC)	220-420 μg/dL (39.4-75.2 μmol/L)	Measures the capacity of transferrin to bind iron; high in iron-deficiency anemia.
Transferrin saturation (TSAT)	30%-50% (0.30-0.50)	Transferrin saturation = (serum iron/TIBC) × 100; a saturation of less than 15% is common in iron-deficiency anemia.
Other Tests		
Red blood cell distribution width (RDW)	11.5%-14.5% (0.115-0.145)	A higher value means the presence of many different sizes of RBCs; the MCV is therefore less reliable.
Reticulocyte count Males Females	 0.5%-15% of RBCs (0.005-0.025) 0.5%-2.5% of RBCs (0.005-0.025)	Should be elevated in patients who are responding to treatment.
Folic acid (plasma)	3.1-12.4 ng/mL or mcg/L (7-28 nmol/L)	Used to determine folic acid deficiency.
Folic acid (RBC)	125-600 ng/mL (283-1360 nmol/L)	Used to determine folic acid deficiency.
Vitamin B_{12}	180-600 pg/mL (133-738 pmol/L)	Used to determine vitamin B_{12} deficiency.
Erythropoietin level	2-25 mIU/mL (2-25 IU/L)	Patients may benefit from erythropoietin therapy if they are anemic and erythropoietin levels are normal or mildly elevated.

Reproduced with permission from Li EC, Hoffman JM. Anemia. In: Chisholm-Burns MA, Wells BG, Schwinghammer TL, Malone PM, Kolesar JM, Rotschafer JC, DiPiro JT, eds. *Pharmacotherapy Principles & Practice*. New York, NY: McGraw-Hill; 2008:975-986.

(10 g/L or 0.62 mmol/L) per week. Patients should be reassessed if hemoglobin values do not increase by 2 g/dL (20 g/L or 1.24 mmol/L) in 3 weeks. Hemoglobin levels should normalize in 6 to 8 weeks, but iron therapy may continue for 6 to 12 months in order to fully replenish iron stores. Iron dosing should be divided into two to three daily doses, depending upon the oral formulation utilized. Maximal absorption is achieved on an empty stomach (1 hour before or 2 hours after a meal); however, patients who cannot tolerate iron on an empty stomach may take it with food. Side effects for oral iron include: dark/discolored stools, abdominal pain, nausea, constipation, and heartburn. Iron may bind to medications causing a decreased absorption of the interacting drug; examples include fluoroquinolones, tetracyclines, and phenytoin. This

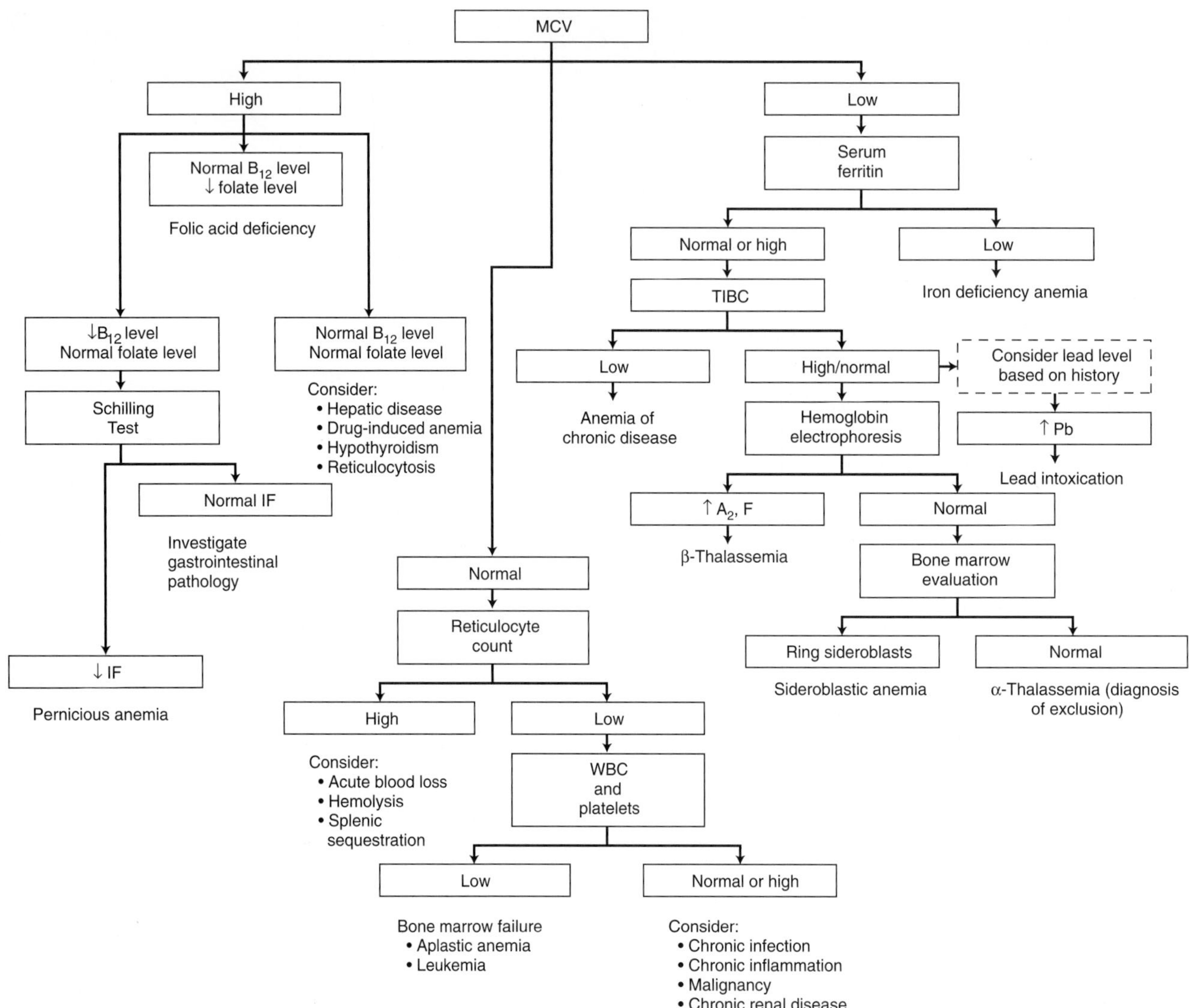

FIGURE 10-1 Algorithm for diagnosis of anemia.

Reproduced with permission from: Ineck B, Mason BJ, Lyons W. Anemias. In: DiPiro JT, Talbert RL, Yee GC, Matzke GR, Wells BG, Posey LM, eds. *Pharmacotherapy: A Pathophysiologic Approach*. 7th ed. New York, NY: McGraw-Hill; 2008:1639-1663.

interaction is avoided if the administration of iron and the interacting drug are separated by 2 to 4 hours.

Parenteral iron therapy is for patients unable to tolerate the oral formulation, noncompliance, or nonresponders (malabsorption).[16,17] Table 10-4 lists the three parenteral formulations of iron. Iron dextran is FDA approved for the treatment of iron deficiency in patients unable to tolerate the oral formulation. Sodium ferric gluconate and iron sucrose are indicated to treat anemia associated with CKD in patient receiving erythropoietin products. Side effects associated with parenteral products are: anaphylaxis (dextran only), arthralgias, arrhythmias, hypotension, flushing, and pruritus.[17-18] A test dose of iron dextran should be given on the first day of therapy and patients should be observed for 1 hour for the hypersensitivity reaction. The remaining iron dextran dose (dose minus test dose) should be given if patients tolerate the test dose.

Vitamin B_{12} and Folic Acid Anemia

Vitamin B_{12} and folic acid anemias are treated by replacing the missing nutrient. Both vitamin B_{12} and folic acid are essential for erythrocyte production and maturation. Replacing these factors allows for normal DNA synthesis and erythropoiesis.

Vitamin B_{12} Anemia The goals of treatment for vitamin B_{12} deficiency include reversal of hematologic manifestations, replacement of body stores, and prevention or resolution of neurologic manifestations. Early treatment is paramount because neurologic damage may be irreversible if the deficiency is not detected and corrected within months. Permanent disabilities range from mild paresthesias and numbness to memory loss and psychosis.

Vitamin B_{12} (cyanacobalamin) administered orally or parenterally is effective in treating vitamin B_{12} anemia.[19-20] Parenteral use is more common because absorption is

TABLE 10-4 **Iron Products (Oral and Intravenous) and Elemental Iron Content**

Salt Form	Brand Name	Elemental Iron Content per Dose Form
Oral		
Ferrous sulfate	Feosol	65 mg/325 mg tablet 60 mg/300 mg tablet
Ferrous sulfate, anhydrous	N/A	65 mg/200 mg tablet
Ferrous gluconate	Fergon	39 mg/325 mg tablet 37 mg/300 mg tablet
Ferrous fumarate	Feostat	33 mg/100 mg capsule
Polysaccharide-iron complex	Niferex	150 mg/capsule 50 mg/tablet
Intravenous		
Iron dextran[a]	InFED	50 mg/mL
Iron sucrose	Venofer	20 mg/mL
Sodium ferric gluconate	Ferrlecit	62.5 mg/5 mL

[a]Dose of iron dextran can be calculated by: dose (mL) = 0.0442 (desired Hgb – observed Hgb) × body weight (0.26 × body weight).

Note: Lean body weight should be used for adults and children weighing more than 15 kg. Actual body weight should be used for children weighing 5 to 15 kg. The dose in milligrams can be calculated based on a standard concentration of 50 mg elemental iron per milliliter. A test dose (0.5 mL over 30 seconds) must be administered to patients receiving their first dose of iron dextran because of an anaphylaxis risk. Patients should be monitored for signs of anaphylaxis for at least 1 hour after the test dose before administering the total dose.

higher and more predictable. Subcutaneous or intramuscular administration may be given. A common oral dosing regimen is 1000 to 2000 μg/d. Parenteral regimens consist of daily injections of 1000 μg for 1 week to saturate vitamin B_{12} stores in the body and resolve clinical manifestations. Parenteral administration can be given weekly for 1 month and monthly thereafter for maintenance. Vitamin B_{12} nasal spray is available for patients in remission following IV vitamin B_{12}, who have no nervous system involvement. The response to therapy is quick, neurologic symptoms and megaloblastic cells disappear within days and hemoglobin levels increase after a week of therapy. Vitamin B_{12} is well tolerated and has minimal adverse effects. Injection site pain, pruritus, fluid retention, rash, and diarrhea have been reported. Drug interactions with omeprazole and ascorbic acid may decrease oral absorption.[21]

Folic Acid Anemia Folic acid deficiency is a common cause of vitamin anemia, largely resulting with pregnancy and excessive alcohol intake. An initial daily dose of oral folic acid 1 mg/d is effective. Resolution of symptoms is prompt, occurring within days of starting therapy. Hemoglobin levels will start to rise after 2 weeks and may take 2 to 4 weeks to resolve the anemia completely. If the underlying deficiency is corrected, folic acid replacement can be discontinued. Folic acid is well tolerated. Nonspecific adverse effects are: allergic reactions, flushing, malaise, and rash.[22-23]

Anemia of Chronic Disease

Anemia of chronic disease (ACD) is a term describing anemia caused by underlying chronic conditions. These chronic conditions include cancer, chronic kidney disease, and other inflammatory disorders. Treatment of ACD is less specific than treatment of other anemias. In patients with anemia from cancer or chronic kidney disease, therapy with epoetin or darbepoetin can increase hemoglobin, decrease transfusions, and improve quality of life.

Chemotherapy Induced Anemia The National Comprehensive Cancer Network (NCCN) recommends an anemia work-up for patients with hemoglobin levels less than 11 g/dL (110 g/L or 6.8 mmol/L). Cancer patients with chemotherapy-related anemia who are symptomatic or asymptomatic with risk factors (extensive transfusion history or myelosuppressive therapy) qualify for treatment with erythropoietic agents such as epoetin-alfa or darbepoetin. Epoetin is recombinant human erythropoietin and darbepoetin is structurally similar to endogenous erythropoietin. Both bind to the same receptor to simulate red blood cell production. Darbepoetin differs from epoetin in that it has a longer half-life due to additional N-linked carbohydrate side chains. The response to erythropoietin products must be monitored closely to prevent adverse effects. Adverse events include hypertension, thrombosis, and tumor progression. Concomitant drugs with the same adverse-event profile may increase a patient's risk for side effects. Patient survival may be decreased if the hemoglobin level is titrated above 11 to 12 g/dL (110-120 g/L or 6.82-7.44 mmol/L). Hemoglobin values should be monitored at least every 2 weeks. The following are recommendations for modification of the erythropoietin agent:

- If hemoglobin levels rise above 1 g/dL (10g/L or 0.62 mmol/L) or greater in 2 weeks, decrease the dose by 25%.
- If hemoglobin levels rise above 12 g/dL (120 g/L or 7.44 mmol/L), hold dose until hemoglobin levels fall below 12 g/dL. Therapy can be restarted after hemoglobin levels fall, but decrease the dose by 25%.
- Increase dose by 50% in nonresponding patients. Nonresponding is defined as patients who do not exhibit at least a 1 g/dL (10 g/L or 0.62 mmol/L) increase in hemoglobin after 4 to 6 weeks. In addition, if their hemoglobin has not increased by 1 g/dL after 8 weeks of therapy, the drug should be discontinued.

Table 10-5 provides dosing recommendations for chemotherapy-related anemia.

Cancer patients may have concurrent iron deficiency anemia secondary to cancer. It is imperative that these patients have iron studies performed to assess adequate iron stores needed to drive hematopoiesis.[8,24-27]

Chronic Kidney Disease Patients with chronic kidney disease progress through five stages of disease based upon glomerular

TABLE 10-5 Erythropoietin Products and Doses for Anemia for Chemotherapy and CKD

	Epoetin-Alfa (Epogen, Procrit)	Darbepoetin-Alfa (Aranesp)
Cancer/chemotherapy dosing regimens	150 units/kg subcutaneously three times per week 40,000 units subcutaneously once every week	2.25 μg/kg subcutaneously once every week 3 μg/kg subcutaneously once every 2 weeks; may increase to 5 μg/kg 200 μg subcutaneous fixed dose every 2 weeks, may increase to 300 μg 300-500 μg every 3 weeks
CKD dosing regimens[a]	50-100 units/kg subcutaneously three times per week	0.45 μg/kg subcutaneously once every week 0.75 μg/kg subcutaneously once every 2 weeks

[a]According to National Kidney Foundation guidelines for the use epoetin in patients with anemia owing to kidney disease, the subcutaneous route is preferred. However, the intravenous route is used commonly in clinical practice.

Reproduced with permission from Li EC, Hoffman JM. Anemia. In: Chisholm-Burns MA, Wells BG, Schwinghammer TL, Malone PM, Kolesar JM, Rotschafer JC, DiPiro JT, eds. *Pharmacotherapy Principles & Practice*. New York, NY: McGraw-Hill; 2008:975-986.

filtration rate (GFR). Anemia is a common development in patients with CKD, and evaluation and treatment should be initiated in patients with stage 3 CKD (GFR less than 60). CKD anemia typically is a normocytic, normochromic anemia that is due to erythropoietin deficiency. Therefore, therapy with epoetin or darbepoetin is effective in treating CKD anemia. The target hemoglobin for CKD patients is similar to the target for chemotherapy anemia, but requires lower doses (see Table 10-5). Epoetin doses should be:

- Decreased by 25% if Hgb increases by greater than 1 g/dL in 2 weeks
- Increased by 25% if Hgb increases by less than 1 g/dL in 4 weeks

It can take up to 6 to 12 weeks to see the maximal effects, so doses should not be changed more frequently than once every 4 weeks.

Iron stores in patients with CKD should be maintained. If iron stores are not maintained, epoetin and darbepoetin will not be effective. Oral iron therapy can be used, but is often ineffective, particularly in dialysis patients.[8,27-28] Therefore, IV iron therapy (see Table 10-4) is used extensively in these patients.

SPECIAL CONSIDERATIONS

Erythropoietin Products

Epoetin-alfa (Epogen, Procrit) and Darbepoetin-alfa (Aranesp) are effective agents in the treatment of anemia. Epoetin-alfa is used in the treatment of anemia associated with human immunodeficiency virus (zidovudine therapy), chronic renal failure, and concurrent chemotherapy in patients with metastatic cancer. Darbepoetin-alfa is used in the treatment of anemia associated with chronic renal failure and treatment of anemia due to concurrent chemotherapy in patients with metastatic cancer. Erythropoietin products are *not* indicated for use in cancer patients under the following conditions:

1. Receiving hormonal therapy, therapeutic biologic products, or radiation therapy unless the patient is also receiving concurrent myelosuppressive chemotherapy.
2. Receiving myelosuppressive therapy when the expected outcome is curative.
3. Anemia due to other factors (eg, iron deficiency, folate deficiency, gastrointestinal bleed).

Erythropoietin products have a pregnancy category C. There are no adequate and well-controlled studies in pregnant women. Contraindications for erythropoietin products are hypersensitivity to the agent, uncontrolled hypertension, and hypersensitivity to albumin or mammalian cell-derived products (epoetin-alfa only). There are several black box warnings for erythropoietin products and they include:

- Increased risk of serious cardiovascular events, thromboembolic events, mortality, and/or tumor progression. A rapid rise in hemoglobin (greater than 1 g/dL over 2 weeks) or maintaining higher hemoglobin levels may contribute to these risks.
- A shortened overall survival and/or increased risk of tumor progression or recurrence has been reported in studies with breast, cervical, head and neck, lymphoid, and non–small-cell lung cancer patients.
- To decrease the risk of cardiovascular and thromboembolic events, use erythropoietin products in cancer patients only for the treatment of anemia related to concurrent chemotherapy and use the lowest dose needed to avoid red blood cell transfusions. Discontinue erythropoietin products following completion of the chemotherapy course. Erythropoietin products are not indicated for patients receiving myelosuppressive therapy when the anticipated outcome is curative.
- An increased risk of death and serious cardiovascular events was reported in chronic renal failure patients administered erythropoietin products to target higher versus lower hemoglobin levels (13.5 vs 11.3 g/dL; 14 vs 10 g/dL) in two clinical studies. Dosing should be individualized to achieve and maintain hemoglobin levels within 10 to 12 g/dL range. Hemoglobin rising greater than 1 g/dL in a 2-week period may contribute to the risk.

CASE Application

1. Patients with symptomatic anemia may present with:
   a. Fatigue
   b. Shortness of breath
   c. Tachycardia
   d. Neurologic manifestations
   e. All of the above

2. Select the nutritional factor that may cause a hypo-productive anemia.
   a. Iron
   b. Cancer
   c. Phenytoin
   d. Chronic kidney disease
   e. Anemia of chronic disease

3. Select the hypo-productive anemia that is caused by destruction of proliferating stem cells.
   a. Chronic kidney disease
   b. Iron
   c. Chemotherapy
   d. Folic acid
   e. Anemia of chronic disease

4. Select the treatment for pernicious anemia.
   a. Oral cyanocobalamin
   b. Parenteral vitamin B_{12}
   c. Iron
   d. Epoetin
   e. Sodium ferric gluconate

5. Select the cause(s) of macrocytic, megaloblastic anemia.
   a. Sickle cell anemia
   b. Hemolysis
   c. Anemia of chronic disease
   d. Iron
   e. Vitamin B_{12}

6. Select the hemoglobin or hematocrit normal range for a 37-year-old male patient.
   a. Hemoglobin 12.3 g/dL
   b. Hematocrit 39%
   c. Hematocrit 44%
   d. Hemoglobin 13.1g/dL
   e. All of the above

7. Select the laboratory test that measures the size of a red blood cell.
   a. Mean corpuscular volume
   b. Hematocrit
   c. Red cell distribution width
   d. Total iron-binding capacity
   e. Red blood cell

8. A patient with a low mean corpuscular volume and low serum ferritin would have what type of anemia?
   a. Low mean corpuscular volume and serum ferritin are not associated with anemia
   b. Iron deficiency anemia
   c. Vitamin B_{12} deficiency anemia
   d. Anemia of chronic disease
   e. Aplastic anemia

9. Select the nonpharmacologic therapy for anemia that exhibits the greatest increase on hemoglobin and hematocrit.
   a. Dietary supplementation with vitamin B_{12}
   b. Dietary supplementation with iron
   c. Dietary supplementation with folic acid
   d. Red blood cell transfusion
   e. All of the above

10. Select the product and dose that would be appropriate for a patient with iron deficiency anemia.
    a. Feosol 325 mg four times per day without food
    b. Niferex capsule 150 mg daily
    c. Niferex 50 mg tablet tid
    d. Feostat 100 mg daily
    e. Fergon 325 mg tid with food

11. Select the iron formulation that may cause the highest rate of anaphylaxis.
    a. Ferrous sulfate
    b. Ferrous gluconate
    c. Iron dextran
    d. Iron sucrose
    e. Sodium ferric gluconate

12. Select the generic name for polysaccharide-iron complex.
    a. Feostat
    b. Niferex
    c. Feosol
    d. InFED
    e. Fergon

13. Calculate the dose of iron dextran in milliliters for a 37-year-old man. Height 6 ft 3 in, weight 80 kg, hemoglobin (observed) 7.0 g/dL, and hemoglobin (desired) 12.0 g/dL.
    a. 367 mL
    b. 410 mL
    c. 514 mL
    d. 574 mL

14. A patient is to receive 300 mL of iron dextran to treat an iron deficiency anemia not corrected by oral therapy. How many milliliters should the patient receive during the first hour?
    a. 50 mL
    b. 100 mL
    c. 30 mL
    d. 0.5 mL
    e. 300 mL

15. Select the disabilities that may occur for vitamin B_{12} deficiency anemia that is not treated appropriately.
    a. Paresthesias
    b. Memory loss
    c. Psychosis
    d. Numbness
    e. All of the above
16. Select the pharmacokinetic variable that differentiates subcutaneous administration of vitamin B_{12} as compared to oral administration of vitamin B_{12}.
    a. Absorption
    b. Distribution
    c. Metabolism
    d. Elimination
    e. All of the above
17. Vitamin B_{12} may be administered via which of the following formulations?
    a. Oral
    b. Subcutaneous
    c. Intramuscular
    d. Nasal
    e. All of the above
18. Causes of anemia of chronic disease include:
    a. Chemotherapy
    b. Rheumatoid arthritis
    c. Chronic kidney disease
    d. Systemic lupus erythematosus
    e. All of the above
19. Select the pharmacokinetic variable(s) that differentiates epoetin-alfa and darbepoetin-alfa.
    a. Absorption
    b. Distribution
    c. Metabolism
    d. Elimination
    e. All of the above
20. Select the target hemoglobin concentration for chronic kidney disease patients receiving epoetin-alfa and darbepoetin-alfa.
    a. 7 g/dL
    b. 8 g/dL
    c. 9 g/dL
    d. 10 g/dL
    e. 11 g/dL
21. What nutritional factor is required to be normal to maximize effectiveness of epoetin-alfa and darbepoetin-alfa?
    a. Vitamin B_{12}
    b. Folic acid
    c. Iron
    d. a and b
    e. b and c

TAKEAWAY POINTS ››

- Anemia is a decline in the concentration of hemoglobin resulting in a reduction of the oxygen-carrying capacity of the blood.
- Lack of oxygen may result in fatigue, lethargy, shortness of breath, headache, edema, and tachycardia. Complications arise when the hemoglobin concentration is below 7 to 7.9 g/dL and include cardiovascular sequelae and hypoxia.
- Drug therapy is a key component to decreased production. Factors leading to hypo-productive anemia are: nutritional (iron, vitamin B_{12}, and folic acid), cancer, and CKD.
- Deficiencies in nutrients such as folic acid and vitamin B_{12} hinder the process of erythrocyte maturation.
- Iron deficiency decreases hemoglobin synthesis and ultimately red blood cells.
- Chemotherapy may cause destruction of proliferating stem cells, thereby decreasing erythrocyte production.
- CKD patients develop anemia because erythropoietin is produced in the kidneys.
- Anemias are classified by RBC size as macrocytic, normocytic, or microcytic. Vitamin B_{12} and folic acid deficiency are macrocytic anemias, iron deficiency is a microcytic anemia, and normocytic anemia is associated with recent blood loss or chronic disease.
- The goal of anemia therapy is to increase the hemoglobin level, which will improve the red cell oxygen-carrying capacity, alleviate symptoms, and prevent anemia complications.
- Treatment of iron-deficiency anemia is oral iron therapy with 200 mg of elemental iron daily.
- Parenteral iron therapy is for patients unable to tolerate the oral formulation, noncompliance, or nonresponders (malabsorption).
- Vitamin B_{12} or folic acid anemias are treated by replacing the missing nutrient.
- Anemia of chronic disease is a term describing anemia caused by underlying chronic conditions. These chronic conditions include cancer, chronic kidney disease, and other inflammatory disorders.
- In patients with anemia from cancer or chronic kidney disease, therapy with epoetin or darbepoetin can increase hemoglobin, decrease transfusions, and improve quality of life.
- Contraindications for erythropoietin products are hypersensitivity to the agent, uncontrolled hypertension, and hypersensitivity to albumin or mammalian cell-derived products (epoetin-alfa only).
- There are several black box warnings for erythropoietin products related to cardiovascular, thromboembolic, and tumor progression risks.

REFERENCES

1. Beutler E, Waalen J. The definition of anemia: what is the lower limit of normal of the blood hemoglobin concentration? *Blood.* 2006;107:1747-1750.
2. Guralnik JM, Eisenstaedt RS, Ferrucci L, et al. Prevalence of anemia in persons 65 years of age and older in the United States: evidence for a high rate of unexplained anemia. *Blood.* 2004;104:2263-2268.
3. Woodman R, Ferrucci L, Guralnik J. Anemia in older adults. *Curr Opin Hematol.* 2005;12:123-128.
4. Eisenstaedt R, Penninx BW, Woodman RC. Anemia in the elderly: current understanding and emerging concepts. *Blood Rev.* 2006;20:213-226.
5. Lozoff B, Georgieff MK. Iron deficiency and brain development. *Semin Pediatr Neurol.* 2006;13:158-165.
6. Gleason G. Iron deficiency anemia finally reaches the global stage of public health. *Nutr Clin Care.* 2002;5:217-219.
7. Groopman JE, Itri LM. Chemotherapy-induced anemia in adults: incidence and treatment. *J Natl Cancer Inst.* 1999;91(19):1616-1634.
8. Weiss G. Pathogenesis and treatment of anemia of chronic disease. *Blood Rev.* 2002;16:87-96.
9. Rodriguez RM, Corwin HL, Gettinger A, et al. Nutritional deficiencies and blunted erythropoietin response as causes of the anemia of critical illness. *J Crit Care.* 2001;16:36-41.
10. Miller CB, Jones RJ, Piantadosi S, et al. Decreased erythropoietin response in patients with the anemia of cancer. *N Engl J Med.* 1990;332:1689-1692.
11. Cazzola M, Ponchio L, de Benedetti F, et al. Defective iron supply for erythropoiesis and adequate endogenous erythropoietin production in the anemia associated with systemic-onset juvenile chronic arthritis. *Blood.* 1996;87:4824-4830.
12. Goodnough LT, Skikne B, Brugnara C. Erythropoietin, iron, and erythropoiesis. *Blood.* 2000;96:823-833.
13. Alleyne M, Horne MK, Miller JL. Individualized treatment for iron-deficiency anemia in adults. *Am J Med.* 2008;121:943-948.
14. Killips S, Bennett JM, Chambers MD. Iron deficiency anemia. *Am Fam Physician.* 2007;75(5):671-678.
15. Hillman RS, Ault KA. Iron deficiency anemia. *Hematology in Clinical Practice.* 4th ed. New York, NY; McGraw Hill: 2005;53-64.
16. Auerbach M, Ballard H, Glaspy J. Clinical update: intravenous iron for anemia. *Lancet.* 2007;369:1502-1504.
17. Auerbach M, Goodnough LT, Picard D, Maniatis A. The role of intravenous iron in anemia management and transfusion avoidance. *Transfusion.* 2008;48:988-1000.
18. Chertow GM, Mason PD, Vaage-Nilsen O, Ahlmen J. Update on adverse drug events associated with parenteral iron. *Nephrol Dial Transplant.* 2006;21:378-382.
19. Elia M. Oral or parenteral therapy for B_{12} deficiency. *Lancet.* 1998;352:1721-1722.
20. Kuzminski AM, Del Giacco EJ, Allen RH, Stabler SP, Lindenbaum J. Effective treatment of cobalamin deficiency with oral cobalamin. *Blood.* 1998;92:1191-1198.
21. Bradford GS, Taylor CT. Omeprazole and vitamin B_{12} deficiency. *Ann Pharmacother.* 1999;33:641-642.
22. Pitkin RM. Folate and neural tube defects. *Am J Clin Nutr.* 2007;85:285S-288S.
23. Institute of Medicine, Food, and Nutrition Board. Dietary Reference Intakes: Thiamin, Riboflavin, Niacin, Vitamin B_6 Folate, Vitamin B_{12} Pantothenic Acid, Biotin, and Choline. Washington DC: National Academy Press, 1998.
24. Bohlius J, Wilson J, Seidemfeld, et al. Erythropoietin or darbepoetin for patients with cancer. *Cochrane Database Syst Rev.* 2006;3:CD003407.
25. Seidenfeld J, Piper M, Flamm C, et al. Epoetin treatment of anemia associated with cancer therapy: a systematic review and meta-analysis of controlled trials. *J Natl Cancer Inst.* 2001;93:1204-1214.
26. Bennett CL, Silver SM, Djulbegovic B, et al. Venous thromboembolism and mortality associated with recombinant erythropoietin and darbepoetin administration for the treatment of cancer-associated anemia. *JAMA.* 2008;299:914-924.
27. Weiss GW, Goodnough LT. Anemia of chronic disease. *N Engl J Med.* 2005;352:1011-1023.
28. NKF-/DOQI clinical practice guidelines and clinical practice recommendations for anemia in chronic kidney disease: 2007 update of hemoglobin target. *Am J Kideny Dis.* 2007;50:471-530.

CHAPTER

11 Immune System

S. Scott Sutton, Philip D. Hall, LeAnn B. Norris, and Charles L. Bennett

FOUNDATION OVERVIEW

The immune system protects the body from invading pathogens and has an amazing ability to evolve and adapt based upon environmental exposure. The immune system is designed to attack and destroy foreign antigens/pathogens; however, the immune system must be able to distinguish self from nonself. Failure to differentiate self from nonself may lead to autoimmune diseases[1] (see Table 11-1 for a list of autoimmune diseases). The immune system includes two functional divisions: (1) innate or nonspecific and (2) adaptive or specific.[2,3] The body uses the innate and adaptive immune responses to kill foreign pathogens. The greatest differences between the responses are in specificity and memory. The adaptive immune response can evolve with each subsequent infection, whereas the innate immune response stays the same with each infection.[2,3] Awareness of immune systems components and consequences of disrupting homeostasis must be understood in order to appropriately dose, administer, and monitor effects of medications given to manipulate immune responses.

INNATE IMMUNE SYSTEM

Physical and chemical defenses compose the innate immune system and are the first line of defense against pathogens.

Physical Defense

The skin is the primary method of physical defense. Alterations in the skin allow for an easy portal of entry for pathogens.[4] Burns and abrasions are common examples that alter the physical defense of the skin; however medications can also alter this nonspecific system (drug-associated Stevens Johnson syndrome—see Table 11-2). The low pH of the stomach serves as a major defense to pathogen entry through the gastrointestinal system. Medications that alter the pH of the stomach may change the gastrointestinal bacterial flora and increase risk of infections. Antisecretory agents such as proton pump inhibitors have been associated with pH changes in the stomach and subsequent development of bacterial infections.[5] The rapid turnover of gastrointestinal cells also limits systemic infection, as cells are frequently sloughed. Cell-cycle antineoplastics that disrupt the sloughing process may leave the patient at increased risk for infections. The respiratory tract has forms of physical defense such as coughing, mucous coating the epithelial cells, and the cilia lining the epithelium of the lungs. The combination of coughing, cilia, and mucus provide a barrier to invasion of the respiratory tract. Disruption of the respiratory physical defense through mechanical ventilation can increase the risk for penetration by a pathogenic organism (pneumonia) or anti-infectives that alter gastrointestinal flora leaving the patient at an increased risk of infection (eg, *Clostridium difficile* infection).[6] Other examples of nonspecific defenses include: normal urine flow, lysozymes in tears and saliva, and the normal flora in the throat, gastrointestinal tract, and genitourinary tract.

Cellular Components Defense

If a pathogen invades and is able to infiltrate through a host's physical defense system, innate immunity (cellular) is used to halt progression of the pathogen. Innate immunity cells include the leukocytes or white blood cells (monocytes, neutrophils, basophils, and eosinophils).[2] Other white blood cells (lymphocytes) are involved in adaptive immunity.[2,3] The innate cells are one of the most widely monitored clinical laboratory tests. Innate cells may be evaluated by ordering a complete blood count (CBC). When a CBC is ordered, part of the laboratory test reports a tally of the total white blood cells (WBCs) in a given volume of blood plus the relative percentages that each cell type contributes to the total. Table 11-3 provides a breakdown of the different types of WBCs and their usual cell counts in peripheral blood for an adult.

Granulocytes

Granulocytes are phagocytes (engulfing cells) and derive their name from the presence of granules within the cytoplasm.[2,3] The granules store lysozymes and other chemicals needed to produce the oxidative and nonoxidative burst to lyse the pathogen. Granulocytic leukocytes include neutrophils, eosinophils, basophils, and monocytes. Granulocytes are formed in large numbers in the bone marrow, undergo numerous steps in the marrow, and are usually released into the peripheral blood in their mature form. Neutrophils, eosinophils, and basophils die in the course of destroying pathogens, yielding pus. In contrast, monocytes do not die when destroying pathogens because they play a critical role in activating the adaptive immune response via antigen presentation.

Neutrophils Neutrophils represent the majority of granulocytes and leukocytes and serve as the primary defense

TABLE 11-1 **Autoimmune Diseases**

An autoimmune disorder is a condition that occurs when the immune system mistakenly attacks and destroys healthy body tissue. A person may have more than one autoimmune disorder at the same time. Examples of autoimmune disorders include:
Addison disease
Hashimoto thyroiditis
Rheumatoid arthritis
Systemic lupus erythematosus
Sjogren syndrome
Multiple sclerosis
Myasthenia gravis
Insulin-dependent diabetes mellitus
Graves disease
Idiopathic thrombocytopenia purpura
Sarcoidosis
Scleroderma

against bacterial infections. Neutrophils, also termed segs or polymorphonuclear cells, migrate from the bloodstream into infected or inflamed tissue. In this migration process known as chemotaxis, neutrophils reach the desired site and adhere to, recognize, and phagocytose pathogens.[2] During phagocytosis, the pathogen is internalized within the phagocyte. The neutrophil releases its granular contents which lead to destruction of the engulfed pathogen. The less mature form of a neutrophil is a band. During an acute infection there is an increase in the percentage of neutrophils as they are released from the bone marrow. Less mature band forms may also be released. These immature neutrophils are still considered active. The appearance of band cells is called a shift to the left. The actions of cytokine medications such as granulocyte colony-stimulating factor (G-CSF) and granulocyte-macrophage colony-stimulating factor (GM-CSF) may intensify neutrophil activity. G-CSF

TABLE 11-2 **Stevens Johnson Syndrome**

Stevens Johnsons Syndrome (SJS) is a rare, serious disorder in which the skin and mucous membranes react severely to a medication or infection. Often SJS begins with flu-like symptoms, followed by a painful red or purplish rash that spreads and blisters, eventually causing the top layer of skin to die and shed. Examples of drug-induced SJS are:
Allopurinol
Nonsteroidal anti-inflammatory drugs (NSAID)
Sulfonamides
Penicillins
Phenytoin
Carbamazepine
Valproic acid
Lamotrigine
Phenobarbital

TABLE 11-3 **Normal White Blood Cell Count and Differential in Adults**

Cell Type	Normal Range
Total white blood cell count	4.4-11.3 × 10^3 cells/mm^3
Polymorphonuclear neutrophils (polys, segs, PMN)	2.3-7.7 × 10^3 cells/mm^3
Band neutrophils (immature neutrophils, bands, stabs)	0-10 × 10^3 cells/mm^3
Eosinophils	0.0-0.7 × 10^3 cells/mm^3
Basophils	0.0-0.2 × 10^3 cells/mm^3
Monocytes	0.3-0.8 × 10^3 cells/mm^3
Lymphocytes	1.6-2.4 × 10^3 cells/mm^3

(filgrastim [Neupogen]) and long-acting G-CSF (pegylated filgrastim [Neulasta]) are granulocyte colony-stimulating factors licensed to prevent chemotherapy-induced neutropenia or to stimulate granulocyte production among patients with severe chronic neutropenia. GM-CSF (sargramostim [Leukine]) is a granulocyte-macrophage colony-stimulating factor licensed to shorten the time to neutrophil recovery in acute myelogenous leukemia and stem cell transplantation.

Eosinophils and Basophils The major role of eosinophils is in host defense against parasitic infections; however, eosinophils can phagocytize, kill, and digest bacteria and yeast, but not as efficiently as neutrophils. Eosinophils account for less than 7% of circulating leukocytes and are present in the intestinal mucosa and lungs, two locations where foreign proteins enter the body.[2,3] Elevations of eosinophil counts are highly suggestive of parasitic infections.[1-3] Along with mast cells, eosinophils play an important role in allergies and allergic asthma.

Basophils are the least common granulocyte, accounting for 0.1% to 0.3% of granulocytes. They contain heparin, histamine, and leukotriene B_4.[7] Along with eosinophils and mast cells, basophils play a role in allergies and allergic asthma. Basophils may also be associated with immediate hypersensitivity and delayed hypersensitivity reactions, and increased chronic inflammation and leukemia.[2,3]

Monocytes Functions of monocytes include removal of necrotic apoptotic tissues, lysis of cancer cells, and antigen presentation.[2] They account for 1% to 10% of circulating leukocytes. Monocytes migrate to tissues (lymph nodes, spleen, liver, lung), where they mature into macrophages.[8] After engulfing pathogens, monocytes/macrophages are transformed into antigen-presenting cells (APC). These transformed macrophages present antigen (lysed pathogens) to CD4(+) helper T lymphocytes; therefore, macrophages and other antigen presenting cells (eg, dendritic cells) activate the adaptive immune response (Figure 11-1). Dendritic cells are the most potent antigen presenting cell; however, they make up less than 1% of circulating leukocytes. Dendritic cells, like macrophages, are found more commonly in tissues (eg, spleen, liver). Tissue

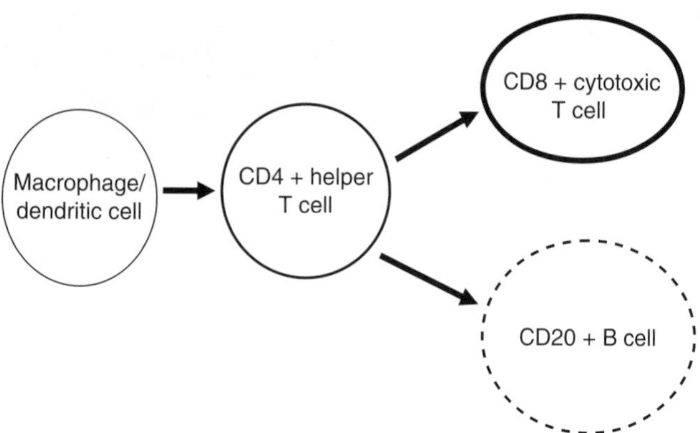

FIGURE 11-1 Activation of the adaptive immune response. Macrophage and/or dendritic cells present antigen to the CD4+ helper T cell. If the CD4+ T cell recognizes the antigen by its T cell receptor (TCR), the CD4+ helper T cell becomes activated to secrete cytokines to stimulate **either** a CD8+ cytotoxic T cell response or a CD20+ B cell response to produce antibody.

macrophages also salvage iron from hemoglobin of old erythrocytes and return iron to transferrin for delivery to bone marrow.

ADAPTIVE IMMUNE SYSTEM

The adaptive immune response consists of two parts, humoral and cell-mediated. The B lymphocytes compose the humoral part, and the T lymphocytes compose the cell-mediated part. T lymphocytes are tailored to defend against infections that are intracellular (viral infections), whereas B lymphocytes secrete antibodies that neutralize pathogens prior to their entry into host cells. Recent research, however, has shown that there is cross talking and interplay between humoral and the cell-mediated immune responses.

Lymphocytes

Lymphocytes make up the second major group of leukocytes. They are characterized by a less granular cytoplasm and large, smooth nuclei. These cells give specificity and memory to the body's defense against foreign invaders.[9] A lymphocyte that has never encountered an antigen it recognizes is referred to as naive. Lymphocytes are not phagocytic, but the T-cells are cytotoxic. Morphologic differentiation of lymphocytes is difficult; visual inspection of a blood smear cannot distinguish between T and B cells. Fortunately, lymphocytes can be distinguished by the presence of lineage-specific membrane proteins, termed clusters of differentiation (CD).[10] Mature T cells express CD4 or CD8, while B lymphocytes express CD20. Identification of the subtype of lymphocyte is not a routine clinical hematology test; they are reported as a total lymphocyte count on the CBC. An exception is the reporting/monitoring of CD4 cells for patients with human immunodeficiency virus (HIV), as low CD4 cell counts are associated with increased risks of opportunistic infections.

TABLE 11-4 **Subtypes of T Lymphocytes**

Surface Marker	Common Name	Comment
CD4(+)	Helper	Plays critical role in up-regulating immune response
CD8(+)	Cytotoxic or suppressor	Cytotoxic: Plays critical role in lysing cells, particularly viral cells Suppressor: Plays critical role in down-regulating the immune response

T Lymphocytes

T lymphocytes are responsible for cell-mediated immunity and are the predominant lymphocyte in circulation and tissue.[10] There are two major subtypes of T lymphocytes: helper and cytotoxic/suppressor (Table 11-4). To activate the adaptive immune response, APCs must present antigen to be recognized by helper T lymphocytes which then activate either cytotoxic T cells or B cell. The role of the T cell is to search and destroy pathogens that infect and replicate intracellularly. When these pathogens enter a cell, they are no longer vulnerable to innate host defenses. Therefore, it is critical that T cells be able to distinguish which cells are infected and which cells are not. In addition to identifying infections, T cells play a prominent role in delayed hypersensitivity reactions (eg, skin reaction to poison ivy, skin tests for tuberculosis, mumps, and *Candida*) and rejection of transplanted organs.[11] In order for a foreign antigen to be recognized by a CD4(+) T lymphocyte, the antigen must be presented by macrophages/dendritic cells in major histocompatibility complex (MHC) II. In contrast, CD8(+) T lymphocytes recognize antigen presented in MHC class I molecules. MHC molecules are often referred to as human leukocyte antigens (HLA).

B lymphocytes

A B lymphocyte recognizes antigen via its antibody or immunoglobulin located on its cell surface. The antibody on the surface can recognize an intact pathogen, such as bacteria, and then present antigen to T cells (ie, acts as an APC). However, the major function of B cells is to produce antibodies to bind to the invading pathogen, a process that first entails activation of the B cell.[10] B cells, once activated by CD4(+) helper T lymphocytes, become a plasma cell that will produce one of five immunoglobulin types: IgA, IgD, IgE, IgG, or IgM. The two antibodies most commonly associated with the development of immunity to foreign proteins, viruses, and bacteria are IgM and IgG. A fraction of the B cells do not differentiate into plasma cells but rather form a pool of memory cells. Memory cells will respond to subsequent encounters with the pathogen, generating a quicker and more vigorous response to the pathogen.[2,10]

One of the most important functions of the adaptive immune response is to produce antibodies or immunoglobulins. IgG is the prevalent immunoglobulin in the serum, and IgG concentrations less than 600 mg/dL (hypogammaglobulinemia) are associated with bacterial infections. IgA is the second most prevalent concentration in the serum, but IgA's most important role relates to its secretion in the respiratory, gastrointestinal, and genitourinary tract. IgM is the first immunoglobulin secreted by a plasma cell, and it is the most efficient activator of complement of the five immunoglobulin subtypes. There are very low concentrations of circulating IgE in serum because the majority of IgE is bound to mast cells. Therefore, IgE plays a critical role in allergic disorders. Clinically, IgE concentrations are measured in IU/mL, and IgE concentrations > 200 IU/mL are associated with allergic disorders. IgD is one of the surface immunoglobulins on B cells, but the function of circulating IgD is unknown. Serum concentrations of the immunoglobulins are:

Isotype	Serum concentration (mg/dL)
IgG	600-1200
IgA	140-260
IgM	70-120

Clinically, only IgG, IgA, and IgM isotypes are determined. IgE concentrations must be ordered separately, usually as IU/mL.

LEUKOCYTE DISORDERS

Patients can suffer from disorders of the white blood cells. Leukocyte disorders can be classified into three major classes: (1) functional, (2) quantitative, and (3) myeloproliferative.

Functional Leukocyte Disorders

Functional white blood cell disorders consist of recognition, signaling, and cytotoxic effects. Examples include hypogammaglobulinemia and chronic granulomatous disease.

Quantitative Leukocyte Disorders

Quantitative leukocyte disorders involve too few or too many white blood cells, however, several terms are used to refer to low numbers of WBCs.[12] Examples are listed in Table 11-5. Key definitions for quantitative disorders include: neutropenia, leukopenia, granulocytopenia, and agranulocytosis.

- Neutropenia is the presence of abnormally low numbers of neutrophils in circulating blood.[13] Neutropenia is a neutrophil count < 1500/mm^3, but one clinically becomes concerned when the neutrophil count falls below 500 cells/mm^3.
- Leukopenia is a total WBC < 3000/mm^3. Leukopenia may be from any cause (neutrophils, lymphocytes, etc), but almost all leukopenia patients are neutropenic since the neutrophils comprise the majority of circulating leukocytes.
- Granulocytopenia is a granulocyte count < 1500 granulocytes/mm^3. Granulocytes consist of neutrophils, eosinophils, and basophils. Because neutrophils comprise the vast majority of circulating granulocytes, granulocytopenia is generally caused by neutropenia.
- Agranulocytosis is defined as a severe form of neutropenia with a total granulocyte count < 500/mm^3. Unfortunately, clinicians use variable definitions when reporting white blood cell dyscrasias. The term agranulocytosis has been used to describe granulocyte counts ranging from < 100 to < 1000/mm^3.

Myeloproliferative Leukocyte Disorders

Myeloproliferative disorders involve an abnormal proliferation of bone marrow cells.[14] Neoplasms of the myeloproliferative stem cells may involve a leukocyte progenitor line. Leukemias are classified as myeloblastic (granulocytic lineage) or lymphoblastic (lymphocytic lineage) and according to whether they primarily affect the very early progenitor cells (acute) or more mature cells (chronic).

- Acute myelogenous (AML)
- Acute lymphocytic (ALL)
- Chronic myelogenous (CML)
- Chronic lymphocytic (CLL)

A lymphoma is a neoplasm of lymphocytic origin but predominates in the lymph nodes rather than the bone marrow. Therefore, patients with lymphomas present with lymphadenopathy. Lymphomas are categorized as Hodgkin and non-Hodgkin lymphoma. Lymphomas can evolve from either T- or B-lymphocyte precursors, and many express CD markers characteristic of mature lymphocytes. Identification of the CD20 marker on B-cell lymphomas provides an opportunity to treat these patients with recombinant antibodies specific to this surface marker (eg, rituximab).

SPECIAL CONSIDERATIONS

The complement system, mannose-binding lectin, and C-reactive protein are also mediators of innate immunity. The complement system consists of more than 30 circulating proteins that play a key role in immune defense. The complement system serves as an adjunct or "complement" to humoral immunity.[15] The four major functions of the complement system include:

1. Direct lysis of pathogens and cells
2. Stimulate chemotaxis
3. Opsonize foreign pathogens for recognition by neutrophils, macrophages, and dendritic cells
4. Clear immune complexes

TABLE 11-5 **Quantitative Leukocyte Disorders**[a]

WBC Abnormality	Cell Count (cells/mm³)	Potential Causes
Neutrophilia	> 12,000	Acute bacterial infection Trauma Myocardial infarction Chronic bacterial infection Epinephrine Lithium G-CSF GM-CSF Glucocorticosteroids
Neutropenia	< 1500	Antineoplastic agents Captopril Cephalosporins Chloramphenicol Ganciclovir Methimazole Penicillin Phenothiazines Procainamide Ticlopidine Tricyclic antidepressants Vancomycin Zidovudine Radiation exposure Overwhelming bacterial infection
Eosinophilia	> 350	Allergic disorders Asthma Parasitic infections Leukemia ACE inhibitors Antibiotics (allergic reaction)
Basophilia	> 300	Chronic inflammation Leukemia
Monocytosis	> 800	Tuberculosis Endocarditis Protozoal infection Leukemia
Lymphocytosis	> 4000	Mononucleosis Viral infections Rubella Varicella Mumps CMV Pertussis Tuberculosis Syphilis Lymphoma
Lymphopenia	< 1000	HIV Radiation Glucocorticosteroids Lymphoma Aplastic anemia

[a]White blood cell counts are sensitive, not specific markers. For example, if a patient has a lymphocyte count < 1000 (lymphopenia), the patient may or may not have HIV or radiation exposure. There are numerous things that may cause a lymphopenia; those listed in the above chart serve as examples.

Abbreviations: CMV, cytomegalovirus; HIV, human immunodeficiency virus; G-CSF, granulocyte colony stimulating factor; GM-CSF, granulocyte-macrophage colony-stimulating factor; WBC, white blood cell.

Complement factors (C3a, C5a) act as chemotactic factors for phagocytic cells. Patients with hereditary deficiencies of complement may have recurrent bacterial infections or autoimmune syndromes. Both mannan-binding lectin and C-reactive protein are acute phase reactants produced by the liver during early stages of infection or inflammation. Acute phase reactants or proteins increase in response to inflammatory stimuli such as tissue injury or infection. C-reactive protein is a plasma protein that can increase up to 1000 times its baseline concentration in inflammatory conditions (eg, infections, autoimmune disorders).[2] Recent clinical evidence suggests that CRP is also released in response to inflammatory markers present within atherosclerotic plaques that lead to cardiovascular disease.[16] Cholesterol medications (HMG-CoA reductase inhibitors/statins) decrease CRP levels, and rosuvastatin was found to decrease cardiovascular disease in patients with elevated CRP levels.

Chemokines play an essential role in linking the innate and adaptive immune response by orchestrating traffic. The chemokine system consists of a group of small polypeptides and their receptors. Chemokines possess four cysteines. Based upon the positions of the cysteines, almost all chemokines fall into one of two categories: (1) CC group or (2) CXC group.[17] The CC group has cysteines that are contiguous and the CXC group has cysteines separated by another amino acid (X). A cell can only respond to a chemokine if the cell possesses a receptor that recognizes the chemokine. An example is maraviroc (Selzentry) used for treatment of CCR5-tropic HIV-1 infection. Maraviroc selectively and reversibly binds to the chemokine receptor (C-C motif receptor 5 [CCR5]) co-receptors located on CD4 cells.[18] CCR5 antagonism prevents interaction between the human CCR5 co-receptor and the gp120 subunit of the viral envelope glycoprotein, thereby inhibiting gp120 conformational change required for fusion of CCR5 HIV fusion with the CD4 cell and subsequent entry.

CASE Application

1. The immune system is designed to attack and destroy foreign antigens and should be able to differentiate self from nonself. Failure to differentiate self from nonself may lead to:
   a. Addison disease
   b. Rheumatoid arthritis
   c. Systemic lupus erythematosus
   d. All of the above

2. Select the nonspecific functional division of the immune system.
   a. Innate
   b. Adaptive
   c. Granulocytes
   d. Lymphocytes
   e. a and b

3. The difference between the innate and adaptive immune system is described by:
   a. Specificity
   b. Memory
   c. Strength
   d. a and b
   e. All of the above

4. Physical and chemical defenses compose the innate immune system and consist of:
   a. Skin
   b. Lymphocytes
   c. Granulocytes
   d. a and c
   e. All of the above

5. Examples of physical defense innate immunity are:
   a. Skin
   b. Stomach pH
   c. Normal flora of GI tract
   d. Coughing
   e. All of the above

6. Select the medication that may cause Stevens Johnson syndrome and in turn alter the skin, leading to an easy portal of entry for bacterial pathogens.
   a. Carbamazepine
   b. Lamotrigine
   c. Loratadine
   d. a and b
   e. All of the above

7. Select the agent(s) that may cause pneumonia by altering the pH of the stomach.
   a. Omeprazole
   b. Ranitidine
   c. Ceftriaxone
   d. a and b
   e. All of the above

8. Select the medication that may alter the normal flora of the gastrointestinal tract leading to infection.
   a. Lansoprazole
   b. Clindamycin
   c. Pantoprazole
   d. a and c
   e. All of the above

9. Select the chemical cell(s) of the innate immune system.
   a. Neutrophils
   b. Eosinophils
   c. Basophils
   d. Granulocytes
   e. All of the above

10. Innate cells may be evaluated clinically by ordering which laboratory test?

    a. C-reactive protein
    b. Chemokines
    c. Complete blood cell count
    d. a and c
    e. All of the above

11. Select the innate cell that represents the majority of granulocytes and serves as the primary defense against bacterial infections.

    a. Lymphocytes
    b. Neutrophils
    c. Monocytes
    d. Eosinophils
    e. Basophils

12. Select the innate cell that is immature.

    a. Basophil
    b. Eosinophil
    c. Band
    d. Neutrophil
    e. Macrophage

13. Select the cell that is part of cell-mediated immunity.

    a. B lymphocyte
    b. Neutrophil
    c. Macrophage
    d. T lymphocyte
    e. Complement

14. B and T lymphocytes may be distinguished from each other by the presence of lineage specific membrane markers termed:

    a. Clusters of differentiation (CD)
    b. Complement
    c. C-reactive protein (CRP)
    d. Chemokines
    e. CCR5 coreceptor

15. A neutrophil count greater than 12,000 cells/mm^3 is termed:

    a. Neutrophilia
    b. Bandemia
    c. Lymphocytosis
    d. a and b
    e. a and c

16. Select the cause(s) of neutrophilia.

    a. Acute bacterial infections
    b. G-CSF
    c. Glucocorticoids
    d. a and c
    e. All of the above

17. Select the drug-induced cause of a neutrophil count less than 1500 cells/mm^3.

    a. Zidovudine
    b. Beta-lactam antibiotics
    c. ACE inhibitors
    d. Ticlopidine
    e. All of the above

18. Select the cause(s) of an eosinophil count greater than 350 cells/mm^3.

    a. Asthma
    b. Parasitic infections
    c. Antibiotics (allergic reaction)
    d. All of the above

19. Human immunodeficiency virus (HIV) is most likely to cause:

    a. Neutrophilia
    b. Eosinophilia
    c. Monocytosis
    d. Lymphocytosis
    e. Lymphopenia

20. A patient that is found to have a granulocyte count less than 500 cells/mm^3 would be classified as:

    a. Lymphopenia
    b. Basophilia
    c. Agranulocytosis
    d. Eosinophilia

21. Which of the following functions is performed by neutrophils?

    a. Antigen presentation to T lymphocytes
    b. Engulfing pathogens
    c. Lysing virally infected cells
    d. Secreting antibody

22. Which of the following cell types can present peptide fragments from an engulfed pathogen in association with MHC class II to T lymphocytes?

    a. Neutrophils
    b. Basophils
    c. Dendritic cell
    d. Eosinophils

23. Which of the following cell types plays a critical role in parasitic infections?

    a. Basophil
    b. Macrophage
    c. Plasma cell
    d. Eosinophil

TAKEAWAY POINTS ››

- The immune system protects the body from invading pathogens and has an amazing ability to evolve and adapt based upon environmental exposure.
- The immune system is designed to attack and destroy foreign antigens/pathogens; however, the immune system must be able to distinguish self from nonself. Failure to differentiate self from nonself may lead to an autoimmune disease.
- The immune system includes two functional divisions: (1) innate or nonspecific and (2) adaptive or specific.
- Physical and chemical defenses compose the innate immune system and are the first line of defense against pathogens.
- The skin is the primary method of physical defense.
- Innate immunity cells include the leukocytes or white blood cells (monocytes, neutrophils, basophils, and eosinophils).
- Granulocytes are phagocytes (engulfing cells) and derive their name from the presence of granules within the cytoplasm.
- Granulocytic leukocytes include neutrophils, eosinophils, and basophils.
- Neutrophils represent the majority of granulocytes and leukocytes and serve as the primary defense against bacterial infections.
- Eosinophils can phagocytize, kill, and digest bacteria and yeast. Elevations of eosinophils counts are highly suggestive of parasitic infections. Along with mast cells, eosinophils control mechanisms associated with allergies and asthma.
- Basophils may be associated with immediate hypersensitivity and delayed hypersensitivity reactions, and increased chronic inflammation and leukemia.
- Monocytes migrate to tissues (lymph nodes, spleen, liver, lung), where they mature into macrophages. Macrophages play a critical role in the adaptive immune response in the eradication of pathogens.
- Macrophages not only engulf and destroy pathogens, but also present antigens from the engulfed pathogen to helper T lymphocytes.
- The adaptive immune response consists of two parts, humoral (B cells) and cell-mediated (T cells).
- CD4(+) helper T lymphocytes up-regulate the immune response by activating either CD8(+) cytotoxic T lymphocytes or CD20(+) B lymphocytes.
- CD8(+) T lymphocytes destroy cells within intracellular infections (eg, viruses).
- B lymphocytes secrete antibodies that neutralize pathogens prior to their entry into host cells.
- Leukocyte disorders can be classified into three major classes: (1) functional, (2) quantitative, and (3) myeloproliferative.
- Patients with neutropenia (neutrophil count less than 1500 cells/mm^3) are particularly vulnerable to bacterial infections.

REFERENCES

1. Chaplin DD. Overview of the human immune response. *J Allergy Clin Immunol.* 2006;117:S430-S435.
2. Delves PJ, Roitt IM. The immune system, first of two parts. *N Engl J Med.* 2000;343:37-49.
3. Medzhitov R, Janeway C. Innate immunity. *N Engl J Med.* 2000;343(5):338-344.
4. Gallo RL, Nizel V. Innate barriers against infection and associated disorders. *Drug Discov Today Dis Mech.* 2008;5(2): 145-152.
5. Herzig SJ, Howell MD, Ngo LH, Marcantonio ER. Acid-suppressive medication use and the risk for hospital-acquired pneumonia. *JAMA.* 2009;301(20):2120-2128.
6. Rennard SI, Romberger DJ. Host defenses and pathogenesis. *Semin Respir Infect.* 2000;15:7-13.
7. Serafin WE, Austen KF. Mediators of immediate hypersensitivity reactions. *N Engl J Med.* 1987;317:30-34.
8. Ganz T, Lehrer RI. Production, distribution, and fate of monocytes and macrophages. In: Beutler E, Coller BS, Lichtman MA, et al. eds. *Williams Hematology.* 6th ed. New York, NY: McGraw Hill; 1999:873-876.
9. Baird SM. Morphology of lymphocytes and plasma cells. In: Beutler E, Coller BS, Lichtman MA, et al. eds. *Williams Hematology.* 6th ed. New York, NY: McGraw Hill; 1999:911-919.
10. Delves PJ, Roitt IM. The immune system, second of two parts. *N Engl J Med.* 2000;343:108-117.
11. Roitt IM, Brostoff J, Male D. *Immunology.* 6th ed. New York, NY: Mosby; 2001:21-100.
12. Toutman WG. Drug induced diseases. In: Anderson PO, Knoben JE, Troutman WG, eds. *Handbook of Clinical Drug Data.* 10th ed. New York, NY: McGraw Hill; 2002:817-829.
13. Dale DC. Neutropenia and neutrophilia. In: Beutler E, Coller BS, Lichtman MA, et al. eds. *Williams Hematology.* 6th ed. New York, NY: McGraw Hill; 1999:823-834.
14. Campbell PJ, Green AR. The myeloproliferative disorders. *N Engl J Med.* 2006;355:2452-2466.
15. Walport MJ. Complement, first of two parts. *N Engl J Med.* 2001;344:1058-1066.
16. Ridker PM, Danielson E, Fonseca FAH, et al. Rosuvastatin to prevent vascular events in men and women with elevated C-reactive protein. *N Engl J Med.* 2008;359:2195-2207.
17. Charo IF, Ransohoff RM. The many roles of chemokines and chemokine receptors in inflammation. *N Engl J Med.* 2006;354:610-621.
18. Gulick RM, Lalezari J, Goodrich J, et al. Maraviroc for previously treated patients with R5 HIV-1 infection. *N Engl J Med.* 2008;359:1429-1441.

CHAPTER

12 Lung Cancer

Philip D. Hall

FOUNDATION OVERVIEW

In 2009, over 215,000 cases of lung cancer were anticipated which represented 15% of all cancer diagnoses. Lung cancer is the second leading cancer diagnosis in men and women behind prostate cancer and breast cancer, respectively, with a slightly higher prevalence of lung cancer diagnosis in men as compared to women. However, the incidence of lung cancer in men is declining while the incidence in women is increasing. In 2009, over 161,000 deaths attributed to lung cancer were anticipated which makes lung cancer the leading cause of death secondary to cancer in both sexes.[1]

There are four major subtypes of lung cancer: small cell, squamous cell, adenocarcinoma, and large cell. Squamous cell, adenocarcinoma, and large cell are collectively referred to as non–small-cell lung cancer (NSCLC). NSCLC represents approximately 85% of the lung cancer diagnoses while small-cell lung cancer (SCLC) represents only approximately 15% of lung cancer diagnoses. Adenocarcinoma represents the most common histology of NSCLC and is associated with a high incidence of distant metastasis at diagnosis. Squamous cell is the second most common histology of NSCLC followed by large cell, the least common histology in NSCLC. An important subtype of adenocarcinoma is bronchoalveolar, which is more responsive to erlotinib. Finally, SCLC is a very aggressive histology but occurs in only 15% of patients with lung cancer. Adenocarcinoma and large-cell lung cancer generally present as peripheral lesions in the lung whereas squamous cell and small cell histologies commonly present as central lesions, often causing hemoptysis or postobstructive pneumonia.[2,3]

Smoking, either voluntary or second-hand cigarette smoke, causes the overwhelming majority of cases of lung cancer. The risk of lung cancer increases with the amount and the duration of smoking. One's smoking history is defined by the packs per day (amount) and duration of smoking (eg, 2 packs per day × 20 years = 40 pack years). The risk of lung cancer decreases after smoke cessation but it remains above the risk of a nonsmoker for the rest of a former smoker's life.[4] Asbestos exposure increases one's risk of lung cancer by fivefold, and it is synergistic with smoking for causing lung cancer. Although the most common lung cancer associated with asbestos exposure is NSCLC; patients with mesothelioma almost always have a history of asbestos exposure. Other risk factors associated with lung cancer include radon exposure, ionizing radiation, a diet low in fruit/vegetables/β-carotene/vitamin E, a family history of lung cancer, and certain occupational exposures (ie, coal, arsenic, nickel, and other mining jobs).

The most common signs and symptoms of lung cancer include cough, increased sputum production, pleuritic chest pain, dyspnea, wheezing, and stridor; however, these symptoms are also common in smokers in general. One's suspicion of lung cancer should increase if the patient experiences hemoptysis. Extrapulmonary symptoms associated with lung cancer include bone pain and/or fracture from bone metastasis, neurologic deficits secondary to brain metastasis, and spinal cord compression secondary to bone metastasis in the spinal vertebrae. Multiple paraneoplastic syndromes, symptoms of lung cancer caused not by direct metastasis to the area but proteins secreted by the lung cancer, can occur in lung cancer (Table 12-1).

Evaluating a patient with suspected lung cancer begins with a complete medical history and physical, then diagnostic imaging of the lung. If the physical examination or the lung imaging is suspicious, then a diagnostic biopsy is undertaken. Generally, bronchoscopy for medial lesions and image-guided biopsy for peripheral lesions, or thoracentesis for patients presenting with pleural effusions establish the diagnosis. Because of the importance of lymphatic spread to prognosis, the patient's lymph nodes must be assessed for staging. In addition to histological type determination, determination of epidermal growth factor receptor (EGFR) and Kirsten-Rous sarcoma virus (*K-ras*) oncogene expression helps to determine treatment options. EGFR is a transmembrane receptor whose expression occurs in the vast majority of individuals with NSCLC. The *K-ras* oncogene mutations promote cell proliferation, and *K-ras* oncogene mutations predict a worse outcome in patients with a variety of tumors including NSCLC.

Accurate staging of patients with lung cancer is critical because it determines appropriate treatment and predicts survival. SCLC is simply staged as limited (confined to one lung and able to fit in a radiation port) or extensive stage (distant metastases or the disease that cannot fit into a radiation port). Extensive-stage SCLC portends a worse prognosis than limited-stage SCLC. In contrast, NSCLC is staged based upon the TNM (tumor, node, and metastasis) staging. It is staged from I to IV with worsening prognosis as the stage increases. In NSCLC, stages I, II, and resectable stage IIIA are considered

TABLE 12-1 **Paraneoplastic Syndromes Associated with Lung Cancer**

Paraneoplastic Syndrome	Comments
Cachexia	Extreme muscle wasting and malnutrition
SIADH	Hyponatremia due to ADH secretion
Hypercalcemia	Caused by PTH-rp secretion; associated with squamous cell histology
Cushing syndrome	Caused by the tumor secreting ACTH
Pulmonary hypertrophic osteoarthropathy	Associated with clubbing of the fingers and toes, and painful swollen joints
Hypercoaguable state	Increased risk of DVTs and PE
Eaton-Lambert syndrome	Upper extremity weakness and diminished reflexes

Abbreviations: ACTH adrenal corticotropin hormone; DVT, deep vein thrombosis; PE, pulmonary embolus; PTH-rp, parathyroid hormone-related peptide; SIADH, syndrome of antidiuretic hormone.

early-stage while unresectable stage IIIB and stage IV are referred to as advanced disease. Stage I has no evident lymph node involvement or distant metastasis. Stages II and III involve lymph nodes with exception of tumors invading the chest wall, diaphragm, mediastinal pleura, pericardium, or tumors within 2 cm of the carina and no lymph node involvement are stage II. The primary differences between stages II and III include the size of the primary tumor with larger masses in stage III and different intrathoracic lymph node chains involved. Stage IIIA disease involves ipsilateral lymph nodes while stage IIIB involves contralateral lymph nodes. Stage IV disease involves distant metastasis. The most common sites for distant metastasis for either NSCLC or SCLC include lymph nodes, bone, bone marrow, liver, brain, and the adrenal glands. Unfortunately, the majority of patients with lung cancer present with unresectable, advanced disease.[2,3]

A key predictor of survival in lung cancer besides staging is performance status (PS). The Eastern Cooperative Oncology Group (ECOG) PS (Table 12-2) delineation ranges from fully active to confinement to bed. Generally, patients with a PS of 3 and 4 are not treated, but offered best supportive care. Other factors utilized to determine treatment options include

TABLE 12-2 **ECOG Performance Status**

Grade	Description
0	Fully active, no restrictions in predisease activities
1	Ambulatory, able to carry out most sedentary work
2	Ambulatory, out of bed < 50% of the day, unable to work
3	In bed < 50% of the day, capable of limited self-care
4	Totally confined to the bed, unable to perform self-care

EGFR and *K-ras* mutation status. In retrospective analysis of clinical trials, it was noted that patients with EGFR mutations are more likely to respond to EGFR tyrosine kinase inhibitors (eg, erlotinib) than those patients whose tumor does not exhibit EGFR mutations. In contrast, *K-ras* mutations are associated with poorer clinical outcomes in patients treated with EGFR tyrosine kinase inhibitors. Interestingly, *K-ras* mutation status does not appear to affect chemotherapy (eg, cisplatin, carboplatin, taxane, etc.) efficacy.

PREVENTION

To reduce the morbidity and mortality of lung cancer, several studies have evaluated various screening methodologies to detect lung cancer at an early stage. The first early detection studies investigated annual or semiannual chest radiography (X-rays) with or without sputum cytology. Unfortunately, none of these trials demonstrated a reduction in lung cancer mortality. Recently, spiral computed tomography (CT) has been investigated for early detection of lung cancer. Preliminary results of nonrandomized trials of annual spiral CT scans are promising; however, we are awaiting the results of the National Lung Screening Trial which compares annual spiral CT scans to chest X-rays in high-risk populations. Until the results of this randomized trial are known, there are no recommendations outside of a clinical trial for screening patients at high-risk of developing lung cancer.[5]

Because of the strong association between smoking and the development of lung cancer, prevention of the initiation of smoking and smoking cessation in current smokers remain the best preventive intervention strategies. The risk of lung cancer for former smokers definitely decreases; however, the risk of developing lung cancer in former smokers never decreases to the level of a nonsmoker.[4]

Based upon epidemiological data about the influence of diet on the risk of developing lung cancer, researchers investigated β-carotene, α-tocopherol, and retinyl palmitate (retinoids) as preventive agents. In males at risk for lung cancer, the α-tocopherol, β-carotene (ATBC) trial compared placebo to β-carotene, α-tocopherol, or the combination of the two. Interestingly, β-carotene increased the risk of lung cancer and mortality in patients taking β-carotene while α-tocopherol had no effect on lung cancer development. The β-carotene and retinol efficacy (CARET) trial investigated the use of placebo or the combination of β-carotene and retinyl palmitate. Again, patients receiving β-carotene and retinyl palmitate had increased mortality compared to placebo. At this time chemoprevention with β-carotene, α-tocopherol, or retinyl palmitate cannot be recommended in patients at high risk for the development of lung cancer.[6,7]

TREATMENT

Non–Small-Cell Lung Cancer

Treatment of NSCLC involves surgery, radiation therapy, and chemotherapy, and their use is dependent on the patient's stage. For stage I disease, resection of the mass offers the best

TABLE 12-3 **Adjuvant Regimens in NSCLC**

Recommended based upon clinical trials
Cisplatin plus vinorelbine × 4 cycles
Cisplatin plus etoposide × 4 cycles
Cisplatin plus vinblastine × 4 cycles
Potential alternative regimens
Carboplatin plus paclitaxel × 4 cycles
Cisplatin plus gemcitabine × 4 cycles
Cisplatin plus docetaxel × 4 cycles

chance for cure. For patients who are not candidates for surgery for stage I NSCLC, radiation therapy can be utilized. The use of adjuvant chemotherapy in stage I NSCLC is controversial. Stage I NSCLC can be divided into IA in which the mass is ≤3 cm or stage IB in which the tumor is < 3 cm, the mass involves the main stem bronchus, or close to the carina. To date adjuvant chemotherapy trials have not demonstrated any survival benefit in patients with stage IA NSCLC so chemotherapy has no role in stage IA disease outside of a clinical trial. Stage IB patients appear to benefit from adjuvant cisplatin-based chemotherapy. For patients with stage II disease (lymph node positive disease), the combination of surgery followed by adjuvant chemotherapy offers patients the best survival. Stage III is divided into IIIA (involvement of ipsilateral and/or subcarinal lymph nodes) and IIIB (involvement of contralateral mediastinal, hilar, ipsilateral or contralateral scalene lymph nodes, or supraclavicular lymph nodes). For stage IIIA, surgery followed by adjuvant chemotherapy offers the greatest benefit. Stage IIIB patients are not resectable. For unresectable stage III patients, concurrent chemoradiation is recommended. In some cases of large masses (< 5 cm) or a specific location (superior sulcus masses), neoadjuvant chemotherapy may be utilized to shrink the tumor and potentially makes the patient a surgical candidate. To date, most of the clinical trials demonstrating a benefit to adjuvant chemotherapy are cisplatin-based (Table 12-3). However, carboplatin plus paclitaxel is an alternative for patients unable to tolerate cisplatin-based regimens.[2]

For patients with stage IV (metastatic) and recurrent disease after primary therapy (eg, surgery and/or adjuvant chemotherapy), chemotherapy offers response rates of 20% to 30% and 1-year survival rates of 30% to 40%. Platinum-based regimens (eg, carboplatin or cisplatin) offer the most benefit, and two-drug regimens offer superior response rates compared to single agent therapy. A meta-analysis comparing the outcomes between the platinums found a survival benefit, although small (11%), in those receiving cisplatin rather than carboplatin.[8] The platinum agents are commonly combined with paclitaxel, docetaxel, gemcitabine, vinorelbine, etoposide, and pemetrexed as first-line regimens in metastatic/recurrent NSCLC (Tables 12-4 and 12-5). No regimen has been proven to be superior to another in randomized trials, so decisions about regimens are based upon adverse events (see Table 12-5) and upon patient toleration of a regimen.[2] In patients with non-squamous cell NSCLC (eg, adenocarcinoma, large-cell carcinoma), cisplatin plus pemetrexed demonstrates benefit over cisplatin plus gemcitabine. In contrast, patient with squamous cell histology had a significant improvement in survival if they received cisplatin plus gemcitabine as compared to cisplatin

TABLE 12-4 **Common Agents Utilized in Lung Cancer**

	Mechanism of Action	Route of Administration	Usual Doses
Cisplatin (Platinol)	Alkylator	IV over 1 h	50-100 mg/m² every 3 wk
Carboplatin (Paraplatin)	Alkylator	IV over 30 min	AUC of 5-7 every 3 wk
Bevacizumab (Avastin)	Anti-VEGF	IV First dose: 90 min Second dose: 60 min Third dose: 30 min	15 mg/kg every 3 wk
Gemcitabine (Gemzar)	Antimetabolite	IV over 30 min	1000 mg/m² on days 1, 8, and 15 every 28 d or 1250 mg/m² on days 1 and 8 every 21 d
Pemetrexed (Alimta)	Antimetabolite (inhibitor of thymidylate synthase)	IV over 10 min	500 mg/m² every 21 d
Docetaxel (Taxotere)	Antimicrotubule	IV over 1 h	75 mg/m² every 21 d
Paclitaxel (Taxol)	Antimicrotubule	IV over 3 h	175 mg/m² every 21 d
Vinorelbine (Navelbine)	Antimicrotubule	IV over 10 min	Monotherapy: 25-30 mg/m² weekly Combination: 30 mg/m² on days 1, 8, and 15 every 28 d
Erlotinib (Tarceva)	EGFR tyrosine kinase inhibitor	Oral	150 mg daily
Topotecan (Hycamtin)	Topoisomerase I inhibitor	IV over 30 min or oral	IV: 1.5 mg/m² on days 1-5 every 21 d Oral: 2.3 mg/m² daily × 5 d every 3 wk
Etoposide (Toposar, Vepesid)	Topoisomerase II inhibitor	IV over 30-60 min or oral	IV: 80-100 mg/m² on days 1-3 Oral: 50 mg/m² daily × 3 wk every 4 wk

Abbreviations: AUC, area-under-the-curve; IV, intravenous.

TABLE 12-5 Common Toxicities of Chemotherapy Utilized in Lung Cancer

Agent	Acute[a]	Delayed[b]	Long Term[c]	Comments
Cisplatin	Severe N/V acute and delayed	Anemia	Mg^{++} and K^+ wasting; nephrotoxicity (cumulative); neurotoxicity (cumulative); ototoxicity	Requires hydration with NS to reduce risk of nephrotoxicity
Carboplatin	Mild to moderate acute and delayed N/V	Myelosuppression (particularly platelets)	Alopecia	Dosed based on AUC to reduce risk of thrombocytopenia
Vinorelbine	Mild N/V	Mild myelosuppression	Mild neurotoxicity	
Vinblastine	Mild N/V	Severe myelosuppression; mucositis		
Docetaxel	Mild N/V	Severe myelosuppression; mucositis	Alopecia; mild neurotoxicity	Must receive dexamethasone premedication to reduce the risk of fluid retention
Paclitaxel	Mild N/V	Severe myelosuppression; arthralgias/myalgias	Neurotoxicity (cumulative); alopecia	Must receive dexamethasone premedication to reduce the risk of hypersensitivity reaction
Gemcitabine	Mild N/V; fever and chills	Elevated transaminases; mild myelosuppression	Alopecia	
Pemetrexed	Mild N/V; rash	Mild myelosuppression		Must receive folate and vitamin B_{12} supplementation to minimize myelosuppression; give dexamethasone 4 mg po bid the day before, the day of, and day after pemetrexed to prevent rash
Topotecan	Mild N/V	Severe myelosuppression; mucositis	Alopecia	
Etoposide	Mild N/V; IV infusion reactions (fever, chills, hypotension, bronchospasm)	Severe myelosuppression; mucositis	Alopecia	

[a]Occurs during the infusion of the drug or within 1 to 3 days of administration.
[b]Occurs 1 to 2 weeks after administration of the agent.
[c]Occurs after multiple cycles of the agent.
Abbreviations: AUC, area-under-the-curve; NS, normal saline; N/V, nausea and vomiting; RBC, red blood cell.

plus pemetrexed.[9] If the patient exhibits EGFR mutation status, the addition of erlotinib may improve outcome. If *K-ras* mutations are found, one should avoid erlotinib.[10]

Bevacizumab is a monoclonal antibody directed against vascular endothelial growth factor (VEGF). VEGF promotes new blood vessel formation. In a phase III trial in patients with previously untreated NSCLC, patients who received chemotherapy plus bevacizumab experienced a 2-month improvement in survival compared to patients who received chemotherapy alone.[11] However, bevacizumab should not be used in squamous cell carcinoma because it is associated with pulmonary hemorrhage in these patients. Other toxicities associated with bevacizumab include gastrointestinal perforation, wound dehiscence, impaired wound healing, hypertension, thromboembolic events, and proteinuria. Because of its effects on wound healing, one should not administer bevacizumab for 42 to 48 days before surgery or 28 days after surgery.[12]

For second-line therapy for NSCLC, single agent docetaxel, pemetrexed, and erlotinib are suitable alternatives. In a randomized controlled trial, patients who progressed on or failed a previous regimen were randomized to either docetaxel or pemetrexed. There were no significant differences in response rates or time to progression, but docetaxel was associated with an increased risk of neutropenia, febrile neutropenia, hospitalizations, infections, and alopecia compared to pemetrexed. Erlotinib is a small-molecule inhibitor of the tyrosine kinase of the EGFR. In phase III trials as second-line or third-line therapy in patients with NSCLC, erlotinib demonstrated a 2-month survival advantage over best supportive care. Erlotinib also exhibits significant activity as first-line therapy of NSCLC. The most common toxicities associated with erlotinib include acneiform rash, dry skin, and diarrhea. In contrast to most of the chemotherapy agents utilized in NSCLC, erlotinib is not associated with myelosuppression.[13]

Small-Cell Lung Cancer

SCLC represents approximately 15% of lung cancer cases. In contrast to NSCLC, surgery has a very minimal role in SCLC, and SCLC is initially very sensitive to chemotherapy with response rates up to 90%. The treatment of choice for limited stage SCLC is chemotherapy with concurrent radiation therapy to the involved lung.[14] This results in 70% to 90% response rate and a survival rate of 14 to 20 months. The most common chemotherapy regimen utilized is cisplatin plus etoposide (see Tables 12-4 and 12-5) for four cycles. If the patient achieves a complete remission from this concurrent chest radiation therapy and chemotherapy, prophylactic cranial irradiation (PCI) is recommended because the development of brain metastases is greater than 30%, and PCI improves overall survival by 5%. For extensive stage SCLC, chemotherapy with cisplatin or carboplatin plus etoposide is used alone. Again, if the patient achieves a complete remission with the chemotherapy regimen, the patient should receive PCI to decrease the incidence of brain metastases and to potentially improve survival.[15]

SCLC patients who relapse or progress after first-line therapy have a median survival of 4 to 5 months. If the SCLC is refractory (relapsed < 3 months since completing first-line therapy), the patient is unlikely to benefit from first-line therapy; so best supportive care or a clinical trial is recommended in these patients. A patient in whom SCLC relapsed greater than 3 months since completing first-line therapy may benefit from second-line therapy. Options in this patient population include a clinical trial, topotecan (a FDA-approved indication), gemcitabine, or taxanes.[3]

SPECIAL CONSIDERATIONS

Generally, cycles of chemotherapy are given every 3 or 4 weeks. In lung cancer, cycles are commonly given for a total of four to six cycles. Patients are generally restaged after every two to three cycles to determine response to the chemotherapy. Chemotherapy is continued if the restaging demonstrates tumor shrinkage or stable disease and the patient is tolerating the treatment. A change in the regimen is considered if the tumor has progressed.

CASE Application

1. A 62-year-old man who has quit smoking 10 years ago comes to clinic asking, "Should I undergo screening for lung cancer?" His past medical history is significant for hypertension and COPD. His social history is significant for a 30-pack year history of smoking and drinks a beer or two a day. What should you advise?
   a. A chest x-ray annually
   b. A chest x-ray annually plus sputum cytology
   c. A spiral CT annually
   d. Enrollment in a clinical trial of lung cancer screening

2. A 60-year-old woman comes into your pharmacy to pick up her prescription for hydrochlorothiazide for hypertension. She asks you about taking vitamin supplements to decrease her risk of lung cancer. Her social history is significant for smoking a pack of cigarettes a day for 25 years, but she stopped a year ago. Based upon this information, you should recommend which of the following?
   a. No supplement is recommended
   b. β-Carotene
   c. Vitamin E plus β-carotene
   d. β-Carotene plus retinyl palmitate

3. A 68-year-old man with recently diagnosed adenocarcinoma of the lung is found to have stage IV disease (liver metastases). At home, he is bedridden due to severe COPD that requires home oxygen. His social history is significant for an 80-pack year history. Which of the following chemotherapy regimens, if any, would be rational?
   a. Cisplatin plus etoposide
   b. Carboplatin plus paclitaxel
   c. Cisplatin plus gemcitabine
   d. Best supportive care

4. A 59-year-old man with recently diagnosed limited-stage small-cell lung cancer comes to clinic for treatment. Which of the following would be rational therapy for this gentleman?
   a. Surgery followed by four cycles of cisplatin plus etoposide
   b. Six cycles of cisplatin plus pemetrexed
   c. Concurrent radiation therapy, cisplatin, and etoposide
   d. Six cycles of carboplatin plus paclitaxel

5. For a patient receiving etoposide, you should counsel the patient about which of the following side effects?
   a. Severe acute nausea and vomiting within hours of receiving etoposide
   b. Myelosuppression about 1 week after receiving etoposide
   c. Neurotoxicity starting after two or more cycles of etoposide
   d. Nephrotoxicity occurring after three or more cycles of etoposide

6. A 61-year-old woman presents to clinic with newly diagnosed squamous cell carcinoma of the lung which metastasize to the liver and bone. The EGFR status reveals no mutations. All of her laboratory values are within normal limits and report that she is extremely active. Based upon this information, which of the following treatments would be rational?
   a. Best supportive care
   b. Erlotinib
   c. Cisplatin plus pemetrexed
   d. Cisplatin plus gemcitabine

7. Which of the following side effects is more common with carboplatin rather than cisplatin?

a. Tingling in the hands and feet
b. A lowered platelet count
c. A rising serum creatinine
d. Nausea and vomiting

8. What is the best treatment option for a 61-year-old man who is chemotherapy naïve and was recently diagnosed with extensive-stage small-cell lung cancer?

a. Cisplatin plus vinorelbine
b. Carboplatin plus paclitaxel
c. Cisplatin plus etoposide
d. Carboplatin, paclitaxel, plus bevacizumab

9. For a patient receiving erlotinib, you should counsel them about which of the following side effects?

a. Rash
b. Myelosuppression
c. Neurotoxicity
d. Alopecia

10. Which of the following factors predicts a favorable chance to respond to erlotinib?

a. Adenocarcinoma histology
b. Squamous histology
c. EGFR mutations present
d. *K-ras* mutations present

11. Which of the following is the trade name of erlotinib?

a. Tarceva
b. Alimta
c. Navelbine
d. Hycamtin

12. A 64-year-old man with a performance status of 1 returns to clinic with relapsed small-cell lung cancer (SCLC), new bone and liver metastases. He completed his previous chemotherapy of carboplatin and etoposide 5 months ago and reports no other medical problems. He and his wife request further treatment if it is reasonable. Based upon this information, which of the following treatments would be rational?

a. Best supportive care
b. Erlotinib
c. Cisplatin, paclitaxel, and bevacizumab
d. Topotecan

13. For a patient receiving gemcitabine, you should counsel them about which of the following side effects?

a. Rash after the first and subsequent doses
b. Fever and chills with 1 to 2 days of the infusion
c. Neurotoxicity after four cycles
d. Severe magnesium and potassium wasting after multiple cycles

14. For a patient receiving bevacizumab, you should closely monitor the patient for which of the following side effects?

a. Nausea and vomiting, myelosuppression (especially thrombocytopenia), and alopecia
b. Fluid retention, severe myelosuppression, and alopecia
c. Hypertension, thromboembolic events, and proteinuria
d. Arthralgias/myalgias, tingling in the hands and feet, and alopecia

15. In which of the following histologies of lung cancer should one avoid bevacizumab due to its association with causing pulmonary hemorrhage in this histology?

a. Adenocarcinoma
b. Large cell
c. Bronchoalveolar
d. Squamous

16. Which of the following is the trade name of bevacizumab?

a. Gemzar
b. Avastin
c. Taxotere
d. VePesid

17. In addition to a short course of dexamethasone, one should ensure that a patient receiving pemetrexed receives which of the following medications?

a. Folate and vitamin B_{12} supplementation
b. Aggressive hydration with normal saline
c. Oral potassium and magnesium supplementation
d. β-Carotene and α-tocopherol supplementation

18. Which of the following is the trade name of pemetrexed?

a. Paraplatin
b. Taxol
c. Alimta
d. Taxotere

19. Which of the following patients with small-cell lung cancer should receive prophylactic cranial irradiation?

a. All patients with limited-stage SCLC.
b. All patients with extensive-stage SCLC.
c. Patients with limited-stage SCLC who achieve a complete response to their chemotherapy regimen.
d. Patients with extensive-stage SCLC who do not respond to their chemotherapy regimen.

20. For a patient receiving docetaxel, you should closely monitor the patient for which of the following side effects?

a. Acneiform rash, dry skin, and diarrhea
b. Fluid retention, severe myelosuppression, mucositis, and alopecia
c. Impaired wound healing, hypertension, proteinuria, and thromboembolic events
d. Severe nausea/vomiting, nephrotoxicity, neurotoxicity, and ototoxicity

TAKEAWAY POINTS ››

- Lung cancer is the second leading cause of cancer in men and women; however, it is the leading cause of cancer deaths in both sexes.
- The leading causes of lung cancer include smoking and asbestos exposure. Unfortunately, this combination of risk factors acts synergistically to increase one's risk of lung cancer.
- There are four major subtypes of lung cancer: adenocarcinoma, large-cell carcinoma, squamous cell, and small cell. Adenocarcinoma, large-cell carcinoma, and squamous cell carcinoma are collectively referred to as non–small-cell lung cancer.
- The best preventive strategy to decrease one's risk of lung cancer is to never smoke or to stop smoking.
- Unfortunately, no attempts at early detection have improved survival to date.
- The treatment of choice for curative-intent in NSCLC is surgery. For inoperable patients with potentially curative intent, radiation therapy may be utilized.
- For unresectable or recurrent NSCLC, chemotherapy results in 6 to 8 week improvement in overall survival.
- Platinum-based (ie, cisplatin, carboplatin) therapy is recommended as the frontline chemotherapy for NSCLC. The platinum is usually combined with a taxane (eg, paclitaxel, docetaxel), gemcitabine, or vinorelbine.
- Bevacizumab may be added to front-line therapy of NSCLC except in patients with squamous cell carcinoma because it increases the risk of bleeding in those patients.
- Second-line therapy for NSCLC includes erlotinib, docetaxel, and pemetrexed.
- The best predictor of response to erlotinib is EGFR mutation status.
- Because of its high propensity to metastasize early, the front-line treatment of either stage of SCLC includes systemic chemotherapy with cisplatin plus etoposide.
- Most patients with SCLC initially respond to chemotherapy but relapse.

REFERENCES

1. Jemal A, Siegel R, Ward E, Hao Y, Xu J, Thun MJ. Cancer statistics. *CA Cancer J Clin.* 2009;59:225-249.
2. National Comprehensive Cancer Network. NCCN clinical practice guidelines in oncology: non-small cell lung cancer, v.2.2009. Available at www.nccn.org/professionals/physicians_gls/PDF/nscl.pdf. Accessed September 30, 2009.
3. National Comprehensive Cancer Network. NCCN clinical practice guidelines in oncology: small cell lung cancer, v.2.2009. Available at www.nccn.org/professionals/physicians_gls/PDF/sclc.pdf. Accessed September 30, 2009.
4. Tong L, Spitz MR, Fueger JJ, Amos CA. Lung carcinoma in former smokers. *Cancer.* 1996;78:1004-1010.
5. Humphrey LL, Teutsch S, Johnson, M. Lung cancer screening with sputum cytologic examination, chest radiography, and computed tomography: an update for the US preventive services task force. *Ann Intern Med.* 2004;140:740-753.
6. Virtamo J, Pietinen P, Huttunen JK, et al. Incidence of cancer and mortality following alpha-tocopherol and beta-carotene supplementation: a post-intervention follow-up. *JAMA.* 2003;290:476-485.
7. Goodman GE, Thornquist MD, Ballmes J, et al. The beta-carotene and retinol efficacy trial: incidence of lung cancer and cardiovascular disease mortality during 6-year follow-up after stopping beta-carotene and retinol supplements. *J Natl Cancer Inst.* 2004;96:1743-1750.
8. Hotta K, Matsuo K, Ueoka H, Kiura K, Tabata M, Tanimoto M. Meta-analysis of randomized clinical trials comparing cisplatin to carboplatin in patients with advanced non-small cell lung cancer. *J Clin Oncol.* 2004;22:3852-3859.
9. Scagliotti GV, Parikh P, von Pawel J, et al. Phase III study comparing cisplatin plus gemcitabine with cisplatin plus pemetrexed in chemotherapy-naïve patients with advanced-stage non-small cell lung cancer. *J Clin Oncol.* 2008;26:3543-3551.
10. Eberhard D, Johnson DE, Amler LC, et al. Mutations in the epidermal growth factor receptor and KRAS are predictive and prognostic indicators in patients with non-small cell lung cancer treated with chemotherapy alone and in combination with erlotinib. *J Clin Oncol.* 2005;23:5900-5909.
11. Sandler A, Gray R, Perry MC, et al. Paclitaxel-carboplatin alone or with bevacizumab for non-small cell lung cancer. *N Engl J Med.* 2006;355:2542-2550.
12. Shord SS, Bressler LR, Tierney LA, Cuellar S, George A. Understanding and managing the possible adverse effects associated with bevacizumab. *Am J Health Syst Pharm.* 2009;66:999-1013.
13. Shepherd FA, Pereira JR, Ciuleanu T, et al. Erlotinib in previously untreated non-small cell lung cancer. *N Engl J Med.* 2005;353:123-132.
14. Pignon JP, Arriagada R, Ihde D, et al. A meta-analysis of thoracic radiotherapy for small cell lung cancer. *N Engl J Med.* 1992;327:1618-1624.
15. Slotman B, Faivre-Finn C, Kramer G, et al. Prophylactic cranial irradiation in extensive stage small cell lung cancer. *N Engl J Med.* 2007;357:664-672.

CHAPTER

13 Prostate Cancer

LeAnn B. Norris

FOUNDATION OVERVIEW

In the United States alone, it is estimated that 192,280 new cases of prostate cancer will be diagnosed and more than 27,360 men will die from this disease in 2009.[1] Although prostate cancer incidence increased during the late 1980s and early 1990s owing to widespread prostate-specific antigen (PSA) screening, deaths from prostate cancer have been declining since 1995.[1]

The widely accepted risk factors for prostate cancer are age, race-ethnicity (African American ancestry), and family history of prostate cancer.[2,3] The disease is rare under the age of 40, but the incidence sharply increases with each subsequent decade, most likely because the individual has had a lifetime exposure to testosterone, a known growth signal for the prostate.[3]

Pathophysiology

The prostate gland is a solid, rounded, heart-shaped organ positioned between the neck of the bladder and the urogenital diaphragm. Adenocarcinoma, the major pathologic cell type, accounts for more than 95% of prostate cancer cases.[4,5] Prostate cancer can be graded systematically according to the histologic appearance of the malignant cell and then grouped into well, moderately, or poorly differentiated grades.[5,6] Gland architecture is examined in two separate specimens and then rated on a scale of 1 (well differentiated) to 5 (poorly differentiated). The grades of each specimen are added together to determine the Gleason score. Groupings for total Gleason score are 2 to 4 for well-differentiated, 5 or 6 for moderately differentiated, and 7 to 10 for poorly differentiated tumors. Poorly differentiated tumors grow rapidly (poor prognosis), while well-differentiated tumors grow slowly (better prognosis).[5,6]

Metastatic spread can occur by lymphatic drainage, hematogenous dissemination, or local extension.[6,7] The pelvic and abdominal lymph node groups are the most common sites of lymph node involvement. Bone metastases from hematogenous spread are the most common sites of distant spread. The lung, liver, brain, and adrenal glands are the most common sites of visceral involvement.

Normal growth and differentiation of the prostate depends on the presence of androgens, specifically dihydrotesterone (DHT).[7,8] The testes and the adrenal glands are the major sources of circulating androgens. Hormonal regulation of androgen synthesis is mediated by a negative feedback loop involving the hypothalamus, pituitary, adrenal glands, and testes. Luteinizing hormone–releasing hormone (LH-RH) released from the hypothalamus stimulates the release of luteinizing hormone (LH) and follicle-stimulating hormone (FSH) from the anterior pituitary gland. LH stimulates the production of testosterone and small amounts of estrogen. FSH acts on the Sertoli cells within the testes to promote the maturation of LH receptors and to produce an androgen-binding protein. Circulating testosterone and estradiol influence the synthesis of the hormones involved in the negative feedback.[9]

Testosterone, the major androgenic hormone, accounts for 95% of the androgen concentration. The primary source of testosterone is the testes; however, 3% to 5% of the testosterone concentration is derived from direct adrenal cortical secretion of testosterone or steroids such as androstenedione.[6-8]

Clinical Presentation/Diagnosis

Prior to the implementation of routine screening, prostate cancers were frequently identified on the investigation of symptoms including urinary hesitancy, retention, painful urination, hematuria, and erectile dysfunction. With the introduction of screening techniques, most prostate cancers are now identified prior to the development of symptoms.[10]

On presentation, most patients with localized disease are asymptomatic. Ureteral dysfunction, frequency, hesitancy, dribbling, and impotence are common symptoms in patients with locally invasive disease. Advanced disease can be accompanied with a variety of symptoms including back pain, spinal cord compression, lower extremity edema, pathologic fractures, anemia, and weight loss.

The information obtained from the diagnostic tests is used to stage the patient. There are two commonly recognized staging classification systems: the International Classification System (tumor, node, metastases; TNM) and the American Urologic System (AUS Stages A-D). The AUS classification is the most commonly used staging system in the United States. Patients are assigned to stages A through D and corresponding subcategories based on size of the tumor (T), local or regional extension, presence of involved lymph node groups (N), and presence of metastases (M).[11]

PREVENTION

Early detection of potentially curable prostate cancers is the goal of prostate cancer screening. Digital rectal examination (DRE) has been recommended for years for the detection of prostate cancer. However, DRE as a single screening method has poor compliance and has had little effect on preventing metastatic prostate cancer.[12]

Prostate specific antigen (PSA) is widely used for prostate cancer screening in the United States.[13] However, PSA may be elevated in men with acute urinary retention, acute prostatitis, and prostatic ischemia or infarction, as well as benign prostatic hyperplasia (BPH), a nearly universal condition in men at risk for prostate cancer. PSA elevations between 4.1 and 10 ng/mL (10 μg/L) cannot distinguish between BPH and prostate cancer, limiting the utility of PSA alone for the early detection of prostate cancer.[14] Neither DRE nor PSA is sensitive or specific enough to be used alone as a screening test. Therefore, the combination of a DRE plus PSA determination is a better method in detecting prostate cancer than DRE alone.

The common approach to prostate cancer screening today involves offering a baseline PSA and DRE at age 40 with annual evaluations beginning at age 50 to all men classified as normal risk with a 10-year or greater life expectancy. Men with an increased risk of prostate cancer, including men of African American ancestry and men with a family history of prostate cancer may begin screening earlier, at age 40 to 45.[15]

Chemoprevention

Currently, the most promising agents for the prevention of prostate cancer are the 5-alpha reductase inhibitors, finasteride and dutasteride.[16-18] These medications work by inhibiting 5-alpha reductase, an enzyme that converts testosterone to its more active form, dihydrotestosterone (DHT), which is involved in prostate epithelial proliferation. Finasteride selectively inhibits the 5-alpha reductase type II isoenzyme, whereas dutasteride inhibits both isoenzymes.[18] Both finasteride and dutasteride falsely lower the PSA in patients and this needs to be accounted for when measuring the PSA in patients on these medications.[16,18] Side effects include sexual dysfunction and breast tenderness. Studies reveal finasteride reduces the rate of prostate cancer, but may actually increase the cancer grade (Gleason grade 7-10) in those who develop prostate cancer. Therefore, finasteride use is debatable and the benefits, side effects, and risks of finasteride should be discussed prior to initiating therapy. Dutasteride is also being investigated as a preventative agent for prostate cancer, but like finasteride, is not currently approved for this indication.[18]

TREATMENT

The initial treatment for prostate cancer depends primarily on the disease stage, the Gleason score, the presence of symptoms, and the life expectancy of the patient.[15] Prostate cancer is usually initially diagnosed by PSA and DRE and confirmed by a biopsy, where the Gleason score is assigned. Asymptomatic patients with a low risk of recurrence, a Gleason score of 2 through 6, and a PSA of less than 10 ng/mL (10 μg/L) may be managed by observation, radiation (external beam or brachytherapy), or radical prostatectomy.

Individuals with moderate disease or a Gleason score of 7 or a PSA ranging from 10 to 20 ng/mL (10-20 μg/L) are considered at intermediate risk for prostate cancer recurrence.[15] Individuals with less than a 10-year expected survival may be offered expectant management, radiation therapy, or radical prostatectomy with or without a pelvic lymph node dissection, and those with a greater than or equal to 10-year life expectancy may be offered either radical prostatectomy with or without a pelvic lymph node dissection or radiation therapy.

The treatment of patients at high risk of recurrence (Gleason score ranging from 8-10, or a PSA value greater than 20 ng/mL, 20 μg/L) should be treated with androgen ablation for 2 to 3 years combined with radiation therapy.

Androgen ablation therapy, with either orchiectomy, an LH-RH agonist alone, or an LH-RH agonist plus an antiandrogen (combined androgen blockade), can be used to provide palliation for patients with advanced (stage D_2) prostate cancer. Secondary hormonal manipulations, cytotoxic chemotherapy, or supportive care is used for the patient who progresses after initial therapy.[19]

Pharmacologic Therapy

LH-RH Agonists

Luteinizing hormone–releasing hormone (LH-RH) agonists are a reversible method of androgen ablation and are as effective as orchiectomy in treating prostate cancer.[20] See Table 13-1 for available LH-RH formulations and dosing. There are no direct comparative trials of the currently available LH-RH agonists, therefore the choice between the three agents is usually made based on cost, physician preference, and dosing schedule.

The most common adverse effects reported with LH-RH agonist therapy include a disease flare during the first week of therapy, hot flashes, erectile impotence, decreased libido, and injection-site reactions.[8] The disease flare is caused by an initial increase in the release of LH and FSH by the LH-RH agonist leading to an initial phase of increased testosterone production, and manifests clinically as either increased bone pain or increased urinary symptoms.[8] Initiating an antiandrogen prior to the administration of the LH-RH agonist and continuing for 2 to 4 weeks is a frequently employed strategy to minimize this initial tumor flare.[9] Additionally, utilizing an antiandrogen with an LH-RH agonist is known as *combined androgen blockade* (CAB) and has been used to maximize androgen deprivation.

Another potentially serious complication of androgen deprivation therapy is a resultant decrease in bone-mineral density leading to an increased risk for osteoporosis. Most clinicians recommend that men starting long-term androgen deprivation therapy should have a baseline bone mineral density assessment and be initiated on a calcium and vitamin D supplement.[9]

Gonadotrophin-Releasing Hormone (GnRH) Antagonists

An alternative to LH-RH agonists is the recently approved GnRH antagonist, degarelix. Degarelix works by binding reversibly to GnRH receptors on cells in the pituitary gland, reducing the production of testosterone to castrate levels. The major advantage of degarelix over LH-RH agonists is the

TABLE 13-1 **LH-RH Agonists and GnRH Antagonists**

Drug	Trade Name	Dose
	LH-RH Agonists	
Leuprolide depot	Lupron	7.5 mg IM monthly 22.5 mg IM every 3 mo 30 mg IM every 4 mo
Leuprolide implant	Viadur	72 mg SQ in abdomen every 12 mo
Goserelin implant	Zoladex	3.6 mg SQ monthly 10.8 mg SQ every 3 mo
Triptorelin depot	Trelstar Depot	3.75 mg every 28 d
Triptorelin LA depot	Trelstar LA	11.25 mg every 84 d
	GnRH Antagonists	
Degarelix	Firmagon	Initial dose: 240 mg SQ × 1 dose (two separate 120 mg injections) Maintenance dose: 80 mg SQ every 28 d

speed at which it can achieve the drop in testosterone levels; castrate levels are achieved in 7 days or less with degarelix, compared to 28 days with leuprolide, eliminating the tumor flare seen and need for antiandrogens, with LH-RH agonists. See Table 13-1 for degarelix dosing information. The most frequently reported adverse reactions were injection sites reactions. Like other methods of androgen supplementation therapy, osteoporosis may develop and calcium and vitamin D supplementation should be considered. Degarelix has not been studied in combination with antiandrogens and routine use of the combination can not be recommended.[21]

Antiandrogens

Three antiandrogens, flutamide, bicalutamide,[19] and nilutamide,[20] are currently available (Table 13-2). For advanced prostate cancer, all currently available antiandrogens are indicated only in combination with androgen-ablation therapy; flutamide and bicalutamide are indicated in combination with an LH-RH agonist, and nilutamide is indicated in combination with orchiectomy.[19] The most common antiandrogen-related adverse effects are listed in Table 13-2. Antiandrogens can reduce the symptoms from the flare phenomenon associated with initiation of LH-RH agonist therapy.[9]

Secondary Therapies

Secondary or salvage therapies for patients who progress after their initial therapy depend on what was used for initial management.[15] For patients initially diagnosed with localized prostate cancer, radiotherapy can be used in the case of failed radical prostatectomy. Alternatively, androgen ablation can be used in patients who progress after either radiation therapy or radical prostatectomy.

In patients treated initially with one hormonal modality, secondary hormonal manipulations may be attempted including adding an antiandrogen to an LH-RH agonist. If the patient initially received combined androgen blockade with an LH-RH

TABLE 13-2 **Comparison of Antiandrogens**

Generic	Brand	Usual Dose	Adverse Effects
Flutamide	Eulexin	750 mg/d (250 mg daily, then 250 mg tid)	Gynecomastia Hot flushes Gastrointestinal disturbances (diarrhea) Liver function test abnormalities Breast tenderness Methemoglobinemia
Bicalutamide	Casodex	50 mg/d	Gynecomastia Hot flushes Gastrointestinal disturbances (diarrhea) Liver function test abnormalities Breast tenderness
Nilutamide	Nilandron	300 mg/d × 1 mo, then 150 mg/d	Gynecomastia Hot flushes Gastrointestinal disturbances (nausea or constipation) Liver function test abnormalities Breast tenderness Visual disturbances (impaired dark adaptation) Alcohol intolerance Interstitial pneumonitis

TABLE 13-3 First Line Chemotherapy Regimens for Metastatic Hormone Refractory Prostate Cancer

Regimen	Usual Dose	Adverse Effects	Dose Adjustments
Docetaxel	75 mg/m² every 3 wk	Fluid retention Alopecia	Do not administer for: AST/ALT > 1.5 × ULN Alk Phos > 2.5 × ULN
Prednisone	5 mg po bid	Mucositis Myelosuppression Hypersensitivity	Assure complete blood count recovery
Estramustine	280 mg tid days 1-5	Edema Gynecomastia	Do not administer for: AST/ALT > 1.5 × ULN Alk Phos > 2.5 × ULN
Docetaxel	60 mg/m² on day 2	Leucopenia Thromboembolic events (increased risk)	Assure complete blood count recovery
Mitoxantrone	12 mg/m² every 3 wk	Myelosuppression Alopecia	EKG prior to initiation
Prednisone	5 mg po bid	Cardiotoxicity Blue/green secretions	Administered with caution in hepatic impairment Assure complete blood count recovery

agonist and an antiandrogen, then androgen withdrawal is the first salvage manipulation.[15] Objective and subjective responses have been noted following the discontinuation of flutamide, bicalutamide, or nilutamide in patients receiving these agents as part of combined androgen ablation with an LH-RH agonist. A potential explanation for response when antiandrogen therapy is discontinued may be mutations in the androgen receptor. These mutations allow antiandrogens such as flutamide, bicalutamide, and nilutamide (or their metabolites) to become agonists and activate the androgen receptor.

Adding an agent that blocks adrenal androgen synthesis, such as aminoglutethimide, at the time that androgens are withdrawn may produce a better response than androgen withdrawal alone. Androgen synthesis inhibitors, such as aminoglutethimide or ketoconazole, can provide symptomatic relief for a short time in approximately 50% of patients with progressive disease despite previous androgen-ablation therapy.[19] Central nervous system effects that include lethargy, ataxia, and dizziness are the major adverse reactions of aminoglutethimide in addition to a self-limiting rash.[19] Adverse effects from ketoconazole include gastrointestinal intolerance, transient rises in liver and renal function tests, and hypoadrenalism. Ketoconazole is combined with replacement doses of hydrocortisone to prevent symptomatic hypoadrenalism.[19]

Supportive care, chemotherapy, or local radiotherapy can be used for palliation in patients who have failed all forms of androgen-ablation manipulations because these patients are considered to have hormone refractory prostate cancer. Skeletal metastases from hematogenous spread are the most common sites of distant spread of prostate cancer and often require palliative therapy. Bisphosphonates may prevent skeletal related events and improve bone mineral density. The dose of pamidronate is 90 mg every month and the approved dose of zoledronic acid is 4 mg every 3 to 4 weeks. Renal function should be monitored in patients receiving zoledronic acid. If a patient's serum creatinine is greater than 3 mg/dL, then zoledronic acid should be avoided. A trial of pamidronate or zoledronic acid can be initiated in prostate cancer patients with metastatic bone pain; if no benefit is observed, the drug may be discontinued.[22]

Chemotherapy

Chemotherapy, with docetaxel and prednisone improves overall survival in patients with hormone-refractory prostate cancer. Docetaxel should be administered at 75 mg/m² every 3 weeks combined with prednisone 5 mg twice a day (Table 13-3).[23] The most common adverse events reported with this regimen are nausea, alopecia, and bone marrow suppression. In addition, fluid retention and peripheral neuropathy, known effects of docetaxel, are observed. Docetaxel is hepatically eliminated; therefore, patients with hepatic impairment may not be eligible for treatment with docetaxel.

The combination of estramustine (280 mg tid, days 1-5) and docetaxel 60 mg/m² on day 2, every 3 weeks also improves survival in hormone refractory metastatic prostate cancer (see Table 13-3).[24] Estramustine causes a decrease in testosterone and a corresponding increase in estrogen, therefore, the adverse effects of estramustine include an increase in thromboembolic events, gynecomastia, and decreased libido. Estramustine is an oral capsule and should be refrigerated. Calcium inhibits the absorption of estramustine. While both the docetaxel/prednisone and the docetaxel/estramustine regimens are effective in hormone refractory prostate cancer, most clinicians prefer the docetaxel/prednisone regimen because of the cardiovascular adverse effects associated with estramustine. In addition, androgen ablation is usually continued when chemotherapy is initiated.[15]

The regimen of mitoxantrone plus prednisone has been shown to be effective in reducing pain from bone metastasis (see Table 13-3). The effectiveness of mitoxantrone after failure of docetaxel-based therapy has not been scientifically evaluated. Many clinicians will treat patients with radiation therapy for palliation of symptoms after failure of docetaxel-based chemotherapy.[15]

CASE Application

1. Which of the following is the most accurate statement pertaining to prostate cancer?
   a. Prostate cancer is the leading cause of cancer death in both men and women.
   b. Age, race-ethnicity, and family history are known risk factors for prostate cancer.
   c. Prostate cancer is related to decreased exposure to testosterone.
   d. Squamous cell carcinoma is the major pathologic cell type of prostate cancer.

2. A prostate cancer with a Gleason score of 7 to 10 is considered:
   a. Poorly differentiated
   b. Differentiated
   c. Moderately differentiated
   d. Well differentiated

3. BD is a 45-year-old African American man with a family history of prostate cancer who presents to his primary care physician for his annual examination. He asks about prostate cancer screening. Which of the following is the most appropriate course of action?
   a. Observation because he is not eligible for prostate cancer due to his age.
   b. Perform a digital rectal examination to determine the size of the prostate.
   c. Draw a PSA level to rule out benign prostatic hyperplasia.
   d. Perform a digital rectal examination and draw a PSA level.

4. AJ is a 60-year-old man with a history of BPH. His most recent DRE was normal, but last PSA was 5.3 ng/mL. AJ is concerned about getting prostate cancer and wants to discuss preventative therapy. Which of the following is the most appropriate recommendation?
   a. Finasteride 5 mg daily
   b. Docetaxel 75 mg/m^2 + Prednisone 5 mg bid
   c. Leuprolide
   d. Surgery

5. SO is a 67–year-old man who was recently diagnosed with prostate cancer and is initiated on leuprolide for androgen ablation. Which of the following agents should be added to his therapy to prevent "tumor flare"?
   a. Bicalutamide
   b. Finasteride
   c. Mitoxantrone
   d. Goserelin

6. Which of the following side effects are associated with flutamide?
   a. Constipation
   b. Increased libido
   c. Rash
   d. Diarrhea

7. Which of the following LH-RH agonists is given subcutaneously every 12 months?
   a. Leuprolide implant (Viadur)
   b. Goserelin implant (Zoladex)
   c. Leuprolide depot (Lupron)
   d. Triptorelin depot (Trelstar Depot)

8. Which of the following LH-RH agonists contains coated pellets and is administered intramuscularly to allow for sustained levels throughout the dosing interval?
   a. Leuprolide implant (Viadur)
   b. Goserelin implant (Zoladex)
   c. Leuprolide depot (Lupron)
   d. Triptorelin depot (Trelstar Depot)

9. TR is a newly diagnosed prostate cancer patient being treated with androgen ablation. Which of the following are appropriate counseling points for a new patient starting on an LH-RH agonist?
   a. Patient may experience side effects such as a loss in libido, hot flushes, and impotence.
   b. Androgen deprivation therapy is associated with osteoporosis and therefore the patient should take a calcium/vitamin D supplement.
   c. Patient may experience worsening symptoms during the first week related to "tumor flare."
   d. All of the above.

10. What is the mechanism of action of Degarelix?
    a. LH-RH agonist
    b. Antiandrogen
    c. Androgen synthesis inhibitor
    d. GnRH antagonist

11. LB is a 63-year-old man with hormone refractory metastatic prostate cancer. He has several other comorbid diseases including CHF, diabetes, and hypertension. Which of the following chemotherapy agents is the most appropriate for this patient?
    a. Estramustine + docetaxel
    b. Mitoxantrone + prednisone
    c. Estramustine + docetaxel + mitoxantrone + prednisone
    d. Docetaxel + prednisone

12. BB is a 69-year-old man with metastatic prostate cancer who is receiving chemotherapy and a bisphosphonate, zoledronic acid. Which of the following tests should be monitored while this patient is on zoledronic acid?
    a. LFTs
    b. Urinalysis and urine culture and sensitivity
    c. Chem-7
    d. PFTs

13. Which of the following side effects is associated with antiandrogen use?
    a. Myelosuppression
    b. Gynecomastia
    c. Increased libido
    d. Rash
14. Which of the following antiandrogens is associated with alcohol intolerance?
    a. Flutamide
    b. Bicalutamide
    c. Nilutamide
    d. Leuprolide
15. Which of the following side effects has been associated with zoledronic acid use?
    a. Osteonecrosis of the jaw
    b. Gastroesophageal reflux disease (GERD)
    c. Diarrhea
    d. Constipation
16. Which of the following patients with prostate cancer can be managed with observation alone?
    a. Patient with a Gleason score of 3 and PSA of 5 ng/mL
    b. Patient with a Gleason score of 8 and PSA of 40 ng/mL
    c. Patient with a Gleason score of 2 and PSA of 15 ng/mL
    d. Patient with a Gleason score of 5 and PSA of 20 ng/mL
17. Which of the following statements is true?
    a. DRE is highly specific and highly sensitive for detecting prostate cancer and may be used alone for diagnosis.
    b. PSA is highly specific and highly sensitive for detecting prostate cancer and may be used alone for diagnosis.
    c. DRE and PSA are highly specific and highly sensitive for detecting prostate cancer and should be used in combination for diagnosis.
    d. Neither DRE nor PSA are highly specific or highly sensitive when used alone for detecting prostate cancer. Therefore, these agents should be used in combination for diagnosis.
18. The use of an antiandrogen and LH-RH agonists is called:
    a. Concurrent chemoprevention
    b. Concurrent chemoradiotherapy
    c. Combined androgen blockade
    d. None of the above
19. Which of the following is considered the primary site of metastases for prostate cancer?
    a. Liver
    b. Brain
    c. Lung
    d. Bone
20. Which of the following is the major pathologic cell type found in 95% of prostate cancers?
    a. Adenocarcinoma
    b. Melanoma
    c. Sarcoma
    d. Carcinoma

TAKEAWAY POINTS ››

- Prostate cancer is the most frequent cancer in American men.
- Risk factors for prostate cancer are age, race-ethnicity (African American ancestry), and family history of prostate cancer.
- Adenocarcinoma is the major pathologic cell type found in 95% of prostate cancer cases.
- Prostate cancer can be graded systematically according to the histologic appearance of the malignant cell and then grouped into well, moderately, or poorly differentiated grades based on the Gleason score.
- Skeletal metastases are the most common site of distant spread of prostate cancer.
- The testes and the adrenal glands are the major sources of circulating androgens.
- Hormonal regulation of androgen synthesis is mediated by a negative feedback loop involving the hypothalamus, pituitary gland, adrenal glands, and testes.
- Ureteral dysfunction, frequency, hesitancy, dribbling, and impotence are common symptoms in patients with prostate cancer.
- The combination of a DRE plus PSA determination is the best method for detecting prostate cancer.
- For prostate cancer screening, a baseline PSA and DRE at age 40 is recommended with annual evaluations beginning at age 50 to all men classified as having a normal risk with a 10-year or greater life expectancy. Men with an increased risk of prostate cancer, including men of African American ancestry, and men with a family history of prostate cancer may begin screening earlier at age 40 to 45.
- 5-alpha reductase inhibitors can be used for the prevention of prostate cancer.
- Prostate cancer managed by observation, radiation (external beam or brachytherapy), radical prostatectomy, androgen ablation, or chemotherapy depending on the stage and grade of the disease.

- Luteinizing hormone–releasing hormone (LH-RH) agonists are a reversible method of androgen ablation and are as effective as orchiectomy in treating prostate cancer.
- "Tumor flare" can be treated with antiandrogens.
- Common side effects of antiandrogens include gynecomastia, hot flushes, gastrointestinal disturbances, and LFT abnormalities.
- Chemotherapy may be used in patients with hormone refractory metastatic prostate cancer.
- Docetaxel and prednisone is the preferred chemotherapy agent in hormone refractory metastatic prostate cancer.
- Bisphosphonates may prevent skeletal related events and improve bone mineral density.

REFERENCES

1. American Cancer Society. *Cancer Facts and Figures 2009.* Atlanta, GA: American Cancer Society; 2009.
2. Thompson IM, Goodman PJ, Tangen CM, et al. The influence of finasteride on the development of prostate cancer. *N Engl J Med.* 2003;349:215-224.
3. Neill MG, Fleshner NE. An update on chemoprevention strategies in prostate cancer for 2006. *Curr Opin Urol.* 2006;16:132-137.
4. Khauli RB. Prostate cancer: diagnostic and therapeutic strategies with emphasis on the role of PSA. *J Med Liban.* 2005;53:95-102.
5. Iczkowski KA. Current prostate biopsy interpretation: criteria for cancer, atypical small acinar proliferation, high-grade prostatic intraepithelial neoplasia, and use of immunostains. *Arch Pathol Lab Med.* 2006;130:835-843.
6. De Marzo AM, Meeker AK, Zha S, et al. Human prostate cancer precursors and pathobiology. *Urology.* 2003;62:55-62.
7. Culig Z. Role of the androgen receptor axis in prostate cancer. *Urology.* 2003;62:21-26.
8. Marks LS. Luteinizing hormone-releasing hormone agonists in the treatment of men with prostate cancer: timing, alternatives, and the 1-year implant. *Urology.* 2003;62:36-42.
9. Sharifi N, Gulley JL, Dahut WL: Androgen deprivation therapy for prostate cancer. *JAMA.* 2005;294:238-244.
10. Cooperberg MR, Moul JW, Carroll PR. The changing face of prostate cancer. *J Clin Oncol.* 2005;23:8146-8151.
11. Labrie F, Dupont A, Cusan L, et al. Combination therapy with flutamide and medical (LHRH agonist) or surgical castration in advanced prostate cancer: 7-year clinical experience. *J Steroid Biochem Mol Biol.* 1990;37:943-950.
12. Galic J, Karner I, Cenan L, et al. Role of screening in detection of clinically localized prostate cancer. *Coll Antropol.* 2003;27 (suppl 1):49-54.
13. Wilson SS, Crawford ED. Screening for prostate cancer: current recommendations. *Urol Clin North Am.* 2004;31:219-226.
14. Gohagan JK, Prorok PC, Kramer BS, et al. The Prostate, Lung, Colorectal, and Ovarian-Cancer Screening Trial of the National-Cancer-Institute. *Cancer.* 1995;75: 1869-1873.
15. The NCCN Clinical Practice Guidelines in Oncology™ Prostate Cancer (Version 2.2009)®. National Comprehensive Cancer Network. Available at NCCN.org. Accessed June 15th, 2009.
16. Thompson IM, Goodman PJ, Tangen CM, et al. The influence of finasteride on the development of prostate cancer. *N Engl J Med.* 2003;349:215-224.
17. Musquera M, Fleshner NE, Finelli A, et al. The REDUCE trial: chemoprevention in prostate cancer using a dual 5-alpha-reductase inhibitor, dutasteride. *Expert Rev Anticancer Ther.* 2008;8:1073-1079.
18. Thorpe JF, Jain S, Marczylo TH, et al. A review of phase III clinical trials of prostate cancer chemoprevention. *Ann R Coll Surg Engl.* 2007;89:207-211.
19. Oh WK. Secondary hormonal therapies in the treatment of prostate cancer. *Urology.* 2002;60:87-92.
20. Maximum androgen blockade in advanced prostate cancer: an overview of the randomised trials. Prostate Cancer Trialists' Collaborative Group. *Lancet.* 2000;355:1491-1498.
21. www.firmagon.com. Accessed June 15, 2009.
22. Posadas EM, Dahut WL, Gulley J. The emerging role of bisphosphonates in prostate cancer. *Am J Ther.* 2004;11: 60-73.
23. Tannock IF, de Wit R, Berry WR, et al. Docetaxel plus prednisone or mitoxantrone plus prednisone for advanced prostate cancer. *N Engl J Med.* 2004;351:1502-1512.
24. Petrylak DP, Tangen CM, Hussain MH, et al. Docetaxel and estramustine compared with mitoxantrone and prednisone for advanced refractory prostate cancer. *N Engl J Med.* 2004;351:1513-1520.

CHAPTER

14 Breast Cancer

Robert K. Sylvester

FOUNDATION OVERVIEW

Breast cancer is the most prevalent malignancy in US women. It was estimated that approximately 192,000 US women were diagnosed with breast cancer in 2009. This number represents approximately 27% of all new cancer cases diagnosed in US women annually. Moreover, in 2009 an estimated 40,000 US women died of breast cancer making it the second leading cause of death from cancer after lung cancer. Breast cancer rarely affects men (2009 US estimates: 1910 new cases, 440 deaths). While breast cancer causes significant morbidity and mortality, death from breast cancer in the United States has been gradually declining since the early 1990s. The implementation of early detection guidelines and effective adjuvant therapy have been identified as approaches resulting in this positive trend.[1,2]

Pathophysiology

Mutations of genes controlling cell proliferation and apoptosis have been established as a primary cause of neoplastic disease. Specific gene mutations (*BRCA1, BRCA2, p53, PTEN*) have been identified in patients with breast cancer. Women with mutations in the tumor suppressor genes *BRCA1* and *BRCA2* have a four- to fivefold increased risk for the development of breast cancer (lifetime risk increases from 12% to 40%-60%).[3-6] In addition, prolonged exposure to estrogen (early menarche, nulliparity, late first pregnancy, late menopause) and age over 50 have been established as risk factors for breast cancer.[7]

Clinical Presentation/Diagnosis

Prior to the development of mammography, breast cancer was often diagnosed after a tissue biopsy of a painless breast mass that was palpated during self or clinical breast examination. The increased survival and improved quality of life for women whose breast cancer was diagnosed before it had spread to lymph nodes (micrometastatic disease) or to distant organs (metastatic disease) led to efforts to increase early detection of localized breast cancers. Since the widespread implementation of screening mammography guidelines in the mid-1980s, the majority of breast cancers are diagnosed after tissue biopsy of a suspicious lesion identified by mammography. The efficacy of mammography to detect breast cancer prior to the development of clinically detectable disease is supported by decreased death rates.[8,9]

After a breast mass is identified, the diagnosis of breast cancer is made by microscopic examination of a tissue biopsy. Breast cancers are categorized by the histologic and biologic characteristics of the cells present in the biopsy specimen. They arise from lobular and ductal epithelial cells and thus classified as adenocarcinomas. Furthermore, adenocarcinomas of the breast are classified as in situ (cancer confined to site of origin) or invasive (cancer that has spread through tissue barriers and invaded surrounding areas). The pathologic description of breast adenocarcinoma also includes the quantification of receptors present on surface of the breast cancer cells. Specifically, the pathology report will specify the level of expression of the estrogen receptor (ER), progesterone receptor (PR), and human epidermal growth factor receptor-2 (HER-2). These biologic markers are prognostic for a patient responding to drugs that target these receptors.[4,5]

Pharmacotherapy Overview

The development of effective pharmacotherapy for breast cancer has evolved considerably since hormonal and cytotoxic chemotherapy agents were first shown effective in the 1970s. Data from clinical research trials established that a patient's individual characteristics (ie, stage of disease, menopausal status, biologic markers, and risk factors for developing cancer) are critical to optimizing pharmacotherapy outcomes.

The stage of a patient's breast cancer is determined by the size of the primary lesion (T), whether regional lymph nodes contain micrometastatic cancer (N), and whether metastatic disease is present (M).[3,4] Stage I breast cancer is characterized by breast tumor ≤ 2 cm and regional lymph nodes that do not contain micrometastatic cancer. Stage II breast cancer exists when regional lymph nodes contain cancer or when the primary lesion is > 5 cm, even though lymph nodes do not contain cancer. Stage III breast cancer exists when either the primary tumor extends into the chest wall or when regional lymph nodes are fixed to surrounding tissue (immobile). Stage IV disease is present when the tumor cells have invaded distant tissue (metastatic disease). Common sites of breast cancer metastases include the bone, liver, and lungs. Survival of women with invasive breast cancer correlates with the stage of disease. Five-year survival rates for women with localized breast cancer (stages I, II), locally advanced breast cancer (stage III), and metastatic breast cancer (stage IV) are 98.1%, 83.1%, and 26%, respectively.[10,11]

The ability of hormonal and cytotoxic chemotherapy agents to slow the growth of metastatic (stage IV) breast cancer was first reported in the 1970s. Since then, seven new classes of antineoplastic drugs to treat breast cancer have been

TABLE 14-1 **Pharmacotherapeutic Classes/Indications for Management of Breast Cancer**

Antineoplastic Class	Effective Drugs	Indications		
		Stage 4 (Metastatic)	Stages 1-3 (Adjuvant)	Prevention
Alkylating agent	Cyclophosphamide (Cytoxan)	√	√	
Anthracycline antibiotics	Doxorubicin (Adriamycin)	√	√	
	Epirubicin (Ellence)	√	√	
Antimetabolites	5-Fluorouracil	√	√	
	Capecitabine (Xeloda)	√		
	Methotrexate	√	√	
	Gemcitabine (Gemzar)			
Microtubule inhibitors Taxanes	Paclitaxel (Taxol)	√	√	
	Albumin-bound paclitaxel	√		
	(Abraxane)	√	√	
	Docetaxel (Taxotere)			
Vinca alkaloid	Vinorelbine (Navelbine)	√		
Epothilone	Ixabepilone (Ixempra)	√		
Monoclonal antibodies	Trastuzumab (Herceptin)	√	√	
	Bevacizumab (Avastin)	√		
Selective estrogen receptor modulators (SERMs)	Tamoxifen (Nolvadex)	√	√	√
	Toremifene (Fareston)	√		
	Raloxifene (Evista)			√
Aromatase inhibitors	Anastrozole (Arimidex)	√	√	
	Letrozole (Femara)	√	√	
	Exemestane (Aromasin)	√	√	
Estrogen receptor antagonist	Fulvestrant (Faslodex)	√		
Signal transduction inhibitor	Lapatinib (Tykerb)	√		

developed. Subsequent research proved that drugs effective in treating patients with metastatic breast cancer were also effective in increasing the overall survival (OS) and disease-free survival (DFS) of women at increased risk of developing metastatic breast cancer following surgery.

The term systemic adjuvant therapy describes the administration of antineoplastic therapy to women after surgical resection of the primary cancer (lumpectomy or modified mastectomy). Systemic adjuvant therapy is administered to eradicate or suppress the growth of breast cancer cells that have spread beyond the breast at the time of surgery. Patients with breast cancers larger than 1 cm or cancer that has spread to lymph nodes at the time of surgery are at increased risk for cancer recurrence. Administration of systemic adjuvant antineoplastic therapy results in significant improvement in patient's DFS and OS.[2,4,5]

The administration of tamoxifen as systemic adjuvant therapy also resulted in the reduction of new breast cancers. Subsequently, two selective estrogen receptor modulators (SERMs) were proven effective in reducing the incidence of breast cancer in women with characteristics placing them at high risk.

Currently, over 20 antineoplastic agents are commonly administered to treat patients with metastatic disease. At least 12 agents are effective in slowing the progression of micrometastatic breast cancer (systemic adjuvant therapy), and two selective estrogen receptor modulators (SERMs) are effective in reducing the risk of women at high risk for developing breast cancer (Table 14-1). The National Comprehensive Cancer Network (NCCN) practice guidelines provide valuable evidence-based recommendations for the use of these agents in the management of breast cancer.[3,4]

PREVENTION

Tamoxifen is a SERM that received the FDA labeled indication for the treatment of metastatic breast cancer in 1977. Twenty-one years later, results from the breast cancer prevention trial documented that tamoxifen was also effective in reducing the risk of breast cancer in women at high risk. SERMs inhibit proliferation of breast cancer by blocking the binding of estrogens to the estrogen receptor. The criterion for defining a woman as being at "high risk" for breast cancer was 1.7% or greater chance of being diagnosed with invasive breast cancer within 5 years. This risk estimate was calculated using a statistical model known as the "Gail model."[12] The Breast Cancer Prevention Trial randomized 13,338 women meeting the "high-risk" criteria to tamoxifen 20 mg tablets daily or placebo for 5 years. After 7 years of follow-up, the incidence of invasive breast cancer in the tamoxifen group was 49% lower than the incidence in the placebo group (43.4/1000 vs 22/1000 women).[13] In 1998 the FDA approved label for Nolvadex (tamoxifen) was amended to include an indication for reduction in risk of invasive breast cancer in women.[14]

In comparison to placebo, tamoxifen was associated with statistically significant increased risks of the following adverse effects: endometrial cancer, bothersome hot flashes, vaginal discharge, and thromboembolic events (deep venous thrombosis and pulmonary emboli) in women aged 50 years and older. Randomized trials evaluating treatment regimens exceeding 5 years did not produce additional benefit, but did document an increase in adverse events. Consequently, the recommended duration of tamoxifen administered to reduce the risk of invasive breast cancer is 5 years.[13]

Raloxifene is a second-generation SERM initially approved by the FDA for treating postmenopausal osteoporosis. Data from studies conducted in postmenopausal women with osteoporosis suggested that it may also reduce the incidence of invasive breast cancer. In addition, raloxifene had the potential advantage of being less likely to cause uterine cancer. These data provided the rationale for the Study of Tamoxifen And Raloxifene (STAR) trial. This clinical trial randomized over 19,000 women at "high risk" to take tamoxifen 20 mg daily or raloxifene 60 mg daily for 5 years. Both agents are manufactured as tablets for oral administration. Study results established that raloxifene is as effective as tamoxifen in reducing the risk of invasive breast cancer and has an improved toxicity profile. Specifically, raloxifene was associated with a significantly lower incidence of thromboembolic events and cataracts. Although raloxifene was associated with a lower incidence of uterine cancer (annual incidence rate 1.25/1000 vs 2/1000 women), the difference was not significant ($P = .07$).[15] These data resulted in the FDA revising the Evista (raloxifene) label in 2007 to include an indication to reduce the risk of invasive breast cancer in postmenopausal women.[16]

In summary, tamoxifen and raloxifene taken for 5 years reduce by approximately 50% the risk of "high-risk" women developing breast cancer. No data have been published establishing that either drug lowers the death rate from breast cancer. While raloxifene has been established as the preferred agent in postmenopausal women because of its superior side effect profile, inadequate data exist to support its use in premenopausal high-risk women. Prior thromboembolic events (ie, deep venous thrombosis, pulmonary emboli, stroke) are contraindications to the administration of tamoxifen and raloxifene for the prevention of breast cancer.[3]

Pharmacists providing care to women taking tamoxifen or raloxifene should routinely assess patients for possible treatment-related adverse reactions. Both drugs are linked to increased risk of deep venous thrombosis, pulmonary embolism, and strokes. The development of any thromboembolic events is a contraindication to continued prophylactic therapy. Tamoxifen has also been associated with increased risk of developing cataracts and endometrial cancer. Consequently, women taking tamoxifen who experience changes in vision should be encouraged to have an ophthalmologic examination; women with an intact uterus reporting vaginal spotting should be recommended to undergo a gynecologic examination.[3,13] Another prominent side effect of tamoxifen is bothersome hot flashes which occur at a rate 12% higher than placebo (81% vs 69%).[13] Various agents have been evaluated for reducing the frequency and severity of tamoxifen-related hot flashes (gabapentin, selective serotonin reuptake inhibitors [SSRIs] and depomedroxyprogesterone acetate).[17,18]

Two studies reported conflicting data regarding the effects of SSRIs on breast cancer recurrence rates in women taking tamoxifen as adjuvant therapy. A US study reported that women taking tamoxifen concomitantly with SSRIs that are strong inhibitors of CYP2D6 (fluoxetine, paroxetine, sertraline) had a statistically significant increase in breast cancer recurrence within 2 years (13.9% vs 7.5%).[19] CYP2D6 is the enzyme responsible for metabolizing tamoxifen to its major active metabolite endoxifen. A Dutch study did not find an association between SSRI therapy and an increased breast cancer recurrence rate in women taking adjuvant tamoxifen therapy.[20] The administration of tamoxifen with fluoxetine, paroxetine, and sertraline should be avoided until further research critically evaluates the effects of different SSRIs on the efficacy of tamoxifen.

TREATMENT

Pharmacotherapy for Patients at Increased Risk of Developing Recurrent Breast Cancer After Surgery (Stages I, II, III)

At the time of lumpectomy or modified mastectomy, a pathologist determines the size of the patient's mass and performs a microscopic evaluation of regional lymph nodes removed at the time of surgery. If any of the patient's lymph nodes contain breast cancer, that patient has micrometastatic disease (positive lymph nodes). Women diagnosed with micrometastatic disease in lymph nodes or a primary breast cancer > 1 cm are at increased risk of subsequently developing metastatic breast cancer.[4,5]

Systemic adjuvant therapy describes the administration of antineoplastic therapy to women at an increased risk of developing metastatic breast cancer after surgery. Adjuvant hormonal, chemotherapy, and trastuzumab regimens have resulted in statistically significant improvement in both the duration of disease-free and overall survival.

The majority of drugs proven effective in treating patients with metastatic disease have also been proven effective in prolonging the DFS and OS of women at risk of disease recurrence (see Table 14-1). A patient's menopausal status and biologic characteristics of the cancer (ER status, HER-2 status) are critical for selecting appropriate systemic adjuvant antineoplastic regimens.[4,5]

Adjuvant Endocrine Therapy

Tamoxifen and aromatase inhibitors (anastrozole, letrozole, and exemestane) are effective systemic adjuvant agents for women with ER+ breast cancer. Tamoxifen has achieved improvements in the DFS and OS of both premenopausal and postmenopausal women. The recommended duration of therapy is 5 years. Continuing tamoxifen beyond 5 years has not been shown to increase benefit, but has been associated with increased risk of adverse events (thromboembolic events, uterine cancer). Adjuvant therapy with aromatase inhibitors is also effective in increasing the DFS and OS of postmenopausal women with ER+ breast cancers. Several different dosing regimens have proven effective. Typically, they are administered for 5 years, either as initial therapy or following 3 to 5 years of tamoxifen.[4,5]

Adjuvant Cytotoxic Chemotherapy

Many combination cytotoxic chemotherapy regimens have been proven effective in prolonging the DFS and OS for women with ER–micrometastatic breast cancers. Combinations of cyclophosphamide, doxorubicin, and a taxane administered for 4 to 6 months are examples of preferred regimens. NCCN breast cancer guidelines are an excellent source for specific adjuvant chemotherapy regimens.[4]

Adjuvant Trastuzumab Therapy

Combination cytotoxic chemotherapy followed by 1 year of trastuzumab has resulted in a significant improvement in the OS of women with HER-2 positive, ER–breast cancer.[4,31]

Pharmacotherapy for Patients with Metastatic Breast Cancer (Stage IV)

Metastatic breast cancer is rarely curable in spite of the availability of drugs that target breast cancer cells in diverse ways. Although at least 50% of women diagnosed with metastatic disease will respond to their initial antineoplastic therapy, most will have progression of the disease within 6 to 8 months. Typically, the duration of remission achieved after subsequent second- and third-line therapies becomes progressively shorter. The median survival of women diagnosed with metastatic breast cancer is approximately 2 years. The biologic characteristics of the breast cancer cells (estrogen receptor and HER-2 status) and the woman's menopausal status are essential in determining the appropriate treatment.[4,5]

If a woman's breast cancer expresses estrogen receptors, endocrine therapy is the initial therapy; if the breast cancer does not express estrogen receptors, cytotoxic chemotherapy is recommended as initial therapy. Trastuzumab is only indicated for women with breast cancers that overexpress HER-2.[4,5,31]

Endocrine Therapy

Three types of endocrine therapy are effective in treating breast cancer. Table 14-2 provides specific dosing regimens and toxicity profiles for these drugs. Sixty to seventy percent of women with ER+ disease respond to initial endocrine treatment. The duration of response is approximately 1 year. A therapeutic trial of several months is recommended since the full therapeutic benefit may not be evident earlier.

TABLE 14-2 Medications That Alter Estrogen Effects and Associated Side Effects

		Dose	Side Effects
SERMs	Tamoxifen (Nolvadex)	20 mg orally daily	Hot flashes Vaginal discharge
	Toremifene (Fareston)	60 mg orally daily	Blood coagulation Endometrial cancer
Aromatase inhibitors	Anastrozole (Arimidex)	1 mg orally daily	Hot flashes Arthralgias
	Letrozole (Femara)	2.5 mg orally daily	Myalgias
	Exemestane (Aromasin)	25 mg orally daily	
Estrogen antagonist	Fulvestrant (Faslodex)	250 mg IM every 28 d	Hot flashes Injection site reactions

When disease progression occurs, a trial of an alternative endocrine treatment is recommended until the disease becomes refractory to hormonal treatments. Patients with hormone refractory ER+ disease are candidates for cytotoxic chemotherapy.[4,5]

SERMs Tamoxifen is the SERM of choice for premenopausal women with ER+ breast cancer. The standard dosage regimen is an oral dose of 20 mg administered daily until the patient experiences disease progression.[4,5] While generally well tolerated, it is imperative that pharmacists counsel women about potential adverse effects and significant drug interactions with paroxetine, fluoxetine, and sertraline as described earlier.

Aromatase Inhibitors Anastrozole, letrozole, and exemestane are aromatase inhibitors (AIs) effective as systemic adjuvant therapy in treating micrometastatic and metastatic breast cancer. Aromatase is an enzyme present in non-ovarian tissues (eg, fat and adrenal gland) and is responsible for producing estradiol in postmenopausal women by converting androgen precursors to estradiol. These agents produce their benefit by depleting estradiol production from non-ovarian tissues in postmenopausal women. The AIs are considered to be therapeutically equivalent. Commonly prescribed dosing regimens and associated side effects are detailed in Table 14-2. Typically, arthralgias and myalgias are reported by 10% to 20% of women 1 to 2 months after beginning therapy.[4,5] A trial with an alternative AI is recommended if a patient develops arthralgias and or myalgias based on reports of individual differences in tolerability.[21]

Pure Estrogen Antagonist Fulvestrant is a pure estrogen antagonist that inhibits ER-mediated gene transcription by binding to and down-regulating estrogen receptors. It is effective in the treatment for postmenopausal women with ER+ metastatic breast cancer whose disease progresses after antiestrogen therapy. Fulvestrant is administered monthly as a 250 mg intramuscular injection. Common side effects include injection site reactions and hot flashes.[22]

Cytotoxic Chemotherapy

Cytotoxic antineoplastic drugs disrupt DNA replication. Their action is nonspecific and disrupts the replication of neoplastic and normal cells, especially normal cells with more rapid growth rates. Cytotoxic chemotherapy agents share many of the same dose-dependent toxicities. Among these are myelosuppression (neutropenia, thrombocytopenia, anemia), alopecia, mucositis, nausea and vomiting. Neutropenia and thrombocytopenia are potentially life threatening. Consequently, it is generally recommended that patient's absolute neutrophil count is > 1500 cells/mm^3 and platelets > 100,000 cells/mm^3 before any additional doses are administered.

These drugs can be administered as single agents or in combination with one or two additional drugs. The administration of single-agent chemotherapy offers the advantage of less toxicity while providing efficacy comparable to combination regimens. The NCCN guidelines identify 9 "preferred" single chemotherapy agents and 10 "preferred" chemotherapy combinations as appropriate for the treatment of metastatic breast cancer.[4] Approximately 50% of women respond to initial chemotherapy treatment. However, progression of disease typically occurs within 8 months. Patients are switched to a chemotherapy agent from another class if the initial chemotherapy agent is not effective or when their disease progresses. Table 14-3 provides specific dosing regimens and toxicity profiles for these agents.[4,5]

Alkylating Agents Numerous alkylating agents provide palliative benefit for women with metastatic breast cancer. Cyclophosphamide has proven superior to other agents in this class by achieving overall response rates (partial plus complete responses) in one-third of treated patients. Subsequently, trials of combinations of cyclophosphamide with other cytotoxic chemotherapy agents resulted in response rates up to 50%. Cyclophosphamide is metabolized to reactive electrophilic alkyl groups that bind to nucleophilic groups on nucleotide bases in DNA, thereby disrupting DNA replication.[5]

Antimetabolites Numerous antimetabolites have been proven effective in providing palliative benefit to patients with metastatic breast cancer. Methotrexate and 5-fluorouracil have long been combined with cyclophosphamide and was the standard of care until doxorubicin combinations resulted in higher response rates.

TABLE 14-3 Cytotoxic Chemotherapy Agents and Associated Side Effects

Chemotherapy Agent	Dosage Regimen	Side Effects[a]
Alkylating Agent		
Cyclophosphamide (Cytoxan)	500-600 mg/m^2 IV 75 mg/m^2 po days 1-14	Nausea, vomiting, rarely hemorrhagic cystitis
Anthracycline Antibiotics		
Doxorubicin (Adriamycin)	50 to 60 mg/m^2 IV	Cardiomyopathy, tissue necrosis if extravasation occurs
Epirubicin (Ellence)	100 mg/m^2 IV	Cardiomyopathy, tissue necrosis if extravasation occurs
Antimetabolites		
5-Fluorouracil	500-600 mg/m^2 IV	Nausea, vomiting, diarrhea
Capecitabine[b] (Xeloda)	2000-2500 mg/m^2 per day po divided twice daily for 14 d	Hand-foot syndrome, diarrhea
Gemcitabine (Gemzar)	600-1000 mg/m^2 IV bolus per week days 1, 8, and 15	Nausea, vomiting, diarrhea
Methotrexate	40 mg/m^2 IV	Nausea, vomiting, diarrhea
Antimicrotubule Agents		
Taxanes		
Paclitaxel[c] (Taxol)	175 mg/m^2 IV over 3 h every 21 d or 80 mg/m^2 IV over 1 h weekly	Hypersensitivity/infusion reactions, nausea, vomiting, diarrhea, peripheral neuropathy, myalgias, arthralgias, elevated ALT/AST
Albumin-bound paclitaxel[c] (Abraxane)	260 mg/m^2 over 30 min every 3 wk	Nausea, vomiting, diarrhea, peripheral neuropathy, myalgias, arthralgias, elevated ALT/AST, hypersensitivity/infusion reactions
Docetaxel[c] (Taxotere)	60-100 mg/m^2 IV over 1 h every 21 d or 30-35 mg/m^2 IV over 0.5 h weekly	Hypersensitivity/infusion reactions, nausea, vomiting, diarrhea, stomatitis, peripheral neuropathy, myalgias, arthralgias, elevated ALT/AST, fluid retention
Vinca alkaloid		
Vinorelbine[c] (Navelbine)	25-30 mg/m^2 IV bolus weekly	Peripheral neuropathy, reactions, nausea, vomiting
Epothilone		
Ixabepilone (Ixempra)	40 mg/m^2 IV over 3 h every 21 d	Hypersensitivity/infusion reactions, nausea, vomiting, diarrhea, peripheral neuropathy, myalgias, arthralgias

[a]Side effects other than common shared toxicities of myelosuppression (neutropenia, thrombocytopenia, anemia), alopecia, and stomatitis.

[b]A dosage reduction of 25% is recommended for patients with creatinine clearances between 30 and 50 mL/min.

[c]Dosage adjustment recommended for patients with hepatic dysfunction characterized by elevated serum bilirubin, alanine or aspartate transaminase; see manufacturer's package insert for specifics.

Methotrexate impedes cell growth by inhibiting dihydrofolate reductase, the enzyme needed to reduce folates to the active form (tetrahydrofolic acid) required for purine and thymidylate synthesis. 5-Fluorouracil is a pyrimidine analogue that is metabolized to fluorodeoxyuridine monophosphate (FdUMP). This metabolite inhibits the enzyme thymidylate synthase which is responsible for thymidine synthesis.[5] Capecitabine is a fluoropyrimidine analog that is administered orally and metabolized to FdUMP, the same active metabolite as 5-fluorouracil. Nonhematologic side effects of note are painful swelling and redness of the hands and feet (hand-foot syndrome), stomatitis (inflammation of mouth), and diarrhea. Patients experiencing painful hand-foot syndrome or stomatitis or more than 4 to 6 stools daily should be instructed to stop taking capecitabine immediately.[23]

The enzyme dihydropyrimidine dehydrogenase (DPD) is responsible for the degradation of 5-fluorouracil to inactive metabolites. Approximately 5% of the population has a DPD deficiency, a contraindication to the administration of capecitabine because of an increased risk of potentially life-threatening mucositis, diarrhea, and myelosuppression. It is also contraindicated in patients with creatinine clearances below 30 mL/min. The ability of 5-fluorouracil and capecitabine to significantly increase warfarin's anticoagulant effects is well documented. Closer monitoring of a patient's INR is required when these drugs are given concomitantly.[23]

Anthracycline Antibiotics Doxorubicin and epirubicin are two anthracycline antibiotics administered as single agents or in combination with other antineoplastic agents as systemic adjuvant treatment or for palliation of symptoms in patients with metastatic breast cancer. They damage DNA by inhibiting the enzyme topoisomerase II that is needed for the normal coiling/uncoiling of DNA and by binding of reactive electrophilic sites on the drugs to nucleophilic nucleotides in DNA.[5]

Cardiomyopathy resulting in congestive heart failure is a dose-related toxicity of anthracyclines. The incidence of cardiomyopathy increases with cumulative doses of both doxorubicin and epirubicin. Therefore, cumulative doses of doxorubicin exceeding 400 mg/m^2 and epirubicin exceeding 900 mg/m^2 should be administered cautiously. These drugs are potent vesicants and can result in severe tissue necrosis at sites of extravasation. They are cleared hepatically. Specific recommendations for dose modification of doxorubicin and epirubicin based on a patient's serum bilirubin and aspartate transaminases are published in the products' FDA approved package insert.[24,25]

Microtubule Inhibitors Microtubules are structures critical to the successful completion of cell division (mitosis). Three subclasses of cytotoxic chemotherapy agents that disrupt normal microtubule function are effective in treating breast cancer. Table 14-3 provides commonly prescribed dosing regimens and associated side effects of these agents.[5]

Taxanes Paclitaxel, albumin-bound paclitaxel, and docetaxel bind to β-tubulin, a protein needed to form microtubules. As a result, taxanes inhibit depolymerization of the microtubules, a terminal phase in cell division. Taxanes are effective agents in treating patients with locally advanced and advanced disease.

A prominent side effect of paclitaxel is the occurrence of infusion-related hypersensitivity reactions. Typically, these reactions are characterized by the onset of symptoms (eg, dyspnea, flushing, tachycardia, chest pain) within 1 hour of administration. These symptoms are attributed to mast cell degranulation caused by Cremophor EL, the surfactant used to increase the solubility of paclitaxel. Premedication with corticosteroids, an H1 and an H2 antagonist, is standard care for any patient receiving paclitaxel.[5,26]

Abraxane, a nanoparticle albumin-bound paclitaxel formulation, is a paclitaxel formulation that does not contain Cremophor EL and does not require premedication. The reported incidence of hypersensitivity reactions are 4% for nanoparticle albumin-bound paclitaxel and 12% for paclitaxel. Paclitaxel is contraindicated in patients with a documented history of a hypersensitivity reaction to Cremophor EL and/or paclitaxel.[26,27]

Docetaxel is contraindicated in patients with a history of severe hypersensitivity reactions. Fluid retention occurs in nearly 25% of patients. Premedication with dexamethasone is recommended to attenuate this adverse effect.[28]

Epothilones Ixabepilone is the prototype semisynthetic analog of epothilone B. It inhibits the depolymerization of microtubules by binding to a β-tubulin site different than the taxane binding site. Ixabepilone should not be administered to patients with alanine aminotransferase or aspartate aminotransferase > 2.5 times the upper limit of normal or bilirubin > 1 times upper limits of normal since there is an increased risk of potentially life-threatening liver toxicity. Cremophor EL is used to increase ixabepilone solubility. Premedication with an H1 and an H2 antagonist an hour prior to administering ixabepilone is recommended in order to minimize hypersensitivity reactions. If a patient develops a hypersensitivity reaction, the addition of dexamethasone to the pretreatment regimen is recommended. Ixabepilone is contraindicated in patients with a history of hypersensitivity reactions to drugs formulated with Cremophor EL.[29]

Vinca Alkaloids Vinorelbine is a semisynthetic vinca alkaloid that impedes mitosis by inhibiting the formation of functioning microtubules. It should be administered with caution to patients with elevated serum bilirubin levels. If a patient's serum bilirubin level is between 2.1 to 3 mg/dL, a 50% dosage reduction is recommended; if a patient's serum bilirubin level exceeds 3 mg/dL, a 70% dosage reduction is recommended.[30]

Monoclonal Antibodies Trastuzumab and bevacizumab are two humanized monoclonal antibodies approved for the treatment of metastatic breast cancer. Table 14-4 provides specific dosing regimens and toxicity profiles of these agents.

Twenty to thirty percent of patients have breast cancers that overexpress the human epidermal growth factor receptor-2 (HER-2). Trastuzumab was developed to bind to the HER-2 receptor. This interaction may cause cell death by several mechanisms. Cell lysis may result from the activation of the complement cascade and/or the enhanced recognition of the antibody-tagged cells by cytotoxic T lymphocytes. Cell growth may also be impeded by the inhibition of normal intracellular

TABLE 14-4 **Monoclonal Antibodies and Associated Side Effects**

Monoclonal Antibody	Dosage Regimen	Side Effects
Targets HER-2		
Trastuzumab (Herceptin)	Initial dose of 4 mg/kg as a 90 min IV infusion followed by subsequent weekly doses of 2 mg/kg as 30 min IV infusions (as tolerated)	Infusion reactions, fever, chills, congestive heart failure, cough, diarrhea, headache
Targets VEGF		
Bevacizumab (Avastin)	10 mg/kg every 2 wk as IV infusion: First infusion: Administer over 90 min Subsequent infusions: Administer second infusion over 60 min if first infusion is tolerated; administer all subsequent infusions over 30 min if infusion over 60 min is tolerated as IV infusion	Infusion reactions, chills, fever, hypertension, proteinuria, thromboembolic events, gastrointestinal perforation

signaling pathways that occurs when the binding of growth factor to growth factor receptor is blocked.[31]

Bevacizumab is a monoclonal antibody developed to bind to and inhibit vascular endothelial growth factor (VEGF). VEGF is the endogenous protein produced by cells to stimulate the growth of blood vessels in the vicinity of its release. The scientific term for this process is angiogenesis. Bevacizumab possesses antiangiogenic activity by binding to and blocking VEGF from binding to cell receptors that stimulate angiogensis.[32]

Signal Transduction Inhibitor Lapatinib is the first signal transduction inhibitor active against breast cancer cells. It is approved to be given with capecitabine as a combination treatment of metastatic breast cancer for patients with HER-2 positive disease that has progressed after therapy with an anthracycline, a taxane, and trastuzumab. It inhibits intracellular tyrosine kinase activity of epidermal growth factor receptor-1 (EGFR-1) and EGFR-2. Lapatinib should be taken at least 1 hour before or after a meal. This instruction is important because lapatinib taken within 1 hour of a meal has resulted in mean AUC increases ranging from 167% to 325%. Lapatinib is extensively metabolized by CYP3A4. Consequently, significant drug interactions can occur when lapatinib is administered concurrently with strong inhibitors or inducers of CYP3A4. It is recommended that concurrent administration of lapatinib with strong CYP3A4 inhibitors (eg, azole antifungal agents, protease inhibitors) and strong CYP3A4 inducers (ie, carbamazepine, dexamethasone, phenytoin, rifampin, phenobarbital) be avoided. If concurrent administration cannot be avoided, it is imperative to cautiously titrate the dose of lapatinib based on patient tolerability. Table 14-5 provides the recommended lapatinib dosing regimen and associated adverse events.[33]

TABLE 14-5 **Signal Transduction Inhibitor and Associated Side Effects**

Signal Transduction Inhibitor	Dosage Regimen	Side Effects
Targets EGFR-1, EGFR-2		
Lapatinib (Tykerb)	1250 mg po once daily at least 1 h before or 1 h after a meal on days 1-21 continuously	Maculopapular rash, diarrhea, decreased left ventricular ejection fraction, rarely severe hepatotoxicity

CASE Application

1. Select the agent that is administered via intramuscular injection for the treatment of metastatic estrogen receptor positive breast cancer.

   a. Anastrozole
   b. Avastin
   c. Herceptin
   d. Faslodex
   e. Femara

2. Which of the following conditions would be a contraindication to administration of tamoxifen for the prevention of breast cancer in a "high-risk" premenopausal patient?

   a. History of deep venous thrombosis
   b. First-degree relative with ER negative breast cancer
   c. History of diabetes mellitus
   d. History of seizures
   e. None of the above

3. A premenopausal woman with ER negative, node positive breast cancer is starting doxorubicin and cyclophosphamide adjuvant treatment. What would you recommend to monitor the most common toxicity associated with this treatment regimen?

   a. An electrocardiogram 1 week after chemotherapy.
   b. A complete blood count including platelets 1 week after chemotherapy.
   c. Serum bilirubin and aspartate transaminase 1 week after chemotherapy.
   d. Urinalysis 1 week after chemotherapy.

4. Select the toxicity that has been associated with the administration of both trastuzumab and bevacizumab.

   a. Myelosuppression
   b. GI perforation
   c. Alopecia
   d. Infusion reactions

5. Select the appropriate premedication regimen that is recommended to be administered prior to the administration of paclitaxel.

   a. Dexamethasone, ranitidine
   b. Ranitidine and diphenhydramine

TABLE 14-4 Monoclonal Antibodies and Associated Side Effects

Monoclonal Antibody	Dosage Regimen	Side Effects
Targets HER-2		
Trastuzumab (Herceptin)	Initial dose of 4 mg/kg as a 90 min IV infusion followed by subsequent weekly doses of 2 mg/kg as 30 min IV infusions (as tolerated)	Infusion reactions, fever, chills, congestive heart failure, cough, diarrhea, headache
Targets VEGF		
Bevacizumab (Avastin)	10 mg/kg every 2 wk as IV infusion: First infusion: Administer over 90 min Subsequent infusions: Administer second infusion over 60 min if first infusion is tolerated; administer all subsequent infusions over 30 min if infusion over 60 min is tolerated as IV infusion	Infusion reactions, chills, fever, hypertension, proteinuria, thromboembolic events, gastrointestinal perforation

signaling pathways that occurs when the binding of growth factor to growth factor receptor is blocked.[31]

Bevacizumab is a monoclonal antibody developed to bind to and inhibit vascular endothelial growth factor (VEGF). VEGF is the endogenous protein produced by cells to stimulate the growth of blood vessels in the vicinity of its release. The scientific term for this process is angiogenesis. Bevacizumab possesses antiangiogenic activity by binding to and blocking VEGF from binding to cell receptors that stimulate angiogensis.[32]

Signal Transduction Inhibitor Lapatinib is the first signal transduction inhibitor active against breast cancer cells. It is approved to be given with capecitabine as a combination treatment of metastatic breast cancer for patients with HER-2 positive disease that has progressed after therapy with an anthracycline, a taxane, and trastuzumab. It inhibits intracellular tyrosine kinase activity of epidermal growth factor receptor-1 (EGFR-1) and EGFR-2. Lapatinib should be taken at least 1 hour before or after a meal. This instruction is important because lapatinib taken within 1 hour of a meal has resulted in mean AUC increases ranging from 167% to 325%. Lapatinib is extensively metabolized by CYP3A4. Consequently, significant drug interactions can occur when lapatinib is administered concurrently with strong inhibitors or inducers of CYP3A4. It is recommended that concurrent administration of lapatinib with strong CYP3A4 inhibitors (eg, azole antifungal agents, protease inhibitors) and strong CYP3A4 inducers (ie, carbamazepine, dexamethasone, phenytoin, rifampin, phenobarbital) be avoided. If concurrent administration cannot be avoided, it is imperative to cautiously titrate the dose of lapatinib based on patient tolerability. Table 14-5 provides the recommended lapatinib dosing regimen and associated adverse events.[33]

TABLE 14-5 Signal Transduction Inhibitor and Associated Side Effects

Signal Transduction Inhibitor	Dosage Regimen	Side Effects
Targets EGFR-1, EGFR-2		
Lapatinib (Tykerb)	1250 mg po once daily at least 1 h before or 1 h after a meal on days 1-21 continuously	Maculopapular rash, diarrhea, decreased left ventricular ejection fraction, rarely severe hepatotoxicity

CASE Application

1. Select the agent that is administered via intramuscular injection for the treatment of metastatic estrogen receptor positive breast cancer.
   a. Anastrozole
   b. Avastin
   c. Herceptin
   d. Faslodex
   e. Femara
2. Which of the following conditions would be a contraindication to administration of tamoxifen for the prevention of breast cancer in a "high-risk" premenopausal patient?
   a. History of deep venous thrombosis
   b. First-degree relative with ER negative breast cancer
   c. History of diabetes mellitus
   d. History of seizures
   e. None of the above
3. A premenopausal woman with ER negative, node positive breast cancer is starting doxorubicin and cyclophosphamide adjuvant treatment. What would you recommend to monitor the most common toxicity associated with this treatment regimen?
   a. An electrocardiogram 1 week after chemotherapy.
   b. A complete blood count including platelets 1 week after chemotherapy.
   c. Serum bilirubin and aspartate transaminase 1 week after chemotherapy.
   d. Urinalysis 1 week after chemotherapy.
4. Select the toxicity that has been associated with the administration of both trastuzumab and bevacizumab.
   a. Myelosuppression
   b. GI perforation
   c. Alopecia
   d. Infusion reactions
5. Select the appropriate premedication regimen that is recommended to be administered prior to the administration of paclitaxel.
   a. Dexamethasone, ranitidine
   b. Ranitidine and diphenhydramine

Methotrexate impedes cell growth by inhibiting dihydrofolate reductase, the enzyme needed to reduce folates to the active form (tetrahydrofolic acid) required for purine and thymidylate synthesis. 5-Fluorouracil is a pyrimidine analogue that is metabolized to fluorodeoxyuridine monophosphate (FdUMP). This metabolite inhibits the enzyme thymidylate synthase which is responsible for thymidine synthesis.[5] Capecitabine is a fluoropyrimidine analog that is administered orally and metabolized to FdUMP, the same active metabolite as 5-fluorouracil. Nonhematologic side effects of note are painful swelling and redness of the hands and feet (hand-foot syndrome), stomatitis (inflammation of mouth), and diarrhea. Patients experiencing painful hand-foot syndrome or stomatitis or more than 4 to 6 stools daily should be instructed to stop taking capecitabine immediately.[23]

The enzyme dihydropyrimidine dehydrogenase (DPD) is responsible for the degradation of 5-fluorouracil to inactive metabolites. Approximately 5% of the population has a DPD deficiency, a contraindication to the administration of capecitabine because of an increased risk of potentially life-threatening mucositis, diarrhea, and myelosuppression. It is also contraindicated in patients with creatinine clearances below 30 mL/min. The ability of 5-fluorouracil and capecitabine to significantly increase warfarin's anticoagulant effects is well documented. Closer monitoring of a patient's INR is required when these drugs are given concomitantly.[23]

Anthracycline Antibiotics Doxorubicin and epirubicin are two anthracycline antibiotics administered as single agents or in combination with other antineoplastic agents as systemic adjuvant treatment or for palliation of symptoms in patients with metastatic breast cancer. They damage DNA by inhibiting the enzyme topoisomerase II that is needed for the normal coiling/uncoiling of DNA and by binding of reactive electrophilic sites on the drugs to nucleophilic nucleotides in DNA.[5]

Cardiomyopathy resulting in congestive heart failure is a dose-related toxicity of anthracyclines. The incidence of cardiomyopathy increases with cumulative doses of both doxorubicin and epirubicin. Therefore, cumulative doses of doxorubicin exceeding 400 mg/m^2 and epirubicin exceeding 900 mg/m^2 should be administered cautiously. These drugs are potent vesicants and can result in severe tissue necrosis at sites of extravasation. They are cleared hepatically. Specific recommendations for dose modification of doxorubicin and epirubicin based on a patient's serum bilirubin and aspartate transaminases are published in the products' FDA approved package insert.[24,25]

Microtubule Inhibitors Microtubules are structures critical to the successful completion of cell division (mitosis). Three subclasses of cytotoxic chemotherapy agents that disrupt normal microtubule function are effective in treating breast cancer. Table 14-3 provides commonly prescribed dosing regimens and associated side effects of these agents.[5]

Taxanes Paclitaxel, albumin-bound paclitaxel, and docetaxel bind to β-tubulin, a protein needed to form microtubules. As a result, taxanes inhibit depolymerization of the microtubules, a terminal phase in cell division. Taxanes are effective agents in treating patients with locally advanced and advanced disease.

A prominent side effect of paclitaxel is the occurrence of infusion-related hypersensitivity reactions. Typically, these reactions are characterized by the onset of symptoms (eg, dyspnea, flushing, tachycardia, chest pain) within 1 hour of administration. These symptoms are attributed to mast cell degranulation caused by Cremophor EL, the surfactant used to increase the solubility of paclitaxel. Premedication with corticosteroids, an H1 and an H2 antagonist, is standard care for any patient receiving paclitaxel.[5,26]

Abraxane, a nanoparticle albumin-bound paclitaxel formulation, is a paclitaxel formulation that does not contain Cremophor EL and does not require premedication. The reported incidence of hypersensitivity reactions are 4% for nanoparticle albumin-bound paclitaxel and 12% for paclitaxel. Paclitaxel is contraindicated in patients with a documented history of a hypersensitivity reaction to Cremophor EL and/or paclitaxel.[26,27]

Docetaxel is contraindicated in patients with a history of severe hypersensitivity reactions. Fluid retention occurs in nearly 25% of patients. Premedication with dexamethasone is recommended to attenuate this adverse effect.[28]

Epothilones Ixabepilone is the prototype semisynthetic analog of epothilone B. It inhibits the depolymerization of microtubules by binding to a β-tubulin site different than the taxane binding site. Ixabepilone should not be administered to patients with alanine aminotransferase or aspartate aminotransferase > 2.5 times the upper limit of normal or bilirubin > 1 times upper limits of normal since there is an increased risk of potentially life-threatening liver toxicity. Cremophor EL is used to increase ixabepilone solubility. Premedication with an H1 and an H2 antagonist an hour prior to administering ixabepilone is recommended in order to minimize hypersensitivity reactions. If a patient develops a hypersensitivity reaction, the addition of dexamethasone to the pretreatment regimen is recommended. Ixabepilone is contraindicated in patients with a history of hypersensitivity reactions to drugs formulated with Cremophor EL.[29]

Vinca Alkaloids Vinorelbine is a semisynthetic vinca alkaloid that impedes mitosis by inhibiting the formation of functioning microtubules. It should be administered with caution to patients with elevated serum bilirubin levels. If a patient's serum bilirubin level is between 2.1 to 3 mg/dL, a 50% dosage reduction is recommended; if a patient's serum bilirubin level exceeds 3 mg/dL, a 70% dosage reduction is recommended.[30]

Monoclonal Antibodies Trastuzumab and bevacizumab are two humanized monoclonal antibodies approved for the treatment of metastatic breast cancer. Table 14-4 provides specific dosing regimens and toxicity profiles of these agents.

Twenty to thirty percent of patients have breast cancers that overexpress the human epidermal growth factor receptor-2 (HER-2). Trastuzumab was developed to bind to the HER-2 receptor. This interaction may cause cell death by several mechanisms. Cell lysis may result from the activation of the complement cascade and/or the enhanced recognition of the antibody-tagged cells by cytotoxic T lymphocytes. Cell growth may also be impeded by the inhibition of normal intracellular

REFERENCES

1. Jemal A, Siegel R, Ward E, et al. Cancer statistics, 2009. *CA Cancer J Clin.* 2009;59:225-249.
2. Berry DA, Cronin KA, Plevritis SK, et al. Effect of screening and adjuvant therapy on mortality from breast cancer. *N Engl J Med.* 2005;353:1784.
3. Breast cancer risk reduction. NCCN Practice Guidelines in Oncology–V.2.2009. Available at: http://www.nccn.org/professionals/physician_gls/PDF/breast_risk.pdf. Accessed August 26, 2009.
4. Breast cancer. NCCN Practice Guidelines in Oncology–V.1.2009. Available at: http://www.nccn.org/professionals/physician_gls/PDF/breast.pdf. Accessed August 26, 2009.
5. Michaud LB, Espirito JL, Esteva FJ. Breast cancer. In: DiPiro JT, Talbert RL, Yee GC, Matzke GR, Wells BG, Posey LM, eds. *Pharmacotherapy: A Pathophysiologic Approach.* 7th ed, chap. 131. http://www.accesspharmacy.com/content.aspx?aID=3218490. Accessed August 31, 2009.
6. Begg CB, Haile RW, Borg A, et al. Variation of breast cancer risk among BRCA1/2 carriers. *JAMA.* 2008;299:194-201.
7. National Cancer Institute Fact Sheet; Bethesda, MD. BRCA1 and BRCA2: cancer risk and genetic testing. Reviewed 5/29/09. Available at: http://www.nci.nih.gov/cancertopics/factsheet/Risk/BRCA. Accessed August 27, 2009.
8. Yager JD, Davidson NE. Estrogen carcinogenesis in breast cancer. *N Engl J Med.* 2006;354:270-282.
9. Dershaw DD. Cancer screening—breast cancer. In: DeVita VT, Lawrence TS, Rosenberg SA, DePinho RA, Weinberg RA, eds. *DeVita, Hellman, and Rosenberg's Cancer: Principles and Practice of Oncology.* 8th ed. Philadelphia, PA: Lippincott Williams & Wilkins; 2008:677-680.
10. Burstein HJ, Harris JR, Morrow M. Malignant tumors of the breast. In: DeVita VT, Lawrence TS, Rosenberg SA, DePinho RA, Weinberg RA, eds. *DeVita, Hellman, and Rosenberg's Cancer: Principles and Practice of Oncology.* 8th ed. Philadelphia, PA: Lippincott Williams & Wilkins, 2008:1612-1616.
11. Ries LAG, Harkins D, Krapcho M, eds. SEER cancer statistics review: 1975-2003. Bethesda, MD. http://seer.cancer.gov/csr/1975_2003/results_merged/sect_04_breast.pdf. Accessed August 25, 2009.
12. Gail MH, Brinton LA, Byar DP, et al. Projecting individualized probabilities of developing breast cancer for white females who are being examined annually. *J Natl Cancer Inst.* 1989;81:1879-1886.
13. Fisher B, Costantino JP, Wickerham L, et al. Tamoxifen for prevention of breast cancer: report of the National Surgical Adjuvant Breast and Bowel Project P-1 Study. *J Natl Cancr Inst.* 1998;90:1371-1388.
14. Nolvadex (tamoxifen citrate) [package insert]. Wilmington, Delaware: AstraZeneca Pharmaceuticals LP; 2006.
15. Vogel VG, Costantino JP, Wickerham L, et al. Effects of Tamoxifen vs raloxifene on the risk of developing invasive breast cancer and other disease outcomes. The NSABP Study of tamoxifen and raloxifene (STAR) P-2 trial. *JAMA.* 2006;295:2727-2741.
16. Evista (raloxifene hydrochloride) [package insert]. Indianapolis, IN: Eli Lilly and Company;2008.
17. Loprinzi CL, Kugler JW, Sloan JA, et al. Venlafazine in management of hot flashes in survivors of breast cancer: a randomized controlled trial. *Lancet.* 2000;356:2059-2063.
18. Stearns V, Slack R, Greep N, et al. Paroxetine is an effective treatment for hot flashes: results from a prospective randomized controlled trial. *J Clin Oncol.* 2005;23:6919-6930.
19. Aubert RE, Stanek EJ, Yao J, et al. Risk of breast cancer recurrence in women initiating tamoxifen with CYP2D6 inhibitors. *J Clin Oncol.* 2009;27:18s (suppl; abstr CRA508).
20. Dezentje V, Van Blijderveen, NJ, Gelderblom H, et al. Concomitant CYP2D6 inhibitor use and tamoxifen adherence in early-stage breast cancer: a pharmacoepidemiologic study. *J Clin Oncol.* 2009;27:18s (suppl; abstr CRA509).
21. Renshaw L, McHugh M, Williams L, et al. Comparison of joint problems as reported by patients in a randomized adjuvant trial of anastrozole and letrozole [abstract 2072]. *Breast Cancer Res Treat.* 2007;106(suppl 1). Available at: www.abstracts2view.com/sabcs07/view.php?nu=SABCS07L_631. Accessed April 6, 2009.
22. Faslodex (fulvestrant) [package insert]. Wilmington, Delaware: AstraZeneca Pharmaceuticals LP;2006.
23. Xeloda (capecitabine) [package insert].Nutley, NJ: Roche Laboratories Inc.; 2006.
24. Adriamycin (doxorubicin HCl) [package insert]. Kalamazoo, MI: Pharmacia & Upjohn Company; 2003.
25. Ellence (epirubicin HCl) [package insert]. Kalamazoo, MI: Pharmacia & Upjohn Company, A subsidiary of Pharmacia Corporation; 2005.
26. Taxol (paclitaxel) [package insert]. Princeton, NJ: Bristol-Myers Squibb Company; 2007.
27. Abraxane (paclitaxel protein-bound particles for injectable suspension) [package insert]. Los Angeles, CA: Abraxis BioScience, Inc.; 2007.
28. Taxotere (docetaxel) [package insert]. Bridgewater, NJ: Sanofi-Aventis U.S. LLC; 2008.
29. Ixempra (ixabepilone) [package insert]. Princeton, NJ: Bristol-Myers Squibb Company; 2009.
30. Navelbine (vinorelbine) [package insert]. Research Triangle Park, NC: GlaxoSmithKline; 2002.
31. Herceptin (trastuzumab) [package insert]. San Francisco, CA: Genentech, Inc.; 2009.
32. Avastin (bevacizumab) [package insert]. San Francisco, CA:Genentech, Inc.; 2009.
33. Tykerb (lapatinib) [package insert]. Research Triangle Park, NC: GlaxoSmithKline; 2008HH.

19. According to STAR trial, which of the following medications are equally effective in decreasing the risk of breast cancer in women meeting criteria for being at high risk of developing breast cancer?

    a. Tamoxifen and raloxifene
    b. Tamoxifen and letrozole
    c. Tamoxifen and anastrozole
    d. Tamoxifen and toremifene
    e. Tamoxifen is the only medication proven effective in reducing the risk of breast cancer

20. Which of the following organizations publishes on their website evidence-based clinical practice guidelines for cancers that affect over 90% of patients with cancer?

    a. The American Cancer Society
    b. The Eastern Cooperative Oncology Group
    c. National Comprehensive Cancer Network—Clinical Practice Guidelines in Oncology
    d. The National Cancer Institute
    e. The American Society of Health-System Pharmacy

21. Arthralgias and myalgias are side effects that patients receiving the following antineoplastic agents are likely to experience.

    a. Docetaxel, ixabepilone, letrozole, exemestane
    b. Paclitaxel, ixabepilone, anastrozole
    c. Anastrozole, exemestane
    d. Letrozole, anastrozole, exemestane
    e. All of the above

22. Stomatitis is an adverse effect that patients administered with which of the following antineoplastic agents may experience?

    a. Doxorubicin, capecitabine, tamoxifen
    b. Paclitaxel, ixabepilone, anastrozole
    c. Methotrexate, capecitabine, cyclophosphamide
    d. Letrozole, paclitaxel, capecitabine
    e. All of the above

23. Which of the following antineoplastic agents is a vesicant?

    a. 5-Fluorouracil
    b. Fulvestrant
    c. Doxorubicin
    d. Methotrexate
    e. All of the above

24. Which of the following antineoplastic agents would not be effective as adjuvant therapy for postmenopausal patients with breast cancer that is ER negative and does not overexpress HER-2?

    a. Cyclophosphamide
    b. Epirubicin
    c. Doxorubicin
    d. Letrozole
    e. All of the above antineoplastic agents have proven to be effective in such patients

25. Which of the following biologic markers are used to determine appropriate pharmacotherapy for breast cancer patients?

    a. Estrogen receptor
    b. HER-2
    c. Progesterone receptor
    d. Estrogen receptor and HER-2
    e. Estrogen receptor, progesterone receptor, and HER-2

TAKEAWAY POINTS ››

- Breast cancer is a prevalent disease. It is the most common cancer diagnosed in American women, the second leading cause of cancer-related death. The lifetime risk for a US woman developing breast cancer is 1:8.
- Over 20 antineoplastic agents representing nine distinct classes of antineoplastic agents are effective in managing breast cancer.
- The selection of an antineoplastic regimen for a patient is individualized based on the size and anatomical location (staging) of the cancer, the patient's menopausal status, and biologic markers (estrogen receptors, HER-2) identified on the breast cancer cells.
- Combination cytotoxic chemotherapy is the preferred treatment regimen for women with breast cancer that is estrogen receptor negative or hormone refractory.
- Myelosuppression is the most common dose-related toxicity associated with cytotoxic chemotherapy.
- Single-agent endocrine therapy with a selective estrogen receptor modulator is the preferred initial treatment for premenopausal women with estrogen receptor positive disease.
- Single-agent endocrine therapy with an aromatase inhibitor is the preferred initial treatment for postmenopausal women with estrogen receptor positive disease.
- The monoclonal antibody trastuzumab, and the signal transduction inhibitor lapatinib are only indicated for the treatment of women who overexpress the human epidermal growth factor-2 (HER-2). Approximately 30% of women with breast cancer overexpress HER-2.
- The administration of antineoplastic effective in treating metastatic breast cancer is palliative, not curative.
- Clinically significant drug interactions have been documented with capecitabine, 5-fluorouracil, tamoxifen, and lapatinib.

12. Select the brand name for letrozole.
    a. Arimidex
    b. Nolvadex
    c. Avastin
    d. Evista
    e. Femara

13. Select the taxane effective in treating advanced breast cancer that is formulated as an albumin nanoparticle product.
    a. Abraxane
    b. Taxol
    c. Docetaxel
    d. Taxotere
    e. None of the above

14. Clinical trials that compared the efficacy of tamoxifen and AIs as adjuvant treatments for patients with breast cancer have established which of these outcomes?
    a. AIs have been better tolerated than tamoxifen.
    b. Sequential hormonal therapy (tamoxifen followed by an AI) has resulted in significantly longer DFS than tamoxifen monotherapy.
    c. Tamoxifen without subsequent AI therapy resulted in superior progression-free survival.
    d. a and b.
    e. a and c are all outcomes documented in clinical trials.

15. A 69-year-old woman is taking anastrozole for ER+/PR+, HER-2 negative stage 4 breast cancer. Upon returning for her third refill, she tells you that she has noticed increased stiffness and joint pain in knees. She started taking ibuprofen 400 mg four times a day and at bedtime without much benefit for the past week. Your recommendation is to:
    a. Increase the ibuprofen dosage to 800 mg four times daily and at bedtime.
    b. The symptoms of joint and muscle pain are likely caused by anastrozole. You offer to call her physician to discuss switching to letrozole or exemestane.
    c. The symptoms are consistent with a hypersensitivity reaction to anastrozole. You recommend she take some diphenhydramine and go to the emergency room for evaluation.
    d. The symptoms have not been associated with anastrozole. She is likely developing rheumatoid arthritis and should be evaluated by her physician.

16. MK is a 63-year-old woman with newly diagnosed metastatic breast cancer is scheduled to receive her first dose of trastuzumab. She is 5 ft 6 inches tall and weighs 175 lb. You receive the following order: trastuzumab 440 mg IV infusion over 1.5 hours. Select the appropriate assessment to discuss with the prescriber.
    a. Trastuzumab causes significant nausea and vomiting warranting premedication with a serotonin antagonist antiemetic. It would be best to call the prescriber and suggest administration of an antiemetic.
    b. Trastuzumab can safely be administered as an IV bolus injection. It would be appropriate to call the prescriber and suggest the order be changed to be administered as an IV bolus injection.
    c. Trastuzumab has been shown effective as an adjuvant treatment but not treatment of metastatic disease. It would be appropriate to call the prescriber and clarify the indication for trastuzumab for this patient.
    d. The recommended initial dose of trastuzumab is 4 mg/kg (320 mg total for this patient). It would be appropriate to call the prescriber and clarify dosage for this patient.
    e. Trastuzumab is ordered appropriately for this patient. No clarification is indicated.

17. A 65-year-old patient brings in her tamoxifen prescription for a refill. Upon reviewing her medication profile you discover that she began taking tamoxifen 20 mg daily in June 2000 for the prevention of breast cancer and she has been having it refilled regularly since then. What, if anything, should you discuss with the patient's physician?
    a. The recommended duration of tamoxifen when prescribed to decrease the risk of breast cancer is 10 years. There is no need to clarify this patient's tamoxifen regimen.
    b. The merits of increasing the dose to 40 mg daily based on results of a recent study documenting superior efficacy of a 40 mg daily dose.
    c. Switching this patient to an AI based on recent studies that have documented improvement in efficacy and tolerability with AIs.
    d. The merits of decreasing the dose to 10 mg daily based on results of a recent study documenting equal efficacy but superior tolerability of a 20 mg daily dose.
    e. The recommended duration of tamoxifen when prescribed to decrease the risk of breast cancer is 5 years.

18. This patient asks you if you could recommend a dietary supplement that has been proven effective in decreasing the risk of breast cancer.
    a. You explain that vitamin A 100 IU daily has been proven effective to decrease the risk of breast cancer.
    b. You explain that vitamin D 200 mg daily has been proven effective to decrease the risk of breast cancer.
    c. You explain that vitamin C 500 IU daily has been proven effective to decrease the risk of breast cancer.
    d. You explain that there is no scientific evidence that supports any dietary supplements are effective in lowering the risk of breast cancer.
    e. You explain that vitamin E 100 IU daily has been proven effective to decrease the risk of breast cancer.

c. Dexamethasone and diphenhydramine
d. Dexamethasone, ranitidine and diphenhydramine

6. A patient taking capecitabine for metastatic breast cancer describes to you the development of tenderness on her hands and feet that make it difficult for her to be on her feet. Select the most appropriate recommendation for this patient.
   a. Her symptoms describe the onset of a known side effect of capecitabine. You recommend she call her physician and describe the onset of these symptoms before taking any more doses of capecitabine.
   b. Her symptoms are classic for individuals with vitamin B_6 deficiency. You recommend she schedule an appointment with her physician to discuss these symptoms.
   c. Her symptoms are commonly caused by capecitabine. You reassure her that there is nothing to worry about and recommend she avoid standing as much as possible while she completes the last week of capecitabine.
   d. Her symptoms are commonly caused by capecitabine. You explain to her the symptoms are self-limiting and easily managed by spraying her hands and feet with benzocaine first aid spray four times daily.

7. A patient presents her prescription for capecitabine to you. Review of her medication profile documents she is also taking 5 mg of warfarin daily for atrial fibrillation and metformin for type 2 diabetes mellitus. Select the appropriate assessment of potential drug interactions for this patient.
   a. Capecitabine has been shown to increase metabolism of warfarin and results in subtherapeutic INRs. More frequent monitoring of this patient's INRs is recommended.
   b. Capecitabine has been shown to decrease metabolism of warfarin and results in elevated INRs and bleeding. More frequent monitoring of this patient's INRs is recommended.
   c. Capecitabine has been shown to decrease metabolism of metformin and results in hypoglycemia. The importance of scheduled blood glucose monitoring and possible need for holding metformin doses needs to be discussed with this patient.
   d. Capecitabine has been shown to increase metabolism of metformin and results in hyperglycemia. The importance of daily blood glucose monitoring and possible need for increasing metformin doses needs to be discussed with this patient.
   e. Metformin has been shown to decrease metabolism of capecitabine and results in the increased severity of capecitabine-induced myelosuppression. A 25% reduction in the dose of capecitabine is indicated.

8. A patient presents a new prescription to you for tamoxifen. Her doctor said he was prescribing it as adjuvant treatment for breast cancer following her surgery last month. You review her medication profile and document that she is also taking metoprolol, hydrochlorothiazide, and Prozac. Select the appropriate assessment of potential drug interactions for this patient.
   a. There are no clinically significant drug interactions to alter her medication regimen.
   b. You explain that a number of SSRIs including Prozac have been documented to decrease the effectiveness of tamoxifen by interfering with its metabolism to an active metabolite. You will call the patient's physician to consider alternative antidepressant options.
   c. You explain that hydrochlorothiazide has been documented to decrease the effectiveness of tamoxifen by interfering with its metabolism to an active metabolite. You will call the patient's physician to consider alternative diuretic.
   d. You explain that metoprolol has been documented to decrease the effectiveness of tamoxifen by interfering with its metabolism to an active metabolite. You will call the patient's physician to consider alternative beta-blocker.

9. Select the statement that accurately describes breast cancer.
   a. The lifetime risk for US women developing breast cancer is 1 in 8.
   b. In the United States, the death rate from breast cancer has decreased since the widespread implementation of screening mammography guidelines.
   c. Breast cancer is the second leading cause of death from cancer in US women.
   d. Pharmacotherapy for metastatic breast cancer is palliative rather than curative.
   e. All of the above.

10. Select the antineoplastic agent associated with an increased incidence of endometrial cancer.
    a. Letrozole
    b. Raloxifene
    c. Toremifene
    d. Fulvestrant
    e. Tamoxifen

11. Which of following conditions would be a contraindication for prescribing an aromatase inhibitor?
    a. The development of arthralgias and myalgias.
    b. A patient with a history of thromboembolic events.
    c. A premenopausal patient.
    d. A postmenopausal patient with a history of thromboembolic events.
    e. There are no contraindications for the administration of aromatase inhibitors.

CHAPTER

15 Colorectal Cancer

Jennifer Baldock and Patrick T. Wong

FOUNDATION OVERVIEW

General Overview

Colorectal cancer (CRC) accounts for the third most common type of cancer and third leading cause of cancer mortality in the United States for both men and women.[1] As with most cancers, CRC is more likely to have better survival outcomes the earlier it is diagnosed. Colon cancer and rectal cancer are usually grouped together in epidemiological studies and share similar pathophysiology, but there are distinct approaches to treatment. Conventional therapies including surgery, radiation, and chemotherapy are still typically used today depending on the stage and type of cancer. Newer therapies are increasingly used that target specific pathways of the cancer's biology.

Pathophysiology

Most CRCs are believed to be a result of an accumulation of genetic mutations that transforms normal epithelial cells into nonmalignant adenomas or polyps, then finally malignant adenocarcinomas. Mutations can originate due to hereditary syndromes or be acquired through lifestyle or environmental risk factors.[2]

Key Definitions

Adenocarcinoma—malignant neoplasm of epithelial cells with glandular or glandlike features.

Adjuvant—in oncology, treatment added after primary therapy, usually a surgery, with the goal to reduce recurrence.

CEA—carcinoembryonic antigen, tumor marker found in the serum for colorectal cancer but is also elevated in other malignant and nonmalignant conditions such as smoking.

Chemoradiation—chemotherapy given concomitantly with radiation, usually with radiosensitizing agents like fluoropyrimidines or platinums.

Microsatellite instability—when microsatellites, repeated sequences of DNA that are usually of a set length, accumulate errors and become longer or shorter than normal.

Neoadjuvant—in oncology, treatment added before primary therapy, usually a surgery, with the goal to improve outcomes of that curative therapy.

TNM staging—method of classifying cancers by T: tumor size, N: lymph node involvement, and M: presence of distant metastases; the combination of these three factors categorizes a cancer into "stages"; the higher the stage number the more widespread the cancer and generally the worse the prognosis.

Epidemiology

CRC is the third most common cancer in both men and women in the United States, making up an estimated 10% of all cancers in 2009 and total 9% of all cancer deaths. Despite these staggering statistics, death rates from CRC have been declining in the past few decades, with an approximate 30% decrease since 1990. Five-year relative survival rates of persons diagnosed with CRC have been significantly increasing over the past 30 years and are most recently estimated at 65% in 2004.[1]

Clinical Presentation/Signs and Symptoms

The clinical presentation of CRCs can be nonspecific which can result in the delay of a diagnosis. Gastrointestinal bleeding, abdominal pain, and change in bowel habits (constipation, abnormal stools) are common at presentation if the patient is symptomatic. Patients sometimes experience significant weight loss, and a partial or complete bowel obstruction may trigger a diagnosis. The pattern of spread to distant sites usually involves the liver and lungs. Liver is more common for colon cancer and lung for rectal cancer.[2]

Diagnosis

The diagnosis of CRC is most commonly accomplished through a colonoscopy and biopsies. A colonoscopy can visualize the entire colon and remove polyps for pathology review. If a full colonoscopy is not possible, for example, due to an obstruction, a postoperative colonoscopy is still recommended to rule out any synchronous tumors that may occur. Barium enemas with flexible sigmoidoscopy can diagnose tumors in the sigmoid colon but could miss any tumors in the remaining two-thirds of the colon. Sometimes a bowel obstruction or other barriers preclude a complete colonoscopy necessitating a radiographic diagnosis.

Both colon and rectal cancers are usually staged clinically using a variety of radiographic, endoscopic, and intraoperative techniques prior to the definitive pathologic staging. The tumor-marker carcinoembryonic antigen (CEA) is not a diagnostic marker, but can be used to monitor response to treatment and recurrence. Staging currently utilizes TNM criteria and this provides both prognostic information and aids treatment decisions. An important component of this staging is the number of lymph nodes resected. Inadequate lymph node sampling can miss advanced disease and should be considered high risk for metastases and tumor recurrence.[2]

Screening

Recommendations are made by various groups for screening and surveillance of CRC. Screening can prevent CRC through early detection and removal of noninvasive adenomatous polyps and can reduce mortality by preventing progression to advanced disease. Current screening methods include stool tests (fecal occult blood tests, stool DNA tests) and structural examinations (flexible sigmoidoscopy [FSIG], colonoscopy, double-contrast barium enema [DCBE], and computed tomographic colonography [CT colonography]).[3] Fecal occult blood tests detect hemoglobin products in the stool through consecutive sampling of three bowel movements. Convenience is limited by only diagnosing active disease. Additionally, aspirin, NSAIDs, vitamin C, red meat, poultry, fish, and some raw vegetables can interact with some versions of this test. Stool tests must be repeated at regular intervals, and require follow up with colonoscopy should they yield abnormal results.[3] It has been reported that the incidence of CRC may be reduced by 20% with stool testing, and mortality from CRC decreased by 15% to 33% over a period of 8 to 13 years.[3,4] FSIG is an endoscopic procedure that can be performed in an outpatient visit with a standard bowel preparation, and usually without sedation. It can reduce mortality from CRC by 60% to 80% over a period of 10 years. However, its drawbacks include limited viewing the rectum, sigmoid, and descending colon, and the need to be followed up by a colonoscopy if adenomas are discovered.[3]

Colonoscopy is also an endoscopic procedure which allows for examination of the entire tract of the bowel. Colonoscopy requires at least a 24-hour liquid diet and bowel preparation as well as procedural sedation. Additionally, removal of adenomatous polyps can be performed during this procedure.[3] Colonoscopy is generally considered the "gold standard" for screening procedures of CRC.

DCBE and CT colonography are less frequently used as screening procedures for CRC due to lack of access to facilities and trained staff to perform the procedures as well as lack of insurance reimbursement for these procedures.[3]

Screening should start at age 50 for average-risk patients and the frequency of screening depends on the method utilized (eg, stool testing should be preformed annually, if stool testing is the screening method utilized; colonoscopy should be performed at least every 10 years, if colonoscopy is the screening method utilized). All abnormal tests should be followed up with a colonoscopy. Persons with above average risk for CRC (history of adenomatous polyps, history of CRC, family history of CRC, inflammatory bowel disease, hereditary syndromes predisposing to CRC) should have more frequent screenings and may benefit from more structural based examinations.[3]

Risk Factors

Obesity has been noted to be a risk factor for the incidence of colon cancer, but disproportionately more for men than women. In a meta-analysis, it was shown that a five-unit increase in BMI correlated with a 30% and 12% increased risk of colon cancer in men and women, respectively. Higher BMI was also significantly associated with rectal cancer in men with a 12% increase per five-unit increase in BMI, but not in women.[5]

Several studies have shown various markers of diabetes (ie, hyperinsulinemia, C-peptide levels) that have been associated with CRC.[6,7] Diabetes has been associated with an increased risk of CRC (relative risk [RR] 1.30), even when the patients studied were controlled for levels of physical activity and body mass index.[8] Due to the association between lack of fiber intake and increase CRC risk, the American Gastroenterological Association recommends a total daily fiber intake of at least 30 to 35 g.[9] A total daily alcohol intake of 30 g or more has been positively associated with a higher risk for CRC (RR 1.16) compared to nondrinkers, over a 6- to 16-year period, in men and women.[10]

Some people may be predisposed to CRC from hereditary conditions such as hereditary non-polyposis colon cancer (HNPCC) or familial adenomatous polyposis (FAP). Screening may be warranted earlier in these patients or even prophylactic surgery in the case of FAP. Other risk factors for CRC include inflammatory bowel disease and smoking.[2,11]

PREVENTION

Aspirin or Nonsteroidal Anti-Inflammatory Drugs (NSAIDs)

Consistent use of aspirin and NSAIDs has been noted to reduce the incidence of colorectal adenoma (RR reductions of 13%-28% and 30%-40%, respectively). Longer-term use and higher doses have been positively associated with greater risk reductions. However, the adverse effects of aspirin (gastrointestinal bleeding and hemorrhagic stroke) and NSAIDs (gastrointestinal bleeding and cardiovascular outcomes) are also increased with longer use and higher doses.[12,13] The US Preventive Services Task Force (USPSTF) and American Cancer Society do not recommend the routine use of these agents for primary prevention of CRC due to the significant risk associated and lack of evidence of decreased mortality from CRC.[14]

Hormone Therapy

Several landmark studies have noted that women who used hormone replacement (estrogen plus progestin) seemed to have lower incidences of CRC than those who did not (RR 0.63).[15,16] However, the USPSTF recommends against combined estrogen and progestin as prevention of any chronic conditions (including CRC) in postmenopausal women due to the associated increased harms.[17]

Other

There are some suggestions in the literature that dietary factors may play a role in the risk of CRC, including protective effects. There have been inconsistencies in the data for supplemental fiber despite the recommendations above. Calcium and magnesium have shown promise and the American College of Gastroenterology recommends calcium supplementation to prevent polyps.[18]

TREATMENT

Colon Cancer

Many early stage colon cancers are resectable and the therapy of choice is surgery. Low risk, localized disease with no lymph node involvement does not usually require adjuvant systemic therapy. Adjuvant chemotherapy is a consideration for higher-risk colon cancer with no nodal or metastatic involvement, for example, high-grade tumors, tumors with microsatellite instability, or inadequate lymph node dissection. Stage III colon cancers, having lymph node involvement, have documented benefit from adjuvant chemotherapy, and therefore 6 months of chemotherapy following surgical resection is recommended. Stage II colon cancers have a less clear documented benefit with adjuvant therapy, although research is currently ongoing. Future guidelines may assist in treatment decisions for these patients. Currently, treatment decisions should be made on a case-by-case basis.[11]

Metastatic disease, unlike most other cancers, will still be surgically resected if the spread is limited. Local therapy for the primary tumor and metastases can translate into long-term remission and survival. Neoadjuvant chemotherapy may be given to shrink unresectable disease with the goal to make the patient eligible for surgery. Metastatic disease almost always warrants the use of systemic therapy.[11]

Chemotherapy usually consists of combination therapy including a fluoropyrimidine, like fluorouracil, or capecitabine. See Table 15-1 for a list of commonly used drugs. If fluorouracil is used, leucovorin is usually added to increase its efficacy, although also increasing toxicity. Historically, fluorouracil was given in bolus regimens (Mayo Clinic and Roswell Park regimens), but are now mostly given as 2-day continuous infusions due to a better safety and perhaps efficacy profile.[19] Oxaliplatin or irinotecan is usually combined with fluoropyrimidine with the addition of other targeted therapies in metastatic disease.[20]

Infusional fluorouracil, leucovorin, and oxaliplatin (FOLFOX) is the recommended regimen for all stage III and some high-risk stage II colon cancers.[11] The MOSAIC trial examined stage II and III colon cancer patients who received a fluorouracil plus leucovorin based therapy with and without the addition of oxaliplatin. The addition of oxaliplatin significantly improved survival in these patients, more prominently so in stage III patients.[21] FOLFOX is also a first-line regimen for metastatic disease. Acute neurotoxicity (cold sensitivity) and cumulative neurotoxicity (peripheral neuropathies) are unique side effects with this regimen and can be dose limiting. Researchers have investigated infusions of calcium and magnesium or planned chemotherapy free holidays to mitigate these effects.

Irinotecan has also shown to increase the efficacy of fluoropyrimidine based therapies. Bolus fluorouracil plus leucovorin when combined with irinotecan (IFL) has shown unacceptable high rates of severe adverse events including fatal diarrhea. Infusional fluorouracil (FOLFIRI) regimens are used in its place.[22] Irinotecan regimens are also considered acceptable first-line therapy for metastatic colon cancer or used as a second-line agent after failing oxaliplatin based therapy.[23,24]

TABLE 15-1 CRC Drug Summary

Drug	Drug Class/MOA	Adverse Effects	Other Considerations
Fluorouracil	Antimetabolite	Bone marrow suppression, mucositis, diarrhea	Infusional less toxic than bolus regimens, contraindicated in DPD deficiency
Capecitabine	Antimetabolite	Fluorouracil toxicities, hand-foot rash	Drug accumulation with renal impairment, oral therapy, contraindicated in DPD deficiency
Oxaliplatin	Platinum agent	Acute cold sensitivity, cumulative peripheral neuropathy, hypersensitivity reactions	Oxaliplatin-free intervals can decrease neurotoxicity; calcium and magnesium infusions may limit neurotoxicity
Irinotecan	Topoisomerase I inhibitor	Early and late diarrhea, dehydration, severe neutropenia	Dose reduction with elevated serum bilirubin, dose reduction in UGT1A1*28 homozygous patients
Bevacizumab	VEGF inhibitor, humanized monoclonal antibody	Bleeding, arterial thrombotic events, impaired wound healing, gastrointestinal perforation	Treat hypertension and monitor for proteinuria. Consider holding dose with uncontrolled elevations.
Cetuximab	EGFR inhibitor, chimeric monoclonal antibody	Infusion reactions, skin rash, electrolyte wasting	*K-Ras* gene mutation leads to tumor insensitivity to EGFR therapy
Panitumumab	EGFR inhibitor, fully human monoclonal antibody	Infusion reactions, skin rash, electrolyte wasting	*K-Ras* gene mutation leads to tumor insensitivity to EGFR therapy

Irinotecan's main toxicity is diarrhea. Early diarrhea occurs due to a cholinergic syndrome and is best treated with an anticholinergic drug such as atropine. Diarrhea can also occur later due to enterohepatic recirculation of irinotecan and its main active metabolite SN-38. Late diarrhea should be treated with an aggressive loperamide regimen, dosed 4 mg at the onset of diarrhea, and 2 mg every 2 hours until diarrhea free for 12 hours. Irinotecan also can cause significant bone marrow suppression.

Substituting orally administered capecitabine for fluorouracil may add to convenience. Most current evidence suggests capecitabine regimens have similar efficacy to fluorouracil based therapy, but with different side effects. Capecitabine has higher rates of palmar-plantar erythrodysesthesias (PPE, or hand-foot rash), GI toxicity, and thrombocytopenia.[25]

Targeted agents are now standard therapy for metastatic colon cancer. Bevacizumab was the first targeted agent approved for use in metastatic colon cancer and works by inhibiting angiogenesis, an important step in tumor biology. Toxicities include bleeding and thrombotic complications, hypertension, proteinuria, and bowel perforation. EGFR1 targeting agents, namely cetuximab and panitumumab, also have activity and are used as part of standard therapy in metastatic disease. EGFR1 agents commonly cause a unique rash described as acneiform, although not caused by bacteria. This rash is best managed with moisturizers, tetracyclines for anti-inflammatory effects, topical antibiotics to prevent superinfections, and in severe cases, corticosteroids. Drying agents like benzoyl peroxide or retinoids should not be used.[26] EGFR agents can also cause infusion reactions that can be serious and fatalities have been reported. This therapy can also cause electrolyte wasting, most commonly hypomagnesemia. Regular monitoring of magnesium, potassium, and calcium is recommended.

Rectal Cancer

Rectal cancer is often treated with a combination of surgery, radiation therapy (RT), chemoradiation, and chemotherapy. Many of the therapies for rectal cancer are the same or similar to colon cancer except for the emphasis on radiation or chemoradiation as a standard modality in treatment. Preoperative chemotherapy may be recommended for 2 to 3 months, and an additional 4 to 6 months of chemotherapy when adjuvant treatment is appropriate. An interesting approach in rectal cancer is the use of radiation sensitizing chemotherapy regimens along with radiation therapy, such as fluorouracil.[27]

SPECIAL CONSIDERATIONS

Pharmacogenetic information is increasingly being used to steer treatment decisions by predicting toxicities or response when treating CRC. Irinotecan and its principle active metabolite, SN-38, are primarily eliminated through glucuronidation by UGT1A1. Homozygous mutant varieties of this gene can significantly decrease clearance of the drug, leading to serious adverse reactions.[28] Similarly, dihydropyrimidine dehydrogenase (DPD) deficiency predicts intolerance to fluoropyrimidines and these agents are contraindicated in patients with known deficiencies.[29] Routine testing for UGT1A1 or DPD polymorphisms is not considered standard and debate remains on the optimal patient for testing. *K-Ras* mutations have shown to predict a lack of response to the EGFR targeting agents cetuximab and panitumumab and testing should be considered for all patients for whom these agents might be used.[30,31]

Alternatively, overexpression or underexpression of EGFR in a particular patient is not a predictor of response to agents targeting that pathway. Instead, the presence of rash as a side effect is the best known predictor for response for these agents.[20]

CASE Application

1. Which of the following statements, if any, is considered *false*?
   a. Colon and rectal cancers are usually grouped together in epidemiological studies.
   b. Colon cancer is the third leading cause of cancer incidence in men in the United States.
   c. Colon cancer is the third leading cause of cancer deaths in women in the United States.
   d. Colon cancer mortality has declined over the past few decades.
   e. None of the above is false.

2. JM is a 55–year-old African American man concerned about colorectal cancer screening. He inquires about screening recommendations for someone of his age. You reply:
   a. CT/PET of chest, abdomen, and pelvis
   b. Digital rectal examination
   c. Flexible sigmoidoscopy
   d. Colonoscopy
   e. CEA blood test

3. Which of the following may decrease a person's risk of colorectal cancer?
   a. Obesity
   b. HNPCC
   c. Hormone replacement therapy (HRT)
   d. Low dietary fiber
   e. Alcoholism

4. According to national guidelines, what is the recommended age to begin screening for colorectal cancer in a person with average risk?
   a. No later than 21 years old
   b. 40 years old
   c. 45 years old
   d. 50 years old
   e. 65 years old

5. Which of the following are signs or symptoms of colon cancer?
   a. Constipation
   b. Abdominal pain
   c. Weight loss
   d. Diarrhea
   e. All of the above

6. During a routine colonoscopy, KG was diagnosed with stage I colon cancer but is otherwise healthy. He is experiencing no symptoms and has no complications from his cancer so far. His oncologist will likely recommend which therapy?
   a. Neoadjuvant chemotherapy
   b. Surgery
   c. Radiation
   d. Adjuvant chemotherapy
   e. All of the above

7. Which of the following regimens is recommended first line for adjuvant treatment of stage III colon cancer?
   a. Fluorouracil plus leucovorin
   b. FOLFOX
   c. FOLFIRI
   d. IFL
   e. Fluorouracil plus radiation

8. Which of the following statements about colorectal cancer is *false*?
   a. Surgery and other local therapies are almost never a valid option.
   b. Colon cancer tends to first spread to the liver.
   c. Survival is significantly worse than early stage disease.
   d. FOLFOX+/– bevacizumab can be used as a first-line therapy.
   e. FOLFIRI+/– bevacizumab can be used as a first-line therapy.

9. Review the following prescription for capecitabine for a female patient with colon cancer who weighs 123 lb and is 65 inches tall (BSA = 1.6 m^2):

   Capecitabine (Xenical) 500 mg tablets. Take 4 tablets po bid 30 minutes after a meal.

   Take medication for 14 days then do not take for 7 days rest period. Repeat cycle every 21 days.

   Qty: 112 tablets; Refills: 2

   Identify an error with the above prescription that will require clarification with the prescriber.

   a. Frequency
   b. Route
   c. Instructions in regards to food
   d. Schedule of 14 days on medicine and 7 days off medicine
   e. Drug name

10. PL is a 67-year-old man with a history of diabetes mellitus (DM) and alcoholism at the clinic for his seventh cycle of oxaliplatin. He is currently taking capecitabine at home. PL's CBC (complete blood count) with differential is all within normal limits. Before preparing the oxaliplatin for infusion, which other parameters would significantly determine if he requires a dose reduction or his dose to be held?

    i. Renal function estimated by creatinine clearance
    ii. Liver function estimated by AST, ALT, total bilirubin
    iii. Assessment of neurotoxicity side effects

    a. i only
    b. ii only
    c. i and ii
    d. i and iii
    e. i, ii, and iii

11. PL is now on day 10 of his capecitabine and oxaliplatin chemotherapy (XELOX or CAPOX). He reports a dry, painful rash on the soles of his feet making it nearly impossible to ambulate and his hands are red and blistered with moist desquamation. Which of the following would you recommend?

    i. Recommend to PL's oncologist that capecitabine is the cause and to hold treatment until dermatologic toxicities resolve.
    ii. Recommend to PL's oncologist that capecitabine is the cause and to finish this current cycle and consider a dose reduction for next cycle.
    iii. Recommend to PL to liberally apply moisturizing creams, avoid constant rubbing or pressure, and/or take pyridoxine (vitamin B_6).

    a. i only
    b. ii only
    c. i and iii
    d. ii and iii
    e. None of the above

12. NK is a 47-year-old woman with stage IV colon cancer who calls your pharmacy 3 days after receiving FOLFIRI (infusional fluorouracil, leucovorin, and irinotecan). She said she picked up some over-the-counter loperamide (Imodium A-D) and is unsure how to take it. She just had a loose bowel movement, and she feels like the urgency has not gone away. What would be the best response?

    i. Loperamide 4 mg now, then 2 mg after each loose stool, not to exceed eight tablets (16 mg) per day
    ii. Loperamide 4 mg now, then 2 mg every 2 hours until diarrhea free for 12 hours
    iii. You should have taken loperamide 2 mg every 6 hours around the clock starting 1 day after irinotecan to prevent diarrhea

    a. i only
    b. ii only

c. i and iii
d. ii and iii
e. None of the above

13. BK is receiving FOLFOX chemotherapy. Which of the following should BK avoid most in the short term for the purpose of avoiding acute neurotoxicity exacerbations caused by oxaliplatin?

a. Direct sunlight
b. Cold
c. Heat
d. Tight fitting clothing
e. OTC acne treatments

14. What of the following is an adverse reaction that is likely to occur with bevacizumab therapy?

a. Hypertension
b. Proteinuria
c. Delayed wound healing
d. Bleeding and thrombotic events
e. All of the above are important adverse reactions to monitor

15. GW is a 58-year-old man with metastatic colon cancer on irinotecan plus cetuximab therapy. When he arrives to the infusion center he is complaining of new "pimples" appearing all over his chest and face. The oncology nurse asks you to counsel him on managing this new finding. Your counselling points would include all of the following *except*:

a. Recommend him to ask his doctor about isotretinoin, give him the FDA approved med guide, and explain about the iPLEDGE program to reduce birth defects.
b. Recommend him to apply moisturizing lotion to the affected areas.
c. Warn him to use sunscreen since direct sunlight can exacerbate his condition.
d. Recommend him to ask his doctor about initiating a tetracycline like doxycycline or minocycline.
e. Reassure him that this side effect actually may be predictive of a positive tumor response to this regimen.

16. Which pair of therapies for colorectal cancer has the highest concerns for hypersensitivity reactions?

a. Irinotecan and bevacizumab
b. Capecitabine and oxaliplatin
c. Panitumumab and fluorouracil
d. Oxaliplatin and cetuximab
e. None of the above causes hypersensitivity reactions

17. UGT1A1*28 mutations have been shown to cause what change in pharmacokinetics?

a. Decreased fluorouracil clearance
b. Increased fluorouracil clearance
c. Decreased irinotecan clearance
d. Increased irinotecan clearance
e. None of the above

18. All of the following would increase the risk of toxicity of fluorouracil *except*:

a. DPD deficiency
b. *K-ras* mutation
c. Choose bolus administration instead of infusional administration
d. Coadminister with leucovorin
e. Increase the dose

19. All of the following brand names or abbreviations are correctly matched with their generic name *except*:

a. 5-FU = fluorouracil
b. CPT-11 = irinotecan
c. Elitek = oxaliplatin
d. Vectibix = panitumumab
e. Avastin = bevacizumab

20. Most cancer therapies are dosed per body surface area. All of the following medications are dose in mg/m^2 *except*:

a. Fluorouracil
b. Oxaliplatin
c. Irinotecan
d. Bevacizumab
e. Cetuximab

TAKEAWAY POINTS »

- CRC is the third leading cause of cancer incidence and cancer death in both men and women in the United States.
- Regular screening for CRC can prevent disease and prevent progression to advanced disease. There are various methods for screening, but all abnormal results should be followed up by a colonoscopy.
- Risk factors for CRC include hereditary predisposition, obesity, diabetes, diet, and alcohol intake.
- Regular use of aspirin and NSAIDs at high doses can reduce the incidence of CRC, but does not decrease mortality and carries significant risk. Primary prevention is not recommended.
- Despite the reduction of incidence in CRC with hormone replacement therapy, use of these drugs for primary prevention of CRC is not recommended due to significant risks.
- Early CRC is often treated with surgery. Adjuvant or neoadjuvant chemotherapy may be considered in stage II CRC and is recommended in stage III disease.

- Metastatic disease is sometimes treated with surgery or other local therapies for limited disease. All metastatic colorectal patients will receive systemic therapy with chemotherapy.
- Fluoropyrimidines are agents in most chemotherapy regimens for both colon and rectal cancer.
- Leucovorin is used with fluorouracil to enhance efficacy, with some increase in toxicity.
- Infusional fluorouracil is preferred over bolus regimens due to lessened toxicity and perhaps better efficacy.
- Oxaliplatin and irinotecan are frequently combined with fluoropyrimidines in colon cancer.
- Agents targeting biological pathways including angiogenesis and EGFR1 are used in CRC.
- Pharmacogenomics in CRC may personalize treatment to predict efficacy and/or toxicities.

REFERENCES

1. Jemal A, Siegel R, Ward E, Hao Y, Xu J, Thun MJ. Cancer statistics, 2009. *CA Cancer J Clin.* 2009;59(4):225-249.
2. Thomas MB, Hoff PM, Wolff RA. Chapter 16. Colorectal cancer. In: Kantarjian HM, Wolff RA, Koller CA, ed. *MD Anderson Manual of Medical Oncology.* New York, NY:McGraw-Hill; 2006.
3. Levin B, Lieberman DA, McFarland B, et al. Screening and surveillance for the early detection of colorectal cancer and adenomatous polyps, 2008: a joint guideline from the American Cancer Society, the US Multi-Society Task Force on Colorectal Cancer, and the American College of Radiology. *CA Cancer J Clin.* 2008;58(3):130-160.
4. Hewitson P, Glasziou P, Irwig L, Towler B, Watson E. Screening for colorectal cancer using the faecal occult blood test, Hemoccult. *Cochrane Database Syst Rev.* 2007;(1):CD001216.
5. Larsson SC, Wolk A. Obesity and colon and rectal cancer risk: a meta-analysis of prospective studies. *Am J Clin Nutr.* 2007;86(3):556-565.
6. Mulholland HG, Murray LJ, Cardwell CR, Cantwell MM. Glycemic index, glycemic load, and risk of digestive tract neoplasms: a systematic review and meta-analysis. *Am J Clin Nutr.* 2009;89(2):568-576.
7. Pisani P. Hyper-insulinaemia and cancer, meta-analyses of epidemiological studies. *Arch Physiol Biochem.* 2008;114(1):63-70.
8. Larsson SC, Orsini N, Wolk A. Diabetes mellitus and risk of colorectal cancer: a meta-analysis. *J Natl Cancer Inst.* 2005;97(22):1679-1687.
9. American Gastroenterological Association medical position statement: impact of dietary fiber on colon cancer occurrence. American College of Gastroenterology. *Gastroenterology.* 2000;118(6):1233-1234.
10. Cho E, Smith-Warner SA, Ritz J, et al. Alcohol intake and colorectal cancer: a pooled analysis of 8 cohort studies. *Ann Intern Med.* 2004;140(8):603-613.
11. NCCN Clinical Practice Guidelines in Oncology: Colon cancer. http://www.nccn.org. Updated c2009. Accessed September 1, 2009.
12. Dube C, Rostom A, Lewin G, et al. The use of aspirin for primary prevention of colorectal cancer: a systematic review prepared for the U.S. Preventive Services Task Force. *Ann Intern Med.* 2007;146(5):365-375.
13. Rostom A, Dube C, Lewin G, et al. Nonsteroidal anti-inflammatory drugs and cyclooxygenase-2 inhibitors for primary prevention of colorectal cancer: a systematic review prepared for the U.S. Preventive Services Task Force. *Ann Intern Med.* 2007;146(5):376-389.
14. Routine aspirin or nonsteroidal anti-inflammatory drugs for the primary prevention of colorectal cancer: recommendation statement. *Am Fam Physician.* 2007;76(1):109-113.
15. Hulley S, Furberg C, Barrett-Connor E, et al. Noncardiovascular disease outcomes during 6.8 years of hormone therapy: Heart and Estrogen/progestin Replacement Study follow-up (HERS II). *JAMA.* 2002;288(1):58-66.
16. Rossouw JE, Anderson GL, Prentice RL, et al. Risks and benefits of estrogen plus progestin in healthy postmenopausal women: principal results from the Women's Health Initiative randomized controlled trial. *JAMA.* 2002;288(3):321-333.
17. U.S. Preventive Services Task Force. Hormone therapy for the prevention of chronic conditions in postmenopausal women: recommendations from the U.S. Preventive Services Task Force. *Ann Intern Med.* 2005;142(10):855-860.
18. Bond JH. Polyp guideline: diagnosis, treatment, and surveillance for patients with colorectal polyps. Practice Parameters Committee of the American College of Gastroenterology. *Am J Gastroenterol.* 2000;95(11):3053-3063.
19. de Gramont A, Bosset JF, Milan C, et al. Randomized trial comparing monthly low-dose leucovorin and fluorouracil bolus with bimonthly high-dose leucovorin and fluorouracil bolus plus continuous infusion for advanced colorectal cancer: a French intergroup study. *J Clin Oncol.* 1997;15(2):808-815.
20. Meyerhardt JA, Mayer RJ. Systemic therapy for colorectal cancer. *N Engl J Med.* 2005;352(5):476-487.
21. Andre T, Boni C, Navarro M, et al. Improved overall survival with oxaliplatin, fluorouracil, and leucovorin as adjuvant treatment in stage II or III colon cancer in the MOSAIC trial. *J Clin Oncol.* 2009;27(19):3109-3116.
22. Fuchs CS, Marshall J, Barrueco J. Randomized, controlled trial of irinotecan plus infusional, bolus, or oral fluoropyrimidines in first-line treatment of metastatic colorectal cancer: updated results from the BICC-C study. *J Clin Oncol.* 2008;26(4):689-690.
23. Colucci G, Gebbia V, Paoletti G, et al. Phase III randomized trial of FOLFIRI versus FOLFOX4 in the treatment of advanced colorectal cancer: a multicenter study of the Gruppo Oncologico Dell'Italia Meridionale. *J Clin Oncol.* 2005;23(22):4866-4875.
24. Tournigand C, Andre T, Achille E, et al. FOLFIRI followed by FOLFOX6 or the reverse sequence in advanced colorectal cancer: a randomized GERCOR study. *J Clin Oncol.* 2004;22(2):229-237.
25. Arkenau HT, Arnold D, Cassidy J, et al. Efficacy of oxaliplatin plus capecitabine or infusional fluorouracil/leucovorin in patients with metastatic colorectal cancer: a pooled analysis of randomized trials. *J Clin Oncol.* 2008;26(36):5910-5917.

26. Melosky B, Burkes R, Rayson D, Alcindor T, Shear N, Lacouture M. Management of skin rash during egfr-targeted monoclonal antibody treatment for gastrointestinal malignancies: Canadian recommendations. *Curr Oncol.* 2009;16(1):16-26.
27. NCCN clinical practice guidelines in oncology: Rectal cancer. http://www.nccn.org. Updated c2009. Accessed September 1, 2009.
28. Toffoli G, Cecchin E, Corona G, et al. The role of UGT1A1*28 polymorphism in the pharmacodynamics and pharmacokinetics of irinotecan in patients with metastatic colorectal cancer. *J Clin Oncol.* 2006;24(19):3061-3068.
29. Mattison LK, Soong R, Diasio RB. Implications of dihydropyrimidine dehydrogenase on 5-fluorouracil pharmacogenetics and pharmacogenomics. *Pharmacogenomics.* 2002;3(4):485-492.
30. Karapetis CS, Khambata-Ford S, Jonker DJ, et al. K-ras mutations and benefit from cetuximab in advanced colorectal cancer. *N Engl J Med.* 2008;359(17):1757-1765.
31. Jimeno A, Messersmith WA, Hirsch FR, Franklin WA, Eckhardt SG. KRAS mutations and sensitivity to epidermal growth factor receptor inhibitors in colorectal cancer: practical application of patient selection. *J Clin Oncol.* 2009;27(7):1130-1136.

CHAPTER

16 Skin and Melanoma

Betty M. Chan

FOUNDATION OVERVIEW

Melanoma is a serious form of skin cancer and is the sixth most common cancer in men and seventh most common cancer in women. In the United States, approximately 68,720 new cases of melanoma were diagnosed in 2009, leading to 8650 deaths. The outcome and survival rate of melanoma is dependent on the stage of the disease at diagnosis (Table 16-1).[1-4]

Melanoma arises from melanocytes located at the epidermal and dermal layers of the skin and the choroids of the eyes. Melanocytes help synthesize melanin, a brown pigment which makes skin tan or brown and protects deeper layers of tissues from ultraviolet radiation damage (eg, sun damage). Melanoma is a result of malignant skin transformation from skin melanocytes or preexisting nevocellular nevi (moles). Although the etiology of melanoma is not fully understood, many risk factors have been identified. Risk for melanoma includes personal or family history of melanoma, presence of multiple atypical moles or dysplastic nevi, previous history of non-melanoma skin cancer (eg, basal cell and squamous cell), and immunosuppression. Incidence of melanoma increases with intermittent intense ultraviolet sun exposure over chronic periods.[5-11]

Normal nevus present as an evenly colored brown, tan, or black spot on the skin. They are round or oval in shape, and appear flat or raised. Nevi are generally less than 6 mm in diameter and stay about the same size, shape, and color. However, any nevi that change size, shape, or color are suspicious and require evaluation by a dermatologist. The ABCDE rule of melanoma is a useful tool to identify suspicious lesions. ***A*** is asymmetry where one-half of the mole does not match the other half; ***B*** is border irregularity where the edges of the mole are often irregular, blurred, ragged, or notched; ***C*** is color where the color of the mole is not uniform, it may appear with different shades of tan or blue-black, and sometimes mixed with colors of red, purple, and white; ***D*** is diameter where lesions are often > 6 mm in diameter, although melanoma can sometimes present with lesions of < 6 mm in diameter; ***E*** is evolving or changing characteristics of a lesion.[5,12]

Classification of Melanoma

Depending on the location and presentation of the lesions, the classification of melanoma can be different. Superficial spreading melanoma is the most common type of melanoma. The lesions arise from a preexisting flat nevus that develops into an irregular and asymmetrical nevus. Nodular melanoma is the second most common type of melanoma. Nodular melanoma has an aggressive and rapid growth pattern. The lesions are uniform in color and are commonly located on the head, neck, and trunk. Lentigo maligna melanomas occur in older individuals and are located on the face. Compared to other melanoma subtypes, lentigo maligna does not metastasize. Acral lentiginous melanoma is the most common type of melanoma in African Americans, Hispanics, and Asians. The lesions are observed on the palms of the hands, soles of the feet, or beneath the nail beds. Uveal melanoma is an ocular melanoma which arises from the pigmented epithelium of the choroids. Uveal melanoma is intraocular lesions reported in adults, with metastases frequently occurring in the liver.[13,14]

Diagnosis and Staging

Suspicious lesions should be evaluated by a dermatologist. A total body skin examination is performed to identify nevi that are suspicious for melanoma. Biopsy of suspicious lesions is the only way to confirm the diagnosis of melanoma.[4,5] Melanomas may be staged by using the American Joint Commission on Cancer (AJCC) TNM staging system, where T stands for tumor, N stands for nodal involvement, and M stands for metastases.[15,16] The two most important prognostic factors influencing staging are the Breslow tumor thickness and the presence or absence of ulceration of the overlying epithelium.[17,18]

PREVENTION

The American Cancer Society recommends practicing sun safety when you are outdoors by remembering to:

1. Protect your skin from sun exposure by wearing clothing. Long-sleeved shirts, long skirts, or long pants offer the most protection. Dark colored clothing offers more protection than light colored clothing. Avoid direct sun exposure between 10 AM to 4 PM when the ultraviolet radiations are the strongest.
2. Wear a hat with a minimum of at least 2- to 3-inch brim to protect sun-exposed areas such as neck, ears, eyes, forehead, nose, and scalp.
3. Use sunscreen and lip balms with sun protection factor (SPF) of 15 or higher on areas where skin is exposed to the sun. Apply sunscreen 20 to 30 minutes prior to sun exposure, and reapply every 2 hours or more frequently if you sweat or swim.

TABLE 16-1 Stages of Melanoma and Mortality

▪ Early stage—Localized disease[a]
▪ Primary tumors ≤ 1 mm in thickness
▪ 5-year survival > 90%
▪ Primary tumors > 1 mm in thickness
▪ 5-year survival rate 50%-90%
▪ Advanced disease
▪ Disease with nodal involvement
▪ 5-year survival rate 20%-70%
▪ Distant metastases[b]
▪ 5-year survival rate < 10%

[a]Majority (80%-85%) of patients.
[b]2%-5% of patients.

4. Wear sunglasses that wrap around the eyes for additional sun protection with at least 99% ultraviolet A and B absorption.

Other recommendations include the avoidance of using tanning beds or sunlamps, a monthly self-examination of the skin to identify any suspicious markings, and annual clinical examination by a dermatologist for high-risk patients.[5,19]

TREATMENT

The treatment and management of melanoma is dependent on the stage and disease involvement. Surgical excision is the primary treatment option for early stage melanoma.[4]

Adjuvant Treatment of Melanoma

High-dose interferon-alfa 2b is FDA approved for adjuvant treatment of melanoma after surgical resection of primary melanoma or any primary melanoma with nodal involvement. The dose of interferon-alfa 2b is 20 million international units (IU)/m^2 intravenously five times weekly for 4 weeks, followed by 10 million international units (IU)/m^2 subcutaneously three times weekly for 48 weeks. Majority of patients (> 80%) develop flu-like symptoms (eg, fever, chills, headache, myalgias, and arthralgias). Premedication with an antipyretic, such as acetaminophen or nonsteroidal anti-inflammatory agent (NSAID), minimizes the risk and severity of fever and chills. Other side effects associated with high-dose interferon-alfa 2b include fatigue, anorexia (can be dose limiting), and neuropsychiatric symptoms (eg, depression, confusion, and somnolence). Other effects associated with interferon include myelosuppression (eg, neutropenia and thrombocytopenia), hepatotoxicity, and thyroid disorders (both hypo and hyperthyroidism).[4,20-24]

Metastatic Treatment of Melanoma

Treatment options for metastatic melanoma are determined based on patients' performance status, whether the lesion is resectable or unresectable, and the presence or absence of distant metastases. Both single agent and combinational chemotherapeutic agents have been used, however, median duration of response remains low (< 1 year).[4]

Single-Agents Chemotherapy

Dacarbazine (DTIC) is an alkylating agent approved for treatment of metastatic melanoma as single or combination therapy. Dacarbazine is dosed at 150 to 250 mg/m^2 intravenous piggyback (IVPB) on days 1 to 5 every 3 to 4 weeks. Response rate with single-agent dacarbazine is 15% to 25%, with duration of response lasting 3 to 6 months.[25-27] Effects associated with dacarbazine are:

- Myelosuppression (eg, leukopenia and thrombocytopenia) is a dose-limiting toxicity.
- Nausea and vomiting can be severe and dacarbazine is classified as a highly emetogenic chemotherapeutic agent.
    - Antiemetic therapy with a 5-HT3 receptor antagonist and a corticosteroid given 30 minutes to 60 minutes prior to dacarbazine is recommended.
- Flu-like symptoms (eg, fever, chills, malaise, myalgias, and arthralgias).
- Local pain and burning sensation at injection site.
- Risk of extravasation (extravasation may lead to severe tissue necrosis around injection site).
- Hepatotoxicity with hepatocellular necrosis and hepatic vein thrombosis.

Temozolomide (Temodar) is an oral alkylating agent structurally similar to dacarbazine. Temozolomide and dacarbazine have demonstrated similar response rates. The dose of temozolomide is 200 mg/m^2/d orally for 5 days; repeat every 28 days up to 12 cycles. Dose-limiting myelosuppression (eg, leukopenia and thrombocytopenia) is associated with temozolomide. Temozolomide is classified as a moderately emetogenic agent. The use of antiemetics prior to drug administration is recommended to minimize the risk of nausea and vomiting. Fatigue, headache, mild elevation of hepatic transaminases, and photosensitivity are also associated with temozolomide.[26,27]

Interleukin-2 (IL-2, Proleukin) is FDA approved for treatment of metastatic melanoma. The dose of IL-2 is 600,000 international units (IU)/kg intravenously every 8 hours for a maximum of 14 doses; repeat after 9 days for a total of 28 doses per course. Treatment with IL-2 is associated with flu-like symptoms and premedication with an antipyretic may decrease symptoms. Vascular or capillary leak syndrome is a dose-limiting toxicity observed with high-dose IL-2. Vascular or capillary leak syndrome may present as weight gain, ascites, arrhythmias, hypotension, oliguria, and pleural effusions. Early intervention with dopamine 1 to 5 μg/kg/min may be necessary to maintain renal perfusion and minimize renal toxicities. Myelosuppression (eg, neutropenia, anemia, and thrombocytopenia), reversible hepatotoxicity, neuropsychiatric symptoms (eg, somnolence, delirium, and confusion) have been observed.[28,29] Continuous neurologic, cardiac, and pulmonary monitoring is recommended during therapy. Avoid concomitant use of:

- nonsteroidal anti-inflammatory agents as they may increase the risk of capillary leak syndrome.
- antihypertensives as IL-2 potentiate the effect of antihypertensives.
- corticosteroids as they may decrease the antitumor effects of IL-2 due to corticosteroids inhibitory effect on the immune system.

Paclitaxel (Taxol) and docetaxel (Taxotere) have been used for treatment of metastatic melanoma, however, response rates are relatively low (6%-18%).[30]

Combination Chemotherapy

Combination chemotherapy regimens are utilized in attempts to improve the treatment and response of metastatic melanoma. Dacarbazine has been used in combination with the Dartmouth regimen (dacarbazine 220 mg/m^2 IVPB on day 1-3, carmustine 150 mg/m^2 IVPB on day 1 of every other cycle, cisplatin 25 mg/m^2 IVPB on days 1-3, and tamoxifen 10 mg po bid with cycle repeat every 3 weeks). Evidence demonstrated equivalent response rates between the Dartmouth regimen and dacarbazine; however, side effects were higher in the combination group. Other combination regimens such as CVD (cisplatin, vinblastine, and dacarbazine) have been used for treatment of metastatic melanoma; however, there is no survival advantage with the use of CVD over dacarbazine.[31-35]

Biochemotherapy

The combination of chemotherapy and biologic agents has been used for the treatment of metastatic melanoma. The most commonly used chemotherapy regimen is the CVD regimen with IL-2 and interferon-alfa 2b.[36] The addition of immunotherapy to combination chemotherapy did not improve quality of response or overall survival, but increased side effects.[37-39]

Follow-up Care

Lifetime annual skin examination is recommended for all patients with melanoma regardless of melanoma stage. Frequency of follow-up surveillance should be individualized and determined based on patients' risk factors, family history, presence of dysplastic nevi, and history of non-melanoma skin cancers. Health care professionals should educate patients to perform monthly self-examination of their skin and suspicious lesions should be evaluated by a health care professional.[4,40,41]

CASE Application

1. Select the risk factor(s) associated with melanoma.
   a. Presence of multiple dysplastic nevi
   b. Presence of genetic factors
   c. Individuals with fair skin type who sunburns easily
   d. All of the above are risk factors associated with melanoma

2. Which of the following statements is true regarding the subtypes of melanoma?
   a. Superficial spreading melanomas are the most common type of melanomas with lesions usually arising from preexisting nevus.
   b. Nodular melanomas are slow-growing lesions that develop and spread in a vertical growth phase pattern.
   c. Lentigo maligna melanomas are more commonly reported in children, with lesions less likely to metastasize.
   d. Uveal melanomas are rare lower extremity malignancies arising from pigmented epithelium of the choroids, with lesions more likely to metastasize to liver.

3. Which of the following is not a part of the ABCDE rule used to identify and evaluate a suspicious lesion?
   a. Asymmetry
   b. Border irregularity
   c. Color of lesions
   d. Depths of the lesions
   e. Evolving or changing characteristics of a lesion

4. Once a suspicious lesion is identified, which is the best method in confirming the diagnosis?
   a. Obtain a complete clinical examination, medical history of patient and family members.
   b. Obtain complete laboratory studies with hematology, electrolytes, liver function test, and LDH.
   c. Consider full-thickness excisional biopsy with 1 to 3 mm margin of normal-appearing skin.
   d. Consider ordering a chest x-ray and a CT scan for confirming diagnosis.

5. Select the American Cancer Society (ACS) recommendation(s) for the prevention and screening of melanoma.
   a. Wear proper protective clothing to cover as much exposed skin as possible (ie, sun glasses, hat with wide brim, long sleeve clothing, etc).
   b. Use sunscreen lotion with an SPF of at least 15 or higher.
   c. Avoid direct sun exposure between 10 AM to 4 PM when ultraviolet rays are the most intense.
   d. Avoid the use of tanning beds or sunlamps to minimize exposure to ultraviolet radiation.
   e. All of the above are recommendations made by ACS for the prevention and screening of melanoma.

6. Select the chemotherapeutic agent regimen used for the treatment of stage IV metastatic melanoma.
   a. CVD regimen
   b. Dacarbazine
   c. Carmustine
   d. a and b
   e. All of the above are chemotherapeutic agent or regimen used for the treatment of stage IV metastatic melanoma

7. Which of the following oral chemotherapeutic agent has been used in the treatment of melanoma?
   a. Capecitabine
   b. Lapatinib
   c. Erlotinib
   d. Procarbazine
   e. Temozolomide

8. Select the side effect(s) associated with the use of high-dose interleukin-2 (IL-2) for the treatment of melanoma.
   a. Flu-like symptoms
   b. Myelosuppression
   c. Constipation
   d. a and b
   e. All of the above

9. CD is a 28-year-old woman who is to start chemotherapy treatment with high-dose interferon-alfa 2b. Select the side effect(s) associated with interferon.
   a. Flu-like symptoms requiring premedication with antipyretic
   b. Fatigue
   c. Depression
   d. Somnolence and confusion
   e. All of the above

10. Select the medication that may be used concurrently with high-dose Aldesleukin *except*:
    a. Dexamethasone
    b. Indomethacin
    c. Losartan
    d. Granisetron

11. Select the side effect(s) associated with dacarbazine.
    i. Leukopenia
    ii. Increased appetite
    iii. Flu-like symptoms

    a. i
    b. i and iii
    c. ii and iii
    d. iii

12. CY is a 25-year-old man with stage IV metastatic melanoma receiving biochemotherapy treatment with cisplatin, vinblastine, dacarbazine, interferon-alfa 2b, and interleukin-2. His laboratory values prior to treatment are within normal limits. Select the supportive care management for CY's biochemotherapy treatment.
    i. Premedication with acetaminophen
    ii. Premedication with dolasetron and dexamethasone
    iii. Premedication with atropine 0.25 mg IV push

    a. ii only
    b. iii only
    c. ii and iii
    d. i and ii
    e. i and iii

13. Which of the following is the correct FDA-approved dosing of dacarbazine when used as single agent for treatment of melanoma?
    a. 375 mg/m^2 IVPB on days 1 and 15 with cycle repeat every 28 days
    b. 20 million IU/m^2 IVPB five times weekly for 4 weeks, then 10 million IU/m^2 subcutaneously three times weekly for 48 weeks
    c. 250 mg/m^2 IVPB on days 1 to 5 with cycle repeat every 21 days
    d. 600,000 IU/kg IVPB every 8 hours for a maximum of 14 doses; repeat after 9 days for a total of 28 doses per course
    e. 150 mg/m^2 po daily for 5 days with cycle repeat every 28 days

14. Which of the following is the correct FDA-approved dosing of Interferon-alfa 2b when used as single agent for treatment of melanoma?
    a. 375 mg/m^2 IVPB on days 1 and 15 with cycle repeat every 28 days
    b. 20 million IU/m^2 IVPB five times weekly for 4 weeks, then 10 million IU/m^2 subcutaneously three times weekly for 48 weeks
    c. 250 mg/m^2 IVPB on days 1 to 5 with cycle repeat every 21 days
    d. 600,000 IU/kg IVPB every 8 hours for a maximum of 14 doses; repeat after 9 days for a total of 28 doses per course
    e. 150 mg/m^2 po daily for 5 days with cycle repeat every 28 days

15. Which of the following is the correct FDA-approved dosing of interleukin-2 when used as single agent for treatment of melanoma?
    a. 375 mg/m^2 IVPB on days 1 and 15 with cycle repeat every 28 days
    b. 20 million IU/m^2 IVPB five times weekly for 4 weeks, then 10 million IU/m^2 subcutaneously three times weekly for 48 weeks
    c. 250 mg/m^2 IVPB on days 1 to 5 with cycle repeat every 21 days
    d. 600,000 IU/kg IVPB every 8 hours for a maximum of 14 doses; repeat after 9 days for a total of 28 doses per course
    e. 150 mg/m^2 po daily for 5 days with cycle repeat every 28 days

16. Select the answer that represents follow-up care recommendations for patients with melanoma.
    a. Annual skin examination and surveillance by a dermatologist for all patients with melanoma regardless of stage of lesions.
    b. Educate patients to perform monthly self-examination of their skin and lymph nodes.
    c. Educate patients about skin cancer prevention including sun protection and proper use of sunscreen with at least SPF of 15 or higher.
    d. All of the above.

17. Select the central nervous system side effect associated with interferon.

    i. Depression
    ii. Confusion
    iii. Somnolence
    iv. Hepatotoxicity

    a. i only
    b. iv only
    c. i, iii, and iv
    d. i, ii, and iii
    e. i and iv

18. Select the parameters that should be monitored with dacarbazine.

    i. Complete blood count
    ii. Liver function tests
    iii. Injection site reactions

    a. i and ii
    b. ii and iii
    c. i, ii, and iii
    d. i and iii

19. Select the receptor antagonists that should be administered with the alkylating agent dacarbazine.

    a. Temozolomide
    b. Interleukin-2
    c. Ondansetron
    d. Cisplatin

20. Select the side effect associated with IL-2 that leads to hypotension and reduced organ perfusion.

    a. Capillary leak syndrome
    b. Myelosuppression
    c. Anemia
    d. Hepatotoxicity
    e. Delirium

TAKEAWAY POINTS ››

- Melanoma is a serious form of skin cancer.
- Risk factors include personal or family history of melanoma, genetic factors, atypical dysplastic nevi, previous history of non-melanoma skin cancer, and individuals who are immunosuppressed.
- Practice sun protective safety measures if you have to be outdoors by wearing sun protective clothing and using sunscreen with an SPF of 15 or higher.
- The ABCDE rule of melanoma identifies clinical features of any suspicious lesions.
- Biopsy is the only way to confirm the diagnosis of melanoma.
- The outcome and survival rate is dependent on stage of disease at diagnosis, outcome is best if melanoma is diagnosed at its earliest stages of disease when 5-year survival rate is > 90%.
- The two most important prognostic factors influencing staging and outcome are the Breslow tumor thickness and the presence or absence of ulceration of the overlying epithelium.
- High-dose interferon-alfa 2b is currently the only FDA approved agent for adjuvant treatment of melanoma.
- Single-agent dacarbazine is standard of care in the treatment of metastatic melanoma.
- Temozolomide has been used in treatment of advanced or metastatic melanoma and has a similar response rate compared to dacarbazine.
- High-dose interleukin-2 has been used in treatment of metastatic melanoma; however, treatment with IL-2 is associated with many severe side effects requiring continuous monitoring.
- NCCN guidelines recommended follow-up care with lifetime annual skin examination for patients with melanoma regardless to stage of lesions.

REFERENCES

1. Jermal A, Siegel R, Ward E, et al. Cancer statistics, 2009. *CA Cancer J Clin*. 2009;59:225-249.
2. Horner MJ, Ries LAG, Krapcho M, et al (eds). *SEER Cancer Statistics Review, 1975-2006*. National Cancer Institute. Bethesda, MD. http://seer.cancer.gov/csr/1975_2006/, based on November 2008 SEER data submission, posted to the SEER web site, 2009. Accessed March 15, 2010.
3. American Cancer Society. Cancer facts and figures 2009. www.cancer.org. Accessed September 10, 2009.
4. Coit DG, Andtbacka R, Bichakjian CK, et al. Melanoma: clinical practice guidelines in oncology. *JNCCN*. 2009;7:250-275.
5. American Cancer Society. Skin cancer–melanoma 2009. www.cancer.org Accessed September 10, 2009.
6. Curtin JA, Fridlyand J, Kageshita T, et al. Distinct sets of genetic alterations in melanoma. *N Engl J Med*. 2005;353:2135-2147.
7. Ferrone CR, Porat LB, Panageas KS, et al. Clinicopathological features of and risk factors for multiple primary melanomas. *JAMA*. 2005;294:1647-1654.
8. Gandini S, Sera F, Cattaruzza MS, et al. Meta-analysis of risk factors for cutaneous melanoma: I. Common and atypical nevi. *Eur J Cancer*. 2005;41:28-44.
9. Gandini S, Sera F, Cattaruzza MS, et al. Meta-analysis of risk factors for cutaneous melanoma: II. Sun exposure. *Eur J Cancer*. 2005;45-60.
10. Gandini S, Sera F, Cattaruzza MS, et al. Meta-analysis of risk factors for cutaneous melanoma: III. Family history, actinic

damage and phenotypic factors. *Eur J Cancer*. 2005;41: 2040-2059.

11. Gallagher RP, Spinelli JJ, Lee TK. Tanning beds, sunlamps, and risk of cutaneous malignant melanoma. *Cancer Epidemiol Biomarkers Prev*. 2005;14:562-566.
12. Abbasi NR, Shaw HM, Rigel DS, et al. Early diagnosis of cutaneous melanoma: revisiting the ABCD criteria. *JAMA*. 2004;292:2771-2776.
13. McGovern VJ, Minhm MC Jr, Bailly C, et al. The classification of malignant melanoma and its histologic reporting. *Cancer*. 1973;32:1446-1457.
14. Clark WH Jr, From L, Bernardino EA, et al. The histogenesis and biologic behavior of primary human malignant melanomas of the skin. *Cancer Res*. 1969;9:705-727.
15. Balch CM, Buzaid AC, Soong SJ, et al. Final version of the American Joint Committee on Cancer Staging System for cutaneous melanoma. *J Clin Oncol*. 2001;19:3635-3648.
16. Balch CM, Soong SJ, Atkins MB, et al. An evidence-based staging system for cutaneous melanoma. *CA Cancer J Clin*. 2004;54:131-149.
17. Balch CM, Soong SJ, Gershenwald JE, et al. Prognostic factors analysis of 17,600 melanoma patients: validation of the American Joint Committee on cancer melanoma staging system. *J Clin Oncol*. 2001;19:3622-3634.
18. Lachiewicz AM, Berwick M, Wiggins CL, et al. Survival differences between patients with scalp or neck melanoma and those with melanoma of other sites in the surveillance, epidemiology, and end results (SEER) program. *Arch Dermatol*. 2008;144:515.
19. American Cancer Society. Cancer prevention & early detection facts & figures 2009. www.cancer.org Accessed September 10, 2009.
20. Kirkwood J, Strawderman M, Ernstoff M, et al. Interferon alfa-2b adjuvant therapy of high-risk resected cutaneous melanoma: the Eastern Cooperative Oncology Group Trial EST 1684. *J Clin Oncol*. 1996;14:7-17.
21. Kirkwood J, Manola J, Ibrahim J, et al. A pooled analysis of eastern cooperative oncology group and intergroup trials of adjuvant high-dose interferon for melanoma. *Clin Cancer Res*. 2004;10:1670-2677.
22. Kirkwood J, Ibrahim J, Sondak V, et al. High- and low-dose interferon alfa-2b in high-risk melanoma: first analysis of intergroup trial E1690/S9111/C9190. *J Clin Oncol*. 2000;18: 2444-2458.
23. Kirkwood J, Ibrahim J, Sosman J, et al. High-dose interferon alfa-2b significantly prolongs relapse-free and overall survival compared with the GM2-KLH/QS-21 vaccine in patients with resected stage IIB-III melanoma: results of intergroup trial E1694/S9512/C509801. *J Clin Oncol*. 2001;19:2370-2380.
24. Fecher LA, Flaherty KT. Where are we with adjuvant therapy of stage III and IV melanoma in 2009. *JNCCN*. 2009;7:295-304.
25. Serrone L, Zeuli M, Sega FM, et al. Dacarbazine-based chemotherapy for metastatic melanoma: thirty-year experience overview. *J Exp Clin Cancer Res*. 2000;19:21-34.
26. Atallah E, Flaherty L. Treatment of metastatic malignant melanoma. *Curr Treat Options Oncol*. 2005;6:185-193.
27. Middleton MR, Grob JJ, Aaronson N, et al. Randomized phase III study of temozolomide versus dacarbazine in the treatment of patients with advanced metastatic malignant melanoma. *J Clin Oncol*. 2000;18:158-166.
28. Atkins MB, Lotze MT, Dutcher JP, et al. High-dose recombinant interleukin 2 therapy for patients with metastatic melanoma: analysis of 270 patients treated between 1985 and 1993. *J Clin Oncol*. 1999;17:2105-2116.
29. Schwartzentruber DJ. High-dose interleukin-2 is an intensive treatment regardless of the venue of administration. *Cancer J*. 2001;7:103-104.
30. Li Y, McClay EF. Systemic chemotherapy for the treatment of metastatic melanoma. *Semin Oncol*. 2002;29:413-426.
31. Chapman PB, Einhorn LH, Meyers ML, et al. Phase III multicenter randomized trial of the Dartmouth regimen versus dacarbazine in patients with metastatic melanoma. *J Clin Oncol*. 1999;17:2745-2751.
32. Legha SS, Ring S, Papadopoulos N, et al. A prospective evaluation of a triple-drug regimen containing cisplatin, vinblastine, and dacarbazine (CVD) for metastatic melanoma. *Cancer*. 1989;64:2024-2029.
33. Rao RD, Holtan SG, Ingle JN, et al. Combination of paclitaxel and carboplatin as second-line therapy for patients with metastatic melanoma. *Cancer*. 2006;106:375-382.
34. Agarwala SS, Keilholz U, Hogg D. Randomized phase III study of paclitaxel plus carboplatin with or without sorafenib as second-line treatment in patients with advanced melanoma [abstract]. *J Clin Oncol*. 2007;25(Supp 1):Abstract 8510.
35. Legha SS, Ring S, Bedikian A, et al. Treatment of metastatic melanoma with combined chemotherapy containing cisplatin, vinblastine, dacarbazine (CVD) and biotherapy using interleukin-2 and interferon-alpha. *Ann Oncol*. 1996;7:827-835.
36. Legha SS, Ring S, Eton O, et al. Development of a biochemotherapy regimen with concurrent administration of cisplatin, vinblastine, dacarbazine, interferon alfa, and interleukin-2 for patients with metastatic melanoma. *J Clin Oncol*. 1998;16: 1752-1759.
37. Eaton O, Legha SS, Bedikian AY, et al. Sequential biochemotherapy versus chemotherapy for metastatic melanoma: result from a phase III randomized trial. *J Clin Oncol*. 2002;20: 2045-2052.
38. Atkins MB, Hsu J, Lee S, et al. Phase III trial comparing concurrent biochemotherapy with cisplatin, vinblastine, dacarbazine, interleukin-2, and interferon alfa-2b with cisplatin, vinblastine, and dacarbazine alone in patients with metastatic malignant melanoma (E3695): a trial coordinated by the Eastern Cooperative Oncology Group. *J Clin Oncol*. 2008;26: 5748-5754.
39. Ives NJ, Stowe RL, Lorigan P, et al. Chemotherapy compared with biochemotherapy for the treatment of metastatic melanoma: a meta-analysis of 18 trials involving 2621 patients. *J Clin Oncol*. 2007;25:5426-5434.
40. Basseres N, Grob JJ, Richard MA, et al. Cost-effectiveness of surveillance of stage I melanoma. A retrospective appraisal based on a 10-year experience in a dermatology department in France. *Dermatology*. 1995;191:199-203.
41. Weiss M, Loprinzi CL, Creagan ET, et al. Utility of follow-up tests for detecting recurrent disease in patients with malignant melanomas. *JAMA*. 1995;274:1703-1705.

CHAPTER

17 Leukemia

David L. DeRemer

FOUNDATION OVERVIEW

Acute Lymphoblastic Leukemia (ALL)

An estimated 5760 new cases of adult lymphoblastic leukemia (ALL) were diagnosed in 2009.[1] Leukemia is the most common malignancy in pediatrics; 80% to 85% of leukemia in children is ALL and represents 2400 new cases diagnosed each year. The peak incidence of adult and pediatric ALL is 50 years and 5 years of age, respectively.[2] The exact cause of ALL is unknown. Less than 5% of cases have been associated with inherited genetic syndromes (Down or Bloom syndrome) or with exposure to ionizing radiation and chemotherapeutic agents. In the development of B cells and T cells, various events occur to develop a competent immune system. In ALL, mutations occur in the development of B- and T-cell progenitors leading to dysregulated proliferation and clonal expansion.[3]

Patients can present with malaise, fever, weight loss, palpitations, bruising, petechiae, bone pain, and lymphadenopathy. Many symptoms will represent malignant cells replacing normal hematopoiesis. Electrolyte disturbances such as hyperkalemia, hyperphosphatemia, hyperuricemia, and hypocalcemia may occur. Patients with acute leukemias may experience tumor lysis syndrome (to be discussed later in this chapter). Upon physical examination, hepatomegaly, splenomegaly, and a mediastinal mass may be noted.[4] Leukocytosis (WBC > 30,000-50,000/μL) confers a poorer prognosis, particularly in B-cell ALL.[5] Other factors which confers poorer prognosis include age (> 30), immunophenotype (B lineage worse), Philadelphia chromosome (Ph+) disease, and CNS disease.[3,5]

Diagnosis is determined by evaluating the following—complete blood count (CBC) with differential, coagulation studies, bone marrow biopsy and aspiration, and lumbar puncture. Cytochemical studies, immunophenotyping, and cytogenetics are performed on bone marrow samples. A lumbar puncture should be performed to assess potential CNS involvement.[4]

TREATMENT

A strong prognostic factor is patient's response to treatment. The primary goal of treatment is to induce and maintain a complete remission (CR). A CR can be induced in 96% to 99% of children and 78% to 93% of adults.[6] Treatment of pediatric ALL is divided into the following phases: induction, consolidation, interim maintenance, delayed intensification, and maintenance. Adult ALL is divided into induction, consolidation, and maintenance. CNS treatment is performed throughout all phases of therapy. Intrathecal therapy consists of methotrexate and cytarabine which can be given alone or in combination.[4] Patients with T-cell ALL have an increased incidence of CNS disease and should receive systemic high-dose methotrexate to penetrate the CNS.[7] Multiple intensive chemotherapy regimens have been shown to provide benefit in adult ALL. Specific agents which are used in the treatment of ALL are summarized in Table 17-1.

Special Populations

Approximately 5% of children and 30% of adult ALL will have Ph+ disease.[2] These patients may receive oral tyrosine kinase inhibitors (TKIs) in combination with traditional chemotherapy.[8,9] These agents will be discussed further in the chronic myelogenous leukemia (CML) section in this chapter. For pediatric patients there is no standard regimen, rather these patients will be enrolled in a clinical trial and must maintain strict adherence to protocol. In older adults (55-65 years) dose reductions may be necessary due to toxicities of adult ALL regimens. Elderly patients rarely achieve a CR and goals of therapy include control of leukemia and maintaining acceptable quality of life.[5]

Acute Myelogenous Leukemia (AML)

According to the estimate of American Cancer Society, in 2009, 12,810 new cases of AML were diagnosed and 9000 people died from this disease.[1] The incidence of AML increases with age and is typically diagnosed in elderly patients and more frequently found in males.[10] Risk factors include ionizing radiation, benzene, and cytotoxic chemotherapy. Specifically, alkylating agents and topoisomerase II inhibitors have been associated with the development of AML.[11] AML arises from a leukemic cell which expands and acquires additional mutations. Genetic alterations lead to AML blasts which are ineffective in generating mature neutrophils, platelets, and red blood cells.[12]

Clinical presentation is nonspecific and related to decreased production of normal hematopoietic cells. Patients will often describe an infection characterized by fatigue and elevated temperature. Other symptoms include weight loss, dyspnea on exertion, bleeding and bruising, joint and bone pain, gingival hypertrophy, and headache.[4] Unlike ALL, AML is less commonly associated with CNS involvement.[13] Metabolic and electrolyte abnormalities are also common. Patients

TABLE 17-1 **Commonly Used Agents in Treatment of ALL**

Agent	Classification	Route of Administration	Adverse Reactions
Asparaginase (*Escherichia coli* strain)	Other	IM/IV/SQ	Allergic reactions, coagulopathy (increased prothrombin time), depression, fatigue, hyperglycemia, pancreatitis, thrombotic events
Cyclophosphamide	Alkylating agent	IV	Alopecia, hemorrhagic cystitis, impairment of fertility, myelosuppression, N/V, secondary malignancies
Cytarabine	Antimetabolite	IV/IT	Cerebellar dysfunction, conjunctivitis, diarrhea, myelosuppression, pulmonary edema, N/V
Daunorubicin	Topoisomerase II inhibitor	IV	Alopecia, cardiotoxicity, discoloration of urine, extravasation, myelosuppression, N/V, secondary malignancies
Doxorubicin	Topoisomerase II inhibitor	IV	Alopecia, cardiotoxicity, discoloration of urine, extravasation, myelosuppression, N/V, secondary malignancies
Mercaptopurine	Antimetabolite	po	Hyperbilirubinemia, increased hepatic transaminases, intrahepatic cholestasis, myelosuppression
Methotrexate	Antimetabolite	IV/IT	IV: Acute renal failure, dermatologic reactions, diarrhea, hepatotoxicity, impaired fertility, mucositis, neurotoxicity IT or high-dose MTX: Headache, motor paralysis of extremities, cranial nerve palsy, seizure
Prednisone	Corticosteroid	po	Cushing's syndrome, diabetes mellitus, fluid retention, insomnia, mood swings, myopathy, osteoporosis, ulcerative esophagitis, wound healing impairment
Vincristine	Antimicrotubule	IV	Alopecia, constipation and paralytic ileus, CNS depression, extravasation, peripheral neuropathy **Note: Do not give intrathecally;** may cause severe neurological toxicity and/or death

Abbreviation: N/V, nausea/vomiting.

may present with hyperuricemia, hyperkalemia, and hyperphosphatemia. A CBC with differential will reveal anemia, thrombocytopenia, and leukopenia or leukocytosis (20% of patients will present with a high WBC).[4]

The diagnostic work-up for AML includes CBC with differential, coagulation studies, examination of a peripheral blood smear, and examination of a bone marrow aspirate and biopsy. Cytochemical studies to determine leukemia lineage (myeloid or lymphoid) and immunophenotyping are also performed. Cytogenetic analysis to determine chromosomal abnormalities assists in diagnosis and prognosis.[4]

TREATMENT

Treatment is immediately initiated following definitive diagnosis. Treatment consists of three phases: induction, post-remission, and refractory/relapsed disease. The goal of induction therapy is to induce a CR with a return of normal hematopoiesis. A CR is defined as achieving a platelet count > 100,000 μL, neutrophil count > 1000 μL, and a bone marrow specimen < 5% blasts.[14] Patients that achieve a CR post-induction have a better prognosis.[12] For the past 30 years, induction therapy has consisted of the combination of cytarabine with an anthracycline (daunorubicin or idarubicin). A common regimen is "7+3" which combines cytarabine (100 mg/m^2 days 1-7) with idarubicin (12 mg/m^2 days 1-3).[15] Patients 60 years of age and older with significant comorbidities should not receive 7+3 due to poor outcomes. These patients may benefit from supportive care or investigational treatment.[12]

Post-remission therapy consists of multiple cycles of high-dose cytarabine (HDAC). The optimal dose (g/m^2) and the number of cycles to be given are controversial. Patients will typically receive 6 to 18 g/m^2 of cytarabine per cycle for 3 to 4 cycles.[12] Toxicities of HDAC include cerebellar dysfunction, pulmonary edema, pericardial effusion, and conjunctivitis.[16,17] Renal function should be closely monitored following HDAC administration since renal dysfunction has correlated to cerebellar dysfunction. For patients who are unable to achieve a CR, refractory/relapsed treatments are available. Cytarabine alone or in combination with fludarabine, mitoxantrone, etoposide, or clofarabine are options. Response rates in the relapsed setting range from 10% to 50% and often have a short duration. Depending on age and cytogenetic risk factors (good, intermediate, or poor) patients may benefit from either an autologous or allogeneic stem cell transplant.[12] Targeted therapy has been attempted in the treatment of AML. Gemtuzumab ozogamicin, an anti-CD33 humanized monoclonal antibody, was indicated for patients ≥ 60 years of age who were not transplant candidates. The CD33 antigen is expressed on leukemic blasts on approximately 80% of AML patients. However in June 2010, the US FDA recommended the withdrawal of gemtuzumab given new concerns with drug safety and lack of clinical benefit.

Acute promyelocytic leukemia (APL or AML-M3) represents approximately 10% of AML cases. In general, APL has a better prognosis than other AML subtypes. Rather than receiving standard 7+3 induction therapy, APL patients should receive an anthracycline with tretinoin. Tretinoin (all-trans retinoic acid, or ATRA) is given orally at 45 mg/m^2, divided into two doses after a full meal.[4] At the initiation of tretinoin, patients need to be monitored for retinoic acid syndrome (or differentiation syndrome, DS). DS is associated with respiratory distress, pleural effusions, pulmonary infiltrates, and fever. This syndrome can be fatal; patients should immediately receive dexamethasone 10 mg IV Q12 for 3 to 5 days to improve symptoms and decrease mortality. Tretinoin may need to be held during this period, but will need to be reinstituted following symptom improvement and continued. Patients should receive tretinoin orally daily ± oral 6-mercaptopurine and methotrexate for maintenance therapy.[18]

SPECIAL CONSIDERATIONS

Supportive care and monitoring is essential in patients with acute leukemias. Patients with high WBC counts are particularly susceptible to tumor lysis syndrome (TLS). Aggressive hydration and diuresis are important in the prevention and management of TLS. TLS is characterized by increased uric acid, hyperphosphatemia, hyperkalemia, hypocalcemia, increased serum creatinine, and decreased urine output. Patients should receive allopurinol to prevent the formation of uric acid. In patients who present with hyperuricemia, rasburicase should be used in select patients. Rasburicase is contraindicated with glucose-6-phosphate dehydrogenase (G6PD) deficiency.[19]

Patients will receive platelet and red cell transfusions as clinically indicated. Also, prophylactic antimicrobial therapy is recommended in patients who may have prolonged neutropenia. The use of colony-stimulating factors (filgrastim, sargramostim) should be considered in older patients to decrease the duration of hospitalization.[4]

Chronic Lymphocytic Leukemia (CLL)

CLL is the most common form of leukemia in the United States and an estimated 15,490 new cases were diagnosed in 2009.[1] The disease is typically diagnosed in the elderly with a median age of onset between 65 and 75.[10] The etiology of CLL is elusive since no causal relationship has been found with exposure of radiation, chemicals, or viral oncogenesis.[20] CLL is thought to arise from a polyclonal expansion of CD5+ B lymphocytes. A majority of patients will be asymptomatic upon diagnosis. Patients with symptoms will most often present with lymphadenopathies. Other symptoms include splenomegaly, hepatomegaly, fever, night sweats, and increased frequency of infections. Laboratory examinations may reveal lymphocytosis, anemia, thrombocytopenia, and hypogammaglobulinemia.[21] The diagnostic workup includes a physical examination, laboratory studies including CBC, bone marrow biopsy and aspirate, immunophenotyping, and cytogenetics.[22]

TREATMENT

CLL is considered incurable and the goals of treatment include palliation and increase duration of life.[20] Standard treatment for CLL may include a period of watchful waiting until progression of disease (eg, high WBC, bulky lymph nodes, symptomatic splenomegaly). Early treatment has not resulted in survival benefit.[23,24] In advanced stages (Rai stage III-IV), treatment is warranted in attempt to obtain disease remission. Both traditional cytotoxic chemotherapy and monoclonal antibodies offer effective treatment options.

Cytotoxic Chemotherapy

Purine analogs are effective agents in treating CLL. Specifically, fludarabine has been shown as monotherapy and in combination to provide benefit. As single-agent therapy, fludarabine is given once daily for 5 days intravenously. Adverse events associated with fludarabine include myelosuppression, autoimmune effects, and neurologic toxicities.[25] Furthermore, patients need to be counseled on documentation of fevers and infection. Due to risk of opportunistic infections patients should receive PCP, antifungal, and antiviral prophylaxis.[26] Oral alkylating agents (cyclophosphamide and chlorambucil) are also a treatment option but have been shown to be inferior to fludarabine.[25] Fludarabine with IV cyclophosphamide has resulted in improved overall survival and complete remission rates when compared to fludarabine alone.[27,28] An additional alkylating agent, bendamustine, which has low cross-resistance with other alkylating agents, was recently approved and is recommended as monotherapy for first-line therapy and in combination for relapsed disease.[29] Bendamustine has been associated with myelosuppression, skin reactions, infections, infusion reactions, and tumor lysis syndrome.

Monoclonal Antibodies

Rituximab is a chimeric monoclonal antibody that targets CD20 surface antigen expressed on B lymphocytes. Single agent weekly rituximab has demonstrated modest clinical benefit and is commonly used in combination regimens.[30] Adverse events associated with rituximab include infusion related reactions, tumor lysis syndrome, flu-like symptoms, skin rash, and cytopenias. Hepatitis B reactivation has been reported in patients treated with rituximab in combination with chemotherapy. As a result, it is recommended that hepatitis B testing be performed prior to the initiation of rituximab.[29]

Alemtuzumab is a humanized monoclonal antibody that targets CD52 antigen expressed on B and T lymphocytes. Severe infusion related reactions are associated with alemtuzumab. Patients should receive acetaminophen and diphenhydramine 30 minutes prior to the initiation of infusion.[31] Due to the infusion related reactions associated with intravenous administration, some investigators sought to improve adverse events with subcutaneous administration.[32] Additional adverse events include pancytopenias, fever, rigors, hypotension, and immunosuppression. Patients who receive alemtuzumab have a significant increased risk of infection. It is recommended that patients receive PCP prophylaxis and herpes viral prophylaxis for a minimum of 2 months following the completion of alemtuzumab in addition to appropriate antifungal prophylaxis.[26] Reactivation of CMV has also been reported and warrants monitoring and preemptive therapy.[31] Alemtuzumab is frequently used as second-line agent, but is recommended as first line in specific patient populations.[29]

Combination Therapy

The combination of fludarabine, cyclophosphamide, and rituximab (FCR regimen) is recommended as first-line regimen following a study which demonstrated superiority over fludarabine and cyclophosphamide (FC) in untreated patients.[33] Multiple rituximab based combinations have demonstrated clinical benefit. Alemtuzumab has also been combined with fludarabine or rituximab for additional treatment options.[34,35]

SPECIAL CONSIDERATIONS

Appropriate supportive care for CLL patients is essential. It is recommended that patients with hypogammaglobulinemia who experience reoccurring infections particularly with encapsulated organisms receive monthly intravenous immunoglobulins (IVIG) 0.3 to 0.5 g/kg. Patients should also be given an annual influenza vaccine and a pneumococcal vaccine every 5 years. Also, patients should receive the appropriate aforementioned antimicrobial prophylaxis secondary to drug toxicities.[29]

Chronic Myelogenous Leukemia (CML)

CML is a myeloproliferative disorder which represents approximately 15% of all adult leukemias with a median age of diagnosis of 66 years.[1,10] The disease results from a translocation of genetic material between the long arms of chromosomes 9 and 22, which is referred to as the Philadelphia chromosome (Ph+). This translocation generates in the *BCR-ABL* fusion gene which encodes a protein that has constitutively active tyrosine kinase activity. The activated tyrosine kinase triggers multiple downstream pathways which lead to cellular proliferation. *BCR-ABL* is found in approximately > 90% of CML patients as well as 15% of patients with ALL.

Patients are often asymptomatic and are diagnosed incidentally. However, some patients will present with symptoms such as early satiety, fatigue, weight loss, night sweats, and bleeding or bruising. Upon physical examination, patients may present with splenomegaly and hepatomegaly.[21] CML has three clinical phases: chronic, accelerated, and blast crisis. Criteria commonly used to define these include the presence of blasts in peripheral blood and bone marrow, peripheral basophilia, thrombocytopenia, clonal evolution, splenomegaly, and anemia. It is recommended as a part of initial evaluation that a physical examination, CBC, platelet count, bone marrow aspirate and biopsy, and cytogenetic analysis be performed.[36]

TREATMENT

Historically, treatment options for CML included busulfan, hydroxyurea, interferon based combinations, and allogeneic stem cell transplants. In 2001, imatinib, an oral tyrosine kinase inhibitor (TKI) targeting *BCR-ABL*, was given FDA accelerated approval following a phase III study demonstrating superiority over interferon-α in combination with cytarabine.[37] Imatinib is considered first-line treatment for chronic phase CML and continues to demonstrate durable response rates.[38] However, *BCR-ABL* kinase mutations have been identified that confer differing levels of resistance to imatinib. Second-generation TKIs (eg, dasatinib, nilotinib) have been developed and offer new treatment options for select patients. See Table 17-2 for a comparison of these agents. Disease monitoring is essential for the evaluation of the efficacy of current therapy and detection of relapse. Goals include achieving a hematologic response (normalization of blood counts), cytogenetic response (decrease number of Ph+ cells), and molecular response (decrease number of BCR-ABL transcripts by quantitative reverse-transcriptase polymerase chain reaction [RT-PCR]).[38]

SPECIAL CONSIDERATIONS

Treatment with oral TKIs is expensive. The average wholesale price of a 1 month supply of imatinib (400 mg/d), dasatinib (100 mg/d), and nilotinib (800 mg/d) are $3420, $4575, and

TABLE 17-2 **Comparison of BCR-ABL Tyrosine Kinase Inhibitors**

	Dose	Indication(s)	Adverse Reactions	Drug Interactions	Contraindications	Reference
Imatinib (Gleevec)	400-800 mg po every day	CML-CP, AP, BP Ph+ALL	Cardiovascular, diarrhea, fluid retention, myelosuppression, nausea, rash	Substrate and inhibitor of CYP3A4	None	40
Dasatinib (Sprycel)	100-140 mg po every day	CML-CP, AP, BP Ph+ALL	Diarrhea, fluid retention, myelosuppression, pleural effusion, rash	Substrate of CYP3A4	None	41
Nilotinib (Tasigna)	300- 400 mg po bid	CML-CP, AP	Elevated bilirubin, and lipase, hypokalemia, hypophosphatemia, increased transaminases, myelosuppression, rash, QT prolongation	Substrate of CYP3A4, inhibits CYP3A4, 2C8, 2C9, 2D6	Hypokalemia, hypomagnesium, long QT interval	42

Abbreviations: CP, chronic phase; AP, accelerated phase; BP, blast phase.

$6700, respectively.[39] For uninsured patients, pharmacists should encourage and assist in patient enrollment into an industry sponsored patient assistance program. Also, pharmacists should emphasize medication adherence, given the importance of these agents.

CASE Application

1. AA is a 58-year-old Caucasian man who reports to his primary care physician complaining of 2-week history of fatigue and fever. A CBC with differential reveals an elevated WBC (50,000 U/L) and profound thrombocytopenia (platelets 30,000 U/L). Patient is diagnosed with acute myeloid leukemia (AML-M5). Initial induction therapy should consist of the following:
   a. Mitoxantrone
   b. Cytarabine + idarubicin
   c. Cytarabine + imatinib
   d. Asparaginase
2. Physician asks you about tumor lysis syndrome (TLS) prevention and management for patient AA, suggestions should include:
   a. Initiating allopurinol
   b. Treating electrolyte disturbances
   c. Aggressive hydration
   d. All of the above
3. TLS is characterized by the following:
   a. Hypocalcemia, hypouricemia, hyperkalemia
   b. Hyperphosphatemia, hyperkalemia, hyperuricemia
   c. Hypercalcemia, hyperkalemia, hypomagnesium
   d. Hypokalemia, hyperphosphatemia, hypouricemia
4. AA achieves complete remission following induction therapy and begins high-dose cytarabine (HDAC). What toxicities should AA be counseled on?
   a. Infusion related reactions, paralytic ileus, cardiotoxicity
   b. Cerebellar toxicity, peripheral neuropathy, infusion related reactions
   c. Nausea, peripheral neuropathy, ocular toxicity
   d. Cerebellar toxicity, nausea, ocular toxicity
5. Which of the following agents is used in the treatment of relapsed AML?
   a. Rituximab (Rituxan)
   b. Mitoxantrone (Novantrone)
   c. Alemtuzumab (Campath)
   d. Imatinib (Gleevec)
6. A newly diagnosed patient with acute promyelocytic leukemia (APL) begins treatment with tretinoin 40 mg orally twice daily. Within 48 hours of the initiation, the patient develops fever, dyspnea, and respiratory distress. Which of the following should be immediately initiated to treat apparent differentiation syndrome (DS)?
   a. Dexamethasone
   b. Acetaminophen
   c. Diphenhydramine
   d. Epinephrine
7. SS is a 55-year-old African American woman newly diagnosed with acute lymphoblastic leukemia (ALL). Her physician has recommended she receive part A hyper-CVAD regimen (cyclophosphamide, vincristine, doxorubicin, and dexamethasone). What baseline examination should she receive prior to initiating doxorubicin on day 4?
   a. CT scan to assess distant site involvement
   b. Lumbar puncture to determine CNS disease
   c. 24-Hour urine collection to determine renal function
   d. MUGA scan to determine left ventricular ejection fraction (LVEF)
8. SS is to receive CNS prophylaxis. Which of the following agents are given intrathecally (IT)?
   a. Cytarabine
   b. Methotrexate
   c. Vincristine
   d. a and b
   e. All of the above
9. You are an oncology pharmacist counseling a parent and their child undergoing treatment for pediatric ALL. Patient will be treated with a Children's Oncology Group (COG) protocol. All of the following adverse events should be discussed with them regarding asparaginase except?
   a. Hyperglycemia
   b. Risk of allergic reactions
   c. Potential for bleeding
   d. Alopecia
10. Which of the following prophylactic agents should be recommended for a CLL patient receiving fludarabine?
    a. Enoxaparin
    b. Sulfamethoxazole/trimethoprim
    c. Pantoprazole
    d. Metronidazole
11. Which of the following statements is false regarding the treatment of chronic lymphocytic leukemia (CLL)?
    a. Early treatment has resulted in improved overall survival.
    b. Fludarabine based therapy has benefit.
    c. Rituximab based combination regimens have demonstrated benefit.
    d. Cyclophosphamide is recommended in CLL.
12. Which of the following agents should be recommended in a CLL patient who is presenting with recurring infections?
    a. Annual influenza vaccine
    b. Monthly intravenous immunoglobulin
    c. Pneumococcal vaccine every 5 years
    d. All of the above

13. Which of the following is true regarding the monoclonal antibody alemtuzumab (Campath)?
    a. Humanized-targets CD33
    b. Chimeric-targets CD52
    c. Humanized-targets CD52
    d. Chimeric-targets CD20

14. Which of the following should be recommended for patients receiving alemtuzumab (Campath)?
    a. Antifungal prophylaxis
    b. Herpes viral prophylaxis
    c. Pegfilgrastim (Neulasta) for neutropenia
    d. a and b
    e. a and c

15. Common adverse events with rituximab (Rituxan) include:
    a. Infusion related reactions
    b. Tumor lysis syndrome
    c. Skin rashes
    d. Hepatitis B reactivation
    e. All of the above

16. The Philadelphia chromosome (Ph+) results from which of the following?
    a. Translocation of chromosomes 9 and 22
    b. Translocation of chromosomes 8 and 21
    c. Inversion of chromosome 16
    d. Translocation of chromosomes 15 and 17

17. Which of the following is a first-line treatment for chronic myelogenous leukemia?
    a. Allogeneic stem cell transplant
    b. Interferon-α + cytarabine
    c. Imatinib (Gleevec)
    d. Sunitinib (Sutent)

18. Select the brand name for dasatinib.
    a. Tasigna
    b. Sprycel
    c. Tarceva
    d. Nexavar

19. Which of the following are adverse events associated with dasatinib?
    a. Pleural effusion
    b. Myelosuppression
    c. Alopecia
    d. a and b
    e. b and c

20. A newly diagnosed patient with CML receives a script for imatinib 400 mg orally daily. Patient is uninsured and has applied for Medicaid. They arrive at your pharmacy asking questions about this medication. What is the best course of action?
    a. Instruct patient to pay with cash.
    b. Refer them back to their physician for alternative agent.
    c. Offer to contact pharmaceutical company for patient assistance program.
    d. Instruct patient to wait on approval for Medicaid and delay therapy.

TAKEAWAY POINTS ››

- The primary goal of treatment is to induce and maintain a complete remission (CR).
- Treatment of pediatric ALL is divided into the following phases: induction, consolidation, interim maintenance, delayed intensification, and maintenance. Adult ALL is divided into induction, consolidation, and maintenance.
- Multiple intensive chemotherapy regimens have been shown to provide benefit in adult ALL.
- CNS treatment is performed throughout all phases of ALL therapy. Intrathecal therapy consists of methotrexate and cytarabine which can be given alone or in combination. Patients with T-cell ALL have an increased incidence of CNS disease and should receive systemic high-dose methotrexate to penetrate the CNS.
- Treatment of AML is immediately initiated following definitive diagnosis. AML treatment consists of three phases: induction, post-remission, and refractory/relapsed disease. The goal of induction therapy is to induce a CR with a return of normal hematopoiesis.
- AML induction therapy has consisted of the combination of cytarabine with an anthracycline (daunorubicin or idarubicin). A common regimen is "7+3" which combines cytarabine at (100 mg/m^2 days 1-7) with idarubicin (12 mg/m^2 days 1-3).
- Post-remission therapy consists of multiple cycles of high-dose cytarabine (HDAC).
- Patients will typically receive 6-18 g/m^2 of cytarabine per cycle in 3 to 4 cycles. Toxicities of HDAC include cerebellar dysfunction, pulmonary edema, pericardial effusion, and conjunctivitis. Renal function should be closely monitored following HDAC administration since renal dysfunction has correlated to cerebellar dysfunction.
- For AML patients who are unable to achieve a CR, refractory/relapsed treatments are available. Cytarabine alone or in combination with fludarabine, mitoxantrone, etoposide, or clofarabine are options.

- Acute promyelocytic leukemia (APL or AML-M3) represents approximately 10% of AML cases. APL has a better prognosis than other AML subtypes. Rather than receiving standard 7+3 induction therapy, APL patients should receive an anthracycline with tretinoin.
- At the initiation of tretinoin, patients need to be monitored for retinoic acid syndrome (or differentiation syndrome, DS). DS is associated with respiratory distress, pleural effusions, pulmonary infiltrates, and fever. This syndrome can be fatal; patients should immediately receive dexamethasone 10 mg IV Q 12 for 3 to 5 days to improve symptoms and decrease mortality.
- CLL is considered incurable and the goals of treatment include palliation and increase duration of life. Standard treatment for CLL may include a period of watchful waiting until progression of disease (eg, high WBC, bulky lymph nodes, symptomatic splenomegaly).
- Fludarabine has been shown as monotherapy and in combination to provide benefit for CLL patients. As single-agent therapy, fludarabine is given once daily for 5 days intravenously. Adverse events associated with fludarabine include myelosuppression, autoimmune effects, and neurologic toxicities.
- Treatment options for CML included busulfan, hydroxyurea, interferon based combinations, and allogeneic stem cell transplants.
- Imatinib is considered first-line treatment for chronic phase CML and continues to demonstrate durable response rates. However, *BCR-ABL* kinase mutations have been identified that confer differing levels of resistance to imatinib. Second-generation TKIs (eg, dasatinib, nilotinib) have been developed and offer new treatment options for select patients.

REFERENCES

1. Jemal A, Siegel R, Ward E, et al. Cancer statistics, 2009. *CA Cancer J Clin*. 2009;59:225-249.
2. Sallan SE. Myths and lesson from the adult/pediatric interface in acute lymphoblastic leukemia. *Hematology Am Soc Hematol Educ Program*. 2006;128-132.
3. Pui CH, Robison LL, Look AT. Acute lymphoblastic leukaemia. *Lancet*. 2008;371:1030-1043.
4. Leather HL, Bickert-Poon B. Acute leukemias. In: DiPiro JT, Talbert RL, Yee G, et al, eds. *Pharmacotherapy: A Pathophysiologic Approach*. 7th ed. New York, NY: McGraw-Hill; 2008.
5. Gokbuget N, Hoelzer D. Treatment of adult acute lymphoblastic leukemia. *Semin Hematol*. 2009;46:64-75.
6. Pui CH, Evans WE. Treatment of acute lymphoblastic leukemia. *N Engl J Med*. 2006;354:166-178.
7. Kantarjian H, Thomas D, O'Brien S, et al. Long-term follow-up results of hyperfractionated cyclophosphamide, vincristine, doxorubicin, and dexamethasone (Hyper-CVAD), a dose-intensive regimen, in adult acute lymphocytic leukemia. *Cancer*. 2004;101:2788-2801.
8. Schultz KR, Aledo A, Bowman WP, et al. Minimal toxicity of imatinib mesylate in combination with intensive chemotherapy for Philadelphia chromosome positive (Ph+) acute lymphoblastic leukemia (ALL) in children: A report of the Children's Oncology Group (COG) AALL0031 protocol for very high risk ALL. *Blood (ASH Annual Meeting Abstracts)*. 2006;108:283.
9. Thomas DA, Faderl S, Cortes J, et al. Treatment of Philadelphia chromosome-positive acute lymphocytic leukemia with hyper-CVAD and imatinib mesylate. *Blood*. 2004;103:4396-4407.
10. Horner MJ, Ries LAG, Krapcho M, et al. SEER Cancer statistics review, 1975-2006. Bethesda, MD: National Cancer Institute. 2008. http://seer.cancer.gov/csr/1975_2006/, based on November 2008 SEER data submission.
11. Smith SM, Le Beau MM, Huo D, et al. Clinical-cytogenetic associations in 306 patients with therapy-related myelodysplasia and myeloid leukemia: the University of Chicago series. *Blood*. 2003;102:43-52.
12. Estey E, Dohner H. Acute myeloid leukaemia. *Lancet*. 2006;368:1894-1907.
13. Dekker AW, Elderson A, Punt K, et al. Meningeal involvement in patients with acute nonlymphocytic leukemia. Incidence, management, and predictive factors. *Cancer*. 1985;56:2078-2082.
14. Cheson BD, Cassileth PA, Head DR, et al. Report of the National Cancer Institute-sponsored workshop on definitions of diagnosis and response in acute myeloid leukemia. *J Clin Oncol*. 1990;8:813-819.
15. Wiernik PH, Banks PL, Case DC Jr., et al. Cytarabine plus idarubicin or daunorubicin as induction and consolidation therapy for previously untreated adult patients with acute myeloid leukemia. *Blood*. 1992;79:313-319.
16. Baker WJ, Royer GL Jr., Weiss RB. Cytarabine and neurologic toxicity. *J Clin Oncol*. 1991;9:679-693.
17. Andersson BS, Cogan BM, Keating MJ, et al. Subacute pulmonary failure complicating therapy with high-dose Ara-C in acute leukemia. *Cancer*. 1985;56:2181-2184.
18. National Comprehensive Cancer Network (NCCN) Practice Guidelines. Acute myeloid leukemia. http://www.nccn.org/professionals/physician_gls/PDF/aml.pdf. Accessed July 29, 2009.
19. Coiffier B, Altman A, Pui CH, et al. Guidelines for the management of pediatric and adult tumor lysis syndrome: an evidence-based review. *J Clin Oncol*. 2008;26:2767-2778.
20. Dighiero G, Hamblin TJ. Chronic lymphocytic leukaemia. *Lancet*. 2008;371:1017-1029.
21. Pick AM, Devetten M, Mcguire TR. Chronic leukemias. In: DiPiro JT, Talbert RL, Yee G, et al, eds. *Pharmacotherapy: A Pathophysiologic Approach*. 7th ed. New York, NY: McGraw-Hill; 2008.
22. Cheson BD, Bennett JM, Grever M, et al. National Cancer Institute-sponsored Working Group guidelines for chronic lymphocytic leukemia: revised guidelines for diagnosis and treatment. *Blood*. 1996;87:4990-4997.
23. Dighiero G, Maloum K, Desablens B, et al. Chlorambucil in indolent chronic lymphocytic leukemia. French Cooperative

Group on Chronic Lymphocytic Leukemia. *N Engl J Med.* 1998;338:1506-1514.

24. Chemotherapeutic options in chronic lymphocytic leukemia: a meta-analysis of the randomized trials. CLL Trialists' Collaborative Group. *J Natl Cancer Inst.* 1999;91:861-868.
25. Rai KR, Peterson BL, Appelbaum FR, et al. Fludarabine compared with chlorambucil as primary therapy for chronic lymphocytic leukemia. *N Engl J Med.* 2000;343:1750-1757.
26. National Comprehensive Cancer Network (NCCN)-Clinical Practice Guidelines in Oncology: prevention and treatment of cancer-related infections. http://www.nccn.org/professionals/physician_gls/PDF/infections.pdf. Accessed October 29, 2009.
27. Eichhorst BF, Busch R, Hopfinger G, et al. Fludarabine plus cyclophosphamide versus fludarabine alone in first-line therapy of younger patients with chronic lymphocytic leukemia. *Blood.* 2006;107:885-891.
28. Catovsky D, Richards S, Matutes E, et al. Assessment of fludarabine plus cyclophosphamide for patients with chronic lymphocytic leukaemia (the LRF CLL4 Trial): a randomised controlled trial. *Lancet.* 2007;370:230-239.
29. National Comprehensive Cancer Network (NCCN)-Clinical Practice Guidelines in Oncology: Non-Hodgkin's Lymphomas. http://www.nccn.org/professionals/physician_gls/PDF/nhl.pdf; 2009.
30. Huhn D, von Schilling C, Wilhelm M, et al. Rituximab therapy of patients with B-cell chronic lymphocytic leukemia. *Blood.* 2001;98:1326-1331.
31. Campath (alemtuzumab) [package insert]. Cambridge, MA: Genzyme Corporation; 2009.
32. Karlsson C, Lundin J, Kimby E, et al. Phase II study of subcutaneous alemtuzumab without dose escalation in patients with advanced-stage, relapsed chronic lymphocytic leukaemia. *Br J Haematol.* 2009;144:78-85.
33. Tam CS, O'Brien S, Wierda W, et al. Long-term results of the fludarabine, cyclophosphamide, and rituximab regimen as initial therapy of chronic lymphocytic leukemia. *Blood.* 2008;112:975-980.
34. Elter T, Borchmann P, Schulz H, et al. Fludarabine in combination with alemtuzumab is effective and feasible in patients with relapsed or refractory B-cell chronic lymphocytic leukemia: results of a phase II trial. *J Clin Oncol.* 2005;23:7024-7031.
35. Faderl S, Thomas DA, O'Brien S, et al. Experience with alemtuzumab plus rituximab in patients with relapsed and refractory lymphoid malignancies. *Blood.* 2003;101:3413-3415.
36. National Comprehensive Cancer Network (NCCN) Practice Guidelines: Chronic myelogenous leukemia. http://www.nccn.org/professionals/physician_gls/PDF/cml.pdf; Accessed July 29, 2009.
37. O'Brien SG, Guilhot F, Larson RA, et al. Imatinib compared with interferon and low-dose cytarabine for newly diagnosed chronic-phase chronic myeloid leukemia. *N Engl J Med.* 2003;348:994-1004.
38. Hochhaus A, O'Brien SG, Guilhot F, et al. Six-year follow-up of patients receiving imatinib for the first-line treatment of chronic myeloid leukemia. *Leukemia.* 2009;23:1054-1061.
39. *Drug Topics Red Book.* Montvale, NJ: Thomson Medical Economics; 2007.
40. Gleevec (imatinib) [package insert]. East Hanover, NJ: Novartis Pharmaceuticals; 2009.
41. Sprycel (dasatinib) [package insert]. Princeton, NJ: Bristol-Myers Squibb Company; 2009.
42. Tasigna (nilotinib) [package insert]. East Hanover, NJ: Novartis Pharmaceuticals; 2010.

CHAPTER

18 Solid Organ Transplantation

Jeong M. Park and Margaret R. Jorgenson

FOUNDATION OVERVIEW

Solid organ transplantation has been accepted as a lifesaving treatment for patients with end-stage kidney, liver, heart, lung, and intestinal disease. The benefit of pancreas or islet cell transplant for type 1 diabetic patients is generally not immediate, however normoglycemia without the need for exogenous insulin following transplantation offers better quality of life and potentially reduces long-term diabetic complications.[1,2] In 2007, 27,578 transplants were performed in the United States. Kidney transplant was most commonly performed followed by liver and heart. However, demand far surpasses supply with about 100,000 people on the waiting list to receive an organ.[3]

The physiologic barrier to solid organ transplant is recognition of the foreign antigens and subsequent orchestrated immune response. When this response is mounted against the allograft, it is referred to as "rejection". There are three types of graft rejection can occur after solid organ transplantation: humoral, acute cellular, and chronic rejection. Humoral rejection is mediated by antibodies against donor antigens present on the vascular endothelium and typically occurs intraoperatively or within days after receiving ABO blood type mismatched or positive crossmatch organ transplant. Avoiding mismatched transplant or desensitizing recipients with donor-specific antibodies may prevent this mode of rejection, but treating humoral rejection remains challenging. Acute cellular rejection is the most common type of rejection and is generally reversible with appropriate treatment. It results from an orchestrated immune response that involves alloantigen presentation by antigen presenting cells that leads to alloreactive T cells. The cytotoxic T cells infiltrate the graft and cause direct tissue damage, whereas the helper T cells produce cytokines to cause subsequent immunological and inflammatory events. Although acute cellular rejection can occur anytime following transplant, the risk is highest in the first several months after transplant. Prevention and treatment of acute cellular rejection is of utmost importance, as it is a significant predictor of chronic rejection. The exact etiology of chronic rejection is unknown. It is a slow process of graft fibrosis and arteriopathy, which results in graft dysfunction, usually manifested years after transplantation. While acute cellular rejection can be treated pharmacologically, the only therapy for chronic rejection is retransplantation.[4]

Signs and symptoms of rejection are nonspecific pain and tenderness over graft site, fever, and lethargy. If left untreated, rejection leads to clinically significant organ dysfunction. The diagnosis of rejection is made based on histological findings from a biopsy specimen of the transplant organ.[4]

PREVENTION OF REJECTION

Immunosuppression Regimen (Table 18-1)

Over the last 30 years, advances in immunosuppression have contributed to the improvement in patient and graft survival rates following solid organ transplantation largely by preventing acute cellular rejection. The goal of immunosuppression after solid organ transplantation is to prevent graft rejection and to minimize the undue side effects such as infection, malignancy, and drug toxicity. In order to achieve this goal, a combination of immunosuppressant drugs with different mechanisms of action are employed at relatively low doses. The mainstay of current maintenance immunosuppressive regimens (the "triple drug regimen") includes a calcineurin inhibitor (cyclosporine or tacrolimus), an antiproliferative agent (azathioprine or mycophenolate) and corticosteroids. Typically these agents are used in high doses in the early weeks post-transplant, with dosages tapering down as the risk of acute cellular rejection decreases. In addition to the maintenance immunosuppression, antibody induction (antithymocyte globulins or interleukin-2 receptor antagonists) can be used at the time of transplant in select patients. Antibody induction therapy has shown to reduce acute cellular rejection rates compared to no induction at all. In an effort to further minimize the negative sequelae of immunosuppression, steroid- and calcineurin inhibitor-sparing regimens are currently being investigated.[5]

Corticosteroids

Corticosteroids are the oldest element of the triple drug regimen and suppress both inflammation and immune activation. Their immunosuppressive effects are exerted on the entire process of immune activation, including antigen presentation by APCs, cytokine release including but not limited to interleukins (such as IL-1, IL-2, IL-6) and tumor necrosis factor α (TNF α), and subsequently lymphocyte proliferation. Typically, doses are higher during the immediate post-transplant period and then are tapered down. Side effects vary by both the dose and the duration of therapy. At high doses, patients can experience neurotoxicity ranging from headache, mood

TABLE 18-1 **Commonly Used Immunosuppressive Agents in Solid Organ Transplantation**

Drug	Brand Name	Generic	Dosage Forms			Indication			TDM
			IV	po	po liquid	Induction	Maintenance	ACR	
Calcineurin Inhibitors									
Cyclosporine	Sandimmune	X	X	X	X		X		X
Cyclosporine (modified)	Neoral Gengraf	X		X	X		X		X
Tacrolimus	Prograf	X	X	X			X		X
Antiproliferatives									
Azathioprine	Imuran	X	X	X			X		
Mycophenolate mofetil	CellCept	X	X	X	X		X		
Mycophenolate sodium	Myfortic			X			X		
Corticosteroids									
Prednisone	Deltasone	X		X	X		X		
Methylprednisolone	Solu-Medrol	X	X	X	X	X	X	X	
mTOR Inhibitors									
Sirolimus	Rapamune			X	X		X		X
IL-2 Receptor Antagonists									
Basiliximab	Simulect		X			X			
Daclizumab	Zenapax		X			X			
Antithymocyte Globulins									
Rabbit ATG	Thymoglobulin		X			X		X	
Equine ATG	Atgam		X			X		X	
Miscellaneous									
Muromonab-CD3	OKT3		X			X		X	

Abbreviations: ACR, acute cellular rejection; ATG, antithymocyte globulin; IL-2, interleukin-2; IV, intravenous; mTOR, mammalian target of rapamycin; po, oral; TDM, therapeutic drug monitoring

disturbance, and insomnia to psychosis, electrolyte disturbances and fluid retention, glucose intolerance, and leukocytosis. The severity of these adverse effects will diminish as the dose is reduced. Long-term use of corticosteroids can lead to cushingoid type effects such as growth suppression, osteoporosis, loss of muscle mass, fragile skin, and lipodystrophy. For these side effects associated with corticosteroids, steroid withdrawal or avoidance immunosuppressive regimens are employed in select patients with good outcomes.[4]

Calcineurin Inhibitors (Cyclosporine or Tacrolimus)

The calcineurin inhibitor is the backbone of the triple drug regimen. Calcineurin, a phosphatase, dephosphorylates nuclear factor of activated T cells (NFAT), which is a required transcription factor in the production of cytokines by T cells. By inhibiting calcineurin, cyclosporine (as cyclosporine-cyclophilin complex) and tacrolimus (as tacrolimus-FKBP12 complex) suppresses synthesis of IL-2, the cytokine that is responsible for lymphocyte activation.

The introduction of cyclosporine (Sandimmune) in the early 1980s improved patient and graft survival rates dramatically.[6] This original formulation was highly dependent on bile acids for absorption, leading to extreme inter- and intra-patient pharmacokinetic variability. The newer modified cyclosporine products (Neoral and Gengraf) improved intra-patient variability, allowing more reliable drug absorption; however, inter-patient pharmacokinetic variability due to gut metabolism persisted. It is important to note that these formulations are not equivalent, and should not be substituted for one another.[7-9]

Tacrolimus (Prograf), also known as FK506, is an alternative calcineurin inhibitor that is widely used in all types of solid organ transplantation.[5] Its use has increased steadily since the FDA approval in the early 1990s. Several multicenter randomized controlled trials and meta-analyses comparing tacrolimus to cyclosporine demonstrated lower acute rejection rates and potentially better graft survival rates with tacrolimus; however, tacrolimus was associated with development of post-transplant diabetes mellitus.[10-12]

Both calcineurin inhibitors demonstrate pharmacokinetic variability and a narrow therapeutic ratio (the window between toxicity and efficacy is small), thus requiring therapeutic drug monitoring. Typically, a trough concentration before the morning dose is monitored and goals vary by type of organ transplant, time elapsed since transplant, concomitant immunosuppression, history of rejection, and complications.

Further aspects of calcineurin inhibitor pharmacokinetics include; poor oral bioavailability, high plasma protein binding (cyclosporine to lipoproteins and tacrolimus to albumin and alpha-1 glycoprotein), extensive intestinal and hepatic metabolism primarily by cytochrome P-450 3A (CYP 3A), and substrates for multiple drug transporters including P-glycoprotein.[7-9,13]

As a class, calcineurin inhibitors have similar adverse effects. Common and significant adverse effects are nephrotoxicity, electrolyte disturbances (hyperkalemia and hypomagnesemia), hypertension, and neurotoxicity (usually manifesting as tremor or headache). These effects are generally dose-dependent, and can complicate diagnosis, especially in renal transplant patients for whom calcineurin inhibitor-induced nephrotoxicity can be confused with renal graft rejection. Adverse effects that are specific to cyclosporine include hyperlipidemia, hyperuricemia, hirsutism, and gingival hyperplasia. Adverse effects that are specific to tacrolimus include hyperglycemia, alopecia, and diarrhea.[7-9,13]

Drug interactions with calcineurin inhibitors can be both pharmacokinetic and pharmacodynamic in nature. Drugs that are inducers or inhibitors of CYP 3A or P-glycoprotein are expected to affect cyclosporine or tacrolimus levels (Table 18-2). While some potent and rapid-acting inhibitors, such as voriconazole, require preemptive calcineurin inhibitor dosage adjustment, other less potent agents, such as fluconazole, can be concomitantly administered with close monitoring of calcineurin-inhibitor levels. Pharmacodynamic interactions include increased nephrotoxicity with concomitant nephrotoxins, such as aminoglycosides and nonsteroidal anti-inflammatory agents (NSAIDs). The calcineurin inhibitors can also block the metabolism of other agents, such as the HMG-CoA reductase inhibitors (or statins), resulting in an increased risk for rhabdomyolysis when used with cyclosporine.[7-9,13]

TABLE 18-2 **Effects of Concomitant Drugs on Cyclosporine, Tacrolimus, and Sirolimus Levels**

Increase Levels	Decrease Levels
Calcium channel blockers	Rifampin
Diltiazem	Phenytoin
Verapamil	Carbamazepine
Nicardipine	St. John's wort (herbal)
Azole antifungals	
Ketoconazole	
Voriconazole	
Itraconazole	
Fluconazole	
Macrolide antibiotics	
Clarithromycin	
Erythromycin	
Grapefruit (food)	

Antiproliferative Agents (Azathioprine, Mycophenolate Mofetil, or Mycophenolate Sodium)

Azathioprine

Azathioprine (Imuran) is an older generation antiproliferative agent that can be used as part of a triple drug immunosuppressive regimen and has other implications such as rheumatoid arthritis. With the availability of more specific mycophenolate products, azathioprine is not commonly used in solid organ transplantation.[5] Azathioprine is a prodrug that is quickly converted in vivo to 6-mercaptopurine, then to the active metabolites 6-thioguanine nucleotides. 6-Thioguanine nucleotides disrupt both the salvage and de novo DNA and RNA synthesis, resulting in nonspecific cell cycle arrest at the G2-M phase. Leukopenia, anemia, and thrombocytopenia are common and often dose-dependent. With the availability of more specific mycophenolate products, azathioprine is not commonly used in solid organ transplantation, although it has a role as an alternative to more teratogenic immunosuppressant agents if a transplant patient becomes pregnant. Less common side effects of azathioprine include hepatotoxicity, pancreatitis, and alopecia. Azathioprine is not metabolized via CYP enzymes, thereby significantly decreasing the risk of drug interactions. However, 6-mercaptopurine is metabolized by xanthine oxidase. This enzyme is inhibited by allopurinol, a drug commonly used to prevent gout. This interaction results in increased production of 6-thioguanine nucleotides, thereby increasing the incidence of pancytopenia.[14]

Mycophenolic Acid Derivatives

Mycophenolate mofetil (CellCept) and mycophenolate sodium (Myfortic) are converted to mycophenolic acid (MPA) in vivo. MPA inhibits inosine monophosphate dehydrogenase (IMPDH), an enzyme required for the de novo synthesis of purines. MPA derivates therefore selectively inhibit lymphocyte proliferation, as these cells are unable to utilize salvage pathways of purine synthesis. MPA undergoes enterohepatic recirculation and is cleared via hepatic glucuronidation as well as renal excretion. MPA derivates should not be administered concurrently with aluminum or magnesium containing antacids (separate by 2 hours) or binding resins such as cholestyramine due to decreased serum levels of MPA. Noticeable adverse effects of both MPA derivatives are gastrointestinal distress, such as diarrhea and bone marrow suppression leading to pancytopenia, although not to the same extent as azathioprine. Mycophenolate sodium was initially touted by the manufacturer as an enteric delayed-release MPA formulation with decreased gastrointestinal side effects. However, this advantage was not evident in clinical trials. Mycophenolate sodium 720 mg is therapeutically equivalent to mycophenolate mofetil 1000 mg.[15,16]

mTOR Inhibitors (Sirolimus)

Sirolimus (Rapamune) is the only mammalian target of rapamycin (mTOR) inhibitor approved for use in solid organ transplantation. The other agent in the class, everolimus, is currently undergoing clinical trials. Blockade of mTOR results in inhibition of lymphocyte proliferation by arresting the G1-S phase of cell cycle. Its greatest utility in clinical practice is to allow sparing of calcineurin inhibitors. Sirolimus is less likely to cause nephrotoxicity than calcineurin inhibitors. However, sirolimus is known to cause hypercholesterolemia and hypertriglyceridemia, leukopenia, anemia, thrombocytopenia, and mouth sores. The most troubling adverse effect is impaired wound healing. Sirolimus has been associated with hepatic artery thrombosis in liver transplant patients and bronchial anastomotic dehiscence in lung transplant patients. Sirolimus is a substrate for CYP 3A and P-glycoprotein with the similar drug interaction potential to calcineurin inhibitors (Table 18-2). Therapeutic drug monitoring was deemed unnecessary during the initial clinical trials, as sirolimus was used primarily as an adjunctive agent. However, the risk of drug interactions and variability in pharmacokinetics warrant monitoring of sirolimus-serum concentrations.[17]

Antibody Induction

There is an increasing trend toward the use of induction therapy with antibodies in most solid organ transplantation, except for liver transplant. Rabbit antithymocyte globulin is the most commonly used antibody in induction, followed by IL-2 receptor antagonists. The use of equine antithymocyte globulin and muromonab-CD3 has decreased significantly in recent years.[5]

Antithymocyte Globulins

Antithymocyte globulins (ATGs) are polyclonal antithymocyte antibodies derived from animals. ATGs interact with lymphocyte surface antigens, including CD2, CD3, CD4, CD8, CD16, CD25, and CD45, thereby depleting the number of circulating T cells. Rabbit ATG (Thymoglobulin) has the more profound lymphopenic effect than equine ATG (Atgam). Residual immunosuppressive effects after rabbit ATG can persist for years. The superior efficacy of rabbit ATG to equine ATG and basiliximab in prevention of acute cellular rejection has been demonstrated in kidney transplant.[18,19] The most common adverse effect of ATGs is cytokine release syndrome. The symptoms include fever, chills, rigors, dyspnea, nausea, vomiting, diarrhea, hypotension or hypertension, malaise, rash, and headache. Slow infusion rates and pretreatment with corticosteroids, acetaminophen, and diphenhydramine can prevent severe cytokine release syndrome. Other common adverse effects are leukopenia, thrombocytopenia, and serum sickness. ATGs may also increase the risk of infections and malignancy.[20,21]

IL-2 Receptor Antagonists

Basiliximab (Simulect) and daclizumab (Zenapax) are monoclonal antibodies (MAb) that bind specifically to the alpha chain (CD25) of the IL-2 receptor and inhibit T-cell activation. Both agents are well tolerated. Basiliximab is a chimeric MAb and daclizumab is a humanized MAb, thereby resulting in low risk of infusion-related reactions. While induction with IL-2 receptor antagonists have shown to lower rejection rates, they have not been studied adequately for treatment of rejection.[22,23]

TREATMENT OF REJECTION

Acute cellular rejection (ACR) is one of the most common complications of solid organ transplantation. The incidence of ACR within 1 year varies depending on the organ transplanted and rejection criteria employed, ranging from 13% in kidney transplant up to 56% in intestinal transplant in 2003. Although corticosteroids remain a primary agent of rejection treatment, the use of antibodies is increasing for this indication.[4]

Steroid Pulses

When treating ACR episodes, large doses of IV corticosteroids are given over a series of days (eg, methylprednisolone 250-1000 mg/dose). This treatment course is commonly referred to as "steroid pulses". Patients receiving steroid pulses are at risk for the aforementioned side effects of corticosteroids.

Antithymocyte Globulins

Antithymocyte globulins (ATGs) are typically used for more severe forms or steroid-resistant ACR. The dose of equine ATG (10-15 mg/kg) is ten times that of rabbit ATG (1.25-1.5 mg/kg) and skin testing is strongly recommended prior to equine ATG.[20,21]

Muromonab-CD3

Muromonab-CD3 (OKT3) is a murine MAb that binds specifically to the CD3 complex on T cells, thus prohibiting antigen recognition and decreasing the number of circulating CD3-positive T cells. The duration of its effects is much shorter than ATGs, lasting approximately 1 week. Muromonab-CD3 is administered as IV push over 1 minute at 5 mg/d for 10 to 14 days. Infusion reactions associated with cytokine release are common and pretreatment with IV corticosteroids is recommended. Vital signs should also be diligently monitored during each infusion. Prior to a second course of muromonab-CD3, flow cytometry should be conducted to test for the presence of human anti-mouse antibodies (HAMA). If these antibodies are present and circulating, the drug will be inactivated prior to exerting its effect.[24]

CASE Application

1. Select the statement that most accurately describes cellular rejection after solid organ transplantation.
   a. An orchestrated immune response that involves alloantigen presentation via antigen presenting cells (APCs) that then leads to alloreactive T lymphocytes.

b. A cytotoxic immune response mediated via preformed antibodies against antigens present on vascular endothelium.
c. A slow process of graft fibrosis and arteriopathy, which results in graft dysfunction.
d. A process which inhibits the entire process of immune activation, including antigen presentation by APCs, the release of cytokines such as IL-1, IL-2, IL-6 and TNF α, and subsequently lymphocyte proliferation.

2. You are counseling a 16-year-old patient who is waiting for a living-related renal transplantation from his brother. The patient states that he has been doing research on the Internet and has heard that acute cellular rejection (ACR) is a major complication of solid organ transplantation. He wants to know if you can inform him of his risk for this complication. You tell him the time period of greatest risk for ACR after transplant is:

a. The first hours to days after transplantation
b. The first several months after transplantation
c. The risk increases with increased time from transplant
d. The risk is the same regardless of time after transplant

3. Select an example of the "triple drug regimen" that describes a common maintenance immunosuppression following solid organ transplantation.

a. Cyclosporine, prednisone, and basiliximab
b. Cyclosporine, tacrolimus, and prednisone
c. Tacrolimus, mycophenolate mofetil, and azathioprine
d. Prednisone, cyclosporine, and mycophenolate sodium

4. Select the drug or drug class that allowed successful solid organ transplant and ushered in the current era of large-scale transplantation and therefore is considered to be the "backbone" of the triple drug immunosuppressive regimen.

a. Corticosteroids
b. Azathioprine
c. IL-2 receptor antagonists
d. Calcineurin inhibitors

5. A patient presents to your pharmacy with a prescription for clarithromycin. He says that his primary care physician prescribed this medication to treat community-acquired pneumonia. You review the patient's medication profile and you see that he received a renal transplant 2 years ago and his immunosuppressive regimen includes tacrolimus, mycophenolate mofetil, and prednisone. Which of the following would be most appropriate as your next course of action?

a. Dispense clarithromycin and counsel on avoiding grape juice.
b. Contact the prescriber about the interactions between clarithromycin and tacrolimus as clarithromycin will inhibit the metabolism of tacrolimus resulting in supratherapeutic levels and toxicity.
c. Contact the prescriber about the interactions between clarithromycin and mycophenolate mofetil as clarithromycin will inhibit the metabolism of mycophenolate mofetil resulting in supratherapeutic levels and toxicity.
d. Recommend an alternative as clarithromycin is not an appropriate therapy for community-acquired pneumonia in an immunosuppressed host.

6. A patient who received a lung transplant a month ago is found to have *Aspergillus* on routine bronchoscopy. The patient's transplant physician wants to begin suppressive treatment with the antifungal voriconazole and is inquiring which of the medications his patient is taking will interact with voriconazole. The patient is currently taking prednisone, cyclosporine, azathioprine, clotrimazole, rabeprazole, co-trimoxazole, valganciclovir, and inhaled amphotericin.

a. Prednisone
b. Azathioprine
c. Cyclosporine
d. Valganciclovir

7. Which of the following best describes the mechanism of the interaction between HMG-CoA reductase inhibitors (or statins) and cyclosporine?

a. Inhibition of CYP 3A4 resulting in increased cyclosporine concentrations in blood
b. Inhibition of CYP 3A4 resulting in increased HMG-CoA reductase inhibitor concentrations in blood
c. Induction of CYP 3A4 resulting in decreased cyclosporine concentrations in blood
d. Concomitant nephrotoxicity, resulting in increased risk of renal failure

8. A patient approaches the counter at your pharmacy. She states that she has mild headache, and would like you to suggest an over-the-counter remedy. She is well known to you, as she received a renal transplant 3 months ago and fills her prescription for tacrolimus at your pharmacy. What would you suggest for her headache?

a. That she proceed immediately to a local emergency room as this might be a symptom of severe tacrolimus toxicity.
b. That she try taking OTC acetaminophen, and alert the transplant physician if the headache does not resolve.
c. That she try taking OTC naproxen, and alert the transplant physician if the headache does not resolve.
d. That she try taking OTC ibuprofen, and alert the transplant physician if the headache does not resolve.

9. Which of the following represents two adverse effects specific to tacrolimus?

a. Diarrhea and leukopenia
b. Alopecia and hyperglycemia

c. Hypertriglyceridemia and nephrotoxicity
d. Hirsutism and gingival hyperplasia

10. Which of the following represents two adverse effects specific to corticosteroids?
    a. Diarrhea and leukopenia
    b. Alopecia and hyperglycemia
    c. Water retention and osteoporosis
    d. Hirsutism and nephrotoxicity

11. Which of the following agents would be most appropriate to prevent a gout flare in a transplant patient who is currently receiving tacrolimus, azathioprine, and prednisone?
    a. Indomethacin
    b. Allopurinol
    c. Diclofenac
    d. Probenecid

12. You are counseling a patient who is being discharged today. He received a living-related renal transplant 5 days ago, and his postoperative course has been uncomplicated except for mild hypertension. When reconciling his home medications, you notice that the medical team has not restarted his home diltiazem. What course of action do you take?
    a. Notify the patient's medical team and request a discharge prescription for amlodipine.
    b. Notify the patient's medical team and instruct the patient to resume his home regimen of diltiazem after discharge.
    c. Notify the patient's medical team and request a discharge prescription for verapamil.
    d. Notify the patient's medical team and request addition of diltiazem at discharge.

13. Which of the following statement is correct about sirolimus?
    a. Sirolimus is not metabolized via cytochrome P-450 enzymes, thus decreasing the propensity for drug interactions.
    b. Sirolimus is less nephrotoxic than calcineurin inhibitors.
    c. Sirolimus is available in many different formulations, thereby facilitating ease of dosing.
    d. Sirolimus does not require therapeutic drug monitoring.

14. Which enzyme or protein does mycophenolic acid inhibit in order to exhibit its immunosuppressive effect?
    a. mTOR
    b. Cyclophilin
    c. FKBP-12
    d. IMPDH

15. A patient presents to the hospital with symptoms concerning for a bowel obstruction. His past medical history is significant for a liver transplant 3 months ago and he receiving Myfortic 720 mg po bid. The physician wants to convert the patient from oral Myfortic to IV due to po intolerance resulting from his bowel obstruction. Which of the following would result in comparable plasma concentrations of mycophenolic acid?
    a. Mycophenolate sodium 720 mg IV bid
    b. Mycophenolate sodium 1000 mg IV bid
    c. Mycophenolate mofetil 720 mg IV bid
    d. Mycophenolate mofetil 1000 mg IV bid

16. Which of the following statements is *incorrect* regarding brand-name and generic tacrolimus?
    a. A sponsor of a generic tacrolimus must complete large, randomized, multiple-center studies of efficacy and safety in the patient population where the drug is intended to be used.
    b. A sponsor of a generic tacrolimus must complete bioequivalence studies.
    c. A generic tacrolimus must demonstrate a peak concentration (C_{max}) and area under the time-concentration curve (AUC) similar to the reference brand-name product.
    d. Monitoring tacrolimus trough concentrations may offer an additional degree of confidence in using generic tacrolimus products.

17. Which of the following is generally considered as a narrow therapeutic ratio drug?
    a. Cyclosporine
    b. Prednisone
    c. Mycophenolate mofetil
    d. Mycophenolate sodium

18. A liver transplant patient presented with elevated liver function tests and she admits to not taking her immunosuppressive regimen for the past week, as she was out of town and forgot her medications. The medical team wants to treat her for acute cellular rejection and wants you to recommend an appropriate agent. Which of the following would treat acute cellular rejection most effectively?
    a. Basiliximab
    b. Muromonab-CD3
    c. Daclizumab
    d. Rituximab

19. Why do patients require flow cytometry prior to administration of a second course of muromonab-CD3?
    a. To evaluate for the presence of antibodies which could make the patient more susceptible to infusion reactions
    b. To evaluate for the presence of antibodies which could result in drug inactivation
    c. To evaluate for the presence of antibodies which could result in heightened immunosuppressive effect

d. To evaluate for the presence of antibodies indicating an episode of humoral rejection

20. During interdisciplinary rounds, the medical resident states that a patient on the transplant service has a low WBC count. The patient received a combined kidney-pancreas transplant for juvenile-onset diabetes mellitus 2 months ago and presented 2 days ago with hyperglycemia and elevated amylase and lipase. Acute cellular rejection of the pancreas transplant was confirmed on a subsequent biopsy. Her rejection episode is being treated with rabbit antithymocyte globulin. Her home immunosuppressive regimen consists of tacrolimus, mycophenolate mofetil, and prednisone. She is receiving antiviral prophylaxis with valganciclovir, antibacterial prophylaxis with trimethoprim-sulfamethoxazole, and antifungal prophylaxis with nystatin. Which of the following approach is most appropriate for this patient's new-onset leukopenia?

    a. Suggest the physician to hold her prednisone until her WBC count normalizes.
    b. Suggest the physician to hold her mycophenolate mofetil until her WBC count normalizes.
    c. Suggest the physician to continue her current therapy, but to closely monitor her WBC count.
    d. Suggest the physician to hold her valganciclovir until her WBC count normalizes.

TAKEAWAY POINTS ››

- To promote allograft and patient survival, solid organ transplantation requires balance between rejection prevention and the adverse sequelae from immunosuppression, such as infection, malignancy, and drug side effects.
- There are three types of allograft rejection: humoral, acute cellular, and chronic.
- Humoral rejection is most commonly encountered in the first days after transplantation and is antibody-mediated.
- Acute cellular rejection is most commonly encountered in the first months after transplantation and is T-lymphocyte mediated.
- Prevention of acute cellular rejection is paramount, as it is a primary risk factor for chronic rejection, which has no treatment and eventually leads to allograft loss.
- Corticosteroids, antithymocyte globulins, and muromonab-CD3 are all indicated for the treatment of acute cellular rejection.
- Treatment of acute cellular rejection results in profound immunosuppressive effects, which in turn places the patient at risk for opportunistic infections and other negative sequelae of immunosuppression.
- Acute cellular rejection is prevented by utilizing a multi-drug immunosuppressive regimen, which maximizes the immunosuppressive effect of each agent while minimizing adverse effects by including drugs with different mechanisms of action and toxicities.
- The gold standard "triple drug" immunosuppressive regimen includes a calcineurin-inhibitor (cyclosporine or tacrolimus), an antiproliferative agent (azathioprine or mycophenolate) and a corticosteroid.
- The discovery and marketing of the first calcineurin inhibitor (cyclosporine) revolutionized solid organ transplantation, significantly decreasing one-year allograft loss and patient mortality.
- Drug interactions with calcineurin inhibitors can be both pharmacokinetic (via CYP 3A and p-glycoprotein) and pharmacodynamic (via common adverse effects).
- Calcineurin inhibitors and sirolimus are considered narrow therapeutic index agents, and therefore serum concentrations are monitored.
- Sirolimus can be used in place of the calcineurin inhibitor or the antiproliferative agent in a triple drug immunosuppressive regimen if a patient has intolerable adverse effects to either of these classes.
- Immunosuppressive agents are associated with various adverse effects, which require close monitoring.
- Pharmacists can play an important role in post-transplant patient care by assessing the appropriateness of their medication therapy, monitoring signs and symptoms of rejection and other negative sequelae of immunosuppression, and educating patients on immunosuppressants and compliance.

REFERENCES

1. Dean PG, Kudva YC, Stegall MD. Long-term benefits of pancreas transplantation. *Curr Opin Organ Transplant.* 2008;13:85-90.
2. Fiorina P, Shapiro AMJ, Ricordi C, et al. The clinical impact of islet transplantation. *Am J Transplant.*2008;8:1990-7.
3. Wolfe RA, Merion RM, Roys EC, et al. Trends in organ donation and transplantation in the United States, 1998-2007. *Am J Transplant.* 2009;9 (Part 2):869-78.
4. Johnson HJ, Schonder KS. Solid-organ transplantation. Chapter 87. In: DiPiro JT, Talbert RL, Yee GC, Matzke GR, Wells BG, Posey LM, eds. *Pharmacotherapy: A Pathophysiologic Approach.* 6th ed. New York, NY: McGraw-Hill; 2005.
5. Meier-Kriesche HU, Li S, Gruessner RWG, et al. Immunosuppression: evolution in practice and trends, 1994-2004. *Am J Transplant.* 2006;6 (Part 2):1111-1131.

6. The Canadian Multicentre Transplant Study Group. A randomized clinical trial of cyclosporine in cadaveric renal transplantation. *N Engl J Med.* 1983;309:809-815.
7. Sandimmune [package insert]. East Hanover, NJ: Norvatis Pharmaceutical Corp; 2008.
8. Neoral [package insert]. East Hanover, NJ: Norvatis Pharmaceutical Corp; 2009.
9. Gengraf [package insert]. North Chicago, IL: Abbott Laboratories; 2009.
10. Webster AC, Woodroffe RC, Taylor RS, et al. Tacrolimus versus ciclosporin as primary immunosuppression for kidney transplant recipients: meta-analysis and meta-regression of randomised trial data. *BMJ.* 1005;331:810-820.
11. McAlister VS, Haddad E, Renouf E, et al. Cyclosporin versus tacrolimus as primary immunosuppressant after liver transplantation: a meta-analysis. *Am J Transplant.* 2006;6:1578-1585.
12. Ye F, Ying-Bin X, Yu-Guo W, et al. Tacrolimus versus cyclosporine microemulsion for heart transplant recipients: a meta-analysis. *J Heart Lung Transplant.* 2009;28:58-66.
13. Prograf [package insert]. Deerfield, IL: Astellas Pharma, Inc; 2009.
14. Imuran [package insert]. San Diego, CA: Prometheus Laboratories, Inc; 2008.
15. CellCept [package insert]. Nutley, NJ: Roche Laboratories, Inc; 2009.
16. Myfortic [package insert]. East Hanover, NJ: Norvatis Pharmaceutical Corp; 2009.
17. Rapamune [package insert]. Philadelphia, PA: Wyeth Pharmaceuticals, Inc; 2009.
18. Brennan DC, Flavin K, Lowell JA, et al. A randomized, double-blinded comparison of Thymoglobulin versus Atgam for induction immunosuppressive therapy in adult renal transplant recipients. *Transplantation.* 1999;67:1011-1018.
19. Brennan DC, Daller JA, Lake KD, et al. Rabbit antithymocyte globulin versus basiliximab in renal transplantation. *N Engl J Med.* 2006;355:1967-1977.
20. Thymoglobulin [package insert]. Cambridge, MA: Genzyme Corp; 2009.
21. Atgam [package insert]. New York, NY: Pfizer & Upjohn Co; 2005.
22. Simulect [package insert]. East Hanover, NJ: Norvatis Pharmaceutical Corp; 2005.
23. Zenapax [package insert]. Nutley, NJ: Roche Laboratories, Inc; 2005.
24. OKT3 [package insert]. Raritan, NJ: Ortho-Biotech; 2004.

PART

3

Infectious Diseases

CHAPTER

19 Antimicrobial Regimen Selection

S. Scott Sutton

FOUNDATION OVERVIEW

Antimicrobials vary in their ability to inhibit or kill different species of bacteria. Antimicrobials that kill many different species of bacteria are called broad-spectrum, whereas antimicrobials that kill a few different species of bacteria are called narrow-spectrum antimicrobials. Empirically treating infectious diseases and monitoring therapy requires knowledge of anti-infective properties, host factors, patient's normal flora, differentiating infection versus colonization, and understanding clinical presentation and diagnostic tests (microbiologic and nonmicrobiologic laboratory studies).[1,2] Broad spectrum anti-infective coverage increases the likelihood of empirically targeting a causative pathogen; unfortunately, the development of secondary infections caused by selection of antimicrobial-resistant pathogens is a common problem. In addition, adverse events may complicate up to 10% of antimicrobial therapy (adverse event rate is higher for select agents).[3,4]

TREATMENT

Antimicrobial Properties

Drug-specific considerations in antimicrobial therapy include spectrum of activity, pharmacokinetic and pharmacodynamic properties, adverse effects, drug interactions, and cost.

Spectrum of Activity

Patients who receive initial antimicrobial therapy that provides coverage against the causative pathogen survive at twice the rate of patients who do not receive adequate therapy initially. Because empiric antimicrobial therapy selection is critical to patient outcomes, broad-spectrum antimicrobials are often utilized because it will increase the likelihood of empirically targeting a causative pathogen. However, if all patients receive broad-spectrum antimicrobials, resistance would become an even more difficult problem. Therefore, it is important to understand the difference in antimicrobial spectrum of activity and select agent(s) that target the pathogens most likely causing the infection. Table 19-1 lists the spectrum of activity for select antimicrobials.

Collateral Damage Collateral damage is defined as the development of resistance occurring in a patient's nontargeted antimicrobial flora that may cause a secondary infection.[5] For example, clindamycin may be utilized to treat gram-positive cocci infections. See Figure 19-1 for a list of gram-positive and gram-negative bacteria. However, clindamycin also readily selects for resistance in a nontargeted organism that may be present in the intestinal tract, *Clostridium difficile*. If several different antimicrobials possess activity against a targeted pathogen, the antimicrobial that is least likely to be associated with collateral damage is preferred.

Antimicrobial Dose

Antimicrobial dosage regimens with the same agent may be different depending upon the infection or pathogen. For example, cefepime (Maxipime) a fourth generation cephalosporin has various dosage regimens based on the site of infection. The usual cefepime dosage range for adults is 1 to 2 g intravenously every 8 to 12 hours.[6] Dosage recommendations for cefepime based upon site of infection are:

Febrile neutropenia: 2 g every 8 hours

Intra-abdominal infections: 2 g every 12 hours

Nosocomial pneumonia: 1 to 2 g every 8 to 12 hours

Community acquired pneumonia: 1 to 2 g every 12 hours

Skin and skin structure: 2 g every 12 hours

Urinary tract infections: 2 g every 12 hours (severe) and 500 to1000 mg every 12 hours (mild-moderate)

Pharmacokinetic and Pharmacodynamic Properties

Integration of pharmacokinetic and pharmacodynamic properties of an agent is important when choosing antimicrobial therapy to ensure efficacy and to prevent resistance.

Pharmacokinetic Properties Pharmacokinetics describes in vivo drug exposure in terms of absorption, distribution, metabolism, and elimination. [7,8]

Bioavailability refers to the amount of antimicrobial that is absorbed orally compared to an equivalent intravenous (IV) dose.[7] Drug factors that affect oral bioavailability include the salt formulation, dosage form, and stability of agent in gastrointestinal tract. Patients manifesting systemic signs of infection such as hypotension or hypoperfusion should receive IV antimicrobials. Patients with a functioning gastrointestinal tract and without hemodynamic instability may receive oral antimicrobials, especially if the agent has good bioavailability. Examples of anti-infectives with good bioavailability include fluoroquinolones, fluconazole, and linezolid. Antimicrobials with poor bioavailability should be administered intravenously for systemic infections (eg, vancomycin—IV vancomycin is utilized

TABLE 19-1 **Drugs of Choice, First Choice, Alternative(s)**

Gram-Positive Cocci

Enterococcus faecalis (generally not as resistant to antibiotics as *Enterococcus faecium*)
Serious infection (endocarditis, meningitis, pyelonephritis with bacteremia)
Ampicillin (or penicillin G) + (gentamicin or streptomycin)
Vancomycin + (gentamicin or streptomycin), linezolid, daptomycin, tigecycline
Urinary tract infection (UTI)
Ampicillin, amoxicillin
Fosfomycin or nitrofurantoin

E. faecium (generally more resistant to antibiotics than *E. faecalis*)
Recommend consultation with infectious disease specialist.
Linezolid, quinupristin/dalfopristin, daptomycin, tigecycline

Staphylococcus aureus/Staphylococcus epidermidis
Methicillin (oxacillin)-sensitive
PRP[a]
FGC,[b,c] trimethoprim-sulfamethoxazole, clindamycin,[d] ampicillin-sulbactam, or amoxicillin-clavulanate
Methicillin (oxacillin)–resistant
Vancomycin ± (gentamicin or rifampin)
Trimethoprim-sulfamethoxazole, doxycycline[e] or clindamycin[d], Line-zolid, quinupristin-dalfopristin, daptomycin, or tigecycline

Streptococcus (groups A, B, C, G, and *Streptococcus bovis*)
Penicillin G[f] or V[g] or ampicillin
FGC,[b,c] erythromycin, azithromycin, clarithromycin,[h]

Streptococcus pneumoniae
Penicillin-sensitive (MIC <0.1 μg/mL)
Penicillin G or V or ampicillin
Erythromycin, FGC,[b,c] doxycycline, azithromycin, clarithromycin[h]
Penicillin intermediate (MIC 0.1-1.0 μg/mL)
High-dose penicillin (12 million units/day for adults) or ceftriaxone[c] or cefotaxime[c]
Levofloxacin,[i] moxifloxacin,[i] gemifloxacin,[i] telithromycin, or vancomycin
Penicillin-resistant (MIC ≥1.0 μg/mL)
Recommend consultation with infectious disease specialist.
Vancomycin ± rifampin
Per sensitivities: TGC,[c,j] telithromycin, levofloxacin,[i] moxifloxacin,[i] or gemifloxacin[i]

Streptococcus, viridans group
Penicillin G ± gentamicin[k]
TGC,[c,j] erythromycin, azithromycin, clarithromycin,[h] or vancomycin ± gentamicin

Gram-Negative Cocci

Moraxella (Branhamella) catarrhalis
Amoxicillin-clavulanate, ampicillin-sulbactam
Trimethoprim-sulfamethoxazole, erythromycin, azithromycin, clarithromycin,[h] doxycycline,[e] SGC,[c,l] TGC,[c,j] or TGC po[c,m]

Neisseria gonorrhoeae (also give concomitant treatment for *Chlamydia trachomatis*)
Disseminated gonococcal infection
Ceftriaxone[c] or cefotaxime[c]
Oral followup: Cefpodoxime,[c] ciprofloxacin,[i] or levofloxacin[i]
Uncomplicated infection
Ceftriaxone[c] or cefotaxime,[c] or cefpodoxime[c]
Ciprofloxacin[i] or levofloxacin[i]
Neisseria meningitides
Penicillin G
TGC[c,j]

Gram-Positive Bacilli

Clostridium perfringens
Penicillin G ± clindamycin
Metronidazole, clindamycin, doxycycline,[e] cefazolin,[c] imipenem,[n] meropenem,[n] or ertapenem[n]

Clostridium difficile
Oral metronidazole
Oral vancomycin

Gram-Negative Bacilli

Acinetobacter spp.
Imipenem or meropenem ± aminoglycoside[o] (amikacin usually most effective)
Ciprofloxacin,[i] ampicillin-sulbactam, colistin, or tigecycline

Bacteroides fragilis (and others)
Metronidazole
BLIC,[p] clindamycin, cephamycins,[c,q] or carbapenem[n]

Enterobacter spp.
Imipenem, meropenem, ertapenem, or cefepime ± aminoglycoside[p]
Ciprofloxacin,[i] levofloxacin,[i] piperacillin-tazobactam, ticarcillinclavulanate, or tigecycline

Escherichia coli
Meningitis
TGC[c,j] or meropenem
Systemic infection
TGC[c,j]
Ampicillin-sulbactam, FGC,[b,c] BL/BLI,[p] fluoroquinolone,[i,n,r] imipenem,[n] meropenem[n]
Urinary tract infection
Most oral agents: check sensitivities
Ampicillin, amoxicillin-clavulanate, doxycyline,[e] or cephalexin[c]
Aminoglycoside,[p] FGC[b,c] nitrofurantoin, fluoroquinolone[i,n,r]

TABLE 19-1 Drugs of Choice, First Choice, Alternative(s) (*Continued*)
Gram-Negative Bacilli (*Continued*)
Gardnerella vaginalis
Metronidazole
Clindamycin
Haemophilus influenzae
Meningitis
Cefotaxime[c] or ceftriaxone[c]
Meropenem[n] or chloramphenicol[s]
Other infections
BLIC,[p] or if β-lactamase-negative, ampicillin or amoxicillin
Trimethoprim-sulfamethoxazole, cefuroxime,[c] azithromycin, clarithromycin,[h] or fluoroquinolone[i,n,r]
Klebsiella pneumoniae
TGC[e,k] (if UTI only: aminoglycoside[p])
Cefuroxime,[e] fluoroquinolone,[b,r] BLIC,[g] imipenem,[o] meropenem,[o] or ertapenem
Legionella spp.
Erythromycin ± rifampin or fluoroquinolone[i,r]
Trimethoprim-sulfamethoxazole, clarithromycin,[h] azithromycin, or doxycycline[e]
Pasteurella multocida
Penicillin G, ampicillin, amoxicillin
Doxycycline,[e] BLIC,[p] trimethoprim-sulfamethoxazole or ceftriaxone[c,j]
Proteus mirabilis
Ampicillin
Trimethoprim-sulfamethoxazole, most antibiotics except PRP[a]
Proteus (indole-positive) (including *Providencia rettgeri, Morganella morganii*, and *Proteus vulgaris*)
TGC[c,h] or fluoroquinolone[f,r]
BLIC,[p] aztreonam,[t] imipenem,[n] or TGC po[c,m]
Providencia stuartii
TGC[c,j] or fluoroquinolone[i,r]
Trimethoprim-sulfamethoxazole, aztreonam,[t] imipenem,[n] meropenem,[n] or ertapenem
Pseudomonas aeruginosa
Cefepime,[c] ceftazidime,[c] piperacillin-tazobactam, or ticarcillinclavulanate plus aminoglycoside[o]
Ciprofloxacin,[i] levofloxacin,[i] aztreonam,[t] imipenem,[n] meropenem,[n] or colistin
UTI only: aminoglycoside[o]
Ciprofloxacin,[i] levofloxacin[i]
Salmonella typhi
Ciprofloxacin,[i] levofloxacin,[i] ceftriaxone,[c] or cefotaxime[c]
Trimethoprim-sulfamethoxazole
Serratia marcescens
Piperacillin-tazobactam, ticarcillin-clavulanate, or TGC[c,j] ± gentamicin
Trimethoprim-sulfamethoxazole, ciprofloxacin,[i] levofloxacin,[i] aztreonam,[t] imipenem,[n] meropenem,[n] or ertapenem
Stenotrophomonas (Xanthomonas) maltophilia
Trimethoprim-sulfamethoxazole
Generally very resistant to all antimicrobials; check sensitivities to ceftazidime,[e] ticarcillin-clavulanate, doxycycline,[e] and minocycline[e]
Miscellaneous Microorganisms
Chlamydia pneumoniae
Doxycycline[e]
Erythromycin, azithromycin, clarithromycin,[h] telithromycin or fluoroquinolone[f,r]
C. trachomatis
Doxycycline[e] or azithromycin
Levofloxacin[i] or ofloxacin[i]
Mycoplasma pneumoniae
Erythromycin, azithromycin, clarithromycin[h]
Doxycycline[e] or fluoroquinolone[f,r]
Spirochetes
Treponema pallidum
Neurosyphilis
Penicillin G
Ceftriaxone[c]
Primary or secondary
Benzathine penicillin G
Doxycycline[e] or ceftriaxone[c]
Borrelia burgdorferi (choice depends on stage of disease)
Ceftriaxone[c] or cefuroxime axetil,[c] doxycycline,[e] amoxicillin
High-dose penicillin, cefotaxime,[c] or azithromycin

[a]Penicillinase-resistant penicillin: nafcillin or oxacillin. [b]First-generation cephalosporins—IV: cefazolin; po: cephalexin, cephradine, or cefadroxil. [c]Some penicillin-allergic patients may react to cephalosporins. [d]Not reliably bactericidal; should not be used for endocarditis. [e]Not for use in pregnant patients or children younger than 8 years old. [f]Either aqueous penicillin G or benzathine penicillin G (pharyngitis only). [g]Only for soft tissue infections or upper respiratory infections (pharyngitis,otitis media). [h]Do not use in pregnant patients. [i]Not for use in pregnant patients or children younger than 18 years old. [j]Third-generation cephalosporins—IV: cefotaxime, ceftriaxone. [k]Gentamicin should be added if tolerance or moderately susceptible (MIC>0.1 g/mL) organisms are encountered; streptomycin is used but can be more toxic. [l]Second-generation cephalosporins—IV: cefuroxime; po: cefaclor, cefditoren, cefprozil, cefuroxime axetil, and loracarbef. [m]Third-generation cephalosporins—po: cefdinir, cefixime, cefetamet, cefpodoxime proxetil, and ceftibuten. [n]Reserve for serious infection. [o]Aminoglycosides: gentamicin, tobramycin, and amikacin; use per sensitivities. [p]β-Lactamase inhibitor combination—IV: ampicillin-sulbactam, piperacillin-tazobactam, ticarcillin-clavulanate; po: amoxicillin-clavulanate. [q]Cefoxitin. [r]IV/po: ciprofloxacin, levofloxacin, and moxifloxacin. [s]Reserve for serious infection when less toxic drugs are not effective. [t]Generally reserved for patients with hypersensitivity reactions to penicillin.

Abbreviations: BLIC, β-lactamase inhibitor combination; BL/BLI, β-lactamase/β-lactamase inhibitor; FGC, first-generation cephalosporin; MIC, minimal inhibitory concentration; po, orally; PRP, penicillinase-resistant penicillin; SGC, second-generation cephalosporin; TGC, third-generation cephalosporin.

Adapted with permission from Burgess DS. Antimicrobial regimen selection. In: DiPiro JT, Talbert RL, Yee GC, Matzke GR, Wells BG, Posey LM, eds. *Pharmacotherapy: A Pathophysiologic Approach*, 7th ed. New York, NY: McGraw-Hill; 2008:1731-1741.

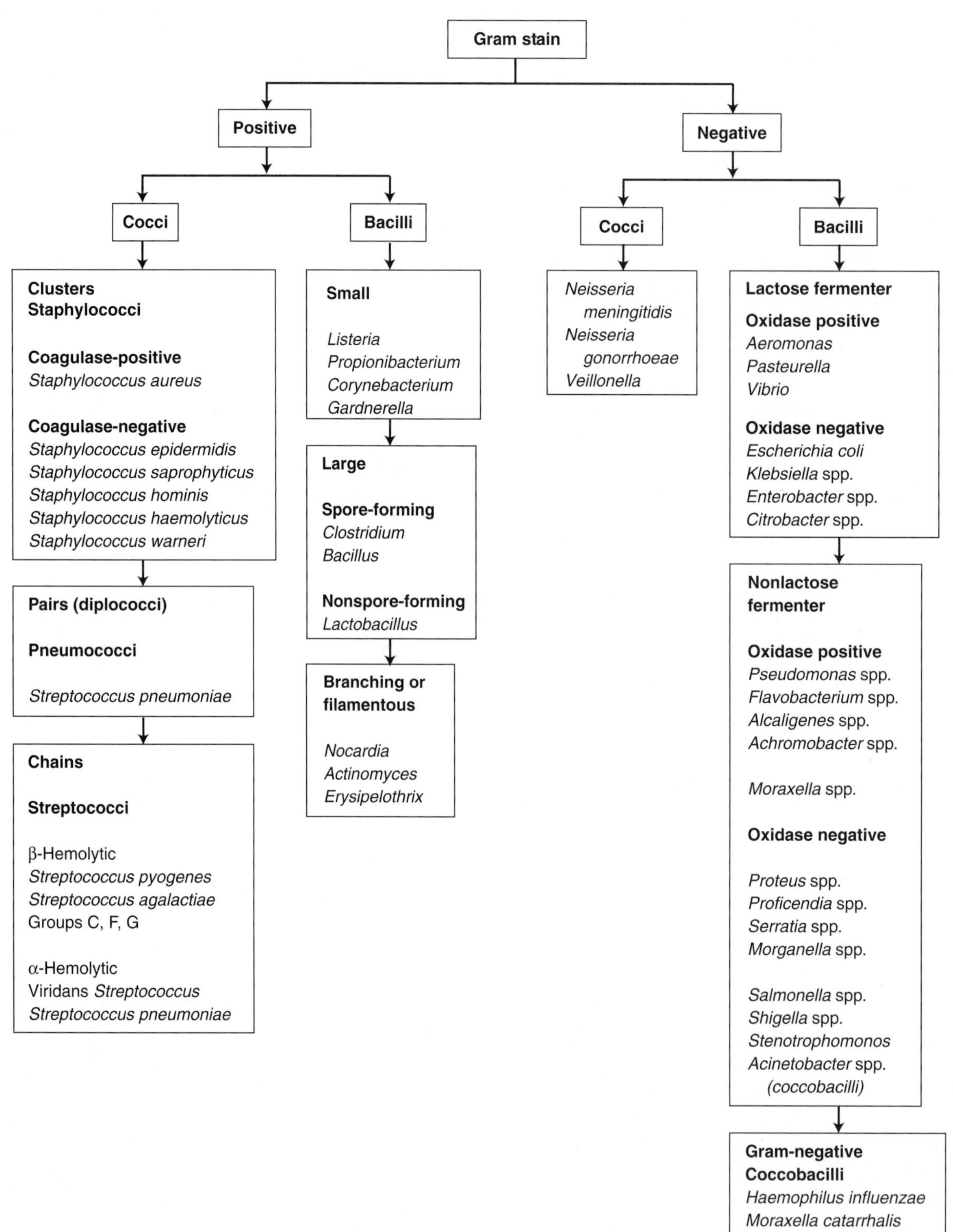

FIGURE 19-1 Bacterial pathogen classification—gram stain and morphologic characteristics.
Reproduced with permission from Rybak MJ, Aeschlimann JR. Laboratory tests to direct antimicrobial pharmacotherapy. In: DiPiro JT, Talbert RL, Yee GC, Matzke GR, Wells BG, Posey LM, eds. *Pharmacotherapy: A Pathophysiologic Approach*, 7th ed. New York, NY: McGraw-Hill; 2008:1715-1730.

for systemic infections, oral vancomycin is utilized to treat *C. difficile* gastrointestinal infections).

Tissue penetration (distribution) relevance varies with the site of infection. The central nervous system (CNS) is one body site where antimicrobial penetration is defined and correlations with clinical outcomes are established.[9] Anti-infectives that do not reach significant concentrations in the cerebrospinal fluid (CSF) should either be avoided or instilled directly. Caution must be utilized when selecting an antimicrobial on the basis of tissue or fluid penetration. Body fluids where drug concentrations are clinically relevant include the CSF, urine, synovial fluid, and peritoneal fluid. Apart from these areas, more attention should be paid to clinical efficacy, antimicrobial spectrum, adverse effects, and cost than to comparative data on penetration.

Oral or parenteral administration of anti-infectives depends on the severity of illness and location of the infection. In sequestered infections, higher concentrations may be required to reach the infected source (meningitis, osteomyelitis, endocarditis, pneumonia) and may require parenteral anti-infectives. Patients treated for upper respiratory tract infections (pharyngitis, bronchitis, sinusitis, and otitis media), skin and soft tissue infections, uncomplicated urinary tract infections, and selected sexually transmitted diseases can receive oral therapy.

Pharmacodynamic Properties Pharmacodynamics (PD) describes the relationship between drug exposure and pharmacologic effect of antibacterial activity or human toxicology.[10] Antimicrobials are categorized based upon their concentration related effects of bacteria. Concentration-dependent PD activity occurs where higher drug concentrations are associated with greater rates and extents of bacterial killing. Concentration-dependent activity is maximized when peak antimicrobial concentrations are high. In contrast, time-dependent activity refers to a minimal increase in the rate or extent of bacterial killing with an increase in dose. Time-dependent activity is maximized when antimicrobials are dosed to maintain blood and/or tissue concentrations above the minimal inhibitory concentration (MIC) in a time-dependent manner. Fluoroquinolones, aminoglycosides, and metronidazole are examples of antimicrobials that exhibit concentration-dependent activity. Beta lactams and glycopeptides exhibit time-dependent activity.

PD properties have been optimized to develop new dosing strategies for antimicrobials. Examples include extended dosing *interval* aminoglycosides and extended *infusion* beta lactam therapy.

- Aminoglycoside antimicrobials (gentamicin, tobramycin, and amikacin) display concentration-dependent activity and may be dosed by *traditional* or *extended interval* methods. *Traditional* dosing in patients with normal renal function is often 1.5 to 2 mg /kg every 8 hours.[7] *Traditional* dosing is monitored by obtaining peaks and troughs after a patient has reached steady state. *Extended interval* dosing is 7 mg/kg every 24, 36, or 48 hours.[11] A 7 mg/kg dose is administered and an aminoglycoside level between 6 to 14 hours after administration is obtained and plotted on the Hartford nomogram to determine the dosing interval. The administration of 7 mg/kg of a medication that has a 2 to 3 hour half-life is a clinical example of utilizing PD properties of aminoglycosides (concentration-dependent activity).
- Beta lactam antimicrobials are often administered intravenously as 30 minute infusions. Examples include piperacillin/tazobactam (Zosyn) 4.5 g IV over 30 minutes every 6 hours and imipenem/cilastatin (Imipenem) 500 mg IV over 30 minutes every 6 hours. In efforts to optimize the time-dependent activity of beta lactams, *extending the infusion interval* is being clinically utilized (piperacillin/tazobactam 3.375 g IV every 8 hours administered as a 4-hour infusion).[12,13] *Extending the infusion interval* allows for the concentration to remain above the MIC for longer periods of time (time-dependent activity).

Antimicrobials are also classified as bactericidal or bacteriostatic. Bactericidal antibiotics kill at least 99.9% of a bacterial population, whereas bacteriostatic antibiotics possess antimicrobial activity but reduce bacterial load to a lower extent. Clinically, bactericidal antibiotics may be necessary to achieve success in infections such as endocarditis or meningitis.

Adverse effects

Antimicrobials with a low propensity of causing adverse events or drug interactions should be selected if possible, particularly for patients with risk factors for a particular complication.[3,4] Risk factors include coadministration of other drugs that are associated with a similar type of adverse event. For example, coadministration of the known nephrotoxin gentamicin with vancomycin increases the risk for nephrotoxicity compared with administration of either drug alone. Other drug interactions may predispose the patient to dose-related toxicity through inhibition of drug metabolism. For example, erythromycin has the potential to prolong cardiac QT intervals in a dose-dependent manner, potentially increasing the risk of sudden cardiac death. Patients prescribed medications that inhibit the metabolism of erythromycin exhibited a five-fold increase in cardiac death versus controls. See Table 19-2 for a list of selected drug interactions with anti-infectives. Examples of selected adverse effects from anti-infectives include:

- Antibiotic associated CNS toxicities (usually when not dose-adjusted for renal function—penicillins, cephalosporins, quinolones, and imipenem).
- Hematologic toxicities (neutropenia) manifested by prolonged use of nafcillin.
- Piperacillin and platelet dysfunction
- Cefotetan and hypoprothrombinemia
- Chloramphenicol and bone marrow suppression
- Trimethoprim and megaloblastic anemia
- Aminoglycosides and nephrotoxicity/ototoxicity
- Photosensitivity and quinolones, tetracyclines, trimethoprim
- *C. difficile* and all antibiotics

Cost

A final consideration with antimicrobial properties in selecting therapy relates to cost. The total cost of antimicrobial therapy includes more than just the acquisition cost of the agent. Many ancillary costs and factors affect the cost of therapy. These include factors such as storage, preparation, distribution, and administration, as well as costs incurred from monitoring for adverse effects and factors such as length of hospitalization, readmissions, and all directly provided health-care goods and services.

TABLE 19-2 Major Drug Interactions with Antimicrobials

Antimicrobial	Other Agent(s)	Mechanism of Action/Effect	Clinical Management
Aminoglycosides	Neuromuscular blocking agents	N: additive adverse effects;	Avoid
	Nephrotoxins (N) or ototoxins (O) (eg, amphotericin B (N) cisplatin (N/O), cyclosporine (N), furosemide (O), NSAIDs (N), radio contrast (N), vancomycin (N)	O: additive adverse effects	Monitor aminoglycoside SDC and renal function
Amphotericin B	Nephrotoxins (eg, aminoglycosides, cidofovir, cyclosporine, foscarnet, pentamidine)	Additive adverse effects	Monitor renal function
Azoles	Cytochrome p450 3a4, 2c9, 2c19 subtrates	Inhibit metabolism/clearance of cytochrome p450 subtrates	See Chap. 28 for specific cytochrome 450 iso-enzyems for the azole antifungals
Chloramphenicol	Phenytoin, tolbutamide, ethanol	Decreased metabolism of other agents	Monitor phenytoin SDC, blood glucose
Foscarnet	Pentamidine IV	Increased risk of severe nephrotoxicity/hypocalcemia	Monitor renal function/serum calcium
Isoniazid	Carbamazepine, phenytoin	Decreased metabolism of other agents (nausea, vomiting, nystagmus, ataxia)	Monitor drug SDC
Macrolides/azalides	Digoxin	Decreased digoxin bioavailability and metabolism	Monitor digoxin SDC; avoid if possible
	Theophylline	Decreased metabolism of theophylline	Monitor theophylline SDC
Metronidazole	Ethanol (drugs containing ethanol)	Disulfiram-like reaction	Avoid
Penicillins and cephalosporins	Probenecid, aspirin	Blocked excretion of β-lactams	Use if prolonged high concentration of β-lactam desirable
Ciprofloxacin/norfloxacin	Theophylline	Decreased metabolism of theophylline	Monitor theophylline
Quinolones	Class Ia and Class III antiarrhythmics	Increased QT interval	Avoid
	Multivalent cations (antacids, iron, sucralfate, zinc, vitamins, dairy, citric acid) didanosine	Decreased absorption of quinolone	Separate by 2 h
Rifampin	Azoles, cyclosporine, methadone propranolol, PIs, oral contraceptives, tacrolimus, warfarin	Increased metabolism of other agent	Avoid if possible
Sulfonamides	Sulfonylureas, phenytoin, warfarin	Decreased metabolism of other agent	Monitor blood glucose, SDC, PT
Tetracyclines	Antacids, iron, calcium, sucralfate	Decreased absorption of tetracycline	Separate by 2 hours
	Digoxin	Decreased digoxin bioavailability and metabolism	Monitor digoxin SDC; avoid if possible

Abbreviations: PI, protease inhibitor; PT, prothrombin time; SDC, serum drug concentrations.

Note: Azalides: azithromycin; Azoles: fluconazole, itraconazole, ketoconazole, and voriconazole; Macrolides: erythromycin, clarithromycin; Protease inhibitors: amprenavir, indinavir, lopinavir/ritonavir, nelfinavir, ritonavir, and saquinavir; Quinolones: ciprofloxacin, gatifloxacin, levofloxacin, moxifloxacin.

Reproduced with permission from Burgess DS. Antimicrobial regimen selection. In: DiPiro JT, Talbert RL, Yee GC, Matzke GR, Wells BG, Posey LM, eds. *Pharmacotherapy: A Pathophysiologic Approach*, 7th ed. New York, NY: McGraw-Hill; 2008:1731-1741.

Host Factors

Host factors should be considered when evaluating a patient for antimicrobial therapy. Important host factors are: drug allergies, age, pregnancy, genetic/metabolic abnormalities, and organ dysfunction.

Allergy

Allergy to an antimicrobial agent generally precludes its use. Assessment of allergy histories must be performed because patients confuse adverse drug effects (gastrointestinal disturbance) with true allergic reactions. Penicillin and penicillin-related compounds are the most commonly cited antimicrobial allergies. Recommendations for administration of cephalosporin antibiotics in penicillin allergic patients depend on the type of reaction.[14-16] Patients with a history of immediate or accelerated reactions (eg, anaphylaxis) to penicillin should not be given cephalosporin antibiotics. Patients with a delayed hypersensitivity reaction (rash) to penicillin may be given cephalosporins under close supervision.

Age

Age is an important factor in determining causative pathogens for certain infections and pharmacokinetic/physiologic factors for certain antibiotics.[17] Causative pathogens in bacterial meningitis differ based upon age. For example, *Listeria monocytogenes* is a possible cause of meningitis in neonates and patients greater than 55 years of age. Pharmacokinetic factors affected by age may alter concentrations of the agent. For example, hepatic functions are not well developed in neonates and the use of chloramphenicol may lead to shock and cardiovascular collapse (gray baby syndrome). This is caused by the inability of the newborn's liver to metabolize and detoxify the drug. Neonates may also develop kernicterus when administered sulfonamides. Physiologic changes in persons older than 65 years of age may impact anti-infective properties. A decrease in the number of nephrons resulting in decreased renal function is a common physiologic change in elderly patients. The decrease in renal function may increase the incidence of side-effects of renally eliminated anti-infectives.

Pregnancy

Antimicrobial agents must be used with caution in pregnant and nursing women. Some agents are known or likely to be teratogenic (eg, metronidazole), and others pose potential threats to the fetus or infant (eg, quinolones, tetracyclines, and sulfonamides).[18] Pharmacokinetic variables also are altered during pregnancy.[19] Both the clearance and volume of distribution are increased during pregnancy. As a result, increased dosages and/or more frequent administration of certain drugs may be required to achieve adequate concentrations.

Metabolic Abnormalities

Inherited or acquired metabolic abnormalities influence infectious diseases therapy. Patients with peripheral vascular disease may not absorb drugs given by intramuscular injection. Other examples include:

- Patients who are phenotypically slow acetylators of isoniazid are at greater risk for peripheral neuropathy.[20]
- Patients with glucose-6-phosphate dehydrogenase (G6PD) deficiency can develop hemolysis when exposed to sulfonamides and dapsone.[4]

Organ Dysfunction

Patients with diminished renal or hepatic function (or both) will accumulate certain drugs unless the dosage is adjusted.[21,22] Recommendations for dosing antibiotics in patients with liver dysfunction are not as formalized as guidelines for patients with renal dysfunction. Antibiotics that should be adjusted in severe liver disease include clindamycin, erythromycin, metronidazole, and rifampin.

Normal Flora

Normal flora is bacteria that are colonized in areas of the human body. Infections arise from normal flora (also called endogenous flora). Knowing what organisms reside where can help guide empirical antimicrobial therapy (Figure 19-2).

Infections acquired from an external source are referred to as exogenous infections. These infections occur as a result of human-to-human transmission, contact with exogenous bacterial populations in the environment, and animal contact. Resistant pathogens such as methicillin-resistant *Staphylococcus aureus* (MRSA) and vancomycin-resistant *Enterococcus* species (VRE) may colonize hospitalized patients. Patients who are colonized with MRSA, VRE, or other multidrug resistant organisms often require different empiric therapy and should be placed in isolation to minimize transmission to other patients.

Patients with a history of recent antimicrobial use may have altered normal flora. If a patient develops a new infection while on therapy, fails therapy, or has received antimicrobials recently, it is prudent to utilize a different class of antimicrobials because of bacterial resistance. Previous hospitalization or home health care utilization are risk factors for the acquisition of exogenous pathogens.

Colonization versus Infection

It is important to differentiate infection from colonization because antimicrobial therapy targeting bacterial colonization is inappropriate and may lead to the development of resistant bacteria. Infection refers to the presence of bacteria that are causing disease. Colonization refers to the presence of bacteria that are not causing disease.

Clinical Presentation

Findings on physical examination, along with the clinical presentation, can help to provide the anatomic location of the infection. Once the anatomic site is identified, the most probable pathogens associated with disease can be determined based upon likely endogenous or exogenous flora.

Fever often accompanies infection and is defined as a rise in body temperature above the normal 98.6°F (37°C). Oral and axillary temperatures may underestimate core temperature by at least 1°F, whereas rectal temperatures best approximate core temperatures. Fever is a host response to bacterial toxins. Fever may also be caused by other infections (eg, fungal or viral), medications (eg, penicillins, cephalosporins, salicylates, phenytoin)[4], trauma, or other medical conditions (autoimmune disease, malignancy, hyperthyroidism). Patients with infections may also present with hypothermia (eg, patients with overwhelming infection, sepsis). Elderly patients may be afebrile, as well as patients with localized infection (eg, uncomplicated urinary tract infections). For some patients, fever may be the only indication of infection. For example, neutropenic

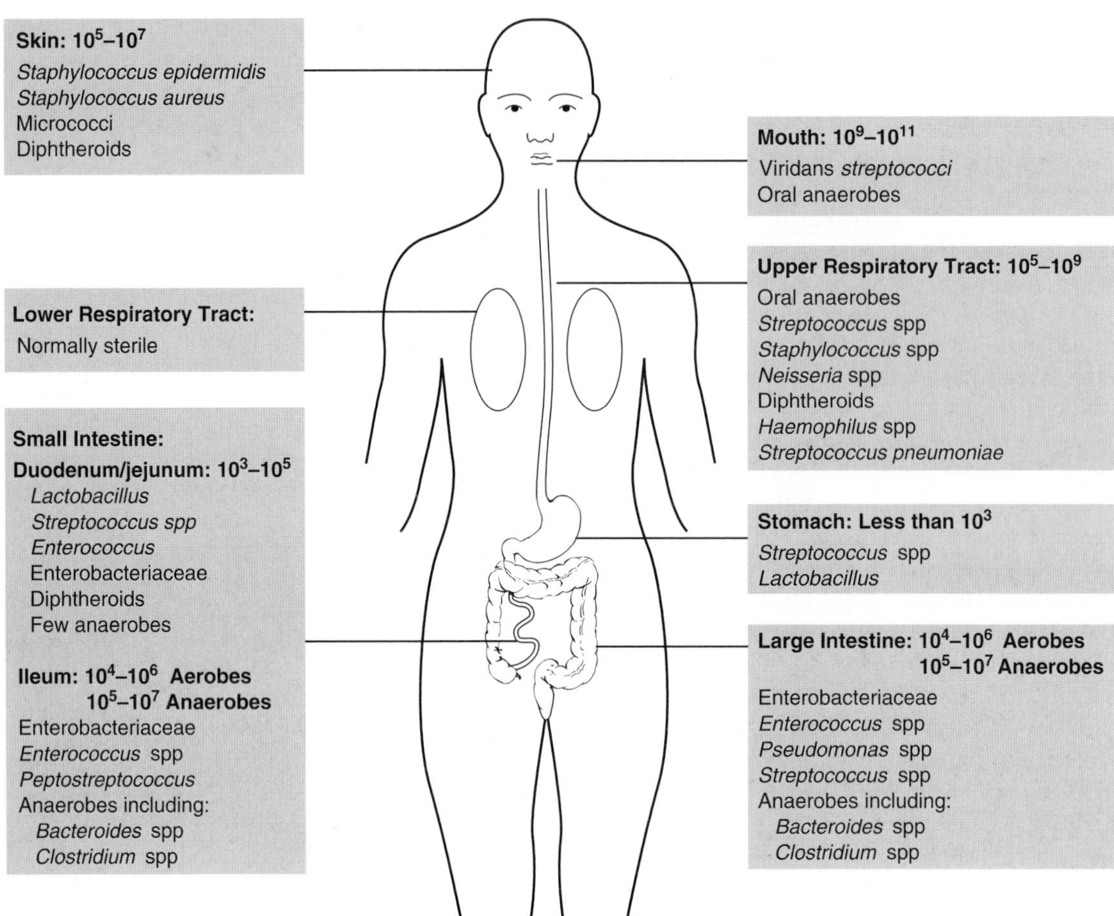

FIGURE 19-2 Normal flora and concentrations of bacteria (organisms per millimeter).
Reproduced with permission from Oliphant CM, Madaras-Kelly K. Antimicrobial regimen selection. In: Chisholm-Burns MA, Schwinghammer TL, Wells BG, Malone PM, Kolesar JM, DiPiro JT, eds. *Pharmacotherapy Principles & Practice*, 2nd ed. New York, NY: McGraw-Hill; 2010:1155-1168

patients may not have the ability to mount normal immune responses to infection and the only finding may be fever.

Diagnosis

Microbiologic studies that allow for direct examination of a specimen may aid in the diagnosis and give an indication of the infecting organism. A gram stain can give rapid information that can be applied immediately to patient care. A gram stain is performed to identify if bacteria are present and to determine morphologic characteristics of bacteria (such as gram-positive or negative, or shape—cocci, bacilli). Figure 19-1 identifies bacterial pathogens as classified by gram stain and morphologic characteristics. The presence of white blood cells on a gram stain indicates inflammation and suggests that the identified bacteria are pathogenic. The gram stain may be useful in judging a sputum specimen's adequacy. For example, the presence of epithelial cells on sputum gram stain suggests that the specimen is either poorly collected or contaminated. A poor specimen can give misleading information with regard to the underlying pathogen and is a waste of laboratory personnel time and patient cost.

Culture and susceptibility testing provides additional information for clinicians to guide therapy. Specimens are placed on culture media that provide the proper growth conditions. Once the bacteria grow on culture media, they can be identified through a variety of biochemical tests. Once a pathogen is identified, susceptibility tests can be performed to various antimicrobial agents. The minimum inhibitory concentration (MIC) is a standard susceptibility test. The MIC is the lowest concentration of antimicrobial that inhibits visible bacterial growth. Breakpoint and MIC values determine if the organism is susceptible (S), intermediate (I), or resistant (R) to an antimicrobial. The breakpoint is the concentration of that antimicrobial that can be achieved in the serum after a normal or standard dose of the antimicrobial. If the MIC is below the breakpoint, the organism is considered to be susceptible to that agent. If the MIC is above the breakpoint, the organism is said to be resistant. Bacterial cultures should be obtained prior to initiating antimicrobial therapy. The decision to culture depends on the sensitivity and specificity of the physical findings, diagnostic examination findings, and whether or not the pathogens are predictable. For example, culture and susceptibility testing usually is not warranted in a young, otherwise healthy woman who presents with signs and symptoms consistent with a urinary tract infection (UTI) because the primary pathogen, *Escherichia coli*, is readily predictable. Cultures need to be interpreted with caution. Poor specimen collection technique can result in misleading information and inappropriate use of antimicrobials.

Common nonmicrobiologic laboratory tests include the white blood cell (WBC) count and differential, erythrocyte sedimentation rate (ESR), and determination of the C-reactive protein level (CRP). In most cases, the WBC count is elevated in response to infection, but it may be normal in localized infections or decreased in overwhelming infection. In response to infection, neutrophils leave the bloodstream and enter the tissue to fight against the offending pathogens (ie, leukocytosis). The ESR and CRP are nonspecific markers of inflammation. They increase as a result of the acute-phase reactant response, which is a response to inflammatory stimuli such as infection or tissue injury. These tests may be used as markers of infectious disease response because they are elevated when the disease is active and usually fall in response to treatment. These tests should not be used to diagnose infection because they may be elevated in noninfectious conditions (autoimmune disorders).

SPECIAL CONSIDERATIONS

Patients must be monitored for a therapeutic response. Culture and susceptibility reports must be reviewed (if obtained) and the therapy changed accordingly. Use of agents with the narrowest spectrum of activity against the identified pathogen is recommended. Patient monitoring should include many of the same parameters to diagnose the infection. The WBC count and temperature should start to normalize. Physical complaints from the patient should diminish (cough, sputum production, shortness of breath). Determinations of serum levels of antimicrobials can be useful in ensuring outcome, preventing adverse events, or both. Anti-infectives that require serum concentration monitoring are the aminoglycosides, flucytosine, and chloramphenicol (vancomycin is often monitored as well). Changes in the volume of distribution can have a significant impact on the efficacy, safety, or both. A low volume of distribution (eg, dehydrated patient) results in higher drug concentrations, whereas a larger than expected volume of distribution (eg, edema) results in low concentrations.

As patients improve clinically, the route of administration of the antimicrobial should be re-evaluated for patients receiving parenteral agents. Streamlining therapy from parenteral to oral should be considered in patients who display clinical improvement, lack of fever for 8 to 24 hours, decreased WBC, and have a functioning gastrointestinal tract. Drugs that exhibit excellent oral bioavailability when compared with IV formulations include the fluoroquinolones, clindamycin, doxycycline, metronidazole, linezolid, and trimethoprim-sulfamethoxazole.

CASE Application

1. Select the antimicrobial that may cause collateral damage by selecting for a nontargeted organism (ie *C. difficile*) leading to a colitis infection.
   a. Clindamycin
   b. Levofloxacin
   c. Ciprofloxacin
   d. b and c
   e. All of the above
2. Select the correct dose of cefepime (Maxipime) for a patient with normal renal function and empirically treated for an infection (at this time the site or source of infection have not been identified).
   a. 1 g IV every 12 hours
   b. 2 g IV every 12 hours
   c. 2 g IV every 8 hours
   d. All of the above
3. Select the antimicrobial pharmacokinetic (PK) property that impacts the dose and/or interval.
   a. Bioavailability
   b. Volume of distribution
   c. Metabolism
   d. Elimination
   e. All of the above
4. Select the factor that may affect the bioavailability of an oral anti-infective.
   a. A medication that is a substrate of the CYP-450 system
   b. Dosage formulation of the anti-infective
   c. A patient that has peripheral vascular disease
   d. A patient that has renal dysfunction
5. Select the factor that would usually necessitate a patient to be given IV anti-infectives.
   a. Fever of 101.9°F
   b. Severe cough
   c. Glucose-6-phosphate dehydrogenase (G6PD) deficiency
   d. Blood pressure of 91/52 mm Hg with signs of hypoperfusion (Baseline blood pressure for patient is 129/86 mm Hg)
6. Select the oral anti-infective(s) that displays good bioavailability.
   a. Fluconazole
   b. Linezolid
   c. Levofloxacin
   d. Vancomycin
   e. a, b, and c
7. Select the infectious disease state that requires excellent tissue penetration (distribution).
   a. Meningitis
   b. Acute cystitis
   c. Bronchitis
   d. a and b
   e. All of the above
8. Select the anti-infective that exhibits the pharmacodynamic property of concentration-dependent activity.
   a. Ceftriaxone
   b. Amoxicillin
   c. Ciprofloxacin
   d. Meropenem

9. Select the anti-infective that exhibits the pharmacodynamic property of time-dependent activity.

   a. Levofloxacin
   b. Doripenem
   c. Amikacin
   d. Metronidazole

10. A patient with a health care-associated pneumonia infection is found to have a multidrug resistant organism (this was found by the culture and susceptibility and the pathogen *Pseudomonas aeruginosa* exhibits a high MIC to all antibiotics). Since the pathogen exhibits a high level resistance, modifications to the dose or interval will be required to achieve successful outcomes. Currently the patient is receiving the beta lactam piperacillin/tazobactam 4.5 g intravenously every 6 hours infused over 30 minutes. Select the factor that may be done to piperacillin/tazobactam that could optimize the pharmacodynamic property.

    a. Increase the infusion time
    b. Increase the dose
    c. Add combination therapy with another beta lactam
    d. All of the above

11. Central nervous system side effects (seizures and mental status changes) are associated with beta lactam and quinolone anti-infectives. A risk factor for development of the central nervous system reactions is:

    a. Duration of therapy
    b. Infusion interval
    c. Bioavailability
    d. Renal dysfunction

12. Select the anti-infective that is associated with the adverse effects of nephrotoxicity and ototoxicity.

    a. Amoxicillin/Clavulanate
    b. Cefpodoxime
    c. Moxifloxacin
    d. Gentamicin

13. Select the anti-infective(s) that is associated with the adverse reaction of antibiotic-associated diarrhea (*C. difficile*).

    a. Augmentin
    b. Levaquin
    c. Cleocin
    d. Vancocin
    e. a, b, and c

14. JG is a patient with an immediate allergic reaction to ticarcillin/clavulanate (Timentin). Select the antimicrobial that JG may take in relation to his allergy.

    a. Piperacillin/tazobactam
    b. Amoxicillin/clavulanate
    c. Ceftriaxone
    d. Aztreonam

15. Select the host factor(s) that may impact antimicrobial therapy.

    a. Age
    b. Pregnancy
    c. Metabolic abnormalities
    d. Organ dysfunction
    e. All of the above

16. Select the risk factor(s) for the acquisition of exogenous pathogens.

    a. Home health care utilization
    b. Pregnancy
    c. Recent antimicrobial use
    d. a and c
    e. All of the above

17. Select the potential cause of a fever.

    a. Infection
    b. Piperacillin
    c. Trauma
    d. Cancer
    e. All of the above

18. Select the information that is revealed by a gram stain.

    a. Minimum inhibitory concentration
    b. Genre and species of the bacteria
    c. Morphologic characteristics of the bacteria
    d. All of the above

19. Select the pathogen(s) that is classified as an atypical organism.

    a. *Escherichia coli*
    b. *Klebsiella pneumoniae*
    c. *Mycoplasma pneumoniae*
    d. All of the above

20. Select the pathogen that represents an exogenous bacteria flora (ie, acquired from the hospital). Characteristics of this pathogen are nonlactose fermenting gram-negative bacilli.

    a. *Neisseria meningitidis*
    b. *Enterobacter cloacae*
    c. *Streptococcus pneumoniae*
    d. *Pseudomonas aeruginosa*

21. Select the penicillin antimicrobial that is broad spectrum and has coverage against nonlactose negative (oxidase-positive) gram-negative bacilli.

    a. Amoxicillin
    b. Nafcillin
    c. Cefepime
    d. Doripenem
    e. Piperacillin/tazobactam

22. Select the pathogen(s) that is part of the normal (endogenous) flora of the large intestine.
    a. *Escherichia coli*
    b. Viridans *streptococci*
    c. *Neisseria meningitidis*
    d. All of the above

23. Select the best answer that represents part of the normal (endogenous) flora of the lower respiratory tract.
    a. Enterobacteriaceae
    b. *Streptococcus pneumoniae*
    c. *Enterococcus* species
    d. Normally sterile

24. Select the drug interaction(s) with aminoglycosides.
    a. Amphotericin B
    b. Vancomycin
    c. Furosemide
    d. Cisplatin
    e. All of the above

25. RL is a patient with a past medical history of iron deficiency anemia. He is being treated with ferrous sulfate. Select the antimicrobial(s) that would have a decreased bioavailability when combined with ferrous sulfate.
    a. Moxifloxacin
    b. Tetracycline
    c. Azithromycin
    d. a and b
    e. All of the above

TAKEAWAY POINTS ››

- Antimicrobials that kill many different species of bacteria are called broad-spectrum, whereas antimicrobials that kill only a few different species of bacteria are called narrow-spectrum antimicrobials.
- Empirically treating infectious diseases and monitoring therapy requires knowledge of anti-infective properties, host factors, patient's normal flora, differentiating infection versus colonization, and understanding clinical presentation and diagnostic tests (microbiologic and nonmicrobiologic laboratory studies).
- It is important to understand the difference in antimicrobial spectrum of activity and select agent(s) that target the pathogens most likely causing the infection.
- Antimicrobial dosage regimens with the same agent may be different depending upon the infection or pathogen.
- Integration of pharmacokinetic and pharmacodynamic properties of an agent is important when choosing antimicrobial therapy to ensure efficacy and to prevent resistance.
- Pharmacokinetics refers to a mathematical method of describing in vivo drug exposure in terms of absorption, distribution, metabolism, and elimination.
- Pharmacodynamics (PD) describes the relationship between drug exposure and pharmacologic effect of antibacterial activity or human toxicology.
- Concentration-dependent PD activity occurs where higher drug concentrations are associated with greater rate and extent of bacterial killing. Fluoroquinolones, aminoglycosides, and metronidazoles are examples of antimicrobials that exhibit concentration-dependent activity.
- Time-dependent activity is maximized when these antimicrobials are dosed to maintain blood and/or tissue concentrations above the minimal inhibitory concentration (MIC) in a time-dependent manner. Beta lactams and glycopeptides exhibit time-dependent activity.
- Antimicrobials with a low propensity of causing adverse events or drug interactions should be selected if possible, particularly for patients with risk factors for a particular complication.
- Host factors should be considered when evaluating a patient for antimicrobial therapy. Important host factors are: drug allergies, age, pregnancy, genetic/metabolic abnormalities, and organ dysfunction.
- Patients with a history of immediate or accelerated reactions (eg, anaphylaxis) to penicillin should not be given cephalosporin antibiotics. Patients with a delayed hypersensitivity reaction (rash) to penicillin may be given cephalosporin under close supervision.
- Normal flora is bacteria that are colonized in areas of the human body. Infections arise from normal flora (also called endogenous flora).
- A gram stain is performed to identify if bacteria are present and to determine morphologic characteristics of bacteria (such as gram-positive or negative, or shape— cocci, bacilli).
- Once a pathogen is identified, susceptibility tests can be performed to various antimicrobial agents. The minimum inhibitory concentration (MIC) is a standard susceptibility test. The MIC is the lowest concentration of antimicrobial that inhibits visible bacterial growth. Breakpoint and MIC values determine if the organism is susceptible (S), intermediate (I), or resistant (R) to an antimicrobial.

REFERENCES

1. Hessen TM, Kaye D. Principles of selection and use of antibacterial agents: in vitro activity and pharmacology. *Infect Dis Clin North Am.* 2000;14:265-279.
2. Slama TG, Amin A, Brunton SA, et al. A clinician's guide to the appropriate and accurate use of antibiotics: The Council for Appropriate and Rational Antibiotic Therapy (CARAT) criteria. *Am J Med.* 2005;118(7A):1S-6S.
3. Gurwitz JH, Field TS, Harrold LR, et al. Incidence and preventability of adverse drug events among older persons in the ambulatory setting. *JAMA.* 2003;289(9):1107-1116.
4. Cunha BA. Antibiotic side effects. *Med Clin North Am.* 2001;85:149-185.
5. Paterson Dl. Collateral damage from cephalosporin or quinolone antibiotic therapy. *Clin Infect Dis.*2004;38(suppl 4):S341-S345.
6. Cefepime [package insert]. Sagent Pharmaceuticals: Schaumburg, IL; January 2008. Accessed October 2009.
7. Winter ME. Part 1: Basic principles. In: *Basic Clinical Pharmacokinetics.* Baltimore, MD: Lippincott Williams & Wilkins; 2004:2-111.
8. Ebert SC. Application of pharmacokinetics and pharmacodynamics for antibiotic selection. *P&To.* 2004:29:244-252.
9. Tunkel AR, Hartman BJ, Kaplan SL, et al. Practice guidelines for the management of bacterial meningitis. *Clin Infect Dis.* 2004;39:1267-1284.
10. Drusano GL. Antimicrobial pharmacodynamics: critical interactions of bug and drug. *Nat Rev Microbiol.* 2004;2(4):289-300.
11. Nicolau DP, Freeman CD, Belliveau PP, et al. Experience with a once-daily aminoglycoside program administered to 2184 adult patients. *Antimicrob Agents Chemother.* 1995;39(3):650-655.
12. Lodise TP, Lomaestro B, Drusano GL. Piperacillin—tazobactam for Pseudomonas aeruginosa infection: clinical implications of an extended infusion dosing strategy. *Clin Infect Dis.* 2007;44(3):357-363.
13. Reese AM, Frei CR, Burgess DS. Pharmacodynamics of intermittent and continuous infusion piperacillin/tazobactam and cefepime against extended-spectrum beta-lactamase producing organisms. *Int J Antimicrob Agents.* 2005;26(2):114-119.
14. Park MA, Li JTC. Diagnosis and management of penicillin allergy. *Mayo Clin Pro.* 2005;80:405-410.
15. Kelkar PS, Li JTC. Cephalosporin allergy. *N Engl J Med.* 2001;345:804-809.
16. Gruchalla RS, Pirmohamed M. Clinical practice. Antibiotic allergy. *N Engl J Med.* 2006;354(6):601-609.
17. Stalam M, Kaye D. Antibiotic agents in the elderly. *Infect Dis Clin North Am.* 2000;14:341-355.
18. Briggs GG, Freeman RK, Yaffe SJ. *Drugs in Pregnancy and Lactation.* 7th ed. Philadelphia, PA: Lippincott Williams & Wilkins; 2005.
19. Anderson GD. Pregnancy-induced changes in pharmacokinetics. *Clin Pharmacokinetic.* 2005;44;989-1008.
20. Weinshilboum R. Inheritance and drug response. *N Engl J Med.* 2003;348:529-537.
21. Livornese LL, Slavin D, Benz RL, et al. Use of antibacterial agents in renal failure. *Infect Dis Clin North Am.* 2000;14:371-389.
22. Tschida SJ, Vance-Bryan K, Zaske DE. Anti-infective agents in hepatic disease. *Med Clin North Am.* 1995;79:895-917.

TABLE 20-3 Antibiotics for the Treatment of Streptococcal Pharyngitis

Antibiotic	Adult Dose	Pediatric Dose	Duration	Comments
Penicillin V (PEN VK)	250 mg 3-4 times daily or 500 mg twice daily	250 mg 2-3 times daily	10 d	Drug of choice, but increasing reports of treatment failure
Penicillin G benzathine (Bicillin LA)	1.2 million units	600,000 units (if under 27 kg)	1 IM dose	Useful for nonadherence or emesis; painful injection
Amoxicillin (Amoxil)	250-500 mg 3 times per day	40-50 mg/kg/d in 3 doses	10 d	Preferred over penicillin for young children (more palatable)
Cephalexin (Keflex)	250-500 mg 4 times daily	25-50 mg/kg/d in 4 doses	10 d	Consider in penicillin allergy (if allergy is delayed reaction)
Azithromycin (Zithromax)	500 mg once daily	12 mg/kg once daily	5 d	Increasing resistance
Clindamycin (Cleocin)	150 mg 4 times daily	20-30 mg/kg/d in 3 doses	10 d	Useful for recurrent infections

with significant pediatric contact are also at increased risk. The signs and symptoms of streptococcal pharyngitis are:

- Sudden onset of sore throat with severe pain on swallowing
- Fever
- Headache, abdominal pain, nausea, vomiting
- Pharyngeal and tonsillar erythema with possible patchy exudates
- Tender, enlarged anterior cervical lymph nodes
- Swollen, red uvula
- Soft palate petechiae
- Scarlatiniform rash

The diagnosis of pharyngitis consists of a throat swab and culture or rapid antigen detection test. These tests should only be performed if there is a clinical suspicion of streptococcal pharyngitis.

TREATMENT

The goals of therapy for streptococcal pharyngitis are to eradicate infection in order to prevent complications, shorten the disease course, and reduce infectivity and spread to close contacts. Sequelae that can be prevented by antibiotics are peritonsillar abscess, cervical lymphadenitis, and rheumatic fever. Antimicrobial therapy is not effective at preventing poststreptococcal glomerulonephritis.

Antibiotics should only be used in cases of laboratory confirmed streptococcal pharyngitis associated with clinical symptoms in order to avoid overtreatment.[18-19] Penicillin is the antibiotic of choice because of its narrow spectrum of activity, documented safety and efficacy, and low cost. Historical studies proving that antibiotics prevented streptococcal complications were performed with penicillin; however, it is presumed other antibiotics are effective for preventing rheumatic heart disease.[20] Recent data suggest that cephalosporins are more effective than penicillin in producing bacteriological and clinical cure and can be considered as first-line options.[21] Table 20-3 lists selected antibiotics used for the treatment of streptococcal pharyngitis.

CASE Application

1. Select the upper respiratory tract infection(s) that may be caused by viruses such as respiratory syncytial virus, influenza virus, rhinovirus, and adenovirus.
   a. Otitis media
   b. Sinusitis
   c. Pharyngitis
   d. Rhinitis
   e. All of the above

2. Select the upper respiratory tract condition that would be defined as the presence of fluid in the middle ear without symptoms of acute illness.
   a. Otitis media with effusion
   b. Sinusitis
   c. Pharyngitis
   d. All of the above

3. Select the bacterial pathogen(s) that cause upper respiratory tract infections.
   a. *Streptococcus pneumoniae*
   b. *Streptococcus pyogenes*
   c. *Haemophilus influenzae*
   d. *Moraxella catarrhalis*
   e. All of the above

4. Select the nonpharmacologic management option(s) for acute otitis media.
   a. Watchful waiting
   b. Tympanostomy tubes
   c. Adenoidectomy
   d. b and c
   e. All of the above

5. Select the pharmacologic management option(s) for acute otitis media in children.
   a. Antibiotics
   b. Acetaminophen
   c. Decongestants

d. Aspirin
e. a and b

6. Select the bacterial resistance mechanism of action that may impact empiric therapy for acute otitis media.
   a. Altered penicillin-binding proteins
   b. Beta lactamase
   c. Penicillinase
   d. b and c
   e. All of the above

7. QW is a 35-year-old-man with a diagnosis of acute bacterial sinusitis. He has a penicillin allergy (delayed reaction—rash). Select the antibiotic that may be used to treat acute bacterial sinusitis in patients with a delayed hypersensitivity reaction to penicillin.
   a. Amoxicillin
   b. Trimethoprim-sulfamethoxazole
   c. Clarithromycin
   d. b and c
   e. All of the above

8. UQ is a 2-year-old child who attends day care and is diagnosed with severe acute bacterial sinusitis. Because the patient is attending a day care and is 2 years of age, penicillin-resistant *S. pneumoniae* is highly suspected. Select the antibiotic regimen that would be recommended to treat this acute bacterial sinusitis infection.
   a. Amoxicillin 45 mg/kg/d in divided doses
   b. Amoxicillin 90 mg/kg/d in divided doses
   c. Trimethoprim-sulfamethoxazole (8 mg/kg trimethoprim) in divided doses
   d. Doxycycline 100 mg in divided doses

9. Select the common side effect(s) for amoxicillin and amoxicillin-clavulanate.
   a. Nausea, vomiting, and diarrhea
   b. Rash
   c. Allergic reactions
   d. All of the above

10. Select the cephalosporin that may be used in the treatment of acute otitis media that has a bitter tasting suspension and has differing bioavailability rates depending upon the oral formulation used.
    a. Ceftin
    b. Vantin
    c. Zithromax
    d. Cleocin

11. Select the parenteral cephalosporin that is often administered intramuscularly as a 3-day regimen for acute otitis media.
    a. Clarithromycin
    b. Amoxicillin-clavulanate
    c. Trimethoprim-sulfamethoxazole
    d. Clindamycin
    e. Ceftriaxone

12. Select the macrolide antibiotic(s) that has CYP-450 3A4 drug interactions.
    a. Biaxin
    b. Bactrim
    c. Pediazole
    d. a and c
    e. All of the above

13. IO is an 11-year-old patient with a diagnosis of acute bacterial sinusitis. IO has been prescribed 10 mg/kg of trimethoprim/sulfamethoxazole. Which component(s) of the antibiotic should the dose is based upon?
    a. Trimethoprim
    b. Sulfamethoxazole
    c. Sulfonamide
    d. All of the above

14. YQ is a 6-year-old patient with a severe case of acute bacterial sinusitis. She has a type I (immediate) allergic reaction to penicillin. Select the antibiotic that may be utilized to treat the sinus infection.
    a. Doxycycline
    b. Moxifloxacin
    c. Clindamycin
    d. Clarithromycin

15. TM is a 7-year-old patient with a diagnosis of strep throat. Select the bacterial pathogen that causes strep throat.
    a. *Streptococcus pyogenes*
    b. Group A *Streptococcus*
    c. Flesh-eating bacteria
    d. All of the above

16. Select the antibiotic to treat strep throat in a 4-year-old child with an immediate penicillin allergy.
    a. Trimethoprim-sulfamethoxazole
    b. Amoxicillin
    c. Cephalexin
    d. Clindamycin

17. Select the antibiotic that may cause an abnormal taste.
    a. Biaxin
    b. Zithromax
    c. Doxycycline
    d. Amoxil

18. Select the antibiotic used in the treatment of upper respiratory tract infections in children less than 8 years of age that can cause photosensitivity.
    a. Doxycycline
    b. Levofloxacin
    c. Moxifloxacin

d. All of the above
e. None of the above

19. Select the brand name of cefuroxime axetil.

a. Vantin
b. Rocephin
c. Ceftin
d. Augmentin

20. Select the viral pathogen(s) that may cause upper respiratory tract infections.

a. *Haemophilus influenzae*
b. Influenza
c. Adenovirus
d. b and c
e. All of the above

TAKEAWAY POINTS ››

- Upper respiratory tract infections include otitis media, sinusitis, pharyngitis, laryngitis (croup), rhinitis, and epiglottitis.
- Most upper respiratory tract infections (URTIs) have a viral etiology and tend to resolve spontaneously; therefore, antibiotics would not be appropriate for the majority of URTIs.
- Otitis media is an inflammation of the middle ear and represents the most common reason for prescribing antibiotics to children.
- Acute otitis media (AOM) is a symptomatic middle ear infection that occurs rapidly with effusion. Otitis media with effusion (OME) is the presence of fluid in the middle ear without symptoms of acute illness. It is important to differentiate between AOM and OME because antibiotics are only useful for AOM.
- Amoxicillin is a drug of choice because of its proven effectiveness in AOM when used in sufficient doses, as well as its excellent safety profile, low cost, good-tasting suspension, and narrow spectrum of activity.
- Bacterial resistance has significantly affected treatment guidelines for AOM (altered binding site of *S. pneumoniae* and beat lactamase production of *H. influenzae* and *M. catarrhalis*).
- Sinusitis is an inflammation and/or infection of the paranasal sinus mucosa.
- Initial management of sinusitis focuses on symptom relief for patients with mild disease lasting less than 10 days. Routine antibiotic use is not recommended for all patients because viral sinusitis is self limiting and bacterial infection often resolves spontaneously. Antibiotic therapy should be reserved for persistent, worsening, or severe cases.
- Amoxicillin is a first-line antibiotic for acute bacterial sinusitis.
- Sinusitis patients that fail treatment with amoxicillin or in patients who have received antibiotic therapy in the previous 4 to 6 weeks, may require improved coverage. Improved coverage of *H. influenzae* and *M. catarrhalis* with either high-dose amoxicillin-clavulanate or a beta-lactamase stable cephalosporin that covers *S. pneumoniae*
- Pharyngitis is an acute throat infection caused by viruses or bacteria.
- Antibiotics should only be used in cases of laboratory confirmed streptococcal pharyngitis associated with clinical symptoms in order to avoid overtreatment.
- Penicillin is the antibiotic of choice because of its narrow spectrum of activity, documented safety and efficacy, and low cost.
- Patients with penicillin allergies require alternative antibiotics for treatment of URTIs and examples include cephalosporins (delayed penicillin-allergic reaction only), macrolides, clindamycin, doxycycline, fluoroquinolones, and trimethoprim-sulfamethoxazole).

REFERENCES

1. Snow V, Mottur-Pilson C, Gonzales R. For the American College of Physicians-American Society of Internal Medicine. Principles of appropriate use for treatment of nonspecific upper respiratory tract infections in adults. *Ann Intern Med.* 2001;134:487-489.
2. Elden LM, Coyte PC. Socioeconomic impact of otitis media in North America. *J Otolaryngol.* 1998;27(suppl 2):9-16.
3. Poole MD. Acute bacterial rhinosinusitis: clinical impact of resistance and susceptibility. *Am J Med.* 2004;117:29S-38S.
4. Gonzales R, Bartlett JG, Besser RE, et al. Principles of appropriate antibiotic use for treatment of nonspecific upper respiratory tract infections in adults: background. *Ann Intern Med.* 2001;134:490-494.
5. American Academy of Pediatrics Subcommittee on Management of Acute Otitis Media. Diagnosis and management of acute otitis media. *Pediatrics.* 2004;113(5):1451-1465.
6. Kaleida PH, Casselbrant ML, Rockette HE, et al. Amoxicillin or myringotomy or both for acute otitis media: results of a randomized controlled trial. *Pediatrics.* 1991;87(4):466-474.
7. Hickner JM, Bartlett JG, Besser RE, et al. Principles of appropriate antibiotic use for acute rhinosinusitis in adults: background. *Ann Inter Med.* 2001;134:498-505.
8. Piccirillo JF. Acute bacterial sinusitis. *N Engl J Med.* 2004;351:902-910.
9. American Academy of Pediatrics. Clinical practice guidelines: management of sinusitis. *Pediatrics.* 2001;108:798-808.

10. Scheid DC, Hamm RM. Acute bacterial sinusitis in adults: Part II. Treatment. *Am Fam Phys*. 2004;70:16997-1704.
11. Lacroix JS, Ricchetti A, Lew D, et al. Symptoms and clinical and radiological signs predicting the presence of pathogenic bacteria in acute rhinosinusitis. *Acta Otolaryngol*. 2002;122(2):192-196.
12. Ioannidis JPA, Lau J. Technical report: evidence for the diagnosis and treatment of acute uncomplicated sinusitis in children: a systematic overview. *Pediatrics*. 2001;108(3):e57.
13. Sinus and Allergy Health Partnership. Antimicrobial treatment guidelines for acute bacterial rhinosinusitis. *Otolaryngol Head Neck Surg*. 2004;130(suppl 1):S1-S45.
14. Sande MA, Gwaltney JM. Acute community-acquired bacterial sinusitis: continuing challenges and current management. *Clin Infect Dis*. 2004;39:S151-S158.
15. Linder JA, Bates DW, Lee GM, Finkelstein JA. Antibiotic treatment of children with sore throat. *JAMA*. 2005;294(18):2315-2322.
16. Linder JA, Stafford RS. Antibiotic treatment of adults with sore throat by community primary care physicians: a national survey, 1989-1999. *JAMA*. 2001;286(10):1181-1186.
17. Shulman ST. Acute streptococcal pharyngitis in pediatric medicine. *Pediatr Drugs*. 2003;5(suppl 1):13-23.
18. Bisno AL, Gerber MA, Gwaltney JM, et al. Practice guidelines for the diagnosis and management of group A streptococcal pharyngitis. *Clin Infect Dis*. 2002;35:113-125.
19. McIsaac WJ, Kellner JD, Aufricht P, et al. Empirical validation of guidelines for the management of pharyngitis in children and adults. *JAMA*. 2004;291:1587-1595.
20. Casey JR, Pichichero ME. Meta-analysis of cephalosporin versus penicillin treatment of group A streptococcal tonsillopharyngitis in children. *Pediatrics*. 2004;113(4):866-882.
21. Casey JR, Pichichero ME. Meta-analysis of cephalosporins versus penicillin for treatment of group A streptococcal tonsillopharyngitis in adults. *Clin Infect Dis*. 2004;38(11):1526-1534.

CHAPTER

21 Lower Respiratory Tract Infections

S. Scott Sutton and John A. Bosso

FOUNDATION OVERVIEW

Respiratory tract infections are a major cause of morbidity and mortality in the United States and represent a common reason for which patients seek medical care. The most common infections involving the lower respiratory tract are bronchitis, bronchiolitis, and pneumonia. Lower respiratory tract infections (LRTIs) in children and adults commonly result from viral or bacterial invasion of lung parenchyma. Viral infections are diagnosed by the recognition of characteristic constellation of clinical signs and symptoms. Treatment of viral LRTI consists largely of supportive care measures. Bacterial LRTIs (in particular bacterial pneumonia) requires expedient, effective, and specific antimicrobial therapy. An appropriate treatment regimen for the patient with a LRTI can be established with the aid of a thorough medical history, physical examination, chest radiograph, knowledge of common bacterial pathogens, and results of properly collected cultures. This chapter will focus on pneumonia; see the special considerations section of this chapter for information on bronchitis and bronchiolitis.

Pneumonia

Pneumonia is inflammation of the lung with consolidation and is the most common infectious cause of death in the United States.[1] Approximately three million cases are diagnosed annually at a cost of more than $20 billion to the health care system. Pneumonia occurs throughout the year and in persons of all ages; however the most severe pneumonia cases are in the very young, the elderly, and the chronically ill. The main classifications of pneumonia are: community-acquired, hospital-acquired (including aspiration), and health care-associated (the term health care-associated pneumonia, as used in this chapter, includes hospital-acquired pneumonia [HAP], ventilator-associated pneumonia [VAP] and other health care-associated pneumonia [HCAP]).

The etiology of bacterial pneumonia varies in accordance with the type of pneumonia. Table 21-1 lists common bacterial pathogens associated with the various classifications of pneumonia.[2-4] Viruses are a common cause of community-acquired pneumonia in adults (often coinfecting with bacteria), and in children (65%). Viral pneumonia in children is frequently caused by respiratory syncytial, influenza or parainfluenza virus.

Pathophysiology

Microorganisms gain access to the lower respiratory tract by three routes.[5] Organisms may enter the lung via:

1. Inhalation of aerosolized particles.
2. The bloodstream from an extrapulmonary site of infection.
3. Aspiration of oropharyngeal secretions. Microaspiration is the major mechanism by which pulmonary pathogens gain access to the normally sterile lungs.

When pulmonary defense mechanisms are functioning optimally, aspirated microorganisms are cleared from the region before infection can become established. Local host defenses of the upper and lower respiratory tract and anatomy of the airway are important in preventing pneumonia. Upper respiratory tract defenses include: mucociliary apparatus of the nasopharynx, nasal hair, normal bacterial flora, IgA antibodies, and complement. Lower respiratory tract defenses include: cough, mucociliary apparatus of the trachea and bronchi, antibodies (IgA, IgM, and IgG), complement, and alveolar macrophages. If microorganisms are not contained/eliminated by host defenses, the pathogen(s) may descend to the alveolar sacs of the lung and infection may ensue.

Microaspiration of oropharyngeal secretion occurs in all people, usually during sleep; however, the normal defense mechanisms described above prevent colonization or infection of the lower respiratory tract in the normal host. This same process may lead to pneumonia in the vulnerable host. A major aspiration of the oropharyngeal or gastric contents may lead to pneumonia or chemical (acid) pneumonitis in the hospitalized and/or compromised host. Dysphagia is a common risk factor for the development of aspiration pneumonia. Dysphagia can be caused by stroke or other neurologic disorders, seizures, or alcoholism. Other factors that may lead or predispose to aspiration pneumonia are: (1) oropharyngeal colonization altered by oral/dental disease; (2) poor oral hygiene; (3) tube feedings; or (4) medications. These factors as well as hospitalization itself may result in colonization of the nasopharynx with organisms from the hospital environment which often exhibit a higher degree of antimicrobial resistance than the usual normal flora. Other risk factors for the development of health care-associated pneumonia include intubation/mechanical ventilation and aspiration.

TABLE 21-1 **Common Bacterial Pathogens by Type of Pneumonia**

Type of Pneumonia	Common Bacterial Pathogens
Community	Typical pathogens *Streptococcus pneumoniae* *Haemophilus influenzae* *Moraxella catarrhalis*
	Atypical pthogens *Mycoplasma pneumoniae* *Chlamydia pneumoniae* *Legionella pneumophila*
Aspiration	Anaerobes[a] *Streptococcus species*
Health care associated (VAP, HAP, HCAP)[b]	Early onset *Streptococcus pneumoniae* *Haemophilus influenzae* *Moraxella catarrhalis*
	Methicillin-susceptible *Staphylococcus aureus* Enterics (ie, *Klebsiella pneumonia, Escherichia coli, Enterobacter* species, *Proteus* species, *Serratia marcescens*)
	Late onset Early onset pathogens plus Multidrug resistant pathogens[c] *Legionella pneumophila*

[a]Anaerobes—*Bacteroides* species, *Fusobacterium* species, and anaerobic gram-positive cocci (eg, *Peptostreptococcus*).

[b]VAP, ventilator-acquired pneumonia; HAP, hospital-acquired pneumonia; HCAP, health care-associated pneumonia.

[c]Multidrug resistant pathogens—*Pseudomonas aeruginosa*, extended spectrum beta-lactamase (ESBL) *Klebsiella pneumoniae, Acinetobacter* species, Methicillin-resistant *Staphylococcus aureus.*

Once breakdown of the local host defenses occurs and organisms invade the lung tissue, an inflammatory response is generated either by the exotoxins produced by the organism or by the immune response to the presence of the organisms. This inflammatory response can remain localized in the lung (and potentially cause tissue damage) or become systemic.

Clinical Presentation

Clinical symptoms associated with pneumonia are both respiratory and nonrespiratory. With increasing age, both respiratory and nonrespiratory symptoms decrease in frequency. Symptoms of pneumonia include:

1. Respiratory: cough (productive or nonproductive), shortness of breath, difficulty breathing
2. Nonrespiratory: fever, fatigue, sweats, headache, myalgias, mental status changes

Signs of pneumonia include:

1. Fever. Temperature may increase or decrease from baseline, but most often is elevated.
2. Respiratory rate is increased. Cyanosis, increased respiratory rate, and use of accessory muscles of respiration are suggestive of severe respiratory compromise.
3. Breath sounds may be diminished.
4. Confusion, lethargy, and disorientation are common in elderly patients.

Scoring systems are available for assessing the severity/mortality of the pneumonia and are used to determine not only severity, but site of care (inpatient or outpatient), and treatment. Examples of the scoring systems include the Pneumonia Severity Index (PSI); Confusion, Urea, Respiratory Rate, and Blood Pressure (CURB); and CURB-65 (those 65 years of age and older).

Diagnosis

Key parameters for the diagnosis of pneumonia include the clinical presentation, diagnostic tests, laboratory tests, and microbiology tests.[3] Key diagnostic tests for pneumonia include: chest x-ray, oxygen saturation, and arterial blood gases. In addition to a constellation of suggestive clinical features, a demonstrable infiltrate by chest radiograph or other imaging technique is required for the diagnosis of pneumonia. The chest x-ray would reveal single or multiple infiltrates in a patient with pneumonia. Oxygen saturation and arterial blood gases would be obtained to evaluate gas exchange in select patients. Laboratory tests obtained to aid in the diagnosis or treatment of patients with pneumonia include: the white blood cell (WBC) count and basic metabolic panel (BMP). Serum creatinine (SCr) is obtained from the basic metabolic panel and needed to dose many antibiotics appropriately. Microbiologic tests that may be utilized in patients with pneumonia include:

1. *Gram stain of respiratory secretions.*[3,6] A sputum gram stain should demonstrate the presence of WBCs and few squamous epithelial cells. It will also reveal if the bacteria are gram-positive or gram-negative and the morphology (eg, cocci or bacilli). For patients with severe pneumonia, bronchoscopy may be performed to obtain tracheal secretions. Tracheal secretions are better culture specimens compared to sputum cultures because they lack oral contamination.
2. *Culture and susceptibility (C&S) tests.*[3,6] C&S tests (sputum and/or blood cultures) may reveal the genera and species of the bacteria and the degree of susceptibility of the bacteria to antimicrobials (susceptible/intermediate/resistant) and, in some institutions, the minimum inhibitory concentration (MIC). C&S reports are not routinely ordered for outpatient pneumonia cases.
3. Serology (IgM and IgG) is useful in determining the presence of atypical pathogens such as *Mycoplasma* and *Chlamydia.*[3]
4. Urinary direct fluorescence antigen is used to diagnose *Legionella pneumophila.*

Health care-associated pneumonia is divided into two subsets, early and late onset. The major difference in early and late onset is time of onset/diagnosis (<5 days vs ≥5 days since admission to hospital). Those with late onset HCAP are at risk for infection with multidrug resistant (MDR) organisms (Figure 21-1) for a host of reasons.[4] Patients with early onset HCAP are usually infected with organisms common to community-acquired pneumonia.

PREVENTION

Prevention of some cases of pneumonia is possible though the use of vaccines and infection control/prevention measures. A polyvalent polysaccharide vaccine is available for one of the leading causes of bacterial pneumonia, *Streptococcus pneumoniae*.[3,7] Influenza vaccine is also effective in preventing pneumonia and should be offered to persons at hospital discharge or during outpatient treatment during the fall and winter.[3,8] Smoking cessation should be a goal as smoking is associated with a substantial risk of pneumococcal bacteremia. Respiratory hygiene measures, including the use of hand hygiene and masks or tissues for patients with cough, should be used in outpatient settings and emergency departments as a means to reduce the spread of respiratory infections. There are also recommendations for preventing health care-associated pneumonia (infection control measures, patients should be kept in semirecumbent position, and enteral nutrition is preferred over parenteral).[4]

TREATMENT

The goal of antimicrobial treatment is to eliminate the patient's symptoms, minimize or prevent complications, and decrease mortality.[2-4] Treatment of bacterial pneumonia involves the empirical use of a relatively broad-spectrum antimicrobial(s) that is effective against probable pathogens. Antimicrobials exhibiting activity against the suspected pathogens without having activity against nontargeted pathogens is preferred. Table 21-1 lists the common bacterial pathogens associated with the different classifications of pneumonia.[2-4] Numerous antimicrobials are available, and the majority are effective in the treatment of bacterial pneumonia. Superiority of one antibiotic over another when both demonstrate similar in vitro activity and tissue distribution characteristics is difficult to define.

The response and outcome of patients with pneumonia depend on the microbial agent involved and the patient status at presentation. Poor prognostic factors include age greater than 65 years; coexisting disease such as diabetes, renal failure, heart failure, or chronic obstructive pulmonary disease (COPD); multiple lobes involved; bacteremia; alcoholism; and neutropenia.[3-4] Most patients with pneumonia improve clinically (decreased temperature and systemic symptoms) 24 to 48 hours after the initiation of effective antibiotic therapy. Chest radiograph resolution lags, taking up to 3 weeks in healthy young adults and 12 weeks in elderly patients and those with complicated infections. Tables 21-2 and 21-3 list recommended empiric treatment options for community-acquired and health care-associated pneumonia. Once the etiology of the pneumonia has been identified on the basis of reliable microbiological methods, antimicrobial therapy should be directed at the pathogen. Antimicrobial treatment of aspiration pneumonia consists of: amoxicillin/clavulanate or clindamycin. Table 21-4 lists key parameters for antimicrobials recommended for treatment of pneumonia.

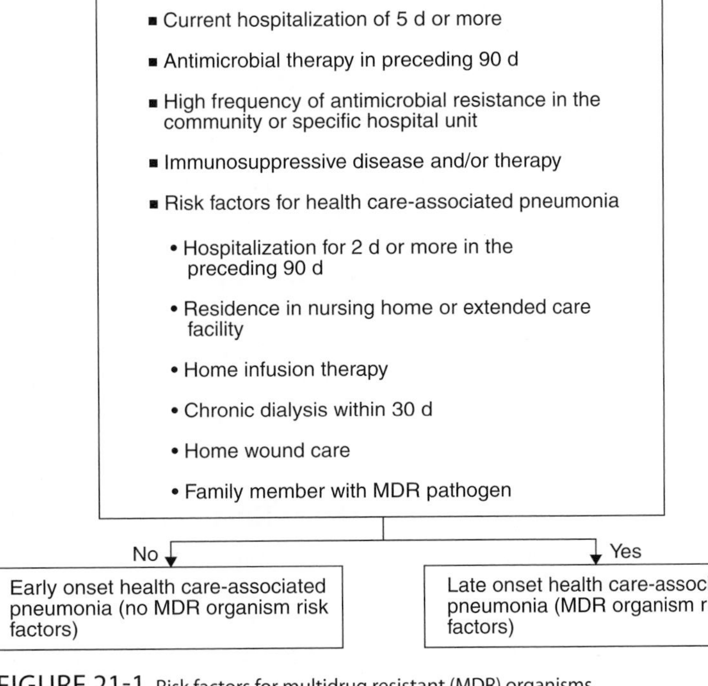

FIGURE 21-1 Risk factors for multidrug resistant (MDR) organisms.

TABLE 21-2 **Empiric Treatment Recommendations for Community-Acquired Pneumonia**

Outpatient Treatment

1. Previously healthy and no use of antimicrobials within the previous 3 mo
   - A macrolide (clarithromycin, azithromycin) *or*
   - Doxycycline

   or
2. Presence of comorbidities (chronic heart, lung, liver, or renal disease; diabetes; alcoholism; malignancy; asplenia; immunosuppressive disease or drug; antimicrobial use within previous 3 mo)
   - Respiratory fluoroquinolone (moxifloxacin, levofloxacin, gemifloxacin) or
   - Beta lactam (high dose amoxicillin 1 g 3 times daily; amoxicillin/clavulanate 2 g 2 times daily; cefpodoxime, cefuroxime) plus a macrolide

   or
3. In regions with high rates of macrolide-resistant *Streptococcus pneumoniae*, consider use of alternative agents listed above (2) for patients previously healthy

Inpatient Treatment (non-Intensive Care Unit)

1. Respiratory fluoroquinolone

   or
2. Beta lactam (ceftriaxone, cefotaxime, ampicillin, ertapenem) plus a macrolide

Inpatient Treatment (Intensive Care Unit Treatment)

1. Beta lactam (ceftriaxone, cefotaxime, ampicillin/sulbactam) plus azithromycin

   or
2. Respiratory fluoroquinolone

Special Concerns

1. *Pseudomonas aeruginosa* is a consideration
   - Antipseudomonal beta lactam (piperacillin/tazobactam, cefepime, imipenem, meropenem, doripenem) plus antipseudomonal fluoroquinolone (ciprofloxacin, levofloxacin)
   - Antipseudomonal beta lactam plus aminoglycoside plus azithromycin
   - Antipseudomonal beta lactam plus aminoglycoside plus respiratory fluoroquinolone

   or
2. Methicillin-resistant *Staphylococcus aureus* (MRSA) is a concern
   - Vancomycin
   - Linezolid

SPECIAL CONSIDERATIONS

Duration of Treatment

The duration of therapy for pneumonia should be kept as short as possible and depends on several factors: type of pneumonia, inpatient or outpatient status, patient comorbidities, bacteremia/sepsis, and the antibiotic chosen. Patients with community-acquired pneumonia (CAP) and aspiration pneumonia should be treated for a minimum of 5 days (range 5-10 days). Antimicrobials indicated for 5 days of treatment include levofloxacin and azithromycin, the duration for all other agents is 7 to 10 days. Patients should be afebrile for 48 to 72 hours and should have no more than one CAP-associated sign of clinical stability (Table 21-5) before discontinuation of treatment. A longer duration of therapy may be needed if initial therapy was not active against the identified pathogen or if it was complicated by extrapulmonary infection (meningitis or endocarditis). Patients with health care-associated pneumonia should be treated for 8 to 21 days, depending on severity of the disease and response to therapy.

TABLE 21-3 **Empiric Treatment Recommendations for Health Care-Associated Pneumonia**

Early Onset

- Ceftriaxone *or*
- Levofloxacin or moxifloxacin *or*
- Ampicillin/Sulbactam *or*
- Ertapenem

Late Onset (combination of three antimicrobials for initial empiric therapy)[a]

- Antipseudomonal beta lactam (piperacillin/tazobactam, cefepime, ceftazidime, imipenem, meropenem, or doripenem) *plus*
- Antipseudomonal fluoroquinolone (ciprofloxacin or levofloxacin) *or*
- Aminoglycoside (amikacin, gentamicin, tobramycin) *plus*
- Vancomycin or linezolid

[a]If *Legionella pneumophila* is suspected, the combination antimicrobial regimen should include a macrolide (eg, azithromycin) or a fluoroquinolone (ciprofloxacin or levofloxacin) should be used rather than an aminoglycoside.

Health Care-Associated Pneumonia

When feasible, a lower respiratory tract culture needs to be collected from all patients before antibiotic therapy for health care-associated pneumonia, but collection of cultures should not delay the initiation of therapy. Negative lower respiratory tract cultures for 72 hours can be used to stop antibiotic therapy. Early, appropriate, broad-spectrum antimicrobial therapy should be prescribed with adequate doses to optimize therapy.

Antibiotic Resistance Issues

Resistance to commonly used antibiotics for pneumonia presents a major consideration in choosing empirical therapy. Resistance patterns vary by geography. Therefore, antibiotic recommendations must be modified on the basis of local susceptibility patterns.

Drug-Resistant *Streptococcus pneumonia*

The emergence of drug-resistant *Streptococcus pneumonia* (DRSP) is well documented but the clinical significance is uncertain. Few well controlled studies have evaluated the impact of in vitro resistance on clinical outcomes of pneumonia caused by DRSP. Current levels of beta-lactam

TABLE 21-4 **Antimicrobials Recommended for Treatment of Pneumonia**

Antibiotic	Indication[a]	Route of Administration (RA); Formulation (F); Dose (D)[b]	Mechanism of Action	Side Effects (SE) and Contraindications (CI)	Excretion (E); Drug Interactions (DI); General Information (GI)
Clarithromycin (Biaxin)	CAP	RA: Oral F: Suspension, tablets, extended release tablets D: 250-500 mg every 12 h; 1000 mg every 24 h (XL)	Inhibits protein synthesis	SE: Headache, rash, abnormal taste, gastrointestinal, *C. diff* CI: Hypersensitivity to macrolide	E: H & R DI: P450 substrate: 3A4 (major); P450 inhibitor: 3A4 (strong), 1A2 (weak) GI: Pregnancy category C.
Azithromycin (Zithromax; Z-pac)	CAP	RA: Oral, IV F: Injection, suspension, tablet D: 250-500 mg every 24 h	Inhibits protein synthesis	SE: Headache, rash, gastrointestinal, *C. diff* CI: Hypersensitivity to macrolide	E: H; use with caution in patients with preexisting liver disease DI: P450 substrate: 3A4 (minor), P450 inhibitor: 3A4 (weak) GI: Pregnancy category B
Doxycycline (Vibramycin and others)	CAP	RA: Oral, IV F: Capsule, tablet, suspension, syrup, injection D: 100 mg every 12 h	Inhibits protein synthesis	SE: Rash (photosensitivity), GI, *C. diff*, BMS (rare), hepatotoxicity (rare), autoimmune disease reported CI: Hypersensitivity to doxycycline/tetracyclines, children ≤ 8 years of age	E: R and feces DI: P450 inhibitor 3A4 (moderate), levels decreased by cations GI: Pregnancy category D
Amoxicillin (Amoxil)	CAP	RA: Oral F: Capsule, tablet, suspension D: 500 mg every 8 h or 875 every 12 h (1000 mg every 8 h for DRSP)	Inhibits bacterial cell wall synthesis	SE: Rash, GI, *C. diff*, BMS (rare), allergic reaction (immediate—anaphylaxis or delayed—rash) CI: Hypersensitivity to amoxicillin or penicillin compounds	E: R (dose reductions required for renal dysfunction) GI: Pregnancy category B; high percentage of patients with infectious mononucleosis develop rash on amoxicillin.
Ampicillin (Principen and others)	CAP	RA: Oral, IV F: Capsule, suspension, injection D: 2 g IV every 6 h	Inhibits bacterial cell wall synthesis	SE: Rash, GI, *C. diff*, BMS (rare), allergic reaction (immediate—anaphylaxis or delayed—rash) CI: Hypersensitivity to amoxicillin or penicillin compounds	E: R (dose reductions required for renal dysfunction) GI: Pregnancy category B; high percentage of patients with infectious mononucleosis develop rash on ampicillin
Amoxicillin/Clavulanate (Augmentin)	CAP; aspiration	RA: Oral F: Suspension, tablet, XR tablet D: 500 mg every 8 h, 875 mg every 12 h, 2000 mg every 12 h	Inhibits bacterial cell wall synthesis; addition of clavulanate extends coverage of amoxicillin to include beta-lactamase producing bacteria[c]	SE: Rash, GI, *C. diff*, BMS (rare), allergic reaction (immediate—anaphylaxis or delayed—rash) CI: Hypersensitivity to amoxicillin or penicillin compounds	E: R (dose reductions required for renal dysfunction) GI: Pregnancy category B; high percentage of patients with infectious mononucleosis develop rash on amoxicillin/clavulanate
Ampicillin/Sulbactam (Unasyn)	CAP	RA: IV F: Injection D: 1.5-3 g every 6 h	Inhibits bacterial cell wall synthesis; addition of sulbactam extends coverage of ampicillin to include beta lactamase- producing bacteria[c]	SE: Rash, GI, *C. diff*, BMS (rare), allergic reaction (immediate—anaphylaxis or delayed—rash) CI: Hypersensitivity to ampicillin or penicillin compounds	E: R (dose reductions required for renal dysfunction) GI: Pregnancy category B; high percentage of patients with infectious mononucleosis develop rash on ampicillin/sulbactam
Piperacillin/Tazobactam (Zosyn)	HCAP	RA: IV F: Injection D: 3.375-4.5 g every 4-6 h	Inhibits bacterial cell wall synthesis; addition of tazobactam extends coverage of piperacillin to include beta lactamase- producing bacteria[c]	SE: Rash, GI, *C. diff*, BMS (rare), allergic reaction (immediate—anaphylaxis or delayed—rash) CI: Hypersensitivity to piperacillin or penicillin compounds	E: R (dose reductions required for renal dysfunction) GI: Pregnancy category B; high percentage of patients with infectious mono-nucleosis develop rash on piperacillin; bleeding

(Continued)

TABLE 21-4 **Antimicrobials Recommended for Treatment of Pneumonia (*Continued*)**

Antibiotic	Indication[a]	Route of Administration (RA); Formulation (F); Dose (D)[b]	Mechanism of Action	Side Effects (SE) and Contraindications (CI)	Excretion (E); Drug Interactions (DI); General Information (GI)
					disorders have been observed, particularly in patients with renal dysfunction, discontinue if thrombocytopenia or bleeding occurs; 4.5 g injection contains 11.17 mEq of sodium, 3.375 g contains 8.38 mEq of sodium
Cefpodoxime (Vantin)	CAP	RA: Oral F: Suspension, tablet D: 200 mg every 12 h	Inhibits bacterial cell wall synthesis	SE: Rash, GI, *C. diff*, BMS (rare), allergic reaction (immediate—anaphylaxis or delayed—rash) CI: Hypersensitivity to cefpodoxime or cephalosporin compounds; if allergic to penicillin: delayed reaction (rash) 8%-10% chance of cross reactions, immediate reaction (anaphylaxis) do not use	E: R (dose reductions required for renal dysfunction); GI: Pregnancy category B
Cefuroxime (Ceftin and others)	CAP	RA: Oral, IV F: Tablet, suspension, injection D: 500 mg every 12 h (po), 750 mg every 8 h (IV)	Inhibits bacterial cell wall synthesis	SE: Rash, GI, *C. diff*, BMS (rare), allergic reaction (immediate—anaphylaxis or delayed—rash) CI: Hypersensitivity to cefuroxime or cephalosporin compounds; if allergic to penicillin: delayed reaction (rash) 8%-10% chance of cross reactions, immediate reaction (anaphylaxis) do not use	E: R (dose reductions required for renal dysfunction) GI: Pregnancy category B; cefuroxime axetil film coated tablets and oral suspension are not bioequivalent and are not substitutable on a mg/mg basis
Ceftriaxone (Rocephin)	CAP	RA: IV F: Injection D: 1-2 g daily	Inhibits bacterial cell wall synthesis	SE: Rash, GI, *C. diff*, BMS (rare), allergic reaction (immediate—anaphylaxis or delayed—rash) CI: Hypersensitivity to ceftriaxone or cephalosporin compounds; if allergic to penicillin: delayed reaction (rash) 8%-10% chance of cross reactions, immediate reaction (anaphylaxis) do not use	E: R (dose reductions *not* required for renal dysfunction), feces GI: Pregnancy category B; do not use in hyperbilirubinemic neonates and concomitant use with calcium containing solutions/products in neonates
Cefotaxime (Claforan)	CAP	RA: IV F: Injection D: 1-2 g every 8 h	Inhibits bacterial cell wall synthesis	SE: Rash, GI, *C. diff*, BMS (rare), allergic reaction (immediate—anaphylaxis or delayed—rash) CI: Hypersensitivity to cefotaxime or cephalosporin compounds; if allergic to penicillin: delayed reaction (rash) 8%-10% chance of cross reactions, immediate reaction (anaphylaxis) do not use	E: R (dose reductions required for renal dysfunction) GI: Pregnancy category B

(*Continued*)

TABLE 21-4 **Antimicrobials Recommended for Treatment of Pneumonia (*Continued*)**

Antibiotic	Indication[a]	Route of Administration (RA); Formulation (F); Dose (D)[b]	Mechanism of Action	Side Effects (SE) and Contraindications (CI)	Excretion (E); Drug Interactions (DI); General Information (GI)
Cefepime (Maxipime)	HCAP	RA: Injection F: IV D: 1-2 g every 8-12 h	Inhibits bacterial cell wall synthesis	SE: Rash, GI, *C. diff*, BMS (rare), allergic reaction (immediate—anaphylaxis or delayed—rash); CI: Hypersensitivity to cefepime or cephalosporin compounds; if allergic to penicillin: delayed reaction (rash) 8%-10% chance of cross reactions, immediate reaction (anaphylaxis) do not use	E: R (dose reductions required for renal dysfunction) GI: Pregnancy category B; may be used for CAP, however since cefepime has activity against *Pseudomonas aeruginosa*, it should be reserved for HCAP, use ceftriaxone or cefotaxime for CAP
Ertapenem (Invanz)	CAP	RA: Injection F: IV D: 1 g daily	Inhibits bacterial cell wall synthesis	SE: Headache, Rash, GI, *C. diff*, BMS (rare), allergic reaction (immediate—anaphylaxis or delayed—rash) CI: Hypersensitivity to ertapenem or carbapenem compounds; if allergic to penicillin: may have a cross reactions	E: R, feces (dose reduction required for renal dysfunction) GI: Pregnancy category B
Imipenem (Primaxin)	HCAP	RA: Injection F: IV D: 500-1000 mg every 6 h	Inhibits bacterial cell wall synthesis	SE: Headache, seizure, rash, GI, *C. diff*, BMS (rare), allergic reaction (immediate—anaphylaxis or delayed—rash) CI: Hypersensitivity to imipenem or carbapenem compounds; if allergic to penicillin: may have a cross reaction	E: R (dose reduction required for renal dysfunction) GI: Pregnancy category C; has been associated with seizures—use with caution in patients with history of seizures
Meropenem (Merrem)	HCAP	RA: Injection F: IV D: 1-2 g every 8 h	Inhibits bacterial cell wall synthesis	SE: Headache, rash, GI, *C. diff*, BMS (rare), allergic reaction (immediate—anaphylaxis or delayed—rash) CI: Hypersensitivity to meropenem or carbapenem compounds; if allergic to penicillin: may have a cross reaction	E: R (dose reduction required for renal dysfunction) GI: Pregnancy category B
Doripenem (Doribax)	HCAP	RA: Injection F: IV D: 500 mg every 8 h	Inhibits bacterial cell wall synthesis	SE: Headache, rash, GI, *C.diff*, BMS (rare), allergic reaction (immediate—anaphylaxis or delayed—rash) CI: Hypersensitivity to doripenem or carbapenem compounds; if allergic to penicillin: may have a cross reaction	E: R (dose reduction required for renal dysfunction) GI: Pregnancy category B; administration is over 1 h (most antimicrobials are administered over 30 min, except for highly resistant bacteria, see Chapter 19); HCAP use is unlabeled/investigational at time of writing
Levofloxacin (Levaquin)	CAP ; HCAP	RA: Oral, injection F: Solution, tablet, IV D: 500-750 mg daily	Inhibits DNA gyrase; inhibits relaxation of supercoiled DNA and promotes breakage of DNA strands	SE: Headache, confusion, mental status changes, GI, *C. diff*, BMS (rare), allergic reaction (immediate or delayed), glucose (hypo or hyperglycemia), photosensitivity	E: R (dose reduction required for renal dysfunction) DI: QTc prolonging agents, cations, rare cases of torsade de pointes reported (use caution in patients with known prolongation of QT interval,

(*Continued*)

TABLE 21-4 **Antimicrobials Recommended for Treatment of Pneumonia (*Continued*)**

Antibiotic	Indication[a]	Route of Administration (RA); Formulation (F); Dose (D)[b]	Mechanism of Action	Side Effects (SE) and Contraindications (CI)	Excretion (E); Drug Interactions (DI); General Information (GI)
				CI: Hypersensitivity to levofloxacin or other quinolones	bradycardia, hypokalemia, hypomagnesemia, or receiving Class 1a or Class III antiarrhythmics GI: Pregnancy category C; black box warning: reports of tendon inflammation and rupture (Achilles tendon); fluoroquinolones have been associated with the development of serious (sometimes fatal), hypoglycemia
Ciprofloxacin (Cipro)	HCAP	RA: Oral, injection F: Suspension, tablet, IV D: Oral: 500-750 mg every 12 h, IV: 400 mg every 8-12 h	Inhibits DNA gyrase; inhibits relaxation of supercoiled DNA and promotes breakage of DNA strands	SE: Headache, confusion, mental status changes, GI, *C. diff*, BMS (rare), allergic reaction (immediate or delayed), glucose (hypo- or hyperglycemia), photosensitivity CI: Hypersensitivity to ciprofloxacin or other quinolones	E: R, feces (dose reduction required for renal dysfunction) DI: Inhibits CYP-450 1A2 (strong) and 3A4 (weak), QTc prolonging agents, cations, theophylline, rare cases of torsade de pointes reported (use caution in patients with known prolongation of QT interval, bradycardia, hypokalemia, hypomagnesemia, or receiving Class 1a or Class III antiarrhythmics; GI: Pregnancy category C; black box warning: reports of tendon inflammation and rupture (Achilles tendon); fluoroquinolones have been associated with the development of serious (sometimes fatal), hypoglycemia
Moxifloxacin (Avelox)	CAP	RA: Oral, injection F: Tablet, IV	Inhibits DNA gyrase; inhibits relaxation of supercoiled DNA and promotes breakage of DNA strands	SE: Headache, confusion, mental status changes, GI, *C. diff*, BMS (rare), allergic reaction (immediate or delayed), glucose (hypo- or hyperglycemia), photosensitivity CI: Hypersensitivity to moxifloxacin or other quinolones	E: R (20%), H, feces DI: QTc prolonging agents, cations, rare cases of torsade de pointes reported (use caution in patients with known prolongation of QT interval, bradycardia, hypokalemia, hypomagnesemia, or receiving Class 1a or Class III antiarrhythmics GI: Pregnancy category C; black box warning; reports of tendon inflammation and rupture (Achilles tendon); fluoroquinolones have been associated with the development of serious (sometimes fatal), hypoglycemia
Gemifloxacin (Factive)	CAP	RA: Oral F: Tablet	Inhibits DNA gyrase; inhibits relaxation of supercoiled DNA and promotes breakage of DNA strands	SE: Headache, confusion, mental status changes, GI, *C. diff*, BMS (rare), allergic reaction (immediate or delayed), glucose (hypo or hyperglycemia), photosensitivity	E: R (dose reduction required for renal dysfunction) DI: QTc prolonging agents, cations, rare cases of torsade de pointes reported (use caution in patients with known

(*Continued*)

TABLE 21-4 **Antimicrobials Recommended for Treatment of Pneumonia (*Continued*)**

Antibiotic	Indication[a]	Route of Administration (RA); Formulation (F); Dose (D)[b]	Mechanism of Action	Side Effects (SE) and Contraindications (CI)	Excretion (E); Drug Interactions (DI); General Information (GI)
				CI: hypersensitivity to gemifloxacin or other quinolones	prolongation of QT interval, bradycardia, hypokalemia, hypomagnesemia, or receiving Class 1a or Class III antiarrhythmics GI: Pregnancy category C; black box warning; reports of tendon inflammation and rupture (Achilles tendon); fluoroquinolones have been associated with the development of serious (sometimes fatal), hypoglycemia
Gentamicin (Garamycin) and Tobramycin (Tobrex)	HCAP	RA: Injection F: IV D: 1-2.5 mg/kg every 8-12 h (conventional) to produce peak of 8-10 mg/L and trough ≤ 2 mg/L, 4-7 mg/kg every 24, 36, 48 h (extended interval) check random level between 6-14 h to determine dosing interval	Inhibits protein synthesis by binding to 30s and 50s ribosomal subunit	SE: Neurotoxicity (vertigo, ataxia), ototoxicity, nephrotoxicity, rash, BMS (rare), GI, *C. diff* CI: Hypersensitivity to gentamicin, tobramycin or other aminoglycosides	E: R (dose modifications required for renal dysfunction) GI: Pregnancy category D; risk factors for nephrotoxicity: preexisting renal impairment, concomitant nephrotoxic drug, advanced age, dehydration; may cause neuromuscular blockade and respiratory paralysis; dosage individualization is critical because of low therapeutic index, initial and periodic plasma drug levels should be determined, particularly in critically ill patients or in disease states known to significantly alter aminoglycoside pharmacokinetics (cystic fibrosis, burns, or major surgery)
Amikacin (Amikin)	HCAP	RA: Injection F: IV D: 5-7.5 mg/kg every 8 h (conventional), 15-20 mg/kg daily	Inhibits protein synthesis by binding to 30s and 50s ribosomal subunit	SE: Neurotoxicity (vertigo, ataxia), ototoxicity, nephrotoxicity, rash, BMS (rare), GI, *C. diff* CI: Hypersensitivity to amikacin or other aminoglycosides	E: R (dose modifications required for renal dysfunction) GI: Pregnancy category D; risk factors for nephrotoxicity: preexisting renal impairment, concomitant nephrotoxic drug, advanced age, dehydration; may cause neuromuscular blockade and respiratory paralysis; dosage individualization is critical because of low therapeutic index, initial and periodic plasma drug levels should be determined, particularly in critically ill patients or in disease states known to significantly alter aminoglycoside pharmacokinetics (cystic fibrosis, burns, or major surgery)

(*Continued*)

TABLE 21-4 **Antimicrobials Recommended for Treatment of Pneumonia (*Continued*)**

Antibiotic	Indication[a]	Route of Administration (RA); Formulation (F); Dose (D)[b]	Mechanism of Action	Side Effects (SE) and Contraindications (CI)	Excretion (E); Drug Interactions (DI); General Information (GI)
Vancomycin (Vancocin)	HCAP	RA: Oral, injection F: Capsule (treatment of *C. diff* only), IV D: Oral:125-250 mg every 6 h, IV: 1-2 g every 12 h to produce trough of 15-20 mg/L or AUC/MIC ratio ≥ 400	Inhibits bacterial cell wall synthesis	SE: Red-man syndrome (rash), BMS (rare, except with high dose), ototoxicity, nephrotoxicity, increase nephrotoxic potential when combined with aminoglycoside CI: Hypersensitivity to vancomycin	E: R (dose modifications required for renal dysfunction) GI: Pregnancy category C, pharmacokinetics may be altered during pregnancy; dosing in dialysis patients is variable, poorly dialyzable by conventional hemodialysis, increased removal with high flux membranes and continuous renal replacement; Red-man syndrome is not an allergic reaction but is associated with too rapid infusion of the drug
Linezolid (Zyvox)	HCAP	RA: Oral, injection F: Suspension, tablet, IV D: 600 mg every 12 h	Inhibits bacterial protein synthesis by binding to 23s ribosomal RNA of the 50s subunit	SE: Headache, GI, *C. diff*, rash, BMS. BMS (including anemia, leucopenia, pancytopenia, and thrombocytopenia may be more common in patients receiving for > 2 wk CI: Hypersensitivity to linezolid, concurrent use if within 2 wk of monoamine oxidase inhibitors, patients with uncontrolled hypertension, taking sympathomimetics, vasopressive agents, or dopaminergic agents unless closely monitored for increase in blood pressure, patients taking antidepressants with serotonin mechanism, meperidine unless closely monitored for serotonin syndrome	E: R (30% parent drug, 50% inactive metabolites), feces DI: Sympathomimetics, antidepressants with serotonin activity, meperidine, tyramine containing foods (hypertensive crisis) GI: Pregnancy category C; monitoring: weekly complete blood count, particularly in patients at increased risk of bleeding, preexisting myelosuppression, on concomitant medications that cause BMS, those requiring more than 2 wk of therapy
Clindamycin (Cleocin)	Aspiration	RA: Oral, injection F: Capsule, solution, IV D: Oral: 300-450 mg every 6-8 h, IV: 600-900 mg every 8 h	Reversibly binds to 50s ribosomal subunit preventing peptide bond formation thus inhibiting bacterial protein synthesis	SE: Rash, GI, *C. diff*, BMS (rare) CI: Hypersensitivity to clindamycin	E: R (10%), H, feces GI: Pregnancy category B; can cause severe and possibly fatal colitis (*C. diff* infection)

[a]Indication lists the type of pneumonia the antimicrobial is recommended for by treatment guidelines. The antimicrobials listed have other indications besides pneumonia.

[b]Adult dose.

[c]Bacteria (eg, *Staphylococcus*, Enterics: *Klebsiella pneumonia, Escherichia coli, Enterobacter* species, *Proteus* species, Serratia marcescens, and gram-negative anaerobes (*Bacteroides fragilis*).

Abbreviations: AUC, area under the curve; BMS, bone marrow suppression; CAP, community-acquired pneumonia; *C. diff*, *Clostridium difficile*; DRSP, drug resistant *Streptococcus pneumonia;* GI, gastrointestinal; H, hepatic; HCAP, health care-associated pneumonia; MIC, minimum inhibitory concentration; R, renal; P450, CYP-450 system.

resistance do not generally result in CAP treatment failures when appropriate agents (amoxicillin, ceftriaxone, cefotaxime) and doses are used. Available data suggest that clinically relevant level of penicillin resistance is a MIC of at least 4 mg/L. Data exist suggesting that resistance to macrolides, ciprofloxacin, and levofloxacin results in clinical

TABLE 21-5 **Criteria for Clinical Stability**

Criteria for Clinical Stability
Temperature less than or equal to 37.8°C
Heart rate less than or equal to 100 bpm
Respiratory rate less than 24 rpm
Systolic blood pressure greater than or equal to 90 mm Hg
Arterial oxygen saturation ≥ 90% or $PO_2 \geq 60$ mm Hg on room air
Ability to maintain oral intake[a]
Normal mental status[a]

[a] Important for discharge or oral switch decision but not necessarily for determination of nonresponse.

failure. Risk factors for infection with beta-lactam resistant *S. pneumonia* include:

- Age < 2 years or > 65 years
- Beta-lactam therapy within the previous 3 months
- Alcoholism
- Various comorbidities (eg, underlying cardiopulmonary disease)
- Immunosuppressive illness or therapy
- Exposure to a child in a day-care center

DRSP is the reason high-dose amoxicillin (1 g every 8 hours) and amoxicillin/clavulanate XR (2 g every 12 hours) is recommended for CAP treatment (see Table 21-2—outpatient treatment section).

Bronchitis / Bronchiolitis

Bronchitis and bronchiolitis are inflammatory conditions of the large and small elements of the tracheobronchial tree. The inflammatory process does not extend to the alveoli. Bronchitis frequently is classified as acute or chronic. Acute bronchitis occurs in individuals of all ages, whereas chronic bronchitis primarily affects adults. Bronchiolitis is a disease of infancy. Acute bronchitis is a self-limiting viral illness. Treatment is symptomatic and supportive. Chronic bronchitis is most often caused by cigarette smoking and leads to excessive sputum production and a smoker's cough. Patients with chronic bronchitis develop exacerbations (acute exacerbations of chronic bronchitis [AECB]). Treatment of AECB may require treatment with bronchodilators and, for more severe cases, antimicrobials. Antimicrobial treatment of AECB consists of agents that have activity against *S. pneumoniae, Haemophilus influenzae, Moraxella catarrhalis, and M. pneumoniae.* Bronchiolitis is an acute viral infection of the lower respiratory tract that affects children. Respiratory syncytial virus (RSV) is the most common cause. Treatment of bronchiolitis is symptomatic and supportive.

Pediatric Bacterial Pneumonia

Pediatric pneumonia is caused by the same bacterial pathogens that cause adult CAP. Fluoroquinolones and tetracyclines should not be used in children. High-dose amoxicillin, amoxicillin-clavulanate, intramuscular ceftriaxone, azithromycin, and clarithromycin are potential agents for use in children.

CASE Application

1. Select the infection(s) that represents lower respiratory tract infections.
   a. Pneumonia
   b. Sinusitis
   c. Bronchitis
   d. a and c
   e. All of the above

2. Select the cause(s) of lower respiratory tract infections.
   a. Bacteria
   b. Virus
   c. *Streptococcus pneumoniae*
   d. Respiratory syncytial virus
   e. All of the above

3. Select the bacterial pathogen that is a common cause of lower respiratory tract infections.
   a. *Haemophilus influenza*
   b. Influenza
   c. Parainfluenza
   d. b and c
   e. All of the above

4. Select the information that is reported by a gram stain.
   a. Presence of white blood cells or epithelial cells
   b. Morphologic characteristic of bacteria
   c. Genera and species of the bacteria
   d. a and b
   e. All of the above

5. Health care-associated pneumonia is divided up into two subsets, early and late onset. Select the factor that is the major difference in early versus late onset.
   a. Severity of illness
   b. Pneumonia severity index score
   c. Time of onset/diagnosis
   d. All of the above

6. Prevention of pneumonia may be achieved by:
   a. Infection control/prevention measures
   b. *Streptococcus pneumoniae* vaccine
   c. Influenza vaccine
   d. All of the above

7. Select the anti-infective that may be used to treat pediatric community-acquired pneumonia.
   a. Levofloxacin
   b. Doxycycline
   c. Ceftriaxone
   d. All of the above

8. Select the atypical pathogen(s) that is a common cause of community-acquired pneumonia (CAP).
   a. *Mycoplasma pneumoniae*
   b. *Chlamydia pneumoniae*
   c. *Moraxella catarrhalis*
   d. a and b
   e. All of the above

9. Select the multidrug resistant pathogen that may cause late-onset health care-associated pneumonia.
   a. *Pseudomonas aeruginosa*
   b. Extended-spectrum beta-lactamase (ESBL) *Klebsiella pneumoniae*
   c. *Acinetobacter* species
   d. Methicillin-resistant *Staphylococcus aureus* (MRSA)
   e. All of the above

10. Select the risk factor(s) for health care-associated pneumonia.
    a. Hospitalization for 2 days or more in the preceding 90 days
    b. Residence in nursing home or extended-care facility
    c. Home infusion therapy
    d. All of the above

11. Select the antimicrobial that is utilized for community-acquired pneumonia, inhibits protein synthesis, and is a strong inhibitor of the CYP-450 3A4 hepatic enzyme.
    a. Azithromycin
    b. Clarithromycin
    c. Amoxicillin
    d. Cefpodoxime

12. Select the antimicrobial that may be used to treat lower respiratory tract infections in pregnant patients.
    a. Clarithromycin
    b. Azithromycin
    c. Doxycycline
    d. Cefuroxime
    e. b and d

13. Select the antimicrobial that has the same oral and IV dose.
    a. Doxycycline
    b. Amoxicillin/clavulanate
    c. Piperacillin/tazobactam
    d. Ceftriaxone
    e. Ciprofloxacin

14. High-dose amoxicillin (1 g every 8 hours) and amoxicillin/clavulanate *XR* (2 g every 12 hours) are recommended in CAP treatment. The increase in dose of the two antimicrobials is recommended because of bacterial resistance. Select the pathogen that requires an increase in the dose of amoxicillin.
    a. Drug-resistant *Streptococcus pneumoniae* (DRSP)
    b. Methicillin-resistant *Staphylococcus aureus* (MRSA)
    c. Extended-spectrum beta-lactamase (ESBL) *Klebsiella pneumoniae*
    d. All of the above

15. Select the antimicrobial(s) that is associated with the side effect of photosensitivity.
    a. Doxycycline
    b. Ciprofloxacin
    c. Cefepime
    d. a and b
    e. All of the above

16. Select the antimicrobials that are often associated with a *Clostridium difficile* infection.
    a. Ciprofloxacin
    b. Clindamycin
    c. Cefotaxime
    d. All of the above

17. Select the side effect that a high percentage of patients with infectious mononucleosis develop when they receive penicillin antimicrobials (amoxicillin, ampicillin, or piperacillin).
    a. Bone marrow suppression (BMS)
    b. Rash
    c. *Clostridium difficile*
    d. Thrombocytopenia

18. Select the antimicrobial that a patient with a delayed allergic hypersensitivity reaction to ampicillin/sulbactam may receive.
    a. Ceftriaxone
    b. Moxifloxacin
    c. Piperacillin/tazobactam
    d. a and b
    e. All of the above

19. Select the penicillin antimicrobial that is combined with a beta-lactamase inhibitor.
    a. Zosyn
    b. Unasyn
    c. Augmentin
    d. All of the above

20. The addition of the beta-lactamase inhibitor sulbactam to ampicillin is done to:
    a. Increase bacterial coverage
    b. Decrease side effects
    c. Improve bioavailability
    d. All of the above

21. Select the salt formation of piperacillin/tazobactam.
    a. Potassium
    b. Hydrochloride
    c. Sodium
    d. All of the above

22. Select the beta-lactam antimicrobial that *does not require* dose or interval reductions in patients with renal dysfunction.
    a. Amoxicillin
    b. Azithromycin
    c. Ceftriaxone

d. Moxifloxacin
e. Cefepime

23. Select the side effect(s) associated with fluoroquinolone antimicrobials.

a. Hypoglycemia
b. *Clostridium difficile* infection
c. Confusion in the elderly
d. QTc prolongation
e. All of the above

24. Aminoglycoside antimicrobials may be dosed via conventional (1-2.5 mg/kg every 8-12 hours) or extended interval (4-7 mg/kg every 24,36, or 48 hours) methods. Select the therapeutic drug monitoring parameter(s) associated with conventional dosing of aminoglycosides.

a. Peak (C_{max}) 8 to 12 μg/mL for serious infections
b. Trough (C_{min}) less than 2 mg/L
c. Random level (between 6-14 hours) of 5 mg/L
d. a and b
e. All of the above

25. Select the brand name of ceftazidime.

a. Zyvox
b. Rocephin
c. Avelox
d. Fortaz
e. Vibramycin

TAKEAWAY POINTS ››

- The most common infections involving the lower respiratory tract are bronchitis, bronchiolitis, and pneumonia.
- The main classifications of pneumonia are: community-acquired and health care-associated (including aspiration pneumonia).
- The etiology of bacterial pneumonia varies in accordance with the type of pneumonia.
- Viruses are a common cause of pneumonia in adults and children (65%).
- Clinical symptoms associated with pneumonia include respiratory and nonrespiratory.
- Key parameters for the diagnosis of pneumonia include the clinical presentation, diagnostic tests, laboratory tests, and microbiology tests.
- Health care-associated pneumonia is divided into two subsets, early and late onset. The major difference in early and late onset is the time of onset after hospitalization.
- Prevention of some cases of pneumonia is possible through the use of vaccines and infection control/prevention measures.
- Treatment of bacterial pneumonia involves the empirical use of a relatively broad spectrum antimicrobial(s) that is effective against probable pathogens. Antimicrobials exhibiting activity against the suspected pathogens without having activity against nontargeted pathogens are preferred.

REFERENCES

1. National Center for Health Statistics. Health, United States, 2006. Available at: http://www.cdc.gov/nchs/fastats/lcod.htm. Accessed October 29, 2009.
2. File TM. Community-acquired pneumonia. *Lancet.* 2003;362:1991-2001.
3. Mandell LA, Wunderink RG, Anzueto A, et al. Infectious Diseases Society of America/American Thoracic Society consensus guidelines of the management of community-acquired pneumonia in adults. *Clin Infect Dis.* 2007:44:S27-72.
4. Niederman MS, Craven DE. Guidelines for the management of adults with hospital-acquired, ventilator-associated, and healthcare-associated pneumonia. *Am J Respir Crit Care Med.* 2005;171:388-416.
5. Mason CM, Nelson S. Pulmonary host defenses and factors predisposing to lung infection. *Clin Chest Med.* 2005;26:11-17.
6. Garcia-Vazquez E, Marcos MA, Mesna J, et al. Assessment of the usefulness of sputum cultures for diagnosis of community-acquired pneumonia using the PORT predictive scoring system. *Arch Intern Med.* 2004;164:1807-11.
7. Jackson LA, Neuzil KM, Yu O, et al. Effectiveness of pneumococcal polysaccharide vaccine in older adults. *N Engl J Med.* 2003;348:1747-1755.
8. Jefferson T, Rivetti D. Rivetti A, et al. Efficacy and effectiveness of influenza vaccine in elderly people: a systematic review. *Lancet.* 2005;366:1165-1174.

CHAPTER

22 Skin and Soft Tissue Infections

S. Scott Sutton, Christopher M. Bland, and Jarrett R. Amsden

FOUNDATION OVERVIEW

Infections of the skin and soft tissues are frequently encountered in acute and ambulatory settings and are among the most common infections seen in clinical practice. Data on the exact incidence of skin and soft tissue infections (SSTIs) are lacking because most infections are believed to be mild and treated in outpatient settings. However, SSTIs can range in severity from mild, superficial, self-limiting infections to severe, deep-seated, life-threatening infections.

The skin serves as a barrier between humans and their environment and functions as a primary defense mechanism against infections. The skin consists of the epidermis, the dermis, and subcutaneous fat. The epidermis is the outermost, nonvascular layer of the skin. The dermis is the layer of skin directly beneath the epidermis. It consists of connective tissue and contains blood vessels and lymphatics, sensory nerve endings, sweat and sebaceous glands, hair follicles, and smooth muscle fibers. Beneath the dermis is a layer of loose connective tissue containing primarily fat cells. This subcutaneous fat layer is of variable thickness over the body. Beneath the subcutaneous fat lies the fascia, which separates the skin from muscle. SSTIs may involve any or all layers of the skin, fascia, and muscle. They may also spread far from the initial site of infection and lead to severe complications, such as sepsis, glomerulonephritis, endocarditis, or osteomyelitis.

Intact skin is generally resistant to bacterial, fungal, and viral infections. In addition to providing a mechanical barrier, its relative dryness, slightly acidic pH, colonizing bacteria, frequent desquamation, and sweat prevent invasion by microorganisms.[1] Conditions that predispose a patient to SSTIs include: 1) high bacterial load, 2) excessive skin moisture, 3) decreased skin perfusion, 4) damage to corneal layer of skin.[2-3] The majority of SSTIs result from disruption of normal host defenses by processes such as skin puncture, abrasion, or underlying disease (eg, diabetes).

Bacterial infections of the skin can be classified as primary or secondary. Primary bacterial infections involve areas of previously healthy skin and are often caused by one or two pathogens. Secondary infections occur in areas of previously damaged skin and are often polymicrobial (Table 22-1). The majority of SSTIs are caused by gram-positive organisms present on the skin surface.[4] *Staphylococcus aureus* (*S. aureus*) and *Streptococcus pyogenes* (also known as group A streptococci (GAS) and flesh-eating bacteria) account for the majority of SSTIs.

Impetigo

Impetigo is a superficial skin infection caused by β-hemolytic *Streptococcus* (includes GAS) and *S. aureus*. Impetigo most often occurs in children, settings of poor hygiene, and crowding during the summer months. The microorganisms colonize the skin and invade through abrasions, insect bites, or other small traumas. Impetigo lesions are numerous, well localized and erythematous. They develop as small or large blisters that rupture, leaving a crust reminiscent of cornflakes. The lesions are rarely painful but often pruritic. Treatment of impetigo consists of soaking the lesions with soap and water, use of skin emollients to dry areas, and antimicrobials. Antimicrobials with activity against group A streptococci (GAS) and the beta-lactamase producing (penicillinase) *S. aureus* (MSSA) are preferred, and include first-generation cephalosporins and penicillinase-stable penicillins (eg, dicloxacillin or nafcillin).[3] Topical mupirocin may be used alone when there are few lesions.[3]

Lymphangitis

Lymphangitis is an inflammation of the lymphatic channel that ensues when a local skin infection is not contained, most often caused by GAS. Lymphangitis is characterized by red linear streaks that extend from the infection site toward regional lymph nodes. The goals of therapy are rapid eradication of infection and prevention of further systemic complications.[5] Because these infections are potentially serious and rapidly progressive, initial treatment should be with IV penicillin G 1 to 2 million units every 4 to 6 hours. Parenteral treatment should be continued for 48 to 72 hours, followed by oral penicillin VK for a total of 10 days. Patients allergic to penicillin may be treated with clindamycin.

Erysipelas

Erysipelas is an infection of the superficial layers of the skin and cutaneous lymphatics. The intense red color and burning pain led to the common name of St. Anthony's fire. The infection is most often caused by GAS. The clinical presentation

TABLE 22-1 Bacterial Classification of Skin and Soft Tissue Infections

Primary Infections	Pathogen
Erysipelas	Group A streptococci
Impetigo	*Staphylococcus aureus*, group A streptococci
Lymphangitis	Group A streptococci, occasionally *S. aureus*
Cellulitis	Group A streptococci, *S. aureus* (including caMRSA; occasionally other gram-positive or negative pathogens)
Necrotizing fasciitis	
Type I	Anaerobes (eg, *Clostridium perfringens*) *Peptostreptococcus*, streptococci, Enterobacteriaceae
Type II	Group A streptococci
Osteomyelitis	
Hematogenous	*S. aureus*
Contiguous	*S. aureus*, streptococci, Enterobacteriaceae, Anaerobes
Vascular insufficiency	*S. aureus*, streptococci, Enterobacteriaceae, Anaerobes
Secondary Infections	
Diabetic foot infections	*S. aureus*, streptococci, Enterobacteriaceae, *Bacteroides* species, *Pseudomonas aeruginosa*
Pressure sores	*S. aureus*, streptococci, Enterobacteriaceae, *Bacteroides* species, *Pseudomonas aeruginosa*
Bite wounds	
Animal	*Pasteurella multocida, S. aureus*, streptococci, *Bacteroides* species
Human	*Eikenella corrodens, S. aureus*, streptococci, *Corynebacterium* species, *Bacteroides* species, *Peptostreptococcus*
Burn wounds	*Pseudomonas aeruginosa*, Enterobacteriaceae, *Acinetobacter* species, *S. acinetobacter aureus*, streptococci

of erysipelas differs from cellulitis in that the lesion has clearly demarcated raised margins. Mild to moderate cases of erysipelas are treated with intramuscular procaine penicillin G or oral penicillin VK daily for 7 to 10 days.[3] Penicillin allergic patients may be treated with clindamycin or a macrolide. Serious erysipelas infections often require treatment with IV penicillin.

Cellulitis

Cellulitis is an acute, infectious process that represents a serious type of SSTI. Cellulitis initially affects the epidermis and dermis and may spread within the superficial fascia. Cellulitis is a serious disease because of the propensity of the infection to spread through the lymphatic tissue and the bloodstream if left untreated. GAS and *S. aureus* are the most frequent etiologic pathogens; however, many etiologic pathogens have been implicated. The rising incidence of infections caused by methicillin-resistant *S. aureus* (MRSA), including community-acquired methicillin-resistant *S. aureus* (caMRSA), is a major concern in the treatment of SSTIs, especially cellulitis. Cellulitis is described as painful and tender with rapidly spreading signs of redness, edema, and heat. The cellulitis lesion has poorly defined margins and is not raised.

The goals of therapy for cellulitis are rapid and successful eradication of the infection and prevention of complications (abscess, osteomyelitis, septic arthritis). Abscesses are usually indicative of *S. aureus* rather than streptococcal species. Nonpharmacological treatment of cellulitis consists of elevating and immobilizing the limb to decrease swelling, sterile saline dressings placed on open lesions, surgical debridement for severe infection, and abscess drainage if present. Pharmacologic treatment of cellulitis is with beta-lactams active against penicillinase-producing strains of *S. aureus*. Examples include dicloxacillin, cephalexin, and amoxicillin-clavulanate. Clindamycin or doxycycline may be used for patients with a penicillin allergy. Table 22-2 lists empiric treatment for cellulitis infections.

caMRSA is rapidly increasing in prevalence in SSTIs (including cellulitis). Treatment of caMRSA is problematic because of the organism's resistance to common antibiotics and the lack of literature documenting effective treatment. caMRSA can be distinguished from health care-associated methicillin-resistant *S. aureus* (haMRSA) by its genetic dissimilarity, drug susceptibility profiles, and toxin production (virulent Panton-Valentine leukocidin toxin). haMRSA is associated with well-defined risk factors (ie, prolonged hospitalization, nursing home, previous antimicrobial use, indwelling catheters, pressure sores, surgery, or dialysis); however, caMRSA risk factors are not well established.[6] caMRSA is susceptible to more antibiotics than haMRSA. Like haMRSA, caMRSA is sensitive to vancomycin, linezolid, daptomycin, tigecycline, and quinupristin/dalfopristin, but caMRSA is also susceptible to trimethoprim-sulfamethoxazole (TMP-SMX), clindamycin, doxycycline, and minocycline.[6] Table 22-2 lists recommended antibiotic regimens for treatment of cellulitis, including caMRSA infections.

Empiric therapy for MRSA in the treatment of cellulitis should be strongly considered in geographical locations with a high incidence of MRSA or in patients with abscesses. The duration of therapy ranges from 7 to 10 days. For complicated cellulitis, begin therapy with IV antibiotics and switch to oral once the patient is afebrile and skin findings begin to resolve.

Necrotizing Fasciitis

Necrotizing fasciitis (NF) is an uncommon, rapidly progressive, life-threatening infection of the subcutaneous tissue and fascia. Although NF risk is higher in patients with underlying

TABLE 22-2 Empiric Antimicrobial Therapy for Cellulitis

Host Factors	Probable Etiologic Bacteria	Mild Infection (Oral)[a]	Moderate—Severe Infection (IV)[a]
Previously healthy[b]	MSSA, GAS	Dicloxacillin 500 mg every 6 h	Nafcillin 1-2 g every 4 h
		Cephalexin 500 mg every 6 h	Cefazolin 1-2 g every 8 h
Injection drug use[b]	MSSA, GAS, gram-negatives, anaerobes	Amoxicillin-clavulanate 500 mg every 8 h or 875 mg every 12 h	Ampicillin-sulbactam 1.5-3 g every 6 h
			Ceftriaxone 1 g daily + clindamycin 600-900 mg every 8 h
			Ertapenem 1 g daily
Immune compromise[b]	MSSA, haMRSA, Gram negatives, *Pseudomonas aeruginosa*	Amoxicillin-clavulanate 500 mg every 8 h or 875 mg every 12 h (*as long as haMRSA or Pseudomonas not suspected*)	Piperacillin-tazobactam 3.375-4.5 g every 4-6 h
			Antipseudomonal carbapenem:
			Imipenem-cilastatin 500 mg every 6 h,
			Meropenem 1 g every 8 h,
			Doripenem 500 mg every 8 h
			Cefepime 2 g every 8-12 h + metronidazole 500 mg every 8 h
			Tigecycline 100 mg load, then 50 mg every 12 h
Special considerations	caMRSA or penicillin allergy	TMP-SMX DS 1-2 tablets every 12 h (*does not cover GAS*)	TMP-SMX 2.5 mg/kg (TMP component) every 12 h (*does not cover GAS*)
		Clindamycin 300-450 mg every 6 h	Clindamycin 600-900 mg every 8 h
		Doxycycline 100 mg every 12 h	Doxycycline 100 mg every 12 h
			Daptomycin 4 mg/kg daily
			Vancomycin 15 mg/kg every 12 h
			Linezolid 600 mg every 12 h

[a]Adult dose with normal renal function.

[b]Include coverage for caMRSA or haMRSA according to patient history and resistance patterns in the area.

Abbreviations: caMRSA, community acquired methicillin-resistant *Staphylococcus aureus*; DS, double strength; GAS, group A streptococci; haMRSA, health care-associated methicillin-resistant *Staphylococcus aureus*; MSSA, methicillin-sensitive *Staphylococcus aureus*; TMP-SMX, trimethoprim-sulfamethoxazole.

diseases (diabetes, alcoholism, cardiac disease, peripheral vascular disease), healthy hosts can become infected as well.[7-8] NF erupts after an initial trauma, which can range from a small abrasion to a deep penetrating wound. The infection begins in the fascia, where bacteria replicate and release toxins that facilitate their spread.[8] There are two types of NF, distinguishable by microbiology, source and severity of illness. Type I NF is polymicrobial and develops after surgery or deep penetrating wounds in the bowel, decubitus ulcer, or injection site in an injection drug user. Type II NF is monomicrobial caused by GAS. Type II occurs after minor trauma such as an insect bite or abrasion.[3] It is more severe than type I because invasive strains of GAS produce toxins that induce erythema, systemic toxicity, multiorgan failure, and shock. The goals of therapy for NF include eradication of infection and reduction of morbidity and mortality. After resuscitation and hemodynamic stabilization, prompt surgical intervention is key in the treatment of NF. Delayed operative debridement increases mortality. Broad-spectrum IV antimicrobial therapy should be initiated immediately in patients with NF regardless of the type. Often a high-dose beta-lactam/beta-lactamase inhibitor or carbapenem is used in combination with clindamycin. Vancomycin, daptomycin, or linezolid should be part of the empiric regimen until MRSA can be excluded. Clindamycin should be added to decrease bacterial toxin production, thereby limiting tissue damage.[3] Clindamycin adds antibacterial activity, particularly in high inoculum bacteria associated with NF. If GAS is identified as the sole causative organism from deep tissue culture, antibiotic therapy can be narrowed to high-dose IV penicillin G plus clindamycin. Antibiotic therapy should be continued until further operative debridements are unnecessary, the patient displays substantial clinical improvement, and fevers have abated for at least 48 to 72 hours.[3] Other possible adjunctive therapies for NF include hyperbaric oxygen (HBO) therapy and intravenous immunoglobulin (IVIG) therapy.

Diabetic Foot Infections

Foot ulcers and related infections are among the most common, severe, and costly complications of diabetes mellitus (DM).

TABLE 22-3 Empiric Pharmacologic Treatment of Diabetic Foot Infection

Infection Severity	PEDIS Grade[a]	General Approach to Therapy	Examples of Empiric Regimens[b]
Uninfected	1	None. Avoid treating uninfected diabetic foot ulcers.	Not applicable.
Mild	2	Oral, narrow-spectrum antibiotics with activity against *Staphylococcus aureus* and streptococcal species. **Include coverage for caMRSA or haMRSA according to patient history and resistance patterns in the area.**	**MRSA not suspected:** Cephalexin 500 mg every 6 h; dicloxacillin 500 mg every 6 h **haMRSA suspected:** Linezolid 600 mg (oral) every 12 h; vancomycin 15 mg/kg every 12 h; daptomycin 4mg/kg daily **caMRSA suspected:** TMP-SMX DS 1-2 tablets every 12 h; doxycycline 100 mg every 12 h; clindamycin 300-450 mg every 6 h
Moderate to severe	3-4	Parenteral, broad spectrum antibiotic therapy. Generally select antibiotics with activity against gram-positive, gram-negative, and anaerobic bacteria. **Include coverage for caMRSA or haMRSA according to patient history and resistance patterns in the area.**	Ceftriaxone 2 g daily + clindamycin 600-900 mg every 8 h[c]; piperacillin-tazobactam 3.375-4.5 g every 4-6 h; imipenem-cilastatin 500 mg every 6 h, meropenem 1 gram every 8 h, doripenem 500 mg every 8 h; fluoroquinolone (ciprofloxacin or levofloxacin) + clindamycin 600-900 mg every 8 h; tigecycline 100 mg load, then 50 mg every 12 h[c] If MRSA suspected, vancomycin, linezolid, daptomycin are indicated in addition to gram-negative and anaerobic coverage

[a]The severity of a patient's infection, based on the PEDIS scale, guides the selection of empiric antimicrobial therapy. While most patients with grade 2 diabetic foot infections can be treated as outpatients with oral antibiotics, all grade 4 and many grade 3 infections require hospitalization and broad spectrum intravenous antibiotics.

[b]Adult dose with normal renal function.

[c]This regimen does not cover *Pseudomonas aeruginosa*.

Abbreviations: caMRSA, community-acquired methicillin-resistant *Staphylococcus aureus*; DS, double strength; haMRSA, health care-associated methicillin-resistant *Staphylococcus aureus*; TMP-SMX, trimethoprim-sulfamethoxazole.

The pathogenesis of diabetic foot infections stems from three factors: neuropathy, angiopathy, and immunopathy.[9-11] Neuropathy develops when high blood glucose levels damage motor, autonomic, and sensory nerves. Angiopathy of large and small vessels also results from high blood glucose levels and results in ischemia and skin breakdown. Diabetic patients develop immunopathy, which predisposes them to infections. Leukocyte function and cell-mediated immunity are compromised in poorly controlled diabetics. Infected diabetics foot ulcers are caused by several different pathogens. Aerobic gram-positive cocci, such as *S. aureus* and GAS, are the predominant pathogens in acutely infected diabetic foot ulcers. However, chronically infected ulcers are polymicrobial and include additional pathogens like Enterobacteriaceae, MRSA, and *Pseudomonas aeruginosa*. Spreading soft tissue infection, osteomyelitis, bacteremia, and sepsis as well as amputation are complications of diabetic foot infections. The goals of therapy are eradication of the infection and avoidance of complications. Comprehensive foot care programs can significantly reduce the rate of diabetic foot infections. Periodic foot examinations with monofilament testing and patient education regarding proper foot care, optimal glycemic control, and smoking cessation are key preventive strategies. Multiple antibiotic options exist for the treatment of diabetic foot infections. Table 22-3 provides examples of antimicrobials that are utilized in the treatment of diabetic foot infections. Duration of treatment ranges from 7 to 28 days or longer, depending upon the severity.

Infected Pressure Sores

Pressure sores, also known as decubitus ulcers or bedsores, are chronic wounds that result from continuous pressure on the tissue overlying a bony prominence. This pressure impedes blood flow to the dermis and subcutaneous fat, resulting in tissue damage and necrosis.[12-13] Pressure sore infections generally are polymicrobial. The goals of therapy for infected pressure sores include resolution of infection, promotion of wound healing, and establishment of effective infection control.[13-14] Prevention is the most effective way to manage pressure sores. Key prevention strategies include monitoring of high-risk patients, reducing skin exposure to pressure and moisture, and promoting good nutritional status. Systemic antimicrobials are indicated for pressure sores associated with spreading cellulitis, osteomyelitis, or bacteremia. Because the infections are polymicrobial, empiric therapy should be broad-spectrum and be given for 10 to 14 days. Mild superficial infections may be treated with topical antimicrobial agents. Table 22-4 lists empiric therapy for pressure sores.

TABLE 22-4 Empiric Therapy for Infected Pressure Sores

Formulation	Antibiotic[a]
Topical	Silver sulfadiazine 1% cream
	Combination antibiotic ointments
Oral[c]	Amoxicillin-clavulanate 500 mg every 8 h or 875 mg every 12 h
	Fluoroquinolone (ciprofloxacin or levofloxacin) + clindamycin 300-450 mg every 6 h[b]
Parenteral[c]	Cefoxitin 1-2 g every 8 h
	Piperacillin-tazobactam 3.375-4.5 g every 4-6 h[b]
	Imipenem-cilastatin 500 mg every 6 h[b]; meropenem 1 g every 8 h[b]; doripenem 500 mg every 8 h[b]
	Fluoroquinolone (ciprofloxacin or levofloxacin) + clindamycin 600-900 mg every 8 h[b]

[a]Include coverage for caMRSA or haMRSA according to patient history and resistance patterns in the area.

[b]Regimens with activity against *Pseudomonas aeruginosa*.

[c]Adult dose with normal renal function.

Infected Bite Wounds

Fifty percent of Americans will be bitten by an animal at least once during their lifetime. Although most of these injuries are minor, approximately 20% will require medical treatment.[3] Dogs represent the most common cause of all bites, followed by cats and humans. However, cat bites have the highest risk of infectious complications.[15] Antibiotic therapy is required *only* when clinical infection is present. However, prophylactic therapy is recommended for wounds at higher risk for infection. These include cat and human bites, deep punctures, bites to the hand, and bites requiring surgical repair.[16-17] The most effective agent for treatment and prophylaxis of human and animal bite-wound infections is amoxicillin-clavulanate. Alternatives for patients with a penicillin allergy include either a fluoroquinolone or TMP-SMX in combination with clindamycin.

Antimicrobial Properties

There are several different antibiotics that may be utilized in the treatment of SSTIs. Certain properties of a drug may influence use of one agent over the other. Key properties such as the side effect profile, drug interactions, formulation, and pregnancy category may influence the selection of a particular antibiotic. See Table 22-5 for properties of antibiotics used for treatment of SSTIs.

SPECIAL CONSIDERATIONS

Folliculitis

Folliculitis is a superficial inflammatory reaction involving the hair follicle. The most familiar form is acne. It can be infectious, caused by pathogens such as: *S. aureus*, *P. aeruginosa*, and *Candida*. Folliculitis often resolves spontaneously. Nonpharmacologic treatment is a warm compress. Pharmacologic treatment, if required, is a topical antibiotic or antifungal. For example, for staphylococcal folliculitis, mupirocin may be utilized.

Furuncles

Furuncles are bacterial infections that have spread to subcutaneous skin layers, but only involve individual follicles. Nonpharmacologic treatment is moist heat to facilitate drainage. Large furuncles require incision and drainage. Pharmacologic treatment is indicated for patients that display cellulitis and fever. Treatment with systemic antibiotics is targeted for *S. aureus* (MSSA) (eg, dicloxacillin, cephalexin, clindamycin). However, with the increasing incidence of caMRSA TMP-SMX or doxycycline may be added until culture results return.

Carbuncles

Carbuncles share all the characteristics of furuncles; however, a carbuncle is larger and involves adjacent follicles and extends into subcutaneous fat. Nonpharmacologic treatment is incision and drainage. Pharmacologic treatment is indicated for patients that display cellulitis and fever. Treatment with systemic antibiotics is targeted for *Staphylococcus* (eg, dicloxacillin, cephalexin, clindamycin). However, with the increasing incidence of caMRSA, TMP-SMX or doxycycline may be added until culture results return.

Cellulitis (Injection Drug Users and Immune Compromised Patients)

Injection-drug use predisposes individuals to a number of infectious complications, including abscess formation and cellulitis at the site of injection.[18-19] The SSTIs are often polymicrobial and include oral flora such as viridans streptococci, GAS, and anaerobes. The incidence of MRSA is also rising in SSTIs in injection-drug users.[20]

Immunocompromised patients are at risk of polymicrobial cellulitis infections. Empiric broad-spectrum antimicrobial coverage, including coverage for haMRSA and *P. aeruginosa*, is appropriate for severe cellulitis or systemic illness in immunocompromised patients. Similarly, HIV patients often have polymicrobic infections and should be treated with broad-spectrum antibiotics.[4] See Table 22-2 for empiric antimicrobial therapy for cellulitis.

Osteomyelitis

Osteomyelitis is an infection of the bone and can be a complication of SSTIs. Gram-positive bacteria (eg, *S. aureus*) are the predominant pathogens seen in osteomyelitis. Osteomyelitis can be divided into three types: (1) hematogenous, (2) contiguous, and (3) secondary to vascular insufficiency.[21] Hematogenous

TABLE 22-5 **Properties of Antimicrobials Used in the Treatment of Skin and Soft Tissue Infections**

Antimicrobial	Formulations	Mechanism of action	Side Effects	Contraindications (CI); Warnings (W)	Drug Interactions (DI); General Information (GI); Monitoring (M)
First Generation Cephalosporins					
Cephalexin (Keflex); Cefazolin (Ancef)	Cephalexin: capsule, tablet, suspension Cefazolin: parenteral	Inhibits bacterial cell wall synthesis by binding to one or more penicillin- binding proteins which inhibits the final transpeptidation step of peptidoglycan synthesis in bacterial cell wall synthesis	CNS (confusion, dizziness), rash, GI, *C. diff*; BMS (rare)	CI: Hypersensitivity to cephalosporins W: Modify dosage in renal dysfunction, use in caution in patients with a delayed penicillin allergy (rash) and avoid in immediate allergic (anaphylaxis/IgE-mediated) penicillin reaction, may be associated with increased INR, especially in nutritionally malnourished patients, prolonged treatment, hepatic or renal disease, use with caution in patients with a history of seizure disorder (high levels, especially in the presence of renal dysfunction, may increase risk of seizures)	DI: Food—peak cephalexin levels are decreased with food, but total absorption is not affected GI: Pregnancy category B, renal elimination M: With prolonged therapy, monitor renal hepatic function periodically, CBC with differential for cytopenias or signs of allergic reaction
Second Generation cephalosporins					
Cefuroxime (Ceftin, Zinacef); Cefoxitin (Apo-cefoxitin)	Cefuroxime axetil: tablet, suspension Cefuroxime sodium: parenteral Cefoxitin: parenteral	Inhibits bacterial cell wall synthesis by binding to one or more penicillin- binding proteins which inhibits the final transpeptidation step of peptidoglycan synthesis in bacterial cell wall synthesis	CNS (confusion, dizziness), rash, GI, *C. diff*; BMS (rare)	CI: IgE-mediated hypersensitivity to cephalosporins or penicillin derivatives W: Modify dosage in renal dysfunction, use with caution in patients with a delayed penicillin allergy (rash) and avoid in immediate allergic (anaphylaxis/IgE-mediated) penicillin reaction, may be associated with increased INR, especially in nutritionally malnourished patients, prolonged treatment, hepatic or renal disease	GI: Pregnancy category B, renal elimination, cefuroxime axetil film-coated tablets and oral suspension are not bioequivalent and are not substitutable on a mg/mg basis M: With prolonged therapy, monitor renal hepatic function periodically, CBC with differential for cytopenias or signs of allergic reaction
Third Generation Cephalosporins					
Cefpodoxime (Vantin); Cefdinir (Omnicef); Ceftriaxone (Rocephin); Cefotaxime (Claforan)	Cefpodoxime: tablet, suspension Cefdinir: capsule, suspension Ceftriaxone: parenteral Cefotaxime: parenteral	Inhibits bacterial cell wall synthesis by binding to one or more penicillin- binding proteins which inhibits the final transpeptidation step of peptidoglycan synthesis in bacterial cell wall synthesis.	CNS (confusion, dizziness), rash, GI, *C. diff*; BMS (rare) Ceftriaxone—biliary toxicities/ obstructions	CI: IgE-mediated hypersensitivity to cephalosporins or penicillin derivatives W: Modify dosage in renal dysfunction (cefpodoxime/ cefotaxime), use with caution in patients with a delayed penicillin allergy (rash) and avoid in immediate allergic (anaphylaxis/ IgE- mediated) penicillin reaction, do not use ceftriaxone in hyperbilirubinemia neonates—particularly those who are premature since ceftriaxone can displace bilirubin from albumin sites, ceftriaxone may complex with calcium causing precipitation—fatal lung and kidney damage has been observed in premature and term neonates	DI: Ceftriaxone—avoid concomitant use with calcium salts (IV) and lactated ringers injection GI: Pregnancy category B, renal elimination (ceftriaxone is 33%-67% eliminated via kidney and does not require dose reduction in renal dysfunction) M: With prolonged therapy, monitor renal hepatic function periodically, CBC with differential for cytopenias or signs of allergic reaction

(*Continued*)

TABLE 22-5 **Properties of Antimicrobials Used in the Treatment of Skin and Soft Tissue Infections (*Continued*)**

Antimicrobial	Formulations	Mechanism of action	Side Effects	Contraindications (CI); Warnings (W)	Drug Interactions (DI); General Information (GI); Monitoring (M)
Penicillin Antimicrobials					
Penicillin (Pen VK, Bicillin CR or Bicillin LA, and Aqueous penicillin G)	Parenteral, oral (tablet, solution)	Inhibits bacterial cell wall synthesis by binding to one or more penicillin- binding proteins which inhibits the final transpeptidation step of peptidoglycan synthesis in bacterial cell wall synthesis	CNS (confusion, dizziness), rash, GI, *C. diff*; BMS (rare)	CI: Hypersensitivity to penicillin W: Use with caution in patients with renal dysfunction (modify dose) or history of seizures, serious and occasionally severe or fatal hypersensitivity reactions have been reported in patients on penicillin therapy, especially with a history of beta-lactam allergies, history of sensitivity to multiple allergens, or previous IgE-mediated reactions (anaphylaxis, urticaria); Bicillin CR (procaine) and Bicillin LA (benzathine) are not interchangeable	GI: Pregnancy category B, renal elimination M: With prolonged therapy, monitor renal function periodically, CBC with differential for neutropenias or signs of allergic reaction
Penicillinase-Stable Penicillins					
Dicloxacillin (Dycill, others); Nafcillin (Unipen)	Dicloxacillin: capsule Nafcillin: parenteral	Interferes with bacterial cell wall synthesis during active multiplication, causing cell wall death and resultant bactericidal activity against susceptible bacteria	CNS (confusion, dizziness), rash, GI, *C. diff*; BMS (rare), renal—acute interstitial nephritis (AIN)	CI: Hypersensitivity to penicillins W: Serious and occasionally severe or fatal hypersensitivity reactions have been reported in patients on penicillin therapy, especially with a history of beta-lactam allergies, history of sensitivity to multiple allergens, or previous IgE-mediated reactions (anaphylaxis, urticaria)	DI: Nafcillin—CYP-450 3A4 inducer GI/GU: Dicloxacillin—Poor oral absorption, pregnancy category B Nafcillin—Primarily eliminated via the liver; biliary and feces; minimal renal elimination (no renal adjustments required) M: With prolonged therapy, monitor renal function periodically (interstitial nephritis), LFT, CBC with differential for neutropenia or signs of allergic reaction
Aminopenicillins					
Amoxicillin (Amoxil, Trimox) Ampicillin (Principen)	Amoxicillin: capsule, suspension Ampicillin: capsule; parenteral	Interferes with bacterial cells wall synthesis during active multiplication, causing cell wall death and resultant bactericidal activity against susceptible bacteria	CNS—rare (confusion, dizziness), rash, GI (high incidence), *C. diff* or superinfections, BMS (rare)	CI: Hypersensitivity to penicillins W: Serious and occasionally severe or fatal hypersensitivity reactions have been reported in patients on penicillin therapy, especially with a history of beta-lactam allergies, history of sensitivity to multiple allergens, or previous IgE-mediated reactions (anaphylaxis, urticaria), high percentage of infectious mononucleosis patients have developed rash while taking ampicillin-class antibiotics	GI/GU: Diarrhea, pregnancy category B, renal elimination M: With prolonged therapy, monitor renal function periodically, CBC with differential for neutropenias or signs of allergic reaction
Beta-Lactam/Beta-Lactamase Inhibitor Combinations					
Amoxicillin-clavulanate (Augmentin); Piperacillin-tazobactam (Zosyn)	Augmentin: suspension, tablet, extended release (XR) tablet; Zosyn: parenteral	Clavulanic acid and tazobactam binds and inhibits beta-lactamases that inactivate amoxicillin or piperacillin	CNS (confusion, dizziness), rash, GI, *C. diff*; BMS (rare)	CI: Hypersensitivity to penicillins W: Use with caution in patients with renal dysfunction (modify dose) or history of seizures, serious and occasionally severe or fatal hypersensitivity reactions have	GI: Pregnancy category B, renal elimination M: With prolonged therapy, monitor renal and hematologic function periodically, signs

(*Continued*)

TABLE 22-5 **Properties of Antimicrobials Used in the Treatment of Skin and Soft Tissue Infections (*Continued*)**

Antimicrobial	Formulations	Mechanism of action	Side Effects	Contraindications (CI); Warnings (W)	Drug Interactions (DI); General Information (GI); Monitoring (M)
Beta- Lactam/Beta- Lactamase Inhibitor Combinations (*Continued*)					
		resulting in amoxicillin or piperacillin having an expanded spectrum of activity. Amoxicillin and piperacillin inhibits bacterial cell wall synthesis by binding to one or more of the penicillin- binding proteins.		been reported in patients on penicillin therapy, especially with a history of beta-lactam allergies, history of sensitivity to multiple allergens, or previous IgE-mediated reactions (anaphylaxis, urticaria), high percentage of infectious mononucleosis patients have developed rash while taking ampicillin-class antibiotics; due to differing content of clavulanate—not all formulations are interchangeable CI for piperacillin only: Bleeding disorders have been observed, particularly in patients with renal dysfunction, discontinue if thrombocytopenia or bleeding occurs due to high sodium load and to adverse effects of high serum concentrations, dosage modifications are required in renal dysfunction	of allergic reaction; piperacillin-tazobactam has 11.17 mEq of sodium in 4.5 g and 8.38 mEq in 3.375 g
Carbapenems					
Imipenem-cilastatin (Primaxin); Meropenem (Merrem); Doripenem (Doribax); Ertapenem (Invanz)	Carbapenems: parenteral	Inhibits bacterial cell wall synthesis by binding to penicillin- binding proteins, which inhibits the final transpeptidation step of peptidoglycan synthesis. Cilastatin prevents renal metabolism of imipenem by inhibition of dehydropeptidase along the brush border of the renal tubules.	CNS (confusion, dizziness), rash, GI, *C. diff*; BMS (rare)	CI: Hypersensitivity to carbapenems W: Dosage reduction required in renal dysfunction has been associated with CNS adverse effects (confusion and seizures), use caution in patients with a history of seizures or hypersensitivity to beta-lactams	GI: Pregnancy category C (imipenem) B (others), renal elimination; ertapenem does not cover *Pseudomonas* species M: With prolonged therapy, monitor renal and hematologic function periodically, signs of allergic reaction
Fluoroquinolones					
Ciprofloxacin (Cipro); Levofloxacin (Levaquin)	Ciprofloxacin: parenteral, suspension, tablet Levofloxacin: parenteral, suspension, tablet	Inhibits DNA gyrase—inhibits relaxation of supercoiled DNA and promotes breakage of double-stranded DNA	Headache, confusion, mental status changes, GI, *C. diff*, BMS (rare), allergic reaction (immediate or delayed), hypoglycemia (early) or hyperglycemia (delayed), photosensitivity	CI: Hypersensitivity to quinolones W: Reports of tendon inflammation and/or rupture (black box warning), CNS stimulation may occur (tremor, restlessness, confusion, and rarely hallucination or seizures); use with caution in patients with CNS disorders; quinolones prolong QTc interval—avoid use in patients with a history of QTc prolongation,	DI: Divalent/trivalent cations, Ciprofloxacin—inhibits CYP-450 1A2 (strong) and 3A4 (weak) GI: Pregnancy category C, renal elimination M: With prolonged therapy, monitor renal and hematologic function periodically, signs of allergic reaction, drug interactions

(*Continued*)

TABLE 22-5 **Properties of Antimicrobials Used in the Treatment of Skin and Soft Tissue Infections (*Continued*)**

Antimicrobial	Formulations	Mechanism of action	Side Effects	Contraindications (CI); Warnings (W)	Drug Interactions (DI); General Information (GI); Monitoring (M)
Fluoroquinolones (*Continued*)					
				uncorrected hypokalemia, hypomagnesemia, or concurrent administration of medications known to prolong QT interval (Class 1a and Class III antiarrhythmics, erythromycin, antipsychotics, tricyclic antidepressants); adverse effects are increased in pediatric patients and should not be considered first-line agents in children (exception is anthrax treatment); dose reduction required in renal dysfunction	
MRSA Antimicrobials					
Clindamycin (Cleocin)	Capsule, solution, parenteral	Reversibly binds to 50s ribosomal subunits preventing peptide bond formation thus inhibiting bacterial protein synthesis	Rash, GI, *C. diff*, BMS (rare), pill esophagitis (rare)	CI: Hypersensitivity to clindamycin W: Dosage adjustment necessary for severe hepatic dysfunction, can cause fatal colitis (*C. diff*)	GI: Pregnancy category B, hepatic metabolism, with prolonged therapy monitor renal and hematologic function periodically, observe for changes in bowel frequency
Doxycycline (Vibramycin, others); Minocycline (Minocin, Dynacin)	Doxycycline: capsule, parenteral, suspension, syrup, tablet Minocycline: capsule, tablet, parenteral	Inhibits protein synthesis by binding with the 30s and 50s ribosomal subunit	Rash (photosensitivity), GI, *C. diff*, BMS (rare), hepatotoxicity (rare), autoimmune disease reported, pill esophagitis (rare)	CI: Hypersensitivity to doxycycline or tetracycline, children ≤ 8 y (except in treatment of anthrax) W: Photosensitivity reaction may occur—avoid prolonged exposure to sunlight or tanning equipment, antianabolic effects may increase blood urea nitrogen (BUN), hepatotoxicity has been reported Minocycline: CNS effects (lightheadedness, vertigo) may occur Outdated tetracycline can cause Fanconi syndrome (renal compromise)	DI: Divalent/trivalent cations, doxycycline—inhibits CYP-450 3A4 (moderate) GI: Pregnancy category D M: Complete blood count, renal, liver function tests periodically with prolonged therapy
Trimethoprim-sulfamethoxazole (Septra, Bactrim)	Parenteral, tablet, suspension	Sulfamethoxazole interferes with bacterial folic acid synthesis and growth via inhibition of dihydrofolic acid formation from para-aminobenzoic acid; trimethoprim inhibits dihydrofolic acid reduction to tetrahydrofolate resulting in inhibition of enzymes of the folic acid pathway	GI, *C. diff*, rash, photosensitivity, hyperkalemia, BMS, hepatitis, renal failure, allergic reaction	CI: Hypersensitivity to any sulfa drug, trimethoprim, megaloblastic anemia due to folate deficiency W: Use with caution in patients with G6PD deficiency, impaired renal or hepatic function or potential folate deficiency (malnourished, chronic anticonvulsant therapy, or elderly), adjust dose in renal impairment, fatalities associated with severe reactions including Stevens-Johnson syndrome, toxic epidermal necrolysis, agranulocytosis, and aplastic anemia—discontinue use at first sign of rash or serious adverse reaction	DI: Sulfamethoxazole—substrate CYP 2C9 (major), 3A4 (minor), inhibits 2C9 (moderate) Trimethoprim— substrate 2C9 (major), 3A4 (major), inhibits 2C8 (moderate), 2C9 (moderate) GI: Pregnancy category C/D, may falsely increase SCr levels due to competitive inhibition for active tubular secretion M: Complete blood count, potassium, serum creatinine, signs/symptoms of allergic reaction

(*Continued*)

TABLE 22-5 **Properties of Antimicrobials Used in the Treatment of Skin and Soft Tissue Infections (*Continued*)**

Antimicrobial	Formulations	Mechanism of action	Side Effects	Contraindications (CI); Warnings (W)	Drug Interactions (DI); General Information (GI); Monitoring (M)
Daptomycin (Cubicin)	Parenteral	Binds to components of the cell membrane and causes rapid depolarization, inhibiting intracellular synthesis of DNA, RNA, and protein	GI, *C. diff*, anemia, BMS, headache, rash, CPK elevation—muscle pain	CI: Hypersensitivity to daptomycin W: Associated with myopathy, discontinue in patients with signs and symptoms of myopathy in conjunction with increase in CPK > 5 times upper limit of normal or in asymptomatic patients with CPK > 10 times upper limit of normal, not indicated for treatment of pneumonia, use caution in renal dysfunction (dosage adjustment required)	GI: Pregnancy category B M: CPK at least weekly (more frequent if on a statin), muscle weakness/pain
Tigecycline (Tygacil)	Parenteral	Binds to 30s ribosomal subunit, inhibiting protein synthesis	GI, *C. diff*, headache, dizziness, rash, BMS, increased LFTs	CI: Hypersensitivity to tigecycline W: Due to structural similarity with tetracyclines, use caution in patients allergic to tetracyclines, other tetracyclines' effects are possible as well—photosensitivity, antianabolic effects, discoloration of teeth	GI: Pregnancy category D, systemic clearance reduced in hepatic impairment—adjust dose in severe hepatic impairment (Child-Pugh C), no dosing adjustment required in renal dysfunction
Linezolid (Zyvox)	Parenteral, tablet, suspension	Inhibits bacterial protein synthesis by binding to 23s ribosomal RNA of the 50s subunit	Headache, GI, *C. diff*, rash, BMS. BMS (including anemia, leukopenia, pancytopenia, and thrombocytopenia) may be more common in patients receiving therapy for > 2 wk	CI: Hypersensitivity to linezolid, concurrent use if within 2 wk of monoamine oxidase inhibitors, patients with uncontrolled hypertension, taking sympathomimetics, vasopressive agents, or dopaminergic agents unless closely monitored for increase in blood pressure, patients taking antidepressants with serotonin mechanism, meperidine unless closely monitored for serotonin syndrome W: Lactic acidosis has been reported with use (rare), myelosuppression has been reported and is more common with >2 wk of therapy but can occur earlier, peripheral and optic neuropathy has been reported, especially with >28 d of therapy. Any neuropathic symptoms require immediate evaluation	DI: Sympathomimetics, antidepressants with serotonin activity, meperidine, tyramine-containing foods (hypertensive crisis) GI: Pregnancy category C M: Weekly complete blood count, particularly in patients at increased risk of bleeding, preexisting myelosuppression, on concomitant medications that cause BMS, those requiring more than 2 wk of therapy
Vancomycin (Vancocin)	Parenteral, capsule (capsule is not absorbed and used for treatment of *C. diff* infections)	Inhibits bacterial cell wall synthesis by blocking glycopeptide polymerization through binding of D-alanyl-D-alanine portion of cell wall precursor	Red-man syndrome (rash), BMS (rare, except with high dose), ototoxicity, nephrotoxicity, increase nephrotoxic potential when combined with aminoglycoside	CI: Hypersensitivity to vancomycin W: May cause nephrotoxicity, usual risk factors are pre-existing renal dysfunction, concurrent nephrotoxic agent, advanced age, and dehydration; ototoxicity is proportional to the amount of drug given and duration of treatment—tinnitus or vertigo may be	GI: Pregnancy category C, reduce dose in renal dysfunction, administer vancomycin by intravenous infusion over at least 60 min, if maculopapular rash appears on the face, neck, trunk, and/or upper extremities (Red-man syndrome), slow infusion

(*Continued*)

TABLE 22-5 **Properties of Antimicrobials Used in the Treatment of Skin and Soft Tissue Infections (*Continued*)**

Antimicrobial	Formulations	Mechanism of action	Side Effects	Contraindications (CI); Warnings (W)	Drug Interactions (DI); General Information (GI); Monitoring (M)
				indications of vestibular injury and impending bilateral irreversible damage	rate to over 1.5-2 h +/– antihistamines M: Renal function, complete blood count, serum vancomycin concentrations, audiogram
Telavancin (Vibativ)	Parenteral	Inhibits bacterial cell wall synthesis by blocking polymerization and cross-linking of peptidoglycan by binding to D-Ala-D-Ala portion of cell wall as well as disruption of cell membrane potential causing changes in cell permeability	Nausea, headache, injection site reaction, metallic/soapy taste, increased serum creatinine, foamy urine	CI: Hypersensitivity to telavancin W: Cardiovascular—may prolong QTc interval; avoid use in patients with a history of QTc prolongation, uncompensated heart failure, severe left ventricular hypertrophy, or concurrent administration of other medications known to prolong the QT interval (including Class Ia and Class III antiarrhythmics, cisapride, erythromycin, antipsychotics, and tricyclic antidepressants). Clinical studies indicate mean maximal QTc prolongation of 12-15 ms at the end of 10 mg/kg infusion. Renal—Nephrotoxicity: may cause nephrotoxicity; usual risk factors include preexisting renal impairment, concomitant nephrotoxic medications, advanced age, and dehydration. Monitor renal function prior to, during, and following therapy. Contains solubilizer cyclodextrin (hydroxypropyl-beta-cyclodextrin) which may accumulate in patients with renal dysfunction.	DI: QTc-prolonging agents—may enhance the adverse/toxic effect of other QTc-prolonging agents. Their effects can be additive, causing life-threatening ventricular arrhythmias. Avoid combination if possible or monitor therapy closely depending on the interacting medication GI: Pregnancy category C, use is not recommended in pregnancy unless risk outweighs benefit and must register with manufacturer, must adjust dose/frequency in renal insufficiency, decreased efficacy in patients with renal insufficiency M: Renal function, complete blood count

Abbreviations: BMS, bone marrow suppression; *C. diff*, *Clostridium difficile*; CNS, central nervous system; CPK, creatine phosphokinase; CYP-450, cytochrome P-450; GI, gastrointestinal; LFT, liver function test.

osteomyelitis most often occurs in children, affects long bones, and is usually with a nonpenetrating trauma or fall. Contiguous osteomyelitis most often occurs in adults, arises from infected adjacent tissues or organs, and is most commonly encountered after surgery. Osteomyelitis due to vascular insufficiency is most commonly seen in older patients with diabetes, affects the lower limbs, and can be more difficult to treat due to decreased blood flow to the area.[21] Empirical therapy (see Table 22-2) should target causative pathogen(s) based on the type of osteomyelitis and patient-specific risk factors. Table 22-6 lists pathogens associated with osteomyelitis. The total duration of antimicrobial therapy is based upon resolution of signs and symptoms as well as clinical imaging, but is typically 4 to 6 weeks.

Outcome Evaluation

Patients receiving antibiotic therapy for SSTIs require monitoring for efficacy and safety. Efficacy is manifested by reductions in temperature, white blood cell count, erythema, edema, and pain. In most cases, resolution of signs and symptoms is rapid in acute SSTI's. The exception is NF, in which the signs and symptoms may worsen owing to toxin release of GAS; however, patients should begin to resolve within 48 to 72 hours of treatment initiation.

TABLE 22-6 **Empirical Therapy for Osteomyelitis**

Type of Osteomyelitis	Probable Etiologic Bacteria	Primary Empirical Regimen(s)	Alternative Empirical Regimen(s)
Hematogenous	*S. aureus* (MSSA or ca-MRSA), *GAS*	**MRSA not suspected:** Nafcillin/oxacillin 1-2 g IV every 4-6 h (adults) Cefazolin 1-2 g IV every 8 h (adults) **MRSA suspected:** Vancomycin 15-20 mg/kg IV every 12 h	**MRSA not suspected or penicillin allergic:** Clindamycin 600-900 mg IV every 8 h **haMRSA suspected:** Daptomycin, linezolid, tigecycline could be considered (not FDA indicated) **caMRSA suspected:** TMP-SMX, doxycycline, or clindamycin can be considered based upon sensitivities
Contiguous	*S. aureus* (MSSA or caMRSA), Streptococci, Enterobacteriaceae, anaerobes	Parenteral, broad spectrum antibiotic therapy. Generally select antibiotics with activity against gram-positive, gram-negative, and anaerobic bacteria that are likely to cause infections of the adjacent skin or organ. **Include coverage for caMRSA or haMRSA according to patient history and resistance patterns in the area.**	Ceftriaxone 2 g daily + clindamycin 600 mg every 8 h[c]; piperacillin/tazobactam 3.375-4.5 g every 4-6 h; imipenem 500 mg every 6 h, meropenem 1 g every 8 h, doripenem 500 mg every 8 h; fluoroquinolone (ciprofloxacin or levofloxacin) + clindamycin 600 mg every 8 h; tigecycline 100 mg load, then 50 mg every 12 h[c] **If MRSA suspected:** Vancomycin, linezolid, daptomycin are indicated in addition to gram-negative and anaerobic coverage
Vascular insufficiency	*S. aureus* (MSSA or caMRSA), Streptococci, Enterobacteriaceae, anaerobes	Parenteral, broad- spectrum antibiotic therapy. Generally select antibiotics with activity against gram-positive, gram-negative, and anaerobic bacteria	Therapy options are similar to those for contiguous osteomyelitis (above)

CASE Application

1. Skin and soft tissue infections (SSTIs) may involve all layers of the skin, fascia, and muscle. Select the part of the skin that represents the outermost nonvascular layer.
   a. Epidermis
   b. Dermis
   c. Subcutaneous fat
   d. Fascia
   e. All of the above

2. Select the most common causative organism(s) for the majority of SSTIs.
   a. *Staphylococcus aureus*
   b. *Streptococcus pyogenes*
   c. *Pseudomonas aeruginosa*
   d. a and b
   e. All of the above

3. Select the answer that is defined as a superficial skin infection caused by β-hemolytic *Streptococcus* and *S. aureus*. Treatment consists of soaking the lesions with soap and water, use of skin emollients to dry areas, and antimicrobials. Topical mupirocin may be used alone when there are few lesions.
   a. Erysipelas
   b. Lymphangitis
   c. Impetigo
   d. Necrotizing fasciitis
   e. All of the above

4. Select the SSTI that may be treated with topical antimicrobials.
   a. Impetigo
   b. Cellulitis
   c. Diabetic foot ulcers
   d. a and c
   e. All of the above

5. CX is a 46-year-old patient diagnosed with lymphangitis. CX has a penicillin allergy, the allergy is a rash. Select the best antimicrobial to treat the lymphangitis in CX.
   a. Penicillin G (IV)
   b. Penicillin VK (oral)
   c. Clindamycin (IV)
   d. Trimethoprim-sulfamethoxazole (IV)
   e. Vancomycin (oral)

6. NV is diagnosed with cellulitis. Pharmacologic treatment of cellulitis is with an antibiotic that is active against penicillinase-producing strains of *S. aureus* (MSSA). Select the penicillin that is active against penicillinase-producing strains of *S. aureus*.

   a. Cephalexin
   b. Amoxicillin
   c. Clindamycin
   d. Doxycycline
   e. Nafcillin

7. Select the patient risk factor(s) for health care-associated MRSA (haMRSA).

   a. Prolonged hospitalization
   b. Nursing home residence
   c. Indwelling catheters
   d. Previous antimicrobial use
   e. All of the above

8. Select the antibiotic that would have activity against caMRSA and haMRSA.

   a. Vancomycin
   b. Clindamycin
   c. Daptomycin
   d. a and c
   e. All of the above

9. Select the antibiotic used in combination treatment of necrotizing fasciitis. This antibiotic is used to decrease bacterial toxin production, thereby limiting tissue damage.

   a. Cleocin
   b. Primaxin
   c. Augmentin
   d. Zosyn

10. Select the factor(s) that are involved in diabetic foot infections.

    a. Angiopathy
    b. Neuropathy
    c. Immunopathy
    d. All of the above

11. Select the factor(s) that may reduce the rate of diabetic foot infections.

    a. Periodic foot examinations
    b. Optimal glycemic control
    c. Smoking cessation
    d. All of the above

12. Select the IV antimicrobial used in the empiric treatment of cellulitis that is active/stable against the penicillinase-producing strains of *S. aureus* and group A streptococci.

    a. Dicloxacillin
    b. Cephalexin
    c. Amoxicillin-clavulanate
    d. Cefazolin

13. PU is a 58-year-old patient diagnosed with cellulitis. It was determined that the most likely pathogens causing the infection were *S. aureus* and group A streptococci. PU has a history of chronic renal insufficiency and the provider would like to use an antibiotic that does not have to be adjusted for renal dysfunction. Select the antibiotic that is *not* required to be adjusted for renal function.

    a. Nafcillin
    b. Ertapenem
    c. Ceftriaxone
    d. a and c
    e. All of the above

14. Select the beta-lactam antibiotic(s) that is (are) renally eliminated and require dose and/or interval modification in renal dysfunction.

    a. Keflex
    b. Ceftin
    c. Unasyn
    d. Zosyn
    e. All of the above

15. TR is a 29-year-old pregnant patient with a diagnosis of cellulitis. Select the antibiotic that may be used to treat systemic infections in a pregnant patient.

    a. Imipenem-cilastatin
    b. Doxycycline
    c. Levofloxacin
    d. Cefazolin

16. Select the antibiotic with the following mechanism of action: binds to components of the cell membrane and causes rapid depolarization, inhibiting intracellular synthesis of DNA, RNA, and protein.

    a. Piperacillin-tazobactam
    b. Imipenem-cilastatin
    c. Clindamycin
    d. Daptomycin
    e. Vancomycin

17. Select the antimicrobial that can alter glucose levels (hyper- or hypoglycemia).

    a. Levofloxacin
    b. Clindamycin
    c. Vancomycin
    d. Daptomycin

18. Select the fluoroquinolone that inhibits the CYP-450 system.
    a. Doxycycline
    b. Levofloxacin
    c. Trimethoprim-sulfamethoxazole
    d. Nafcillin
    e. Ciprofloxacin

19. Fluoroquinolones may prolong the QTc interval. Select the risk factor(s) for prolonged QTc interval.
    a. Uncorrected hypokalemia
    b. Concurrent administration of a medication known to prolong QTc interval
    c. Uncorrected hypomagnesemia
    d. a and c
    e. All of the above

20. Select the antimicrobial utilized to treat SSTIs that may cause photosensitivity.
    a. Ciprofloxacin
    b. Doxycycline
    c. Levofloxacin
    d. a and c
    e. All of the above

21. Select the parameter(s) that should be monitored with daptomycin.
    a. CPK
    b. Muscle weakness
    c. Serum creatinine
    d. All of the above

22. BD is a 24-year-old man with no known drug allergies who was initially treated with vancomycin for his cellulitis. His abscess culture after appropriate incision/drainage revealed caMRSA. He has clinically improved enough to receive oral antibiotics. Which of the following is an appropriate step-down antibiotic for BD?
    a. Cephalexin
    b. Amoxicillin-clavulanate
    c. Ceftriaxone
    d. Trimethoprim-sulfamethoxazole

23. Select the antimicrobial that may cause thrombocytopenia, especially with more than 2 weeks of therapy.
    a. Cleocin
    b. Zyvox
    c. Cubicin
    d. Tygacil

24. Which of the following is a reasonable duration of antimicrobial therapy for treating osteomyelitis?
    a. 1 week
    b. 2 weeks
    c. 3 weeks
    d. 6 weeks

25. Which of the following carbapenem antibiotics does *not* have coverage against *P. aeruginosa*?
    a. Ertapenem
    b. Doripenem
    c. Imipenem-cilastatin
    d. Meropenem

TAKEAWAY POINTS ››

- SSTIs can range in severity from mild, superficial, self-limiting infections to severe, deep-seated, life-threatening infections.
- The skin serves as a barrier between humans and their environment and functions as a primary defense mechanism against infections. The skin consists of the epidermis, the dermis, and subcutaneous fat.
- SSTIs may involve any or all layers of the skin, fascia, and the muscle. They may also spread far from the initial site of infection and lead to severe complications, such as sepsis, glomerulonephritis, endocarditis, or osteomyelitis.
- The majority of SSTIs result from disruption of normal host defenses by processes such as skin puncture, abrasion, or underlying disease (eg, diabetes).
- *Staphylococcus aureus* (*S. aureus*) and *Streptococcus pyogenes* (also known as group A streptococci and flesh-eating bacteria) account for the majority of SSTIs.
- Impetigo is a superficial skin infection caused by β-hemolytic *Streptococcus* and *S. aureus* and treated with first-generation cephalosporins or penicillinase-stable penicillins. Topical mupirocin may be used alone when there are few lesions.
- Lymphangitis is an inflammation of the lymphatic channel that ensues when a local skin infection is not contained, most often caused by GAS and treated with penicillin.
- Erysipelas is an infection of the superficial layers of the skin and cutaneous lymphatics. The intense red color and burning pain led to the common name of St. Anthony's fire. Erysipelas is treated with penicillin.

- Cellulitis is an acute, infectious process that represents a serious type of SSTI.
- Pharmacologic treatment of cellulitis is with beta-lactams active against penicillinase-producing strains of *S. aureus*. Examples include: dicloxacillin, cephalexin, and amoxicillin-clavulanate. Clindamycin or doxycycline may be used for patients with a penicillin allergy.
- Community-acquired methicillin-resistant *S. aureus* (caMRSA) is rapidly increasing in prevalence in SSTIs (including cellulitis).
- Necrotizing fasciitis (NF) is an uncommon, rapidly progressive, life-threatening infection of the subcutaneous tissue and fascia.
- Prompt surgical intervention is key in the treatment of NF.
- A high-dose beta-lactam/beta-lactamase inhibitor or carbapenem is used in combination with clindamycin to treat NF. Vancomycin, daptomycin, or linezolid should be included until MRSA is excluded.
- Foot ulcers and related infections are among the most common, severe, and costly complications of diabetes mellitus (DM).
- Chronically infected ulcers are polymicrobial and include additional pathogens like Enterobacteriaceae, MRSA, and *P. aeruginosa*.
- Osteomyelitis is most often due to *S. aureus*, but the patient's age, predisposing factors, type, and locations of the infection may change the primary pathogens and increase the number of potential pathogens (polymicrobial).
- Several different antibiotics may be utilized in the treatment of SSTIs. Properties of an antibiotic influence the use of one agent over the other. Key properties such as the side effect profile, drug interactions, formulation, and pregnancy category may influence the selection of an antibiotic.

REFERENCES

1. Dieffenbach CW, Tramont EC. Innate (general or nonspecific) host defense mechanisms. In: Mandell GL, Bennett JE, Dolin R, eds. *Principles and Practice of Infectious Diseases.* 6th ed. Philadelphia, PA: Elsevier; 2005:34-41.
2. Yagupski P. Bacteriologic aspects of skin and soft tissue infections. *Pediatr Ann.* 1993;22:217-224.
3. Stevens DL, Bisno AL, Chambers HF, et al. Practice guidelines for the diagnosis and management of skin and soft tissue infections. *Clin Infect Dis.* 2005;41:1373-1406.
4. Fung HB, Chang JY, Kuczynski S. A practical guide to the treatment of complicated skin and soft tissue infections. *Drugs.* 2003;63:1459-1480.
5. Pasternak MS, Swartz MN. Lymphadenitis and lymphangitis. In: Mandell GL, Bennett JE, Dolin E, eds. *Principles and Practice of Infectious Diseases.* 6th ed. New York, NY: Churchill Livingstone, 2006:1204-1214.
6. Rybak JM, LaPlante KL. Community-associated methicillin-resistant Staphylococcus aureus: a review. *Pharmacotherapy.* 2005;25(1):74-85.
7. Kaul R, McGeer A, Low D, et al. Population-based surveillance for group A streptococcal necrotizing fasciitis: clinical features, prognostic indicators, and microbiologic analysis of seventy-seven cases. *Am J Med.* 1997;103:18-24.
8. Wong C, Wang Y. The diagnosis of necrotizing fasciitis. *Curr Opin Infect Dis.* 2005;18:101-106.
9. Calhoun JH, Overgaard KA, Stevens CM, et al. Diabetic foot ulcers and infections: current concepts. *Adv Skin Wound Care.* 2002;15:31-45.
10. Lipsky BA, Berendt AR, Deery G, et al. Diagnosis and treatment of diabetic foot infections. *Clin Infect Dis.* 2004;39:885-910.
11. Williams DT, Hilton JR, Harding KG. Diagnosing foot infection in diabetes. *Clin Infect Dis.* 2004;39(2):S83-S86.
12. Thomas DR. Prevention and treatment of pressure ulcers: what works? What doesn't? *Cleveland Clin J Med.* 2001;68(8):704-707.
13. Livesley NJ, Chow AW. Pressure ulcers in elderly individuals. *Clin Infect Dis.* 2002;35:1390-1396.
14. Cannon BC, Cannon JP. Management of pressure ulcers. *Am J Health Syst Pharm.* 2004;61:1895-1907.
15. Morgan M. Hospital management of animal and human bites. *J Hosp Infect.* 2005;61:1-10
16. Bower MG. Managing dog, cat, and human bite wounds. *Nurse Pract.* 2001;26(4):36-38,41,42,45.
17. Taplitz RA. Managing bite wounds. *Postgrad Med.* 2004;116(2):49-55.
18. Centers for Disease Control and Prevention. Soft tissue infections among injection drug users: San Francisco, California—1996-2000. *MMWR Morb Mort Wkly Rep.* 2001;50:381-384.
19. Binswanger IA, Kral AH, Bluthenthal RN, et al. High prevalence of abscess and cellulitis among community-recruited injection drug users in San Francisco. *Clin Infect Dis.* 2000;30:579-581.
20. Bassetti S, Battegav M. Staphylococcus aureus infections in injection drug users: Risk factors and prevention strategies. *Infection.* 2004;32:163-169.
21. Lew DP, Waldvogel FA. Osteomyelitis. *Lancet.* 2004; 364:369-379

CHAPTER

23 Urinary Tract Infections

Daniel G. Dauner

FOUNDATION OVERVIEW

Urinary tract infections (UTIs) account for at least 7 million outpatient visits and 1 million hospital admissions annually in the United States (US). Total costs associated with UTIs are significant, exceeding $1.6 billion for ambulatory women with UTIs.[1,2]

UTIs can occur in all people, but certain factors increase the likelihood of exposure to uropathogens. These factors include age, sex, pregnancy, diabetes, the presence of a urinary catheter, and vaginal intercourse.[3] The overall self-reported annual incidence is 12.1% among women and 3% among men. Peak incidence among women (18.6%) occurs during ages 20 to 24 and peak incidence among men (7.3%) occurs in those 85 years and older.[2]

UTIs are divided into cystitis (lower tract and bladder) and pyelonephritis (upper tract and kidneys). Cystitis symptoms include dysuria, frequency, urgency, and occasionally suprapubic tenderness. Pyelonephritis is characterized as cystitis plus fever, flank pain, nausea, and vomiting.[1,4-5] Uncomplicated UTIs are infections occurring in women of childbearing age with structurally and neurologically normal urinary tracts. Complicated UTIs occur in urinary tracts with functional or structural abnormalities. In general, UTIs in men, pregnant women, children, and patients who are hospitalized or in health care-associated settings are considered complicated. These infections are more likely to be caused by resistant organisms.[5]

A UTI diagnosis requires a symptomatic patient with a positive urinalysis and urine culture. A urinalysis will identify pyuria, which is defined as ≥10 leukocytes/mm^3 of urine. Pyuria is nonspecific, and patients with pyuria may not have an infection. Urine in the bladder is normally sterile. Patients with a UTI usually have ≥10^5 bacteria/mL identified by culture.[6] Any organism, including fungi and viruses, colonizing the urinary tract can cause a UTI, but most are caused by bacteria.[3] The majority of uncomplicated UTIs are caused by gram-negative bacteria, with *Escherichia coli* being isolated in 70% to 95% of cultures. The most common gram-positive bacteria isolated are *Staphylococcus saprophyticus* and enterococci (Table 23-1).[7]

Asymptomatic bacteriuria is defined as the isolation of a specified quantitative count of bacteria in an appropriately collected urine specimen obtained from a person without symptoms or signs referable to urinary infection.[8] The diagnosis of asymptomatic bacteriuria should be based on results of a urine culture. Pyuria accompanying asymptomatic bacteriuria is not an indication for therapy. Pregnant women should be screened for bacteriuria by urine culture at least once during early pregnancy (12-16 weeks gestation) or at their first prenatal visit. All positive urine cultures, including asymptomatic bacteriuria, should be treated in pregnant women. Screening for and treatment of asymptomatic bacteriuria before transurethral resection of the prostate is recommended.[8,9]

PREVENTION

The following regimens are recommended for prophylaxis of recurrent UTIs.

- Nitrofurantoin 50 mg orally daily
- One-half trimethoprim-sulfamethoxazole (TMP-SMX) single-strength (SS) tablet (Trimethoprim 40 mg-sulfamethoxazole 200 mg) orally daily[1,6]

Recurrent UTI is defined as at least three UTIs in 12 months, without evidence of structural abnormalities. Prophylaxis should be considered in all renal transplant patients to prevent infection of the graft.[6] Systemic antimicrobial prophylaxis should not be routinely used in patients with foley catheters because of concern about selection of antimicrobial resistance.

TREATMENT

There are four responses of bacteriuria to antimicrobial therapy: cure, persistence, relapse, and reinfection. Bacteriologic cure is defined as negative urine cultures while on therapy and during the follow-up period (usually 1-2 weeks). Bacteriologic persistence is defined as persistence of bacteriuria after 48 hours of therapy. Sites of persistence within the urinary tract are the renal parenchyma, calculi, and the prostate. Bacteriologic relapse is defined as recurrence of bacteriuria 1 to 2 weeks post therapy by the same infecting bacteria. Relapse is often associated with renal infection, structural abnormalities, or chronic bacterial prostatitis. Reinfection occurs after the initial sterilization of the urine and is defined as the development of bacteriuria during therapy or at any time thereafter. Reinfection can be due to the same organism, different serotype of the same organism, or a different organism.[6]

There are many antimicrobials effective for the treatment of UTIs. There is no evidence to support any superiority of

TABLE 23-1 Bacterial Causes of UTIs[7]

	Uncomplicated (%)	Complicated (%)
Gram-Negative		
Escherichia coli	70-95	21-54
Proteus mirabilis	1-2	1-10
Klebsiella spp	1-2	2-17
Citrobacter spp	<1	5
Enterobacter spp	<1	2-10
Pseudomonas aeruginosa	<1	2-19
Other	<1	6-20
Gram-Positive		
Staphylococcus saprophyticus	5-10	1-4
Enterococci	1-2	1-23
Group B streptococci	<1	1-4
Staphylococcus aureus	<1	1-2
Other	<1	2

bactericidal medications over bacteriostatic medications for the treatment of UTIs. Bactericidal agents may be more beneficial in the treatment of relapsing UTIs. Nonpharmacological treatment options include hydration, urine acidification, and urinary analgesics. There is no evidence that hydration improves the results of appropriate antimicrobial therapy, and continuous hydration is inconvenient. Urinary acidification is frequently difficult to achieve. Urinary analgesics, such as phenazopyridine, have little place in the routine treatment of symptomatic infections.[6]

Three days of therapy at standard doses is effective treatment for uncomplicated lower UTIs in women. TMP-SMX is the recommended first-line therapy. Trimethoprim alone can be used in patients allergic to sulfa drugs. Due to increasing resistance to TMP-SMX among *E. coli* isolates, ciprofloxacin could be considered as first-line therapy.[6] *E. coli* resistance rates for ampicillin, TMP-SMX, ciprofloxacin, and nitrofurantoin are 37%, 22%, 5%, and 1%, respectively.[10-11] It is important to know your local sensitivity patterns when making treatment recommendations. Nitrofurantoin is an antibiotic used specifically for uncomplicated UTIs. It is not indicated for the treatment of pyelonephritis or perinephric abscesses and contraindicated in patients with a creatinine clearance less than 60 mL/min.[12-13] Ciprofloxacin and levofloxacin are the two fluoroquinolones indicated for UTIs.[14-15] Moxifloxacin is metabolized in the liver via glucuronide and sulfate conjugation, and it is not indicated for the treatment of UTIs.[16]

Table 23-2 summarizes the IDSA guidelines for treatment of uncomplicated acute bacterial cystitis and acute pyelonephritis.[17-18] Short-course therapy is not appropriate for women with a history of UTIs caused by antibiotic-resistant bacteria, 7 days or symptoms, complicated UTIs, or male UTIs. These patients should receive 7 to 14 days of therapy.[6,18] Pyelonephritis should be treated for 14 days. Severely ill patients with pyelonephritis may need to be hospitalized and require IV antimicrobial therapy. Appropriate IV antimicrobial therapy includes gentamicin, piperacillin-tazobactam, ceftriaxone, or a parenteral fluoroquinolone.[6]

Special Populations

UTIs in men are considered complicated. Urine cultures should be obtained in men because the causative organism is not as predictable as in women.[6,18] Initial therapy should be for 10 to 14 days.[18-19] Short-course therapy (3 days) has not been adequately studied in men and is not recommended.[6,18] Prostatitis should be treated for 4 weeks in order to reduce the risk of developing chronic prostatitis.[6,18-19]

The most important factors influencing the prevalence of UTIs in children are age and gender. In newborns, the rate for premature infants (2.9%) exceeds that for full-term

TABLE 23-2 Oral Recommendations for the Treatment of UTIs

Indication	Antibiotic	Dose (mg)	Frequency	Duration (d)
Acute cystitis[a]	TMP-SMX	1 DS tablet	bid	3
	Ciprofloxacin	250	bid	3
	Levofloxacin	250	Daily	3
	Amoxicillin	500	tid	3
	Amoxicillin/Clavulanic acid	500	tid	3
	Trimethoprim	100	bid	3
	Nitrofurantoin (Macrobid)	100	bid	3
Acute pyelonephritis	TMP-SMX	1 DS tablet	bid	14
	Ciprofloxacin	500	bid	14
	Levofloxacin	250-500	Daily	14
	Amoxicillin/Clavulanic acid	500	tid	14

[a]Acute cystitis is an uncomplicated UTI that occurs in females. Remember that all male UTIs are complicated.
Abbreviation: DS, double strength.

CASE Application

1. A 13-day-old former 35-week gestational age baby presents to the emergency room with a temperature of 102°F. The mother reports the baby has been feeding less, is constipated, and is very irritable. Which symptom is *not* a common symptom of meningitis in a neonate?

   a. Temperature of 102°F
   b. Decreased feeding
   c. Constipation
   d. Irritable appearance

2. The emergency physician is unable to obtain CSF after multiple attempts. Based on clinical findings, the team believes that the 13-day-old former 35-week gestational age baby may have meningitis. What is the best therapy to begin in this baby before sending her to a pediatric hospital?

   a. Ampicillin and gentamicin
   b. Ceftriaxone and gentamicin
   c. Vancomycin and cefotaxime
   d. Ampicillin and ceftriaxone

3. When the 13-day-old former 35-week gestational age baby is examined at the pediatric hospital, she is also noted to have some lesions. The team will be sending cultures of the lesions as well as HSV PCR of the CSF. Which of the following is an appropriate pharmacologic approach in this patient?

   a. Wait for the cultures and PCR results to come back, then modify therapy if needed.
   b. Change antibiotic therapy to ceftriaxone and vancomycin.
   c. Add IV acyclovir to the current antibiotic regimen.
   d. Add oral voriconazole therapy to the current antibiotic regimen.

4. If a neonate is begun on acyclovir for herpes simplex virus associated encephalitis, which of the following should be monitored?

   a. Serum creatinine
   b. Neutrophil count
   c. Urine output
   d. All should be routinely monitored

5. Which of the following explains the pharmacokinetic differences between a neonate and an adult with regards to gentamicin?

   a. Increased volume of distribution and increased clearance
   b. Increased volume of distribution and decreased clearance
   c. Decreased volume of distribution and increased clearance
   d. Decreased volume of distribution and decreased clearance

6. Which of the following patients are *not* recommended to receive a vaccine against *S. pneumoniae.*

   a. Healthy infants
   b. A 40-year-old with chronic obstructive pulmonary disease (COPD)
   c. A healthy 55-year-old
   d. A 35-year-old asplenic patient

7. What is the recommended route of administration for ampicillin for the treatment of bacterial meningitis?

   a. IV
   b. Oral
   c. Intramuscular
   d. Any of the above are reasonable

8. Which of the following is *not* common with bacterial meningitis?

   a. CSF WBC 5000 cells/ mm^3
   b. CSF WBC with 70% lymphocytes
   c. CSF glucose 23 mg/dL
   d. CSF protein of 250 mg/dL

9. Which of the following is correct regarding bacterial meningitis?

   a. A bacteria will be identified in majority of the cases.
   b. The likelihood of a bacteria being identified is unchanged if a patient receives antibiotics prior to CSF cultures.
   c. CSF cultures are not reliable for diagnosis.
   d. There is no role for blood cultures in the diagnosis of bacterial meningitis.

10. For which of the following agents is nephrotoxicity *not* one of the more common side effects that are monitored?

    a. IV gentamicin
    b. IV ceftriaxone
    c. IV vancomycin
    d. IV acyclovir

11. Which of the following vaccines is recommended to be given as part of routine child-care to otherwise healthy infants?

    a. MCV4
    b. MPSV4
    c. PCV13
    d. PPSV23

12. A 7-year-old patient with no significant past medical history presents to your hospital with fever, severe headache, photophobia, and neck pain. The physician does a lumbar puncture and sends the CSF collections to the laboratory. Based upon clinical diagnosis the patient

is suspected to have bacterial meningitis. Which of the following are likely pathogens associated with bacterial meningitis in this patient?

a. *Streptococcus pneumoniae* and *H. influenzae*
b. *Neisseria meningitidis* and *L. monocytogenes*
c. *Listeria monocytogenes* and group B *Streptococcus*
d. *Streptococcus pneumoniae* and *N. meningitidis*

13. Which of the following is consistent with the recommended empiric antibiotic therapy for a 7-year-old with bacterial meningitis.

a. Ceftriaxone
b. Ceftriaxone and ampicillin
c. Cefotaxime and vancomycin
d. Ampicillin and gentamicin

14. If the 7-year-old is determined to have *S. pneumoniae* meningitis, what chemoprophylaxis is suggested for close contacts?

a. Ceftriaxone
b. Rifampin
c. Ciprofloxacin
d. No chemoprophylaxis is indicated

15. What is the purpose of adding vancomycin to empiric therapy for bacterial meningitis in a 4-year-old patient?

a. To provide coverage against resistant *L. monocytogenes*
b. To provide coverage against resistant *S. pneumoniae*
c. To provide coverage against resistant *N. meningitidis*
d. Vancomycin is not needed in a 4-year-old with bacterial meningitis because *S. aureus* is unlikely

16. Which meningococcal vaccine would be suggested for outbreak control of A, C, Y, or W135?

a. MCV4
b. MPSV4
c. Either MCV4 or MPSV4 can be used
d. Neither MCV4 or MPSV4 are used for outbreak control

17. Which of the following groups has dexamethasone demonstrated a mortality benefit?

a. A 2-week-old with group B *Streptococcus* meningitis
b. A 17-year-old with *N. meningitidis* meningitis
c. A 35-year-old with *S. pneumoniae* meningitis
d. It has not demonstrated clear benefit for any type of bacterial meningitis

18. A 70-year-old man presents with fever, nausea, vomiting, severe headache, and extreme photophobia. CSF results: WBC 2500 cells/mm^3, 87% neutrophils, glucose 37 mg/dL, and protein 240 mg/dL. What type of CNS infection is his clinical picture most consistent with?

a. Bacterial meningitis
b. Aseptic meningitis
c. Viral encephalitis
d. Any of the above

19. Which of the following is consistent with the recommended antibacterial therapy for a 78-year-old patient with bacterial meningitis?

a. Vancomycin and ceftriaxone
b. Vancomycin, ceftriaxone, and ampicillin
c. Ampicillin and ceftriaxone
d. Ceftriaxone

20. Which of the following patients should *not* receive the varicella vaccine?

a. A 32-year-old with AIDS
b. A 1-year-old with primary immunodeficiency
c. A 25-year-old pregnant woman
d. The vaccine is contraindicated in all of these patients

21. Which of the following persons should receive the MPSV4 vaccine?

a. A 60-year-old who just had his spleen removed after a traumatic car accident
b. A 5-year-old with sickle cell disease
c. A 25-year-old microbiologist that works with *N. meningitidis*
d. A 33-year-old traveling to the meningitis belt

TAKEAWAY POINTS ››

- Bacterial meningitis is a serious infection that causes significant morbidity and mortality.
- Preventative measures against meningitis include preventative perinatal care and appropriate routine vaccinations.
- Pneumococcal conjugate vaccine should be given to all infants beginning between 6 and 8 weeks of age.
- Pneumococcal polysaccharide 23 valent vaccine should be given to any patient over 2 years old that (1) has a chronic disease (including adult asthma), (2) is immunocompromised, or (3) is an adult and smokes.
- Varicella and measles, mumps and rubella vaccines should not be given to persons who are immunocompromised, pregnant, or allergic to anything included in the vaccines (including neomycin or gelatin).
- MCV4 should not be given to patients that have a history of Guillain-Barré syndrome if they are not at considered high risk for meningococcal disease.
- Prompt empiric IV antibiotic therapy is necessary when bacterial meningitis is suspected.
- Antibiotic therapy should be chosen based upon common age-related pathogens.

- Ampicillin with either gentamicin or cefotaxime is recommended to cover the group B *Streptococcus*, *E. coli*, and *L. monocytogenes* that are likely in neonates.
- Vancomycin and either ceftriaxone or cefotaxime are recommended for empiric therapy against *S. pneumoniae* and *N. meningitidis* in older infants, children, and adults.
- In addition to the common bacteria that cause meningitis in adults, *L. monocytogenes*, is possible in older adults, as such ampicillin should be added to therapy in patients older than 50 years.
- Controversy exists regarding whether dexamethasone should be used in pediatric bacterial meningitis since *H. influenzae* is now uncommon.
- Dexamethasone has shown to improve mortality and other clinical outcomes in adult patients with pneumococcal meningitis.
- If dexamethasone is used, it should be given before or with the first dose of antibiotics.
- Viral meningitis is commonly caused by enterovirus and is usually self-limiting.
- When herpes simplex is considered as a possible cause of a CNS infection IV acyclovir should be started.
- Chemoprophylaxis with rifampin, ceftriaxone, or ciprofloxacin is recommended for certain *N. meningitidis* contacts.
- No chemoprophylaxis is recommended for contacts of patients with *S. pneumoniae* meningitis.

REFERENCES

1. Nicolosi A, Hauser WA, Beghi E, et al. Epidemiology of central nervous system infections in Olmsted County, Minnesota, 1950-1981. *J Infect Dis*. 1986;154:399-408.
2. Huttunen P, Lappalainen M, Salo E, et al. Differential diagnosis of acute central nervous system infections in children using modern microbiological methods. *Acta Paediatr.* 2009;98:1300-1306.
3. Holt DE, Halket S, de Louvois J, et al. Neonatal meningitis in England and Wales: 10 years on. *Arch Dis Child Fetal Neonatal Ed.* 2001;84:F85-F89.
4. Loughlin AM, Marchant CD, and Lett SM. The changing epidemiology of invasive bacterial infections in Massachusetts children 1984 through 1991. *American Journal of Public Health.*1995;85:392-394.
5. van de Beek D, de Gans J, Spanjaard L, et al. Clinical features and prognostic factors in adults with bacterial meningitis. *N Engl J Med.* 2004;351:1849-1859.
6. Nigrovic LE, Kuppermann N, Malley R. Bacterial meningitis study group of the Pediatric Emergency Medicine Collaborative Research Committee of the American Academy of Pediatrics. Children with bacterial meningitis presenting to the emergency department during the pneumococcal conjugate vaccine era. *Academic Emergency Medicine.* 2008; 15:522-528.
7. Galiza EP, Heath PT. Improving the outcome of neonatal meningitis. *Current Opinion in Infectious Diseases.* 2009;22:229-234.
8. Theodoridou MN, Vasilopoulou VA, Atsali EE, et al. Meningitis registry of hospitalized cases in children: epidemiological patterns of acute bacterial meningitis throughout a 32-year period. *BMC Infectious Diseases.* 2007;7:101.
9. Cabellos C, Verdaguer R, Olmo M, et al. Community-acquired bacterial meningitis in elderly patients: experience over 30 years. *Medicine.* 2009;88:115-119.
10. Leib SL, Täuber MG. Pathogenesis of bacterial meningitis. *Infect Dis Clin North Am.* 1999;13(3):527-548.
11. Romero JR, Newland JG. Viral meningitis and encephalitis: traditional and emerging viral agents. *Semin Pediatr Infect Dis.* 2003;14:72-82.
12. Tyler KL. Emerging viral infections of the central nervous system. *Arch Neurol.* 2009;66:939-948.
13. Tunkel AR, Glaser CA, Bloch KC, et al. The management of encephalitis: clinical practice guidelines by The Infectious Diseases Society of America. *Clin Infect Dis.* 2008;47:303-327.
14. Weil AA, Glaser CA, Amad Z, et al. Patients with suspected herpes simplex encephalitis: rethinking an initial negative polymerase chain reaction result. *Clin Infect Dis.* 2002;34:1154-1157.
15. Kupila L, Vuorinen T, Vainionpää R, et al. Etiology of aseptic meningitis and encephalitis in an adult population. *Neurology.* 2006;66:75-80.
16. Kennedy PGE. Viral encephalitis: causes, differential diagnosis, and management. *J Neurol Neurosurg Psychiatry.* 2004;75 (suppl I):110-115.
17. Irani DN. Aseptic meningitis and viral myelitis. *Neurol Clin.* 2008;26:635-655.
18. Tunkel AR, Hartman BJ, Kaplan SL, et al. Practice guidelines for the management of bacterial meningitis. *Clin Infect Dis.* 2004;39:1267-1284
19. World Health Organization. WHO-recommended standards for surveillance of selected vaccine-preventable diseases. Geneva 2003. Available at: http://www.who.int/vaccines-documents/DocsPDF06/843.pdf. Accessed January 6, 2010.
20. Negrini B, Kelleher KJ, Wald ER. Cerebrospinal fluid findings in aseptic versus bacterial meningitis. *Pediatrics.* 2000;105:316-319
21. Schrag S, Gorwitz R, Fultz-Butts K, et al. Prevention of perinatal group B streptococcal disease. Revised guidelines from CDC. *MMWR Recomm Rep.* 2002; 51:1-22.
22. Centers for Disease Control and Prevention. *Epidemiology and Prevention of Vaccine-Preventable Diseases.* In: Atkinson W, Wolfe S, Hamborsky J, McIntyre L, eds. 11th ed. Washington, DC: Public Health Foundation; 2009. Avaiable at: www.cdc.gov/vaccines/pubs/pinkbook/default.htm. Accessed August 30, 2010.
23. Wormser GP, Dattwyler RJ, Shapiro ED, et al. The clinical assessment, treatment, and prevention of Lyme disease, human granulocytic anaplasmosis, and babesiosis. *Clin Infect Dis.* 2006; 43:1089-1134.
24. Centers for Disease Control and Prevention. Pneumococcal PCR-based serotyping. http://www.cdc.gov/ncidod/biotech/strep/pcr.htm. Accessed January 6, 2010.

25. Hsu HE, Shutt KA, Moore MR, et al. Effect of pneumococcal conjugate vaccine on pneumococcal meningitis. *N Engl J Med.* 2009;360:244-256.
26. Centers for Disease Control and Prevention. Emergence of Massachusetts, 2001-2006. *MMWR Weekly.* 2007;56:1077-1080.
27. Vardakas KZ, Matthaiou DK, Falagas ME. Adjunctive dexamethasone therapy for bacterial meningitis in adults: a meta-analysis of randomized controlled trials. *Eur J Neurol.* 2009;16:662-673.
28. Rybak M, Lomaestro B, Rotschafer JC, et al. Vancomycin therapeutic monitoring: review and recommendations from the ASHP, IDSA and SIDP Task Force. *Am J Health-Syst Pharm.* 2009; 66:82-98.
29. Bradley JS, Wassel RT, Lee L, Nambiar S. Intravenous ceftriaxone and calcium in the neonate: assessing the risk for cardiopulmonary adverse events. *Pediatr.* 2009;123:e609-e613.
30. American Academy of Pediatrics. *2006 Red Book: Report of the Committee on Infectious Diseases.* In: Pickering LK, ed. 27th ed. Elk Grove Village, IL: American Academy of Pediatrics; 2006.
31. American Academy of Pediatrics Committee on Infectious Diseases. The use of systemic fluoroquinolones. *Pediatr.* 2006;118:1287-1292.

CHAPTER

25 Sepsis and Septic Shock

April D. Miller and S. Scott Sutton

FOUNDATION OVERVIEW

Sepsis is the leading cause of morbidity and mortality for critically ill patients, and the tenth leading cause of death overall.[1] There are 660,000 to 750,000 cases of sepsis annually. Care of septic patients costs $17 billion in the United States per year ($22,000-$50,000 per patient).[2] Sepsis is a continuum of physiologic stages characterized by infection, systemic inflammation, and hypoperfusion with widespread tissue injury. The American College of Chest Physicians and the Society of Critical Care Medicine developed definitions to utilize for sepsis (Table 25-1).[3] Risk factors for sepsis include extremes of age, cancer, immunodeficiency, chronic organ failure, genetic factors (male, and non-white ethnic origin in North America), bacteremic patients, and polymorphisms in genes that regulate immunity. Pulmonary, gastrointestinal, genitourinary, and bloodstream infections account for the majority of sepsis cases.[4]

Gram-positive and gram-negative bacteria, fungal species, and viruses cause sepsis. Gram-positive infections account for 30% to 50% of sepsis and septic shock cases. The percentages of gram-negative, polymicrobial, and viral sepsis cases are 25%, 25%, and 4%, respectively.[4-7] Multidrug resistant bacteria are responsible for approximately 25% of sepsis cases, are difficult to treat, and increase mortality. The rate of fungal sepsis increased 200% from 1979 to 2000.

The development of sepsis is complex and multifactorial.[8,9] The normal host response to infection is designed to localize and control bacterial invasion and initiate repair of injured tissue through phagocytic cells and inflammatory mediators. The key factor in the development of sepsis is inflammation, which is intended to be a local and contained response to infection or injury. Infection or injury is controlled through pro- and anti-inflammatory mediators. Systemic responses ensue when equilibrium in the inflammatory process is lost.

The clinical presentation of sepsis varies and the rate of development of clinical manifestations may differ from patient to patient (see Tables 25-1 and 25-2 for definitions related to sepsis and the systemic inflammatory response syndrome criteria).[3,10] Microbiologic cultures should be obtained before anti-infective therapy is initiated, however, antibiotic therapy should not be delayed until the return of Gram stain or culture data.[3] Cultures take 6 to 48 hours for results to be returned and may be negative (no growth of bacterial organisms). Negative cultures do not rule out infection.

Recognition and treatment of sepsis complications, particularly organ failure is essential to improve outcomes. The cumulative burden of sepsis complications is the leading factor in determining mortality.[11] The risk of death increases 20% with failure of each additional organ. Severe sepsis averages two failed organs, with a mortality rate of 40%. The most common complications are disseminated intravascular coagulation (DIC), acute respiratory distress syndrome (ARDS), acute renal failure (ARF), and hemodynamic compromise.

TREATMENT

The primary treatment goal of sepsis is to prevent morbidity and mortality. Treatment is aimed at early goal-directed resuscitation; reducing or eliminating organ failure; treating and eliminating the source of infection; avoiding adverse reactions of treatment; and providing cost-effective therapy. The speed and appropriateness of therapy administered in the initial hours after sepsis develops influence outcome, as is the case for acute myocardial infarction and cerebrovascular accidents. Pertinent issues in the management of septic patients are: (1) early goal-directed resuscitation of septic patients during the first 6 hours after recognition; (2) early administration of broad-spectrum anti-infective therapy; (3) activated protein C in patients with severe sepsis and high risk of death (Acute Physiology, Age, and Chronic Health Evaluation II [APACHE II] score greater than 25); (4) hydrocortisone for septic shock patients refractory to resuscitation and vasopressors; (5) glycemic control using continuous or intermittent insulin to maintain a glucose level less than 150 mg/dL (8.3 mmol/L); (6) adjunctive therapies: nutrition, deep vein thrombosis prophylaxis, stress ulcer prophylaxis, and sedation for mechanically ventilated patients[3] (Figure 25-1).

Early Goal-Directed Resuscitation

Early goal-directed resuscitation decreases 28-day mortality in septic patients.[12] The use of protocols aimed at resuscitation also improve outcomes. Crystalloid (such as 0.9% sodium chloride or lactated Ringers solutions) or colloid fluids (5% albumin or 6% hetastarch) are used for resuscitation, and clinical studies comparing the fluids found them to be equivalent.[13] Crystalloid solutions require more volume, which may lead to more edema (utilize caution in patients at risk for fluid overload, eg, congestive heart failure and ARDS); however, colloids

TABLE 25-1 **American College of Chest Physicians/ Society of Critical Care Medicine Definitions Related to Sepsis**

Condition	Definition
Bacteremia (fungemia)	Presence of viable bacteria (fungi) within the bloodstream
Infection	Inflammatory response to invasion of normally sterile host tissue by the microorganisms
Systemic inflammatory response syndrome (SIRS)	Systemic inflammatory response to a variety of clinical insults that can be either infectious or noninfectious
Sepsis	SIRS secondary to an infection
Severe sepsis	Sepsis associated with organ dysfunction, hypoperfusion, or hypotension
Septic shock	Sepsis with persistent hypotension despite fluid resuscitation
Multiple-organ dysfunction syndrome (MODS)	Presence of altered organ function requiring intervention to maintain homeostasis

Modified from Kang-Birken SL, Dipiro JT. Sepsis and septic shock, In: DiPiro JT, Talbert RL, Yee GC, Matzke GR, Wells BG, Posey LM, eds. *Pharmacotherapy: A Pathophysiologic Approach,* 7th ed. New York, NY: McGraw-Hill; 2008:1943-1955.

are significantly more expensive. Administer a fluid challenge to hypovolemic patients (hypotension or lactic acidosis) using either crystalloids 500 to 1000 mL or colloids 300 to 500 mL. Infuse over 30 minutes and repeat based on response (increase in blood pressure and urine output). More aggressive fluid rates and volumes and blood transfusion may be needed in patients with severe hypoperfusion.

When fluid resuscitation does not provide adequate arterial pressure and organ perfusion, vasopressors and/or inotropic agents should be initiated.[3, 12] Vasopressors are recommended in patients with a mean arterial pressure (MAP) lower than 65 mm Hg, after failed treatment with crystalloids.[14] Dopamine and norepinephrine are recommended as first-line vasopressors in patients with shock refractory to fluid resuscitation. In patients with myocardial dysfunction, inotropic therapy with dobutamine is recommended. Vasopressors and inotropes are effective in treating life-threatening hypotension and improving cardiac index, but complications such as tachycardia and myocardial ischemia require slow titration of the

TABLE 25-2 **Systemic Inflammatory Response Criteria**

Temperature	>38°C (100.4°F) *or* <36°C (96.8°F)
Heart rate	>90 beats/min
Respiratory rate	>20 breaths/minute *or* $PaCO_2$< 32 mm Hg
White blood cells	>12,000 cells/mm^3 *or* <4000 cells/mm^3 *or* >10% bands

adrenergic agents to restore MAP without impairing stroke volume. These agents may also cause peripheral hypoperfusion and necrosis, impair gut motility, and lead to hypoperfusion or ischemia.

Early Administration of Broad-Spectrum Anti-Infective Therapy

Appropriate empiric anti-infective therapy decreases 28-day mortality compared to inappropriate empiric therapy (24% vs 39%).[15, 16] Anti-infective regimens should be broad-spectrum since there is little margin for error. Administer broad-spectrum anti-infectives for initial therapy, as early as possible and within first hour of recognition of sepsis. If possible, appropriate cultures should be obtained prior to initiating antimicrobial therapy. Empiric anti-infective therapy should include one, two, or three drugs, depending on the site of infection and causative pathogens. Anti-infective clinical trials in sepsis and septic shock patients are scarce and have not demonstrated differences among agents. Therefore, factors that determine selection are site of infection, causative pathogens, community- or nosocomial-acquired infection, immune status of patient, patient history (underlying disease, previous cultures or infections, and drug intolerance), cost and antibiotic susceptibility and resistance profile for the institution.[3] Clinicians should be cognizant of growing prevalence of bacterial resistance in community and healthcare setting. Pharmaocokinetics of agents may be altered beacause septic patients may have altered volume of distribution due to initial resuscitation. Reevaluate the initial regimen daily to optimize activity, prevent development of resistance, reduce toxicity, and decrease costs. Initiate step-down therapy based on microbiologic cultures to prevent resistance and reduce toxicity and cost. Monotherapy is equivalent to combination therapy once a causative pathogen has been identified. Empiric therapy includes combination regimens to ensure coverage of causative organisms. Table 25-3 and Figure 25-1 provide guidelines to selecting appropriate empiric coverage. Average duration of anti-infective therapy for septic patients is 7 to 10 days. However, the durations vary depending on the site of infection and response to therapy. In addition to antimicrobial therapy, an anatomical site for infection should be identified. If feasible and indicated, this source should be contained (ie, removal of infected devices, tissue debridement, abscess drainage).[17]

Activated Protein C in Patients with Severe Sepsis and High Risk of Death

Recombinant human activated protein C (drotrecogin alfa) is recommended for patients at a high risk of death (Acute Physiology and Chronic Health Evaluation [APACHE] II score greater than or equal to 25, multiple organ failure, or septic shock) and no absolute contraindications related to bleeding.[3] Drotrecogin alfa has antithrombotic, anti-inflammatory, and profibrinolytic properties. The Recombinant Human Activated Protein C Worldwide Evaluation in Severe Sepsis (PROWESS) trial evaluated the effects of a 96-hour

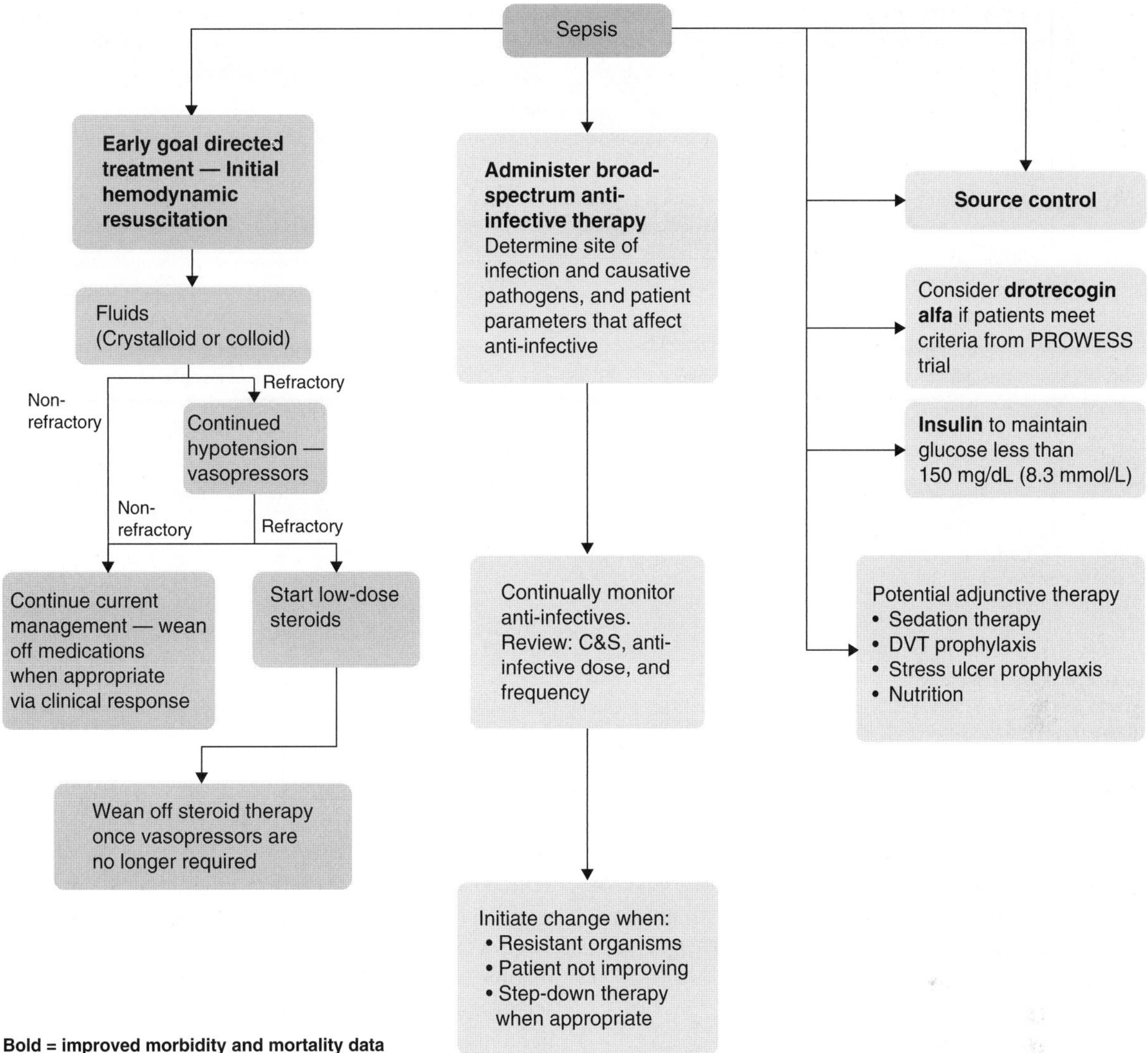

FIGURE 25-1 Therapeutic approach to sepsis.

Reproduced with permission from Sutton SS. Sepsis and septic shock. In: Chisholm-Burns MA, Schwinghammer TL, Wells BG, Malone PM, Kolesar JM, DiPiro JT, eds. *Pharmacotherapy Principles & Practice*. 2nd ed. New York, NY: McGraw-Hill; 2010:1347-1359.

continuous infusion of drotrecogin alfa.[18] Drotrecogin alfa decreased 28-day mortality compared to placebo (30.8% vs 24.7%). A higher incidence of serious bleeding occurred during the 28-day period in the drotrecogin alfa group (3.5%) than in the placebo group (2.0%). An additional open-label study, (ENHANCE) demonstrated that early (within the first 24 hours) administration of drotrecogin alfa is associated with improved outcomes.[19]

Drotrecogin alfa is not recommended for severe sepsis patients at low risk for death (APACHE score <20). The Drotrecogin Alfa (Activated) for Adults with Severe Sepsis and a Low Risk of Death (ADDRESS) trial evaluated the effects of a 96-hour continuous infusion of drotrecogin alfa in patients with low risk of death.[20] There were no statistically significant differences between drotrecogin alfa and placebo in 28-day mortality (18.5% vs 17.0%). As in previous trials, the rate of serious bleeding was higher for drotrecogin alfa during the 96-hour infusion at the end of the 28-day study period.

Hydrocortisone for Septic Shock Patients Refractory to Resuscitation and Vasopressors

Stress-induced adrenal insufficiency complicates 9% to 24% of septic patients and is associated with increased mortality.[3] Sepsis patients with shock refractory to resuscitation and vasopressors should receive IV hydrocortisone 200 to 300 mg per day in three or four divided doses.[3] Patients should be weaned from steroid therapy when vasopressors are no longer required. Previously, the adrenocorticotropic hormone (ACTH) stimulation test was recommended to identify candidates for hydrocortisone therapy. Its use in sepsis is no longer recommended.

Glycemic Control

Glycemic control improves survival in postoperative surgical patients and is recommended in septic patients. Following initial stabilization of septic patients, maintain

TABLE 25-3 Empirical Intravenous Antimicrobial Regimens in Sepsis

Infection (Site or Type)	Community-Acquired	Hospital-Acquired
Urinary tract	Third-generation cephalosporin (ceftriaxone) *or* fluoroquinolone (levofloxacin or ciprofloxacin)	Antipseudomonal penicillin *or* antipseudomonal cephalosporin *or* antipseudomonal carbapenem *plus* aminoglycoside
Community-acquired pneumonia	Third-generation cephalosporin *plus* a macrolide or doxycycline	
Health care-associated, ventilator-associated, or nosocomial pneumonia (early onset; no risk factors for MDR pathogens)		Third-generation cephalosporin *or* fluoroquinolone or ampicillin-sulbactam *or* ertapenem
Health care-associated, ventilator-associated, or nosocomial pneumonia (late onset and/or MDR pathogen risk factors)		Antipseudomonal penicillin *or* antipseudomonal cephalosporin *or* antipseudomonal carbapenem *plus* aminoglycoside *or* antipseudomonal fluoroquinolone *plus* vancomycin or linezolid
Intra-abdominal	Ampicillin-sulbactam *or* fluoroquinolone *plus* metronidazole	Piperacillin-tazobactam *or* imipenem or meropenem *or* cefepime *plus* metronidazole *or* ciprofloxacin or levofloxacin *plus* metronidazole
Skin and soft-tissue: Catheter-related Unknown source of infection	Nafcillin or cefazolin	Ceftriaxone ± vancomycin Vancomycin antipseudomonal penicillin ± antipseudomonal cephalosporin or antipseudomonal carbapenem *plus* aminoglycoside *plus* vancomycin

Abbreviation: MDR, multidrug resistant.

Reproduced with permission from Sutton SS. Sepsis and septic shock. In: Chisholm-Burns MA, Schwinghammer TL, Wells BG, Malone PM, Kolesar JM, DiPiro JT, eds. *Pharmacotherapy Principles & Practice*. 2nd ed. New York, NY: McGraw-Hill; 2010:1347-1359.

blood glucose levels less than 150 mg/dL.[3] Septic patients with high glucose levels should receive insulin with frequent blood glucose monitoring (every 1 to 2 hours until glucose values and insulin infusion rates are stable, then every 4 hours).

Adjunctive Therapy

Adjunctive therapy for patients with sepsis consists of enteral nutrition, deep vein thrombosis prophylaxis, stress ulcer prophylaxis, and sedation in agitated patients. Enteral nutrition is recommended in septic patients to meet the increased energy and protein requirements. Protein requirements are increased from 1.5 to 2.5 g/kg /d. Nonprotein caloric requirements range from 25 to 40 kcal/kg/d.

Deep vein thrombosis (DVT) and stress ulcer prophylaxis (SUP) are recommended for septic patients. Low-dose unfractionated heparin or low-molecular-weight heparin (such as enoxaparin or dalteparin) may be utilized.[21] Patients with contraindications to heparin therapy should receive mechanical prophylaxis using graduated compression stockings or intermittent compression devices.

Patients with severe sepsis and septic shock have risk factors placing them at high risk for stress ulcers, including coagulopathy, mechanical ventilation, hypotension, and in some patients, corticosteroid therapy.[22] Histamine-receptor antagonists (such as ranitidine) are more efficacious than sucralfate.[23] Proton pump inhibitors (such as omeprazole) have demonstrated equivalence to histamine-receptor antagonists.[24] The benefit of prophylaxis must be weighed against the potential effect of an increased stomach pH and development of ventilator-associated pneumonia.

Critically ill patients may require sedation when complex ventilator settings are used or when patients are difficult to ventilate.[3] Patients with progressive hypoxia leading to ARDS frequently require uncomfortable modes of mechanical ventilation. Mechanically ventilated patients should receive sedation by a protocol that includes a daily interruption or lightening of a sedative infusion until the patient is awake.[25, 26] The utilization of sedation protocols decreases the duration of mechanical ventilation, length of hospitalization, and tracheostomy rates.

CASE Application

1. Select the phrase that most accurately describes sepsis.
   a. Presence of bacteria in the bloodstream
   b. Systemic inflammatory response to a physiologic insult
   c. Persistent hypotension and altered organ function
   d. Systemic inflammatory response due to an infection

2. Select the phrase that most accurately describes severe sepsis.
   a. Bacteremia with a high colony count
   b. Bacteremia with the systemic inflammatory response syndrome (SIRS)
   c. Bacteremia with the systemic inflammatory response syndrome (SIRS) and organ dysfunction
   d. Bacteremia with the systemic inflammatory response syndrome (SIRS), organ dysfunction, and immune failure

3. Which of the following organisms cause sepsis?
   a. Gram-positive bacteria
   b. Gram-negative bacteria
   c. Viruses
   d. a and b
   e. All of the above

4. TK is a 32-year-old woman admitted to the intensive care unit with possible sepsis secondary to pneumonia. Her vitals signs are temperature 38.1°C, heart rate 80 beats per minute, and a respiratory rate 16 breaths per minute. She also has a white blood cell count of 15,500 cells/mm^3. Based on this information, does TK have sepsis?
   a. Yes, TK has sepsis because she has an infection source but meets no SIRS criteria.
   b. Yes, TK has sepsis because she has an infection source and meets two SIRS criteria.
   c. No, TK does not have sepsis because she has an infection source but does not have any organ failure.
   d. No, TK does not have sepsis because she does not have positive cultures.

5. Which of the following can help reduce or prevent the morbidity and mortality associated with sepsis?
   a. Preventing organ failures
   b. Early goal-directed resuscitation
   c. Eliminating the infection source
   d. All of the above

6. XJ is a 29-year-old woman who presents with severe sepsis including hypotension and decreased urine output. She has no significant past medical history. Select the appropriate initial regimen for early fluid resuscitation in XJ.
   a. 5% dextrose 500 mL
   b. 5% albumin 1000 mL
   c. 0.9% sodium chloride 1000 mL
   d. 0.45% sodium chloride 1000 mL

7. A patient with hypotension secondary to sepsis has a history of congestive heart failure and fluid overload. Select the appropriate colloid therapy for this patient.
   a. 5% albumin 500 mL
   b. 5% dextrose 500 mL
   c. 0.9% sodium chloride 500 mL
   d. 0.45% sodium chloride 500 mL

8. KT is a 65-year-old man with a history of end-state renal disease on hemodialysis admitted with severe sepsis likely secondary to an infected dialysis catheter. Which of the following represents the best order of events to manage KT sepsis?
   a. Drotrecogin alfa, fluids, microbiologic cultures, antimicrobial therapy
   b. Drotrecogin alfa, antimicrobial therapy, microbiologic cultures, fluids
   c. Fluids, microbiologic cultures, antimicrobial therapy, drotrecogin alfa
   d. Fluids, antimicrobial therapy, microbiologic cultures, drotrecogin alfa

9. What therapy should be administered within 1 hour of the recognition of sepsis?
   a. Broad-spectrum antimicrobial therapy
   b. Corticosteroids in patients with documented adrenal insufficiency
   c. Drotrecogin alfa therapy
   d. Vasopressor therapy

10. SL is a 32-year-old man with sepsis secondary to an intra-abdominal abscess. He has no significant past medical history and currently has been fluid resuscitated with a mean arterial pressure (MAP) of 70 mm Hg. What is the best treatment plan for SL?
    a. Ampicillin/sulbactam 3 g IV every 6 hours and transfer to the intensive care unit
    b. Ampicillin/sulbactam 3 g IV every 6 hours and surgical drainage of the abscess
    c. Amoxicillin/clavulanic acid 875 mg po every 12 hours and transfer to the intensive care unit
    d. Amoxicillin/clavulanic acid 875 mg po every 12 hours and surgical drainage of the abscess

11. Select the most appropriate duration of antimicrobial therapy in a patient with sepsis.
    a. 1 to 3 days
    b. 3 to 5 days
    c. 7 to 10 days
    d. 24 to 28 days

12. Which of the following is an absolute contraindication to therapy with drotrecogin alfa?
    a. Elevated endogenous levels of protein C
    b. Previous therapy with drotrecogin alfa
    c. High risk of death from sepsis
    d. Increased risk of bleeding

13. Select the brand name for drotrecogin alfa.
    a. Activated protein C
    b. Xigris
    c. Levophed
    d. Solu-Medrol

14. Identify the type of patient who is the best candidate for therapy with drotrecogin alfa.
    a. Severe sepsis and a low risk of death
    b. Severe sepsis and a high risk of death
    c. a and b
    d. None of the above

15. Which corticosteroid should be used to treat patients with septic shock refractory to vasopressor therapy?
    a. Prednisone
    b. Hydrocortisone
    c. Methylprednisolone
    d. Dexamethasone

16. What is the brand name for hydrocortisone?
    a. Deltasone
    b. Sterapred
    c. Solu-Medrol
    d. Solu-Cortef

17. What is the goal blood glucose for patients with sepsis?
    a. 80 to 110 mg/dL
    b. <120 mg/dL
    c. <150 mg/dL
    d. <200 mg/dL

18. Select the most appropriate regimen for glycemic control in a patient with sepsis.
    a. Metformin 1000 mg po bid
    b. Sitagliptin 100 mg po daily
    c. Insulin glargine 50 units qhs
    d. Insulin infusion

19. Which of the following nutrition regimens is (are) appropriate in a patient with severe sepsis secondary to pneumonia?
    a. Continuous tube feeding via a nasoduodenal tube
    b. Parenteral nutrition via a central IV catheter
    c. Parenteral nutrition via a peripheral IV catheter
    d. a and b
    e. b and c

20. Which of the following is a risk factor for stress-induced gastrointestinal bleeding?
    a. Mechanical ventilation
    b. Corticosteroid therapy
    c. Warfarin therapy
    d. All of the above

TAKEAWAY POINTS ››

- Sepsis is a serious illness and the number one cause of death in critically ill patients.
- Sepsis is defined as the systemic inflammatory response syndrome (SIRS) secondary to infection.
- SIRS criteria include hypo/hyperthermia, leucocytosis/leukocytopenia, tachypnea, and tachycardia.
- The majority of sepsis cases occur as a result of bacterial infection. Viruses and fungi account for only a minority of cases.
- Early goal-directed resuscitation with IV fluids is essential to improving morbidity and mortality in sepsis.
- Either crystalloids (0.9% sodium chloride, lactated ringers) or colloids (5% albumin, 6% hetastarch) can be used as fluids for resuscitation.
- Broad-spectrum, empiric antimicrobial therapy should be administered within 1 hour of the recognition of sepsis. If the source of sepsis is known, initial therapy may be narrowed.
- Once pathogen(s) have been identified, antimicrobial therapy can be tailored to specific organisms. Therapy should typically be continued for 7 to 10 days.
- Activated protein C (drotrecogin alfa) should be used in patients without contraindications and with two or more sepsis-induced organ dysfunctions and/or APACHE II scores ≥ 25.
- Patients with shock and hypotension refractory to fluid resuscitation and vasopressors should receive hydrocortisone 200 to 300 mg/d in three divided doses.
- The optimal target for blood glucose in sepsis patients is 150 mg/dL.
- Patients with sepsis should receive adjunctive therapies including enteral nutrition, deep vein thrombosis prophylaxis, and stress ulcer prophylaxis.

REFERENCES

1. Linde-Zwirble WT, Angus DC. Severe sepsis epidemiology: sampling, selection, and society. *Crit Care.* Aug 2004;8(4):222-226.
2. Angus DC, Linde-Zwirble WT, Lidicker J, Clermont G, Carcillo J, Pinsky MR. Epidemiology of severe sepsis in the United States: analysis of incidence, outcome, and associated costs of care. *Crit Care Med.* Jul 2001;29(7):1303-1310.
3. Dellinger RP, Levy MM, Carlet JM, et al. Surviving Sepsis Campaign: international guidelines for management of severe sepsis and septic shock: 2008. *Crit Care Med.* Jan 2008;36(1):296-327.
4. Vincent JL, Sakr Y, Sprung CL, et al. Sepsis in European intensive care units: results of the SOAP study. *Crit Care Med.* Feb 2006;34(2):344-353.
5. Harbarth S, Garbino J, Pugin J, Romand JA, Lew D, Pittet D. Inappropriate initial antimicrobial therapy and its effect on survival in a clinical trial of immunomodulating therapy for severe sepsis. *Am J Med.* Nov 2003;115(7):529-535.
6. Valles J, Rello J, Ochagavia A, Garnacho J, Alcala MA. Community-acquired bloodstream infection in critically ill adult patients: impact of shock and inappropriate antibiotic therapy on survival. *Chest.* May 2003;123(5):1615-1624.
7. Garnacho-Montero J, Garcia-Garmendia JL, Barrero-Almodovar A, Jimenez-Jimenez FJ, Perez-Paredes C, Ortiz-Leyba C. Impact of adequate empirical antibiotic therapy on the outcome of patients admitted to the intensive care unit with sepsis. *Crit Care Med.* Dec 2003;31(12):2742-2751.
8. Annane D, Bellissant E, Cavaillon JM. Septic shock. *Lancet.* Jan 1-7 2005;365(9453):63-78.
9. Cohen J. The immunopathogenesis of sepsis. *Nature.* Dec 19-26 2002;420(6917):885-891.
10. Levy MM, Fink MP, Marshall JC, et al. 2001 SCCM/ESICM/ACCP/ATS/SIS International Sepsis Definitions Conference. *Crit Care Med.* Apr 2003;31(4):1250-1256.

11. Guidet B, Aegerter P, Gauzit R, Meshaka P, Dreyfuss D. Incidence and impact of organ dysfunctions associated with sepsis. *Chest.* Mar 2005;127(3):942-951.
12. Rivers E, Nguyen B, Havstad S, et al. Early goal-directed therapy in the treatment of severe sepsis and septic shock. *N Engl J Med.* Nov 8 2001;345(19):1368-1377.
13. Finfer S, Bellomo R, Boyce N, French J, Myburgh J, Norton R. A comparison of albumin and saline for fluid resuscitation in the intensive care unit. *N Engl J Med.* May 27 2004;350(22):2247-2256.
14. Hollenberg SM, Ahrens TS, Annane D, et al. Practice parameters for hemodynamic support of sepsis in adult patients: 2004 update. *Crit Care Med.* Sep 2004;32(9):1928-1948.
15. Kumar A, Roberts D, Wood KE, et al. Duration of hypotension before initiation of effective antimicrobial therapy is the critical determinant of survival in human septic shock. *Crit Care Med.* Jun 2006;34(6):1589-1596.
16. Morrell M, Fraser VJ, Kollef MH. Delaying the empiric treatment of candida bloodstream infection until positive blood culture results are obtained: a potential risk factor for hospital mortality. *Antimicrob Agents Chemother.* Sep 2005;49(9):3640-3645.
17. Jimenez MF, Marshall JC. Source control in the management of sepsis. *Intensive Care Med.* 2001;27 (suppl 1):S49-S62.
18. Bernard GR, Vincent JL, Laterre PF, et al. Efficacy and safety of recombinant human activated protein C for severe sepsis. *N Engl J Med.* Mar 8 2001;344(10):699-709.
19. Vincent JL, Bernard GR, Beale R, et al. Drotrecogin alfa (activated) treatment in severe sepsis from the global open-label trial ENHANCE: further evidence for survival and safety and implications for early treatment. *Crit Care Med.* Oct 2005;33(10):2266-2277.
20. Abraham E, Laterre PF, Garg R, et al. Drotrecogin alfa (activated) for adults with severe sepsis and a low risk of death. *N Engl J Med.* Sep 29 2005;353(13):1332-1341.
21. Geerts W, Cook D, Selby R, Etchells E. Venous thromboembolism and its prevention in critical care. *J Crit Care.* Jun 2002;17(2):95-104.
22. Cook DJ, Fuller HD, Guyatt GH, et al. Risk factors for gastrointestinal bleeding in critically ill patients. Canadian Critical Care Trials Group. *N Engl J Med.* Feb 10 1994;330(6):377-381.
23. Cook D, Guyatt G, Marshall J, et al. A comparison of sucralfate and ranitidine for the prevention of upper gastrointestinal bleeding in patients requiring mechanical ventilation. Canadian Critical Care Trials Group. *N Engl J Med.* Mar 19 1998;338(12):791-797.
24. Conrad SA, Gabrielli A, Margolis B, et al. Randomized, double-blind comparison of immediate-release omeprazole oral suspension versus intravenous cimetidine for the prevention of upper gastrointestinal bleeding in critically ill patients. *Crit Care Med.* Apr 2005;33(4):760-765.
25. De Jonghe B, Cook D, Appere-De-Vecchi C, Guyatt G, Meade M, Outin H. Using and understanding sedation scoring systems: a systematic review. *Intensive Care Med.* Mar 2000;26(3):275-285.
26. Kress JP, Pohlman AS, O'Connor MF, Hall JB. Daily interruption of sedative infusions in critically ill patients undergoing mechanical ventilation. *N Engl J Med.* May 18 2000;342(20):1471-1477.

CHAPTER

26 Human Immunodeficiency Virus and Acquired Immunodeficiency Syndrome (HIV/AIDS)

P. Brandon Bookstaver and Carmen M. Faulkner

FOUNDATION OVERVIEW

Incidence/Prevalence

The disease that came to be known as acquired immunodeficiency syndrome (AIDS) was first reported in 1981 in cohort of young homosexual males affected by *Pneumocystis carinii* (now *jiroveci*) pneumonia.[1] The retrovirus now known as human immunodeficiency virus (HIV) was isolated in 1983 and determined to be the cause of AIDS.[2] Disease progression of HIV ultimately leads to the development of AIDS. Diagnosis of AIDS is based on the presence of an AIDS-defining condition or specific laboratory data as detailed later in the chapter.

Since 1981, 25 million deaths have been attributed to AIDS. Globally, there were an estimated 36 million people living with HIV in 2007 with an estimated 2.7 million new infections occurring annually.[3] At the end of 2006, an estimated 1.1 million persons in the United States (US) were living with HIV infection, with an estimated 21% undiagnosed. Fifty-six thousand new (HIV or AIDS) infections were diagnosed in the United States for 2006.[4]

Pathogenesis

HIV infects cells that express CD4 receptors (T-helper lymphocytes, monocytes, macrophages, dendritic cells, and brain microglia). The glycoprotein (gp) 160 on HIV interacts with CD4 and binds via the gp120 subunit of gp160. HIV then binds chemokine coreceptors (CCR5 and CXCR4). CD4 and coreceptor attachment of HIV to the target cell promotes membrane fusion via gp 41, a subunit of gp160, and then internalization of HIV genetic material and enzymes to begin the replication process. The virus is uncoated and reverse transcription of viral RNA to DNA begins via the enzyme reverse transcriptase. Once the DNA is transcribed, the proviral DNA is integrated in host cell DNA via the enzyme integrase. Once integrated, the transcription of DNA occurs within the nucleus causing nuclear release of viral genomic RNA and mRNA. Translation of the RNA and mRNA into viral proteins occurs and are then assembled by viral protease and packaged into a budding virion. Protease is responsible for cleaving a precursor polypeptide (gag-pol) into functional proteins that are necessary to produce mature, infectious virus. Once mature, the virus will infect other susceptible cells causing ongoing immune system destruction with approximately 10 billion new viruses produced each day. The rapid and complex HIV replication process is prone to mistakes causing numerous mutations, which allows the virus to evade the immune response and allows antiretroviral resistance to evolve.[5]

Clinical Presentation/Diagnosis

There are three primary modes of transmission for HIV: sexual (vaginal, anal, or oral), parenteral, and perinatal. Once infected, 40% to 90% of patients will have an acute retroviral syndrome which closely mimics a mononucleosis-like illness with fever, pharyngitis, lymphadenopathy, weight loss, night sweats, diarrhea, and nausea. Symptoms typically occur 2 to 6 weeks after exposure and can persist for 2 to 10 weeks. Acute infection is associated with a high viral load and a decrease in CD4 cells, but after several weeks an immune response is mounted, the viral load decreases and symptoms will begin to resolve. Since the acute symptoms of primary HIV infection are nonspecific, the diagnosis can be difficult.[6] After the symptoms of acute infection subside, patients infected with HIV are often asymptomatic for several years, usually until their CD4 levels decrease to 200 μL or less, at which time they are diagnosed with AIDS.

HIV infection is diagnosed by a reactive enzyme-linked immunosorbent assay (ELISA) and positive confirmatory test, typically a Western blot analysis. False negative ELISA tests may occur and are typically attributed to new infection since antibody production minimally takes 3 to 4 weeks after initial exposure and sometimes up to 6 months. Once diagnosed a patient should receive additional counseling, a complete medical history, and a baseline physical and laboratory evaluation (Table 26-1). Once HIV is diagnosed and a baseline evaluation is complete, HIV progression is routinely monitored by viral load, which quantifies viremia by measuring copies of viral RNA, and CD4 cell count. A CD4 count of ≤ 200 μL, CD4 percentage of < 14%, or development of an AIDS-defining condition indicates an AIDS diagnosis.

TABLE 26-1 **CDC Recommendations for Baseline Laboratory Evaluation of Newly Diagnosed HIV Patient**[7]

- CD4 T-cell count
- Plasma HIV RNA (viral load)
- Complete blood count
- Complete chemistry profile including transaminase levels
- Urinalysis
- Syphilis screening test (eg, RPR, VDRL, or treponema EIA)
- Tuberculin skin test (TST) or interferon-γ release assay (IGRA) (unless history of prior disease or positive tests)
- Anti-*Toxoplasma gondii* IgG
- Hepatitis A, B, and C serologies
- Pap smear (women)
- Fasting blood glucose and serum lipids at risk for cardiovascular disease and for baseline evaluation prior to initiation of combination antiretroviral therapy
- Genotypic resistance testing in patients with pretreatment HIV RNA >1000 copies/mL, regardless if therapy will be immediately initiated
  - Patients with HIV RNA levels of 500-1000 copies/mL, resistance testing also can be considered, but amplification is not always successful

AIDS-defining conditions include but are not limited to: *Pneumocystis jiroveci* pneumonia, *Mycobacterium avium* complex, esophageal candidiasis, and Kaposi sarcoma.[7] An AIDS diagnosis is forever, regardless of restoration of immune status or increase in CD4 cell count.

PREVENTION

Currently, there are no effective strategies that will cure HIV infection, therefore prevention of virus acquisition is key. Prevention strategies differ based on the mode of transmission. Sexual transmission predominately occurs by receptive anal or vaginal intercourse; however transmission can occur through any sexual contact including oral. Abstinence is the only 100% effective way to prevent sexual transmission of HIV, however barrier methods (male and female condoms, dental dam), reducing or eliminating high-risk behaviors like anal intercourse and decreasing the number of sexual partners can reduce the risk of transmission. Coinfection with other sexually transmitted diseases (STDs) can increase the risk of transmission, so treating other STDs can reduce transmission rates. Any person engaging in any high-risk behavior or having multiple sexual partners should be routinely screened for HIV and other STDs.[8]

Parenteral transmission includes intravenous (IV) drug injection with used needles or shared paraphernalia, needlestick exposure in the health care setting, receipt of contaminated blood products or organs. Prevention of parenteral transmission include stopping IV drug abuse, obtaining clean needles and not reusing any paraphernalia, and using personal protective equipment (PPE) in the health care setting when obtaining blood or injecting medication in a patient. The risk of HIV transmission secondary to receipt of blood products or organs has been dramatically reduced due to rigorous and updated screening mechanisms.[9,10]

Perinatal transmission can be dramatically reduced by screening all pregnant mothers for HIV during the pregnancy and providing antiretroviral therapy to those infected. Mothers with HIV should not breast-feed, because HIV can be transmitted through breast milk.[11]

TREATMENT

Highly active antiretroviral therapy (HAART) has revolutionized treatment for patients diagnosed with HIV/AIDS, leading to a decreased incidence of opportunistic infections, increasing life expectancy to nearly 80% of normal, and improved overall quality of life.[12] Historically, treatment regimens have been quite complex carrying a high-pill burden and less than favorable adverse effect profiles. Research and development in this area now makes it possible for many treatment-naïve patients, those with no previous exposure to antiretrovirals, to have the option of a single pill taken once daily. Since the discovery of the first antiretroviral, the nucleoside-reverse transcriptase inhibitor (NRTI), zidovudine (Retrovir, AZT) in 1981, five additional antiretroviral classes have been approved for therapy: nonnucleoside reverse transcriptase inhibitors (NNRTIs), protease inhibitors (PIs), fusion inhibitors, integrase inhibitors, and CCR5-receptor antagonists.[2,7] The initial step of viral entry into the CD4 cell is inhibited by fusion inhibitors (bind to portion of gp 41 on the viral surface) and CCR5-receptor antagonists (bind to CCR5 protein on CD4 cell to prevent virion binding). NRTIs target reverse transcriptase causing termination of DNA chain elongation acting as false nucleoside analogues. NNRTIs also act at the site of reverse transcriptase, binding to and inhibiting enzymatic activity, preventing viral conversion from RNA to DNA. Viral DNA integration into CD4 DNA is inhibited by integrase inhibitors, targeting the enzyme by the same name (integrase). The final step prior to viral budding from the CD4 cell is a viral "packaging" step, which is inhibited by the PIs. Current International AIDS Society (IAS) and Department of Health and Human Services (DHHS) guidelines recommend a backbone of therapy with two NRTIs plus either the NNRTI, efavirenz (Sustiva, EFV) or a PI boosted with ritonavir (Norvir, RTV) for treatment-naïve patients.[7,13] Fusion inhibitors, integrase inhibitors, and CCR5-receptor antagonists are recommended primarily in treatment experienced patients.[7,13] The question of when to initiate HAART has a quite dynamic answer. Based on existing data, guidelines support that all patients with a CD4 count < 350 cells/mm^3 or those with symptomatic disease regardless of viral load (HIV RNA) or CD4 count should be offered the opportunity to initiate treatment.[7,13] Tables 26-2 and 26-3 summarize treatment initiation recommendations.

TABLE 26-2 Recommendations on When to Initiate Antiretroviral Therapy[7,13]

Condition and/or Laboratory Data	Treatment Decision (IAS Guidelines)	Treatment Decision (DHHS Guidelines)
CD4 < 350 cells/mm^3	Treat	Treat
CD4 > 350 cells/mm^3	Defer; individualize therapy[a]	Defer; patient-clinician decision
AIDS-defining illness	Treat	Treat
HIV-associated nephropathy	Consider treatment	Treat
Coinfected with HBV	Consider treatment	Treat
Pregnancy	Treat	Treat

[a]Strongly consider in HIV RNA>100,000 copies/mL; CD4 decrease 100 cells/mm^3 in 12 months; excessive sexually transmitted infections.

Therapy should be individualized based on a number of patient factors including preexisting comorbid conditions, potential drug-drug interactions, socio-economic status, and long-term ARV effects. Drug-drug interactions are an especially important consideration facilitating treatment and dosing modifications. Many antiretrovirals have clinically relevant drug interactions, especially the PIs and NNRTIs that are metabolized through the CYP 3A4 system. Common drug interactions are listed by agent in the 2008 DHHS guidelines; all regimens should be evaluated for interaction potential when new ARV therapies are initiated.[13] Adherence to therapy is the cornerstone for successful outcomes in suppressing the HIV virus, helping to prevent opportunistic diseases and disease progression. As such, patients' desire and willingness to actively engage in their treatment and maintain adherence to therapy must be evaluated and confirmed prior to initiating treatment. Resistance testing is also recommended prior to initiating ARV therapy, as up to 10% of patients may be initially infected with a resistant strain.[7,13] In the treatment of all patients, having three active agents in the regimen, not counting ritonavir boosting as an individual agent, is associated with increased viral suppression and CD4+ cell count. Thus, in treatment experienced patients or those who have developed resistance, agent selection should be based on resistance profiles and those that will provide the best chance of success. Table 26-4 summarizes antiretroviral-specific dosing information, primary adverse effects, and clinical pearls.

TABLE 26-3 Antiretroviral Treatment Recommendations for Treatment-Naive Patients[7,13]

Antiretroviral Class	Treatment (IAS Guidelines)	Treatment (DHHS Guidelines)
NRTI	*Pref:* TFV + FTC or ABC + 3TC Alt: ZDV + 3TC	*Pref:* TFV + FTC Alt: ABC + 3TC
NNRTI	*Pref:* EFV Alt: NVP	*Pref:* EFV Alt: NVP
PI	*Pref:* LPV/r; ATV/r; DRV/r; FPV/r; SQV/r	*Pref:* ATV/r; DRV/r; LPV/r; FPV/r Alt: ATV; FPV/r; SQV/r

Abbreviation: r, ritonavir boosting.

SPECIAL POPULATIONS

Pediatrics

Initiation of therapy in children early in the disease course appears to be favorable in helping to slow disease progression. All children >1 year of age with AIDS or symptomatic disease should be initiated on therapy. Additionally children 1 to 5 years of age with a CD4 percentage <25% and children >5 years with a CD4 count <350 cells/mm^3 should also be initiated on HAART. Those with mild or asymptomatic disease should be considered for therapy with a high viral load (HIV RNA>100,000 copies/mL). Treatment principles are similar to those of adults, with a backbone therapy of two NRTIs plus either a boosted PI or NNRTI. Typically, zidovudine is recommended as one of the two NRTIs in the backbone as it is the most highly researched antiretroviral in this population. All antiretrovirals with an indication for pediatric use are noted in Table 26-4. Additionally, peripartum use of zidovudine is typically recommended over nelfinavir to reduce transmission in neonates from delivery of HIV-positive mothers.[14]

Renal and Hepatic Insufficiency

Preexisting renal and hepatic insufficiency should be strongly considered when choosing patient-specific antiretroviral therapy. Antiretrovirals such as tenofovir may cause nephrotoxicity, and thus should be used with caution in those with progressive renal disease. All protease inhibitors, specifically when boosted with ritonavir, should be used with caution in those with hepatic dysfunction. Dosing of all NRTIs except abacavir should be modified in patients with moderate to severe renal dysfunction. Specific dosing recommendations are detailed in Table 26-4.[7,13]

Postexposure Prophylaxis

Evaluation of possible HIV exposure should occur without delay. Given a substantial nonoccupational exposure risk from a patient known to be HIV positive, patients evaluated within 72 hours of exposure should be provided postexposure prophylaxis (PEP). Guidelines recommend that the NRTI backbone be chosen from either lamivudine or emtricitabine plus zidovudine or tenofovir in combination with efavirenz. Using lopinavir/ritonavir in combination with zidovudine plus lamivudine or emtricitabine is also an option. These regimens can be modified if resistance patterns of the potentially transmitted virus are known. Occupational exposure is handled similarly in regards to treatment options, with each institution being required to have specific guidelines for PEP and reporting.[9]

TABLE 26-4 **Antiretroviral Therapy Review**[7,12,13]

<table>
<tr><th>Antiretroviral</th><th>Adult Dosing Information</th><th>Adverse Drug Effects</th><th>Clinical Pearls and Notes</th></tr>
<tr><td colspan="4">Nucleoside/tide Reverse Transcriptase Inhibitors
Class-wide adverse effects: lactic acidosis, hepatic steatosis, lipodystrophy (atrophy and fat accumulation), hyperlipidemia</td></tr>
<tr><td>Abacavir (ABC)
(Ziagen)
(Epizicom with 3TC)
(Trizivir with ZDV + 3TC)</td><td>Dose: 300 mg bid; 600 mg daily
Renal: None
Hepatic: Mild impairment ↓ dose 200 mg bid; caution in moderate to severe impairment</td><td>Hypersensitivity reaction (3%-9%)—fever, rash, respiratory distress, GI, malaise, SOB; increased risk of MI</td><td>Available: 300 mg tablet; 20 mg/mL suspension
Notes: HLA-B*5701 screening recommended as risk determinant for hypersensitivity reaction only NRTI with no dose adjustment for renal dysfunction

*Pediatric indication</td></tr>
<tr><td>Didanosine (ddI)
(Videx EC)</td><td>Dose: >60 kg: 400 mg daily; <60 kg: 250 mg daily
Renal:<table><tr><td>CrCl</td><td>>60</td><td><60</td></tr><tr><td>30-59</td><td>200 mg</td><td>125 mg</td></tr><tr><td>10-29</td><td>125 mg</td><td>100 mg</td></tr><tr><td><10 or HD</td><td>125 mg</td><td>75 mg</td></tr></table>Hepatic: No adjustment</td><td>Pancreatitis, peripheral neuropathy, nausea, optic neuritis/retinal changes</td><td>Available: 125, 200, 250, and 400 mg EC tablets
Notes: Avoid in combination with d4T (increased toxicity); EFV + TFV (decrease in CD4 counts); take on empty stomach (food decreases C_{max} 43%)

*Pediatric indication</td></tr>
<tr><td>Emtricitabine (FTC)
(Emtriva)
(Truvada with TDF)
(Atripla with EFV and TDF)</td><td>Dose: 200 mg capsule daily; 240 mg solution daily
Renal:<table><tr><td>CrCl</td><td>Caps</td><td>Soln</td></tr><tr><td>30-49</td><td>200 mg every 48</td><td>120 mg every 24</td></tr><tr><td>15-29</td><td>200 mg every 72</td><td>80 mg every 24</td></tr><tr><td><15 or HD</td><td>200 mg every 96</td><td>60 mg every 24</td></tr></table>Hepatic: No adjustment</td><td>Generally well tolerated; hyperpigmentation of palms/soles (dark complexion)</td><td>Available: 200 mg capsule; 10 mg/mL solution
Notes: Anti-HBV activity—withdrawal/development of resistance may cause HBV flares

*Pediatric indication</td></tr>
<tr><td>Lamivudine (3TC)
(Epivir)
(Epizicom with ABC)
(Combivir with AZT)
(Trizivir with AZT + ABC)</td><td>Dose: 150 mg bid; 300 mg daily
Renal:<table><tr><td>CrCl</td><td>Dose</td></tr><tr><td>30-49</td><td>150 mg daily</td></tr><tr><td>15-29</td><td>150 mg × 1; 100 mg daily</td></tr><tr><td>5-14</td><td>150 mg × 1; 50 mg daily</td></tr><tr><td><5 or HD</td><td>50 mg × 1; 25 mg daily</td></tr></table>Hepatic: None</td><td>Generally well tolerated; pancreatitis in children; mitochondrial toxicities > FTC</td><td>Available: 150, 300 mg tablets; 10 mg/mL oral solution
Notes: Anti-HBV activity—withdrawal/development of resistance may cause HBV flares

*Pediatric indication</td></tr>
<tr><td>Stavudine (d4T)
(Zerit)</td><td>Dose: >60 kg: 40 mg bid; <60 kg: 30 mg bid
Renal:<table><tr><td>CrCl</td><td>>60</td><td><60</td></tr><tr><td>26-50</td><td>20 mg every 12</td><td>15 mg every 12</td></tr><tr><td>10-25 and HD</td><td>20 mg every 24</td><td>15 mg every 24</td></tr></table>Hepatic: None</td><td>Fatal lactic acidosis, lipodystrophies, peripheral neuropathies, hyperlipidemia, development of DM, rapid neuromuscular weakness</td><td>Available: 15, 20, 30, and 40 mg capsules; 1 mg/mL oral solution
Notes: Avoid in combination with ddI (increased toxicity; AZT [antagonism])

*Pediatric indication</td></tr>
</table>

(Continued)

TABLE 26-4 **Antiretroviral Therapy Review[7,12,13] (*Continued*)**

Antiretroviral	Adult Dosing Information	Adverse Drug Effects	Clinical Pearls and Notes
Zidovudine (AZT, ZDV) (Retrovir) (Combivir with 3TC) (Trizivir with 3TC + ABC)	*Dose:* 300 mg bid; 200 mg tid *Renal:* Severe (HD) = 100 mg every 6-8 h *Hepatic:* Caution in moderate-severe impairment, dose adjustment may be necessary	BMS (macrocytic anemia, neutropenia), N/V, asthenia, myopathy, hyperpigmentation of nail beds/mucosa, lipodystrophy, lactic acidosis	*Available:*100 mg capsule; 300 mg tablet; 10 mg/mL oral solution; 10 mg/mL IV solution *Notes:* Avoid in combination with d4T (antagonism) **Pediatric indication*
Tenofovir (TDF) (Viread) (Truvada with FTC) (Atripla with EFV + FTC)	*Dose:* 300 mg daily *Renal:* CrCl: Dose 30-49: 300 mg every 48 10-29: 300 mg twice a week <10 or HD: 300 mg every 7 d *Hepatic:* None	Nephrotoxicity (including Fanconi-like syndrome), asthenia, HA, diarrhea, N/V, flatulence	*Available:* 300 mg tablet *Notes:* Anti-HBV activity—withdrawal/development of resistance may cause HBV flares
Nonnucleoside Reverse Transcriptase Inhibitors (NNRTIs)			
Class-wide effects: rash, drug interactions with 3A4 inducers/inhibitors/substrates, long half-life means stepwise discontinuation			
Efavirenz (EFV) (Sustiva) (Atripla with FTC + TDF)	*Dose:* 600 mg at bedtime *Renal:* None *Hepatic:* None, caution in severe hepatic impairment	Rash, CNS effects (dizziness, HA, insomnia, vivid dreams/nightmares, inability to concentrate), HTG	*Available:* 50, 100, 200 mg capsules; 600 mg tablet *Notes:* Administering drug at bedtime limits CNS effects while awake; take on empty stomach (food increase C_{max} 40-80%) **Pediatric indication*
Nevirapine (NVP) (Viramune)	*Dose:* 200 mg daily × 14 d, then 200 mg bid *Renal:* None *Hepatic:* None, caution in severe hepatic impairment	Rash (4%-7%), SJS, hepatotoxicity, transaminitis, fever	*Available:* 200 mg tablet; 10 mg/mL suspension *Notes:* Risk of hepatotoxicity increased in ♀ CD4 > 250; ♂ CD4>400); 2-wk run-in dose decreases risk of rash development **Pediatric indication*
Etravirine (TMC125, ETR) (Intelence)	*Dose:* 200 mg daily *Renal:* None *Hepatic:* None, caution in severe hepatic impairment	Rash (15%), (SJS), N/V, HA, peripheral neuropathy	*Available:* 100 mg tablet *Notes:* Second-generation NNRTI. not currently recommended in treatment-naïve patients
Delavirdine (DLV) (Rescriptor)	*Dose:* 400 mg tid *Renal:* None *Hepatic:* None, caution in severe hepatic impairment	Rash (SJS), transaminitis, HA, fat redistribution	*Available:* 100, 200 mg tablets; 100 mg tablet can be dispersed in >3 oz to produce slurry *Notes:* Possesses inferior potency and HIV activity compared to other NNRTI, availability in the United States is limited due to manufacturer reduced production
Protease Inhibitors			
Class-wide adverse effects: GI, ↑ bleeding in hemophiliacs, hyperlipidemia (including HTG), DM, hepatotoxicity, drug interactions with 3A4 inhibitors/substrates			
Amprenavir (APV) (Agenerase)	*Dose:* 1400 mg bid *Renal:* Avoid in patients with ESRD *Hepatic:* Avoid in patients with hepatic failure	Rash, GI, oral paresthesias, HLD, HTG, fat maldistribution	*Available:* 15 mg/mL oral solution *Notes:* Solution contains PEG; CI in children <4, hepatic/renal failure; virtually replaced by FPV; only solution still available and limited in United States due to manufacturer reduced production **Pediatric indication*

(*Continued*)

TABLE 26-4 **Antiretroviral Therapy Review[7,12,13] (*Continued*)**

Antiretroviral	Adult Dosing Information	Adverse Drug Effects	Clinical Pearls and Notes
Fosamprenavir (fAPV, FPV) (Lexiva)	*Dose:* Treatment naïve: FPV 1400 mg bid; FPV 1400 mg + RTV 200 mg daily; FPV 700 mg + RTV 100 mg bid PI-experienced: FPV 700 mg + RTV 100 mg BID *Renal:* None *Hepatic:* Child-Pugh: 5-8 — 700 mg bid; 9-12 — Not rec.	Rash, GI, oral paresthesias, HLD, HTG, fat maldistribution	*Available:* 700 mg tablet; 50 mg/mL suspension *Notes:* Caution in sulfa allergic patients; pro-drug of APV; better tolerated than APV **Pediatric indication*
Atazanavir (ATV) (Reyataz)	*Dose:* 400 mg daily; ATV 300 mg + RTV 100 mg daily *Renal:* None *Hepatic:* Child-Pugh: 7-9 — 300 mg daily; >9 — Not rec.	Indirect hyperbilirubinemia, rash, prolonged PR interval, fat maldistribution	*Available:* 100, 150, 200 mg capsules *Notes:* Hyperbilirubinemia can serve as an indirect marker of adherence **Pediatric indication*
Indinavir (IDV) (Crixivan)	*Dose:* 800 mg every 8 h; IDV 800 mg + RTV 100 mg or 200 mg bid *Renal:* None *Hepatic:* Dose reduction in mild/moderate hepatic impairment to 600 mg every 8 h	Nephrolithiasis, urolithiasis, asymptomatic hyperbilirubinemia, musculoskeletal pain, hemolytic anemia	*Available:* 200, 333, 400 mg capsules *Notes:* Take on empty stomach (food decreases AUC 77% and C_{max} 87%); take 1.5 L fluid intake every 24 h
Lopinavir/Ritonavir (LPV/r, LPV/RTV) (Kaletra)	*Dose:* LPV 400 mg/100 mg bid; or 800 mg/200 mg daily in treatment naïve is an option *Renal:* None *Hepatic:* Caution in moderate to severe hepatic impairment	N/V/D (diarrhea can be treatment limiting)—higher with daily dosing, asthenia, hyperlipidemia (specifically HTG), transaminitis	*Available:* LPV/RTV 200/50 mg tablets (note 133/33 mg capsules no longer manufactured); LPV/RTV 400/100 mg per 5 mL oral solution *Notes:* Take solution with food (increase AUC 80% and C_{max} 54%), solution contains 42% ethyl alcohol, store solution under refrigeration, 60-d expiration at room temperature **Pediatric indication*
Nelfinavir (NFV) (Viracept)	*Dose:* 1250 mg bid; 750 mg tid *Renal:* None *Hepatic:* Caution in moderate to severe hepatic impairment	Diarrhea, flatulence, nausea, rash, transaminitis, phenylketonuria (w/ powder)	*Available:* 250, 625 mg tablets; 50 mg/g oral powder *Notes:* 1g powder contains 11.2 mg phenylalanine **Pediatric indication*
Ritonavir (RTV) (Norvir)	*Dose:* 100-400 mg per day daily/bid as PI booster *Renal:* None *Hepatic:* Caution in moderate to severe hepatic impairment	N/V/D, pancreatitis, hyperlipidemia (HTG), new onset diabetes, taste perversion, hepatitis	*Available:* 100 mg caps; 600 mg/7.5mL oral solution *Notes:* Food: Capsules ↑ 13% AUC; take with food if possible—primarily for GI; refrigerate capsules; 30-day expiration at room temperature; *do not* refrigerate solution **Pediatric indication*
Saquinavir (SQV) (Invirase)	*Dose:* SQV 1000 mg + RTV 100 mg bid *Renal:* None *Hepatic:* Caution in moderate to severe hepatic impairment	Hepatotoxicity, transaminitis, GI intolerance	*Available:* 200 mg capsules; 500 mg tablet *Notes:* Least effect on lipids of all PIs; higher pill burden and GI effects make this agent less preferred

(Continued)

TABLE 26-4 Antiretroviral Therapy Review[7,12,13] (*Continued*)

Antiretroviral	Adult Dosing Information	Adverse Drug Effects	Clinical Pearls and Notes
Tipranavir (TPV) (Aptivus)	*Dose:* TPV 500 mg + RTV 200 mg bid *Renal:* None *Hepatic:* Caution in moderate to severe hepatic impairment	Rash, hepatitis, transminitis, diarrhea, intracranial hemorrhage	*Available:* 250 mg capsules *Notes:* Caution in sulfa allergic patients; take with food (increased bioavailability); refrigerate stable for 60 d at room temperature; risk of rash increased in young women on oral contraceptives **Pediatric indication*
Darunavir (DRV) (Prezista)	*Dose:* DRV 600 mg + RTV 100 mg bid *Renal:* None *Hepatic:* Caution in moderate to severe hepatic impairment	Rash (SJS) ~ 7%, new onset DM, diarrhea, nausea, tansaminitis	*Available:* 300 mg tablet *Notes:* Caution in sulfa allergic patients; take with food (increased AUC and C_{max} by 30%) **Pediatric indication*
Fusion Inhibitors			
Enfuvirtide (T-20, ENF) (Fuzeon)	*Dose:* 90 mg SC bid *Renal:* None *Hepatic:* None	Injection site reaction, increased risk of bacterial pneumonia, hypersensitivity reaction	*Available:* 90 mg/mL syringes *Notes:* Reconstituted syringe stable for 24 h under refrigeration **Pediatric indication*
Integrase Inhibitors			
Raltegravir (MK-0518, RAL) (Isentress)	*Dose:* 400 mg bid *Renal:* None *Hepatic:* None	GI, transaminitis	*Available:* 400 mg tablet *Notes:* Relatively well-tolerated agent
CCR5 Receptor Antagonists			
Maraviroc (MVC) (Selzentry, Celsentri in Europe)	*Dose:* 300 mg bid; 150 mg bid in combination with 3A4 inhibitors; 600 mg bid in combo with 3A4 inducers *Renal:* None *Hepatic:* None, caution in severe hepatic dysfunction	Hepatotoxicity, respiratory distress (coughing), GI, dizziness, musculoskeletal	*Available:* 150 mg, 300 mg tablets *Notes:* Patients receiving both 3A4 inducers/inhibitors, should be dosed as if receiving inducer (600 mg bid), tropism testing required to detect presence of CCR5-tropic virus prior to use

Abbreviations: AUC, area under the curve; HA, headache; HLD, hyperlipidemia; HTG, hypertriglyceridemia; N/V, nausea/vomiting; PIs, protease inhibitors.

HIV AND UPDATES

HIV treatment frequently changes and requires consistent updating. Treatment guidelines are frequency modified and new medications/product labeling are common occurrences with HIV. See Table 26-5 for a list of approved HIV treatment medications and commonly used abbreviations. Please refer to www.cdc.gov/hiv or www.aidsinfo.nih.gov for up to date information on HIV treatment.

CASE Application

1. Select the statement that *most* accurately describes HIV.
   a. A DNA virus
   b. An RNA virus
   c. An RNA retrovirus
   d. A parasite
2. What is the primary mode of HIV transmission globally?
   a. Contaminated blood and tissue products
   b. Casual contact with an HIV-infected person
   c. Homosexual contact
   d. Heterosexual contact
3. What is the primary mode of HIV transmission in the United States?
   a. Heterosexual contact
   b. Homosexual contact
   c. Casual contact with an HIV-infected person
   d. Contaminated blood and tissue products
4. When is a person living with HIV classified as having an AIDS diagnosis?
   a. Diagnosis of *Pneumocystis jiroveci* pneumonia
   b. CD4 count decreases to 350 μL
   c. HIV viral load of > 100,000 copies/mL
   d. a and b only
   e. All of the above
5. LF is a 31-year-old man recently diagnosed with HIV. He presents to the HIV clinic for the first time and is eager to start treatment. What is your most appropriate course of action?
   a. Immediately begin therapy with a triple drug regimen
   b. Counsel the patient regarding HIV, transmission, prevention of transmission to others, answer his questions, and schedule another follow-up visit
   c. Obtain baseline labs and schedule another follow-up visit
   d. a and b only
   e. b and c only

TABLE 26-5 **Antiretroviral Table with Abbreviations**[2,7,12,13]

Generic Name (Abbreviation)	Brand Name	Manufacturer	Approval Date
Protease Inhibitors (PIs)			
Amprenavir (APV)	Agenerase	GSK	1999; withdrawn 2007
Atazanavir (ATV)	Reyataz	BMS	2003
Darunavir (TMC114/DRV)	Prezista	Tibotec	2006
Fosamprenavir (fAMP, FPV)	Lexiva (US); Telzir (Europe)	GSK	2003
Indinavir (IDV)	Crixivan	Merck	1996
Lopinavir/Ritonavir (rLPV; or LPV/RTV)	Kaletra	Abbott	2000; Meltrex formulation 2005
Nelfinavir (NFV)	Viracept	Pfizer	1997
Ritonavir (RTV)	Norvir	Abbott	1996
Saquinavir (SQV)	Invirase (hard gel); Fortovase (soft gel)	Roche	1995 1997; withdrawn 2005
Tipranavir (TPV)	Aptivus	BI	2005
Nucleoside/tide Reverse Transcriptase Inhibitors (NRTIs)			
Abacavir (ABC)	Ziagen	GSK	1998
Didanosine (ddI)	Videx	BMS	1991; Videx EC 2000
Emtricitabine (FTC)	Emtriva	Gilead	2003
Lamivudine (3TC)	Epivir	GSK	1995
Stavudine (d4T)	Zerit	BMS	1994
Tenofovir DF (TDF/TFV)	Viread	Gilead	2002
Zalcitabine (ddC)	Hivid	Roche	1992; withdrawn 2006
Zidovudine (AZT, ZDV)	Retrovir	GSK	1987
Nonnucleoside Reverse Transcriptase Inhibitors (NNRTIs)			
Delavirdine (DLV)	Rescriptor	Pfizer	1997
Efavirenz (EFV)	Susctiva (US); Stocrin (non-US)	BMS	1998
Etravirine (ETV, TMC125)	Intelence	Tibotec	2008
Nevirapine (NVP)	Viramune	BI	1996
Fusion Inhibitors			
Enfuvirtide (T-20)	Fuzeon	Roche/Trimeris	2003
CCR5 Antagonist			
Maraviroc (MVC)	Selzentry (US); Celsentri (elsewhere)	Pfizer	2007
Integrase Inhibitors			
Raltegravir (RAL)	Isentress	Merck	2007
Fixed-Dose Combinations			
Lamivudine/Abacavir	Epzicom (US); Kivexa (Europe)	GSK	2004
Tenofovir/Emtricitabine	Truvada	Gilead	2004
Tenofovir/Emtricitabine/Efavirenz	Atripla	Gilead and BMS	2006
Zidovudine/Lamivudine	Combivir	GSK	1997
Zidovudine/Lamivudine/Abacavir	Trizivir	GSK	2000

6. Select the most common signs of symptoms of primary HIV infection in an adult patient.
   a. Mononucleosis-like illness (fever, sore-throat, fatigue, weight loss)
   b. GI upset (nausea, vomiting, diarrhea)
   c. Lymphadenopathy
   d. Night sweats
   e. All of the above

7. Which of the following statements about HIV prevention is *true*?
   a. Condoms are 100% effective in preventing HIV transmission
   b. All pregnant women should be screened for HIV
   c. Only pregnant women who engage in high-risk behaviors should be screened for HIV
   d. IV drug abusers can reuse/share syringe hubs as long as a new needle is used
   e. None of these statements is true

8. Which of the following are targets for currently available HIV medications?
   a. Reverse transcriptase, protease, and integrase
   b. Reverse transcriptase, protease, and proviral DNA
   c. Reverse transcriptase, mRNA, protease, and integrase
   d. Reverse transcriptase, protease, mRNA, and proviral DNA

9. A health care worker has a higher risk of contracting HIV from a HIV-positive patient if:
   a. The health care worker has a deep needlestick injury and the patient has an undetectable viral load
   b. The health care worker has a superficial needlestick injury and the patient has an undetectable viral load
   c. The health care worker has a deep needlestick injury and the patient has a high viral load
   d. The health care worker has a superficial needlestick injury and the patient has a high viral load

10. One of the primary goals of HIV therapy is:
   a. Complete eradication of the virus
   b. Maintain CD4 count at the level it was when treatment began
   c. Durable and maximal suppression of HIV replication
   d. None of the above

11. A patient presents to the hospital with a 2-week history of a mono-like illness. All of her laboratory tests are within normal limits or are negative including her ELISA. The patient reports being sexually active with multiple partners. The most appropriate course of action is:
   a. Inform her that she does not have HIV and discharge home
   b. Inform her that she does not have HIV, but counsel her on HIV and STD prevention
   c. Inform her that she will need to complete a follow-up ELISA in 6 months
   d. Inform her that she will need to complete a follow-up ELISA in 6 months, and counsel her on HIV and STD prevention

12. In a patient receiving zidovudine therapy, which of the following could you expect to be elevated on laboratory evaluation?
   a. Blood urea nitrogen (BUN)
   b. Mean corpuscular volume (MCV)
   c. Serum creatinine
   d. Potassium

13. A treatment experienced patient receiving atazanavir therapy should avoid the addition of which of the following medications:
   a. Omeprazole
   b. Metronidazole
   c. Pravastatin
   d. Metoprolol

14. Which of the following treatment regimens would be considered appropriate in a treatment-naïve patient?
   a. Maraviroc + efavirenz + nevirapine
   b. Raltegravir + abacavir +indinavir + ritonavir
   c. Tenofovir + zidovudine + abacavir
   d. Lamviudine + zidovudine + lopinavir + ritonavir

15. In a patient with a history of acute chronic pancreatitis, which of the following medications should be avoided?
   a. Didanosine
   b. Darunavir
   c. Tenofovir
   d. Enfuvirtide

16. Which of the following properties are true of efavirenz?
   a. Should be taken with a high-fat meal.
   b. Is a common cause of vivid dreams and hallucinations.
   c. Is the NNRTI of choice in pregnancy.
   d. a and b

17. Which of the following antiretrovirals is/are available in an injectable form?
   a. Zidovudine
   b. Etravirine
   c. Enfuvirtide
   d. Darunavir
   e. a and c

18. Which of the following patients would be at highest risk for developing hepatotoxicity secondary to nevirapine therapy?
   a. A 31-year-old woman with a CD4+ count equal to 91 cells/mm^3
   b. A 21-year-old man with CD4+ count equal to 270 cells/mm^3
   c. A 50-year-old man with CD4+ count equal to 260 cells/mm^3
   d. A 25-year-old woman with CD4+ count equal to 265 cells/mm^3

19. Which of the following combinations of antiretrovirals should be avoided?
   a. Didanosine and stavudine
   b. Tenofovir and efavirenz
   c. Lamivudine and zidovudine
   d. Fosamprenavir and ritonavir

20. Which of the following antiretrovirals should be used with caution in patients with documented sulfa allergy?
   a. Fosamprenavir
   b. Tipranavir
   c. Darunavir
   d. a and b
   e. All of the above

21. Dosing of Selzentry (maraviroc) should be increased to 600 mg twice daily when combined with which of the following medications?
   a. Ketoconazole
   b. Clarithromycin
   c. Rifampin
   d. Warfarin

TAKEAWAY POINTS ››

- HIV is an RNA retrovirus affecting over 36 million patients globally.
- The three primary modes of transmission for HIV are sexual, parenteral, and perinatal.
- Viral load and CD4 cell counts are the primary laboratory tests used to monitor HIV progression.
- Symptoms of acute HIV mimic a mononucleosis-like illness with fever, pharyngitis, lymphadenopathy, weight loss, night sweats, diarrhea, and nausea.
- HIV infection is diagnosed by a reactive enzyme-linked immunosorbent assay (ELISA) and positive confirmatory test, typically a Western blot analysis.
- HIV antibody production minimally takes 3 to 4 weeks after initial exposure and sometimes up to 6 months.
- Currently there is no cure for HIV infection.
- Abstinence is the only 100% effective way to prevent sexual transmission of HIV.
- Barrier methods, reducing or eliminating high-risk behaviors like anal intercourse and decreasing the number of sexual partners can reduce the risk of sexual transmission.
- Perinatal transmission can be dramatically reduced if HIV-positive mothers appropriately take antiretroviral therapy and do not breast-feed
- Highly active antiretroviral therapy (HAART) has greatly decreased the incidence of opportunistic infections, increased life expectancy and quality of life.
- All patients with a CD4+ count <350 cells/mm^3 should be offered therapy.
- The backbone of therapy in treatment-naïve patients should consist of two nucleoside reverse transcriptase inhibitors (NRTI) plus either an nonnucleoside reverse transcriptase inhibitor (NNRTI) or boosted protease inhibitor (PI).
- Adherence, short- and long-term adverse effects, and drug-drug interactions are only a few of the important factors in patient-specific drug selection.
- At least three active agents, excluding ritonavir as a boosting agent, should be the goal of every regimen.
- Ritonavir is given at a low-dose in combination with other PIs as a "boosting" agent due to its potent CYP 3A4 inhibition.
- Primary adverse effects of the NRTI class include mitochondrial toxicities such as lipodystrophy, lactic acidosis, and hepatosteatosis.
- Thymidine analogues, zidovudine, stavudine, and didanosine have the greatest potential for mitochondrial effects.
- The PIs are all substrates of the CYP 3A system and associated with significant drug interactions.
- Treatment should always be initiated in pregnancy and specific agents such as efavirenz should be avoided due to teratogenic effects.
- Nonoccupational postexposure prophylaxis should be offered to patients at high-risk who present within 72 hours of exposure.

REFERENCES

1. Centers for Disease Control and Prevention. Pneumocystis pneumonia—Los Angeles. *MMWR*. 1981;30;250-52.
2. Fauci, A. HIV and AIDS: 20 years of science. *Nature Medicine*. 2003;9(7):839-843.
3. UNAIDS. The Global HIV Challenge—2008 Report on the Global AIDS Epidemic. Available at http://www.unaids.org. Accessed July 17, 2009.
4. Centers for Disease Control. HIV prevalence estimates—United States, 2006. *MMWR*. 2008;57(39):1073-1076.
5. Stevenson, M. HIV-1 pathogenesis. *Nature Medicine*. 2003;9(7):853-860.
6. Kassutto, S, Rosenberg ES. Primary HIV Type 1 Infection. *CID*. 2004;38;1447-1453.
7. Panel on Antiretroviral Guidelines for Adults and Adolescents. Guidelines for the use of antiretroviral agents in HIV-1-infected adults and adolescents. Department of Health and Human Services. November 3, 2008; 1-139. Available at http://www.aidsinfo.nih.gov/ContentFiles/AdultandAdolescentGL.pdf.
8. Simon V, Ho DD, Abdool Karim Q. HIV/AIDS epidemiology, pathogenesis, prevention, and treatment. *Lancet*. 2006;368:489-504.
9. Panlilo AL, Cardo DM, Grohskopf LA, Heneine W, Ross CS. Updated U.S. Public Health Service Guidelines for the Management of Occupational Exposures to HIV and Recommendations for Postexposure Prophylaxis. *MMWR*. 2005;54(RR09):1-17.
10. Centers for Disease Control and Prevention Divisions of HIV/AIDS Prevention. Basic information preventing transmission. 2008. Available at http://www.cdc.gov/hiv/topics/basic/index.htm#prevention. Accessed July 17, 2009.
11. Public Health Service Task Force. Recommendations for use of antiretroviral drugs in pregnant HIV-infected women for maternal health and interventions to reduce perinatal HIV transmission in the United States: living document. April 29, 2009. Available at http://www.AIDSinfo.NIH.gov. Accessed July 17, 2009.
12. Antiretroviral therapy cohort collaboration. *Lancet*. 2008;372:293-299.
13. Hammer SM, et al. International AIDS Society HIV/AIDS 2008 Treatment Guidelines. *JAMA*. 2008;300:555-570.
14. Working Group on Antiretroviral Therapy and Medical Management of HIV-Infected Children. *Guidelines for the use of antiretroviral agents in pediatric HIV infection*. February 23, 2009;1-139. Available at http://aidsinfo.nih.gov/ContentFiles/PediatricGuidelines.pdf. Accessed August 12, 2009.

CHAPTER

27 Tuberculosis

Kristen Cook

FOUNDATION OVERVIEW

Tuberculosis (TB) remains one of the top 10 causes of death in the world with 9.27 million new cases and approximately 1.7 million deaths in 2007.[1-2] The highest TB incidence occurs in Asia and Africa (86%).[1] The incidence is lower in the United States with 13,299 TB cases in 2007 and rates continue to decline in the United States.[3] The HIV-positive population has a significantly higher incidence than the general population and deserves additional attention for TB.[4]

Tuberculosis is caused by *Mycobacterium tuberculosis*, an acid-fast bacillus (AFB). Acid-fast bacteria retain their staining color after being washed with acid-alcohol washes.[5] Transmission of TB is person to person through inhalation of droplet nuclei in the air. The majority of patients infected with *M. tuberculosis* do not develop active, symptomatic, contagious disease; they are said to have latent tuberculosis infection.[6] Approximately 10% of those patients will go on to have active disease if not treated. Risk is highest in the first 2 years after infection.[6-7] Cell-mediated immunity is the body's main defense against TB.[6]

TB's main site of infection is pulmonary. Clinical presentation of pulmonary TB includes: productive cough, fever, weight loss, night sweats, and hemoptysis.[6] Extrapulmonary TB can develop in sites including: genitourinary, skeletal, central nervous system, pericardial system.[6] Disseminated TB can also occur in several parts of the body. Immunosuppression puts people at higher risk for forms of TB other than pulmonary.[6]

Targeted tuberculin skin testing is used to identify patients with TB infection. The Mantoux test is where tuberculin purified protein derivative (PPD) is injected intradermally on the inner portion of the forearm.[6] The induration at the injection should be read within 48 to 72 hours.[6] The size of the induration and the patient's risk determine whether the test is read as positive.[6] Patients who have previously received the bacillus Calmette-Guerin vaccine in another country can have a positive skin test due to the vaccine.[6] This vaccination is not recommended for most of the US population.[6] The QuantiFERON TB-Gold test measures the level of interferon gamma released in a blood sample in response to PPD.[8] This test can provide more rapid diagnosis confirmation than skin testing.[8] Sputum cultures, chest radiographs, and drug susceptibilities are obtained at first suspicion of active disease.[6]

TREATMENT

The goals of TB treatment include: controlling the spread of TB, reducing the development of drug resistance, and preventing relapse to active disease.[9] A four-drug regimen comprised of isoniazid, pyrazinamide, rifampin, and ethambutol is initiated in suspected active TB infection.[9] The combination therapy prevents selecting out drug-resistant organisms. Typical treatment for active disease includes an initial 2 month phase of four drugs and a continuation phase of 4 months (18 weeks) with two drugs.[9] First-line drug treatment regimens for TB recommended by the Center for Disease Control and Prevention are listed in Table 27-1. This continuation phase is extended to 7 months in the following patient groups: cavitary pulmonary TB with positive-sputum culture at the end of 2-month initial phase, if the initial phase did not include pyrazinamide, and those taking isoniazid-rifapentine once-weekly regimens who have positive-sputum cultures at the end of initial phase.[9] Directly observed therapy is recommended in patients receiving regimens of five times per week or less.[9] Ethambutol can be safely discontinued after drug susceptibility reveals the TB is susceptible to isoniazid and rifampin.[9] Baseline laboratory values before initiating treatment include: liver function tests, creatinine, bilirubin, and platelets. Routine monitoring of these parameters is not needed unless they are abnormal initially or clinical situation warrants rechecking.[9] For example, if any symptoms of liver toxicity are found at follow-up visits, this situation would warrant rechecking of baseline labs. Treatment in children is generally the same regimens as in adults with the exception that ethambutol is not included.[9]

Latent TB infection treatment should not be initiated until active disease has been ruled out. Latent TB infection is recommended to be treated with isoniazid monotherapy for 9 months unless contraindicated.[7] Acceptable latent TB infection treatment regimens are shown in Table 27-2. In children daily or twice-weekly isoniazid for 9 months is the preferred regimen.[7] Baseline laboratory monitoring is not always indicated for patients receiving latent TB therapy.[7] Patients taking isoniazid for treatment of latent disease who are over the age of 35 should have baseline liver function tests.[10] This group is at higher risk for liver toxicity.[10] The following populations should have the same baseline and routine laboratory monitoring as listed above in the active disease section: HIV-positive patients, pregnant women, postpartum women (3 months of delivery), chronic liver disease, and regular alcohol users.[7]

TABLE 27-1 First-Line Regimens for Active Pulmonary Tuberculosis

Drugs	Frequency	Time	Drugs	Frequency	Interval
Isoniazid, Rifampin, Pyrazinamide, Ethambutol	7 d/wk or 5 d/wk	8 wk	Isoniazid, Rifampin Isoniazid, Rifapentine[a]	7 d/wk or 5 d/wk or twice weekly[b] Once weekly	18 wk
Isoniazid, Rifampin, Pyrazinamide, Ethambutol	5-7 d/wk for 2 wk then twice weekly	8 wk	Isoniazid, Rifampin Isoniazid, Rifapentine[a]	Twice weekly[b] Once weekly	18 wk
Isoniazid, Rifampin, Pyrazinamide, Ethambutol	3 d/wk	8 wk	Isoniazid, Rifampin	3 d/ wk	18 wk
Isoniazid, Rifampin, Ethambutol	7 d/wk or 5 d/wk	8 wk	Isoniazid, Rifampin	7 d/wk or 5 d/wk or twice weekly	18 wk

[a]Should not be used in HIV-positive patients.

[b]Twice weekly rifampin in the continuation phase of treatment is not recommended for HIV-positive patients with CD4 counts <100 cells/m^3.

Reproduced with permission from Centers for Disease Control and Prevention. Treatment of tuberculosis, American Thoracic Society, CDC, and Infectious Diseases Society of America. *MMWR*. 2003;52(No. RR-11):1-63.

Outcome Evaluation

Effectiveness of TB therapy is determined by AFB smears and cultures. Sputum cultures should be sent for AFB staining and microscopic examination every 1 to 2 weeks until two consecutive smears are negative. This provides early evidence of a response to treatment. If sputum cultures continue to be positive after 2 months, drug susceptibility testing should be repeated, and serum concentration of the drugs should be checked.

Patient nonadherence is a serious problem with TB therapy. The most effective way to achieve adherence is with directly observed therapy (DOT). DOT also provides opportunities to observe the patient for toxicity, thus improving overall care.

Hepatotoxicity

Hepatotoxicity should be suspected in patients whose transaminases exceed five times the upper limit of normal or whose bilirubin is significantly elevated and in patients with symptoms such as nausea, vomiting, and jaundice. At this point, the offending agent(s) should be discontinued.

TABLE 27-2 Treatment Regimens for Latent Tuberculosis

Drug	Length of Treatment	Adult Dose
Isoniazid[a]	9 mo	300 mg daily
Isoniazid	9 mo	900 mg twice weekly
Isoniazid[b]	6 mo	300 mg daily
Isoniazid[b]	6 mo	900 mg twice weekly
Rifampin	4 mo	600 mg daily

[a]Preferred regimen

[b]Not recommended in HIV-positive patients

Reproduced with permission from Centers for Disease Control and Prevention. Targeted tuberculin testing and treatment of latent tuberculosis infection. *MMWR*. 2000;49(No. RR-6):1-6.

Specific Agents

Isoniazid

Isoniazid is a first-line agent against latent TB and also one of the first-line drugs in combination therapy for active TB. Isoniazid (INH) inhibits production of mycolic acids, which form a large part of the mycobacterial cell wall.[11] Metabolism of isoniazid occurs by acetylation and may be affected by genetic differences in slow and fast acetylators.[11] Currently there are no recommendations in testing for genetic differences that affect treatment. Dosing is typically 300 mg once daily or 900 mg for the once, twice, and three times weekly regimens in adults.[9] Caution should be used with this agent in patients with significant liver disease.[9] Pyridoxine (vitamin B6) 25 to 50 mg daily is recommended to be taken with isoniazid to help prevent drug-induced peripheral neuropathy.[9] Adverse effects of isoniazid include: rash, neuropathy, gastrointestinal upset, and hepatotoxicity.[9] Isoniazid-induced hepatitis is rare, but rates are increased in the elderly, pregnant women, postpartum women, alcohol abusers, patients with underlying liver disease, and when used in combination with rifampin.[9-12] Isoniazid should be discontinued immediately and not used again with confirmation of INH-induced hepatitis.[9] Ten to twenty percent of patients will have benign liver function tests elevations if all patients were monitored.[11]

Rifamycins

Rifampin is a first-line agent against active TB, when used in combination. Rifampin inhibits DNA-dependent RNA polymerase in bacterial cells.[11,13] Dosing is 600 mg for once daily and twice or three times weekly regimens in adults.[9] Rifabutin and rifapentine are other rifamycins which can be used in place of rifampin.[9] All three rifamycins have drug interactions with significant induction of cytochrome P-450, however rifabutin is a less potent enzyme inducer.[9] Rifampin, rifabutin, and rifapentine can significantly induce cytochrome P-450 and increases metabolism of several drugs including: oral anticoagulants, anticonvulsants, antiretrovirals, cyclosporine, oral contraceptives, and others.[11,13] The alternative rifamycins can also be used with intolerance to rifampin.[9] Adverse reactions to rifamycins include: pruritus, rash, gastrointestinal upset, flu-like syndrome, and rare hepatotoxicity.[9,13] Rifamycins also give urine, sweat, and tears a harmless reddish-orange color.[11]

Pyrazinamide

Pyrazinamide (PZA) is a first-line agent for active TB, when used in combination. PZA exerts its effects against dormant organisms inside macrophages.[9] Mechanism of action is uknown.[14] Dosing is 20 to 25 mg/kg/d in adults rounded to the nearest 500 mg tablets.[9] PZA is contraindicated in patients with severe liver disease and acute gout attacks. Caution should be taken in those with a history of gout.[14] Adverse reactions include: hepatotoxicity, gastrointestinal upset, and hyperuricemia.[11,14] Baseline liver function tests should be performed in patients with preexisting liver disease and if used with rifampin. [9,14]

Ethambutol

Ethambutol is a first-line treatment of active tuberculosis, when used in combination. Ethambutol targets mycobacterial arabinosyl transferase to inhibit cell wall production.[11] Ethambutol is added to the TB regimen to prevent rifampin resistance. Dosing in adults is 15 to 20 mg/kg/d rounded to the nearest dose using whole tablets (100 mg, 400 mg).[9] Dose adjustments are required for renal dysfunction.[9,15] Ethambutol is contraindicated in patients with optic neuritis as well as with those who would have difficulty determining visual acuity (children).[15] Ethambutol can cause retrobulbar neuritis, which presents as decreased visual acuity or red-green color blindness.[9,15] This can occur in one or both eyes and typically at higher doses.[9] Patients should have baseline visual acuity and color blindness assessed as well as continued monitoring for this adverse effect.[9]

Special Populations

Immunocompromised

All patients diagnosed with HIV should receive TB testing at diagnosis.[4] Patients with HIV and other immunocompromised hosts may be managed with chemotherapeutic agents similar to those utilized in immunocompetent individuals, although treatment is extended to 9 months. Highly intermittent regimens (twice or once weekly) are not recommended for HIV-positive TB patients.

HIV-positive patients can have a paradoxical reaction when antiretroviral therapy is initiated in TB-positive patients.[4] It is possibly thought to be a recovery of the immune response. It is often an exaggerated inflammatory response and self-limited. It can be treated with nonsteroidal anti-inflammatory or corticosteroids.[4]

Drug interactions with rifamycins are important in this patient population. Interactions among rifamycins, HIV-protease inhibitors, and nonnucleoside reverse transcriptase inhibitors are common and require dose and frequency modifications. Rifabutin provides an alternative rifamycin in this case but careful attention still must be paid to drug adjustments.[16]

Pregnant/Breastfeeding

Drug therapy is warranted in pregnant women with active TB. Treatment in pregnant patients with latent TB is more controversial. Patients with latent TB who are HIV positive or who have recently been infected with latent TB infection should be considered for treatment.[7] All pregnant and postpartum women should have baseline liver function tests before therapy initiation due to physiological increased risk for hepatotoxicity.[9] The first-line drug regimen in pregnancy consists of isoniazid, rifampin, and ethambutol. Pyrazinamide is not recommended due to potential concerns for safety in this population.[9] Known teratogens that should not be used include several second-line drugs: streptomycin, kanamycin, amikacin, and capreomycin.[9] Patients taking TB therapy can breastfeed.[9]

Multidrug Resistant TB

There are no standardized treatment regimens for multidrug resistant (MDR) TB. Treatment of MDR-TB is based on the patient's previous drug therapy, exposure history, geographic resistance patterns, and drug-susceptibility data. One important principle in multidrug resistant TB is to never change one drug at a time.[9] Two or more new drugs should be added to a regimen to lessen the likelihood of further resistance development.[9]

Treatment of MDR-TB consists of second-line antituberculosis drugs. Examples of second-line agents are cycloserine, ethionamide, streptomycin, amikacin/kanamycin, capreomycin, p-Aminosalicylic acid (PAS), and select fluoroquinolones.

CASE Application

1. JK is a 32-year-old HIV-negative new patient at the clinic you work at. He receives a Mantoux skin test that returns positive 2 days later. He was born in the United States and works as a prison guard. He injects heroin on a regular basis. His chest x-ray comes back normal, he has no symptoms of tuberculosis, and his smear culture is negative. What type of drug therapy would be appropriate for this patient?

   a. Isoniazid 300 mg daily × 9 months
   b. Rifampin 100 mg daily × 4 months
   c. No drug therapy needed
   d. Isoniazid 300 mg and rifampin 600 mg × 6 months
   e. Isoniazid, rifampin, ethambutol, and pyrazinamide

2. BCG vaccine should be given to which patient in the United States?

   a. A 10-year-old child
   b. A 2-month-old infant
   c. A 65-year-old man
   d. A 6-month-old infant
   e. None of the above

3. Which of the following is *not* a counseling point on rifampin?
   a. This medication can cause your body secretions to be an orange-red color.
   b. This medication can decrease the effectiveness of your oral contraceptives.
   c. This medication can cause you to need a decrease in your warfarin dose.
   d. This medication may cause gastrointestinal upset.
   e. This medication can cause your phenytoin concentrations to go down.

4. RS is a 25-year-old Hispanic woman who is recently diagnosed with active tuberculosis. Her physician asks what drug regimen you would recommend to treat her disease. She does not have any contraindications to any of the tuberculosis medications. You do not have susceptibility testing back yet.
   a. INH, RIF, PZA × 8 weeks, then INH, RIF × 18 weeks
   b. INH × 9 months
   c. INH, RIF × 9 months
   d. INH, RIF, EMB, FQ × 8 weeks, then INH, RIF × 18 weeks
   e. INH, RIF, EMB, PZA × 8 weeks, then INH, RIF × 18 weeks

5. Which of the following is true regarding acid-fast bacteria?
   a. They cause the majority of bacterial infectious diseases.
   b. *Mycobacterium tuberculosis* is the only type of acid-fast bacteria.
   c. Cultures of acid-fast bacteria grow faster than other bacteria.
   d. They retain their stained color even with acid-alcohol washes.

6. Select the primary method for transmission of tuberculosis.
   a. Inhalation
   b. Exposure to blood and/or bodily fluids
   c. Exposure to dead birds
   d. Hospitalization

7. What time period is the risk highest for conversion to active disease in those patients with latent tuberculosis infection?
   a. 10 years after exposure
   b. 8 years after exposure
   c. 6 years after exposure
   d. 4 years after exposure
   e. 2 years after exposure

8. Which of the following is *not* a sign/symptom of pulmonary tuberculosis?
   a. Weight loss
   b. Productive cough
   c. Headache
   d. Fever
   e. Night sweats

9. How long after a Mantoux skin test for TB infection is placed should it be read?
   a. 12 hours
   b. 24 hours
   c. 48 hours
   d. 96 hours
   e. 120 hours

10. Which patient group should get drug-susceptibility testing?
    a. All latent tuberculosis patients
    b. Latent tuberculosis patients over age 35
    c. All active tuberculosis disease patients
    d. Active tuberculosis patients over age 35
    e. Foreign-born cases of latent and active tuberculosis

11. Which medication is typically not included in the first-line regimen for children with active TB disease?
    a. Isoniazid
    b. Rifampin
    c. Pyrazinamide
    d. Ethambutol

12. The addition of which of the following drugs necessitates follow-up liver function tests in a patient being treated for latent TB infection?
    a. Naproxen
    b. Multivitamin
    c. Sertraline
    d. Acetaminophen
    e. Lisinopril

13. What is the preferred regimen for treating latent tuberculosis infection in adults?
    a. Isoniazid 300 mg daily × 6 months
    b. Isoniazid 300 mg daily × 9 months
    c. Rifampin 600 mg daily × 6 months
    d. Rifampin 600 mg daily × 9 months

14. Which of the following group or groups are at higher risk for hepatotoxicity related to their TB treatment regimens?
    a. Pregnant
    b. Postpartum
    c. Drinks 2 beers daily
    d. 65-year-olds
    e. All of the above

15. Which of the following is *not* a second-line agent for treatment of active TB disease?
    a. Streptomycin
    b. Ciprofloxacin
    c. Amoxicillin
    d. Capreomycin
    e. Ethionamide

16. The addition of pyridoxine (vitamin B6) helps protect against which isoniazid toxicity?
    a. Hepatotoxicity
    b. Peripheral neuropathy
    c. Gastrointestinal upset
    d. Rash

17. Which rifamycin has the least drug interaction?
    a. Rifampin
    b. Rifabutin
    c. Rifapentine
    d. Rocephin

18. Which of the following is an appropriate test of monitoring ethambutol toxicity?
    a. Creatinine
    b. Foot examination
    c. Snellen visual chart examination
    d. Complete blood count
    e. Triglycerides

19. Which of the following is a contraindication to pyrazinamide therapy?
    a. Acute gout attacks
    b. Chronic obstructive pulmonary disease
    c. Rheumatoid arthritis
    d. Asthma

20. Which of the following first-line TB drugs is recommended not to be given in pregnant patients?
    a. Isoniazid
    b. Rifampin
    c. Ethambutol
    d. Pyrazinamide

TAKEAWAY POINTS ››

- Tuberculosis is a common disease that causes significant morbidity and mortality, especially in the HIV-positive population.
- TB is caused by *M. tuberculosis*, an acid-fast bacilli and is a public health concern worldwide.
- Tuberculosis is transmitted by inhalation and not all people who are exposed develop active tuberculosis.
- The majority of patients exposed with competent immune systems develop latent TB infection. Latent TB infection is not contagious.
- Latent TB infection should be treated with INH to prevent people from converting to active disease later on in life. The risk for active disease is greatest 2 years after exposure.
- Mantoux skin tests are used to identify patients who have TB infection. The skin tests need to be read within 48 to 72 hours of placement.
- Common symptoms of active pulmonary TB include productive cough, night sweats, fever, fatigue, weight loss, and hemoptysis. Pulmonary TB is the most common type of active tuberculosis disease.
- The following diagnostic test should be done when active TB is suspected: chest x-ray, culture, and drug susceptibility.
- Drug treatment for active tuberculosis typically includes isoniazid, rifampin, ethambutol, and pyrazinamide for the first 2 months and isoniazid and rifampin for an extra 4 month continuation phase.
- HIV-positive patients typically have this continuation phase last for 7 months.
- Directly observed therapy is recommended for any regimen in which meds are given five times per week or less.
- Multi drug resistant tuberculosis treatment has no standard treatment regimen recommended.
- MDR-TB treatment is based on the patient's previous drug therapy, exposure history, patterns of resistance in area, and drug susceptibility data.
- Isoniazid should be used with caution in patients with preexisting liver disease as it can cause hepatotoxicity.
- Isoniazid hepatotoxicity is rare but increased in the following circumstances: rifampin use, increasing age, pregnant women, postpartum women, alcohol abusers, and underlying liver disease.
- Pyridoxine is given with isoniazid to help prevent peripheral neuropathy caused by isoniazid.
- Rifamycins induce cytochrome P450 significantly and can decrease the concentration of several medications. Rifabutin is often the preferred rifamycin in patients on antiretroviral regimens.
- All patients diagnosed with HIV should receive skin testing for tuberculosis.
- Pregnant women with active TB disease should receive treatment at time of diagnosis. Pyrazinamide is not included in TB treatment regimens of pregnant patients.

REFERENCES

1. World Health Organization. Global Tuberculosis Control: Epidemiology, Strategy, Financing: WHO Report 2009. Geneva, Switzerland.
2. World Health Organization. *The Global Burden of Disease: 2004 Update*. Geneva, Switzerland; 2008
3. CDC. *Reported Tuberculosis in the United States, 2007*. Atlanta, GA: U.S. Department of Health and Human Services, CDC; September 2008.
4. Centers for Disease Control and Prevention. Guidelines for prevention and treatment of opportunistic infection in

HIV infected adolescents and adults. *MMWR.* Early Release 2009;58:19-28.

5. Daniels R. *Delmars Guide to Laboratory and Diagnostic Tests.* Acid fast bacterial culture and stain, sputum. 2002. STAT REF! Online Medical Library. Available at http://online.statref.com/document.aspx?fxid=59&docid=25. Accessed August 30, 2009.
6. Diagnostic Standards and Classification of Tuberculosis in Adults and Children. This official statement of the American Thoracic Society and the Centers for Disease Control and Prevention was adopted by the ATS Board of Directors, July 1999. This statement was endorsed by the Council of the Infectious Disease Society of America, September 1999. *Am J Respir Crit Care Med.* 2000;161(4 Pt 1):1376-1395.
7. Centers for Disease Control and Prevention. Targeted tuberculin testing and treatment of latent tuberculosis infection. *MMWR.* 2000;49(No. RR-6): 1-6.
8. Centers for Disease Control and Prevention. Guidelines for using the QuantiFERON-TB Gold test for detecting Mycobacterium tuberculosis infection, United States. *MMWE Recomm Rep.* 2005;54(RR-15):49-55.
9. Centers for Disease Control and Prevention. Treatment of Tuberculosis, American Thoracic Society, CDC, and Infectious Diseases Society of America. *MMWR.* 2003;52(No. RR-11):1-63.
10. Isoniazid [package insert]. Pomona, NY: Barr Laboratories; 1998.
11. Chambers H: Antimycobacterial drugs. In: Katzung B, ed. *Basic and Clinical Pharmacology.* 8th ed. New York, NY: McGraw-Hill, 2001; 803-813.
12. Fountain F, Tolley E, Chrisman C, et al.. Isoniazid hepatotoxicity associated with treatment of latent tuberculosis infection. *Chest.* 2005;128:116-123.
13. Rifampin [package insert]. Philadelphia, PA: Lannett Company; 2007.
14. Pyrazinamide [package insert]. Atlanta, GA: Mikart Inc; 1994.
15. Ethambutol [package insert]. Eatontown, NJ: West-ward Pharmaceutical Corp; 2005.
16. Centers for Disease Control and Prevention. *Managing drug interactions in the treatment of HIV-related tuberculosis.* Atlanta, GA: Centers for Disease Control and Prevention; 2007.

CHAPTER

28 Invasive Fungal Infections

Douglas Slain

FOUNDATION OVERVIEW

Invasive fungal infections are associated with significant morbidity and mortality and occur most frequently in immunocompromised patients.[1] *Candida* species represent the fourth most common cause of bloodstream infections in hospitalized patients.[2] Over the past decade, the field of clinical mycology has changed dramatically and there has been a doubling of licensed medications available for systemic fungal infections. Advances in medical technology, including organ and bone marrow transplantation, cytotoxic chemotherapy, the widespread use of indwelling IV catheters, and the increased use of broad-spectrum antibiotics have contributed to the increase of fungal infections.

Fungi are eukaryotic organisms that exist in two basic forms, yeasts and molds (moulds).[3] Figure 28-1 displays how pathogenic fungi can be grouped based on their morphological characteristics. Yeasts are unicellular in nature whereas molds are filamentous. Some fungal organisms exist in both forms and are referred to as dimorphic fungi. Dimorphic fungi exist as molds in the environment and convert to parasitic yeast in the human body. Common dimorphic fungi that cause invasive infection are *Blastomyces dermatitidis*, *Histoplasma capsulatum*, and *Coccidioides immitis*.[3,4] Exposure to these organisms occurs in certain regions of the country and as such are termed endemic fungi.

The most common invasive fungal infections are caused by yeasts (*Candida* species).[5] Examples of *Candida* species include *C. albicans*, *C. glabrata*, *C. parapsilosis C. tropicalis*, *C. krusei, and C. lusitaniae*.[3,5] *Candida* are normal inhabitants of mucocutaneous surfaces of the human body and frequently colonize the female genital tract, gastrointestinal (GI) tract, and skin. These organisms can cause infections if they overwhelm host defenses and get into sterile areas. A classic example is seen with a proliferation in the number of *Candida* in the GI tract after broad-spectrum antibiotic use. Common invasive infections include bloodstream infections (candidemia) and/or invasive candidiasis (eg, peritonitis and hepato-splenic).[5] Risk factors for invasive candidiasis include neutropenia, diabetes, immunodeficiency diseases, high-dose corticosteroids, immunosuppressants, antineoplastic agents, total parenteral nutrition, receipt of antibiotics, surgery, and burns.

Cryptococcus neoformans is an encapsulated yeast found in soil or bird excrement that causes invasive infections less frequently than *Candida*.[3,6] *Cryptococcus neoformans* most often causes meningitis and respiratory infections in immunocompromised patients.

Molds cause fewer infections than yeasts because they affect patients with severely suppressed immune systems.[7] The most common molds that cause clinical infections are the *Aspergillus* species. Mortality from aspergillosis is very high.[8] *Aspergillus* is a ubiquitous mold that grows well on a variety of substrates, including soil, water, decaying vegetation, and organic debris. Common species of *Aspergillosis* infections are: (1) *Aspergillus fumigatus*, (2) *Aspergillus flavus*, and (3) *Aspergillus niger*. The term aspergillosis may be broadly defined as a spectrum of diseases attributed to allergy, colonization, or tissue invasion.

Diagnosis

Invasive fungal infections are often suspected in patients that show continued signs of infection despite broad-spectrum antibiotic therapy. This is especially true in immunocompromised patients. *Candida* and *Cryptococcus* may be isolated in a culture of body fluid like blood or cerebral spinal fluid (CSF).[9] Generally, fungi may take longer to grow in specimen cultures than bacteria. India ink is a stain that helps to identify the capsule of *Cryptococcus neoformans*.[6]

Diagnosis of molds and the endemic fungi may involve identifying organisms in blood or tissue. Serologic antibody testing or antigen detection may also be used in the diagnosis.[4,9] Two examples are the *Histoplasma capsulatum* antigen assay and the galactomannan antigen assay which is used in the diagnosis of aspergillosis. Computed tomography (CT) is a radiologic test that is often used to provide a better diagnostic yield than conventional x-rays. A classic finding in pulmonary aspergillosis is the "halo" and "crescent" signs.[8]

PREVENTION

Prophylactic use of antifungal agents has been employed for preventing serious fungal infections in bone marrow transplant (BMT) or hematopoietic stem cell transplantation (HSCT), high-risk leukemias, liver, and lung transplant patients.[10,11] The primary preventative agents have been oral or IV azoles (fluconazole or posaconazole). Some medical institutions use IV echinocandins or inhaled amphotericin B (lung transplants). Another preventative use of antifungals is the practice of secondary prophylaxis (suppression) of cryptococcal disease in HIV patients.[6] After a patient is treated for cryptococcal disease, they receive oral fluconazole 200 mg daily lifelong or until immune reconstitution.

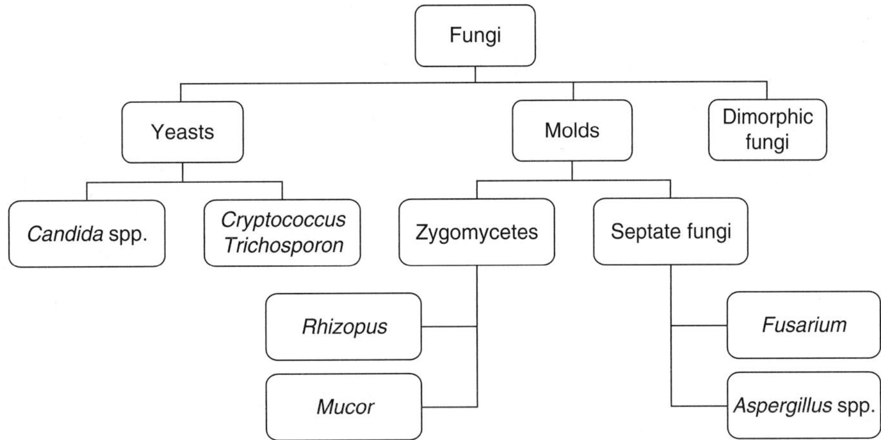

FIGURE 28-1 Morphologically, pathogenic fungi can be grouped as either filamentous molds or unicellular yeasts. Molds grow as multicellular branching, thread-like filaments (hyphae) that are either septate (divided by transverse walls) or coenocytic (multinucleate without cross walls).
Reproduced with permission from: Carver PL. Invasive fungal infections. In: DiPiro JT, Talbert RL, Yee GC, Matzke GR, Wells BG, Posey LM, eds. *Pharmacotherapy: A Pathophysiologic Approach*. 7th ed. New York, NY: McGraw-Hill; 2008:1973-2002.

TREATMENT

The approach to antifungal therapy for invasive fungal infections is determined by the type of fungal infection (yeast vs mold), severity of clinical presentation, patient's underlying immunosuppression, susceptibility data, potential toxicities, and drug interactions. Antifungals are associated with significant drug interactions and toxicities, especially with prolonged treatment courses. A majority of patients are treated empirically for invasive candidiasis before conclusive evidence of infection is available to direct therapy. Empiric therapy for invasive candidiasis should be considered in patients with persistent, unexplained fever and host deficits that predispose patients to candidemia (broad-spectrum antibiotics, presence of central venous catheter, patients with severe organ dysfunction or on dialysis, patients with neutropenia). Response to antifungal therapy for patients with invasive candidiasis is more rapid than for endemic fungal infections. Resolution of fever and sterilization of cultures are indications of response to fungal therapy.

Amphotericin B

Amphotericin B is a polyene antifungal that binds to fungal cell membrane ergosterol and promotes enhanced permeability leading to fungal cell death.[12] Amphotericin B is regarded as the gold standard systemic antifungal because of its fungicidal activity and broad spectrum of antifungal activity (molds and yeasts). Amphotericin B is administered intravenously and available as an injection (eg, 50 mg powder for reconstitution). The conventional formulation of amphotericin B is the desoxycholate (deoxycholate) formulation. This formulation must be prepared in dextrose 5% to facilitate the proper micellular dispersion.[13] Lipid-based (liposomal) formulations are also available and include liposomal, lipid-complex, and lipid colloidal dispersion formulations. All formulations of amphotericin B are nephrotoxic and can be associated with infusion-related toxicities (fever, chills, and rigors). Premedication with acetaminophen and diphenhydramine may help lessen infusion-related toxicities.[14] Administration of normal saline boluses before (and sometimes after) amphotericin B infusions may help ameliorate the nephrotoxicity.[15] The lipid-based agents appear less nephrotoxic than the conventional formulation of amphotericin B.[16] Unfortunately liposomal products are considerably more expensive than conventional amphotericin B. The liposomal formulation (AmBisome) has a lower rate of infusion-related reactions than other amphotericin B formulations.[17] Despite the improved safety profile; lipid-based amphotericin B formulations have not improved patient survival rates. Lipid-based formulations are dosed at 3 to 6 mg/kg versus the 0.5 to 1.5 mg/kg dose of conventional amphotericin B.[12,16] Amphotericin B is the treatment of choice for pregnant patients with fungal infections, because the other classes of antifungal agents have displayed some risk of teratogenicity (categories C and D). Anaphylaxis has been reported with amphotericin B products; therefore the drug should be administered under close clinical observation. Other key drug parameters for amphotericin B products include:

- Avoid use with other nephrotoxic medications
- Drug-induced renal toxicity usually improves with interrupting therapy, decreasing dosage, or increasing dosing interval
- Electrolyte wasting is associated with amphotericin products (hypokalemia, hypomagnesemia)

Flucytosine

Flucytosine (5-flucytosine, 5-FC, Ancobon) is a pyrimidine analog that penetrates fungal cells and is converted to 5-fluorouracil which interferes with fungal RNA and protein synthesis. Flucytosine is used as adjunctive treatment of systemic fungal infections (eg, susceptible strains of *Candida* or *Cryptococcus*). 5-FC is not used as monotherapy because resistance rapidly develops. The drug is available as an oral capsule and has good absorption and distribution (penetrates well into the CSF).[18] 5-FC is associated with causing bone marrow suppression (black box warning) leading to blood dyscrasias including neutropenia, thrombocytopenia, and anemia.[12] Gastrointestinal adverse effects are also common. Flucytosine is dosed 50 to 150 mg/kg in divided doses every 6 hours in patients with a CrCl greater than 40 mL/min. Use with extreme caution in patients with renal dysfunction and adjust dose as required. Peak serum concentrations should be monitored in all patients (particularly those with a CrCl less than 10 mL/min). Peak levels should not exceed 100 μg/mL.

Azole Antifungals

Azole antifungals interfere with the fungal enzyme 14α-demethylase thereby decreasing ergosterol synthesis and inhibiting cell membrane formation. Azoles are *well tolerated, but* are associated with cytochrome P-450 drug interactions and occasionally hepatotoxicity.[18,19] Most of the drug interactions are due to enzyme inhibition of CYP 3A4 metabolism. Itraconazole and voriconazole are also substrates of some of the P-450 isoenzymes and can have their metabolism affected by other drugs (Table 28-1).

Fluconazole (Diflucan) is the most commonly used triazole antifungal and is used for candidiasis, cryptococcal meningitis, and antifungal prophylaxis in allogenic bone marrow transplants. Fluconazole is well tolerated, available in oral (tablet and suspension) and IV formulations, and has a lower rate of drug interactions compared to other triazoles. Fluconazole penetrates into the CSF (thus used for meningitis) and is eliminated renally (dosage adjustments are required for renal dysfunction).[18] Fluconazole is effective against *Cryptococcus* and most *Candida* species (*C. albicans*, *C. parapsilosis*, and *C. tropicalis*), but is inactive against molds and *C. krusei*. Fluconazole's susceptibility to *C. glabrata* is usually defined as "susceptible-dose-dependent" (S-DD), meaning that larger dose may be needed to achieve cure in serious infections.[5] The daily dose for fluconazole is the same for oral and IV administration and depends upon the type of fungal infection (400-800 mg daily for candidemia, 150 mg for vaginal candidiasis; 400 mg for cryptococcosis [step-down therapy from amphotericin B + flucytosine]).

Despite having activity against *Candida* species and some molds including *Aspergillus*, itraconazole (Sporanox) is not used much because of its lack of predictable pharmacokinetics (eg, bioavailability). The capsule formulation of itraconazole displays wide interpatient oral absorption.[20] The bioavailability may be enhanced by administering itraconazole with cola, meals, or nutritional supplements and by avoiding concomitant acid-suppressing agents (eg, proton pump inhibitors, H2 antagonists, antacids). A newer oral solution provides more predictable absorption.[21] Due to differences in bioavailability; oral capsules and oral solution cannot be used interchangeably. An IV formulation with a cyclodextrin carrier molecule is available to reach approximate steady-state concentrations more rapidly.[22] Itraconazole can display negative inotropic effects and should be used with caution in patients with left ventricular dysfunction or a history of heart failure (black box warning). The daily dose of itraconazole depends upon the type of fungal infection (eg, 200-400 mg daily for aspergillosis; 200 mg daily for endemic fungal infections; 100-200 mg daily for esophageal candidiasis). Trough serum concentrations may be performed to assure therapeutic levels, especially in the face of oral therapy. Itraconazole has largely been relegated to treating the endemic fungi infections.[23]

Voriconazole (VFEND) is an analog of fluconazole that has a broader spectrum of activity against *Candida* species. In addition, the drug has good activity against *Aspergillus* and has become a drug of first choice for invasive aspergillosis.[24] Voriconazole

TABLE 28-1 **Drug Interactions, Administration, and Dietary Recommendations for Azole Antifungals**

Azole Antifungal	Drug Interactions (CYP 450)	Administration
Fluconazole (Diflucan)	I: 1A2 (weak); 2C9 (strong); 2C19 (strong); 3A4 (moderate)	Take with or without regard to meals
Itraconazole (Sporanox)	S: 3A4 (major)	Capsule: Absorption enhanced by food and possibly gastric acidity. Cola drinks have been shown to increase the absorption of the capsules in patients with achlorhydria or those taking H-2 receptor antagonists
	I: 3A4 (strong)	Solution: Take on an empty stomach
		Capsules and oral solutions are not interchangeable; doses greater than 200 mg are given in two divided doses
Voriconazole (Vfend)	S: 2C9 (major); 2C19 (major); 3A4 (minor); I: 2C9 (weak); 2C19 (weak); 3A4 (moderate)	Oral: Should be taken 1 h before or 1 h after a meal
		Dietary: Tablets contain lactose—avoid in lactose intolerance; suspension contains sucrose—use caution in sucrose/fructose malabsorption
Posaconazole (Noxafil)	I: 3A4 (strong)	Administer with food; food and/or nutritional supplement increases absorption; fasting states do not provide sufficient absorption to ensure adequate plasma concentration.

I, inhibitor of CYP isoenzyme; S, substrate of CYP isoenzyme.

is subject to a large number of drug interactions and has been associated with reversible visual disturbances.[25] Voriconazole drug interactions are dose dependent, as they exhibit unpredictable nonlinear pharmacokinetics; thus, drug interactions are more difficult to predict and manage. Studies indicate that CYP 2C19 is significantly involved in the metabolism of voriconazole. This enzyme exhibits genetic polymorphism; about 3% to 5% of Caucasians and 12% to 23% of Asians are expected to be poor metabolizers of voriconazole. Voriconazole is available in both oral and cyclodextrin IV formulations. There are concerns about the IV cyclodextrin carrier accumulating in and exacerbating renal failure. Visual changes, including blurred vision, changes in visual acuity, color perception, and photophobia, are commonly associated with treatment. Patients should be warned to avoid tasks which depend on vision, including operating machinery or driving. Changes are reversible on discontinuation following brief exposure (less than 28 days). The daily dose of voriconazole depends upon the type of fungal infection (aspergillosis 6 mg/kg every 12 hours on day 1 followed by 4 mg/kg every 12 hours; esophageal candidiasis 200 mg every 12 hours). Patients with mild-moderate hepatic dysfunction (Child Pugh class A and B) should receive a normal loading dose followed by 2 mg/kg every 12 hours. Voriconazole should only be used in severe hepatic dysfunction when the benefits outweigh the risks. In patients with CrCl less than 50 mL/min, accumulation of the IV vehicle cyclodextrin occurs. After the initial IV loading dose, oral voriconazole should be administered to these patients, unless an assessment of the benefit: risk to the patient justifies the use of IV voriconazole.

Posaconazole (Noxafil) is approved for prophylaxis of *Candida* and *Aspergillus* infections in high-risk neutropenic patients and in the treatment of oropharyngeal candidasis.[26] Posaconazole is available in an oral suspension and has a variable absorption. The absorption can be enhanced by administering with meals or nutritional supplements and by avoiding concomitant acid-suppressing agents.[27] The dose of posaconazole depends upon the type of fungal infection. Posaconazole is dosed 200 mg tid for prophylaxis (*Aspergillus* and *Candida*) and 400 mg twice daily for treatment of *Candida* infections.

Echinocandins

There are three echinocandin antifungals and they are caspofungin (Cancidas), micafungin (Mycamine), and anidulafungin (Eraxis). Echinocandins inhibit the fungal enzyme (1, 3) β-D-glucan synthase; which inhibits the formation (1, 3) β-D-glucan fibrils, which are essential components for outer cell walls of some fungi.[28] These agents are effective against most *Candida* species and *Aspergillus* species. Echinocandins are well-tolerated with minimal drug interaction potential. Echinocandins are available as parenteral formulations and do not require dosage adjustments in patients with renal insufficiency.[28]The dose of caspofungin is 70 mg daily on day 1, followed by 50 mg daily. Patients with a Child-Pugh score of 7 to 9 should be given a maintenance dose of 35 mg/d, instead of 50 mg/d. The dose of micafungin is 50 to 150 mg daily depending upon the indication and the dose of anidulafungin is 50 to 200 mg daily depending upon the indication.

Special Considerations

There are studies with all of the antifungal agents in children; amphotericin B, fluconazole, and echinocandins are recommended in neonatal candidiasis.[5] Amphotericin B carries a pregnancy category B, whereas most azoles, echinocandins and flucytosine all carry category C status.[29] Voriconazole is category D.[25,29] Clinicians must weigh the potential benefit/risks of therapy in pregnant patients when using azoles, echinocandins and flucytosine.

CASE Application

1. Which one of the following adjunctive measures is used to lessen the occurrence of nephrotoxicity associated with amphotericin B?
   a. Test dose of amphotericin B
   b. Diphenhydramine premedication
   c. Normal saline boluses
   d. Furosemide
   e. All of the above

2. Which of one of the following organisms is most likely to manifest a positive India ink stain on a cerebral spinal fluid sample?
   a. *Candida albicans*
   b. *Candida glabrata*
   c. *Aspergillus fumigatus*
   d. *Cryptococcus neoformans*
   e. All of the above

3. When preparing an IV formulation of amphotericin B deoxycholate (desoxycholate), the lyophilized amphotericin B powder must first be reconstituted with sterile water. What type of IV fluid must the reconstituted amphotericin B be placed in for IV administration?
   a. 0.9% sodium chloride
   b. 5% dextrose in water
   c. Lactated Ringers solution
   d. Any of the above solutions

4. Which of the following agents is not recommended as therapy for invasive aspergillosis?
   a. Amphotericin B
   b. Fluconazole
   c. Voriconazole
   d. Liposomal amphotericin B

5. Which one of the following antifungal agents is most associated with causing neutropenia and bone marrow suppression?
   a. Fluconazole
   b. Amphotericin B
   c. Voriconazole
   d. Flucytosine

6. Lipid-based or liposomal amphotericin B formulations have what advantage over conventional amphotericin B (desoxycholate)?
   a. Less expensive than conventional amphotericin B
   b. Decreased mortality
   c. Decreased rates of nephrotoxicity
   d. More efficacious than conventional amphotericin B

7. Which antifungal preparation carries a relative contraindication against use in patients with severe renal insufficiency (due to risk of renal complications from a carrier molecule) ?
   a. IV fluconazole
   b. IV voriconazole
   c. Oral itraconazole
   d. IV caspofungin
   e. Oral voriconazole

8. A patient with a histoplasmosis infection is to be discharged from the hospital and started on oral itraconazole capsules. Which one of the following statements would you tell the patient about his medication to maximize the oral absorption?
   a. Take with food and avoid concomitant use of antacids
   b. Take on an empty stomach
   c. Food will not affect the oral absorption
   d. Do not take this with cola

9. A patient is to receive home infusion therapy with liposomal amphotericin B. What laboratory values should be monitored?
   a. Serum creatinine
   b. Serum potassium
   c. Serum magnesium
   d. All of the above

10. Which of the following antifungal agents has been shown to cause visual acuity side effects?
    a. Amphotericin B
    b. Flucytosine
    c. Fluconazole
    d. Voriconazole
    e. Caspofungin

11. A 54-year-old man with leukemia developed neutropenia 10 days ago after a chemotherapy course. His absolute neutrophil count (ANC) is 200, and he has been febrile for 7 days despite empiric bacterial therapy with imipenem and vancomycin. He was ordered amphotericin B 5 days ago. His CrCl has diminished to < 30 mL/min. Which one of the following antifungal agents would be the best option for a febrile neutropenic patient with renal insufficiency? The provider would like a broad-spectrum antifungal that covers yeasts and molds and an agent that does not affect the kidneys as much as conventional amphotericin B.
    a. Liposomal amphotericin B
    b. Fluconazole
    c. Caspofungin
    d. Posaconazole
    e. a and c.

12. A 58-year-old febrile woman in the surgical intensive care unit has one out of two blood culture bottles growing yeast. A urine sample collected 2 days ago is growing *C. glabrata*. What is the best empiric decision for this patient?
    a. Start fluconazole 400 mg daily
    b. Wait for a susceptibility report and then start with a sensitive antifungal agent
    c. The one out of two blood bottles and the urine culture do not require therapy
    d. Initiate caspofungin 70 mg × 1 dose, then 50 mg daily

13. Genetic variability in cytochrome P-450 CYP 2C19 has been linked to significant interpatient pharmacokinetic differences for which antifungal agent?
    a. Fluconazole
    b. Voriconazole
    c. Micafungin
    d. Flucytosine

14. A 55-year-old man is to be treated for invasive aspergillosis. He is not obese and weighs 100 kg. What amphotericin B formulation dose(s) would be appropriate for this patient?
    a. Amphotericin B desoxycholate 80 mg
    b. Amphotericin B desoxycholate 400 mg
    c. Liposomal amphotericin B 400 mg
    d. a and c
    e. None of the above

15. The fungal cell wall component (1, 3) β-D-glucan is not a key structure in *C. neoformans* and therefore explains the poor activity of what class of antifungal agents for *Cryptococcus*?
    a. Triazoles
    b. Amphotericin B
    c. Echinocandins
    d. 5-Flucytosine
    e. None of the above

16. What drug interaction would be exhibited by adding fluconazole to a person's medication regimen that includes warfarin (stabilized at an INR of 2.5)?
    a. Fluconazole and warfarin concentrations would both be reduced
    b. An increase in INR would be expected
    c. Warfarin cytochrome P-450 metabolism would be induced
    d. An interaction would not be expected

17. BK is a 40-year-old HIV-positive patient. He develops CSF culture-positive cryptococcal meningitis. He has no hepatic or renal insufficiency and his complete

blood count is within normal limits. Select the preferred antifungal regimen for a patient with cryptococcal meningitis?

a. Amphotericin B desoxycholate + flucytosine
b. Amphotericin B desoxycholate
c. Liposomal amphotericin B
d. Fluconazole
e. Micafungin

18. Which antifungal agent is only available as an oral formulation?

a. Amphotericin B lipid-complex
b. Voriconazole
c. Posaconazole
d. Anidulafungin
e. None of the above

19. Which antifungal agent has the greatest 24-hour urinary excretion percentage?

a. Amphotericin B desoxycholate
b. Fluconazole
c. Voriconazole
d. Caspofungin

20. At the end of a 10-week course of treatment for cryptococcal meningitis (CSF-sterilized) in an HIV-positive patient, what is generally recommended in terms of cryptococcal infection?

a. Once-weekly doses of azithromycin
b. Four weeks of fluconazole oral therapy
c. Indefinite low-dose suppressive fluconazole therapy
d. No further antifungal therapy is needed

TAKEAWAY POINTS ››

- Invasive fungal infections are associated with high morbidity and mortality in immunocompromised patients.
- Amphotericin B desoxycholate has been the gold standard antifungal agent due to broad-spectrum and fungicidal killing.
- Amphotericin B desoxycholate is associated with significant infusion-related reactions and nephrotoxicity.
- Lipid-based (liposomal) formulations of amphotericin B have a lower rate of nephrotoxicity. Some formulations have less infusion-related reactions than amphotericin B desoxycholate.
- Lipid-based formulations are given in a higher mg/kg dosage than amphotericin B desoxycholate.
- Flucytosine is adjunctive therapy used in combination with amphotericin B to treat cryptococcal meningitis. Once patients are stable, step-down therapy to an oral azole may be utilized.
- Flucytosine can cause blood dyscrasias.
- All azole antifungal agents are subject to cytochrome P-450 drug interactions. Fluconazole has less interaction potential than voriconazole or itraconazole.
- Fluconazole has excellent activity against *C. albicans* but may be less effective against *C. glabrata* and other *Candida* species.
- Oral itraconazole and posaconazole are not well absorbed and benefit from coadministration with food or acidic beverages. Acid-suppressing agents (proton pump inhibitors and H_2-antagonists) may decrease absorption of these azoles.
- Voriconazole and amphotericin B are the drugs of first choice for invasive aspergillosis.
- IV voriconazole is formulated with a cyclodextrin-carrier molecule that may accumulate in renal insufficiency.
- Echinocandins are well tolerated and have excellent activity against most *Candida* species.
- Echinocandins do not have very good activity against dimorphic fungal pathogens or molds with the exception of *Aspergillus* species.

REFERENCES

1. Caston-Osorio JJ, Rivero A, Torre-Cisneros J. Epidemiology of invasive fungal infection. *Int J Antimicrob Agents.* 2008;32 (suppl 2): S103- S109.
2. Wisplinghoff H, Bischoff T, Tallent SM, et al. Nosocomial bloodstream infections in US hospitals: analysis of 24,179 cases from a prospective nationwide surveillance study. *Clin Infect Dis.* 2004;39:309-317.
3. Pfaller MA, Wenzel RP. The epidemiology of fungal infections. In: Anaissie EJ, McGinnis MR, Pfaller MA, eds. *Clinical Mycology.* Philadelphia, PA: Churchill Livingstone; 2003.
4. Wheat J. Approach to the diagnosis of the endemic mycoses. *Clin Chest Med.* 2009;30:379-389.
5. Pappas PG, Kauffman CA, Andes D, et al. Clinical practice guidelines for the management of candidiasis: 2009 update by the Infectious Diseases Society of America. *Clin Infect Dis.* 2009; 48:503-535.
6. Saag MS, Graybill RJ, Larsen RA, et al. Practice guidelines for the management of cryptococcal disease. Infectious Diseases Society of America. *Clin Infect Dis.* 2000; 30:710-718.
7. Neofytos D, Horn D, Anaissie E, et al. Epidemiology and outcome of invasive fungal infection in adult hematopoietic stem cell transplant recipients: analysis of Multicenter Prospective Antifungal Therapy (PATH) Alliance registry. *Clin Infect Dis.* 2009;48:265-273.

8. Walsh TJ, Anaissie EJ, Denning DW, et al. Treatment of aspergillosis: clinical practice guidelines of the Infectious Diseases Society of America. *Clin Infect Dis.* 2008;46:327-360.
9. Wheat J. Approach to the diagnosis of invasive aspergillosis and candidiasis. *Clin Chest Med.* 2009;30:367-377.
10. Goodman JL, Winston DJ, Greenfield RA, et al. A controlled trial of fluconazole to prevent fungal infections in patients undergoing bone marrow transplantation. *N Engl J Med.* 1992;326:845-851.
11. Silveira FP, Husain S. Fungal infections in solid organ transplantation. *Med Mycol.* 2007;45:305-320.
12. Chen SCA, Sorrell TC. Antifungal agents. *Med J Aust.* 2007; 187:404-409.
13. Fungizone (amphotericin B desoxycholate) injection [package insert]. Princeton, NJ: Apothecon; September 1993.
14. Goodwin SD, Cleary JD, Walawander CA, et al. Pretreatment regimens for adverse events related to infusions of amphotericin B. *Clin Infect Dis.* 1995;20:755-761.
15. Branch RA. Prevention of amphotericin B-induced renal impairment. A review on the use of sodium supplementation. *Arch Intern Med.* 1988;148:2389-2394.
16. Slain D. Lipid-based amphotericin B for the treatment of fungal infections. *Pharmacotherapy.* 1999;19:306-323.
17. Wingard JR, White MH, Anaissie E, et al. A randomized, double-blind comparative trial evaluating the safety of liposomal amphotericin B versus amphotericin B lipid complex in the empirical treatment of febrile neutropenia. L Amph/ABLC Collaborative Study Group. *Clin Infect Dis.* 2000;31:1155-1163.
18. Dodds-Ashley ES, Lewis R, Lewis J, et al. Pharmacology of systemic antifungal agents. *Clin Infect* Dis. 2006;43 (Suppl 1): S28-S39.
19. Brüggemann RJ, Alffenaar JW, Blijlevens NM, et al. Clinical relevance of the pharmacokinetic interactions of azole antifungal drugs with other coadministered agents. *Clin Infect Dis.* 2009;48(10):1441-1458.
20. Poirier JM, Berlioz F, Isnard F, Cheymol G. Marked intra- and inter-patient variability of itraconazole steady state plasma concentrations. *Therapie.* 1996;51:163-167.
21. Cartledge JD, Midgely J, Gazzard BG. Itraconazole solution: higher serum drug concentrations and better clinical response rates than the capsule formulation in acquired immunodeficiency syndrome patients with candidiasis. *J Clin Path.* 1997;50:477-480.
22. Sporanox (itraconazole) injection [package insert]. Raritan, NJ: Ortho Biotech; July 2004.
23. Goldman M, Johnson PC, Sarosi GA. Fungal pneumonias. The endemic mycoses. *Clin Chest Med.* 1999;20:507-519.
24. Herbrecht R, Denning DW, Patterson TF, et al. Voriconazole versus amphotericin B for primary therapy of invasive aspergillosis. *N Engl J Med.* 2002;347:408-415.
25. V fend (voriconazole) injection [package insert]. New York, NY: Pfizer Pharmaceuticals; March 2008.
26. Noxafil (posaconazole) oral suspension [package insert]. Kenilworth, NJ: Schering-Plough Corp; February 2009.
27. Krishna G, Moton A, Ma L, et al. Pharmacokinetics and absorption of posaconazole oral suspension under various gastric conditions in healthy volunteers. *Antimicrob Agents Chemother.* 2009;53:958-966.
28. Sucher AJ, Chahine EB, Balcer HE. Echinocandins: The newest class of antifungal. *Ann Pharmacother.* 2009;43:1647-1657.
29. Briggs GG, Freeman RK, Yaffe SJ, eds. *Drugs in Pregnancy and Lactation.* 7th ed. Philadelphia, PA: Lippincott Williams & Wilkins; 2005.

CHAPTER

29 Sexually Transmitted Diseases

Winter J. Smith

FOUNDATION OVERVIEW

Sexually transmitted diseases (STDs) collectively describe a wide range of infections that are acquired through sexual contact and have a major impact on public health and the utilization of health care resources.[1] Sexually transmitted diseases are associated with symptomatic disease, infertility, and deleterious effects on pregnancy and childbirth, among other complications.[1,2] Approximately 19 million new STD cases occur annually, almost half of these cases occurring in patients 15 to 24 years of age.[3] The estimated annual cost of STDs to the US health care system was over $15 billion in 2007.[1]

Four major STDs will be reviewed in this chapter: chlamydia, gonorrhea, genital herpes, and syphilis.

Chlamydia

Chlamydial genital infection is the most frequently reported infectious disease in the United States, with highest prevalence in persons aged 25 or younger.[1,2] Chlamydial genital infection is caused by *Chlamydia trachomatis*, an obligate intracellular pathogen and the most common bacterium responsible for STDs.[4] Infection is transmissible through vaginal, anal, or oral sex.

Chlamydia typically manifests as cervicitis in women and urethritis in men; however, asymptomatic infection is common, occurring in up to 70% of women and 50% of men.[2,4] In symptomatic disease, women may present with mucopurulent vaginal discharge, postcoital bleeding, and urethral infection.[4] Symptoms in men include dysuria and urethral discharge.[4] Without appropriate and timely treatment, complications such as pelvic inflammatory disease (PID), ectopic pregnancy, premature delivery, and infertility can result.[2,5]

A number of testing methods are available for diagnosis of chlamydia including cell culture, antigen-based tests, molecular methods such as nucleic acid hybridization (DNA probing), and nucleic acid amplification tests (NAATs).[4] Nucleic acid amplification tests have become the tests of choice for diagnosing chlamydial genital infection due to their high sensitivity and specificity and FDA-cleared use for a wide range of specimen types.[2,4]

Gonorrhea

Gonorrhea is the second most commonly reported bacterial STD, with an estimated 600,000 new cases each year.[2] Infection risk is highest in women younger than 25 years of age.[2] Infection is caused by *Neisseria gonorrhoeae*, a gram-negative *Diplococcus*, and is transmissible through contact with genitals, mouth, or anus. After contact is made, the organism attaches to mucosal epithelium causing a strong neutrophil response with pus production.[6]

Gonococcal infection typically causes cervicitis in women and urethritis in men.[7] In men, symptoms include dysuria and urethral discharge which becomes purulent within days.[6] Because of the early presentation and discomfort associated with symptoms in men, treatment is often sought early enough to prevent complications.[2] Women with gonorrhea are generally asymptomatic or have only minor symptoms.[2,6] Symptoms usually occur within 10 days in those who develop them and include vaginal discharge, dysuria, and vaginal bleeding (sometimes postcoital).[6] Asymptomatic infection in women can lead to PID, ectopic pregnancy, tubal scarring, and infertility.[2] In both men and women, gonorrhea can cause increased susceptibility to and transmission of human immunodeficiency virus (HIV) infection.[8]

In symptomatic men, a urethral specimen Gram stain showing neutrophils and gram-negative diplococci can be considered diagnostic, but a negative Gram stain is not sufficient to rule out infection in asymptomatic men.[2] Other diagnostic tests for gonococcal urethritis and cervicitis include culture, nucleic acid hybridization, and NAATs.[2] Nucleic acid amplification tests offer the widest range of specimen types for diagnosis.[2] Nonculture diagnostic tests cannot provide antibiotic susceptibility results, which may be necessary in cases of infection that persists after treatment.[2]

Genital Herpes

Genital herpes affects at least 50 million persons in the United States.[2] The overall percentage of US adults aged 20 to 29 with genital herpes was 10%, according to 2003-2006 data, a decrease from 17% in 1988 to 1994.[9] Genital herpes is a chronic, lifelong viral infection due to double-stranded DNA viruses of the *Herpesviridae* family.[10] Two types of virus cause clinical disease: herpes simplex virus-1 (HSV-1) and HSV-2. While most genital herpes is due to HSV-2, cases of genital herpes due to HSV-1 are increasing. Type of herpes virus (HSV-1 vs HSV-2) does not impact treatment recommendations.[2,10] Genital herpes is transmissible through sexual contact as well as oral sex, and most transmission is from those who are not aware that they are infected.[10] The HSV viruses enter the body through skin or mucosa, and then begin replication at the entry site. Subsequent skin cell damage causes epithelial detachment and blister formation. The viruses then penetrate the dermis and enter peripheral sensory nerves, where they lie dormant between outbreaks (recurrences).[10]

During the first episode of genital herpes, clusters of papular and vesicular lesions on the external genitalia are accompanied by pain, itching, and burning. Involvement may also include perianal, buttock, and thigh areas. Within 2 to 3 weeks, lesions typically transform into ulcers before healing.[10] In most patients, recurrences are within 1 year of the first episode and are associated with fewer lesions and milder pain. The lesions usually heal within 5 to 10 days without antiviral therapy. The rate of recurrence generally decreases over time.[10]

The diagnosis of genital herpes can be made through virologic and/or serologic tests.[2,10] Virologic tests detect the presence of the virus using specimens from genital lesions, while serologic tests detect antibodies to HSV viruses.[2,10] Additionally, some serologic tests can distinguish between HSV-1 and HSV-2 viruses.[10]

Syphilis

Rates of syphilis infection have varied over time and reached the lowest point of 2.1 cases per 100,000 persons in 2000.[11] Since that nadir, rates have almost doubled to a reported 3.8 cases per 100,000 persons in 2007.[1] The highest rates of syphilis infection are among 25 to 29 year olds and more than 60% of new cases occur in men who have sex with men (MSM).[11,12] Syphilitic disease is caused by *Treponema pallidum*, a spiral-shaped bacterium.[11] Syphilis is transmissible through vaginal and anal intercourse, oral sex, and kissing at or near infectious lesion. The disease can also be transmitted in utero.[11] After contact, *T. pallidum* enters the host through compromised skin or intact mucosa.[11]

After acquisition of *T. pallidum*, untreated syphilitic disease passes through a series of four stages: primary syphilis, secondary syphilis, latent syphilis, and tertiary syphilis.[11] Neurosyphilis can occur at any stage of the disease.[11]

The characteristic lesion of primary syphilis is the chancre (ulcer). The chancre is usually painless and appears at the site of *T. pallidum* entrance into the body approximately 3 weeks after transmission.[11,13] Regional lymphadenopathy may also develop 7 to 10 days after the chancre appears.[11] In secondary syphilis a diffuse rash, classically affecting the palms and soles, appears approximately 8 weeks after transmission. Other systemic symptoms may also be present.[11,13] Latent syphilis refers to patients with a positive serologic diagnosis for syphilis, but no clinical symptoms.[11] This stage occurs after secondary syphilis symptoms have subsided and there are two possible outcomes: progression to tertiary syphilis or clinical cure.[11] Tertiary syphilis encompasses the long-term complications of syphilitic disease such as granulomatous disease (also called gummatous syphilis) and cardiovascular syphilis. Tertiary syphilis is now uncommon due to antibiotic treatment and is not transmissible.[11] Central nervous system (CNS) involvement can present at any stage of syphilis.[11] Early neurosyphilis occurs within first few years of infection and usually coexists with primary or secondary syphilis.[14] The meninges and cerebrospinal fluid (CSF) are primarily affected. Early neurosyphilis can present with symptomatic meningitis or be asymptomatic.[14] Late neurosyphilis occurs years to decades after the initial infection and represents a tertiary manifestation of syphilis.[14] Symptoms include general paresis, dementia, and sensory ataxia with incontinence and pain.[14]

Treponema pallidum cannot be cultured, so indirect diagnostic techniques must be used.[12] Serologic testing, including treponemal and nontreponemal tests, provides a presumptive diagnosis and is the standard method of detecting primary, secondary, latent, and tertiary syphilis in the United States.[2,11] Nontreponemal tests, such as the venereal disease research laboratory (VDRL) and rapid plasma reagin (RPR) are used for initial syphilis screening.[11] Nontreponemal tests should be confirmed by treponemal-specific tests (such as the *T. pallidum* particle agglutination or fluorescent treponemal antibody absorption test) due to the rate of false-positive results.[2,11] Since there is no single diagnostic test for neurosyphilis, a combination of clinical manifestations, CSF evaluation, and serologic tests are typically used.[2] Detection of an elevated leukocyte count with lymphocyte predominance and increased protein upon CSF evaluation is suggestive of syphilis.[11] The VDRL-CSF is the standard serologic test (CSF specimen) for neurosyphilis.[2]

PREVENTION

Because STDs are highly transmissible and can lead to serious complications, effective preventative strategies are essential. Goals of prevention include the avoidance of disease transmission to partners and children as well as prevention of long-term disease complications.[2] There are currently no available vaccines for chlamydia, gonorrhea, genital herpes, or syphilis.[5] The most reliable methods to prevent transmission of these STDs are abstinence, monogamy with an uninfected partner, and barrier methods (condoms).[2] Condom use and STD/HIV counseling have been shown to be effective in reducing the acquisition and transmission of STDs.[2,5,15] Diaphragms cannot be relied upon, and hormonal contraception, hysterectomy, and surgical sterilization are not effective preventative measures.[2] Of great concern is the prevention of perinatal transmission. Chlamydia, gonorrhea, genital herpes, and syphilis can all be passed by mothers to children during childbirth (vertical transmission).[2,4,10,11] Syphilis can also be passed to the unborn fetus in utero.[2,11] Specific strategies to prevent perinatal STD transmission are discussed in the treatment section of this chapter.

TREATMENT

Treatment for STDs is indicated at time of diagnosis and/or symptom presentation.[2] Patients who seek treatment for STDs should be also be screened for HIV infection.[2] Goals of therapy include symptom resolution, prevention of disease transmission, and prevention of long-term disease complications. [2,4,7,10,11] For gonorrhea, chlamydia, and syphilis, disease eradication is also a goal of therapy.[2,4,7,11] Since genital herpes cannot be eradicated, goals of therapy include viral suppression and decreased frequency and severity of recurrences.[2,10] Antimicrobial therapies for individual STDs will be reviewed in this section, however, specific dose and regimen information is presented in Table 29-1.

TABLE 29-1 **Adult Treatment Regimens for Select Sexually Transmitted Diseases (STDs)**[2,22]

Infection	Recommended Regimen(s)	Alternative Regimen(s)
Chlamydia	■ Azithromycin 1 g po × 1 dose ■ Doxycycline 100 mg po bid × 7 d	■ Erythromycin base 500 mg po qid × 7 d ■ EES 800 mg po qid × 7 d ■ Ofloxacin 300 mg po bid × 7 d[a] ■ Levofloxacin 500 mg po once daily × 7 d[a]
Gonorrhea[b, c]	■ Ceftriaxone 125 mg IM × 1 dose ■ Cefixime 400 mg po × 1 dose	Other single-dose cephalosporin regimens: ■ Ceftizoxime 500 mg IM ■ Cefoxitin 2 g IM + probenecid 1 g po ■ Cefotaxime 500 mg IM
Genital herpes[d]	First episode: ■ Acyclovir 400 mg po tid × 7-10 d ■ Acyclovir 200 mg po five times daily × 7-10 d ■ Famciclovir 250 mg po tid × 7-10 d ■ Valacyclovir 1 g po bid × 7-10 d	n/a
	Recurrence: ■ Acyclovir 400 mg po tid × 5 d ■ Acyclovir 800 mg po bid × 5 d ■ Acyclovir 800 mg po tid × 2 d ■ Famciclovir 125 mg po bid × 5 d ■ Famciclovir 1000 mg po bid × 1 d ■ Valacyclovir 500 mg po bid × 3 d ■ Valacyclovir 1 g po once daily × 5 d	n/a
	Suppressive therapy: ■ Acyclovir 400 mg po bid ■ Famciclovir 250 mg po bid ■ Valacyclovir 500 mg po once daily ■ Valacyclovir 1 g po once daily	n/a
Syphilis	Primary and secondary syphilis: ■ Benzathine penicillin G, 2.4 MU IM × 1 dose	Primary and secondary syphilis—PCN allergy[e]: ■ Doxycycline 100 mg po bid × 14 d[a] ■ Tetracycline 500 mg po qid × 14 d[a] ■ Ceftriaxone 1 g IV/IM once daily × 8-10 d
	Early latent syphilis: ■ Benzathine penicillin G, 2.4 MU IM × 1 dose	Early latent syphilis—PCN allergy: ■ Same as primary and secondary syphilis
	Late latent syphilis (or unknown duration): ■ Benzathine penicillin G, 2.4 MU IM once weekly × 3 d (7.2 million units total)	Late latent syphilis (or unknown duration)—PCN allergy: ■ Doxycycline 100 mg po bid × 28 d[a] ■ Tetracycline 500 mg po qid × 28 d[a]
	Tertiary syphilis (not including neurosyphilis): ■ Benzathine penicillin G, 2.4 MU IM once weekly × 3 d (7.2 million units total)	Tertiary syphilis (not including neurosyphilis)—PCN allergy: ■ Same as late latent syphilis

(Continued)

TABLE 29-1 **Adult Treatment Regimens for Select Sexually Transmitted Diseases (STDs)[2,22] (*Continued*)**

Infection	Recommended Regimen(s)	Alternative Regimen(s)
	Neurosyphilis:	Neurosyphilis:
	■ Aqueous crystalline penicillin G, 18-24 MU IV daily (3-4 MU IV every 4 hours or by CI) × 10-14 d	■ Procaine penicillin 2.4 MU IM once daily × 10-14 d + probenecid 500 mg po qid × 10-14 d
		PCN allergy[e]:
		■ Ceftriaxone 2 g IV/IM once daily × 10-14 d

[a]Fluoroquinolones and tetracyclines are generally not recommended for use during pregnancy.
[b]Regimens are for uncomplicated gonococcal infections of the cervix, urethra, and rectum only.
[c]Fluoroquinolones are no longer recommended for the treatment of gonorrhea in the United States due to increasing rates of fluoroquinolone-resistant *N. gonorrhoeae*.
[d]The use of topical antiviral agents (eg, acyclovir ointment) is discouraged, as it offers minimal clinical benefit.
[e]The possibility of cross-allergenicity between ceftriaxone and penicillin exists and desensitization may be necessary.
Abbreviations: bid, twice daily; CI, continuous infusion; EES, erythromycin ethylsuccinate; IM, intramuscularly; IV, intravenously; MU, million units; PCN, penicillin; po, orally; qid, four times daily; tid, three times daily.

Treatment Agents for Chlamydia

Azithromycin and doxycycline are the drugs of choice for the treatment of chlamydia. Erythromycin, ofloxacin, and levofloxacin are alternatives. Because azithromycin is administered in a single dose, it may have advantages over doxycycline in patients with compliance difficulties. Erythromycin may be less effective than the azithromycin and doxycycline due to frequency of gastrointestinal side effects associated with its use.[2] Because coinfection with *C. trachomatis* and *N. gonorrhoeae* commonly occurs, presumptive therapy for gonorrhea should be considered when treating chlamydia.[2]

Azithromycin and Erythromycin

Azithromycin and erythromycin, both macrolide antibiotics, work intracellularly by binding to the 23S component of the 50S ribosomal subunit, thereby inhibiting RNA-dependent protein synthesis. Their effects can be bacteriostatic or bactericidal.[16] Gastrointestinal side effects such as nausea, vomiting, and diarrhea, can be observed with all macrolides, but are more commonly encountered with erythromycin. Prolongation of the QTc interval also may occur, but is infrequent with azithromycin use. Erythromycin is metabolized by the cytochrome P450 3A4 (CYP 3A4) enzyme system and drug interactions are possible. Azithromycin is associated with fewer drug interactions because it is metabolized by CYP 3A4 to a lesser extent. Azithromycin's long half-life allows less frequent dosing than erythromycin.[16]

Doxycycline and Tetracycline

Doxycycline and tetracycline are tetracycline antibiotics that reversibly bind to the 30S bacterial ribosomal subunit, ultimately inhibiting bacterial protein synthesis. This intracellular mechanism of action results in primarily bacteriostatic effects.[17] Dose-related gastrointestinal side effects can occur, but are least common with doxycycline. The calcium-binding effects of tetracyclines cause permanent darkening of teeth in children and effects on developing bone. For this reason, tetracyclines are contraindicated in pregnancy (pregnancy category D) and in children under the age of eight.[17] Photosensitivity can also occur with the tetracyclines, but can be decreased by using skin protective measures.[17] Tetracyclines bind multivalent cations (calcium, aluminum, magnesium, iron, etc.), causing interactions with foods and vitamins that decrease antibiotic absorption. Patients should be instructed to separate cation-containing products from tetracycline antibiotics.[17]

Ofloxacin and Levofloxacin

Ofloxacin and levofloxacin are fluoroquinolone antibiotics that exhibit bactericidal action due to their effects on bacterial DNA. Fluoroquinolones bind and stabilize DNA complexes with topoisomerase II and topoisomerase IV enzymes, causing DNA strand breakage and subsequent cell death.[18] Gastrointestinal side effects and CNS effects (dizziness and headache) have been associated with their use.[18] Prolongation of the QTc interval can also occur, although generally less frequently than with macrolides. Caution should be used when administering fluoroquinolones with other QTc interval-prolonging drugs.[18] Fluoroquinolones have the potential to cause dysglycemia (hypo- or hyperglycemia), and this adverse effect has been most commonly reported in patients with underlying diabetes mellitus.[18] Arthropathy and tendon injury may be experienced in specific populations. Arthropathy is most common in patients under 30 years old and presents as joint pain, swelling, and stiffness of the knees.[18] Tendon injury generally occurs in older persons and is associated with additional risk factors. Clinical manifestations include severe and sudden pain, most often affecting the Achilles tendon.[18] Fluoroquinolones have not adequately been studied in pregnancy (pregnancy category C), and their use is generally discouraged. Fluoroquinolones should not be used as first-line antimicrobial agents in children younger than 18 years of age. Although emerging data suggests these agents can possibly be safely administered to children, extreme caution is advised. Use of fluoroquinolones in children should be limited to life threatening or difficult to treat infections where the benefits of therapy outweigh the risks.[18-20]

Treatment Agents for Gonorrhea

Therapy for gonococcal urethritis and cervicitis is complicated by the ability of *N. gonorrhoeae* to develop resistance to antimicrobials.[7,8,21,22] Recently, the Centers for Disease Control and Prevention (CDC) revised their treatment recommendations, no longer recommending the use of fluoroquinolones due to the emergence of fluoroquinolone-resistant *N. gonorrhoeae*.[22] Presumptive therapy for chlamydia should be considered when treating gonorrhea since coinfection with *C. trachomatis* and *N. gonorrhoeae* is common.[2]

Cephalosporins

Currently, cephalosporins represent the only antibiotic class available in the United States that is recommended for the treatment of gonorrhea.[22] Along with penicillins, carbapenems, and monobactams, cephalosporins are members of the beta-lactam antibiotic group. Beta-lactams bind and inactivate a family of enzymes, called penicillin-binding proteins, which are required for bacterial cell wall synthesis. This action causes cell death and is bactericidal.[23,24] Cephalosporins are generally well tolerated. The potential for cross-allergenicity with cephalosporins exists in patients with penicillin allergy, and is most common with first- and second-generation cephalosporins. While penicillin allergy (hypersensitivity) is reported in up to 10% of the general population, the frequency of a life-threatening reaction (anaphylaxis) is much less (0.01%-0.05%).[23]

Treatment Agents for Genital Herpes

The antiviral agents recommended for the management of genital herpes are acyclovir, famciclovir, valacyclovir.[2] These drugs inhibit viral DNA replication by competitively inhibiting viral DNA polymerase. Subsequent incorporation of the drug into the growing viral DNA chain causes chain termination.[25] Famciclovir has a lower affinity for viral DNA polymerase than acyclovir, but has a longer intracellular half-life.[25] Valacyclovir is a prodrug of acyclovir that has increased oral bioavailability.[25] Acyclovir, famciclovir, and valacyclovir are very well tolerated overall. Neurologic toxicity has been reported with acyclovir and valacyclovir administration due to drug accumulation in renal failure.[25]

Antiviral therapy does not eradicate latent herpes viral infection, but aids in disease management. Therapy is divided into three approaches: treatment for the initial episode, intermittent therapy for recurrence, and daily suppressive therapy.[2] All treatment approaches provide symptom improvement during genital herpes episodes. Daily suppressive therapy also reduces the frequency and severity of recurrences and decreases HSV viral shedding, thereby reducing the risk of disease transmission.[2,10] Daily suppressive therapy is associated with an improved quality of life in patients who have frequent recurrences.[2] Use of topical antiviral therapy (eg, acyclovir ointment) is discouraged due to limited clinical benefit.[2]

Treatment Agents for Syphilis

Parenteral penicillin is the drug of choice for syphilis. Tetracyclines and cephalosporins (reviewed earlier) are alternative therapies.[2] Penicillins are beta-lactam antimicrobials with the same mechanism of action as cephalosporins.[26]

Parenteral Penicillin Preparations

Three parenteral penicillin preparations are used for the treatment of syphilis: aqueous crystalline penicillin G, procaine penicillin, and benzathine penicillin G.[2] Aqueous crystalline penicillin G is used in the treatment of neurosyphilis and is administered intravenously. Its short half-life necessitates administration every 4 hours or by continuous infusion.[26] Procaine penicillin, with the addition of oral probenecid, is an alternative for the treatment of neurosyphilis and is administered intramuscularly. The addition of procaine delays intramuscular drug absorption, allowing for less frequent administration—as infrequently as once daily.[26] Benzathine penicillin G is used in the treatment of primary, secondary, latent, and tertiary syphilis. It is administered intramuscularly. Penicillin is released slowly after intramuscular administration of the benzathine preparation, providing sustained concentrations and allowing for single-dose therapy or once weekly dosing.[26] Other parenteral penicillin preparations exist, and health care professionals should be aware of their differences in order to avoid mix-ups and inappropriate therapy. The inadvertent administration of a procaine-benzathine penicillin mix (Bicillin C-R) instead of benzathine penicillin (Bicillin L-A) to patients with syphilis has been reported.[27] Bicillin C-R contains only half the dose of benzathine penicillin recommended for the treatment of syphilis and is inappropriate therapy for this indication.[27] Penicillins are well tolerated, as are other beta-lactam antibiotics. Neither procaine nor benzathine penicillin should be administered intravenously due to the potential for cardiorespiratory arrest and death.[26] As mentioned previously, up to 10% of the population reports a penicillin allergy, but life-threatening reactions are much less common. Penicillin desensitization may be considered in certain patients with a confirmed or suspected penicillin allergy who require penicillin therapy.[2,23]

Jarisch-Herxheimer Reaction

An acute febrile reaction may occur within hours of initiation of therapy for syphilis.[2,11] This reaction, which occurs due to the release of cytokines from dying *T. pallidum* organisms, is most common in patients with early syphilis. Symptoms such as myalgia, headache, and tachycardia may accompany the fever. The reaction usually subsides within a 24-hour period. Analgesics and antipyretics may provide symptomatic improvement, but have not been shown to be effective for prevention. Complications of the Jarisch-Herxheimer reaction include induction of early labor and fetal distress in pregnant women.[11]

Special Populations

Pregnancy

The treatment of STDs in pregnancy can decrease pregnancy complications and prevent disease transmission to the child.[28]

Chlamydia Treating pregnant women for chlamydial infection usually prevents transmission to infants during birth.[2] Doxycycline and fluoroquinolones should generally be avoided during pregnancy, and azithromycin or amoxicillin (500 mg po tid × 7 days) are recommended.[2] Both azithromycin and amoxicillin are classified in pregnancy category B.

Gonorrhea Spontaneous abortion, preterm labor, and postpartum infection are associated with untreated *N. gonorrhoeae* infection. The disease is also transmissible to the newborn, commonly manifesting as a scalp abscess, ophthalmic infection, or disseminated gonococcal disease.[28] Cephalosporin treatment is recommended for gonococcal infection during preganancy.[2] The recommended cephalosporins are classified in pregnancy category B.

Genital Herpes Herpes transmission from an infected mother can cause symptomatic disease in the neonate. The risk of transmission is highest in mothers who have the initial outbreak at the time of delivery. Although a lower risk, transmission also occurs in mothers who have a disease recurrence at the time of delivery. The risk in a mother with recurrent disease but no visible lesions is thought to be low.[28] Use of antiviral therapy late in pregnancy decreases herpes recurrences near term as well as transmission to the neonate.[28] Acyclovir, famciclovir, and valacyclovir are classified in pregnancy category B.

Syphilis In addition to transmission during delivery, syphilis can be transmitted in utero during pregnancy. Exposure to syphilis before birth can lead to preterm labor, fetal death, and neonatal infection.[28] Penicillin regimens, appropriate for the stage of disease, are recommended for the treatment of syphilis in pregnant women.[2] No proven alternatives to penicillin exist for the treatment of syphilis during pregnancy. It is recommended that pregnant patients with a penicillin allergy undergo desensitization and subsequent treatment with penicillin.[2]

Children

Children, including neonates and infants, who are diagnosed with congenital or acquired STDs should be treated according to guideline recommendations.[2] In children who acquire STDs after the neonatal period and for which a nonsexual explanation does not exist, the possibility of sexual abuse and/or assault should be considered.[2]

Adolescents

In general, pharmacologic treatment for STDs in adolescent patients is the same as in adults. As with adults, appropriate education and counseling on STD risk reduction are important components of the treatment plan.[2,29]

HIV Infection

Because severe or prolonged herpes episodes may occur in immunocompromised patients, doses for patients with HIV infection are typically higher and/or treatment durations longer than in patients who are HIV-negative.[2] Treatment guidelines should be consulted for specific recommendations.[2] Patients infected with HIV and diagnosed with chlamydia, gonorrhea, or syphilis should be treated in the same manner as patients who are HIV negative.[2]

POSTEXPOSURE PROPHYLAXIS

Postexposure prophylaxis is not recommended for chlamydia, gonorrhea, genital herpes, or syphilis infections.[2] However, patients diagnosed with these STDs are encouraged to inform their sexual partner(s) of the diagnosis so that they may seek treatment. In some cases, evaluation and treatment of sexual partners may be facilitated by health care providers or public health authorities.[2]

SPECIAL CONSIDERATIONS

Although not specifically reviewed in this chapter, practitioners should also be familiar with treatment and prevention recommendations for genital human papillomavirus (HPV). Most HPV infections are asymptomatic and self-resolving; however, persistent infection can lead to cervical cancer in women as well as anogenital cancer in men and women.[2,30] Topical therapies are available for symptomatic infections (ie, genital and anal warts).[2] Additionally, a quadrivalent HPV vaccine (GARDASIL) is approved for the prevention of HPV-related cancer in females ages 9 to 26.[30]

CASE Application

1. Complications of chlamydia genital infection include which of the following?
   a. Granulomatous and cardiovascular disease
   b. Vesicular lesions on the external genitalia
   c. Pelvic inflammatory disease and infertility
   d. General paresis, dementia, and sensory ataxia

2. TD is 27-year-old man who presents to a local STD clinic with complaints of painful urination and urethral discharge over the past 4 days. He is sexually active, reporting three partners within the past 30 days. He has no known drug allergies. A diagnosis of chlamydia is made. Select the most appropriate therapy for TD.
   a. Doxycycline
   b. Azithromycin + cefixime
   c. Ceftizoxime
   d. Acyclovir + ofloxacin

3. Which of the following is a contraindication to doxycycline therapy?
   a. Age less than 8 years
   b. Concomitant use of QTc interval-prolonging drugs
   c. Diabetes mellitus
   d. Documented penicillin allergy

4. JM is a 23-year-old woman who is 28 weeks pregnant. She presents to her primary care physician (PCP) with symptoms of dysuria and unusual vaginal discharge. A diagnosis of chlamydia is made. Assuming no drug allergies, select the most appropriate therapy for JM.
   a. Doxycycline
   b. Amoxicillin
   c. Cefixime
   d. Levofloxacin

5. Which of the following represents an adverse effect associated with fluoroquinolone use?
   a. Permanent tooth darkening
   b. Neurologic toxicity
   c. Dysglycemia
   d. Jarisch-Herxheimer reaction

6. Which of the following is true regarding gonococcal urethritis and/or cervicitis?
   a. Women older than 25 years are at the highest risk of infection.
   b. Men are typically asymptomatic or have minor symptoms.
   c. Increased transmission of HIV infection is associated with gonococcal infection.
   d. Antibiotic susceptibility data can be obtained using nonculture diagnostic tests for gonorrhea.

7. The presence of gram-negative diplococci on Gram stain is suggestive of which organism?
   a. *Treponema pallidum*
   b. *Chlamydia trachomatis*
   c. Herpes simplex virus-2
   d. *Neisseria gonorrhoeae*

8. AF is a 19-year-old college student who is considering becoming sexually active. During her annual Pap smear she asks her gynecologist for information on STD and pregnancy prevention. Which of the following statements is true regarding STD prevention?
   a. Vaccines are currently available for chlamydia, gonorrhea, and syphilis.
   b. Diaphragm use is a reliable method of STD prevention.
   c. Hormonal contraception is effective in preventing pregnancy and STDs.
   d. Condom use reduces the acquisition and transmission of STDs.

9. Select the mechanism of action for cephalosporin antibiotics.
   a. Bind to the 30S bacterial ribosomal subunit, ultimately inhibiting bacterial protein synthesis
   b. Bind and inactivate a family of enzymes required for bacterial cell wall synthesis, causing cell death
   c. Bind and stabilize DNA complexes with topoisomerase II and topoisomerase IV enzymes, causing DNA-strand breakage and cell death
   d. Bind to the 23S component of the 50S ribosomal subunit, inhibiting RNA-dependent protein synthesis

10. SA is a 33-year-old man with no known drug allergies who presents to the local STD clinic with complaints of extreme pain on urination and urethral discharge for 2 days. A diagnosis of gonococcal urethritis is made. Select the most appropriate therapy for SA.
    a. Ceftriaxone
    b. Benzathine penicillin
    c. Azithromycin
    d. Levofloxacin

11. Which of the following *does not* describe a current goal of therapy for genital herpes infection?
    a. Disease eradication
    b. Viral suppression
    c. Transmission prevention
    d. Decrease recurrence frequency

12. Which of the following is true regarding genital herpes infection?
    a. Genital herpes is an acute, self-limiting disease.
    b. Genital lesions are typically vesicular in nature and accompanied by pain, itching, and burning.
    c. The rate of recurrence increases over time in most patients.
    d. It is important to determine virus type (HSV-1 or HSV-2), as this impacts therapy selection.

13. Which of the following is true regarding genital herpes infection and pregnancy?
    a. The risk of herpes transmission is lowest in mothers who have the initial outbreak at the time of delivery.
    b. Acyclovir, famciclovir, and valacyclovir are classified in pregnancy category D.
    c. Use of antiviral therapy late in pregnancy decreases herpes transmission to the neonate.
    d. Transmission risk in a mother with recurrent disease but no visible lesions is high.

14. HF is a 29-year-old woman who was diagnosed with genital herpes 6 years ago. She reports approximately one to two recurrences each year since diagnosis. Recently she has experienced an increase in outbreaks, having three in a 6-month period. The decision is made to

start HF on daily suppressive therapy. Select the most appropriate therapy for HF.

a. Valacyclovir po
b. Erythromycin ointment
c. Tetracycline po
d. Acyclovir ointment

15. Which of the following is true regarding the stages of syphilis infection?

a. The characteristic lesion of primary syphilis is a diffuse rash, usually affecting the palms and soles.
b. Manifestations of latent syphilis include regional lymphadenopathy and meningitis.
c. Tertiary syphilis is highly transmissible.
d. Neurosyphilis can present at any stage of syphilis.

16. Which of the following is true regarding the diagnosis of syphilis?

a. The diagnosis of syphilis is made through direct techniques such as culture.
b. Serologic testing is the standard method of detecting primary, secondary, latent, and tertiary syphilis in the United States.
c. The VDRL-CSF is the standard serologic test for secondary syphilis.
d. Nontreponemal serologic testing alone is sufficient for a definitive diagnosis of syphilis.

17. Select the brand name for benzathine penicillin.

a. Bicillin C-R
b. Wycillin
c. Bicillin L-A
d. Pen-VK

18. TP is a 26-year-old woman who is 31 weeks pregnant. She visits her obstetrician-gynecologist because of a sore throat, generalized weakness, and a rash on her palms and soles for the past week. Testing is performed and a diagnosis of secondary syphilis is made. The treating physician requests pharmacist consultation because the patient is allergic to penicillin. Select the most appropriate therapy for TP.

a. Doxycycline
b. Cefoxitin + probenecid
c. Levofloxacin
d. Desensitization + benzathine penicillin G

19. The Jarisch-Herxheimer reaction is an acute febrile reaction associated with therapy for which STD?

a. Genital herpes
b. Gonorrhea
c. Chlamydia
d. Syphilis

20. Which of the following is true regarding the treatment of STDs in special populations?

a. The treatment of STDs in pregnancy can decrease pregnancy complications and prevent disease transmission to the child.
b. Children diagnosed with congenital or acquired STDs should not be treated until they reach 2 years of age due to antimicrobial toxicities.
c. In general, adolescent patients require lower doses of recommended antimicrobials for the treatment of STDs.
d. Management of genital herpes in patients with HIV infection is the same as the management in patient who are HIV-negative.

TAKEAWAY POINTS ››

- STDs are acquired through sexual contact and associated with symptomatic disease, infertility, and deleterious effects on pregnancy and childbirth.
- Effective STD preventative measures include abstinence, monogamy with an uninfected partner, and barrier methods (condoms).
- Chlamydia and gonorrhea are the first and second most common bacterial STDs and typically present as cervicitis in women and urethritis in men. However, asymptomatic infection is common.
- Recommended agents for the treatment of chlamydia are azithromycin and doxycycline. Erythromycin, ofloxacin, and levofloxacin are alternatives.
- Cephalosporins are the recommended agents for the treatment of gonorrhea. Fluoroquinolones are no longer recommended due to the emergence of resistance.
- Because coinfection with chlamydia and gonorrhea is common, therapy for both infections should be considered when one of the infections is diagnosed.
- Genital herpes is a chronic, lifelong viral infection characterized by an initial episode followed by periodic recurrences. The typical disease manifestation includes clusters of painful papular and vesicular lesions on the external genitalia.
- Genital herpes cannot be cured, but antiviral therapy decreases the frequency and severity of recurrences as well as the risk of disease transmission.
- Four stages are associated with syphilitic disease: primary syphilis, secondary syphilis, latent syphilis, and tertiary syphilis. Neurosyphilis can occur at any stage of the disease. Distinct clinical manifestations are associated with each stage of disease as well as neurosyphilis.
- Penicillin is the drug of choice for syphilis treatment. Different preparations and regimens are recommended depending on the stage of disease.
- Patients with penicillin allergy who require penicillin therapy (eg, for syphilis in pregnancy) should be desensitized and subsequently treated with penicillin.
- Treatment of STDs during pregnancy can decrease complications and prevent disease transmission to the child.
- Tetracyclines and fluoroquinolones should be avoided in pregnancy.

REFERENCES

1. Trends in reportable sexually transmitted diseases in the United States, 2007: Atlanta, US Department of Health and Human Services; 2007.
2. Workowski KA, Berman SM. Sexually transmitted diseases treatment guidelines, 2006. *MMWR Recomm Rep*. 2006;55:1-94.
3. Weinstock H, Berman S, Cates W Jr. Sexually transmitted diseases among American youth: incidence and prevalence estimates, 2000. *Perspect Sex Reprod Health*. 2004;36:6-10.
4. Bebear C, de Barbeyrac B. Genital Chlamydia trachomatis infections. *Clin Microbiol Infect*. 2009;15:4-10.
5. Starnbach MN, Roan NR. Conquering sexually transmitted diseases. *Nat Rev Immunol*. 2008;8:313-317.
6. Handsfield HH, Sparling PF. Neisseria gonorrhoeae. In: Mandell GL, Bennett JE, Dolin R, eds. *Mandell, Douglas, and Bennett's: Principles and Practice of Infectious Diseases*. 6th ed. Philadelphia, PA: Elsevier; 2005.
7. Newman LM, Moran JS, Workowski KA. Update on the management of gonorrhea in adults in the United States. *Clin Infect Dis*. 2007;44(suppl 3):S84-S101.
8. Workowski KA, Berman SM, Douglas JM Jr. Emerging antimicrobial resistance in Neisseria gonorrhoeae: urgent need to strengthen prevention strategies. *Ann Intern Med*. 2008;148:606-613.
9. QuickStats: Percentage of Adults Aged 20-29 Years with Genital Herpes Infection, by Race/Ethnicity - National Health and Nutrition Examination Survey, United States, 1988-1994, 1999-2002, and 2003-2006. *MMWR Morb Mortal Wkly Rep*. 2009;58:173.
10. Gupta R, Warren T, Wald A. Genital herpes. *Lancet*. 2007;370:2127-2137.
11. Kent ME, Romanelli F. Reexamining syphilis: an update on epidemiology, clinical manifestations, and management. *Ann Pharmacother*. 2008;42:226-236.
12. Daskalakis D. Syphilis: continuing public health and diagnostic challenges. *Curr HIV/AIDS Rep*. 2008;5:72-77.
13. Lee V, Kinghorn G. Syphilis: an update. *Clin Med*. 2008;8:330-333.
14. Marra CM. Neurosyphilis. *Curr Neurol Neurosci Rep*. 2004;4:435-440.
15. Warner L, Stone KM, Macaluso M, Buehler JW, Austin HD. Condom use and risk of gonorrhea and Chlamydia: a systematic review of design and measurement factors assessed in epidemiologic studies. *Sex Transm Dis*. 2006;33:36-51.
16. Dang V, Nanda N, Cooper TW, Greenfield RA, Bronze MS. Antimicrobial Symposium Part VII - Macrolides, azalides, ketolides, lincosamides, and streptogramins. *J Okla State Med Assoc*. 2007;100:75-81.
17. Vincent S, Bronze MS, Cooper TW, Greenfied RA. Antimicrobial Symposium Part X - Tetracycline and glycylcycline antimicrobials. *J Okla State Med Assoc*. 2007;100:241-247.
18. Vincent S, Machado L, Cooper TW, Bronze MS, Greenfield RA. Antimicrobial Symposium Part IX - Quinolone antimicrobials. *J Okla State Med Assoc*. 2007;100:149-156.
19. Leibovitz E. The use of fluoroquinolones in children. *Curr Opin Pediatr*. 2006;18:64-70.
20. Sabharwal V, Marchant CD. Fluoroquinolone use in children. *Pediatr Infect Dis J*. 2006;25:257-258.
21. Tapsall JW. Neisseria gonorrhoeae and emerging resistance to extended spectrum cephalosporins. *Curr Opin Infect Dis*. 2009;22:87-91.
22. Update to CDC's sexually transmitted diseases treatment guidelines, 2006: fluoroquinolones no longer recommended for treatment of gonococcal infections. *MMWR Morb Mortal Wkly Rep*. 2007;56:332-336.
23. Cooper TW, Gibbs WJ, Bronze MS, Greenfield RA. Antimicrobial Symposium Part II - Introduction to the beta-lactam antibiotics. *J Okla State Med Assoc*. 2006;99:516-520.
24. Cooper TW, Gibbs WJ, Bronze MS, Greenfield RA. Antimicrobial Symposium Part IV - Cephalosporins. *J Okla State Med Assoc*. 2006;99:579-583.
25. Lockhart SM, Salvaggio MR, Bronze MS, Greenfield RA. Antimicrobial Symposium Part XIV - Antiviral agents other than antiretrovirals: therapy for herpesvirus infections, viral hepatitis, and influenza. *J Okla State Med Assoc*. 2007;100:388-395.
26. Gibbs WJ, Cooper TW, Bronze MS, Greenfield RA. Antimicrobial Symposium Part III - Penicillins. *J Okla State Med Assoc*. 2006;99:551-556.
27. Inadvertent use of Bicillin C-R to treat syphilis infection—Los Angeles, California, 1999-2004. *MMWR Morb Mortal Wkly Rep*. 2005;54:217-219.
28. Hollier LM, Workowski K. Treatment of sexually transmitted infections in pregnancy. *Clin Perinatol*. 2005;32:629-656.
29. Branson BM, Handsfield HH, Lampe MA, et al. Revised recommendations for HIV testing of adults, adolescents, and pregnant women in health-care settings. *MMWR Recomm Rep*. 2006;55:1-17.
30. Markowitz LE, Dunne EF, Saraiya M, Lawson HW, Chesson H, Unger ER. Quadrivalent Human Papillomavirus Vaccine: Recommendations of the Advisory Committee on Immunization Practices (ACIP). *MMWR Recomm Rep*. 2007;56:1-24.

CHAPTER

30 Influenza

S. Scott Sutton and P. Brandon Bookstaver

FOUNDATION OVERVIEW

Influenza causes significant morbidity and mortality, particularly among young children and the elderly. Seasonal influenza epidemics result in 25 to 50 million influenza cases, approximately 200,000 hospitalizations, and more than 30,000 deaths each year in the United States.[1-3] Influenza infection can occur at any time during the year with the highest rates of illness occurring between December and March.[4] Influenza A and B are the two types of influenza viruses that cause disease in humans. Influenza A viruses are categorized into different subtypes based upon presence of two surface antigens—hemagglutinin and neuraminidase.[1-2] Immunity to influenza virus occurs as a result of the development of antibody directed at the surface antigens.

The route of influenza transmission is person-to-person via inhalation of respiratory droplets. The incubation period for influenza ranges between 1 and 4 days, with an average of 2 days.[1,4-5] Classic signs and symptoms of influenza include rapid onset of fever, myalgia, headache, malaise, nonproductive cough, sore throat, and rhinitis. Signs and symptoms typically resolve in 3 to 7 days; however, cough and malaise may persist for more than 2 weeks. Nausea, vomiting, and otitis media are commonly reported in children. The gold standard for the diagnosis of influenza is viral culture. The clinical utility of the viral culture is limited because of the length of time to receive results. Tests such as the rapid antigen and point-of-care (POC) tests, direct fluorescence antibody (DFA) test, and the reverse transcriptase polymerase chain reaction (RT-PCR) assay may be used for rapid detection of the influenza virus.[2]

PREVENTION

Annual vaccination is the most effective prevention of influenza. Vaccination should be administered to any person who wishes to reduce the likelihood of becoming ill with influenza or transmitting influenza to others.[1-2] Emphasis should be placed upon vaccinating certain groups at higher risk of influenza infection and influenza related complications (Table 30-1). The trivalent influenza vaccine and the live-attenuated influenza vaccine are the commercially available vaccines. Both vaccines are grown in hens eggs, are trivalent, and contain equivalent strains (influenza A H1N1, influenza A H3N2, and influenza B).[1,6-8] See Table 30-2 for a comparison of influenza vaccines.

Trivalent Influenza Vaccine

Trivalent influenza vaccine (TIV) is approved for use in people 6 months of age and older.[7-8] TIV is administered intramuscularly and made with killed influenza viruses. TIV cannot cause signs and symptoms of influenza or influenza-like illness. The most frequent adverse effect associated with TIV is injection site soreness that may last up to 48 hours. TIV may cause fever and malaise in those who have not previously been exposed to the viral antigens in the vaccine.[1,7-13]

Live-Attenuated Influenza Vaccine

Live-attenuated influenza vaccine (LAIV) is a live, weakened virus approved for intranasal administration in healthy, non-pregnant persons between 2 and 49 years of age.[6] Advantages of LAIV include ease of administration and the potential induction of broad mucosal and systemic immune response. Adverse events associated with LAIV administration include runny nose, congestion, sore throat, and headache. LAIV should not be given to those who are immunocompromised or those with close contact to immunocompromised persons who require a restricted environment.[14-22]

Contraindications

TIV or LAIV should not be administered to a person with hypersensitivity to eggs. Allergic type reactions (hives, systemic anaphylaxis) rarely occur after influenza vaccination; however, when allergic reactions occur it is likely a result of residual egg protein in the vaccine.[1-2,23] Table 30-3 lists contraindications for LAIV or TIV.

Guillain-Barre Syndrome (GBS) has been linked to influenza vaccination; however, there is insufficient evidence to establish causality.[1,6-8] Vaccination (TIV or LAIV) should be avoided in persons who experienced GBS within 6 weeks of receiving a previous influenza vaccine and are not at high risk for influenza complications.[25]

Special Populations

Pregnant women, regardless of trimester, should receive annual influenza vaccination with TIV but not with LAIV.[6-8,24] TIV is also safe for breast-feeding mothers. Immunocompromised hosts should receive annual vaccination with TIV but not LAIV.[6-8] Children 6 months of age and greater should receive annual influenza vaccination.[1] Children greater than

TABLE 30-1 Target Groups for Vaccination and Persons at High Risk of Influenza Complications[1]

Target Groups
▪ All persons who want to reduce the risk of becoming ill with influenza or transmitting it to others
▪ Children aged 6 mo to 18 y
▪ All persons more than 50 y of age
▪ Adults at risk for medical complications of influenza
▪ Persons who live with or care for perons at high risk for influenza-related complications, including contacts of children less than 6 mo of age
Persons at High Risk of Complications From Influenza
▪ Unvaccinated infants aged 12-24 mo
▪ Persons with:
▪ Asthma or other chronic pulmonary diseases, such as cystic fibrosis in children or chronic obstructive pulmonary disease in adults
▪ Hemodynamically significant cardiac disease
▪ Immunosuppressive disorders or who are receiving immunosuppressive therapy
▪ HIV
▪ Sickle cell anemia and other hemoglobinopathies
▪ Diseases that require long-term aspirin therapy, such as rheumatoid arthritis or Kawasaki disease
▪ Chronic renal dysfunction
▪ Cancer
▪ Chronic metabolic disease, such as diabetes mellitus
▪ Neuromuscular disorders, seizure disorders, or cognitive dysfunction that may compromise handling of respiratory secretions
▪ Adults aged more than 65 y of age
▪ Residents of any age of nursing homes or other long-term care institutions

6 months of age may receive TIV and children greater than 24 months of age may receive LAIV.[1-2,6-8] Multidose vials and a few of the single-dose preparations of TIV contain trace to small amounts of the preservative thimerosal. No scientifically persuasive evidence is linked between thimerosal and autism.[1-2]

TREATMENT

The four goals of therapy for influenza are: control symptoms, prevent complications, decrease work and/or school absenteeism, and prevent the spread of infection.[1-2] Treatment options for influenza consist of neuraminidase inhibitors and the adamantanes. Antiviral drugs shorten the duration of illness (1 day), provide symptom control, and are most effective if started within 48 hours of the onset of illness.[1-2] Adjunctive agents may be used concomitantly with the antiviral drugs and include acetaminophen for fever or antihistamines for rhinitis.

Adamantanes

Amantadine and rimantadine are adamantanes that have activity against influenza A only. Rapid emergence of resistance is a problem with these agents because cross-resistance is conferred by a single point mutation. Ninety-two percent of the circulating influenza A viruses are resistant to the adamantanes, which is why these agents are not currently recommended as monotherapy for treatment of influenza in the United States.[26] Central nervous system toxicity is the primary adverse reaction to adamantanes. Rimantadine causes fewer central nervous system side effects than amantadine.

TABLE 30-2 Comparison of Live-Attenuated Influenza Vaccine (LAIV) With Trivalent Inactivated Influenza Vaccine (TIV)[1,2]

Factor	LAIV	TIV
Route of administration	Intranasal spray	Intramuscular injection
Type of vaccine	Live-attenuated virus	Killed virus
Number of included virus strains	Three (two influenza A, one influenza B)	Three (two influenza A, one influenza B)
Vaccine virus strains updated	Annually	Annually
Frequency of administration	Annually	Annually
Approved age	Persons aged 2-49 y (healthy, nonpregnant)	Persons >6 mo of age
Interval between 2 doses recommended for children aged ≥ 6 mo-8 y who are receiving influenza vaccine for the first time	4 wk	4 wk
Can be administered to children with asthma or children aged 2-4 y with wheezing during the preceding year	No	Yes
Can be administered to family members or close contacts of immunosuppressed persons not requiring a protected environment	Yes	Yes
Can be administered to family members or close contacts of immunosuppressed persons requiring a protected environment (eg, hematopoietic stem cell transplant recipient)	No	Yes
Can be simultaneously administered with other vaccines	Yes[a]	Yes[a]
If not simultaneously administered, can be administered within 4 wk of another live vaccine	Prudent to space 4 wk apart	Yes
If not simultaneously administered, can be administered within 4 wk of an inactivated vaccine	Yes	Yes

[a]LAIV coadministration has been evaluated systematically only among children aged 12 to 15 months who received measles, mumps, and rubella vaccine or varicella vaccine. TIV coadministration has been evaluated systematically only among adults who received pneumococcal polysaccharide or zoster vaccine.

TABLE 30-3 **Persons Who Should Not Receive Influenza Vaccine[1,2]**

TIV
▪ Persons known to have anaphylactic hypersensitivity to eggs.
▪ Persons with moderate to severe acute febrile illness usually should not be vaccinated until their symptoms have abated. Minor illnesses with or without fever do not contraindicate use of influenza vaccine.
▪ Persons who experienced Guillain-Barre syndrome within 6 wk following a previous dose of TIV is considered to be a precaution for use of TIV.
LAIV
▪ Persons with a history of hypersensitivity to any components of LAIV or to eggs.
▪ Persons less than 2 y of age or more than 49 y of age.
▪ Persons with any of the underlying medical conditions that serve as an indication for routine influenza vaccination.
▪ Asthma
▪ Reactive airway disease
▪ Chronic disorders of pulmonary system
▪ Chronic disorders of cardiovascular system (except hypertension)
▪ Metabolic diseases (eg, diabetes)
▪ Renal dysfunction
▪ Hemoglobinopathies
▪ Known or suspected immunodeficiency
▪ Children aged 2-4 y whose parents or caregivers report that a health care provider has told them during the preceding 12 mo that their child had wheezing or asthma, or whose medical record indicates a wheezing episode has occurred in the preceding 12 mo.
▪ Children or adolescents receiving aspirin or other salicylates.
▪ Persons with a history of Guillain-Barre syndrome after influenza vaccination.
▪ Pregnant women.

Neuraminidase Inhibitors

Oseltamivir and zanamivir are neuraminidase inhibitors that have activity against both influenza A and B viruses. Without neuraminidase, release of the virus from infected cells is impaired, and thus, viral replication is decreased. Oseltamivir is approved for treatment in those more than 1 year of age, while zanamivir is approved for treatment in those older than 7 years of age. The recommended dosages vary by agent and age. The duration of treatment is 5 days. Most seasonal influenza A (H1N1) virus strains tested from the United States and other countries are now resistant to oseltamivir. The Centers for Disease Control (CDC) issued interim recommendations for antiviral treatment and chemoprophylaxis of influenza in December 2008, and these should be consulted for guidance pending recommendations from the ACIP. Influenza treatment may change frequently because of resistance. Please refer to www.cdc.gov/flu for the most up-to-date treatment recommendations.

Adverse effects of neuraminidase inhibitors are typically mild, although more serious side effects have been described. Zanamivir can cause bronchospasm and a decline in respiratory function in patients with asthma and other chronic respiratory disorders. Oseltamivir can also cause nausea and vomiting but these side effects have not generally resulted in discontinuation of therapy. The manufacturer of oseltamivir notified healt care professionals and the FDA of post marketing reports of self-injury and delirium in patients (primarily children) receiving the drug for treatment of influenza. Most of these reports came from Japan, where the drug is used more commonly than in the United States. However, a subsequent study has not demonstrated a causal association between neuraminidase inhibitors and abnormal behavior.

Special Populations

Inadequate data exist regarding the use of adamantanes or the neuraminidase inhibitors in immunocompromised patients. No clinical studies have been conducted evaluating the safety and efficacy of adamantanes or the neuraminidase inhibitors during pregnancy. All of the agents are pregnancy category C. Both the adamantanes and the neuraminidase inhibitors are excreted in breast milk and should be avoided by mothers who are breast-feeding their infants.

POSTEXPOSURE PROPHYLAXIS

The two classes of antiviral drugs for influenza prophylaxis are the adamantanes and the neuraminidase inhibitors (because of high-level resistance, the adamantanes are not recommended as monotherapy). Antiviral drugs used for prophylaxis should be considered adjuncts and not a replacement for annual vaccination with TIV or LAIV.

SPECIAL CONSIDERATIONS

Influenza antiviral drugs should not be administered for 2 weeks after administration of LAIV because the antiviral drugs inhibit influenza virus replication and LAIV should not be administered until 48 hours after influenza antiviral therapy has been stopped. No contraindication exists for concomitant use of TIV and influenza antiviral drugs.

Novel 2009 H1N1 (2009 Swine Flu)

Novel 2009 H1N1 (referred to as "swine flu" previously) is a new strain of influenza virus. This new influenza strain was first detected in April 2009. On June 11, 2009, the World Health Organization (WHO) signaled that a pandemic of 2009 H1N1 flu was underway. This virus was originally referred to as "swine flu" because laboratory testing showed that many of the genes in this new virus were very similar to influenza viruses that normally occur in pigs (swine) in North America. But further study has shown that this new virus is very different from what normally circulates in North American pigs. A 2009 H1N1 vaccine is currently in production.

There are everyday actions that can help prevent the spread of germs that cause respiratory illnesses like influenza. Take these everyday steps to protect your health:

- Cover your nose and mouth with a tissue when you cough or sneeze. Throw the tissue in the trash after you use it.

- Wash your hands often with soap and water. If soap and water are not available, use an alcohol-based hand rub.
- Avoid touching your eyes, nose, or mouth. Germs spread this way.
- Try to avoid close contact with sick people.
- If you are sick with flu-like illness, CDC recommends that you stay home for at least 24 hours after your fever is gone except to get medical care or for other necessities. (Your fever should be gone without the use of a fever-reducing medicine.) Keep away from others as much as possible to keep from making others sick.

Influenza information may change frequenlty because of resistance or new information. Please refer to www.cdc.gov/flu for the most up-to-date recommendations for the novel 2009 H1N1 and seasonal influenza.

CASE Application

1. Select the statement that most accurately describes influenza.
   a. A bacterial illness caused by *Haemophilus influenzae.*
   b. A viral illness caused by respiratory syncytial virus (RSV).
   c. A viral illness caused by rhinovirus.
   d. A viral illness caused by influenza A and B.
   e. A bacterial illness caused by *Streptococcus pneumoniae.*

2. ZC is a 35-year-old woman. She does not have a significant past medical history and is currently taking a multivitamin and calcium supplementation. She has a 3-year-old child. Based upon the information provided, provide influenza vaccination recommendations.
   a. ZC is too young and influenza only affects the elderly and young children. Vaccination not recommended.
   b. ZC does not have comorbidites that place her at risk for influenza complications. Vaccination not recommended.
   c. ZC has a child that is at risk for influenza complications. Vaccination recommended for ZC.
   d. ZC has a child that is at risk for influenza complications. Vaccination recommended for ZC and her 3-year-old child.

3. Select the primary method for transmission of seasonal influenza.
   a. Inhalation
   b. Exposure to blood and/or bodily fluids
   c. Exposure to dead birds
   d. All of the above

4. Select the classic signs and symptoms of influenza.
   a. Rapid onset of fever
   b. Myalgia
   c. Headache
   d. Nonproductive cough
   e. All of the above

5. BC is a 28-month-old child with no significant past medical history. BC has not had a wheezing episode in the last 12 months. Select the best statement as it relates to influenza vaccination.
   a. BC should be vaccinated with TIV.
   b. BC should be vaccinated with LAIV.
   c. BC should be vaccinated with TIV or LAIV.
   d. BC should be administered oseltamivir for prophylaxis.
   e. BC does not meet criteria for vaccination.

6. Select the agent that is administered via intramuscular injection for influenza prevention or postexposure prophylaxis.
   a. TIV
   b. LAIV
   c. Zanamivir
   d. Amantadine
   e. All of the above

7. XW is a 28-year-old pregnant patient. She is currently receiving amoxicillin for a urinary tract infection caused by *Escherichia coli*. She comes to your pharmacy wanting an influenza vaccination. She hates shots and prefers not to receive any injection. During last year's influenza season she received treatment with oseltamivir. Select the appropriate agent for influenza vaccination for XW.
   a. LAIV
   b. TIV
   c. Oseltamivir
   d. Rimantadine
   e. Any of the above agents may be used

8. Which of the following condition(s) would be a contraindication for receiving LAIV?
   a. Diabetes mellitus
   b. Development of Guillain-Barre syndrome (GBS) within 6 weeks of receiving previous influenza vaccine
   c. Egg allergy
   d. Recently received amantadine (within 48 hours)
   e. All of the above

9. Which of the following condition(s) would be a contraindication for receiving TIV?
   a. Diabetes mellitus
   b. Egg allergy
   c. Recently received amantadine (within 48 hours)
   d. Concerned about development of autism from thimerosal in TIV
   e. All of the above

10. Adamantanes have activity against which influenza types?
   a. Influenza A
   b. Influenza B
   c. Influenza C
   d. All of the above

11. Select the brand name for zanamivir.
    a. Relenza
    b. Tamiflu
    c. FluMist
    d. Flumadine
    e. Symmetrel

12. Select the anti-influenza agent that is formulated as a Rotadisk inhaler.
    a. Rimantadine
    b. Amantadine
    c. Oseltamivir
    d. Zanamivir
    e. LAIV

13. YQ is a 59-year-old man with a past medical history significant for chronic obstructive pulmonary disease, diabetes mellitus, hypertension, and hyperlipidemia. YQ wanted to receive influenza vaccination, but the United States has a short supply of TIV. YQ's physician recommended postexposure prophylaxis if he is exposed to influenza. If YQ is exposed to influenza, which agent should be used as postexposure prophylaxis?
    a. Amantadine
    b. Rimantadine
    c. Oseltamivir
    d. Zanamivir
    e. LAIV

14. A patient presents to your pharmacy to ask a question about influenza symptom resolution. She was diagnosed with influenza B. She still has cough and malaise. What should you discuss with the patient?
    a. Influenza symptoms will disappear within 48 hours. If you are still having symptoms, see your provider.
    b. Influenza symptoms typically last 3 to 7 days. Cough and malaise may last up to 2 weeks. If your symptoms have increased/worsened, you may need to see your provider.
    c. Influenza does not cause a cough. Patient should be counseled to see provider.
    d. As long as a patient does not have a fever, there is no need to worry. Cough and malaise symptoms will go away.

15. The best agent for prevention of influenza is:
    a. TIV
    b. LAIV
    c. Adamantanes
    d. a and b
    e. b and c

16. Influenza vaccination emphasis should be placed upon:
    a. Patients at high risk of complications
    b. Children 6 months to 18 years
    c. People more than 50 years of age
    d. All of the above

17. Select the most common adverse reaction of TIV.
    a. Injection site soreness
    b. Birth defects
    c. Bronchospasm
    d. Guillain-Barre syndrome
    e. Autism

18. Select the following patient(s) that should receive influenza vaccination.
    a. Pregnant patients
    b. Children 18 to 24 months of age
    c. Diabetes
    d. A 65-year-old healthy man
    e. All of the above

19. LWS is a 28-year-old man returning home from a military tour of duty from overseas. LWS is an OEF (operation enduring freedom) veteran. He received LAIV 7 days ago. Today he presents with symptoms of influenza. Select the reason LWS could develop influenza symptoms, even if he received the appropriate vaccine.
    a. LAIV is a live virus and can cause influenza.
    b. LWS was not a candidate for influenza vaccination; therefore, he should not have received LAIV.
    c. LWS does not have influenza. He has the common cold.
    d. Influenza vaccines are not 100% effective.
    e. LWS should have received TIV.

20. Select the two surface antigens that categorize influenza A.
    a. Hemagglutinin
    b. Thimerosal
    c. Neuraminidase
    d. Guillain-Barre syndrome
    e. a and c

21. Select the common cause of influenza.
    a. Influenza A
    b. Influenza B
    c. *Haemophilus influenzae*
    d. *Streptococcus pneumoniae*
    e. a and b

22. TK is a 32-year-old HIV-positive patient. He does not want to develop influenza and would like to be vaccinated since he is immunocompromised. Select the appropriate vaccination for TK.
    a. LAIV
    b. Oseltamivir
    c. TIV
    d. Amantadine
    e. Immunocompromised patients should not be vaccinated

TAKEAWAY POINTS ››

- Influenza is a viral illness associated with a high morbidity/mortality and hospitalization rates in children and elderly patients.
- The primary route of influenza transmission is person-to-person via inhalation of respiratory droplets.
- Classic signs and symptoms include abrupt onset of fever, muscle pain, headache, malaise, nonproductive cough, sore throat, and rhinitis.
- Annual influenza vaccination is the primary mechanism for prevention.
- TIV and LAIV are the two commercially available vaccines for prevention of influenza.
- TIV can be administered to persons greater than 6 months of age.
- TIV should not be administered to patients with egg allergy, patients who experience GBS within 6 weeks of receiving influenza vaccine, and persons with moderate to severe febrile illness.
- LAIV can be administered to healthy persons between 2 and 49 years of age.
- LAIV should not be administered to patients with an egg allergy, patients less than 2 years of age, patients more than 49 years of age, persons with COPD, asthma, diabetes, cardiovascular or renal disease, children with a wheezing and / or asthma episode in the preceding 12 months, children or adolescents receiving aspirin or other salicylates, persons with a history of Guillain-Barre syndrome after influenza vaccination, or pregnant women.
- Antiviral drugs (adamantanes and neuraminidase inhibitors) for prophylaxis should be considered adjuncts to vaccine and are not replacements for annual vaccination.
- Neuraminidase inhibitors are the agents of choice for treatment of influenza. They are most effective if started within 48 hours of the onset of illness.

REFERENCES

1. Fiore AE, Shay DK, Broder K, et al. Prevention and control of influenza: recommendations of the Advisory Committee on Immunization Practices (ACIP). *MMWR*. 2009;58:1-52.
2. Harper SA, Bradley JS, Englund JA, et al. Seasonal influenza in adults and children—diagnosis, treatment, chemoprophylaxis, and institutional management: clinical practice guidelines of the infectious diseases society of America. *Clin Infect Dis*. 2009;48:1003-1032.
3. Thompson WW, Shay DK, Weintraub E, et al. Influenza-associated hospitalizations in the United States. *JAMA*. 2004;292:1333-1340.
4. Brankston G, Gitterman L, Hirji Z, Lemieux C, Gardam M. Transmission of influenza A in human beings. *Lancet Infect Dis*. 2007;7:257-265.
5. Leekha S, Zitterkopf NL, Espy MJ, et al. Duration of influenza A virus shedding in hospitalized patients and implications for infection control. *Infect Control Epidemiol*. 2007;28:1071-1076.
6. FluMist [package insert]. Gaithersburg, MD: MedImmune Vaccines, Inc; 2007.
7. Fluzone [package insert]. Swiftwater, PA: Sanofi-Pasteur, Inc; 2006.
8. Fluvirin [package insert]. Emeryville, CA: Novartis Vaccines and Diagnostics, Inc; 2006.
9. France EK, Jackson L. Vaccine Safety Datalink Team. Safety of the trivalent inactivated influenza vaccine among children: a population-based study. *Arch Pediatr Adolesc Med*. 2004;158:1031-1036.
10. Hambidge SJ, Glanz JM, France EK. Safety of inactivated influenza vaccine in children 6 to 23 months old. *JAMA*. 2006;296:1990-1997.
11. Neuzil KM, Dupont WD, Wright PF, Edwards KM. Efficacy of inactivated and cold-adapted vaccines against influenza A infection, 1985 to 1990: the pediatric experience. *Pediatr Infect Dis J*. 2001;20:733-740.
12. Barry DW, Mayner RE, Hochstein HD, et al. Comparative trial of influenza vaccines. Adverse reactions in children and adults. *Am J Epidemiol*. 1976;104:47-59.
13. Zangwill KM, Droge J, Mendelman P, et al. Prospective, randomized, placebo-controlled evaluation of the safety and immunogenicity of three lots of intranasal trivalent influenza vaccine among young children. *Pediatr Infect Dis J*. 2001;20:740-746.
14. Besikari T, Fleming DM, Aristequi JF, et al. Safety, efficacy, and effectiveness of cold-adapted influenza vaccine-trivalent against community-acquired, culture confirmed influenza in young children attending day care. *Pediatrics*. 2006;118:2298-2312.
15. Redding G, Walker RE, Hessel C, et al. Safety and tolerability of cold-adapted influenza virus vaccine in children and adolescents with asthma. *Pediatr Infect Dis J*. 2002;21:44-48.
16. Bergen R, Black S, Shinefield H, et al. Safety of cold-adapted live attenuated influenza vaccine in a large cohort of children and adolescents. *Pediatr Infect Dis*. 2004;23:128-144.
17. Belshe RB, Edwards KM, Vesikari T, et al. Live attenuated versus inactivated influenza vaccine in infants and young children. *N Engl J Med*. 2007;356:729-731.
18. Nichol KL, Mendelman PM, Mallon KP, et al. Effectiveness of live, attenuated intranasal influenza virus vaccine in healthy, working adults: a randomized controlled trial. *JAMA*. 1999;282:137-144.
19. Izurieta HS, Haber P, Wise RP, et al. Adverse events reported following live, cold-adapted, intranasal influenza vaccine. *JAMA*. 2005;294:2720-2725.
20. Govaert TM, Dinant GJ, Aretz K, et al. Adverse reactions to influenza vaccine in elderly people: randomized double blind placebo controlled trial. *BMJ*. 1993;307:988-990.
21. Margolis KL, Nichol KL, Poland GA, et al. Frequency of adverse reactions to influenza vaccine in the elderly.

A randomized, placebo-controlled trial. *JAMA.* 1990;264:1139-1141.
22. Jackons LA, Holmes SJ, Mendelman PM, et al. Safety of a trivalent live attenuated intranasal influenza vaccine, FluMist, administered in addition to parenteral trivalent inactivated influenza vaccine to seniors with chronic medical conditions. *Vaccine.* 1999;17:1905-1909.
23. Pool V, Iskander J. Saftey of influenza vaccination during pregnancy. *Am J Obstet Gynecol.* 2006;194:1200.
24. Zeiger RS. Current issues with influenza vaccination in egg allergy. *J Allergy Clin Immunol.* 2002;110:834-840.
25. Lasky T, Terracciano GJ, Magder L, et al. The Guillain-Barre syndrome and the 1992-1993 and the 1993-1994 influenza vaccines. *N Engl J Med.* 1998;339:1797-1802.
26. England JA, Champlin RE, Wyde PR, et al. Common emergence of amantidine- and rimantidine-resistant influenza A viruses in symptomatic immunocompromised adults. *Clin Infect Dis.* 1998;26:1418-1424.

PART

4

Renal and Nutritional Disorders

CHAPTER

31 Acid–Base Disorders

Kurt A. Wargo

FOUNDATION OVERVIEW

Acid–base pathophysiology often creates a mindset of frustration among not only student pharmacists, but many other health care providers as well, who have difficulty grasping the concepts.[1] While the complexity of the concepts is certainly quite daunting, having a basic understanding will allow you to optimize the care of many critically ill patients.

When discussing any complicated process, it is best to start from a reference point, one that can be referred to whenever confusion arises. For acid–base disturbances, that reference point is the bicarbonate–carbon dioxide buffer system, shown in Equation 31-1.[2]

$$CO_2 + H_2O \leftrightarrow H_2CO_3 \leftrightarrow H^+ + HCO_3^- \qquad \text{(Equation 31-1)}$$

This simple buffering equation holds the foundation for all acid–base physiology within the human body. The processes that occur in the body drive this equation either to the left or the right in order to maintain a neutral pH. Think in terms of the left side of the equation occurring in the lungs and the right side occurring in the kidneys. Anytime the body loses hydrogen ions, the equation shifts to the right. That is to say, the lungs retain more CO_2 in order to convert it into carbonic acid, which is then converted to hydrogen ions and bicarbonate, thereby replacing the lost hydrogen ions. Likewise, anytime an extra hydrogen ion is gained, the equation shifts to the left and the respiratory center is activated to increase ventilation in an effort to get rid of excess acid (CO_2). However, an important point needs to be made here; CO_2 and HCO_3^- are excreted independent of one another. If excess CO_2 exists in the body, it cannot be excreted in the kidneys; rather it must be exhaled by the lungs. Similarly, if there is an increase in H^+, the body cannot convert it to CO_2 for excretion in the lungs; it must be excreted by the kidneys.

From this equation all acid–base disturbances can be explained. Metabolic acidosis results from either an excess in H^+ or a deficiency in HCO_3^-. On the other hand, metabolic alkalosis results from an excess in HCO_3^- or a deficiency in H^+. Respiratory acidosis results from an excess in arterial carbon dioxide ($Paco_2$), whereas respiratory alkalosis results from a deficiency in $Paco_2$. The determination of all acid–base disturbances can be done through evaluation of electrolyte panels, arterial blood gasses (ABG), and patient assessment.

Two final concepts that need to be discussed are the compensatory response that occurs in response to the primary acid–base disorder, as well as mixed acid–base disorders. Primary metabolic disorders can be seen as disturbances in the serum bicarbonate level, with compensation occurring via the respiratory route and reflected in the $Paco_2$. Likewise, all respiratory disturbances will be reflected in the $Paco_2$ level, with compensation occurring metabolically as reflected in the serum bicarbonate level. Sometimes it may be unclear which disturbance is the primary problem by simply evaluating the laboratory values; thus it is crucial to assess the patient in order to get a good history of their present illness to determine which acid–base disorder may be primary. Unfortunately, some acid–base disorders are not as clear as others and may actually be mixed disorders. However, this chapter will provide a stepwise approach to assessing ABGs and will provide actual case examples in order to familiarize you with the concepts of acid–base disorders. At the completion, you will have the tools necessary to assess *any* ABG that may be encountered in clinical practice.

STEPWISE APPROACH TO ASSESSING ACID–BASE DISORDERS

In order to interpret acid–base disorders, a basic understanding of the general concepts is necessary. Many hospital laboratories report ranges in normal laboratory values, such as pH 7.35 to 7.45 and $Paco_2$ 35 to 45 mm Hg. What is important to understand is that under normal physiologic conditions, the human body attempts to maintain homeostasis by keeping the pH and $Paco_2$ as close as possible to 7.40 and 40 mm Hg, respectively. Therefore, any variation from those values should be considered abnormal for the purposes of blood gas evaluation. Serum bicarbonate levels, on the other hand, may vary from 22 to 28 mEq/L on a daily basis, based upon a number of metabolic variables. In general terms, it is best to always keep in mind that *acidosis* is defined as the existence of a pH <7.40, whereas an *alkalosis* is defined as having a pH >7.40.

When presented with an ABG, your task is to determine the primary acid–base disturbance and whether compensation has occurred. *Compensation* is a process that the body undergoes in an effort to maintain homeostasis (pH = 7.40). For any respiratory abnormality, the body will compensate metabolically with changes in serum HCO_3^- through renal regulation. This compensation may take 3 to 5 days to completely occur. On the other hand, for any metabolic disorder, the body compensates through pulmonary regulation of $Paco_2$. This compensation occurs much more rapidly than metabolic compensation, taking minutes to begin, with full compensation seen in hours. An example will help to enhance understanding of this concept.

When undergoing strenuous exercise, a number of changes occur within the body. First, as muscles become deprived of oxygen they begin to undergo anaerobic metabolism, producing lactic acid as a byproduct, thereby creating a metabolic acidosis. In an effort to compensate and maintain a normal pH, the respiratory rate increases, thereby causing CO_2 to be ventilated out of the body, resulting in respiratory alkalosis. Therefore, if an ABG were drawn during the exercise activity, low HCO_3^- with an increased anion gap, as well as a low $PaCO_2$ should be seen. Although, the pH may be slightly acidic depending on the level of exercise, the respiratory center will continue to compensate in order to prevent severe metabolic acidosis.

Determining the primary acid–base disturbance and whether or not compensation has occurred is not an easy task; however, if a stepwise approach is utilized, outlined in Figure 31-1, both simple and complex acid–base disorders can be determined. First, and most important, is the assessment of the patient in order to determine what may be physiologically occurring at that moment in time. At the same time, assessment of the pH points one in the direction of a primary acidosis (pH <7.40) or alkalosis (pH >7.40). Second, assessment of $Paco_2$ and HCO_3^- will allow you to determine the primary disturbance and whether compensation has occurred. Third, if a metabolic acidosis is present, you must calculate an anion gap in an effort to further differentiate the cause of the disturbance and better determine treatment options. Finally, check to see if the patient is compensating for the primary disorder.

Example: A patient with community-acquired pneumonia presents with a pH of 7.46, $Paco_2$ of 32 mm Hg, and serum HCO_3^- of 26 mEq/L. Using the first step, assessment of the patient, it is determined that the patient has a pulmonary process occurring (pneumonia). In addition, through assessment of the pH, it is evident that this patient has an alkalosis, as the pH is >7.40. Next, assessment of both the $PaCO_2$ and the HCO_3^-, in the second step, must be done in order to determine which is causing the acid–base abnormality. In this case, the $PaCO_2$ is lower than normal and the HCO_3^- is normal, indicating the major driving force for the pH to increase is respiratory alkalosis. It does not appear that the patient is compensating for the primary respiratory problem, as the bicarbonate is normal; although, the patient would not have had time to compensate for the acute respiratory alkalosis. Treatment of the patient's underlying pneumonia with antimicrobials (if bacterial in origin) should resolve this acid–base disturbance.

There are five acid–base disturbances that can occur in the human body, Table 31-1: metabolic acidosis, metabolic alkalosis, respiratory acidosis and respiratory alkalosis, and mixed

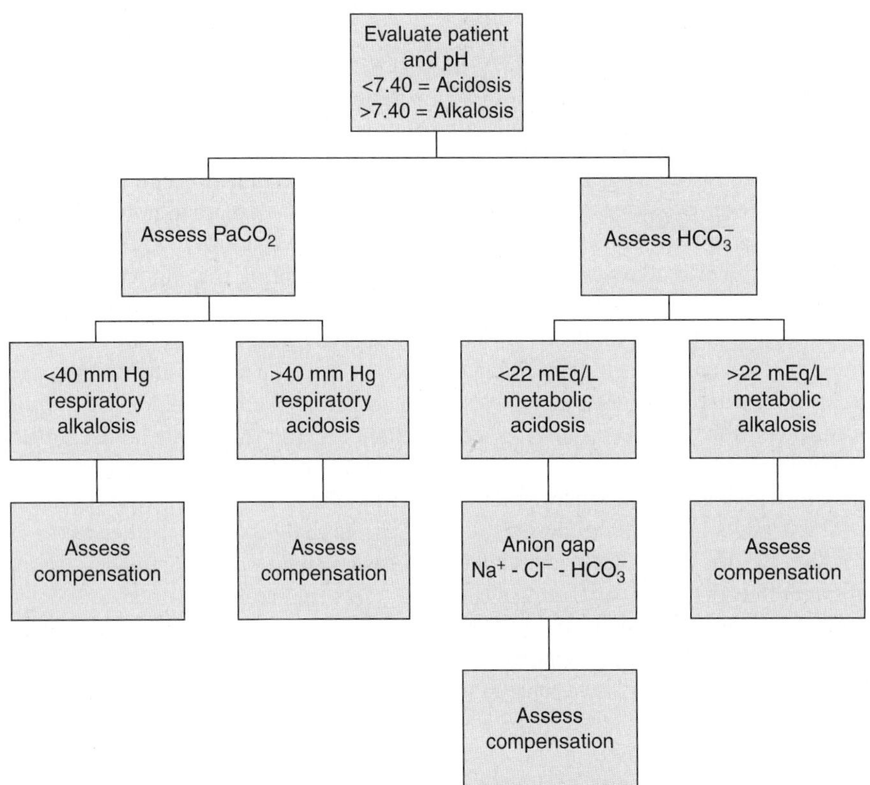

FIGURE 31-1 Stepwise approach to assessing acid–base disturbances.[1]

TABLE 31-1 **Causes of Various Acid–Base Disorders**[2]

Metabolic Acidosis				
Normal Anion Gap	**Increased Anion Gap**	**Metabolic Alkalosis**	**Respiratory Acidosis**	**Respiratory Alkalosis**
Drugs	Ketoacidosis	Drugs	Drugs	Drugs
Acetazolamide	Alcoholism	Corticosteroids	Aminoglycosides	Catecholamines
Amphotericin B	Starvation	Diuretics	Anesthetics	Methylphenidate
Cholestyramine	Diabetic	Volume contraction	Beta-blockers	Nicotine
Lithium	Ingestions	Vomiting or NG suction	Sedatives	Salicylates
Topiramate	Methano	Alkali administration	Opioids	Central nervous system diseases
Zonisamide	Ethylene glycol	Hypokalemia	Neuromuscular blocking agents	Anxiety/panic disorders
Diarrhea	Salicylates	Hyperaldosteronism	Neuromuscular diseases	Pneumonia
Renal tubular acidosis	Lactic acidosis		Central nervous system diseases	Pulmonary embolism
Lead poisoning	Metformin		Pneumonia	Tissue hypoxia/severe anemia
Saline infusions	Lorazepam		Restrictive airway diseases	Thyrotoxicosis
Adrenal insufficiency	Isoniazid		COPD	
	NRTIs (nucleoside reverse transcriptase inhibitors)		Obesity	
			Ascites	
			Hypothyroidism	
	Uremia			

acid–base disturbances. If the stepwise approach to assessing ABGs is used, all of these disturbances can be discovered.

Metabolic Acidosis

Case 1[3]

A 58-year-old woman presented with a 4-day history of lethargy, anorexia, abdominal pain, and nausea. Her medical history was positive for type 2 diabetes, for which she was taking metformin 500 mg twice daily, and osteoarthritis of the knees, for which she had recently been started on rofecoxib (unknown dose). Her laboratory values on admission were the following: Electrolytes: sodium 140 mEq/L (136-145 mEq/L); potassium 4.4 mEq/L (3.5-5 mEq/L); chloride 100 mEq/L (98-106 mEq/L); bicarbonate 5 mEq/L (22-28 mEq/L); blood urea nitrogen 77 mg/dL (10-20 mg/dL); creatinine 9 mg/dL (0.5-1.2 mg/dL); glucose 112 mg/dL (70-110 mg/dL); lactic acid 178 mg/dL (5-20 mg/dL). Arterial blood gas: pH 6.8; $Paco_2$ 20 mm Hg; Pao_2 77 mm Hg.

Metabolic acidosis can be divided into that which is caused by an increased amount of unmeasured anions (increased anion gap metabolic acidosis) and that which is caused by a normal anion gap. In the case of an increased anion gap, several variables can lead to an increase in unmeasured anions. A useful way to remember the potential causes is through the use of the mnemonic "KILU", where "K" signifies *ketoacidosis* (caused by diabetes, starvation, and chronic alcoholism), "I" signifies *ingestions* (typically from salicylates, ethylene glycol, and methanol), "L" signifies *lactic acidosis*, and "U" signifies *uremia.*[1] Some refer to the mnemonic "MUDPILES" (methanol, uremia, DKA, paraldehyde, INH/Iron, lactic acid, ethylene glycol/ethanol, salicylates) for elevated anion gap metabolic acidosis, though we developed the mnemonic KILU because it is more physiologic and refers to items which are pertinent to today's practice of medicine. When faced with a serum electrolyte panel that reveals a lower than normal serum HCO_3^-, indicating a metabolic acidosis, an anion gap must be calculated by subtracting the difference in serum concentrations of the major cation, sodium (Na^+) and anions chloride (Cl^-) and bicarbonate (HCO_3^-), see Equation 31-2.[2,4]

$$\text{Anion gap} = ([Na^+] - [Cl^-] - [HCO_3^-]) \qquad \text{(Equation 31-2)}$$

Under normal circumstances, the anion gap should be 8 to 16 mEq/L; however, negatively charged proteins, specifically albumin, can have a significant impact on the anion gap, such that a 1 g/dL drop in albumin will lower the anion gap by 2.5 mEq/L.[2,4] If the albumin of a patient is known, the *normal* anion gap can be calculated by multiplying the serum albumin by 3. This proves to be crucial when calculating the *delta gap*, which is the difference between the observed and the expected anion gap, Equation 31-3.[5] The delta gap is used, whenever an increased anion gap is observed, in order to determine what the bicarbonate level would be, in the absence of unmeasured anions. That is, the result of the delta gap is added back to the measured bicarbonate, resulting in the serum bicarbonate without an anion gap, Equation 31-3. This is especially useful in determining if treatment with sodium bicarbonate should be given to correct the acidosis.

From the Equation 31-2, the following can be calculated:

$$\begin{aligned}\text{Anion gap} &= 140\text{ mEq/L} - 100\text{ mEq/L} - 5\text{ mEq/L}\\ &= 35\text{ mEq/L} \qquad \text{(Equation 31-3)}\end{aligned}$$

Expected anion gap = 12 mEq/L (no albumin is provided)

Based upon this case example, the increased anion gap is secondary to unmeasured anions, in this case lactic acid, secondary to metformin therapy in the setting of acute kidney injury. Therefore, if the pH were >6.9, it may be inappropriate to administer sodium bicarbonate; however, due to the severity of the acidosis, the administration would be justified. To complete this case example, it is necessary to assess the $Paco_2$ in order to determine respiratory compensation. In this case it is lower than 40 mm Hg, therefore the patient has been appropriately compensated for the metabolic acidosis with a respiratory alkalosis.

Metformin is an extremely rare cause of lactic acidosis, particular care should be taken when using it in patients where renal blood flow has been altered, such as in acute kidney injury, sepsis, contrasted studies, and acutely decompensated heart failure. More commonly, isoniazid and nucleoside reverse transcriptase inhibitors, such as didanosine and stavudine, cause lactic acidosis. Another type of lactic acidosis, D-lactic acidosis (the "D" isomer of lactic acid), can rarely be encountered in practice as well. This type of lactic acidosis is caused by intravenous (IV) infusions of products containing the excipient propylene glycol, such as IV lorazepam and IV diazepam, and typically occurs after high doses of continuous infusions.[6] Typical presentation is an increased osmolar gap, increased anion gap, and renal failure.[7] Although propylene glycol can cause either a lactic acidosis or D-lactic acidosis, the D-isomer is not detected in the routine assay, and thus lactic acidosis may or may not be identified.[7] In these patients, it is still recommended to check a lactic acid level or determine the osmolar gap, which if elevated, would indicate the presence of D-lactic acid.

Case 2[8]

A 42-year-old man with HIV is admitted to the hospital with headache and fever. He is diagnosed with cryptococcal meningitis and initiated on amphotericin B and flucytosine. One week later, the patient is found to be confused and the following laboratory values were drawn: Electrolytes: sodium 152 mEq/L; potassium 3.4 mEq/L; chloride 120 mEq/L; bicarbonate 20 mEq/L; blood urea nitrogen 32 mg/dL; creatinine 1.4 mg/dL; glucose 112 mg/dL. Arterial blood gas: pH 7.30; $Paco_2$ 36; Pao_2 85

Normal anion gap metabolic acidosis is a result of either bicarbonate loss or inadequate buffering.[2] The most common cause of bicarbonate loss is excessive diarrhea, but can also be seen in proximal (type 2) renal tubular acidosis (RTA). Because stool has a basic pH, large volume diarrhea can result in a loss of HCO_3^-, resulting in a normal anion gap acidosis. In type 2 RTA, there is a disruption in the proximal tubular reabsorption of HCO_3^-, resulting in lower serum HCO_3^- levels. Medications such as carbonic anhydrase inhibitors and ifosfamide are common iatrogenic causes of type 2 RTA. One common mnemonic used to recall causes for normal gap metabolic acidosis is USED CAR: *u*reteral diversion, *s*aline infusion, *e*xogenous acid, *d*iarrhea, *c*arbonic anhydrase inhibitors, *a*drenal insufficiency, *r*enal tubular acidosis.

Inadequate buffering in a normal anion gap acidosis, is a result of decreased distal H^+ secretion by luminal H^+-ATPase pumps in the collecting duct of the kidneys, defined as distal RTA (type 1).[2] This decreased secretion of H^+ results in the inability to establish normally acidic urine and therefore a urine pH that is typically above 5.3. Another mechanism of type 1 RTA is secondary to increased permeability of the luminal membrane, resulting in back diffusion of secreted H^+ and distal secretion of K^+. Amphotericin B is an agent which inserts into the cell membranes and creates pores which decrease the membrane permeability. The net result is H^+ retention and K^+ excretion resulting in normal anion gap acidosis and hypokalemia.[9]

In Case 2, the first step in the approach to evaluating ABGs leads the reader to determine the patient has a metabolic process occurring with the cryptococcal meningitis, and no reason to suspect a respiratory problem. In addition to evaluating the patient, evaluation of the pH reveals an acidosis is present. When assessing the metabolic component of the ABG, it is discovered the patient has a lower than normal HCO_3^-, indicating a metabolic acidosis is present. Evaluation of the respiratory component of the ABG shows that the $Paco_2$ is lower than normal, indicating a respiratory alkalosis may be present due to compensation. Therefore, we determine that the patient has a metabolic acidosis with respiratory compensation. The next step, according to our approach, is to calculate an anion gap because of the presence of a metabolic acidosis. When this is calculated, it is determined that a normal anion gap is present (12 mEq/L). Therefore, it is evident that the acid–base disturbance present is a normal gap metabolic acidosis with appropriate respiratory compensation.

Metabolic Alkalosis

Case 3[10]

A 65-year-old man is admitted to the hospital for abdominal pain and diarrhea. He has a history of chronic constipation for which he takes lactulose. Three weeks prior to admission, an exploratory laparotomy revealed no obstruction. He then developed pneumonia and received 5 days of gatifloxacin. Five days prior to admission he developed large-volume, watery diarrhea, without nausea or vomiting. He had the following laboratory values upon admission: Electrolytes: sodium 143 mEq/L; potassium 3.3 mEq/L; chloride 102 mEq/L; bicarbonate 33 mEq/L; urea nitrogen 19 mg/dL; creatinine 1 mg/dL; glucose 109 mg/dL. Arterial blood gas: pH 7.44; $Paco_2$ 42 mm Hg; Pao_2 53 mm Hg. *Clostridium difficile* toxin: negative × 3.

Metabolic alkalosis is characterized by a pH >7.40 and HCO_3^- >28 mEq/L. Causes of metabolic alkalosis can be divided into gastrointestinal loss of H^+, renal loss of H^+, intracellular shift of H^+, or retention of HCO_3^-.[2] Gastrointestinal loss of H^+ usually is a result of vomiting and nasogastric (NG) suctioning, or through antacid use. Renal H^+ loss is associated with a number of conditions including diseases of mineralocorticoid excess, such as primary hyperaldosteronism or Cushing disease.

In these conditions, the presence of hypokalemia exists, which acts as a stimulus for H^+ secretion and HCO_3^- reabsorption. Diuretics also promote renal H^+ loss through distal secretion. This condition, referred to as "contraction alkalosis," occurs secondary to increased production of aldosterone and reabsorption of Na^+ and HCO_3^- in the proximal tubule, in response to hypovolemia. Additionally, diuretics can cause hypokalemia that may result in the previously mentioned H^+ secretion and HCO_3^- reabsorption. In addition to diuretic use, vomiting can also lead to a condition of contraction alkalosis where Na^+, Cl^-, and H_2O are lost without HCO_3^-. Finally, retention of bicarbonate, due to excessive administration of sodium bicarbonate, can also result in metabolic alkalosis.

Because the most common causes of metabolic alkalosis include vomiting, NG suction, and diuretics, the usual treatment involves administration of IV fluids containing NaCl.[2] However, in some cases, patients may be resistant to administration of IV NaCl, usually due to edematous states or hypokalemia. In those patients, withholding conventional diuretics and possibly administering a carbonic anhydrase inhibitor, acetazolamide, is recommended.

In the case above, the stepwise approach indicates the patient currently has a metabolic process occurring (large volume diarrhea), as well as a pH that shows alkalosis. The second step of the approach demonstrates that the $Paco_2$ is slightly higher than normal, representing a potential respiratory acidosis, with an HCO_3^- that is higher than normal, demonstrating a metabolic alkalosis. Because the pH is elevated, this leads us to the conclusion that the patient has metabolic alkalosis with and respiratory compensation. It is puzzling, however, that this patient has had large amounts of diarrhea and has an alkalosis, a state in which one would normally expect to see metabolic acidosis (through loss of bicarbonate in the stool). Nevertheless, upon closer examination, the etiology becomes clear. The metabolic alkalosis that was present in this patient was most likely a result of hypokalemia combined with lactulose therapy. Lactulose creates an acidic stool, thereby converting ammonia (NH_3) into ammonium (NH_4^+) for excretion. Therefore, the patient was losing H^+ through diarrhea, in a way that was analogous to vomiting or NG suctioning. The patient was given IV fluids, lactulose therapy was discontinued, and the metabolic alkalosis resolved.

Respiratory Acidosis

Case 4[11]

An 89-year-old man with a history of heart failure and chronic kidney disease (baseline creatinine 1.6 mg/dL) was being treated in the hospital for a left femoral neck fracture. While in the hospital, he developed a urinary tract infection with *Pseudomonas aeruginosa*, and began to experience decreased mental status, a temperature of 103°F (39°C), and a white blood cell count (WBC) of 41,000 cells/mm^3. At that time he was on room air and his ABG showed pH 7.43, $Paco_2$ 19 mm Hg, Pao_2 57 mm Hg. Therapy with gentamicin was begun and the patient's WBC began to drop and his mental status began to improve. Days later he began to experience acute kidney injury secondary to gentamicin as evidenced by a serum creatinine of 4.5 mg/dL and a gentamicin trough of 6 mg/dL, therefore gentamicin was discontinued. His mental status began to deteriorate and he began to go into respiratory failure. The ABG revealed pH 7.19, $Paco_2$ 57 mm Hg, and Pao_2 59 mm Hg. After 3 days of mechanical ventilation, the patient improved and was extubated.

Respiratory acidosis is characterized by a pH <7.40, and results from retention of $Paco_2$; therefore an elevated $Paco_2$ should be evident. Acutely, respiratory acidosis is most commonly associated with severe asthma exacerbations, pneumonia, pulmonary edema, and suppression of the respiratory center secondary to medications such as opioids, benzodiazepines, paralytics, and neuromuscular blockers.[2] Chronic respiratory acidosis is most commonly associated with chronic obstructive pulmonary disease (COPD) and extreme obesity. Because the renal compensation may take days, through secretion of H^+, acute respiratory acidosis must be treated by removal of the offending agent, or treating the underlying cause. Supplemental oxygenation may be required in severe cases.

In the case presented, the stepwise approach demonstrates the patient has a pulmonary process occurring (respiratory failure), as well as a pH that is acidotic.[11] Evaluation of the $Paco_2$ from the time of respiratory failure indicates a respiratory acidosis. Although the HCO_3^- is not available for assessment, one would not expect to see much of a change from normal, as metabolic compensation would take several days to occur. Through assessment of the patient we know a pulmonary process is occurring at this moment in time; therefore, it is clear the patient has a primary respiratory acidosis, with no evidence of metabolic compensation. The authors believed the acute respiratory failure was secondary to a rare adverse effect of gentamicin therapy, neuromuscular blockade. After gentamicin was discontinued and mechanical ventilation was employed, the patient improved. While it is rare, aminoglycosides have been associated with neuromuscular blockade, an adverse effect of which all clinicians should be cognizant, although more commonly seen with gentamicin and neomycin than with tobramycin and amikacin.

Respiratory Alkalosis / Mixed Acid–Base Disorders

Case 5[12]

A 58-year-old schizophrenic man was brought to the hospital because of strange behavior. He was completely disoriented and provided no history. The following laboratory values were collected: Electrolytes: sodium 139 mEq/L; potassium 4.7 mEq/L; chloride 90 mEq/L; bicarbonate 14 mEq/L; urea nitrogen 18 mg/dL; creatinine 1 mg/dL; glucose 100 mg/dL. Arterial blood gas: pH 7.49; $Paco_2$ 15 mm Hg; Pao_2 169 (2 L nasal O_2).

Respiratory alkalosis is characterized by a pH >7.40 and hyperventilation resulting in a lower than normal $Paco_2$. This is commonly seen during states of hypoxia, such as in pneumonia, pulmonary thromboembolism, heart failure, and severe anemia.[2] Other causes include psychogenic hyperventilation, pregnancy, hepatic failure, salicylate overdose, fever, infections, cerebrovascular events, and drugs such as catecholamines, methylphenidate, nicotine, and progesterone. Treatment of respiratory alkalosis should be solely aimed at correcting the underlying cause.

The case provided above is complicated, in the sense that it is a mixed acid–base disorder. If the stepwise approach is used, we see the patient's pH is elevated, indicating alkalosis. Unfortunately, it is difficult to assess the patient due to his current mental status; therefore we must rely exclusively upon laboratory values. The $Paco_2$ is markedly decreased, indicating a respiratory alkalosis. Furthermore, the Hco_3^- is also markedly decreased indicating metabolic acidosis. After recognizing a metabolic acidosis, the next step is calculation of the anion gap, which in this case is 35 mEq/L, strikingly elevated. At first glance it is difficult to ascertain which came first, though one might simply state the patient has a metabolic acidosis with respiratory compensation. However, upon further laboratory analysis, it was noted that his salicylate level was extremely elevated. The classic presentation of salicylate overdose involves respiratory alkalosis followed by an increased anion gap metabolic acidosis. A family member then brought in an empty bottle of *Alka-Seltzer* that was found near the patient's bedside, which contains aspirin. Thus, the patient experienced respiratory alkalosis and an increased anion gap acidosis secondary to aspirin overdose.

CONCLUSION

Acid–base pathophysiology can be complicated and overwhelming to both the novice and the experienced clinician alike. Recalling the five major disorders that can occur and utilizing this stepwise approach proposed in this manuscript will help clinicians at any level of training assess and develop treatment options for any acid–base disturbance encountered in practice.

CASE Application

Questions 1 and 2 pertain to the following case.

A 58-year-old woman is in the intensive care unit, intubated after a recent abdominal surgery. While in the operating room, she received more than 10 L of fluid and blood products, but has been aggressively diuresed since that time. In the past 3 days she has generated 8 L of urine output, her BUN and Cr have increased to 40 mg/dL and 1.5 mg/dL, respectively, and her blood pressure has decreased to 100/60 mm Hg. This morning her ABG shows the following: pH 7.51, $Paco_2$ 46 mm Hg, and HCO_3 35 mEq/L.

1. Which of the primary acid–base disturbance is present in this patient?
   a. Metabolic acidosis
   b. Metabolic alkalosis
   c. Respiratory acidosis
   d. Respiratory alkalosis

2. Has the patient been appropriately compensated for the primary disorder?
   a. Yes, the $Paco_2$ is elevated, indicating appropriate compensation.
   b. Yes, the Hco_3 is elevated, indicating appropriate compensation.
   c. No, the Hco_3 is low, indicating the patient has not yet compensated.
   d. No, the $Paco_2$ is low, indicating the patient has not yet compensated.

3. Which of the following acid–base disturbances would *most likely* be exhibited in a person with chronic obstructive pulmonary disease (COPD)?
   a. Metabolic alkalosis with respiratory acidosis compensation
   b. Respiratory alkalosis with metabolic acidosis compensation
   c. Respiratory acidosis with metabolic alkalosis compensation
   d. Metabolic acidosis with respiratory alkalosis compensation

4. Which of the following acid–base disturbances would you expect to see in an acute asthma exacerbation?
   a. Respiratory acidosis
   b. Respiratory alkalosis
   c. Metabolic acidosis
   d. Metabolic alkalosis

5. A patient presents to the emergency department unconscious, after ingesting a bottle of lorazepam. What acid–base disturbance would you expect to see?
   a. Increased anion gap metabolic acidosis
   b. Respiratory alkalosis
   c. Metabolic alkalosis
   d. Respiratory acidosis

Questions 6 and 7 pertain to the following case.

A 62-year-old woman has been hospitalized in the ICU for several weeks. She has had a complicated hospital course with pneumonia and sepsis, requiring prolonged courses of antibiotics. Over the past few days, she began spiking fevers and is having a lot of diarrhea. Her stool was positive for *C. difficile* by polymerase chain reaction. Laboratory values include Na 142 mEq/L, Cl 110 mEq/L, HCO_3 18 mEq/L, albumin 4.5 g/dL, pH 7.32, and $PaCO_2$ 33 mm Hg.

6. What is the *most likely primary* acid–base disturbance?
   a. Increased anion gap metabolic acidosis
   b. Normal anion gap metabolic acidosis
   c. Metabolic alkalosis
   d. Respiratory acidosis
   e. Respiratory alkalosis

7. Has the patient been appropriately compensated for the primary disorder?
   a. No, the $Paco_2$ is elevated, indicating the patient has not yet been compensated.
   b. Yes, the Hco_3 is elevated, indicating appropriate compensation.
   c. No, the Hco_3 is low, indicating the patient has not yet been compensated.
   d. Yes, the $Paco_2$ is low, indicating appropriate compensation.

Questions 8 and 9 pertain to the following case.

An 18-year-old man with no known medical history is brought to the emergency department (ED) in a difficult-to-arouse state. His parents report he has been complaining of a vague abdominal pain earlier in the morning, and then began vomiting and urinating frequently in the hours before admission. Urine and blood were positive for ketones. The following laboratory values were taken: Na 142 mEq/L, K 4.5 mEq/L, Cl 100 mEq/L, HCO_3 10 mEq/L, glucose 795 mg/dL, pH 7.26, and $Paco_2$ 23 mm Hg.

8. What is the *most likely primary* acid–base disturbance?
   a. Increased anion gap metabolic acidosis
   b. Normal anion gap metabolic acidosis
   c. Metabolic alkalosis
   d. Respiratory acidosis
   e. Respiratory alkalosis

9. Has the patient been appropriately compensated for the primary disorder?
   a. Yes, the $Paco_2$ is elevated, indicating appropriate compensation.
   b. Yes, the $Paco_2$ is low, indicating appropriate compensation.
   c. Yes, the Hco_3 is elevated, indicating appropriate compensation.
   d. Yes, the Hco_3 is low, indicating appropriate compensation.

Questions 10 and 11 pertain to the following case.

A 27-year-old man with no medical history is admitted after being "found down" at a party after drinking a lot of alcohol over a 30-minute time period. Upon arrival to the ER, he was neurologically unresponsive and had the following laboratory values: pH 7.15, Pao_2 55, $Paco_2$ 60 mm Hg, Hco_3 25 mEq/L, Na 132 mEq/L, Cl 95 mEq/L, and albumin 4.2 g/dL. Urine drug screen is positive for benzodiazepines.

10. What is the *primary* acid–base disturbance?
    a. Increased anion gap metabolic acidosis
    b. Normal anion gap metabolic acidosis
    c. Metabolic alkalosis
    d. Respiratory acidosis
    e. Respiratory alkalosis

11. Has the patient been appropriately compensated for the primary acid–base disorder?
    a. Yes, the $Paco_2$ is elevated, indicating appropriate compensation.
    b. Yes, the $Paco_2$ is low, indicating appropriate compensation.
    c. Yes, the Hco_3 is elevated, indicating appropriate compensation.
    d. Yes, the Hco_3 is low, indicating appropriate compensation.
    e. Unsure, it is too soon after the acute respiratory event to assess metabolic compensation at this time.

Questions 12 and 13 pertain to the following case.

A 45-year-old woman with previous peptic ulcer disease was admitted with persistent vomiting. She looked dehydrated, with dry mucus membranes and skin tenting. Her blood results were Na 141 mEq/L, K 2.6 mEq/L, Cl 87 mEq/L, pH 7.51, $Paco_2$ 50 mm Hg, and Hco_3 40 mEq/L.

12. What is the primary acid–base disorder?
    a. Increased anion gap metabolic acidosis
    b. Normal anion gap metabolic acidosis
    c. Metabolic alkalosis
    d. Respiratory acidosis
    e. Respiratory alkalosis

13. Has the patient been appropriately compensated for the primary acid–base disorder?
    a. Yes, the $Paco_2$ is elevated, indicating appropriate compensation.
    b. Yes, the $Paco_2$ is low, indicating appropriate compensation.
    c. Yes, the Hco_3 is elevated, indicating appropriate compensation.
    d. Yes, the Hco_3 is low, indicating appropriate compensation.

Questions 14 and 15 pertain to the following case.

A 55-year-old man was admitted to the hospital with a 3-day history of persistent vomiting. The following laboratory values are taken: pH 7.40, $Paco_2$ 40 mm Hg, Hco_3 24 mEq/L, Na 149 mEq/L, Cl 100 mEq/L, BUN 110 mg/dL, and Cr 8.7 mg/dL.

14. What would you *expect* the pH, $PaCO_2$, and HCO_3 to be in a patient who has persistent vomiting? (↑, ↓, N)
    a. pH ↑; $Paco_2$ ↓; HCO_3 ↑
    b. pH ↓; $Paco_2$ ↓; HCO_3 ↓

c. pH ↑; $Paco_2$ N; HCO_3 ↑
d. pH ↓; $Paco_2$ N; HCO_3 ↓

15. What acid–base disturbance would you expect in this patient who has uremia?
    a. Increased anion gap metabolic acidosis
    b. Normal anion gap metabolic acidosis
    c. Metabolic alkalosis
    d. Respiratory acidosis
    e. Respiratory alkalosis

16. A 55-year-old woman with a history of severe chronic obstructive pulmonary disease is admitted after several days of worsening shortness of breath. Recently, she was discharged from the hospital with a similar episode and was doing fine until 3 days before admission, when she developed a productive cough, requiring an increase in her home O_2 and more frequent metered-dose inhaler use. What would you *expect* the pH, $Paco_2$, and HCO_3 to be in this patient (↑, ↓, N)?
    a. pH ↑; $Paco_2$ ↓; HCO_3 ↑
    b. pH ↓; $Paco_2$ ↑; HCO_3 ↑
    c. pH ↑; $Paco_2$ N; HCO_3 ↑
    d. pH ↓; $Paco_2$ N; HCO_3 ↓

17. What acid–base disturbance would you expect to see in a person hiking up Mount Everest?
    a. Increased anion gap metabolic acidosis
    b. Normal anion gap metabolic acidosis
    c. Metabolic alkalosis
    d. Respiratory acidosis
    e. Respiratory alkalosis

Match the following diseases to the *primary* acid–base disturbance.

18. Diabetic ketoacidosis
19. Severe anemia
20. Furosemide administration
    a. Metabolic acidosis
    b. Metabolic alkalosis
    c. Respiratory acidosis
    d. Respiratory alkalosis

TAKEAWAY POINTS ››

- Acid–base disorders are primarily due to either metabolic or respiratory problems, as manifested by disorders in HCO_3^- or $Paco_2$; however a combination of the two may also result in an acid–base disorder.
- Acidosis is defined by a pH <7.40, whereas alkalosis is defined by a pH >7.40.
- Respiratory acidosis occurs when the $Paco_2$ >40 mm Hg, while respiratory alkalosis occurs when the $Paco_2$ <40 mm Hg.
- Metabolic acidosis occurs when the HCO_3^- <22 mEq/L, whereas metabolic alkalosis occurs when it is >28 mEq/L.
- Metabolic acidosis is further characterized based upon the anion gap ($[Na^+] - [Cl^-] - [HCO_3^-]$).
- Increased anion gap metabolic acidosis is caused by "KILU," while normal anion gap acidosis is caused by "USED CAR."
- A stepwise approach should be employed when assessing acid–base disturbances:
  1. Evaluate the patient. Do they have a pulmonary process occurring at that particular point in time, or a metabolic one?
  2. Evaluate pH. Is the patient acidotic or alkalotic?
  3. Evaluate $Paco_2$. Is it less than or greater than 40 mm Hg? Assess possible causes.
  4. Evaluate HCO_3^-.
     a. Is it <22 mEq/L? If so, check the anion gap. If the gap is elevated, check the delta gap, and add the result to the HCO_3^-, to reveal the true level (if all the anions were removed).
     b. Is it >28 mEq/L? Assess causes of metabolic alkalosis.
  5. Evaluate compensation.

REFERENCES

1. Wargo KA, Centor RM. ABCs of ABGs: a guide to interpreting acid-base disorders. *Hosp Pharm.* 2008;43:808-815.
2. Rose BD, Post TW. *Clinical Physiology of Acid-Base and Electrolyte Disorders.* 5th ed. New York, NY: McGraw-Hill; 2001.
3. Price G. Metformin lactic acidosis, acute renal failure and rofecoxib. *Br J Anaesth.* 2003;91:909-910.
4. Narins RG, Emmett M. Simple and mixed acid-base disorders: a practical approach. *Medicine.* 1980;59(3):161-187.
5. Wrenn K. The delta (delta) gap: an approach to mixed acid-base disorders. *Ann Emerg Med.* 1990;19(11):1310.
6. Neale BW, Mesler EL, Young M, Rebuck JA, Weise WJ. Propylene glycol-induced lactic acidosis in a patient with normal

renal function: a proposed mechanism and monitoring recommendations. *Ann Pharmacother*. 2005;39(10):1732-1736.
7. Zar T, Graeber C, Perazella MA. Recognition, treatment, and prevention of propylene glycol toxicity. *Semin Dial.* 2007;20(3):217-219.
8. Centor RM. A 42-year old man with HIV. http://www.medscape.com/viewarticle/547710. Accessed March 3 2007.
9. Sawaya BP, Briggs JP, Schnermann J. Amphotericin B nephrotoxicity: the adverse consequences of altered membrane properties. *J Am Soc Nephrol.* 1995;6(2):154-164.
10. Centor RM. Why is the bicarb 33? http://medrants.com/inex.php/archives/2715. Accessed March 13 2007.
11. Brownsberger RJ, Morrelli HF. Neuromuscular blockade due to gentamicin sulfate. *West J Med*. 1988;148(2):215.
12. Centor RM. A 58-year old disoriented, schizophrenic man. Available at http://www.medscape.com/viewarticle/537148. Accessed March 13 2007.

CHAPTER

32 Enteral Nutrition

Laurajo Ryan

FOUNDATION OVERVIEW

When a patient cannot ingest the necessary nutrients by eating food, either because of illness, injury, surgery, dysphagia, or changes in absorption, enteral nutrition (EN) can be used to fill the void. Enteral nutrition refers to the act of taking nutrients into the body through the gastrointestinal (GI) tract. In medical terms, we typically think of EN as supplying specialized nutrition support via tube feedings. Parenteral nutrition (see Chapter 33) provides nutrition intravenously, entirely bypassing the GI tract. In general, if the GI system is functional, it is preferable to use enteral nutrition rather than parenteral feedings.[1]

Enteral nutrition is used in various clinical situations. It may be used to provide nutrition acutely when a patient cannot ingest or absorb adequate nutrition from oral intake or to provide nutrition during periods of extended illness. In general, if an otherwise well-nourished patient cannot take food by mouth for 7 to 14 days, EN should be considered. Enteral nutrition may be the only means of energy intake, or may be used as a supplement to food when oral intake alone is insufficient. Enteral feedings are preferred to parenteral feedings (provision of nutrients through the venous system) for several reasons. Enteral feedings make use of a functional or partially functional gut; reducing the risk of gut atrophy. Enteral nutrition also reduces the risk of infection by removing the need for venous access, and it is also less costly than parenteral nutrition.[2]

TREATMENT

The decision to initiate enteral nutrition therapy must be based on determination of risk to benefit. The potential benefit for the patient must outweigh the risks of tube placement as well as risk of complications. There are a variety of factors that must be considered when initiating EN in any patient. These issues are discussed below.

Route of Administration

Several considerations dictate the route of administration. The level of GI dysfunction and disease state determines where nutrients should enter the GI tract. Feeding should be initiated at the highest level of functional gut, consistent with the patient's disease. This will maximize the nutrient absorption as well as maintain the gut function at the highest level possible. Patients with gastroparesis or other motility disorders may benefit from tube placement in the jejunum or duodenum as opposed to the stomach. Another consideration is anticipated length of treatment; short-term therapy is typically achieved through use of a nasogastric, orogastric, nasoenteric, or oroenteric tube, but longer therapy usually requires percutaneous placement (Table 32-1).[3] With nasogastric tubes, placement is often made at bedside. The feeding tube which is quite flexible and soft at room or body temperature becomes rigid when iced, easing placement.

Tubes

The type of enteral feed as well as the route of feeding is determined by the level at which the normal process has broken down. For instance, in a patient whose jaw is wired shut, the mouth is the portion of the GI tract that needs to be bypassed, so a nasogastric tube would be appropriate, whereas a patient with gastric cancer may require feeding at the level of the duodenum, bypassing the stomach completely.

The tubes used for EN are classified by their external diameter, which is measured in French units (Fr); 1 French unit equals 0.33 mm. The inner lumen size is dependent upon the material used; the smallest practical size is used for patient comfort. While small-bore tubes are more likely to become clogged, they are preferred for oral or nasal feedings. Larger nasogastric or orogastric tubes are typically reserved for suctioning or decompression.

Administration Methods

For critically ill patients, continuous feeds are usually the preferred method of administration. Most patients tolerate continuous feeds better than intermittent or bolus regimens, but continuous feeding regimens are restrictive. They require that the patient remain attached to the feeding source, which in the case of ambulatory patients is extremely limiting. Continuous feeds may also need to be interrupted for medication administration. Intermittent feedings provide more flexibility as they are scheduled for specific times and durations. Bolus feeds mimic meals as a relatively large amount of formula is provided over a short amount of time. Initially, bolus feeds are not tolerated as well as other methods, but many patients who are on long-term EN come to accept them as their diet is advanced.

Contraindications

Enteral nutrition is contraindicated in patients with a mechanical bowel obstruction and GI ischemia, and is a relative contraindication in acute GI bleeding. Feeds should also be held in those with intractable nausea and vomiting.

TABLE 32-1 **Enteral Feeding Routes**

Tube	Type/Insertion Technique	Clinical Uses	Potential Complications
Nasogastric	Placed into the stomach through the nose Position verified by injecting air and auscultation or by x-ray	Short-term (up to 4 wk) or longer periods with intermittent insertion; bolus feeding simpler, but continuous drip with pump better tolerated	Aspiration; ulceration of nasal and esophageal tissues, leading to stricture
Nasoduodenal	Placed into the duodenum through the nose, usually endoscopically	Short-term clinical situations where gastric emptying is impaired Requires continuous drip with pump Decreased aspiration risk compared to gastric insertion	Spontaneous pulling back into stomach (position verified by aspirating content, pH > 6) Diarrhea common, fiber-containing formulas may help
Nasojejunal	Placed into the jejunum through the nose, usually endoscopically	Short-term clinical situations where gastric emptying is impaired Requires continuous drip with pump	Spontaneous pulling back into stomach Diarrhea common, fiber-containing formulas may help
Gastronomy	Percutaneous endoscopic gastrostomy (PEG) Endoscopic placement directly into the stomach	Long-term clinical situations, swallowing disorders, or impaired small-bowel absorption requiring continuous drip	Aspiration; irritation around tube exit site; peritoneal leak; balloon migration and obstruction of pylorus
Jejunostomy	Percutaneous endoscopic jejunostomy (PEJ) Endoscopic placement directly into the jejunum	Long-term clinical situations where gastric emptying is impaired Requires continuous drip with pump; direct endoscopic placement (PEJ) is the most comfortable for patient	Clogging or displacement of tube; jejunal fistula if large-bore tube used; diarrhea from dumping; irritation of surgical anchoring suture
Combined gastrojejunostomy	Double-lumen line, one lumen in stomach for gastric suction, the other in the jejunum to provide nutrition	Used for patients with impaired gastric emptying and at high risk for aspiration or patients with acute pancreatitis or proximal leaks	Clogging, especially of small bore jejunal tube

Note: All small tubes are at risk for clogging, especially if used for crushed medications. In long-term enteral patients, gastrostomy and jejunostomy tubes can be exchanged for a low-profile ""button" (access port) once the tract is established.

Adapted from Table 79-3 by Bruce R. Bistrian, David F. Driscoll in *Harrison's Principles of Internal Medicine*, 17ed.

REGIMEN SELECTION

The choice of nutritional products must be made on an individual basis, taking into account not only nutritional requirements (Table 32-2), but individual patient preferences as well.

Fluid Requirements

Daily fluid requirements vary by age and body weight (Table 32-3). Individual requirements can diverge from these estimations dramatically in those that are acutely ill, as the formulas do not account for fluid losses from sources such as diarrhea, vomiting, nasogastric suction, or wound drainage. These most basic calculations also cannot account for fluid retention in diseases such as heart, renal, or hepatic failure.

Assessment of the fluid needs of each patient must be made on an individual basis, and all sources of fluid intake (oral intake, tube feeding, intravenous infusion) must be taken into account.

Energy Requirements

Adult energy requirements in well-nourished adults on bed rest average 30 to 35 kcal/kg. Critical illness, trauma (burns especially), catabolic states such as some cancers, and preexisting malnutrition can increase energy requirements, while those with chronic illnesses or wasting with a loss of lean body tissue may have significantly lower energy requirements.

Enteral formulas are available commercially with a caloric density of 0.5 to 2.0 kcal/ mL, while most standard formulas are around 1 kcal/mL. The availability of various caloric densities is useful for those with fluid restrictions, or those unable to tolerate more concentrated feedings.

Proteins and Amino Acids

In patients who require nutritional support, at least 1 g protein per kilogram body weight per day is recommended. This level of protein repletion can minimize protein loss and muscle wasting. Up to 1.5 g/kg may be recommended in malnourished patients or those in catabolic states, reserving 1 g/kg or less for those with renal or hepatic failure.

Protein in enteral nutritional formulas is provided in several different forms. Standard enteral formulas (also known as polymeric formulas) are appropriate for those who do not have any difficulty with digestion, because they contain intact proteins. These proteins are most often derived from milk, meat, egg, or soybeans sources. For those unable to digest intact proteins, the proteins may be hydrolyzed to peptides or specific amino acids. Smaller molecular forms of protein provide higher osmolar loads. Many products contain combinations of proteins forms.

TABLE 32-2 Enteral Formula Components

Formula	Carbohydrate	Protein	Fat	Indication	Comments
Standard polymeric	Corn syrup solids Hydrolyzed corn starch Sucrose Fructose	Casein Whey Soy protein Egg white	Corn oil Soybean oil Canola oil MCT	Patients with functional GI tract	Isotonic 1-2 kcal/mL
Elemental or peptide based	Hydrolyzed corn starch Maltodextrin Fructose	Hydrolyzed casein Hydrolyzed whey Hydrolyzed soy protein Hydrolyzed lactalbumin Crystalline amino acids	Corn oil Soybean oil Canola oil MCT	Patients who cannot digest intact proteins	
High protein			Patients who require ≥1.5 g/kg protein daily		
Modular formulas			Those who need supplementation of specific nutrient (protein, fat, or carbohydrate) to supplement other EN formula		

Essential amino acids are those that must be provided by the diet and cannot be synthesized in the body. Conditionally, essential amino acids are those that can become depleted. Essentially the body's production of these amino acids cannot keep up with the demand. Therefore, in times of high demand, conditionally essential amino acids must be supplemented by the diet.

Glutamine and arginine may become conditionally essential amino acids in times of physiological stress such as trauma or infection, and are often present in EN formulas used for critical illness even though clinical trials have not shown consistent benefit.[4]

Carbohydrates

Carbohydrates provide the majority of calories in EN; usually 40% to 60%. These calories are provided as monosaccharides and polysaccharides depending on the formulation. Polysaccharides are preferred in patients who have the ability to digest them; kcal/kcal monosaccharides are more osmotically active than polysaccharides, increasing the osmolality of the formulation.

Care must be taken in those with insulin resistance or diabetes to minimize glucose excursions, which expose the patient to hyper or hypoglycemia and may complicate the course of recovery.

Most enteral formulae are lactose free. This is important because of the high prevalence of lactase deficiency in the population. There is also decreased lactase production during critical illness, which decreases the tolerability of lactose-containing products.

TABLE 32-3 Daily Maintenance Fluid Requirements

Age	Weight	Calculation
Neonates	1-10 kg	100 mL/kg body weight
Child	10-20 kg	1000 mL + 50 mL/kg >10 kg
Adult	>20 kg	1500 mL + 20 mL/kg >20 kg

Lipids

Most enteral nutrition products derive 30% to 40% of their calories from fat, although specialty products with different levels are available. Lipid content is usually derived from corn, soybean, or canola oil. Medium-chain triglycerides (MCT) are available in elemental formulas and are easier to digest than lipids in standard formulas; they may be especially beneficial for those with hepatic failure.

Fiber

Fiber requirements for EN patients are driven by several factors. Enteral nutrition products containing fiber may be beneficial for those who experience GI intolerance to EN such as diarrhea or constipation. Fiber supplementation may also help maintain GI function in those on long-term EN, but may be inappropriate for patients at risk for GI obstruction.

Disease-Specific Therapy

Patients with chronic renal disease, particularly those with nephrotic syndrome, are at risk of protein malnutrition. Malnutrition risk must be balanced with the possible benefit of protein restriction (potential decrease in disease progression) depending on disease stage. This is done by providing enteral feeds with low protein and high amino acid content. Formulas for dialysis patients have higher protein content (closer to usual protein diet) to replace protein lost during dialysis. All renal preparations are calorically dense to decrease fluid load and have low electrolyte content.

Hepatic disease causes irregularities in protein metabolism and synthesis which can not only lead to protein malnutrition, but to hepatic encephalopathy from accumulation of nitrogenous waste, particularly from aromatic amino acids (AAA). Hepatic patients tend to have low levels of branched chain amino acids (BCAA) and high levels of aromatic AAA.

Formulations high in BCAA and low in AAA are available; the results of randomized clinical trials using these products are mixed.

Trauma patients are in a state of catabolism with high caloric needs; the products for these patients are calorically dense and provide high levels of nitrogen to prevent protein malnutrition.

Malnutrition in pulmonary disease is common, and many advanced COPD patients are in a hypermetabolic state. Carbohydrate metabolism produces more CO_2 than fat or protein metabolism. Pulmonary formulations provide a lower percent of calories from carbohydrate and higher percent from fat (approximately 50%) when compared to a standard nutritional product to help ease this strain on the respiratory system.

DRUG ADMINISTRATION

As pharmacists, some of the most common questions that arise regarding EN surround the medications that can and cannot be administered via feeding tubes.

When drugs are administered orally, they are delivered directly to the stomach. Once in the stomach, medications must contend with a relatively low pH environment. Many drugs have been designed with this in mind; bypassing the stomach may delay or decrease drug dissolution.

When administering drugs via feeding tube, special attention must be paid to timing of drugs versus timing of feedings, especially in those receiving continuous feedings. In those on continuous feeding regimens, feeding should be held at least 15 minute prior to and after drug administration. A few drugs require administration on an empty stomach. In those cases feeding needs to be stopped 1 to 2 hours before and after drug administration.

The size of the feeding tube also needs to be taken into account. While very narrow tubes may be more comfortable for the patient, they are more likely to clog with drug administration. Flushing with 30 mL of water (10-15 mL for children) both before and after drug administration can minimize clogging. When administering drugs that are provided in tablet form, special attention needs to be paid to whether or not the tablet is crushable. Numerous lists of "do not crush" drugs have been published, and the package insert for the specific drug will also provide this information. Tablets that can be crushed must be ground to a fine powder and mixed with 15 to 30 mL of water (or other solvent, check package insert) for tube administration. It is imperative to verify "crushability" of each specific medication. Crushing delayed-release medications will result in a bolus effect and the outcome can be deadly.[5] Some capsules can be opened, and the intact beads administered via the feeding tubes, but with small-bore tubes, the granules may clog the tube. Intuitively, liquid medication would be more appropriate for tube administration than other forms, but this is not always the case, as some liquid medications may cause GI intolerance (especially those containing sorbitol); primarily when administered to the small intestine rather than the stomach. In addition, liquid medications are likely to have physical incompatibilities with the EN product itself, becoming insoluble in the GI tract or clog the feeding tube; diluting the liquid prior to administration may avoid this complication.[6]

One of the most well-known drug–tube feed interactions is phenytoin. When phenytoin is administered in the presence of EN products, drug absorption may be decreased by up to 75%. When phenytoin is administered to patients receiving EN, consistent timing between feeds and drug administration must be maintained. Vigilant patient monitoring is also required to minimize toxicity and maintain therapeutic phenytoin concentrations.

Another drug that requires vigilant monitoring in those receiving EN is warfarin. Many EN products have above the adequate intake level (90-120 μg/d) of vitamin K; most products contain approximately 200 μg/1000 kcal. Warfarin resistance is commonly reported in those using EN.

Aside from some of the more obvious interactions, drugs administered via tube feedings often cause diarrhea, especially liquid medications that contain sorbitol and those with high osmolality.

COMPLICATIONS

Many complications of EN are a direct result of mechanical problems related to the feeding process itself, while others are GI or metabolic complications, which may be related to the specific formula being used, or to the patient's disease state.

Gastrointestinal

Motility disorders, both constipation and diarrhea, are frequent adverse effects of EN. Diarrhea from malabsorption, medication, or bacterial overgrowth is common. Less commonly, diarrhea may be caused by administration of a hypertonic formula. It can often be managed by the use of continuous drip versus intermittent feedings or by using a formula that contains fiber. Likewise, constipation may be caused by drugs, or it may be precipitated by low volume status, obstruction, or low fiber intake.

Nausea and vomiting, also commonly seen in EN, is believed to be a result of high gastric residual (high volume of formula left in the stomach). In acute situations, gastric residuals are commonly monitored every 4 to 6 hours, or prior to the next scheduled feeding time. High gastric residual is also considered a culprit in aspiration.

Aspiration

Aspiration is a frequent complication of tube feeding. The risks for aspiration increase with delayed gastric emptying (and subsequent high gastric residual), impaired lower esophageal sphincter tone, inhibition of cough reflex, decreased consciousness, and mechanical ventilation. All patients should be evaluated for risk of aspiration.[3]

The most serious complication of aspiration and of EN itself is aspiration pneumonia. This is a chemical pneumonitis initially, as gastric pH is not conducive to bacterial growth. The ubiquitous use of proton pump inhibitors and H_2 blockers may contribute to bacterial involvement early in the infection process.

Risks of aspiration can be minimized by elevating the head of the bed to 30° to 45° during feeding and for at least 30 to 60 minutes after feeding. The use of continuous feeding versus intermittent or bolus feeds and regular assessment for correct tube placement can also decrease the risk of aspiration as can duodenal tube placement.

Metabolic

Metabolic complications seen with EN include hyperglycemia, fluid and electrolyte imbalances. These complications are more common in the critically ill patient than in patients managed long-term on EN.

Mechanical

By far the most common mechanical complication seen in EN is clogging of the feeding tube. This may be due to incorrect medication administration such as insufficient flushing of the tube or crushing/mixing of tablets. Malfunctioning feeding tubes and physical irritation from the tube itself may complicate therapy.

CASE Application

1. Which of the following routes of supplemental nutrition would be most appropriate for a patient who is malnourished secondary to facial trauma?
   a. Parenteral nutrition
   b. Nasojejunal enteral nutrition
   c. Percutaneous gastric enteral nutrition
   d. Nasoduodenal enteral nutrition

2. While administering medications via nasogastric tubes:
   a. The medication must be compatible with basic fluids.
   b. Tablets must be fully crushed and mixed with 15 to 30 mL of water.
   c. The tube must be flushed with 250 mL of water before and after medication administration.
   d. Capsule beads should be crushed and mixed with 15 to 30 mL of water.

3. When phenytoin is administered to patient receiving tube feeds:
   a. The acidic medium of the jejunum degrades the phenytoin to inactive products.
   b. The basic medium of the duodenum degrades the phenytoin to inactive products.
   c. Phenytoin must be administered very slowly with enteral nutrition.
   d. Administration with enteral nutrition products may decrease drug absorption.

4. When administering drugs via enteral feeding tube:
   a. Liquid medications are always preferable to solid dosage forms.
   b. As long as tablets are crushed very finely they will retain their pharmacokinetic properties.
   c. All drugs that a patient receives should be given simultaneously to minimize feeding interruptions.
   d. Liquid medications may interact with nutritional formula and clog the feeding tube.

5. Which of the following statements is correct?
   a. Modular formulas contain a balanced mixture of carbohydrates and lipids.
   b. Calorically dense formulas provide nutrition targeted to a specific disease state.
   c. Elemental formulas contain intact proteins and polysaccharides.
   d. Standard formulas contain intact proteins.

6. Aspiration risks during enteral nutrition feedings are increased by:
   a. Feeding in an elevated or upright position
   b. High gastric residual prior to feeding
   c. Continuous feeding regimens
   d. High-protein modular feeding

7. Aspiration pneumonia:
   a. Is usually polymicrobial
   b. Is usually preceded by a bacterial infection
   c. Is a chemical pneumonia initially
   d. Is decreased by H_2 blockers

8. Which of the following factors is most important for initial selection of an enteral formulation?
   a. Formula osmolality
   b. Cost of formulation
   c. Location of tube
   d. Nutritional needs

9. Enteral nutrition may be contraindicated in which of the following situations?
   a. Gastrointestinal bleeding
   b. Gastric cancer
   c. Short bowel syndrome
   d. Colostomy

10. MJ is a hospitalized man who weighs 78 kg and has a BMI of 24 kg/m^2. What is his calculated daily fluid requirement?
    a. 2160 mL
    b. 2660 mL
    c. 3160 mL
    d. 3660 mL

11. Which of the following daily calorie counts would be most appropriate for MJ?
    a. 1500 kcal
    b. 2000 kcal
    c. 2500 kcal
    d. 3000 kcal

12. Which of the following is a common complication of enteral nutrition therapy?
    a. Weight loss
    b. Diarrhea
    c. Weight gain
    d. Hypoglycemia

13. Fluid retention associated with enteral nutrition is a problem that is commonly encountered in all of the following disease states *except*:
    a. Heart failure
    b. Respiratory distress
    c. Renal insufficiency
    d. Hepatic failure

14. ED is a 62-year-old woman with type 2 diabetes and end stage renal disease who requires enteral nutrition. She was recently placed on hemodialysis therapy 3 times/wk. Please select the most appropriate nutrition combination.
    a. Low protein, high carbohydrate
    b. Low protein, low carbohydrate
    c. Moderate protein, moderate carbohydrate
    d. High protein, high carbohydrate

15. Patients with hepatic encephalopathy may benefit from nutritional formulations containing:
    a. High branched chain amino acids, low aromatic amino acids.
    b. Low branched chain amino acids, low aromatic amino acids.
    c. High protein, low amino acids.
    d. Protein and amino acid content does not affect hepatic encephalopathy.

16. TR is a 72-year-old man with diabetes and COPD. He is currently hospitalized and on a ventilator for community-acquired pneumonia. Which of the following regimens would be most appropriate dietary therapy?
    a. 50% carbohydrate, 30% fat, 20% protein
    b. 65% carbohydrate, 30% fat, 35% protein
    c. 35% carbohydrate, 25% fat, 40% protein
    d. 35% carbohydrate, 50% fat, 15% protein

17. TR (from Question 16) has been in your facility on the ventilator for 4 days and the resident asks how the risk of aspiration can be decreased. Which of the following methods in *not* an appropriate intervention for this patient?
    a. Elevating head of the bed during and after feedings
    b. Initiating continuous feedings rather than intermittent bolus feedings
    c. Placing gastric tube and stopping proton-pump inhibitor use
    d. Placing duodenal tube instead of gastric tube

18. Fiber in enteral formulations:
    a. Decreases tolerability in most patients
    b. May increase diarrhea
    c. May increase constipation
    d. May contribute to GI obstruction

19. Which of the following tubes are correctly matched to their preferred use or tube type?
    a. Nasogastric tube, long-term use
    b. Orogastric tube, small bore
    c. Percutaneous gastric tube, short-term use
    d. Nasojejunal tube, large bore

20. All of the following patient groups have increased metabolic needs *except*:
    a. Type 1 diabetics
    b. Trauma patients
    c. Burn patients
    d. Critically ill patients

TAKEAWAY POINTS ››

- Enteral nutrition is preferred to parenteral nutrition in those with a functional gut.
- Enteral nutrition should be provided at the highest gut level consistent with the patient's disease state.
- Transnasal tube insertion is appropriate for short-term enteral nutrition.
- Nausea, vomiting, diarrhea, and constipation are common adverse effects of enteral nutrition feeding.
- Aspiration pneumonia is the most devastating complication that is commonly encountered with enteral nutrition.
- Risk for aspiration is increased with decreased mental status, prolonged supine position, and bolus feeding regimens.
- Standard enteral formulas provide proteins in their intact form that must be hydrolyzed in the gut.
- Fluid content of enteral nutrition feeds must be individualized based on the disease state and patient-specific parameters.

REFERENCES

1. Zaloga GP. Parenteral nutrition in adult inpatients with functioning gastrointestinal tracts: assessment of outcomes. *Lancet.* 2006;367:1101-1111.
2. ASPEN Board of Directors and the Clinical Guidelines Task Force. Guidelines for the use of parenteral and enteral nutrition in adult and pediatric patients. *J Parenter Enteral Nutr.* 2002;26(suppl):1SA-138SA.
3. Bankhead R, Boullata J, Brantley S, et al. Clinical guidelines for the use of parenteral and enteral nutrition in adult and pediatric patients. *J Parenter Enteral Nutr.* 2009;33:122-167.
4. Garrel D, Patenaude J, Nedelec B. Decreased mortality and infectious morbidity in adult burn patients given enteral glutamine supplements: a prospective, controlled, randomized clinical trial. *Crit Care Med.* 2003;31:2444-2449.
5. Schier JG, Howland MA, Hoffman RS, Nelson LS. Fatality from administration of labetalol and crushed extended-release nifedipine. *Ann Pharmacother.* 2003;37:1420-1423.
6. Madigan SM, Courtney DE, MaCauley D. The solution was the problem. *Clin Nutr.* 2002;21:531-532.

CHAPTER

33 Parenteral Nutrition

Sarah J. Miller

FOUNDATION OVERVIEW

Parenteral nutrition (PN) involves delivery of nutrients by the intravenous (IV) route. The term total parenteral nutrition (TPN) implies that all of the patient's nutritional needs are being met by this route even though the term is often used when patient is receiving both oral feedings or tube feedings (enteral nutrition or EN) and IV feedings simultaneously.

Parenteral nutrition may be delivered by either the central (CPN) or peripheral (PPN) route. When delivered centrally, the feeding catheter is typically placed into the subclavian vein with the tip of the catheter near the opening of the right atrium. For PPN, the catheter is placed into a peripheral vein; because hypertonic solutions of PN can cause phlebitis when administered peripherally, the osmolality of PPN solutions is usually limited to about 900 mOsm/L. Peripherally inserted central catheters (PICC lines) are often utilized for PN administration. PICC lines provide central venous access through which hypertonic PN formula may be administered.

Parenteral nutrition is preferred over EN only when EN cannot be used safely. Parenteral nutrition is indicated in situations when EN is not possible or feasible. When to start PN in these situations is patient and situation specific and is sometimes controversial. In a previously well-nourished patient in the intensive care unit (ICU), PN may be delayed and therefore no feedings delivered for 7 to 10 days. In the ICU patient who was malnourished prior to hospitalization, PN should be started earlier in a course of illness precluding EN.[1,2] Typically, if resumption of EN is anticipated within 5 to 7 days, PN should not be initiated as it is unlikely to improve outcomes, is expensive, and is associated with potentially significant adverse events. See Table 33-1 for a list of more common situations in which PN is indicated. Central PN may be used long term; patients with short bowel syndrome may receive home PN for decades. On the other hand, PPN is usually a short-term therapy lasting no more than 7 to 10 days.

COMPONENTS AND DESIGNING A REGIMEN

Parenteral nutrition solutions contain both macrosubstrates and microsubstrates. Macrosubstrates consist of a carbohydrate source, lipid emulsion, and amino acid solution. Microsubstrates include electrolytes, vitamins, and trace elements.

Fluid

Fluid requirements of PN patients can vary widely. Some fluid-restricted patients may receive as little as 1000 or 1250 mL of PN per day. Typical PN volumes for patients without fluid restrictions are 1500 to 3000 mL/d. In the hospital, PN is most commonly infused continuously over 24 hours. In the home setting, PN may be cycled over a shorter period of time (eg, 12-16 hours), often at night, to allow the patient more freedom in mobility.

Dextrose

The carbohydrate source of most PN solutions is dextrose. Intravenous dextrose provides 3.4 kcal/g. Stock solutions of 10%, 20%, 30%, 50%, and 70% dextrose are commonly used in compounding.

Lipid

Intravenous lipid emulsions contain fat, glycerol, and phospholipid. When calculating calories from IV lipid emulsions, the following caloric densities are used: 10% emulsion – 1.1 kcal/mL; 20% emulsion – 2 kcal/mL; 30% emulsion – 2.9 kcal/mL.

Amino Acids

Standard amino acid solutions (Aminosyn, Travasol, FreAmine, Novamine) contain both essential and nonessential amino acids and are supplied by the manufacturer in concentrations ranging from 2.75% to 20%. Some of these products contain standard concentrations of electrolytes already added, whereas others do not. Specialized amino acid formulations designed for pediatrics (TrophAmine, Aminosyn-PF) are widely utilized. Specialized amino acid formulations designed for adults with renal failure, hepatic failure, and stress are expensive and clinically useful only uncommonly. Amino acid solutions provide 4 kcal/g. In past decades, a patient's total caloric content of PN was based on nonprotein calories with additional calories from protein supplemented. Currently, the trend is to calculate patients' caloric needs based on both protein and nonprotein calories.

Macrosubstrate Provision Recommendations

Following development of the techniques for administration of CPN in the late 1960s, the philosophy of "more is better" reigned for more than a decade. As adverse events associated

TABLE 33-1 **Indications for Parenteral Nutrition**

Indications
Bowel obstruction Physical/mechanical (eg, tumor compressing intestinal lumen) Functional (eg, postoperative ileus)
Major small bowel resection (eg, short bowel syndrome) Adult patients with > 100 cm small bowel distal to the ligament of Treitz without a colon Adult patients with > 50 cm of small bowel if the colon is intact
Diffuse peritonitis
Gastrointestinal fistulas if enteral nutrition cannot be provided above or below the fistula
Pancreatitis—if patients have failed enteral nutrition beyond the ligament of Treitz or cannot receive enteral nutrition (eg, due to obstruction)
Severe intractable vomiting
Severe intractable diarrhea
Preoperative nutrition support in patients with moderate to severe malnutrition who cannot tolerate enteral nutrition and in whom surgery can be delayed safely for at least 7 d

Reproduced with permission from: Kraft MD, Btaiche IF. Parenteral nutrition. In: Chisholm-Burns MA, Wells BG, Schwinghammer TL, et al, eds. *Pharmacotherapy Principles & Practice.* New York, NY: McGraw-Hill; 2008:1493-1510.

with overfeeding became evident, provision of energy in the form of dextrose and lipid became more conservative. Most guidelines now call for provision of energy via PN for adults between 20 and 35 total kcal (including protein kcal) per kg body weight per day (kcal/kg/d).[3,4] New guidelines for calorie provision in the obese critically ill patients are shown in Table 33-2.[1] Calories should be divided between dextrose and lipid (as well as protein) such that dextrose does not exceed 7 g/kg/d and lipid does not exceed 2.5 g/kg/d.[3,4] Lipid kilocalories typically make up about 15% to 30% of nonprotein kilocalories. Note that propofol, a medication used in the intensive care unit for sedation, is compounded in a 10% lipid emulsion; these lipid kilocalories should be taken into account when calculating total kilocalories in a patient's regimen. Likewise, many medications are compounded in dextrose 5% which may provide significant calories.

Amino acids are generally supplied in PN solutions at amounts of up to about 2 g/kg/d.[3,4] New guidelines for critical care patients with body mass index (BMI) <30 kg/m^2 call for 1.2 to 2 g/kg actual body weight per day or perhaps higher in burn and trauma patients.[1] Protein guidelines for critically ill obese patients are given in Table 33-2.[1] Although formerly parenteral products containing extra amounts of branched chain amino acids and decreased amounts of aromatic amino acids were promoted for patients experiencing hepatic encephalopathy, these products are rarely used today. Patients receiving hemodialysis or continuous renal replacement therapy may require up to 2.5 g protein per kg body weight per day to account for protein losses through the dialysis process itself.[1]

TABLE 33-2 **Guidelines for Calorie and Protein Provision in the Obese, Critically Ill Patients**

BMI	Calorie Recommendation per Day	Protein Recommendation per Day
30-40	22-25 kcal/kg ideal body weight	≥ 2 g/kg ideal body weight
30-40	11-14 kcal/kg actual body weight	
≥40	22-25 kcal/kg ideal body weight	≥ 2.5 g/kg ideal body weight
≥40	11-14 kcal/kg actual body weight	

Note: There are no recommendations in these guidelines[1] for proteins based on actual body weight in obese patients.

Electrolytes, Vitamins, and Trace Elements

The electrolytes, vitamins, and trace elements commonly included in PN solutions are listed in Table 33-3.

Other Additives

Medications most commonly added to PN formulations are listed in Table 33-4.

ORDERING, COMPOUNDING, LABELING, AND ADMINISTRATION

Hospitals administering PN solutions should utilize an order form.[4,5] Compounding of PN solutions may occur by a manual system (ie, not using a pump and utilizing volumes of macrosubstrates supplied by the manufacturers) or by using an automated compounder by which volumes of the various macrosubstrates can be more tightly controlled. Some health care institutions outsource PN compounding to entities outside the institution. Sterility in compounding PN is important because these solutions may support microbial growth and may hang for up to 24 hours.[6] Some hospitals prefer standardized PN solutions (ie, a limited number of concentrations and amounts of macrosubstrates available for ordering by the prescriber), whereas other hospitals more closely customize formulas to individual patients.[5]

PN solutions may be compounded as a combination of dextrose, amino acids, lipid, and additives in a single container. These are referred to as three-in-one emulsions or total nutrient admixtures (TNA). Another method for administration mixes dextrose and amino acids together; the lipid emulsion is then piggybacked onto a primary IV line. Whereas TNA or dextrose plus amino acid solutions can hang for 24 hours, lipid emulsion alone should only hang for 12 hours due to the higher potential of microbial growth in the isotonic environment of lipid emulsion which has a pH near the physiologic range.

Addition of electrolytes, particularly calcium and phosphate, to PN solutions must be done with care. Calcium and phosphate can form a precipitate if added in large quantities. Factors affecting calcium/phosphate solubility include temperature, pH, and amino acid concentration of the solution.[7] When compounding PN, it is typically recommended to add phosphate first, and then to add calcium near the end of the compounding sequence when the volume of the PN is maximized.[4]

Total nutrient admixtures present other stability concerns. Destabilization of the negative charge on the surface of lipid emulsion globules in the admixture can lead to creaming

TABLE 33-3 Electrolytes, Vitamins, and Trace Elements Commonly Included in PN Solutions

Electrolytes
Sodium (from sodium chloride, sodium acetate, sodium phosphate)
Potassium (from potassium chloride, potassium acetate, potassium phosphate)
Magnesium (from magnesium sulfate, magnesium chloride)
Calcium (from calcium gluconate, calcium chloride)
Phosphorus (from potassium phosphate, sodium phosphate)
Chloride (from potassium chloride, sodium chloride, calcium chloride, magnesium chloride)
Acetate (from sodium acetate, potassium acetate)
Vitamins
Vitamin A
Vitamin D
Vitamin E
Vitamin K
Thiamine
Riboflavin
Niacin
Pyridoxine
Vitamin B_{12}
Folic acid
Pantothenic acid
Biotin
Vitamin C
Trace elements
Zinc
Copper[a]
Chromium
Manganese[a]
Selenium

[a]Copper and manganese are commonly omitted with cholestasis, that is, if serum total bilirubin exceeds about 5 mg/dL

or cracking of the emulsion. A creamed emulsion can be made homogeneous again by gently inverting the bag containing the emulsion several times; such an emulsion may be safely administered to a patient. On the other hand, gentle inversion of a cracked emulsion does not result in the emulsion returning to its initial state and cannot be safely administered to a patient.

Dextrose/amino acid solutions can be administered through a 0.22-μm filter; such filters remove particulates as well as microorganisms introduced into the solution during the compounding process. Total nutrient admixtures cannot be administered through 0.22-μm filters because lipid globules within these admixtures are larger than 0.22 μm. Thus, TNA should be administered through 1.2 μm filters which remove particulates but not smaller microbes.

Parenteral nutrition labels should include daily amounts of components.[4] This should decrease errors, particularly when transferring a patient from one health care setting to another

TABLE 33-4 Medications Most Commonly Added to PN

Medication
Regular insulin
Histamine$_2$-receptor antagonists
Heparin[a]
Hydrocortisone[a]
Iron dextran[b]

[a]Sometimes added to PPN to help prevent thrombophlebitis.
[b]Can be added to dextrose/amino acid solutions but is incompatible with TNA

(eg, hospital to home or vice versa). Listing concentrations and amounts per liter of components may lead to more errors due to misinterpretation as compared to listing amounts per day.

COMPLICATIONS AND MONITORING

Metabolic

Parenteral nutrition can be associated with various metabolic complications. Hyperglycemia is common; because this complication can be associated with poorer outcomes, it is important to avoid extremes of high blood sugars, and blood sugar is typically monitored several times daily at initiation of PN. Frequency of blood sugar monitoring can be decreased when stability is demonstrated. Regular insulin is frequently added to PN solutions, and subcutaneous sliding scale insulin is also frequently administered. Use of long-acting insulin, such as insulin glargine, may be useful in selected patients on PN, although this use is problematic if the PN is unexpectedly discontinued or held. Separate insulin drips are frequently utilized in ICU patients receiving PN. Hypoglycemia can occur when PN is abruptly discontinued. Although this is not commonly a problem, some institutions cut the rate of PN in half for an hour or so before discontinuing. Home PN patients often run their solution at lower rates for the first and last hours of their daily infusion cycle.

Abnormalities of electrolytes are frequently seen in PN patients. Hypophosphatemia, hypokalemia, and hypomagnesemia may require increases in the amounts of these electrolytes added to the PN, additional bolus dosages, or both. These electrolyte abnormalities, especially hypophosphatemia, can be associated with the so-called refeeding syndrome in chronically malnourished patients. These electrolytes should be monitored at least twice a week upon initiation of PN; frequency of monitoring can be cut back when levels have demonstrated stability. Hyperphosphatemia, hyperkalemia, and hypermagnesemia occur primarily during renal insufficiency and require decreasing these electrolytes in the PN solution. Mild hyponatremia is common in PN patients. Addition of more sodium to the PN is not always appropriate; the patient could already be fluid-overloaded and thus the decreased serum sodium is due to dilution. Acid–base imbalances are not typically secondary to PN therapy itself. Acetate in PN solutions is converted to bicarbonate in the liver. Decreasing the acetate to chloride ratio in the PN may help correct metabolic alkalosis, whereas increasing this ratio may be helpful in metabolic acidosis.

Hypertriglyceridemia, defined as a serum triglyceride concentration above 400 to 500 mg/dL, may occur in patients receiving IV lipid. Hypertriglyceridemia of this magnitude can be associated with increased risk of pancreatitis. With hypertriglyceridemia in this range, generally the amount of lipid emulsion infused is decreased. Triglycerides should be measured prior to initiation of lipid emulsion, after a day of administration, and approximately weekly thereafter in hospitalized patients. Caution is warranted if lipid emulsion is completely withheld in patients receiving PN for more than a couple of weeks; essential fatty acid deficiency could develop if there is no intake of fat.

Liver function abnormalities have been associated with PN therapy. Two general patterns have been described. The first pattern, characterized by elevation of aspartate and alanine aminotransferase, typically occurs within a few days of initiation of PN and is associated with hepatic steatosis, or fat accumulation in the liver. This pattern is seen in patients being overfed especially with dextrose. The second pattern is cholestasis characterized by an increase in alkaline phosphatase and total bilirubin. This pattern tends to develop after two or more weeks of PN in adult patients. Liver function tests should be monitored weekly in hospitalized patients receiving PN.

Mechanical

Mechanical complications of PN include problems with insertion of the central venous catheter such as pneumothorax (punctured lung). Catheter occlusion or thrombosis may also occur. Occlusion may be treated by infusion of a thrombolytic agent or hydrochloric acid, depending on the nature of the occlusion.

Infectious

Catheter-related infections are common in patients receiving PN. Such infections present with symptoms such as fever, chills, and rigors. Because placement of a permanent central venous catheter is expensive and invasive, attempts to salvage infected catheters are frequently made in long-term home PN patients where IV access sites may also be limited. Administration of IV antibiotics and/or placement of a small amount of antibiotic as an antibiotic lock of the catheter may be utilized. Most catheter-related infections are secondary to gram-positive bacteria, although gram-negative bacteria or fungi may also be culprits. Typically, fungal infection requires catheter removal and replacement.

CASE Application

1. VB is a 54-year-old man who underwent small bowel resection for bowel necrosis. He is receiving PN and has required a nasogastric tube for suction. He develops metabolic alkalosis. Which one of the following is the most appropriate adjustment to VB's PN solution?

   a. Add sodium bicarbonate
   b. Decrease acetate and increase chloride
   c. Increase acetate and decrease chloride
   d. Increase sodium and chloride

2. Which one of the following statements is most correct regarding macrosubstrates found in PN solutions?

   a. Dextrose and amino acids can be mixed together by the manufacturer, heat sterilized, and then shipped to hospitals.
   b. Glycerin and amino acids can be mixed together by the manufacturer, heat sterilized, and then shipped to hospitals.
   c. Premixed PN solutions containing dextrose, amino acid, and fat all in a single chamber are available from various manufacturers.
   d. Combinations of dextrose and amino acid solution must be used within 24 hours of mixing, even if they are stored in the refrigerator.

3. A patient is receiving ProcalAmine postoperatively at 125 mL/h. ProcalAmine contains 3% final concentration of glycerin and 3% final concentration of amino acid. Glycerin provides 4.3 kcal/mL. How many calories and how much protein is provided per day by this solution?

   a. 747 kcal and 90 g amino acid
   b. 666 kcal and 90g amino acid
   c. 720 kcal and 60 g amino acid
   d. 747 kcal and 60 g amino acid

4. Which one of the following amino acid profiles best describes a specialty formulation for use in patients with hepatic encephalopathy compared to standard amino acid formulations?

   a. Higher in branched chain amino acids, same level of aromatic amino acids
   b. Higher in branched chain amino acids, lower in aromatic amino acids
   c. Higher in essential amino acids, lower in nonessential amino acids
   d. Fortified with dipeptides containing glutamine

5. HO is a 63-year-old woman with cancer cachexia. She has lost 10% of her body weight since her diagnosis with colon cancer about 6 months ago. Her cancer treatments are causing severe nausea and vomiting. The physician wants to start PN. The dietitian expresses concern regarding refeeding syndrome. Which electrolyte abnormality is the hallmark of this syndrome?

   a. Hypermagnesemia
   b. Hypercalcemia
   c. Hyponatremia
   d. Hypophosphatemia

6. A national shortage of IV multivitamin products leads a hospital to ration this product in patients receiving PN. Ten days after receiving PN with minimal multivitamins,

TE develops congestive heart failure symptoms that are diagnosed as wet beriberi. Deficiency of which vitamin is causing TE's symptoms?

a. Vitamin B_{12}
b. Vitamin K
c. Folic acid
d. Thiamine

7. Which one of the following increases the solubility of calcium and phosphate in a PN solution?

a. Increased temperature
b. Increased pH
c. Use of calcium chloride instead of calcium gluconate
d. Increased amino acid concentration in the PN

8. A hospital is transitioning from use of dextrose/amino acid solutions plus piggybacked lipid for PN to a system utilizing TNA. Which one of the following best describes proper use of final filters in this setting?

a. A switch from use of 0.22 μm filters to use of 1.2 μm filters is appropriate.
b. A switch from use of 1.2 μm filters to use of 0.22 μm filters is appropriate.
c. No switch in filtration practices is necessary; use of 0.22 μm filters may continue.
d. Switching from the current 0.22 μm filters to no filters is most appropriate.

9. PW is a 46-year-old man receiving PN because of intolerance to enteral feeding following multiple trauma. He is receiving 150 g of protein each day. A 24-hour urine collection for urea nitrogen (UUN) yields a value of 20 g. What is the estimated nitrogen balance in grams per day for this patient?

a. +4
b. 0
c. −10
d. −120

10. SR is a 26-year-old mechanically ventilated woman receiving propofol for sedation. The drug is provided as 10 mg/mL propofol and is being delivered at 100 mg/h. Propofol is commercially provided in a 10% lipid emulsion vehicle. How many grams per day of lipid is SR receiving via the propofol infusion?

a. 2.4
b. 4.8
c. 24
d. 48

11. Which one of the following statements is true regarding TNA?

a. A cracked TNA may be safely administered to a patient, but a creamed TNA is unsafe for administration.
b. A creamed TNA may be safely administered to a patient, but a cracked TNA is unsafe for administration.
c. Neither a creamed nor a cracked TNA may be safely administered to a patient.
d. Both creamed and cracked TNA may be safely administered to a patient after rehomogenization.

12. Which one of the following would be most likely to cause instability when added to a TNA?

a. Famotidine
b. Regular insulin
c. Iron dextran
d. Copper

13. AZ is to receive cycled PN over 16 h/d at home. The PN is to be infused at half the goal rate for the first and last hours of the 16-hour cycle. If the final concentration of amino acid in the solution is 5%, what goal rate of PN (in mL/h) will supply about 80 g of protein per day?

a. 77
b. 87
c. 97
d. 107

14. Which of the following most closely reflects the current recommendation for the optimal goal blood glucose range for a critically ill PN patient?

a. 70 to 100 mg/dL
b. 80 to 110 mg/dL
c. 110 to 150 mg/dL
d. 180 to 240 mg/dL

15. Which one of the following statements is most correct regarding markers of nutritional status in the hospitalized patient?

a. Albumin, because of its short half-life, is a good marker of the adequacy of a nutritional regimen when followed serially over several days.
b. Prealbumin has a short half-life and can be useful as a marker of nutritional status.
c. Transferrin is a very specific marker of overall nutritional status and reflects nutritional status over a period of several days.
d. To adequately assess nutritional status, albumin, prealbumin, and transferrin should all be monitored weekly.

16. NJ is a 53-year-old woman who is receiving PN following a bowel resection for mesenteric ischemia. She is receiving a dextrose/amino acid solution with final concentrations of 15% dextrose and 5% amino acid. This solution is being administered at 75 mL/h continuously over 24 hours. She is also receiving 250 mL of 20% lipid each day. Renal function is normal. NJ weighs 60 kg, which is near her ideal body weight of 62 kg. Which of the following best describes the amount of kcal, protein, and dextrose that NJ is receiving?

a. Calories are excessive, but the amounts of protein and dextrose are within recommended ranges.
b. The amounts of dextrose and protein are lower than recommended ranges as is the amount of calories.
c. Protein is below the recommended range, but calories and dextrose are adequate.
d. The number of calories, as well as the amounts of protein and dextrose, are within recommended ranges.

17. Which one of the following vitamins commonly included in PN solutions could interfere with warfarin anticoagulation?

a. Vitamin D
b. Vitamin K
c. Thiamine
d. Vitamin B_6

18. Which of the following trace elements is least commonly included in PN solutions?

a. Iodide
b. Zinc
c. Manganese
d. Copper

19. What is the most common cause for hospitalization in patients receiving home PN?

a. Metabolic bone disease
b. Catheter-related sepsis
c. Trace element deficiency
d. Hyperglycemia

20. HM is a 63-year-old critically ill, morbidly obese man (BMI 42 kg/m^2) with severe acute pancreatitis in whom enteral nutrition has failed. On day 7 of hospitalization, PN is initiated. HM weighs 150 kg; ideal body weight is 82 kg. The PN regimen consists of 1800 kcal/d and 205 g protein per day. What is the most appropriate assessment of this PN regimen?

a. Appropriate calories and protein
b. Appropriate calories; too much protein
c. Appropriate protein; too many calories
d. Too few calories; too much protein

TAKEAWAY POINTS ››

- PN is a potentially lifesaving modality of feeding for the patient with severe gastrointestinal compromise precluding adequate oral or enteral feeding.
- EN is preferred over PN if EN can be administered safely, mainly due to a lesser chance of infectious complications with EN.
- PN may be delivered through either a central or peripheral venous access. Peripheral delivery is limited by the osmolality of solution that can be administered by this route.
- In patients for whom PN is appropriate, timing of PN can be controversial. In general, patients who are previously malnourished should be started on PN sooner than those who are not previously malnourished.
- Caloric contribution of the major macrosubstrates used in PN is as follows: dextrose 3.4 kcal/g, lipid emulsion 20% 2 kcal/mL, amino acid 4 kcal/g.
- Calories are generally provided via PN at 20 to 35 kcal/kg/d. For the obese patient, recommendations call for 11 to 14 kcal/kg actual body weight or 22 to 25 kcal/kg ideal body weight.
- Dextrose is generally limited to <7 g/kg/d. Lipid is generally limited to <2.5 g/kg/d.
- Amino acids are generally administered at 1.2 to 2 g/kg/d. Higher amounts (2-2.5 g/kg ideal body weight per day) are appropriate for obese patients. Patients receiving renal replacement therapy also require higher amounts of amino acid.
- Standard amino acid formulations are appropriate for most patients; specialized amino acid formulations (eg, hepatic, renal, stress formulas) are more expensive and rarely indicated.
- Total nutrient admixtures are inherently less stable than dextrose/amino acid solutions. A TNA that has creamed may be administered to a patient after redispersion, whereas a cracked TNA should never be administered to a patient.

REFERENCES

1. McClave SA, Martindale RG, Vanek VW, et al. Guidelines for the provision and assessment of nutrition support therapy in the adult critically ill patient: Society of Critical Care Medicine (SCCM) and American Society for Parenteral and Enteral Nutrition (A.S.P.E.N.). *JPEN J Parenter Enteral Nutr.* 2009;33:277-316.
2. Critical Care Nutrition. Clinical practice guidelines. Available at: http://www.criticalcarenutrition.com/index.php?option=com_content&task=view&id=17&Itemid=100. Accessed on October 26, 2009.
3. A.S.P.E.N. Board of Directors and the Clinical Task Force. Guidelines for the use of parenteral and enteral nutrition in adult and pediatric patients. *JPEN J Parenter Enteral Nutr.* 2002;26(suppl):1SA-138SA.

4. Task Force for the Revision of Safe Practices for Parenteral Nutrition. Safe practices for parenteral nutrition. *JPEN J Parenter Enteral Nutr.* 2004;28(suppl):S39-S70.
5. A.S.P.E.N. Board of Directors and Task Force on Standardization of Parenteral Nutrition Solutions. A.S.P.E.N. statement on parenteral nutrition standardization. *JPEN J Parenter Enteral Nutr.* 2007;31:441-448.
6. O'Grady NP, Alexander M, Dellinger EP, et al. Guidelines for the prevention of intravenous catheter-related infections. *MMWR Morb Mortal Wkly Rep.* 2002;55(RR10):1-26.
7. Trissel LA. Calcium chloride. *Handbook on Injectable Drugs.* 15th ed. Bethesda, MD: American Society of Health-Systems Pharmacists; 2009: 240-244.

CHAPTER

34 Electrolyte Disorders

Kendrea M. Jones, Kathryn K. Neill, T. Scott Warmack

FOUNDATION OVERVIEW

Throughout the body, electrolytes are involved in numerous metabolic and homeostatic processes. Abnormalities are associated with excessive or reduced intake, altered absorption and excretion, or changes in hormonal and neurological homeostasis. Signs and symptoms of electrolyte disorders range from asymptomatic to life-threatening, depending on the speed of onset and degree of electrolyte loss or excess. The goals of therapy for electrolyte disorders are to prevent the development and/or treat life-threatening complications, identify and treat the underlying cause of the disturbance, correct concomitant abnormal electrolyte findings, and attain a normal electrolyte concentration while preventing overcorrection. The rapidity of development, severity of symptoms present, concomitant medical conditions, medications, dietary factors, and considerations for patient compliance should all be considered when selecting a treatment strategy. This chapter provides a review of the pathophysiology, clinical manifestations, and treatment of the most common electrolyte disorders. Listed in Table 34-1 are the normal serum concentrations of the common electrolytes.

SODIUM DISORDERS

General Overview

Sodium is the major extracellular cation and responsible for the majority of the extracellular fluid osmolality. Under normal conditions, the serum sodium concentration is kept between 135 and 145 mEq/L. Disorders of sodium balance are the most common electrolyte disturbances encountered in clinical practice and occur in both inpatient and ambulatory patients.[1] Hyponatremia can be classified by the patient's serum osmolality and volume status (Figure 34-1).[2] Hypernatremia always causes hypertonicity, and can be classified by the patient's volume status (Figure 34-2).[2] Common causes of sodium disorders are listed in Table 34-2.

Pathophysiology

Maintenance of extracellular fluid tonicity and sodium concentration is controlled by homeostatic mechanisms that regulate the intake and excretion of free water. Antidiuretic hormone (ADH), also known as arginine vasopressin, plays a major role in determining serum sodium concentration by regulating the renal handling of water. ADH and the thirst mechanism are efficient at maintaining a normal serum osmolality despite large variations in sodium and water intake. While a loss or excess of total body sodium may occur, sodium disorders are primarily caused by abnormalities of water metabolism.[3]

When brain cells are threatened with swelling from hyponatremia or shrinkage from hypernatremia, adaptive measures are taken to maintain normal cell volume. In sodium disorders, intracellular electrolytes and organic osmolyte concentrations are altered to reduce osmotic fluid shifts between the extracellular and intracellular space. This adaptive process normalizes cell volume and is responsible for the relatively mild symptoms seen in chronic sodium disorders.[4] It is also responsible for life-threatening complications that arise from correcting serum sodium too quickly in chronic sodium disorders.

Signs and Symptoms

Clinical manifestations of sodium disorders are related to central nervous system dysfunction. Cases can range from asymptomatic to life threatening. Symptoms are more apparent when the change in serum sodium is large or develops rapidly. Symptoms associated with sodium disorders are listed in Table 34-3.

TREATMENT OF HYPONATREMIA

Serum sodium should be corrected at a rate that improves symptoms but does not place the patient at risk for osmotic demyelination. In patients with chronic hyponatremia (>48 hours), neurologic complications can be avoided by limiting the correction rate to 10 to 12 mEq/L in 24 hours or 18 mEq/L in 48 hours. A correction rate of 2 to 4 mEq/L within 2 to 4 hours may be beneficial in patients with severe symptoms such as seizures.[5] Available intravenous solutions are listed in Table 34-4.[2]

Hypovolemic Hypotonic Hyponatremia

The cornerstone of therapy for hypovolemic hyponatremia is isotonic (0.9%) saline infusion. Additionally, specific therapies for underlying causes should be initiated. Due to a high rate of reoccurrence, thiazide diuretics should be permanently discontinued. Gastrointestinal losses can be treated with antiemetics and antidiarrheals as appropriate.[5]

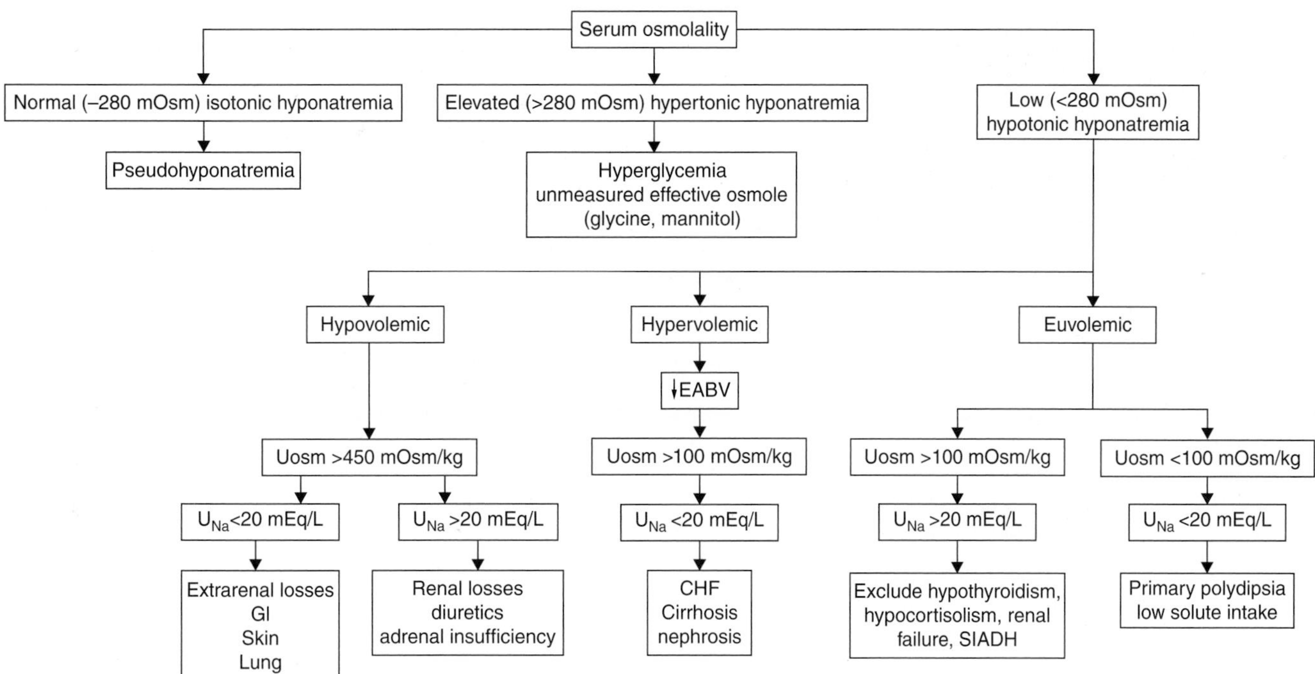

FIGURE 34-1 Diagnosis of hyponatremia.

Reprinted with permission from Coyle JD, Joy MS. Disorders of sodium and water homeostasis. In: DiPiro JT, Talbert RL, Yee GC, et al, eds. *Pharmacotherapy: A Pathophysiologic Approach*. 7th ed. Available at: http://www.accesspharmacy.com/content.aspx?aID=3183025.

Isovolemic Hypotonic Hyponatremia

Fluid restriction is generally considered the cornerstone of therapy for mild or moderate cases of isovolemic hyponatremia. Patients with SIADH should have fluid restricted to 1 L/d to ensure a negative fluid balance of 500 mL daily.[6] Dietary intake should be relatively high unless otherwise contraindicated, to augment free water excretion. Medications associated with SIADH should be discontinued. Pharmacologic therapy is reserved for patients not responding to fluid restriction. Demeclocycline is the preferred agent.[5] It interferes with the action of ADH in the collecting duct and increases water excretion.[7] Demeclocycline should be given orally in doses of 600 to 1200 mg/d in divided doses. Because of its delayed onset, doses should not be increased for 3 to 4 days.[8] Adverse effects include reversible azotemia and nephrotoxicity, especially in patients with renal insufficiency.[9] Lithium has a similar renal effect, but is less efficacious than demeclocycline and is poorly tolerated.[10] Recently approved vasopressin receptor antagonists represent a new treatment option for isovolemic hyponatremia.[11,12] Developed agents include oral agents (tolvaptan, satavaptan, and lixivaptan) and the intravenous agent, conivaptan. However, clinical experience is needed to establish their role in therapy.[5] Acute symptomatic SIADH should be treated with hypertonic (3%) saline. Intravenous furosemide 20 to 40 mg can be added to treat or prevent volume overload.[5]

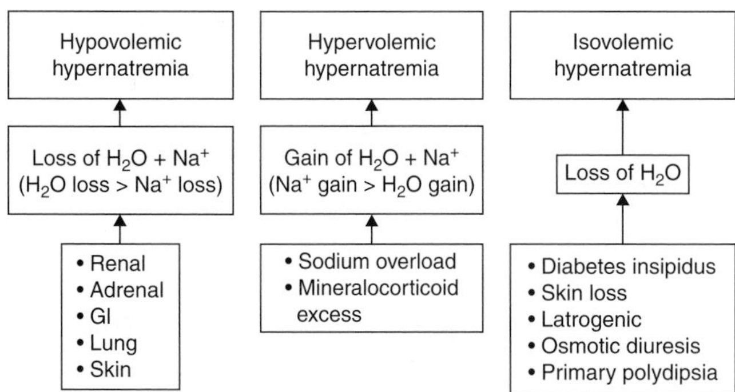

FIGURE 34-2 Diagnosis of hypernatremia.

Reprinted with permission from Coyle JD, Joy MS. Disorders of sodium and water homeostasis. In: DiPiro JT, Talbert RL, Yee GC, et al, eds. *Pharmacotherapy: A Pathophysiologic Approach*. 7th ed. Available at: http://www.accesspharmacy.com/content.aspx?aID=3183025.

Hypervolemic Hypotonic Hyponatremia

The cornerstone of therapy for hyponatremia associated with edema is dietary sodium restriction and diuretic therapy.[5] Vasopressin receptor blockers represent a new treatment option for the treatment of hypervolemic hyponatremia.[13] As with isovolemic hyponatremia, further studies are needed to determine their place in therapy.[5]

TABLE 34-1 **Electrolyte Serum Concentrations**

Electrolytes	Normal Values
Sodium (Na)	135-145 mEq/L
Potassium (K)	3.5-5.0 mEq/L
Magnesium (Mg)	1.4-1.8 mEq/L
Calcium (Ca)	8.5-10.5 mg/dL
Phosphate (PO_4)	2.6-4.5 mg/dL

TABLE 34-2 **Causes and Contributing Factors for Electrolyte Disorders**

Electrolyte	Decreased	Increased
Sodium	*Hypovolemic hypotonic hyponatremia* Excessive sweating GI losses Renal losses *Isovolemic hypotonic hyponatremia* SIADH secondary to malignancy, pulmonary disease, CNS disorders, iatrogenic sources *Hypervolemic hypotonic hyponatremia* Cirrhosis Congestive heart failure	*Hypovolemic hypernatremia* Dermal losses Vomiting NG suction Lactulose Osmotic diuresis—hyperglycemia, mannitol Loop diuretics *Isovolemic hypernatremia* Insensible water loss Diabetes insipidus *Hypervolemic hypernatremia* Hypertonic saline
Potassium	Poor dietary intake β-Agonists Loop and thiazide diuretics Penicillins Sorbitol Theophylline Caffeine Insulin overdose Mineralocorticoids Amphotericin B Cisplatin Aminoglycosides	Dietary noncompliance Spironolactone Amiloride Triamterene Angiotensin-converting enzyme inhibitors Renal insufficiency Metabolic acidosis
Magnesium	Alcoholism Protein malnutrition Malabsorptive disease Vomiting Laxative abuse Diarrhea Bartter syndrome Amphotericin B Aminoglycosides Loop and thiazide diuretics Hyperthyroidism Hypercalcemia	Renal insufficiency Treatment of eclampsia Cathartics Lithium therapy Hypothyroidism Milk-alkali syndrome Addison disease Diabetic ketoacidosis
Calcium	Decreased parathyroid activity Vitamin D deficiency Hyperphosphatemia Hypoalbuminemia Hypomagnesemia Loop diuretics Glucocorticoids Calcitonin Phenobarbital Phenytoin	Malignancy Increased parathyroid activity Thiazide diuretics Lithium Excessive calcium intake Paget disease Increased thyroid activity Adrenal insufficiency Sarcoidosis
Phosphate	Renal tubular dysfunction Increased parathyroid activity Refeeding syndrome Insulin and dextrose treatment for hyperkalemia Alcoholism Malnutrition Phosphate binders Decreased vitamin D intake	Chronic kidney disease Tumor lysis syndrome Rhabdomyolysis Septic shock Excessive phosphate administration Increased vitamin D intake

TABLE 34-3 Signs and Symptoms of Electrolyte Disorders

Electrolyte	Low	High
Sodium	Disorientation Headache Lethargy Malaise Nausea Restlessness Coma Respiratory arrest Seizures	Anorexia Weakness Nausea Restlessness Vomiting Altered mental status Coma Irritability Lethargy
Potassium	Muscle cramps Weakness Malaise Myalgias Impaired muscle function ECG changes Arrhythmias	Palpitations ECG changes Arrhythmias
Magnesium	Tetany Muscular fasciculation Convulsions Trousseau and/or Chvostek sign Palpitations ECG changes Arrhythmias Hypertension	Hypotension Flushing ECG changes Complete heart block, asystole Sedation Coma Hypotonia/hyporeflexia Paralysis Respiratory failure
Calcium	Paresthesia Muscle cramps Tetany Laryngeal spasm Depression Confusion Memory loss Brittle nails Hair loss Eczema Seizures Myocardial infarction Arrhythmias Hypotension	Nausea Vomiting Abdominal pain Dyspepsia Anorexia Acute pancreatitis Lethargy Obtundation Ataxia Coma ECG changes Arrhythmias Hypertension Polyuria/polydipsia Nephrolithiasis Renal dysfunction
Phosphate	Arrhythmias Respiratory failure Myalgias Confusion Hallucinations Weakness Platelet/WBC dysfunction Hemolysis	Calcium-phosphate precipitation

TREATMENT OF HYPERNATREMIA

Treatment should correct serum sodium at a rate sufficient to alleviate symptoms and not place the patient at risk for cerebral edema. In patients with chronic hypernatremia, neurologic complications can be avoided by not exceeding a correction rate of 0.5 mEq/L/h. Sodium correction should be limited to 10 mEq/L/d.[14] A faster correction rate of 1 mEq/L/h may be beneficial in patients with acute hypernatremia.[15]

Hypovolemic Hypernatremia

Patients with hemodynamic instability should first receive normal saline until volume status is restored and vital signs are stable. Subsequently, the patient should be switched to hypotonic fluids to correct serum sodium.[16] Oral or enteral replacement with hypotonic fluids is the preferred route. Intravenous is appropriate when oral replacement is not possible.[14]

Isovolemic Hypernatremia

Access to free water or replacement with intravenous hypotonic fluids is the cornerstone of therapy for isovolemic hypernatremia. Patients with central diabetes insipidus require exogenous ADH.[3] Desmopressin is the drug of choice and is typically initiated at a dose of 10 μg intranasally in the evening.[14] Most adults require a dose of 10 μg twice daily. Desmopressin is also available in injectable and oral forms. Injectable desmopressin is given at a dose of 2 to 4 μg daily in two divided doses. The initial dose of oral desmopressin is 0.05 mg orally twice daily, with doses ranging from 0.1 to 1.2 mg daily in divided doses. Since unsuppressed ADH activity can cause water intoxication from excess water retention, patients should be monitored for signs and symptoms of hyponatremia and hypervolemia.[3] Thiazide diuretics and sodium restriction are used in nephrogenic diabetes insipidus to cause modest volume depletion. This results in proximal tubule sodium and water reabsorption and diminishes water delivery to the collecting tubules. The overall effect is a reduction in water excretion.[17] Medications used to treat diabetes insipidus are listed in Table 34-5.

Hypervolemic Hypernatremia

Treatment consists of 5% dextrose infusion with loop diuretics added to promote renal sodium excretion.[14] Since this disorder is commonly iatrogenic and develops within a few hours, rapid correction of serum sodium is safe and appropriate.

POTASSIUM DISORDERS

General Overview

Potassium is the most plentiful intracellular cation in the body. Total body stores of potassium are estimated at 3,000 to 4,000 mEq with approximately 2% being distributed in the extracellular compartment. Potassium homeostasis is maintained through intra- and extracellular shifting, predominantly regulated by the sodium-potassium-adenosine triphosphatase (Na^+-K-ATPase) pump[18]; therefore, serum potassium concentrations do not accurately reflect the total body content. Potassium is responsible for many cellular functions, including protein synthesis, cellular metabolism, and conduction of the electrical action potential.[19] The normal range for serum potassium concentration is 3.5 to 5.0 mEq/L.[20]

TABLE 34-4 Intravenous Replacement Solutions

Solution	Dextrose (g/dL)	[Na^+] (mEq/L)	[Cl^-] (mEq/L)	Tonicity	Distribution % ECF	Distribution % ICF	Free Water/L
D_5W	5	0	0	Hypotonic	40	60	1000 mL
0.45% Sodium chloride	0	77	77	Hypotonic	73	37	500 mL
0.9% Sodium chloride	0	154	154	Isotonic	100	0	0 mL
3% Sodium chloride[a]	0	513	513	Hypertonic	100	0	−2331 mL

[a]This solution will result in osmotic removal of water from the intracellular space.

Abbreviations: Cl^-, chloride; D_5W, 5% dextrose in water; ECF, extracellular fluid; ICF, intracellular fluid; Na^+, sodium.

Reprinted with permission from Coyle JD, Joy MS. Disorders of sodium and water homeostasis. In: DiPiro JT, Talbert RL, Yee GC, et al, eds. *Pharmacotherapy: A Pathophysiologic Approach.* 7th ed. Available at: http://www.accesspharmacy.com/content.aspx?aID=3183025.

Pathophysiology

Maintenance of the normal range for potassium is affected by diet, acid–base balance, aldosterone, insulin, catecholamines, tonicity of body fluids, and GI and renal excretion.[21] The recommended daily intake of potassium is 50 mEq/d. The primary route of potassium elimination is the kidney, though small amounts are excreted via the GI tract. Hypokalemia is the finding of a serum potassium concentration <3.5 mEq/L and can be classified as mild (serum potassium 3-3.5 mEq/L), moderate (2.5-3 mEq/L), or severe (<2.5 mEq/L).[22] It is caused by a total body deficit of potassium when there is insufficient intake of potassium in the diet or excessive loss through the renal or GI tracts. Hypokalemia caused by the intracellular shift of serum potassium is known as *false hypokalemia* because there is no true deficit in total body content. Hypokalemia is commonly iatrogenic with the most common causes being loop and thiazide diuretics.[23] Increased gastrointestinal loss of potassium is also a common cause. Hypomagnesemia contributes to the development of hypokalemia by increasing renal potassium wasting and decreasing the intracellular uptake of potassium. If both disorders are present, hypomagnesemia should be addressed first to facilitate correction of the potassium deficiency.

Hyperkalemia is defined as a serum potassium concentration >5.5 mEq/L and can be classified as mild (5.5-6 mEq/L), moderate (6.1-6.9 mEq/L), or severe (>7 mEq/L).[24] It is caused by excessive potassium intake in comparison to potassium elimination or when the compartmental distribution of potassium is disrupted. Elevated serum potassium resulting from cellular shifts is known as *false hyperkalemia* since there is no true excess in total body potassium. Hyperkalemia is commonly associated with acute or chronic kidney disease, especially if patients are noncompliant with dietary restrictions. Potassium disorders are commonly induced by drugs.[25] Causes of potassium disorders are listed in Table 34-2.

TABLE 34-5 Central and Nephrogenic Diabetes Insipidus Treatment

Drug	Indication	Dose
Desmopressin acetate	Central and nephrogenic	5-20 µg intranasally every 12-24 h
Chlorpropamide	Central	125-250 mg po daily
Carbamazepine	Central	100-300 mg po bid
Clofibrate	Central	500 mg po qid
Hydrochlorothiazide	Central and nephrogenic	25 mg po every 12-24 h
Amiloride	Lithium-related nephrogenic	5-10 mg po daily
Indomethacin	Central and nephrogenic	50 mg po every 8-12 h

Reprinted with permission from Coyle JD, Joy MS. Disorders of sodium and water homeostasis. In: DiPiro JT, Talbert RL, Yee GC, et al, eds. *Pharmacotherapy: A Pathophysiologic Approach.* 7th ed. Available: http://www.accesspharmacy.com/content.aspx?aID=3183025.

Signs and Symptoms

Patients with potassium disorders are often asymptomatic; however, alterations in serum potassium concentration can affect neuromuscular, cardiac, and smooth muscle tissue. Signs and symptoms of potassium disorders are listed in Table 34-3.

TREATMENT

Hypokalemia

The treatment options for hypokalemia consist of increased dietary intake of potassium-rich foods, oral potassium supplements, and intravenous (IV) potassium. A general rule for replacement is that there is a total body potassium deficit of 100 to 400 mEq for every 1 mEq/L decrease in the serum potassium concentration below the normal range. However, a patient's renal function, acid–base status, concomitant medications, or disease processes must all be considered before recommending an estimated dose for replacement. For patients with concomitant hypomagnesemia, the magnesium deficit should be corrected to prevent refractory hypokalemia.

Dietary Potassium

Dietary supplementation is recommended for patients with low-normal serum potassium concentrations and may be considered for those with serum potassium concentrations of 3 to 3.5 mEq/L.[26]

Oral Potassium Replacement

Oral potassium supplements are preferred whenever possible, especially for asymptomatic patients. It should be given to patients with potassium concentrations of 3 to 3.5 mEq/L who have underlying risk for cardiac arrhythmias. Patients with serum potassium concentrations below 3 mEq/L should receive supplementation to target a goal of 4 to 4.5 mEq/L.[26] Of the three salt forms available, chloride is used more frequently because it is effective for common causes of hypokalemia. Phosphate should be reserved for patients with concomitant hypophosphatemia, and bicarbonate is advantageous for patients with concurrent metabolic acidosis. In stable patients receiving preventative supplementation, serum potassium and magnesium concentrations and renal function parameters should be obtained every 1 to 2 months. Hospitalized patients being treated for mild hypokalemia should be monitored every 2 to 3 days. When more aggressive replacement is warranted, the potassium concentration should be obtained 1 to 2 hours following the administration of an immediate-release oral dose to allow time for absorption and distribution. Oral potassium replacement may result in nausea, vomiting, and GI erosions.

Intravenous Potassium Replacement

Intravenous potassium can be used in patients with severe deficiency, those exhibiting severe symptoms such as ECG changes, or patients unable to tolerate oral supplements. Intravenous therapy is more likely to cause hyperkalemia and may cause damage to the veins and infusion site pain. Typically, 10 to 20 mEq of potassium is diluted in 100 mL of 0.9% sodium chloride and administered through a peripheral vein over 1 hour. Patients should be monitored for burning pain and phlebitis at the injection site. Larger amounts can be diluted in larger total volumes and infused at a rate not exceeding 40 mEq/h for severe hypokalemia. For intravenous infusion rates exceeding 10 mEq/h, ECG monitoring is recommended. These infusions should employ a central venous line due to the risk of pain and peripheral venous sclerosis. After each 30 to 40 mEq infusion, the serum potassium concentration should be reevaluated to guide further dosing needs. Following completion of the infusion, at least 30 minutes should elapse before drawing the serum level to allow time for potassium distribution. Observing recommendations regarding the amount, site (peripheral or central), and rate of potassium infusion is instrumental in preventing untoward effects of potassium replacement.

Alternative Therapies

Potassium-sparing diuretics such as spironolactone, triamterene, and amiloride are alternatives to chronic exogenous potassium. They may be particularly useful when patients are concomitantly receiving potassium-depleting medications.

Hyperkalemia

Along with addressing underlying causes, the treatment options for hyperkalemia consist of dietary restriction, pharmacotherapy, and hemodialysis. Asymptomatic patients with mild hyperkalemia may be managed with dietary education and careful monitoring of potassium concentration. A loop diuretic may be added to increase urinary potassium elimination. For patients unable to tolerate loop diuretics, a cation-exchange resin like sodium polystyrene sulfonate (SPS) may be administered orally or rectally. In patients with severe hyperkalemia or acute ECG changes, intravenous calcium is administered for stabilization of the cardiac membrane and hemodynamics. Calcium gluconate is preferred over calcium chloride due to an increased risk of tissue necrosis with the chloride salt if extravasation occurs. Concomitantly, an additional therapy should be instituted to shift potassium intracellularly and attain a serum potassium concentration <5.5 mEq/L. Sodium bicarbonate, insulin and dextrose, and albuterol are available options. Comorbid disease processes may influence the choice of therapy. Sodium bicarbonate is advantageous for patients with concomitant metabolic acidosis; however, the effects on potassium-lowering are significantly delayed in patients with advanced renal insufficiency. Additionally, renal patients are at increased risk of sodium and volume overload. Insulin and dextrose administration does not adversely impact volume status, but blood glucose levels must be monitored carefully. Beta-agonists have a dual mechanism for lowering potassium by stimulating the Na^+-K^+-ATPase pump and stimulating increased secretion of pancreatic insulin, but the effects can be unpredictable secondary to variable bioavailability of inhaled agents. Finally, excess potassium is removed from the body with diuretics, a resin binder, or hemodialysis.[27,28] Dosing information and utility of available therapies for potassium disorders is described in Tables 34-6 and 34-7.

Adverse effects associated with treatment of hyperkalemia include hypo- or hyperglycemia from administration of insulin and dextrose, SPS-induced diarrhea, cardiac excitability from albuterol, volume depletion or electrolyte abnormalities following diuretic therapy, and hypercalcemia from intravenous calcium. Additionally, skin necrosis may occur if calcium extravasates.

During emergent treatment, the serum potassium concentration should be evaluated hourly, and ECG monitored continuously until the serum concentration is <5 mEq/L and ECG changes have resolved. Patients who receive SPS and are asymptomatic should have serum potassium concentrations obtained within 4 hours to guide the need for readministration.

MAGNESIUM

General Overview

Magnesium is the second most abundant intracellular cation and is mainly distributed in bone and muscle. The normal range for the serum magnesium concentration is 1.4 to 1.8 mEq/L, or 1.7 to 2.3 mg/dL. Magnesium is responsible for many physiologic functions including protein synthesis, function of the cell membrane and mitochondria, and secretion of parathyroid hormone (PTH).[29] Magnesium abnormalities are common because allocation of magnesium between extracellular and intracellular compartments is not hormonally regulated. It is estimated that up to 65% of intensive care unit patients

TABLE 34-6 Available Treatment Modalities for Hypokalemia

Source	Utility
Dietary	
Dried fruits—figs, dates, prunes	Food sources are often insufficient for replacement and may cause increased weight
Nuts	
Vegetables—lima beans, spinach, potatoes	
Fruits—bananas, cantaloupe, oranges	
Meats—beef, pork, lamb	
Potassium chloride salt substitutes	
Oral Replacement	
Controlled-release tablets	Microencapsulated formulations cause fewer GI erosions than wax-matrix tablets
Elixir	Elixir is inexpensive and works quickly but poor taste often results in poor compliance
Effervescent tablets	
Chloride, phosphate, bicarbonate salts	Chloride salts are most effective for most causes of hypokalemia; bicarbonate is useful for hypokalemia with concomitant metabolic acidosis
Intravenous Replacement	
Chloride, phosphate, bicarbonate salts	Most useful in severe deficiency; requires continuous monitoring at rates >10 mEq/h; concentrations >10 mEq/L should be administered via a central line to avoid pain and vein necrosis
Potassium-Sparing Diuretics	
Spironolactone, triamterene, amiloride	Used as alternatives to exogenous supplementation; may be especially useful when administered concomitantly with potassium-depleting medications

have hypomagnesemia.[30] Compared with hypomagnesemia, hypermagnesemia is rare. Serum magnesium concentrations outside the normal range can result in significant alterations in neuromuscular and cardiovascular activity. These changes can have life-threatening consequences including cardiac arrhythmias and paralysis.

Pathophysiology

Like other electrolytes, magnesium homeostasis is dependent upon the balance of intake versus output with approximately 30% to 40% of dietary magnesium absorbed in the small bowel. Renal reabsorption of magnesium occurs predominantly in the loop of Henle, with only about 20% of filtered magnesium reabsorbed in the proximal tubule.[19] Like potassium, magnesium is principally located intracellularly; therefore, the serum concentration may not accurately reflect the total body content. The recommended daily intake of magnesium is approximately 310 mg/d for women and 400 mg/d for men.

Hypomagnesemia is usually associated with decreased absorption secondary to small bowel disease or increased renal

TABLE 34-7 Available Treatment Modalities for Hyperkalemia

Therapy	Dose	Route	Onset/Duration	Monitoring	Physiologic Effect
Albuterol	10-20 mg	Inhalation	30 min/1-2 h	Palpitations/heart rate	Increases intracellular K^+ uptake
Calcium	1 g	IV	1-2 min/10-30 min	Serum calcium, ECG	Increases cardiac membrane potential
Furosemide	20-40 mg	IV	5-15 min/4-6 h	Urine output, serum chemistry	Increases renal K+ elimination
Insulin	5-10 U	IV	30 min/2-6 h	Hourly blood glucose	Increases intracellular K^+ uptake
Dextrose	25 g	IV	30 min/2-6 h	Hourly blood glucose	Increases intracellular K^+ uptake following insulin release
Sodium bicarbonate	50-100 mEq	IV	30 min/2-6 h	Volume status, pH, serum chemistry	Increases intracellular K^+ concentration
Sodium polystyrene sulfonate	15-60 g	po or PR	1 h/–	Stool output	Increases K^+ elimination by exchanging Na^+ for K^+
Hemodialysis	4 h	–	Immediate	Volume status, serum chemistry	Increases K^+ elimination

elimination as occurs with diuretic therapy.[30,31] Hypermagnesemia occurs when magnesium intake is greater than relative elimination by the kidney. Causes of magnesium disorders are listed in Table 34-2.

Signs and Symptoms

Signs and symptoms that typically manifest in the setting of magnesium disorders involve the neuromuscular and cardiovascular systems and are listed in Table 34-3.[31] Hypomagnesemia (serum magnesium concentration <1.4 mEq/L) is commonly asymptomatic. Concomitant electrolyte abnormalities, such as hypokalemia and hypocalcemia, are often associated with hypomagnesemia and complicate the discrimination of symptoms specific to hypomagnesemia. Hypermagnesemia (serum magnesium concentration >2 mEq/L) is an uncommon finding, and symptoms often do not present until the serum magnesium concentration exceeds 4 mEq/L.[29]

TREATMENT

Hypomagnesemia

The treatment of hypomagnesemia can be accomplished by supplementation via oral, intramuscular (IM), or IV routes. The selection of a route of delivery is dependent on the severity of deficiency and associated signs and symptoms. Because approximately half of the dose administered is eliminated in the urine, magnesium replacement should occur over several days. A description of magnesium replacement strategies is described in Table 34-8. Ongoing supplementation may be necessary if the patient is unable to ingest maintenance requirements of magnesium or has ongoing losses.[31] Empiric dosing should be reduced by half for patients with renal insufficiency.

Oral Magnesium Replacement

Oral magnesium supplementation can be given to patients with magnesium concentrations >1 mEq/L who are asymptomatic. Available products include magnesium-containing antacids or laxatives as well as magnesium oxide. Diarrhea is the most common side effect of oral replacement and more likely with large doses. Usual oral dosing is 400 to 800 mg tid or qid. In hospitalized patients, serum magnesium concentrations should be evaluated at least daily until released from the hospital.

Intramuscular Magnesium Replacement

Because IM administration is painful, it should be limited to patients with limited IV access who warrant more aggressive replacement than can be accomplished with oral supplementation.

Intravenous Magnesium Replacement

Patients with severe magnesium deficiency (<1 mEq/L) or signs and symptoms of hypomagnesemia should receive IV repletion until signs and symptoms resolve. IV administration is associated with rate-related flushing and sweating. Bolus administration should be avoided if possible, and IV solutions should be diluted to 20% before infusion to prevent sclerosis of the vein.[29] Serum magnesium concentrations should be monitored hourly until symptoms resolve and the serum concentration is at least 1.5 mEq/L. For the next 24 hours, serum magnesium concentration should be obtained every 6 to 12 hours, and then daily, once the concentration has returned to normal.

Hypermagnesemia

The treatment of hypermagnesemia is typically addressed in three ways: reduction of intake, enhanced elimination, and antagonism of the adverse effects of elevated magnesium concentrations. Patient-specific therapy is dependent upon associated signs and symptoms of hypermagnesemia. Education regarding magnesium-rich foods, beverages, and over-the-counter products is essential to prevent recurrent episodes of hypermagnesemia. Available therapies for acute treatment include intravenous calcium and forced diuresis using saline and loop diuretics.[29] Dialysis patients may require emergency hemodialysis using a magnesium-free dialysate. Adverse effects of hypermagnesemia treatment are similar to those of hyperkalemia.

Intravenous Calcium

Intravenous calcium can be employed to antagonize the neuromuscular and cardiac signs and symptoms of hypermagnesemia. Because the effect is transient, doses may need to be repeated as

TABLE 34-8 Magnesium Replacement

Serum Magnesium Concentration	<1 mEq/L		>1 mEq/L and <1.5 mEq/L
Symptoms	Life-threatening (seizures, arrhythmias)	Asymptomatic	Asymptomatic
Day 1	2 g magnesium sulfate[a] followed by 1 mEq/kg IV over 24 h	1 mEq/kg/d continuously or IM every 4 h × 5 doses	1 mEq/kg/d continuous IV or divided IM doses, *or* Milk of magnesia 5 mL qid, or Magnesium-based antacid 15 mL tid, *or* Magnesium oxide tablets 400 mg qid
Days 2-5	0.5 mEq/kg/d in maintenance fluids	0.5 mEq/kg/d as continuous IV or divided IM doses	May increase magnesium oxide tablets to 800 mg qid as tolerated; monitor need for continued supplementation

[a]Initial replacement given over 5 to 60 minutes. For torsades de pointes with cardiac arrest, shorten to 5 to 20 minutes IV push. For seizures, give over 10 minutes.

frequently as hourly until the signs and symptoms resolve and the magnesium concentration returns to normal. The typical dose is 100 to 200 mg of elemental calcium. If life-threatening adverse effects of elevated serum magnesium are present, additional care measures such as ventilatory and hemodynamic support may be required. Continuous ECG and hourly serum magnesium concentrations should be monitored until symptoms resolve and the serum magnesium concentration is <4 mg/dL.

Forced Diuresis

Diuresis to enhance magnesium elimination can be employed in patients without kidney dysfunction. This is usually accomplished via administration of saline accompanied by an intravenous loop diuretic such as furosemide, similar to hyperkalemia treatment. Patients with chronic renal insufficiency may require continued administration of diuretic therapy to maintain normal electrolyte concentrations. Urine output and signs and symptoms of volume overload should be monitored closely.

CALCIUM DISORDERS

Pathophysiology

Calcium is involved in numerous processes including propagation of neuromuscular activity, regulation of the blood coagulation cascade, bone and tooth metabolism, and endocrine and exocrine function.[32] Under normal conditions, the total serum calcium concentration is 8.5 to 10.5 mg/dL. Only 0.5% of calcium stores may be found in the extracellular fluid (ECF), while 99% of calcium stores are found in skeletal bone. ECF calcium is transported in three different forms: bound to plasma proteins, mostly albumin (45%); ionized or free state (40%); and bound to small anions including phosphates, citrates, and bicarbonates (6%).[33] The unbound or ionized calcium is the physiologically active form and regulated through complex interactions between parathyroid hormone (PTH), vitamin D, and serum phosphate levels.[34]

Any disease state or factor that alters albumin concentrations or its affinity to bind to calcium may change the concentration of serum calcium in the ionized form. The total calcium concentration may not accurately reflect the metabolically active or free concentration. Despite decreased levels of albumin, ionized calcium concentration may actually remain normal. The serum total calcium concentration falls approximately 0.8 mg/dL for every 1 g/dL fall in serum albumin below 4 g/dL. Thus, in patients with hypoalbuminemia, total serum calcium concentration should be corrected using the following equation:

Corrected calcium = [(4 − albumin) × 0.8 mg/dL] + measured calcium.

If a laboratory can reliably measure an ionized calcium concentration (reference range 1.12-1.3 mmol/L),[35] many clinicians prefer this measure in patients with hypoalbuminemia and acid–base disturbances.[36]

Hormonal Regulation of Calcium and Phosphate

The three major hormones that regulate serum calcium and phosphate concentrations are parathyroid hormone (PTH), vitamin D, and calcitonin (Table 34-9.).[34,37] PTH is released from the parathyroid gland in response to reduction in serum-ionized calcium. Upon release, it acts on the kidneys to stimulate reabsorption of calcium in the distal tubule and increases intestinal absorption of calcium by increasing renal production of 1-25-dihydroxycholecalciferol (1,25-DHCC or calcitriol), the active form of vitamin D. In addition, it stimulates osteoclast and osteoblast activity to increase calcium mobilization from skeletal bone. PTH acts in the kidneys to increase phosphate excretion by blocking renal reabsorption.

Vitamin D refers to a group of closely related sterols that are hormones, not vitamins. Vitamin D_2 and vitamin D_3 can be ingested in the diet or formed as a result of ultraviolet radiation of the skin, converting 7-dehydrocholesterol (D_2) to cholecalciferol (D_3). Cholecalciferol must be converted to calcitriol via hepatic and renal hydroxylation. Active vitamin D increases calcium and phosphate levels by increasing intestinal absorption and renal reabsorption. Additionally, vitamin D regulates the synthesis and release of PTH. Calcitonin is released in response to increased ionized calcium concentrations. It inhibits

TABLE 34-9 **Hormonal Regulation of Calcium and Phosphate**

Hormone	Effects on Calcium	Effects on Phosphate
PTH	• Promotes absorption of calcium by intestine • Mobilizes Ca^{2+} salts from the bones by activating osteoclasts • Increases Ca^{2+} reabsorption in the distal tubules • Stimulates the release of vitamin D *Net effect:* ↑ Serum calcium levels	• Decrease PO_4 reabsorption in the proximal tubule *Net effect:* ↓serum phosphate levels
Vitamin D	• Increases intestinal absorption of calcium • Facilitates reabsorption of calcium in the proximal tubules • Activates osteoclasts to mobilize calcium from bone *Net effect:* ↑ Serum calcium levels	• Increases intestinal absorption of phosphate • Facilitates reabsorption of phosphate in the proximal tubules *Net effect:* ↑ Serum phosphate levels
Calcitonin	• Inhibits osteoclasts and stimulates osteoblasts • Increases renal excretion of Ca^{2+} *Net effect:* ↓Serum calcium levels	

osteoclast activity and decreases calcium levels.[34,37] An alteration in any of these hormones may result in calcium and phosphate abnormalities.

Causes of Calcium Disorders

The most common causes of hypocalcemia are due to hypoparathyroidsim and vitamin D deficiency seen in rickets, GI disorders, and chronic kidney disease. The most common causes of hypercalcemia are malignancy and primary hyperparathyroidism. Malignancy-associated hypercalcemia may be caused by tumor invasion of bone leading to osteolysis and calcium release from the bone, tumor production of PTH-like substances, or substances that increase osteoclast development and activity.[38] Primary hyperparathyroidism is characterized by inappropriate release of PTH from the parathyroid gland resulting in increased calcium levels. Additionally, these patients may experience increased production of calcitriol. Other causes of calcium disorders are listed in Table 34-2.

Signs and Symptoms

Patients with acute hypocalcemia exhibit symptoms associated with the neuromuscular system. Chronic hypocalcemia is associated with CNS and dermatological disturbances.[35] Chvostek and Trousseau signs may be observed on physical examination. Chvostek sign is the unilateral twitch of the facial muscles when the facial nerve is slightly tapped. Trousseau sign is a carpal spasm that occurs when a blood pressure cuff is compressed on the upper arm.[37] Patients with hypercalcemia, especially those with a serum calcium level >14 mg/dL, may present with GI symptoms, including acute pancreatitis. In addition to GI symptoms, hypercalcemia may be associated with neuromuscular, cardiovascular, or renal manifestations. Common symptoms of calcium disorders are listed in Table 34-3. Renal insufficiency is associated with an increased calcium-phosphate product (usually >55 mg/dL) which may lead to soft-tissue calcification and deposits in the coronary arteries, myocardial fibers, and aortic valves.[39] Increased serum calcium levels may inhibit antidiuretic hormone's affects on the collecting ducts, leading to polyuria and polydipsia. Chronic hypercalcemia may cause renal tubular dysfunction.

TREATMENT

Hypocalcemia

In patients with hypocalcemia due to hypoalbuminemia, an ionized calcium should be obtained and treatment based on the level. Acute symptomatic hypocalcemia requires intravenous administration of calcium until signs and symptoms resolve. Administration of 100 to 300 mg of elemental calcium over 10 minutes will usually alleviate symptoms.[37] Intravenous calcium is available in two salt forms: calcium gluconate (1g Ca gluconate = 90 mg elemental calcium) and calcium chloride (1 g of Ca chloride = 270 mg elemental calcium).[37] Calcium gluconate administration is preferred over calcium chloride because it is associated with less risk of tissue necrosis.[35] Rapid administration of calcium may result in cardiac dysfunction. Additionally, intravenous calcium should not be administered with bicarbonate or phosphate containing solutions due to the risk of precipitation. Bolus doses of calcium only last about 2 hours, and ionized calcium and magnesium levels should be monitored closely after IV administration.[32,35]

TABLE 34-10 **Calcium Products**

Calcium Salt	Calcium Content per Gram	
	mg	mEq
Acetate	250	12.7
Carbonate	400	20
Chloride	270	13.5
Citrate	211	10.6
Glubionate	64	3.2
Gluconate	90	4.5
Lactate	130	6.5
Phosphate tribasic	390	19.3

Patients with chronic or asymptomatic hypocalcemia due to hypoparathyroidism or vitamin D deficiency may be managed with oral calcium salts or vitamin D replacement. Calcium replacement may begin with 1 to 3 g/d of elemental calcium and progress to a maintenance dose of 2 to 8 g/d in divided doses. Numerous oral calcium-containing products are available, with calcium carbonate containing more elemental calcium and being the least expensive. A complete list of oral calcium supplements are listed in Table 34-10. Calcium carbonate requires an acidic environment for absorption.[35,37] Adverse effects of calcium salts include GI upset, constipation, and hypercalcemia.[37]

Vitamin D supplementation should be reserved for patients with vitamin D deficiency. Several different products are available including: ergocalciferol, calcitriol, paricalcitriol, doxercalciferol. Usual oral dosage ranges from 0.5 to 3 μg daily, with adjustments made every 4 weeks. In patients with reduced hepatic metabolism, calcitriol is preferred.[37]

Hypercalcemia

Hypercalcemia treatment involves definitive treatment of primary hyperparathyroidism or malignancy. In patients with drug-induced hypercalcemia, the offending agent should be discontinued. The initial treatment for hypercalcemia in patients without severe renal dysfunction is volume expansion with saline-containing fluids and loop diuretics to enhance urinary excretion of calcium. Loop diuretics block calcium reabsorption in the ascending limb of the loop of Henle. Calcitonin is an alternative treatment that increases renal excretion of calcium by inhibiting bone resorption. It has a rapid onset of action but an unpredictable effect on serum calcium levels. Calcitonin may be administered intramuscularly, subcutaneously, intranasally,

TABLE 34-11 **Treatment of Hypercalcemia**

Drug	Starting Dose	Initial Response	Contraindications	Adverse Effects
NS ± electrolytes	200-300 mL/h	24-48 h	Renal insufficiency; chronic heart failure	Electrolyte abnormalities; fluid overload
Loop diuretics	40-80 mg IV every 1-4 h	NA		Electrolyte abnormalities
Calcitonin	4 U/kg every 12 h SQ/IM 10-12 U/h IV	1-2 h		Facial flushing, N/V, allergic reaction
Pamidronate	30-90 mg IV over 2-24 h	2 d	Renal insufficiency	Fever
Etidronate	7.5 mg/kg IV over 2 h	2 d	Renal insufficiency	Fever
Zoledronate	4-8 mg IV over 15 min	1-2 d	Renal insufficiency	Fever, fatigue, skeletal pain
Gallium nitrate	200 mg/m^2 daily	Variable	Severe renal insufficiency	Nephrotoxicity; hypophosphatemia; N/V/D; metallic taste
Mithramycin	25 μg/kg IV over 4-6 h	12 h	Decreased liver function; renal insufficiency, thrombocytopenia	Nausea/vomiting; stomatitis; thrombocytopenia; nephrotoxicity; hepatotoxicity
Glucocorticoids	40-60 mg po prednisone equivalents	Variable	Serious infections	Hyperglycemia, osteoporosis; infection

Abbreviation: NS, normal saline.

Reprinted with permission from Pai AB, Rohrscheib M, Joy MS. Disorders of calcium and phosphorus homeostasis. In DiPiro JT, Talbert RL, Yee GC, et al, eds. *Pharmacotherapy: A Pathophysiologic Approach*. 7th ed. Available at: http://www.accesspharmacy.com/content.aspx?aID=3183287.

or intravenously. Intravenous calcitonin is associated with an infusion-related syndrome and is therefore not preferred. Due to rare allergic reactions, a test dose should be administered prior to initiating therapy.

Bisphosphonates are first-line treatment in prevention and treatment of malignancy-induced hypercalcemia.[38,40] They lower calcium levels by inhibiting bone resorption and the formation of osteoclast. The onset of action of bisphosphonates may be slow, so saline hydration with loop diuretics or calcitonin may be necessary if a rapid decline in calcium levels is warranted. Intravenous therapy is associated with fever, and serum creatinine monitoring is recommended for all bisphosphonate therapy. Bisphosphonates are contraindicated in patients with a creatinine clearance <30 mL/min. Osteonecrosis of the jaw is a severe complication of bisphosphonate therapy, most commonly seen in patients with multiple myeloma.[38]

Gallium nitrate reduces serum calcium levels by inhibiting bone resorption. Due to its adverse effects, it is reserved for patients with hypercalcemia of malignancy that is unresponsive to hydration and other therapies. Mithramycin (plicamycin) is an antibiotic that inhibits osteoclast activity. It is recommended for short-term use due to adverse effects including renal and hepatotoxicity and platelet dysfunction. Glucocorticoids may be effective in treatment of hypercalcemia associated with malignancy, sarcoidosis, and syndromes of increased vitamin A and D. Glucocorticoids increase bone resorption, decrease osteoblast proliferation, and reduce estrogen and testosterone levels. Glucocorticoid therapy is not preferred due to its slow onset of action in lowering calcium levels and numerous adverse effects. Potassium and magnesium serum levels should be monitored closely in all patients receiving treatment for hypercalcemia.[37]

A list of the most commonly used agents for the management of hypercalcemia may be found in Table 34-11.

PHOSPHATE DISORDERS

Many of the factors that regulate serum calcium levels also influence serum phosphate levels (see Table 34-9). Phosphate is a major intracellular anion, and normal serum concentrations are 2.6 to 4.5 mg/dL. Phosphate is involved in numerous functions including regulation of enzymatic reactions and metabolism of protein, fats, and carbohydrates. It is a major component of phospholipid membranes of all cells and 2,3 diphosphoglycerate, which regulates the oxygen-carrying capacity of hemoglobin. In addition, it is required for the formation of high-energy bonds in ATP production.[37] The majority of dietary phosphate is absorbed in the small intestine, and absorption may be increased by 1,25-DHCC. In the kidneys, the elimination of phosphate is dependent on both glomerular filtration and reabsorption in the proximal tubule.[37]

Causes of Hypo- and Hyperphosphatemia

Phosphate disorders are commonly caused by disorders of excretion, altered intake, and cellular shifting. Common disorders associated with hypo- and hyperphosphatemia are listed in Table 34-2.

Signs and Symptoms

Symptoms of hypophosphatemia may present as the serum phosphate level falls below 2 mg/dL. Most of the symptoms are due to decreased formation of ATP and depletion of 2,3-DPG, which increases the affinity of oxygen for hemoglobin, leading to tissue hypoxia. Symptoms of hypophosphatemia are listed in Table 34-3. The most common clinical manifestation of hyperphosphatemia is hypocalcemia due to the formation of a calcium-phosphate precipitate, which may lead to tetany. Patients with a serum calcium and phosphate product that exceeds 55 mg/dL are at increased risk for precipitate formation and soft tissue calcification.[39]

TREATMENT

Hypophosphatemia

Administration of phosphate is key to preventing hypophosphatemia in hospitalized patients at risk, including patients with a history of alcoholism or receiving parenteral nutrition.

Asymptomatic, mild hypophosphatemia may be treated with oral phosphate supplementation. Oral phosphate supplements are associated with diarrhea and unpredictable absorption. Severe, symptomatic hypophosphatemia should be treated with intravenous phosphate administration; which are available as a potassium or sodium salt. One millimole of potassium phosphate contains 1.47 mEq of potassium, and 1 mmol of sodium phosphate contains 1.33 mEq of sodium. Potassium phosphate is reserved for patients with concomitant hypokalemia. Usually, 15 to 45 mmols of phosphorus is infused over 4 to 6 hours to reduce infusion-related adverse effects and formation of a calcium-phosphate precipitate.[35] The available therapies for hypophosphatemia are listed in Table 34-12.

Hyperphosphatemia

Elevated serum phosphate is common in chronic kidney disease. Dietary restriction of phosphate intake is key to preventing and treating hyperphosphatemia. If tetany is present, intravenous calcium is required to increase serum calcium levels. The mainstay of pharmacological treatment of hyperphosphatemia is phosphate binders administered with each meal and snack to bind dietary phosphate (Table 34-13). Oral calcium supplements are considered first-line therapy for long-term treatment. Calcium carbonate and calcium acetate are two commonly used agents and are adjusted based on phosphate levels. Recently, concerns have risen that calcium-based salts may be associated with increased risk of vascular calcification and hypercalcemia.[41] Aluminum-containing antacids also bind phosphate in the intestines and may be more beneficial for acute management of hyperphosphatemia. Long-term use should be avoided because of the risk of aluminum intoxication. Sevelamer is a noncalcium-, nonaluminum-containing phosphate binder. It is more costly than calcium products, but efficacious in patients with persistent hyperphosphatemia secondary to chronic kidney disease. After approximately 5 days, it will decrease dietary absorption of phosphate, with peak effects seen in 2 weeks.

Lanthanum carbonate is another noncalcium, nonaluminum-containing phosphate binder that dissociates in the upper GI tract to lanthanum ions (La^{3+}) which bind to dietary phosphate. This results in insoluble lanthanum-phosphate complexes and a net decrease in serum phosphate.[41]

Antacids and lanthanum may bind to some drugs in the GI tract and decrease their absorption. Therefore, patients should be counseled not to take interacting medications within 2 hours of antacids or lanthanum.

TABLE 34-12 Pharmacological Treatment of Hypophosphatemia

Product	PO_4^- (mmol)	Na^+ (mEq)	K^+ (mEq)
Oral Therapy			
Neutra-Phos cap/packet	8	7.1	7.1
Neutra-Phos-K	8	0	14.2
K-Phos Original tab	3.6	0	3.7
K-Phos MF tab	4	2.9	1.1
K-Phos Neutral tab	8	13	1.1
K-Phos No. 2 tab	8	5.8	2.3
Phospho-Soda	16	32	0
Uro-KP-Neutral tab	8	10.8	1.3
Intravenous Therapy			
Sodium phosphate	3 mmol/mL	4 mEq/mL	4.4 mEq/mL
Potassium phosphate	3 mmol/mL		

Note: 250 mg elemental phosphorus = ~ 8 mmol phosphate.

TABLE 34-13 Oral Phosphate Binders

Phosphate Binder	Advantages	Disadvantages
Aluminum salts	High efficacy	Aluminum toxicity
Calcium carbonate	Aluminum free Inexpensive	pH influences efficacy Hypercalcemia Constipation Drug interactions
Calcium acetate	Aluminum free Absorption less dependent on pH Reduced calcium content than carbonate Lower cost than newer agents	Hypercalcemia Constipation Drug interactions
Sevelamer	Calcium and aluminum free Increased efficacy over calcium products	Expensive Bind fat-soluble vitamins pH influences efficacy Drug interactions
Lanthanum carbonate	Calcium and aluminum free Chewable Increased efficacy Lower pill burden	Expensive Drug interactions

MONITORING

In general, patients receiving treatment for electrolyte disorders should be monitored aggressively when these agents are initiated and during titration. Once a stable dose is achieved, patients with normal renal function should have serum concentrations evaluated at least monthly. Patients with renal insufficiency should be evaluated more frequently.

PREVENTION

Prevention of electrolyte disorders involves proper dietary intake, careful monitoring of patients receiving medications which contribute to alterations in serum concentrations, and aggressive monitoring and treatment of disease processes which alter electrolyte homeostasis.

SPECIAL POPULATIONS

Aside from patients with concomitant disease processes or electrolyte disorders which influence the choice of salt for replacement or guide the selection of therapy for lowering serum concentrations, there are no recommendations of note for special populations.

CASE Application

1. A 72-year-old man is admitted for a low level of serum sodium at a routine check-up. The patient states he feels fine. Past medical history includes chronic obstructive pulmonary disease, depression, gout, and hypertension. Current medications are albuterol, allopurinol, lisinopril, and sertraline. Physical examination is unremarkable. Pertinent laboratory values include serum sodium of 123 mEq/L, urinary sodium of 90 mEq/L, and a urine osmolarity of 585 mOsm/L. The patient is diagnosed with SIADH. The most appropriate treatment to correct this patient's sodium abnormality includes:
   a. 3% Saline infusion
   b. Demeclocycline
   c. Stopping the offending agent and fluid restriction
   d. Normal saline infusion
2. A medication commonly associated with SIADH is:
   a. Hydrochlorothiazide
   b. Furosemide
   c. Lithium
   d. Sertraline
3. A 68-year-old woman is brought to the hospital because of progressive drowsiness and syncope. She complains of diarrhea for the past 3 days. She is lethargic but has no focal neurologic deficits. Past medical history is significant for lung cancer, depression, hypertension, GERD, and osteoarthritis. Medications include acetaminophen, hydrochlorothiazide, fluoxetine, ranitidine, and magnesium oxide. Physical examination reveals a blood pressure of 96/56 mm Hg, pulse of 110 beats/min, dry mucous membranes, and reduced skin turgor. Laboratory value is significant for serum sodium of 125 mEq/L. The most appropriate treatment to correct this patient's sodium abnormality includes:
   a. 3% Saline infusion
   b. Demeclocycline
   c. Fluid restriction of <1000 mL/d
   d. Normal saline infusion
4. A 54-year-old man is admitted to the hospital from the outpatient clinic with abdominal swelling, weight gain, and abnormal laboratory values. Medical history is significant for cirrhosis and hepatitis C. Medications include furosemide and propranolol. His physical examination is significant for distended abdomen with shifting dullness. Significant laboratory values include serum sodium of 124 mEq/L, INR of 1.9, and albumin of 2.1. The most appropriate treatment to correct this patient's sodium abnormality includes:
   a. 3% Saline with IV furosemide
   b. Fluid restriction
   c. Normal saline infusion
   d. Sodium restriction and diuretics
5. An 82-year-old man was brought to the emergency department by his daughter for worsening confusion and diarrhea. The daughter reports he has had poor oral intake over the last week. Medical history is significant for hypertension, stroke, reflux, and chronic constipation. Medications include aspirin, lactulose, lisinopril, omeprazole, and simvastatin. His physical examination is significant for orthostatic hypotension, tachycardia, and dry mucous membranes. Significant laboratory values include serum sodium of 162 mEq/L, BUN of 66, and serum creatinine of 2.5. Appropriate initial treatment for this patient would include:
   a. 0.45% Saline infusion
   b. 5% Dextrose infusion
   c. Desmopressin
   d. Normal saline infusion
6. A 39-year-old man presents to the emergency department with abnormal laboratory values from a local psychiatric hospital. He is 4 days post neurosurgical repair of intraventricular hemorrhage secondary to bilateral self-enucleation. He is currently constrained to the hospital bed and hallucinating. Medical history includes hypertension and schizophrenia. Medications include haloperidol, fluphenazine, and benztropine. Physical examination is normal. Pertinent laboratory values include sodium of 158 mEq/L and urine osmolarity of 76 mOsm/kg.

Urine output was 6500 mL over the last 24 hours. The patient is admitted for the treatment of central diabetes insipidus. The most appropriate treatment to correct this patient's sodium abnormality includes:

a. Desmopressin
b. Free access to water
c. Hydrochlorothiazide
d. Normal saline infusion

7. What is the drug of choice for lithium-induced diabetes insipidus when lithium must be continued?

a. Amiloride
b. Desmopressin
c. Hydrochlorothiazide
d. Indomethacin

8. Which is *not* an expected side effect of potassium replacement?

a. Irritation of the vein
b. Constipation
c. Nausea/vomiting
d. Cardiac arrhythmias
e. Dyspepsia

9. A 66-year-old man is seen for annual follow-up. He has a history of hypertension, type 2 diabetes, coronary artery disease, and heart failure. Current medications include spironolactone 25 mg daily, lisinopril 20 mg daily, metoprolol 100 mg twice daily, furosemide 40 mg daily, simvastatin 40 mg daily, metformin 500 mg twice daily, and aspirin 81 mg daily. Laboratory values reveal Na 141, K 5.6, BUN 11, SCr 1.1, Phos 3.5, and Mg 2.2. Patient has no complaints at this time. What is the most likely cause of this patient's hyperkalemia?

a. Spironolactone
b. Metoprolol
c. Metformin
d. Furosemide
e. Simvastatin

10. Which hyperkalemia treatment results in a reduction in total body potassium?

a. IV sodium bicarbonate
b. IV Insulin and dextrose
c. IV calcium
d. PO sodium polystyrene sulfonate (SPS)
e. Nebulized albuterol

11. Which statement best describes a mechanism of potassium homeostasis?

a. Insulin decreases the intracellular uptake of potassium.
b. Aldosterone increases potassium excretion.
c. Calcitonin increases the tubular reabsorption of potassium.
d. Increasing the plasma pH decreases the uptake of potassium into the cells.
e. β-Receptor stimulation increases movement of potassium extracellularly.

12. A 48-year-old man presents to the ambulatory clinic with complaints of palpitations over the past few days. Current medications are ramipril 10 mg daily, aspirin 325 mg daily, and omeprazole 20 mg daily. Vitals are blood pressure 152/90 mm Hg, pulse 90, temp 98.6°F, and respiratory rate 14 breaths/min. Laboratory values reveal Na 141, K 5.9, Cl 101, HCO_3 25, BUN 12, SCr 1.1, and glucose 115. ECG showed peaked T waves. Which is the most appropriate initial management for this patient's hyperkalemia?

a. PO sodium polystyrene sulfonate (SPS)
b. IV calcium
c. IV sodium bicarbonate
d. Nebulized albuterol
e. IV insulin and dextrose

13. Which is *not* an expected symptom of hypermagnesemia?

a. Hypotension
b. Flushing
c. Coma
d. ECG changes
e. Diarrhea

14. Which commonly causes hypomagnesemia?

a. Amphotericin b
b. Amiloride
c. Lithium
d. Lisinopril
e. Omeprazole

15. Loop diuretics are commonly associated with all except:

a. Hypokalemia
b. Hypocalcemia
c. Hypermagnesemia
d. Hypomagnesemia

16. Which statement most accurately describes hormonal regulation of calcium and phosphate homeostasis?

a. Vitamin D reduces calcium and phosphate levels.
b. Calcitonin decreases calcium levels.
c. Parathyroid hormone (PTH) decreases calcium levels and increases phosphate levels.

17. A 55-year-old woman with a past medical history of multiple myeloma is admitted to the hospital with nausea, abdominal pain, and severe constipation. Current laboratory values are Na 140, K 4.2, Cl 103, CO_2 24, BUN 13, SCr 0.9, Glu 123, Mg 2.2, Ca 11.5, Phos 4, albumin 1.3. She is currently receiving normal saline and furosemide 20 mg IV q4h with adequate urine output. Select the best treatment to prevent recurrence of her hypercalcemia.

a. Intranasal calcitonin
b. IV potassium phosphate
c. Sevelamer
d. IV pamidronate 90 mg

18. Which adverse effect may be associated with pamidronate therapy?

a. Constipation
b. Tachycardia
c. Osteonecrosis of the jaw

19. A patient with hyperparathyroidism is admitted to the medical intensive care unit with pneumonia and respiratory distress, requiring mechanical ventilation. Current laboratory values are Na 144, K 3.4, Cl 105, CO_2 24, BUN 16, SCr 0.9, Glu 130, Mg 1.9, Ca 9, Phos 0.8, and albumin 4. Select the best medication to manage this patient's phosphate disorder.

a. IV sodium phosphate
b. IV potassium phosphate
c. IV calcium chloride
d. PO Neutra-Phos

20. A 70-year-old man on hemodialysis with Stage 5 chronic kidney disease (CKD) presents to the nephrology clinic for routine follow-up. Past medical history includes ESRD, hypertension, and type II diabetes. Current medications include amlodipine 10 mg daily, lisinopril 20 mg daily, glipizide 10 mg daily, aspirin 325 mg daily. Current laboratory values are BUN 60, SCr 4.5, Ca 9, Phos 8, and albumin 2. Which is the best initial management of this patient's hyperphosphatemia?

a. Calcium acetate
b. Sevelamer
c. Discontinuation of lisinopril
d. Calcium carbonate

21. Patients should be counseled to take a phosphate binder:

a. With meals to reduce phosphate absorption
b. With meals to increase phosphate absorption
c. With meals to reduce GI side effects
d. Between meals to reduce food–drug interactions

22. Which electrolyte abnormalities commonly occur in patients with chronic kidney disease?

i. Hyperkalemia
ii. Hyperphosphatemia
iii. Hypomagnesemia

a. i only
b. iii only
c. i and ii
d. ii and iii
e. i, ii, and iii

TAKEAWAY POINTS ››

- To avoid possibly fatal neurologic consequences, chronic sodium disorders should be corrected slowly in patients without life-threatening symptoms.
- Medications are a common cause of hyponatremia. Thiazide diuretics cause hypovolemic hyponatremia. Antidepressants, chemotherapy, and anticonvulsants may be the cause of SIADH.
- Normal saline is used to restore volume and correct serum sodium in hypovolemic hyponatremia.
- Hypertonic saline is reserved for hyponatremic patients with life-threatening symptoms.
- Fluid restriction is the mainstay of therapy for patients with isovolemic hyponatremia.
- Patients with hypovolemic and isovolemic hypernatremia require free water to correct serum sodium. Patients with central diabetes insipidus require exogenous ADH.
- Thiazides and NSAIDs are useful for the treatment of nephrogenic diabetes insipidus.
- Amiloride is useful in lithium-induced nephrogenic diabetes insipidus.
- Intravenous potassium replacement at a rate >10 mEq/h requires ECG monitoring.
- It is necessary to correct concomitant hypomagnesemia in order to successfully treat hypokalemia.
- Hyperkalemia and hypermagnesemia commonly occur in patients with renal disease.
- Hypokalemia is commonly induced by drugs.
- Hypomagnesemia is typically caused by excessive GI or renal elimination.
- Serum calcium and phosphate levels are regulated by PTH, vitamin D, and calcitonin.
- Classic signs and symptoms of calcium and phosphate disorders involve neurological, neuromuscular, renal, cardiac, and dermatological manifestations.
- Hypercalcemia is most commonly managed with volume expansion, diuretics, and bisphosphonates.
- Hyperphosphatemia commonly occurs in patients with renal disease and may be treated with phosphate binders.

REFERENCES

1. Reynolds RM, Padfield PL, Seckl JR. Disorders of sodium balance. *BMJ*. 2006;332:702-705.
2. Coyle JD, Joy MS. Disorders of sodium and water homeostasis. In: DiPiro JT, Talbert RL, Yee GC, et al, eds. *Pharmacotherapy: A Pathophysiologic Approach*. 7th ed. Available at: http://www.accesspharmacy.com/content.aspx?aID=3183025.
3. Rose DR, Post TW. *Clinical Physiology of Acid-Base and Electrolyte Disorders*. 5th ed. New York, NY: McGraw-Hill; 2001.
4. Andreoli TE. Water: normal balance, hyponatremia, and hypernatremia. *Ren Fail*. 2000;22:711-735.
5. Verbalis JG, Goldsmith SR, Greenberg A, Schrier RW, Sterns RH. Hyponatremia treatment guidelines 2007: expert panel recommendations. *Am J Med*. 2007;120:S1-S21.
6. Smith DM, McKenna K, Thompson CJ. Hyponatremia. *Clin Endocrinol*. 2000;52:667-678.
7. Androgué HJ, Madias NE. Hyponatremia. *N Engl J Med*. 2000;342:1581-1589.
8. Cawley MJ. Hyponatremia: current treatment strategies and the role of vasopressin antagonists. *Ann Pharmacother*. 2007;41:840-850.
9. Miller PD, Linas SL, Schrier RW. Plasma demeclocycline levels and nephrotoxicity. Correlation in hyponatremic cirrhotic patients. *JAMA*. 1980;243:2513-2515.
10. Forrest JN, Jr, Cox M, Hong C, Momson G, Bia M, Singer I. Superiority of demeclocycline over lithium in the treatment of chronic syndrome of inappropriate secretion of antidiuretic hormone. *N Engl J Med*. 1978;298:173-177.
11. Zeltser D, Rosansky S, van Rensburg H, et al. Assessment of the efficacy and safety of intravenous conivaptan in euvolemic and hypervolemic hyponatremia. *Am J Nephrol*. 2007;27:447-457.
12. Schrier RW, Gross P, Gheorghiade M, et al. Tolvaptan, a selective oral vasopressin V2-receptor antagonist, for hyponatremia. *N Engl J Med*. 2006;355:2099-2112.
13. Udelson JE, Smith WB, Hendrix GH, et al. Acute hemodynamic effects of conivaptan, a dual V(1A) and V(2) vasopressin receptor antagonist, in patients with advanced heart failure. *Circulation*. 2001;104:2417-2423.
14. Androgué HJ, Madias NE. Hypernatremia. *N Engl J Med*. 2000;342:1493-1499.
15. Weiss-Guillet EM, Takala J, Jakob SM. Diagnosis and management of electrolyte emergencies. *Best Pract Res Clin Endocrinol Metab*. 2003;17:623-651.
16. Kumar S, Berl T. Sodium. *Lancet*. 1998;352:220-228.
17. Earley LE, Orloff J. The mechanism of antidiuresis associated with the administration of hydrochlorothiazide to patients with vasopressin-resistant diabetes insipidus. *J Clin Invest*. 1962;41:1988.
18. Greenlee M, Wingo CS, McDonough AA, Youn JH, Kone BC. Narrative review: evolving concepts in potassium homeostasis and hypokalemia. *Ann Intern Med*. 2009;150:619-625.
19. Peterson LN, Levi M. Disorders of potassium metabolism. In: Schrier RW, ed. *Renal and Electrolyte Disorders*. 6th ed. Philadelphia, PA: Lippincott Williams & Wilkins; 2003:171-215.
20. Schaefer TJ, Wolford RW. Disorders of potassium. *Emerg Med Clin North Am*. 2005;23:723-747.
21. Sharma K, Cox M. Potassium homeostasis. In: Szerlip HM, Goldfarb S, eds. *Workshops in Fluid and Electrolyte Disorders*. New York, NY: Churchill Livingstone; 1993:71-96.
22. Gennari FJ. Hypokalemia. *N Engl J Med*. 1998;339:451-458.
23. Weiner ID, Wingo CS. Hypokalemia—consequences, causes, and correction. *J Am Soc Nephrol*. 1997;8:1179-1188.
24. Weiner ID, Wingo CS. Hyperkalemia: a potential silent killer. *J Am Soc Nephrol*. 1998;9:1535-1543.
25. Perazella MA. Drug-induced hyperkalemia: old culprits and new offenders. *Am J Med*. 2000;109:307-314.
26. Cohn JN, Kowey PR, Whelton PKK, Prisant LM. New guidelines for potassium replacement in clinical practice: a contemporary review by the National Council on Potassium in Clinical Practice. *Arch Intern Med*. 2000;160: 2429-2436.
27. Weisberg LS. Management of severe hyperkalemia. *Crit Care Med*. 2008;36:3246-3251.
28. Hollander-Rodriguez JC, Calvert JF. Hyperkalemia. *Am Fam Physician*. 2006;73:283-290.
29. Brophy Donald F, Gehr Todd W. Disorders of potassium and magnesium homeostasis. In: DiPiro JT, Talbert RL, Yee GC, et al, eds. *Pharmacotherapy: A Pathophysiologic Approach*. 7th ed. Available at: http://www.accesspharmacy.com/content.aspx?aID=3193873.
30. Tong GM, Rude RK. Magnesium deficiency in critical illness. *J Intensive Care Med*. 2005;20:3-17.
31. Topf JM, Murray PT. Hypomagnesemia and hypermagnesemia. *Rev Endocr Metab Disord*. 2003;4:195-206.
32. Arlyan Ce, Sosa JA. Assessment and management of patients with abnormal calcium. *Crit Care Med*. 2004;32(suppl):S146-S154.
33. Lau A, Chan LN. Electrolytes, other minerals, and trace elements. In: Lee M, ed. *Basic Skills in Interpreting Laboratory Data*. 4th ed, Bethesda, MD: American Society of Health-System Pharmacists; 2009;119.
34. Moe SM. Disorders of calcium, phosphorus, and magnesium. *Prim Care*. 2008;35:215-232.
35. Kraft MD, Btaiche IF, Sacks GS, Kudsk KA. Treatment of electrolyte disorders in adult patients in the intensive care unit. *AJHP*. 2005;62:1663-1682.
36. Slomp J, van der Voort PH, Gerritsen RT, et al. Albumin-adjusted calcium is not suitable for diagnosis of hyper- and hypocalcemia in critically ill. *Crit Care Med*. 2003;31: 1389-1393.
37. Pai AB, Rohrscheib M, Joy MS. Disorders of calcium and phosphorus homeostasis. In: DiPiro JT, Talbert RL, Yee GC, et al, eds. *Pharmacotherapy: A Pathophysiologic Approach*. 7th ed. Available at: http://www.accesspharmacy.com/content.aspx?aID=3183287.
38. Lumachi F, Brunello A, Roma A, Basso U. Cancer-induced hypercalcemia. *Anticancer Res*. 2009;29:1551-1556.
39. Bailie GR, Massry SG. Clinical practice guidelines for bone metabolism and disease in chronic kidney disease: an overview. *Pharmacotherapy*. 2005;25:1687-1707.
40. Mehrotra B. Bisphosphonates—role in cancer therapies. *J Oral Maxillofac Surg*. 2009;67:S19-S26.
41. Hutchison AJ. Oral phosphate binders. *Kidney Int*. 2009;75:906-914.

CHAPTER

35 Estimating Renal Function

Danny McNatty

FOUNDATION OVERVIEW

Estimating renal function is of great importance for patients taking renally eliminated medications. The glomerular filtration rate (GFR) is an effective indicator of renal function and normal values are approximately 130 mL/min/1.73 m^2 for men and 120 mL/min/1.73 m^2 for women.[1] GFR cannot be directly measured; therefore other measurements must be used to approximate renal function. The gold standard for approximating GFR is the inulin clearance method.[2] Inulin is filtered by the glomerulus and is not secreted or reabsorbed, making it an ideal agent for approximating GFR. GFR approximation via inulin clearance is rarely done because it is costly, invasive, and requires a great deal of technical expertise.[3] Other markers used to estimate GFR include iothalamate, iohexol, and ethylenediaminetetraacetic acid. Like inulin, these agents are expensive and have limited availability, making them impractical in the clinical setting.

Numerous methods have been developed to estimate GFR. A clinician must balance ease of use and accuracy to determine the best method for estimating GFR in the clinical setting.

Serum Creatinine

Creatinine is an endogenous substance that is eliminated primarily by glomerular filtration and serves an important role in estimating renal function. Creatinine is not as precise as inulin because it undergoes some tubular secretion. The range of serum creatinine (SCr) is approximately 0.6 to 1.2 mg/dL in normal, healthy adults.[4] SCr is affected by age, gender, race, diet, muscle mass, and certain drugs; therefore, SCr is not used alone in predicting GFR.[2] Muscle mass is a particularly important consideration when analyzing SCr values. Creatinine is a by-product of creatine metabolism and is influenced by the amount of muscle mass present in a patient.[2] Patients with low muscle mass would be expected to have lower SCr values. Low muscle mass can occur in elderly, cachectic (eg, acquired immunodeficiency patients), or individuals with limited muscle use (eg, spinal cord injury).

Urinary Clearance of Creatinine

GFR can be estimated via the combination of a timed urine collection and blood sampling of creatinine. The most common time interval utilized is a 24-hour urine collection. This practice has decreased due to the difficulty with accurate collection and data indicating the 24-hour urine collection is equivalent to mathematical equations in estimating GFR.[2,5]

Creatinine Clearance and GFR Prediction Equations

Equations estimating GFR based on SCr, age, weight, and race are more accurate than SCr alone.[2] The Cockcroft-Gault method calculates a creatinine clearance (CrCl) and is a widely used equation to estimate GFR.[6]

$$\text{CrCl (mL/min)} = \frac{[(140 - \text{age}) \times \text{ideal body weight (kg)}]\ [0.85\ \text{(for women)}]}{(72 \times \text{SCr})}$$

If a patient's actual body weight is below the ideal body weight (IBW), then the actual body weight should be used when calculating CrCl. The Cockcroft-Gault equation may be used for determining drug dosing in obese patients; however, it becomes less accurate in obese patients.

$$\text{Ideal body weight (IBW) (men)} = 50\ \text{kg} + (2.3\ \text{kg} \times \text{height in inches over 5 ft})$$

$$\text{Ideal body weight (women)} = 45.5\ \text{kg} + (2.3\ \text{kg} \times \text{height in inches over 5 ft})$$

Cockcroft and Gault published this equation in 1976, using data primarily from healthy men. The equation has subsequently been validated in other patient populations. In clinical practice it is customary to round the SCr up to 1.0 mg/dL in patients with actual values <1.0 mg/dL (eg, patients with low muscle mass or age >65).

The Modification of Diet in Renal Disease (MDRD) equation is another calculation utilized to estimate GFR; however, this method is not as common as CrCl.[7]

$$\text{GFR (mL/min)} = 186 \times (\text{Scr})^{-1.154} \times (\text{age})^{-0.203} \times 0.742\ \text{(if patient is woman)} \times 1.210\ \text{(if patient is African American)}$$

The MDRD was originally validated in patients with chronic kidney disease, but was subsequently validated in a large group of patients. MDRD factors race into the equation accounting for increased muscle mass (and therefore SCr) in African American patients.

When dosing medications based on renal function, either Cockcroft-Gault or MDRD are appropriate; however, most pharmacokinetic studies used the Cockcroft-Gault method

and the National Kidney Foundation recommends employing Cockcroft-Gault in guiding dosage adjustments.[8]

SPECIAL CONSIDERATIONS

Children

The Cockcroft-Gault and MDRD equations are not validated in children and therefore should be used with caution when estimating renal function in pediatrics. The most common equation used to estimate renal function in children is the Schwartz equation.[9]

Schwartz GFR (mL/min) = [length (in cm) × k]/Scr, where k = 0.45 (age <1 year), 0.55 (age 1-13 years), 0.7 (adolescent male), 0.55 (adolescent female).

The Schwartz equation is convenient and provides a relatively good estimate of GFR in the pediatric population. Height (length) is used in the Schwartz equation as it has been shown to be proportional to muscle mass.[2]

Unstable Renal Function

Using traditional methods for estimating GFR can be problematic in patients with rapidly changing renal function. Serum creatinine levels do not correlate well with GFR because there can be a lag in the rise and fall of serum creatinine during acute kidney injury. Equations such as Cockcroft-Gault and MDRD overestimate GFR during periods of renal function decline and underestimate GFR during periods of recovery. If a serum creatinine doubles within 24 hours the GFR is likely close to zero.[3] Numerous equations have been developed in an attempt to accurately estimate renal function in this patient population. The most commonly accepted is the Jelliffe equation.[10] Clinical judgment must be used to adjust medication dosages in patients with rapidly changing renal function as even the Jelliffe equation has limited supporting data. The effect of unstable renal function on drug clearance and the potential ramifications of overdosing or underdosing the patient must be considered before making a decision regarding renal dose-adjustment.

CASE Application

1. AR is a 50-year-old Caucasian woman who is 63 in tall and weighs 165 lb. Her current serum creatinine is 1.6 mg/dL. What is her ideal body weight (IBW)?
    a. 125 lb
    b. 115 lb
    c. 135 lb
    d. 165 lb

2. What is AR's creatinine clearance as estimated by the Cockcroft-Gault equation?
    a. 41 mL/min
    b. 34 mL/min
    c. 50 mL/min
    d. 58 mL/min

3. What is AR's GFR as estimated by the MDRD equation?
    a. 25 mL/min
    b. 35 mL/min
    c. 45 mL/min
    d. 55 mL/min

4. TM is a 79-year-old African American man who is 71 in tall and weighs 254 lb. His current serum creatinine is 1.2 mg/dL. What is his ideal body weight (IBW)?
    a. 145 lb
    b. 156 lb
    c. 166 lb
    d. 254 lb

5. What is TM's creatinine clearance as estimated by the Cockcroft-Gault equation?
    a. 69 mL/min
    b. 45 mL/min
    c. 81 mL/min
    d. 53 mL/min

6. What is TM's GFR as estimated by the MDRD equation?
    a. 45 mL/min
    b. 55 mL/min
    c. 65 mL/min
    d. 75 mL/min

7. AB is a 4-year-old girl who is 42 in tall and weighs 50 lb. Her current serum creatinine is 0.6 mg/dL. What is AB's estimated GFR based on the Schwartz equation?
    a. ~30 mL/min
    b. ~60 mL/min
    c. ~80 mL/min
    d. ~100 mL/min

8. DW is a 6-month-old infant who is 25 in long and weighs 15 lb. His current serum creatinine is 0.4 mg/dL. What is DW's estimated GFR based on the Schwartz equation?
    a. 60 mL/min
    b. 70 mL/min
    c. 80 mL/min
    d. 90 mL/min

9. Which of the following factors independent from GFR affect serum creatinine?
    a. Age
    b. Diet
    c. Gender
    d. Race
    e. All of the above

10. Which of the following patients would be most likely to have a baseline serum creatinine of <0.8?
    a. A 24-year-old man in very good health
    b. A 35-year-old man adhering to the Atkins diet
    c. A 93-year-old woman who is wheelchair bound
    e. A bodybuilder taking creatine supplements

11. Which of the following is considered the gold standard for measurement of GFR?
    a. Cockcroft-Gault equation
    b. MDRD equation
    c. 24-hour urine creatinine
    d. Inulin clearance

12. Which of the following factors are important to consider when dosing a medication based on renal function?
    a. The extent to which the drug is renally eliminated
    b. The potential for drug toxicity
    c. The manufacturer-recommended dosing guidelines for the agent
    d. All of the above are important factors to consider

13. RT is a 50-year-old man who is admitted with serum creatinine of 1.1 mg/dL. Twenty-four hours later, his serum creatinine is 2.0 mg/dL. RT is on several medications that need to be dose-adjusted for renal function. What is the most appropriate course of action?
    a. Calculate RT's GFR using the MDRD equation and dose adjust based on the result.
    b. Calculate RT's CrCl using the Cockcroft-Gault equation and dose-adjust based on the result.
    c. Discontinue all of RT's medications until his renal function improves.
    d. Assess each of RT's medications and use clinical judgment to determine the best course of action, balancing the risk of treatment failure and drug toxicity.

14. TY is an 88-year-old man who weighs 70 kg and is 71 in tall. His current serum creatinine is 0.5. What is his creatinine clearance as estimated by the Cockcroft-Gault equation?
    a. 101 mL/min
    b. 51 mL/min
    c. 92 mL/min
    d. 46 mL/min

15. FW is a 33-year-old woman with a serum creatinine of 1.3 mg/dL. She is 64 in tall and weighs 118 lb. She has no past medical history. Which of the following methods is the most appropriate way to estimate her renal function?
    a. Schwartz equation.
    b. MDRD equation.
    c. Cockcroft-Gault equation.
    d. Both b and c are appropriate.
    e. All of the above are appropriate.

16. QR is a 32-year-old Caucasian woman who is 67 in tall and weighs 88 lb. Her current serum creatinine is 0.8 mg/dL. What is QRs IBW?
    a. 135 lb
    b. 125 lb
    c. 145 lb
    d. 85 lb

17. What is QRs CrCl as estimated by the Cockcroft-Gault equation?
    a. 98 mL/min
    b. 115 mL/min
    c. 64 mL/min
    d. 75 mL/min

18. What is QRs GFR as estimated by the MDRD equation?
    a. 54 mL/min
    b. 66 mL/min
    c. 75 mL/min
    d. 88 mL/min

19. Select the normal serum creatinine for an adult patient.
    a. 0.3 mg/dL
    b. 0.7 mg/dL
    c. 1.7 mg/dL
    d. 2.0 mg/dL

20. Select the weight that should be used to calculate the CrCl via the Cockcroft-Gault method.
    a. Ideal body weight
    b. Actual body weight
    c. Adjusted body weight
    d. All of the above

TAKEAWAY POINTS ››

- The GFR is the best indicator of renal function; however, since it cannot be readily measured, surrogate markers must be used to estimate GFR.
- Inulin clearance is the gold standard for estimating GFR since it is filtered by the glomerulus. Inulin is rarely used in clinical practice due to cost and need for technical expertise.
- Serum creatinine is affected by several factors including age, gender, race, diet, muscle mass, and certain drugs.
- The most practical way to estimate renal function is to use GFR and CrCl estimation equations.
- The MDRD and Cockcroft-Gault equations provide a reasonable estimate of GFR in most patients with stable renal function.

- Both the Cockcroft-Gault and the MDRD equations are *estimates* of renal function.
- In children with stable renal function, the Schwartz equation can be used to estimate GFR.
- In patients with unstable renal function, the standard equations used to estimate GFR become very inaccurate and clinical judgment must be used to assess renal function.

REFERENCES

1. Stevens LA, Coresh J, Greene T, Levey AS. Assessing kidney function—measured and estimated glomerular filtration rate. *N Engl J Med.* 2006;354:2473-2483.
2. National Kidney Foundation. K/DOQI Clinical practice guidelines for chronic kidney disease: evaluation, classification, and stratification. *Am J Kidney Dis.* 2002;39(suppl 1):S1-S266.
3. Frequently asked questions about GFR estimates. National Kidney Foundation Web site. Available at: http://www.kidney.org/professionals/KLS/GFR.cfm#faq. Accessed July 15, 2009.
4. Jones CA, McQuillan GM, Kusek JW, et al. Serum creatinine levels in the US population: Third National Health and Nutrition Examination Survey. *Am J Kidney Dis.* 1998;32:992-999.
5. Lemann J, Bidani AK, Bain RP, Lewis EJ, Rohde RD. Use of the serum creatinine to estimate glomerular filtration rate in health and early diabetic nephropathy. *Am J Kidney Dis.* 1990;16:236-243.
6. Cockcroft DW, Gault MH. Prediction of creatinine clearance from serum creatinine. *Nephron.* 1976;16:31-41.
7. Levey AS, Bosch JP, Lewis JB, Greene T, Rogers N, Roth D. A more accurate method to estimate glomerular filtration rate from serum creatinine: a new prediction equation. *Ann Intern Med.* 1999;130:461-470.
8. Pharmacists and authorized drug prescribers: creatinine standardization recommendations. National Kidney Disease Education Program Web site. Available at: http://www.nkdep.nih.gov/labprofessionals/pharmacists_and_authorized_drug_prescribers.htm. Accessed July 15, 2009.
9. Schwartz GJ, Brion LP, Spitzer A. The use of plasma creatinine concentration for estimating glomerular filtration rate in infants, children, and adolescents. *Pediatr Clin North Am.* 1987;34:571-590.
10. Jelliffe RW. Estimation of creatinine clearance in patients with unstable renal function, without a urine specimen. *Am J Nephrol.* 2002;22(4):320-324.

CHAPTER

36 Acute Kidney Injury

Sarah R. Tomasello

FOUNDATION OVERVIEW

The kidneys are particularly vulnerable to certain types of injury for a number of reasons. First, they are dependent upon the heart and vasculature to deliver sufficient blood supply to drive glomerular filtration (GFR). Secondly, they are major excretory organs, exposed to numerous endogenous and exogenous substances that are eliminated from the body via the urine. Acute kidney injury (AKI) can occur due to a variety of localized or systemic disease states, toxicity from chemicals or medicinal agents, or as the result of poor perfusion or outlet obstruction. It may be difficult to evaluate and diagnose because more than one type of damage may occur simultaneously, or one type of damage may occur secondary to another type. Although the incidence of AKI is greatest in hospitalized patients, it may also occur in patients residing in the community. Acute kidney injury is also very interesting because, in many cases, if the cause is identified and stopped promptly there may not be any permanent damage to the kidney. More severe, prolonged, or untreated injury can ultimately lead to permanent damage and even complete loss of kidney function.

The kidneys have an incredible reserve capacity. Although a single insult may be sufficient to cause AKI, in many cases it is a combination of two or more factors that ultimately overwhelm the kidneys' ability to maintain GFR. Factors such as the presence of underlying chronic kidney disease (CKD), as well as the severity, extent, multiplicity, and duration of the injuries/insults, will determine how much damage (if any) will result and possibly persist.

Definition

There is no exact definition for AKI. Generally, the diagnosis is considered when there has been a relatively sudden and significant decrease in kidney function. Serum creatinine (SCr) is a metabolic byproduct of muscle metabolism and unless there is a significant change in muscle mass the serum concentration of an individual should remain relatively constant. An increase in the SCr concentration is generally the result of accumulation due to a decrease in the GFR. As chronic kidney disease may result in a higher baseline SCr value, the diagnosis of AKI is based on the change in SCr from baseline as well in changes in urine production.

Incidence

The incidence of AKI in the United States appears to be increasing. A community-based study showed an increase in cases of AKI from 323 cases per 100,000 in 1988 to 522 cases per 100,000 in 2002.[1] There has also been an increase in hospital-acquired AKI[2] with recent incidence estimated to be >7% in patients undergoing surgical procedures.[3] The incidence of AKI in the community setting has been difficult to evaluate.[1] The variation in the definition of AKI and the use of SCr concentration to define AKI as the primary marker of kidney function are particularly problematic in an aging population.[4,5] As the incidence of AKI is highest in the critical care setting, there is more information and data compiled about the presentation, clinical course, and outcomes in this population.[6,7,8] It is estimated that two-thirds of all patients admitted to the intensive care unit will develop AKI.[8] In response, a classification system has been developed to predict the severity of AKI and permanence of damage.[9] This method utilizes the SCr concentration, the calculated eGFR, and the urine output to categorize AKI into one of five strata using the acronym RIFLE: *r*isk, *i*njury, *f*ailure, *l*oss and *e*nd-stage renal disease. The first three categories rate the severity of kidney injury, while the last two categories refer to the long-term clinical outcomes of partial or complete loss of kidney function. The RIFLE criteria is a relatively new tool for predicting the outcome of an episode of AKI. Although it has not been validated for predicting all outcomes of AKI,[6] it does offer a systematic approach to assess a very unpredictable disease state.

PROGNOSES AND OUTCOMES

Due to the variability of factors such as the location, severity, and extent of the damage, as well as duration of time until the discontinuation/reversal of the cause, it is often difficult to predict the outcome of an episode of AKI. Generally, patients who do not have intrinsic AKI and do not have serious comorbidities have better outcomes. They may experience an episode of pre-renal or post-renal AKI, have a rapid and complete recovery, and return to baseline kidney function if diagnosed promptly and treatment/supportive care attenuates the damage quickly. In contrast, those who have significant comorbidities, who present later in the course of AKI, or who experience an intrinsic type of AKI[10] may have a more complicated recovery and a greater likelihood of long-term/permanent loss of kidney function. An estimated 13% to 20% of patients who experience AKI during acute hospitalization will be dialysis dependent upon discharge.[11,12]

PATHOPHYSIOLOGY AND CLASSIFICATION OF AKI

Acute kidney injury can be classified into three basic categories; pre-renal AKI, intrinsic AKI, and post-renal AKI based on the location and type of damage.

Pre-Renal Acute Kidney Injury

The term "pre-renal" implies that the damage or defect causing AKI occurs before the kidney, or without damage to the kidney itself. Pre-renal AKI results from insufficient pressure in the Bowman capsule to drive glomerular filtration. This decrease in pressure may result from systemic changes, such as dehydration, a decrease in cardiac output, or hypotension. This decrease in pressure may also stem from a localized decrease in perfusion caused by significant renal artery stenosis or thromboembolism. A decrease in blood flow/pressure to the kidneys will result in a decrease in intraglomerular pressure, a decrease in GFR, and hypoxia/ischemia within the kidneys. While transient hypotension/poor perfusion would not be likely to cause AKI, such an insult could result in AKI if there were underlying risk factors, or if the insult were pronounced or sustained.

It should be noted that pre-renal AKI can occur with normal/elevated systemic blood pressure and total body fluid overload. The important factor is not the total body fluid volume, but the effective intravascular blood volume (EABV). Patients with disorders such as heart failure, significant renal artery stenosis, nephrotic range proteinuria, or advanced liver disease may present with normal or even elevated blood pressure. These disorders can cause an increase in total body water with a decrease in the EABV secondary to decreased cardiac output and/or the fluid shift from the intravascular to extravascular compartment. Although such patients may appear fluid overloaded (presenting with edema, rales, ascites, etc), the decrease in EABV will result in a decreased perfusion to the kidney and may result in pre-renal AKI as described above.

The term "functional pre-renal AKI" describes a subtype of pre-renal AKI. The mechanism of injury is still hypoperfusion and intraglomerular hypotension; however the pathophysiology is occurring at the microscopic level of the glomerulus. As noted, intraglomerular pressure is dependent on the pressure of the blood flow entering the Bowman capsule (via the afferent arteriole) as well as the pressure of the blood flow leaving the Bowman capsule (via the efferent arteriole) (Figure 36-1). The tone of the afferent arteriole is maintained by vasodilatory prostaglandins such as PGE_2 and prostacyclin (PGI_2).[13] Agents such as nonsteroidal anti-inflammatory agents (NSAIDs) that inhibit prostaglandin synthesis may cause vasoconstriction of the afferent arteriole and therefore decrease the pressure in the Bowman capsule (Figure 36-2). Other agents that can cause

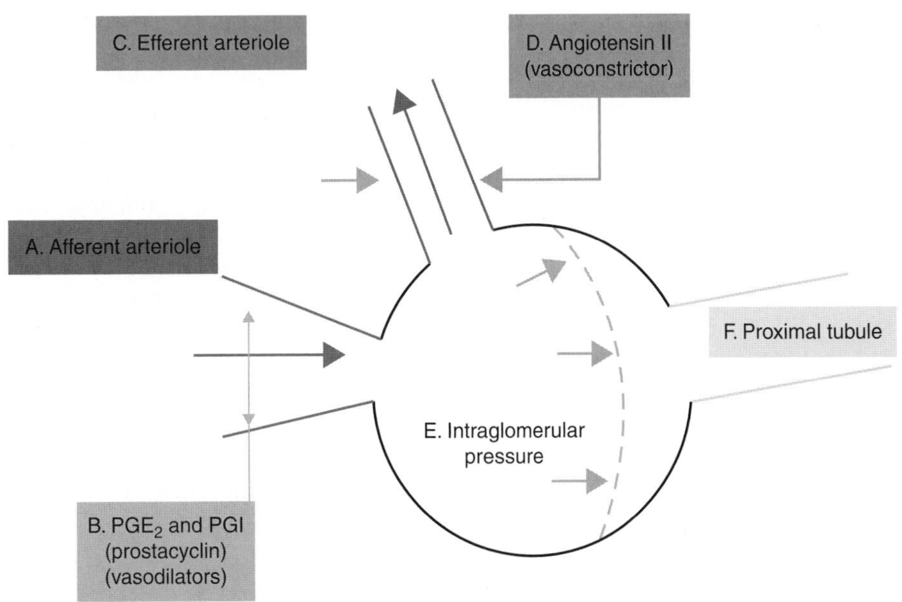

FIGURE 36-1 Physiology and regulation of intraglomerular pressure. Intraglomerular pressure (E), and therefore glomerular filtration rate, depend on the pressure in Bowman capsule. A. Blood enters the glomerulus via the afferent arteriole. B. Vasodilatory prostaglandins (PGE2 and prostacyclin) maintain appropriate vascular tone of the afferent arteriole. Substances that cannot pass through the glomerulus into the proximal tubule (F) are returned to systemic circulation via the efferent arteriole (C). Angiotensin II (D) acts to vasoconstrict the efferent arteriole to maintain pressure in Bowman capsule.

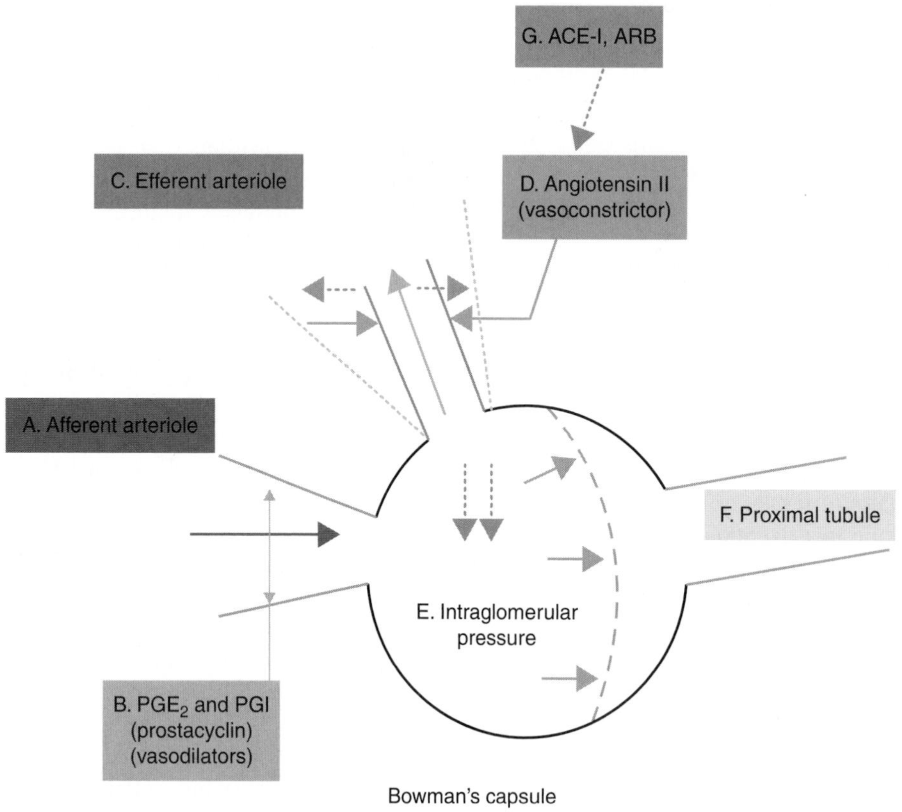

FIGURE 36-2 The effect of angiotensin-converting enzyme inhibitors or angiotensin receptor blockers (G) on the regulation of intraglomerular pressure. By inhibiting angiotensin II, these agents cause vasodilation of the efferent arteriole and a subsequent decrease in intraglomerular pressure.

vasoconstriction of the afferent arteriole include cyclosporine and tacrolimus by a slightly different mechanism.[13] The tone in the efferent arteriole is maintained by the vasoconstrictive properties of angiotensin II. Agents that decrease the production of angiotensin II or antagonize its effects (angiotensin-converting enzyme inhibitors, angiotensin II receptor antagonists) will therefore cause the efferent arteriole to vasodilate and cause decreased pressure in the Bowman capsule (Figure 36-3). Signs and symptoms will be consistent with pre-renal AKI, as the decreased perfusion to the glomeruli causes activation of the renin-angiotensin-aldosterone axis with subsequent increases in sodium and water reabsorption.

Intrinsic-Acute Kidney Injury

Intrinsic AKI is the result of direct damage to one or more areas of the kidney, including the glomerulus, the tubules, or the interstitium. Examples include glomerulonephritis, acute tubular necrosis, and acute interstitial nephritis.

Glomerulonephritis

Glomerulonephritis (GN) occurs as the result of either an immune-mediated process or another precipitating event such as an acute infection that causes inflammation and direct damage to the glomerulus. Deposits of immune complexes may accumulate and damage the glomerulus causing filtering defects. Large molecules such as proteins and blood cells pass through the glomerulus into the proximal tubule and may be visualized on microscopic urinalysis. Although an acute infection or diseases involving the production of immune complexes may cause AKI,[14] GN is more commonly associated with CKD.

Acute Tubular Necrosis

Acute tubular necrosis (ATN) is the most commonly encountered form of intrinsic AKI, particularly in hospitalized patients.[7,11,15] Acute tubular necrosis signifies the death of tubular epithelial cells, which slough off and may then be visualized in the urine. In fact, this cellular debris, described as "muddy brown casts" is very specific to ATN and is important to the diagnosis. There are two basic mechanisms that can destroy the tubular epithelial cells, prolonged ischemia, or the direct toxic effects of a substance. Prolonged ischemia may be viewed as an extreme form of pre-renal acute renal failure, and indeed, ATN may develop as a consequence of a pre-renal ARF that could not be reversed in a timely manner. This fact may make the diagnosis process more difficult. The second cause of ATN is a direct toxic effect. Some commonly used medicinal and diagnostic agents such as aminoglycosides, cisplatin, and radio-contrast media may cause tubular cell apoptosis by a direct toxic effect.[16]

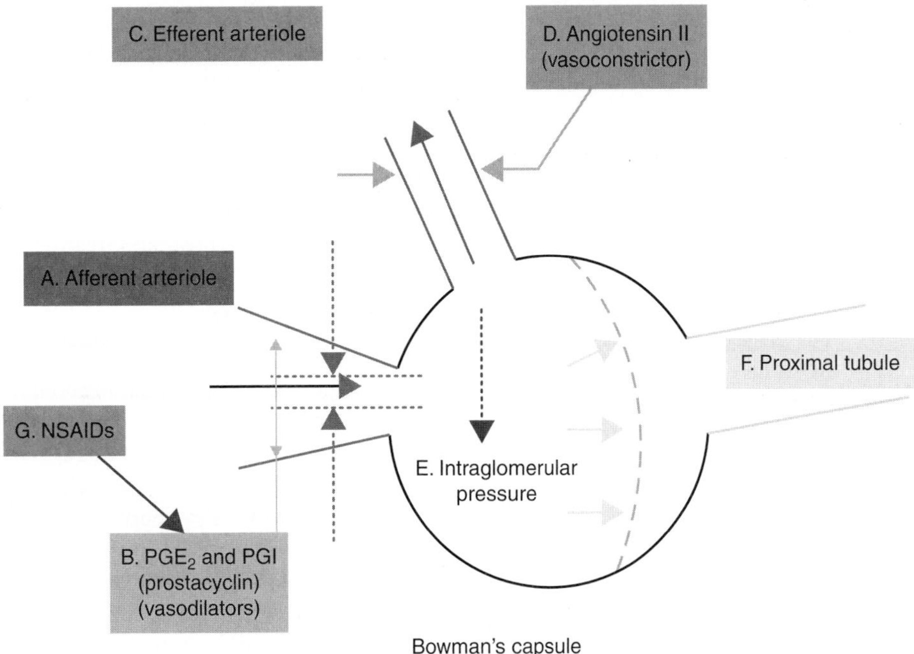

FIGURE 36-3 The effect of nonsteroidal anti-inflammatory agents (G) on the regulation of intraglomerular pressure. By inhibiting the synthesis of vasodilatory prostaglandins (PGE_2 and prostacyclin) these agents cause vasoconstriction of the afferent arteriole and a subsequent decrease in the intraglomerular pressure.

Acute Interstitial Nephritis

Acute interstitial nephritis (AIN) is a very interesting disease for pharmacists as it is a hypersensitivity reaction manifesting itself predominantly in the kidneys. It is commonly caused by pharmacotherapy and less commonly triggered by an infection.[17] The first agent that was most often associated with AIN was methacillin.[18] In fact, antimicrobial agents and other agents commonly associated with drug allergy often are the cause of AIN. As AIN is often a drug-induced disease, a thorough medication history should be completed to gather information regarding the use of agents that are more likely to cause an allergic reaction. Because the hypersensitivity reaction causes an inflammatory response in the interstitium of the kidney, it is imperative that the causative agent be identified and discontinued as soon as possible. Table 36-1 lists examples of pharmacotherapeutic agents that can cause acute interstitial nephritis as well as other intrinsic AKI.

TABLE 36-1 Examples of Pharmacotherapeutic Agents[a] Associated with Intrinsic Acute Kidney Injury[13,16,19]

Acute Glomerulonephritis	Acute Tubular Necrosis	Acute Interstitial Nephritis
Gold compounds	Amphotericin B	Ciprofloxacin
Lithium	Cisplatin	Levofloxacin
	Bisphosphonates (IV)	Agents that contain a sulfonamide moiety
	Tenofovir	Penicillins
	Pentamidine	Cephalosporins
	Sucrose (IV immunoglobulin)	Nonsteroidal anti-inflammatory agents
	Radio contrast media[a]	

[a]Diagnostic agent.

Post-Renal Acute Kidney Injury

There are a variety of substances and situations that can cause an obstruction of urine flow at any portion of the urinary tract from the tubules, ureters, bladder, to the urethra. The formation of calculi ("kidney stones"), precipitation of crystals, benign or malignant masses, misplaced indwelling catheters, or hypertrophic prostatic disease can partially or completely block urine flow. The impedance of urine excretion, complete or partial, will result in backflow of urine into the kidney. This reverse pressure can damage the kidneys, causing AKI or, if left untreated, may result in CKD. As with pre-renal AKI, post-renal AKI may resolve completely or cause significant long-term kidney damage depending on the duration of the insult and quick reversal and supportive care.

Urine Output

In addition to qualifying the type of AKI, it is important to quantify and qualify the urine output. Knowing the amount of urine produced in 24 hours provides information about the extent and type of the damage, as well as the prognosis and complications. It is important to assess the total fluid input as well as the output to determine the kidney's ability to maintain homeostasis. Anuria, defined as < 50 mL/d of urine suggests that the patient's renal clearance is severely decreased and complications of hyperkalemia, hypertension, and acid–base disorders may ensue. Oliguria, defined as 50 to 400 mL of urine in 24 hours, may make fluid and electrolyte management slightly more manageable, although patients with oliguria/anuria have a worse prognosis than those patients who produce >400mL/24 h of urine.[7,11] In some cases, the urine volume may remain relatively normal or even increased (nonoliguria). Polyuria (generally defined as urine output >1.5 to 2 L/d) can occur and may seem paradoxical. The urinalysis (U/A) will show very dilute urine, with an increased amount of sodium, and the FeNa will be increased. The copious urine production with increased sodium excretion signifies the ability to perform filtration through the glomerulus with a relative inability of the damaged tubules to appropriately reabsorb sodium and water. In fact, due to the inability to reabsorb substances properly, this situation may actually lead to electrolyte losses such as hypokalemia and hypomagnesemia.

DIAGNOSIS

The process of differentiating between different types of AKI involves evaluation of the past medical history, medication history, and physical examination findings, as well as evaluation of laboratory values and other diagnostic tests. While the following paragraphs describe each facet of the evaluation in detail, Table 36-2 is a summary of this information.

In many instances, AKI may be asymptomatic, especially if the patient presents early or if the symptoms are masked by other medical conditions. Generally, the first noticeable signs of AKI are an increase in blood urea nitrogen (BUN) and SCr concentrations with or without changes in urination or urine volume. It is important to note that the SCr concentration rises as creatinine accumulates in the body secondary to a decreased GFR caused by kidney damage. For this reason the investigation for the causes of AKI must target the days (possibly weeks) before the SCr concentration began to rise. Diagnosing and classifying AKI may be very difficult if there is little or no knowledge regarding the patient's baseline SCr concentration, and past medical and medication history. Also, by the very nature of AKI, renal function cannot be easily quantified using only traditional methods as the SCr concentrations are not at steady state. This can complicate the management of pharmacotherapeutic agents that would require dose adjustment for decreased kidney function.

Presentation

The timely evaluation and diagnosis of AKI is extremely important for optimal outcomes.[19] Hospital-acquired AKI may be somewhat easier to evaluate than community-acquired AKI, as more information may be available about baseline kidney function, recent medications, and comorbidities. This being noted, hospitalized patients may be exposed to more medications and circumstances that can cause AKI making the determination of a specific cause(s) more challenging. In either situation, obtaining as much information as possible about the patient and the circumstances that led to the onset of AKI will facilitate prompt diagnosis and treatment.

Patient History

Ideally, the clinician can obtain information regarding past history to gain useful information about the etiology, type, and extent of the AKI and the patient's current kidney function. A past medical history of certain diseases such as diabetes mellitus, hypertension, or any type of chronic kidney disease may be risk factors for the development of AKI. Any recent surgical procedure should be reviewed and evaluated for potential contributing factors such as blood loss, hypotension, or the use of radio contrast media. The social and occupational history should be reviewed for potential causes of AKI such as exposure to environmental toxins or illicit drug use. Drug allergies should be reviewed and compared to any recent changes in pharmacotherapy. A thorough medication history should be obtained to rule out drug-induced causes.

Review of Systems and Physical Examination

The physical findings during the initial examination must be interpreted carefully. Both the interval of time that has elapsed since the insult to the kidneys as well as any treatments or events that have been initiated should be considered. Additionally, other comorbid disease states or treatments can confound assessment of parameters related to AKI.

Laboratory and Diagnostic Studies

Generally, the first noticeable signs of AKI are elevations of blood urea nitrogen (BUN), SCr concentrations, and possibly changes in urine output. Perhaps the first step in assessing these parameters is to rule out other causes of the abnormalities. Both the BUN and SCr concentrations are dependent on the steady state homeostasis of muscle synthesis and breakdown. There are certain circumstances that may cause an increase and confound the interpretation of BUN and SCr. Diseases or drug therapy that can cause muscle breakdown can elevate the serum concentrations of these parameters. The use of corticosteroids, diets high in protein or protein supplements, and rhabdomyolysis can cause elevated serum concentrations with normal kidney function. Likewise, BUN and SCr concentrations may be decreased in situations of malnutrition or muscle wasting. Additionally, there are several therapeutic agents that can interfere with the laboratory assay used to quantify the SCr concentration, such as cefazolin, cephalexin, and ascorbic acid.[20] Cases of isolated elevations in the BUN or SCr concentrations not resulting from a decreased GFR are termed "pseudorenal failure."

In addition to assessing and quantifying renal function, the BUN and SCr can be useful in differentiating between

TABLE 36-2 **Examples of Signs and Symptoms Indicative of Each Type of AKI**

	Pre-Renal	GN	ATN	AIN	Post-Renal
CC/HPI	Dehydration, blood loss, infection, hypotension	Vasculitis/ inflammation, (ie, arthralgias, myalgias)	Infection, hospitalization, procedure with IV contrast, muscular damage	Infection, new medications	Difficulty urinating, decreased force of stream or intermittent stream
PMH (CKD, HTN, DM)	Heart failure, renal artery stenosis, severe liver disease	Systemic immune disorder			Genitourinary or GI masses, lithotripsy
PSH	Recent surgery—blood loss, hypotension		Procedure with IV contrast		Recent urinary catheter, TURP
Allergies				PCN, sulfa	
Meds	Diuretics, ACE-I, ARBs, cyclosporine, tacrolimus, NSAIDs	Gold	Radio contrast media, aminoglycosides cisplatin, amphotericin	Penicillins, cephalosporins	Finasteride, tamsulosin, TCAs
Vitals	Low BP, tachycardia			+/− Increased temperature	
ROS	Decreased urination, syncopal episode, thirst, blood loss	Unusual arthralgias, myalgias, viral illness			Decreased urination, decreased force of stream, pain on urination
Physical examination	Dehydration/Decreased EABV		Prolonged pre-renal state	Possible rash/ urticaria	Enlarged prostate, palpable abdominal masses, indwelling bladder catheter
Laboratory values	BUN:SCr>15 (AST/ALT abnormalities in hepatic dysfunction)	WBC serum markers of immune activation		Increased WBC, eosinophilia	Elevated PSA, elevated urate concentration
U/A	No sediment, SpGr>1.013 uOsom>350 mOsm/Kg	Active sediment + protein	Active sediment, muddy brown casts SpGr <1.013 uOsom <250 mOsm/kg	Active sediment, +WBC, +/−eosinophils	Active sediment, variable crystalluria
Urine electrolytes	Na <20 mEq/L FeNa<1%		Na>20 mEq/L FeNa >1%-2%		
Urine output	Scant urine		Anuria, oliguric or polyuric		Anuria or decreased force of stream or painful urination
Tests	Echo: decreased EF				KUB: hydronephrosis

Abbreviations: TURP, transurethral resection of prostate; EABV, effective arteriole blood volume; PSA, prostate-specific antigen; Echo, echocardiogram; EF, ejection fraction; KUB, ultrasound of kidney ureters and bladder.

pre-renal and non–pre-renal causes of AKI. Although both parameters may be elevated in any type of AKI, the ratio of BUN to SCr is increased, generally >15 in pre-renal AKI. In response to hypoxia or poor perfusion, the kidney will compensate by increasing the amount of water that is reabsorbed in the proximal tubule. An increased amount of urea (not creatinine) will be absorbed with the water due to passive diffusion resulting is the disproportionate rise of BUN compared to SCr.

Analysis of Urine

Obtaining and analyzing a urine sample is important in classifying the type of AKI. The results should be interpreted with careful consideration of the clinical characteristics of the patient as well as any treatments or confounding factors that may influence the results. Numerous factors may affect the evaluation of the results including; the presence of more than one type of AKI, or the use of diuretics or hyper-osmolar agents such as mannitol or radio contrast media. While there are a number of tests that can be performed, the first step is usually a urinalysis. This test comprises three basic components: macroscopic, microscopic, and chemical analysis. Many findings from a urinalysis may be nonspecific especially in the case of post-renal obstructive AKI. The urinalysis may however, be particularly useful in differentiating between pre-renal and intrinsic damage, especially acute tubular necrosis (Table 36-3). In addition to the U/A, urine electrolyte analysis should be performed. This test provides information about the

TABLE 36-3 Comparison of Laboratory Results Between Pre-renal and Acute Tubular Necrosis Types of Acute Kidney Injury[18,23]

Laboratory Test	Pre-Renal AKI	ATN
Color of urine	Dark, concentrated	Pale, clear
Volume of urine	Scant	Varies (anuria to polyuria)
Urine sediment	Bland (no cells/casts)	Active (cells, casts, etc)
Urine sodium	<20 mEq/L	>40 mEq/L
FeNa	<1%	>2%
Urine:serum osmolality	>1.5	<1.5
BUN:SCr	>15-20	<15
		"Muddy brown casts"[a]

[a]Casts of tubular epithelial cells sloughed off and excreted in urine.

sodium, chloride, and potassium excretion in the urine. Evaluating the urine sodium concentration and percent excreted (FeNa) is particularly helpful in differentiating between a pre-renal AKI and ATN. In a pre-renal state, the kidneys should excrete very little sodium as a compensatory mechanism to increase water reabsorption and restore EABV. The FeNa is often calculated as a more accurate means of determining the kidneys' ability to reabsorb sodium, as it takes into account the decrease in urinary sodium excretion due to a decrease in creatinine excretion. Under normal conditions, the kidneys excrete approximately 1% to 2% of the total sodium intake (normal FeNa value). In a pre-renal AKI, the FeNa should be lower than 1% as the kidneys should reabsorb more sodium to absorb more water. In contrast, a FeNa of greater than 1% in ATN as the tubules are not able to reabsorb the sodium as efficiently. The expected urine findings would be oliguria/anuria, decreased urinary sodium concentration and low FeNa, a high specific gravity, and high urine osmolality. In contrast, in ATN the damaged tubules are unable to reabsorb sodium and water and therefore the urinary sodium concentration and FeNa will generally be higher than normal and both the specific gravity and osmolality will be lower than normal.

In general, a urine sample of a patient with pre-renal AKI should not contain cells or casts or other particulate matter. The presence of these substances in the urine may be used to rule out a pre-renal AKI and may be consistent with another type of AKI. Unfortunately, the presence of white blood cells, red blood cells, protein, and casts (with the exception of muddy brown casts) is not uncommon in many other types of AKI including any of the intrinsic forms as well as in post-renal obstructive AKI. Eosinophilia may be caused by a hypersensitivity reaction, supporting the diagnosis of possible AIN. While not very sensitive or specific, the presence of any eosinophils in the urine may indicate AIN[21] and careful review of the drug history and infections should be pursued. Serum urate concentrations may be helpful if post-renal obstruction from uric acid crystallization is suspected. Other crystals or calculi may be indicative of oversaturation and/or precipitation of particular compounds.

A diagnostic test that is helpful to detect a post-renal obstructive AKI is an ultrasound of the kidney, ureters, and bladder (often referred to as a "KUB").This test measures the size of the kidneys and can detect the presence of abdominal masses, free air, and fluid collections. Fluid around the kidneys is called hydronephrosis and often signifies reverse flow of urine due to a post-renal obstructive AKI.

In some cases, a kidney biopsy may be used to determine the exact type of AKI. This procedure is invasive and is contraindicated in many patients, such as those with uncontrolled hypertension, bleeding diatheses, or those with a solitary kidney. Because this procedure has risks, it is generally reserved for situations in which the diagnosis is undetermined by other, less invasive means, and/or the findings will result in different treatment plans.

Prevention

The best treatment of AKI is *prevention*! Strategies to protect high-risk patients should include the judicious use (or complete avoidance) of known nephrotoxins and maintaining optimal fluid status.

Many agents have been investigated to prevent ATN caused by the administration of radio contrast media (also called contrast-induced nephropathy, CIN). It was thought that agents that cause vasodilation of the renal vasculature and/or act as antioxidants could be nephroprotective. Unfortunately, there are no clear data to identify any specific agents to prevent CIN. Recent guidelines[22] recommend intravenous hydration with isotonic fluids prior to the administration of radio contrast media. Other agents that have been studied and found to be potentially helpful in reducing the incidence of CIN include theophylline and *N*-acetylcysteine[23] (Table 36-4).

TABLE 36-4 Strategies to Prevent Contrast-Induced Nephropathy[18,23]

Minimize volume of contrast utilized
Use agents that are iso-osmolar or low osmolar
Discontinue/avoid the use of nephrotoxins or agents that can alter kidney perfusion ▪ Diuretics, ACE-I, ARB, NSAIDs, aminoglycosides
Hydration: *normal saline* preferred ▪ 1 mL/kg/h up to 150 mL/h ▪ Begin 3-6 h preprocedure and continue for at least 8 h post-exposure
Other potentially beneficial therapies: ▪ *N*-acetylcysteine: 600-1200 mg po every 12 h. First dose preprocedure ▪ Theophylline: 200 mg IV or po in various regimens. First dose preprocedure ▪ Sodium bicarbonate 150 mEq/L IV infusion instead of normal saline: various regimens beginning 1-6 h preprocedure

Abbreviations: ACE-I, angiotensin-converting enzyme inhibitor; ARB, angiotensin receptor blocker; NSAIDs, nonsteroidal anti-inflammatory agents; po, oral; IV, intravenous.

The guidelines allow for the discretionary use of these agents given the potential benefit and the low risk of adverse events when used for this indication. It appears that fenoldopam and dopamine are ineffective or even harmful in this situation and should generally be avoided.[24,25] If the use of a radio-labeled product is deemed necessary, an iso-osmolar or low osmolar agent should be used in the lowest possible dose.

Treatment of Established AKI

For all cases of AKI the first treatment should be supportive care consisting of proper fluid and electrolyte management, acid–base balance, and vigilant protection of the vulnerable kidneys from further insult. Identifying the cause of AKI and stopping/minimizing the damage is imperative in preserving renal function.

Pre-Renal Acute Kidney Injury

Improving perfusion to the kidneys and optimizing intraglomerular pressure is imperative to mitigating kidney damage. If allowed to persist, hypoxia and ischemia may cause acute tubular necrosis. Efforts to improve perfusion and glomerular pressure may include optimizing cardiac output, appropriate volume repletion, and discontinuation/monitoring of agents that can negatively affect EABV or intraglomerular pressure (diuretics, ACE, ARB, calcineurin inhibitors, NSAIDs). Efforts to restore EABV might include the administration of isotonic fluids, blood products, inotropes, or the use of vasopressors to maintain systemic blood pressure, as indicated by the cause of the injury. Judicious use of colloid solutions in conjunction with diuretics may be beneficial in cases of total body fluid overload with a decrease in EABV such as heart failure, liver failure, or nephrotic syndrome.

Glomerulonephritis

There are many causes and types of GN. As the damage in the glomerulus causes inflammation, corticosteroids or other immunosuppressive agents may be helpful in certain situations. The exact agent/regimen should be determined depending on the exact type of GN.

Acute Interstitial Nephritis

As AIN is the result of an inflammatory process, there is some evidence that corticosteroids may be used early in the process to quell the inflammation and therefore limit damage to the kidney.[26,27] This treatment is not standard of care, and underlying disease states (such as infection, diabetes) should be considered.

Acute Tubular Necrosis

Once ATN has developed, there is little that can be done to further recovery other than supportive care and protecting the kidneys from additional insults. Please refer to the "Supportive care" section below.

Post-Renal Acute Kidney Injury

As with pre-renal AKI, the most important treatment for post-renal AKI is to identify and reverse/discontinue the cause. Depending on the etiology, there may be specific treatments or pharmacologic agents that can be employed. For example, if the obstruction is caused by prostatic hypertrophy, agents such as tamsulosin may be beneficial. If the obstruction is caused by a neoplasm pressing on the ureter, a ureteral stent might be placed to maintain patency. If the obstruction is caused in part by the anticholinergic effects of a tricyclic antidepressant used for neuropathic pain, an alternative agent to treat neuropathic pain should be tried.

Fluid and Electrolytes

Although studies have shown that patients with oliguric or anuric AKI have increased morbidity and mortality,[7,11] it is unclear whether the use of diuretics to enhance urine production actually confers better outcomes for patients.[28,29] It is clear however, that judicious use of diuretics allows for pharmacologic control of fluid and electrolytes (and perhaps drug elimination) and may postpone/avoid the need for renal replacement therapy. The patient's total fluid volume as well as an estimation of EABV must be considered before diuretics are instituted. Fluid management may be particularly difficult in heart failure, cirrhosis, and nephrotic syndrome. It is precarious to use diuretics in conditions that cause an increase in total body water with a decrease in effective blood volume, such as heart failure, nephrotic syndrome, or advanced liver disease. In this type of situation the diuretic helps to eliminate water from the intravascular space. However, due to capillary leak syndrome, third-spacing, loss of intravascular oncotic pressure, the fluid is slow to redistribute from the tissue back into the vasculature and hypotension and an exacerbation of AKI may ensue. For this reason the removal of fluid should be carefully monitored.

Fluid overload may occur rapidly as kidney function declines. The administration of intravenous fluids for volume expansion, resuscitation, and blood pressure support can cause a rapid accumulation. Additionally, many patients with AKI are critically ill and may require the administration of numerous intravenous medications that add significantly to the total daily fluid intake. Provided that the patient is not hyponatremic, a sodium restriction of 2 to 3 g/d may be applied. Diuretics should be used judiciously to remove excess fluid, with careful consideration of EABV. Most patients with AKI are prone to hyperkalemia. For this reason, diuretics that antagonize aldosterone (spironolactone, eplerenone), and those that inhibit potassium secretion (triamterene) are often avoided. Thiazide-type diuretics have been shown to be less effective as monotherapy in patients with decreased kidney function. They are, however, often used in combination with a loop diuretic to provide synergistic natriuresis and diuresis. By blocking sodium reabsorption in loop of Henle (blocking the Na-K-Cl transporter) there is a greater delivery of sodium to the distal tubule. By blocking sodium reabsorption in the distal tubule first, the excretion of sodium is greater than what could have been achieved by loop or thiazide alone.

Any of the loop diuretics can be utilized in AKI. Although there may be a perception that one agent is more effective than another, they all have similar efficacy when given in equipotent doses. There are differences in the oral bioavailability, and care should be taken when converting patients from intravenous to oral preparations. Generally, ethacrynic acid has been reserved for patients with an allergy to sulfa moieties. In patients with oliguria/anuria, higher doses may be required as the flow of water and sodium reaching the tubules is decreased. Initial bolus, intravenous doses are used and then titrated based on response. While higher doses are often needed to achieve the desired effect, ototoxicity is a dose-dependent adverse reaction and the risk:benefit ratio should be considered. In an effort to limit toxicity and enhance receptor blockade, continuous infusions of loop diuretics can be utilized. Another strategy that has shown mixed results is the administration of albumin as an osmotic agent before or concomitantly with furosemide to mobilize fluid from the extravascular compartment into the vasculature to be excreted in the urine.[30]

Electrolyte Abnormalities

Depending on the type of ARF and the remaining urine output, electrolyte homeostasis may be affected. Generally, electrolytes such as potassium, sodium, magnesium, and phosphorus will all accumulate in pre-renal ARF (generally low urine output). In cases of intrinsic or post-renal ARF, the effect on electrolytes may vary depending on the urine output as well as the exact location of the damage. ATN may cause drastic losses of potassium, magnesium, and even phosphorus, as the tubules are unable to reabsorb the substances appropriately.

Hyperkalemia

The accumulation of potassium in AKI is common and potentially life threatening. All of the potassium in the serum passes freely through the glomeruli and then is completely reabsorbed into systemic circulation throughout the tubules. The majority of potassium in the body is excreted by the distal tubule under the control of aldosterone while only a small portion is excreted from the colon in the feces. Dietary potassium restriction of <2 g/d is often initiated in oliguric or anuric states to prevent accumulation. Once hyperkalemia develops (or is suspected) an electrocardiogram should be completed immediately to evaluate cardiac effects. Irregularities such as peaked T waves or widened QRS complexes connote a potential life-threatening situation and emergent treatment of hyperkalemia should be initiated.

The first agent that should be given is 1g of intravenous calcium (either chloride or gluconate) over 2 to 5 minutes. Calcium antagonizes the excitatory effects of potassium on the heart. The next steps involve shifting potassium from the extracellular to intracellular fluid. While this can be achieved by different means, the most common first approach is to administer 10 U of regular human insulin with 25 g of dextrose, IV push over 2 to 5 minutes. Insulin acts to stimulate Na^+/K^+-ATPase receptors to exchange more potassium into the cell and more sodium outside the cell. Although beta-2 agonists have the same action, the excitatory effects on the beta-2 receptors in the heart may be deleterious. Sodium bicarbonate can also be utilized to cause an intracellular shift of potassium. This agent is generally reserved for patients with an underlying acidosis or in situations when the patient has been hypoxic and presumably in an anaerobic metabolic state. Doses of 50 mEq/L sodium bicarbonate can be given by intravenous injection over 2 to 5 minutes in life-threatening situations. While these interventions antagonize the effect of potassium on the myocardium (calcium) or force extracellular potassium into cells, the only way to remove potassium from the body is through the urine, feces, or renal replacement therapy ("dialysis"). If the patient has urine output, loop diuretics (and hydration if appropriate) can be utilized to enhance potassium excretion. Sodium polystyrene sulfonate in sorbitol can be given orally or as a retention enema to bind potassium in the gastrointestinal tract to be excreted in the feces. This agent is an exchange resin, binding potassium ions in exchange for sodium ions. For this reason it should be used with caution in patients with heart failure or cirrhosis as it may enhance fluid overload. Renal replacement therapy is generally a last line treatment option unless the patient already has vascular or peritoneal access for this type of therapy

Renal Replacement Therapy

Renal replacement therapy (RRT), the general term used to refer to any renal dialytic/hemofiltration therapy, is reserved for specific indications. The acronym "AEIOU" is used to remember these indications: *a*cid/base abnormalities, *e*lectrolyte imbalances, *i*ntoxications, fluid *o*verload, and *u*remia (Table 36-5). Any RRT can be used as supportive therapy depending on the hemodynamic stability of the patient, the resources available, as well as other patient factors. Hemodialysis provides solute and water clearance. However, patients must be hemodynamically stable to withstand the rapid fluid shifts caused by this therapy. Continuous renal replacement therapies (CRRT) provide excellent clearance as they run continuously, utilizing slower blood flow and fluid rates and add additional solute clearance due to increased convective clearance. These therapies are generally reserved for patients who are hemodynamically unstable and in an intensive care setting with individualized nursing care. Although not as common, peritoneal dialysis can be used during acute renal failure,[31,32] provided there are no contraindications (ie, recent abdominal surgery, intra-abdominal infections, ascites).

INDIVIDUALIZING DRUG DOSAGE IN AKI

Pharmacokinetic parameters may be altered due to kidney dysfunction or the use of RRT. Absorption and bioavailability from enteral sources may be diminished secondary to edema and decreased motility in the gastrointestinal tract. Volume of distribution may fluctuate due to edema or fluid removal. While metabolism and excretion of substances in the kidney may be altered, other organs may be more active to compensate. One strategy to avoid dosage adjustment is to identify alternative

TABLE 36-5 "AEIOU"—The Acronym Used to Remember the Indications for Acute Renal Replacement Therapy

A	*A*cid–base abnormalities Metabolic acidosis is the most common disorder seen and can predispose patients to cardiac arrhythmias.
E	*E*lectrolyte abnormalities Hyperkalemia is the most common abnormality seen as the kidneys are responsible for ~95% of the total body elimination. Hyperkalemia can be life threatening, leading to fatal arrhythmias.
I	*I*ntoxication or *i*ngestion Whether toxic concentrations are intentional, accidental, or simply a consequence of decreased elimination, renal replacement therapy may be employed to remove compounds that have a low molecular weight. Volume of distribution and protein binding may not preclude clearance with dialysis under toxic conditions.
O	*O*verload—*fluid* overload Pulmonary edema is a life-threatening situation that can occur quickly.
U	*U*remia Uremia is a clinical syndrome that occurs due to the accumulation of all of the substances that the body cannot eliminate in severe kidney insufficiency. While all of the toxic substances have not been identified, metabolic wastes, drugs, and other substances may cause symptoms such as intractable nausea/vomiting and pruritus, pericarditis, asterixis, obtundation, and seizures.

agents that do not require dose adjustment for kidney dysfunction. While this is not always possible, it avoids the problem of inefficacy or toxicity when the exact kidney function is uncertain. In any case, all medications should be reviewed and evaluated for the potential to cause toxicity if accumulation occurs due AKI.

The SCr concentration is not at steady state in AKI and therefore is of limited use to assess renal function. Although a quick calculation can be used as a basis for determining kidney function, clinical factors and professional judgment should be used in conjunction with common formulas used to quantify renal function. The trend in SCr concentrations and the urine output should be utilized to predict current function as well as function in the hours to come.

The SCr concentration should not be used to determine kidney function during RRT. The fluctuations in this value reflect the creatinine clearance achieved by the RRT as well as the patient's own clearance. Determining appropriate drug doses during RRT is confounded by numerous factors. Primary literature may provide information regarding dosing regimens successfully employed during RRT. Review articles that compile dosing recommendations for frequently prescribed agents (such as antibiotics) may be especially helpful.[33]

While there are a number of formulas that can be utilized to predict drug dosing during RRT, it is very important to consider clinical factors and use professional judgment before making a final recommendation regarding drug dosing. Factors that can alter drug clearance include the flow rates of blood, dialysate and other solutions, the amount of ultrafiltration (fluid removal) achieved, residual urine output, and the specific dialyzer pore size. Another important consideration is the amount of time RRT was actually employed. Many times RRT may be interrupted due to clotting within the system or if the patient becomes hemodynamically unstable. With all of the variables involved, it may be impossible to accurately predict drug clearance. When a drug is deemed necessary (no alternative appropriate), a thorough risk:benefit analysis should be conducted. The risk of subtherapeutic concentrations versus dose-related toxicity must be weighed. Reference texts often recommend initial doses based on a CrCl of 10 to 50 mL/min.[34,35] Once the drug is initiated, therapeutic drug monitoring of serum concentrations may be useful if available. Whether serum concentrations are available/useful or not, the clinician must rely on careful monitoring for objective and subjective signs and symptoms of toxicity/inefficacy to assess the safety and efficacy of the regimen.

PROGNOSES AND OUTCOMES

The mortality rate of AKI is highly dependent upon the etiology, severity, and duration of the damage. Pre-renal AKI is generally reversible, and most patients regain independent kidney function.[36,37] Patients with hospital-acquired AKI in the intensive care setting have a poor prognosis, with an estimated mortality rate >60%.[7] Prognostic factors that are associated with an increased mortality rate include oliguria/anuria, advanced age, organ failure, increased disease severity scores,[7,11] thrombocytopenia,[7] and Caucasian race.[38] Interestingly, while a history of CKD is considered a risk factor for the development of AKI, some studies have found that it is associated with a decreased mortality rate.[7,15] Although the exact reason for this unexpected finding is still unknown, it is may be related to the variation in the definition of AKI, including the use of SCr concentration in the diagnostic criteria.[39]

CONCLUSION

Acute kidney injury can develop from a variety of insults and can result in permanent damage and loss of renal function. Identifying patients at risk for AKI may help to prevent and/or minimize injury. Once AKI is established, it is imperative to stop the injury and support the patient. Support treatments address fluid and electrolyte management, acid–base balance, and protecting the kidneys from further insult or damage. Drug dosing and monitoring should be individualized for the patient's clinical status. Factors that should be considered include dialytic modalities used, urine output, and pharmacokinetic alterations caused by the decrease in renal function (or other comorbid conditions/states). The risk/benefit of any therapy should be carefully evaluated and the patient should be monitored closely for signs of toxicity or adverse events.

CASE Application

1. HL is a 69-year-old woman who presents to the emergency room complaining of severe nausea and vomiting for 3 days. On admission her serum creatinine is 2.0 mg/dL (her baseline is 0.8 mg/dL). She has not been able to eat or drink for 3 days and has lost 2.5 kg. Her medications on admission include hydrochlorothiazide 25 mg po every day, lisinopril 10 mg po every day. Which of the following statements is *false* regarding HL at this time?
   a. Nausea and vomiting may have caused a decrease in her effective arterial blood volume leading to pre-renal AKI.
   b. HL should not receive radio contrast media unless absolutely necessary until her kidneys recover.
   c. Hydrochlorothiazide may have caused vasoconstriction of the afferent arteriole leading to pre-renal AKI.
   d. Lisinopril should be discontinued until HL's kidney function returns near her baseline.
   e. HL's weight loss suggests fluid volume depletion.

2. Which of the following findings are most consistent with the diagnosis of pre-renal AKI?
   a. Specific gravity 1.029, FeNa 0.72%, uOsmol 550 mOsm/kg
   b. Specific gravity 1.013, FeNa 1.72%, uOsmol 350 mOsm/L
   c. Specific gravity 1.009, FeNa 2.02%, uOsmol 213 mOsm/L
   d. Urinalysis: 1+ protein, 10 to 15 RBC, 10 to 15 WBC
   e. Urinalysis: 3+ protein, no RBC, no WBC

3. A patient in the intensive care unit develops AKI. You review the medications the patient has been taking to evaluate for drug-induced AKI. Which of the following agents would be *most likely* to cause AIN?
   a. Labetalol
   b. Diltiazem
   c. Cefazolin
   d. Fentanyl
   e. Propofol

4. Which of the following statements is *true* regarding the use of diuretics in patients with oliguric AKI?
   a. Diuretics may increase urine output and reverse kidney damage.
   b. Diuretics should never be used in AKI as they may cause dehydration and exacerbate AKI.
   c. Diuretics can be used in very high doses as there are no toxicities to be concerned with.
   d. Thiazides and potassium-sparing diuretics are the preferred agents in AKI.
   e. Diuretics may improve urine output and help manage fluid and electrolyte abnormalities.

5. Which of the following agents can cause constriction of the *afferent* arteriole?
   a. Nonsteroidal anti-inflammatory agents (NSAIDs)
   b. Calcineurin inhibitors
   c. Angiotensin-converting enzyme inhibitors (ACE-I)
   d. a and b only
   e. a, b, and c

6. Which of the following combinations would be most effective to enhance urine production in a patient who has oliguric ARF secondary to ATN?
   a. Furosemide and ethacrynic acid
   b. Triamterene and hydrochlorothiazide
   c. Bumetanide and spironolactone
   d. Furosemide and metolazone
   e. Spironolactone and metolazone

7. A patient with anuric acute tubular necrosis has a serum potassium concentration of 6.5 mEq/L with associated electrocardiogram changes of peaked T waves. Which intervention should be initiated first?
   a. Regular insulin 10 U and 25 g of dextrose IV push over 2 to 5 minutes
   b. Sodium bicarbonate 50 mEq IV push over 2 to 5 minutes
   c. Calcium chloride 1 g IV push over 2 to 5 minutes
   d. Sodium polystyrene sulfonate 15 g po
   e. Furosemide 80 mg IV push over 2 to 5 minutes

8. PH is a 68-year-old man who was admitted to the hospital yesterday with an acute myocardial infarction. The cardiologists want to perform a cardiac catheterization with radio contrast dye. Which of the following regimens would be best as prophylaxis for contrast-induced nephropathy in this patient?
   a. *N*-acetylcysteine 150 mg/kg IV for 6 hours preprocedure.
   b. Sodium chloride 0.9% IV infusion 6 hours before and 6 hours after.
   c. Theophylline 200 mg po every 12 hours, two doses before, two doses after.
   d. Dopamine 0.5 μg/kg/min IV infusion 6 hours before and 6 hours after.
   e. No prophylaxis is recommended.

9. Which of the following circumstances can lead to acute tubular necrosis?
   a. Administration of a direct nephrotoxin
   b. Prolonged hypotension
   c. Prolonged pre-renal AKI
   d. a and b only
   e. a, b, and c

10. Which of the following statements is *true* regarding drug dosing in AKI?
    a. All patients should be dosed for a creatinine clearance <10 mL/min.

b. Pharmacokinetic parameters do not usually change so dose adjustment is not needed.
c. Although elimination may be decreased, the volume of distribution should remain unchanged in AKI.
d. The estimation of kidney function should include urine output.
e. All drugs should be monitored by serum levels to ensure safety and efficacy.

11. Which of the following urinalysis findings would be *most indicative* of acute glomerulonephritis (GN)?

a. SpGr <1.003
b. Muddy brown casts
c. pH 8.0
d. Eosinophils
e. Protein

12. Which of the following statements is *true* regarding urine volume?

a. Anuria is defined as <50 mL of urine per day.
b. Oliguria is defined as <50 mL of urine per day.
c. Polyuria is defined as <50 mL of urine per day.
d. Anuria is defined as no urea in the urine.
e. Polyuria is defined as >1 g of proteinuria per day.

13. Please identify the correct interpretation of the acronym "AEIOU" as it relates to the initiation of acute RRT.

a. A, *a*cid–base imbalance; E, *E*KG changes; I, *i*nflammation; O, *o*btundation, U, *u*remia
b. A, *a*cute distress; e, *e*lectrolyte disturbance; I, *i*nflammation O, *o*vert proteinuria, U, *u*remia
c. A, *a*cid–base imbalance, E, *e*lectrolyte disturbance; I, *i*ngestion/*i*ntoxication; O, fluid *o*verload; U, *u*remia
d. A, *a*cid–base imbalance; E, *E*KG abnormality; I, *i*ngestion/*i*ntoxication; O, *o*liguria; U, *u*remia
e. A, *a*nuria; E, *e*lectrolyte disturbance; I, *i*ngestion/*i*ntoxication; O, fluid *o*verload; U, *u*remia

14. JT is a 24-year-old woman brought to the hospital by her roommate. She states that she has been having diarrhea and vomiting for 3 days. She reports a 3 kg weight loss and cannot keep down anything, even water. In the emergency department her BP is 96/46 mm Hg, HR 120 beats/min, temp is 102.6°F, weight is 48 kg. On examination her mucous membranes are dry, she has no peripheral edema. She does not recall the last time that she urinated but thinks it may have been yesterday. Which of the following findings would you expect from her serum and urine laboratory analysis?

a. SpGr 1.016, 2+protein, light-yellow urine, many WBC and RBCs
b. SpGr 1.035, 0 protein, hazy-red urine, granular casts, FeNa >2%
c. SpGr 1.016, 2+protein, light-yellow urine, many WBC and RBCs
d. SpGr 1.005, 0 protein, hazy-red urine, granular casts, FeNa >1%
e. SpGr 1.035, 0 protein, dark yellow urine, no casts, FeNa <1%

15. Which of the following statements is *true* regarding the blood urea nitrogen (BUN) to serum creatinine (SCr) ratio?

a. In situations of dehydration the BUN:SCr will be <10.
b. In situations of dehydration the BUN:SCr will be >15.
c. In situations of volume overload the BUN:SCr will be <10.
d. In situations of volume overload the BUN:SCr will be >15.
e. In situations of glomerulonephritis the BUN:SCr will be <5.

16. PL is a 38-year-old man brought to the emergency department (ED) after being found at the bottom of the stairs to his apartment. Apparently, he was intoxicated, fell down the stairs, and lay there, unconscious, for approximately 6 hours. In the ED he was diagnosed with rhabdomyolysis. Which of the following statements are *true* regarding his situation?

a. Rhabdomyolysis may cause acute interstitial nephritis.
b. Rhabdomyolysis may cause acute tubular necrosis.
c. Rhabdomyolysis may cause eosinophilia and eosinophiluria.
d. PL should undergo renal replacement therapy for his intoxication.
e. Acute tubular necrosis is associated with a very good prognosis.

17. Hyperkalemia may result from AKI and can lead to which one of the following life-threatening complications?

a. Seizures
b. Arrhythmias
c. Hypertension
e. Acidosis
f. Encephalopathy

18. AB is a 60-year-old man with a history of chronic kidney disease and heart failure. His baseline SCr is 1.6mg/dL with a corresponding CrCl of approximately 50mL/min. Today he is brought by ambulance to the emergency room with dyspnea at rest and lower extremity edema all the way up to his thighs. His laboratory analysis shows SCr of 3.2 mg/dL and he does not recall urinating at all in the past 24 hours. Which of the following statements is *true* regarding the estimation of AB's kidney function today?

a. His CrCl is essentially zero as his is not making urine.
b. His CrCl is approximately 25mL/min.
c. His CrCl is still approximately 50mL/min.
d. He has AKI and so we cannot estimate his CrCl.
e. Wait to calculate the CrCl until after giving diuretics.

19. CG is a 58-year-old woman with a history of stage 4 ovarian cancer. She has metastases in her colon, abdominal cavity, liver, and bone. Recently she has undergone chemotherapy and radiation as palliative treatment. She is admitted due to 1-week history of fatigue, malaise, nausea, vomiting, and she notes that she has not urinated for days. Upon examination the doctor notes that her bladder is palpable and distended. Which of the following tests would be best to confirm a post-renal obstruction in this patient?
    a. MRI with contrast media
    b. CT abdomen with contrast media
    c. X-ray of the abdomen
    d. Ultrasound of the kidneys, ureters, and bladder
    e. MRI of the bladder without contrast

20. Which of the following agents may be used to treat acute interstitial nephritis?
    a. Prednisone
    b. Furosemide
    c. Lisinopril
    d. Ibuprofen
    e. Metformin

TAKEAWAY POINTS ››

- The best treatment for AKI is prevention.
- Acute kidney injury can result in permanent kidney damage and CKD.
- The first step in treating AKI is to identify the cause and stop/reverse it.
- Unnecessary exposure to nephrotoxins should be avoided during AKI.
- Supportive care includes management of fluid and electrolyte abnormalities, acid–base balance, blood pressure support/control, nutrition support, avoidance of potential nephrotoxins/further insults, and proper drug dosing.
- Diuretic therapy may be used to enhance fluid and electrolyte excretion.
- Targeted pharmacotherapy may be considered for AIN and GN.
- Drug dosing should be individualized for each patient and close monitoring is necessary.

REFERENCES

1. Hsu CY, McCulloch CE, Fan D, Ordonez JD, Chertow GM, Go AS. Community-based incidence of acute renal failure. *Kidney Int.* 2007;72:208-212.
2. Chertow GM, Burdick E, Honour M, Bonventre JV, Bates DW. Acute kidney injury, mortality, length of stay, and costs in hospitalized patients. *J Am Soc Nephrol.* 2005;16:3365-3370.
3. Abelha FJ, Botelho M, Fernandes V, Barros H. Determinants of postoperative acute kidney injury. *Crit Care.* 2009;13(3):R79. Available at: http://ccforum.com/content/13/3/R79. Accessed September 25, 2009.
4. Cockcroft DW, Gault MH. Prediction of creatinine clearance from serum creatinine. *Nephron.* 1976;16:31-41.
5. Levey AS, Bosch JP, Lewis JB, Greene T, Rogers N, Roth D. A more accurate method to estimate glomerular filtration rate from serum creatinine: a new prediction equation. Modification of Diet in Renal Disease Study Group. *Ann Intern Med.* 1999;130:461-470.
6. Ali T, Khan I, Simpson W, et al. Incidence and outcomes in acute kidney injury: a comprehensive population-based study. *JASN.* 2007;18(4):1292-1298.
7. Chertow GM, Soroko SH, Paganini EP, et al. Mortality after acute renal failure: models for prognostic stratification and risk adjustment. *Kidney Int.* 2006;70:1120-1126.
8. Hoste EA, Schurgens M. Epidemiology of acute kidney injury: how big is the problem? *Crit Care Med.* 2008;36(4):s146-s151.
9. Bellomo R, Chapman M, Finfer S, et al. Low-dose dopamine in patients with early renal dysfunction: a placebo-controlled randomised trial. Australia and New Zealand Intensive Care Society (ANZICS) Clinical Trials Group. *Lancet.* 2000:356:2139-2143.
10. Lewers DT, Mathew TH, Maher JF, Schreiner GE. Long-term follow-up of renal function and histology after acute tubular necrosis. *Annals Internal Med.* 1970:73:523-529.
11. Uchino S, Kellum JA, Bellomo R, et al. Acute renal failure in critically ill patients: a multinational, multicenter study. *JAMA.* 2005;294:813-818.
12. Bagshaw SM, Laupland KB, Doig CJ, et al. Prognosis for long-term survival and renal recovery in critically ill patients with severe acute renal failure: a population based study. *J Am Soc Nephrol.* 2007;18:1292-1298.
13. Clarkson MR, Friedwald JJ, Eustace JA, Rabb H. Acute kidney injury, Chapter 29. In: Brenner BM, ed. *Brenner and Rector's The Kidney.* 8th ed. Philadelphia, PA: Saunders/Elsevier; 2007.
14. Zeledon JI, McKelvey RL, Servilla KS, et al. Glomerulonephritis causing acute renal failure during the course of bacterial infections. *Int Urol & Nephrol.* 2008;40(2)461-470.
15. Waikar SS, Curhan GC, Wald R, McCarthy EP, Chertow GM. Declining mortality in patients with acute renal failure, 1988-2002. *J Am Soc Nephrol.* 2006;17:1143-1150.
16. Coffman TM. Kidney failure due to therapeutic agents. In: Greenberg A, ed. *Primer of Kidney Diseases.* 4th ed. New York, NY: National Kidney Foundation; 2005:293-300.
17. Verma N, Arunabh S, Brady TM, Charytan C. Acute interstitial nephritis secondary to infectious mononucleosis. *Clin Neph.* 2002;58:151-154.
18. Hewitt WL, Finegold SM, Monzon OT. Untoward side effects associated with methacillin therapy. *Antimicrob Agents Chemother.* 1961;1:765-772.

19. Mehta RL, McDonald B, Gabbai F, et al. Nephrology consultation in acute renal failure: does timing matter? *Am J Med.* 2002;113:456-461.
20. Ravel R. Renal function tests, Chapter 13. *Clinical Laboratory Medicine: Clinical Application of Laboratory Data.* 6th ed. St Louis MO: Mosby-Year Book; 1995.
21. Ruffing KA, Hoppes P, Blend D, Cugino A, Jarjoura D, Whittier FC. Eosinophils in urine revisited. *Clin Nephrol.* 1994;41(3):163-166.
22. McCullough PA, Stacul F, Davidson C, et al. Overview. Contrast induced nephropathy consensus guidelines. *Am J Cardiol.* 2006;98(6a):2k-4k. Accessible online at: http://www.ajconline.org/. Accessed September 25, 2009.
23. Meschi M, Detrenis S, Musini S, Strada E, Savazzi G. Facts and fallacies concerning the prevention of contrast medium-induced nephropathy. *Crit Care Med.* 2006;34(8)2060-2068.
24. Friedrich JO, Adhikari N, Herridge MS, Beyene J. Meta analysis: low-dose dopamine increases urine output but does not prevent renal dysfunction or death. *Ann Int Med.* 2005;142(7):510-524.
25. Lauschke A, Teichgraber UK, Frei U, Eckardt KU. "Low-dose" dopamine worsens renal perfusion in patients with acute renal failure. *Kidney Int.* 2006;69:1669-1674.
26. Pusey CD, Saltissi D, Bloodworth L, et al. Drug associated acute interstitial nephritis: clinical and pathological features and the response to high dose steroid therapy. *Quarterly J Med.* 1983;52(206):194-211.
27. Kodner CM, Kudrimoti A. Diagnosis and management of acute interstitial nephritis. *Am Family Phys.* 2003;67(12):2527-2534.
28. Minuth AN, Terrell JB, Suki WN. Acute renal failure: a study of the course and prognosis of 104 patients and the role of furosemide. *Am J Med Sci.* 1976;271(3):317-324.
29. Mehta RL, Pascual MT, Soroko S, Chertow GM; The PICARD Study Group. Diuretics, mortality, and nonrecovery of renal function in acute renal failure. *JAMA.* 2002;28(20):2547-2553.
30. Chalasani N, Gorski JC, Horlander J, Sr, et al. Effects of albumin/furosemide mixtures on responses to furosemide in hypoalbuminemic patients. *J Am Soc Nephrol.* 2001;12:1010-1016.
31. Gabriel DP, Nascimento GV, Cacmori JT, et al. Peritoneal dialysis in acute renal failure. *Renal Failure.* 2006;28(6):451-456.
32. Gabriel DP, Caramori JT, Martin LC, Barretti P, Balbi AL. Continuous peritoneal dialysis compared with daily hemodialysis in patients with acute kidney injury. *Peritoneal Dial Int.* 2009;29(suppl 2):s62-s71.
33. Choi G, Gomersall CD, Tian Q. Principles of antibacterial dosing in continuous renal replacement therapy. *Crit Care Med.* 2009;37(7):2268-2282.
34. Subach RA, Marx MA. Drug dosing in acute renal failure: the role of renal replacement therapy in altering drug pharmacokinetics. *Adv Renal Replace Ther.* 1998;5:141-147.
35. Aronoff GR, Bennett WM, Bern GS, et al, eds. *Drug Prescribing in Renal Failure.* 5th ed. Philadelphia, PA: American College of Physicians; 2002.
36. Barrentes F, Feng Y, Ivanov O, et al. Acute kidney injury predicts outcomes of non-critically ill patients. *Mayo Clin Proc.* 2009;84(5)410-416.
37. Liano F, Pascual J. Outcomes in acute renal failure. *Semin Nephrol.* 1998;18(5):541-550.
38. Waikar SS, Curhan GC, Ayanian JZ, Chertow GM. Race and mortality after acute renal failure. *J Am Soc Nephrol.* 2007;18:2740-2748.
39. Waikar SS, Liu KD, Chertow GM. Diagnosis, epidemiology and outcomes of acute kidney injury. *Clin J Am Soc Nephrol.* 2008;3:844-861.

PART

5 Gastrointestinal Disorders

CHAPTER

37 Liver Cirrhosis and Complications

Julie M. Sease

FOUNDATION OVERVIEW

The term cirrhosis refers to the histological findings of regenerative hepatic nodules surrounded by fibrous bands (collagenous scars) in the liver.[1] These abnormal findings are caused by chronic liver injury and can lead to portal hypertension, esophageal varices, ascites, spontaneous bacterial peritonitis, hepatic encephalopathy, hepatorenal syndrome, hepatopulmonary syndrome, hepatocellular carcinoma, thrombocytopenia, and coagulopathies. While the exact prevalence of cirrhosis worldwide is difficult to determine for a number of reasons, a reasonable estimate is that up to 1% of populations are afflicted with the histological abnormalities that define cirrhosis. In the United States, liver disease is currently ranked 12th among the leading causes of death.[2] Alcoholism and hepatitis C are the most common causes of cirrhosis in the western world.[1] Other causes include hepatitis B, nonalcoholic steatohepatitis, primary biliary cirrhosis, primary sclerosing cholangitis, hemochromatosis, Wilson disease, and alpha-1-antitrypsin deficiency. Liver injury has been linked to nearly 1000 drugs.[3] Examples of common drugs which may cause liver injury include amiodarone, HMG-CoA reductase inhibitors, highly active antiretroviral therapy, ketoconazole, nicotinic acid, acetaminophen, retinol, rifampin, isoniazid, phenytoin, valproic acid, azathioprine, estrogens, and oral contraceptives. Usually, drug-induced liver disease resembles acute hepatitis, cholestatic liver disease or mixed hepatitis/cholestasis, but may also resemble fibrosis and cirrhosis (eg, methotrexate).

Cirrhosis is an advanced state of liver fibrosis.[1] Fibrosis is, in essence, the encapsulation or replacement of injured tissue by scar tissue. In cirrhosis, fibrosis is accompanied by a distortion of the hepatic vasculature. It leads to shunting of the hepatic blood supply from the portal vein and hepatic artery directly to hepatic outflow the central vein. This shunting compromises exchange between hepatic sinusoids and hepatocytes, which normally execute the expected functions of the liver (Figure 37-1). The major consequences of cirrhosis include impaired hepatocyte function, portal hypertension, and hepatocellular carcinoma. Portal hypertension can manifest as ascites, gastric or esophageal varices, and hepatic encephalopathy. Cirrhosis may be clinically silent or may include a variety of symptoms. Some of the possible symptoms of uncompensated cirrhosis include jaundice, spider angiomata, splenomegaly, ascites, palmar erythema, gynecomastia, hypogonadism, anorexia, fatigue, weight loss, muscle wasting, and type 2 diabetes.

Abnormal liver enzyme levels may signal liver damage.[4] Both acute and chronic liver injury lead to increases in serum concentrations of aspartate aminotransferase (AST) and alanine aminotransferase (ALT). ALT elevation is more specific for liver damage than AST elevation as AST is also present in the heart, skeletal muscle, kidneys, brain, and red blood cells. Marked elevations (greater than 10 times normal) in AST and ALT are typically associated with acute hepatic injury such as with toxic liver injury or acute viral hepatitis. Cirrhosis and chronic hepatitis may also cause elevations in AST and ALT, but typically not to the same degree as acute insults, or AST and ALT may test within the normal range in patients with cirrhosis or another chronic liver disease. An AST/ALT ratio greater than one can be found in 79% of patients who have cirrhosis. Elevations in alkaline phosphatase (alk phos) may accompany liver disease, particularly in cases of obstructive diseases such as primary biliary cirrhosis or primary sclerosing cholangitis. Alk phos is not specific to the liver either. It is also present in a number of other tissues. Because of its lack of specificity but high sensitivity for liver disease, gamma-glutamyl transpeptidase is often tested for elevation in an effort to identify causes for elevations in alk phos. Elevations in conjugated bilirubin may accompany cirrhosis. Though also nonspecific for liver disease, decreased serum albumin and increased prothrombin time are possible findings in end-stage liver disease and may be useful monitoring tests for hepatic synthetic capacity.

QUANTIFICATION OF LIVER DYSFUNCTION AND DRUG DOSE ADJUSTMENT

The Child-Pugh classification system (Table 37-1) is one means of quantifying the myriad effects of the cirrhotic process on laboratory and clinical manifestations.[5] Recommended drug dosing adjustments for patients in liver failure, when available, are normally based upon Child-Pugh score. The model for end-stage liver disease (MELD) scoring system is now the accepted classification scheme used by the United Network for Organ Sharing (UNOS) in the allocation livers for transplantation and is less subjective than the Child-Pugh

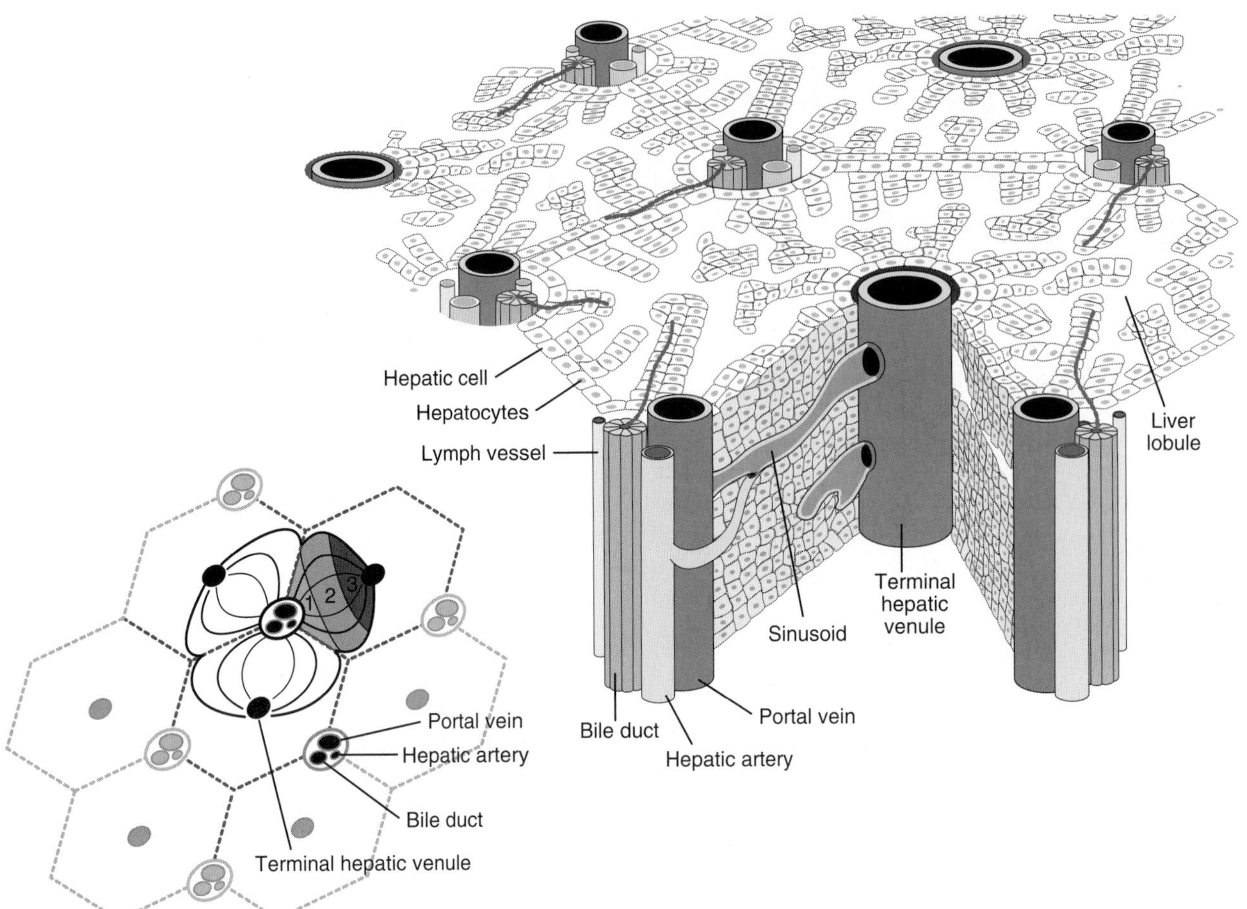

FIGURE 37-1 The hepatic lobule. The numbers 1, 2, and 3 indicate the three functional zones based on relative oxygen supply, 1 being the highest.

Reproduced with permission from Sease JM, Timm EG, Stragand JJ. Portal hypertension and cirrhosis. In: DiPiro JT, Talbert RL, Yee GC, Matzke GR, Wells BG, Posey LM, eds. *Pharmacotherapy: A Pathophysiologic Approach*. 7th ed. New York, NY: McGraw-Hill; 2008:633-649.

TABLE 37-1 Citeria and Scoring for the Child-Pugh Grading of Chronic Liver Disease

Score	1	2	3
Total bilirubin (mg/dL)	1-2	2-3	> 3
Albumin (g/dL)	> 3.5	2.8-3.5	< 2.8
Ascites	None	Mild	Moderate
Encephalopathy (grade)	None	1 and 2	3 and 4
Prothrombin time (seconds prolonged)	1-4	4-6	> 6

Grade A, < 7 points; Grade B, 7-9 points; Grade C, 10-15 points.

system.[6] The MELD scoring calculation is as follows: MELD score = 0.957 × Log_e(creatinine mg/dL) + 0.378 × Log_e(bilirubin mg/dL) + 1.120 × Log_e(INR) + 0.643.[7] The number is then multiplied by 10 and rounded to the nearest whole number.

Understanding the possible effects of cirrhosis on drug effect and clearance begins with understanding hepatic drug elimination. Hepatic drug elimination is dependent upon blood flow, drug binding in blood, and intrinsic clearance (the activity of enzymes and transporters involved in the hepatic elimination of drugs).[8] The clearance of high hepatic extraction ratio ($E_H > 0.7$) drugs is dependent on blood flow while the clearance of low hepatic extraction ratio ($E_H < 0.3$) drugs is dependent on binding of drug to blood components or enzyme/transporter activity. Unfortunately, the extraction ratio of drugs is not always known.

Cirrhosis affects the pharmacokinetics of drugs eliminated by hepatic metabolism or biliary excretion by reducing their blood/plasma clearance.[8] It appears to affect drug elimination through multiple factors, especially hepatocellular dysfunction and portal-systemic shunting. In liver disease, phase I oxidative metabolism is affected to a greater extent than phase II conjugation reactions like glucuronidation, though phase II reactions may also be affected in severe hepatic dysfunction. Further complicating matters, chronic liver disease is associated with nonuniform reductions in oxidative metabolism as it affects the different cytochrome P450 enzymes to varying extents. Liver dysfunction may also decrease plasma protein binding of some drugs influencing the processes of distribution

TABLE 37-2 **General Drug Dosage Adjustment Guidelines for Hepatic Dysfunction**[8]

1	The oral bioavailability of relatively high hepatic extraction ratio drugs can be greatly increased and therefore dosage should be reduced accordingly.
2	Pharmacokinetic evaluation of low hepatic extraction and highly plasma protein bound drugs should be based on unbound concentrations and dosage adjustment may be necessary even though total blood/plasma concentrations are within the normal range.
3	Dosage adjustment of low hepatic extraction ratio/low plasma protein bound drugs should be aimed at maintaining normal total (bound plus unbound) plasma concentrations.
4	Elimination of drugs partly excreted unchanged by the kidneys will be impaired in patients with hepatorenal syndrome. Creatinine clearance significantly overestimates glomerular filtration rate in these patients.
5	Volume of distribution of hydrophilic drugs may be increased in patients with cirrhosis and edema or ascites. Loading doses of these drugs may need to be increased if a rapid effect of the drug is required. Renal function should also be taken into consideration.
6	Extreme caution is recommended when using drugs with a narrow therapeutic index.

and elimination. Additionally, patients with cirrhosis may exhibit pharmacodynamic changes unrelated to pharmacokinetic alterations. The most important of these pharmacodynamic changes are a decreased therapeutic effect to β-blockers and diuretics and an increased sensitivity to opioid analgesics, anxiolytics, and sedatives. Patients with cirrhosis are more sensitive to the adverse effects of nonsteroidal anti-inflammatory drugs on the kidneys. The hepatorenal syndrome that may accompany chronic liver disease further complicates drug dosing as well as the fact that renal function estimations using serum creatinine measurements are often inaccurate in patients with severe liver disease. Some medications contain dosage adjustment recommendations based on the Child-Pugh score, but many do not. When no recommendations for dosage adjustment in patients with hepatic dysfunction based on their Child-Pugh score are available, some general considerations may be helpful (Table 37-2) and the manufacturer's prescribing information should be consulted for recommendations (if any) in patients with hepatic dysfunction.

TREATMENT OF CIRRHOSIS COMPLICATIONS

Portal Hypertension and Esophageal Varices

Fibrotic changes within the hepatic sinusoids during cirrhosis lead to an increase in the pressure gradient between portal venous and central venous pressures. This increased pressure gradient results in the creation of gastrointestinal and esophageal varices. Esophageal and gastric varices arise after the hepatic venous pressure gradient (HVPG) of 8 to 10 mm Hg is reached and bleeding can occur from these varices once the gradient rises above 12 mm Hg.[9] Varices occur because of the body's need to find collateral outlets to relieve the increased pressure of portal hypertension. Other outlets, besides esophageal and gastric varices, include retroperitoneal vessels, the hemorrhoidal venous plexus, a recanalized umbilical vein, and intrahepatic shunts. The management of varices involves three strategies: (1) primary prophylaxis (prevention of the first bleeding episode); (2) treatment of acute variceal hemorrhage; and (3) secondary prophylaxis (prevention of rebleeding in patients who have previously bled).[10] Recommendations for the management of portal hypertension and variceal bleeding are listed in Table 37-3.[11]

The mainstay of primary prophylaxis is the use of nonselective orally administered β-adrenergic blocking agents such as propranolol or nadolol.[9] These agents reduce portal pressure by reducing portal venous inflow via two mechanisms:

TABLE 37-3 **Table of Therapeutic Recommendations: Variceal Bleeding in Portal Hypertension**[11]

Recommendation	Notes
Prevention of variceal bleeding in patients found to have varices Propranolol 20 mg po bid *or* Nadolol 40 mg po daily	Titrate β-blocker to maximal tolerated dose or 55 to 60 beats per minute. Nadolol is renally eliminated and dosing adjustments are required in patients with renal dysfunction. Endoscopic variceal ligation may be used instead of drug therapy in the case of medium/large varices and high risk of bleeding (Child B/C or red wale markings on varices).
Treatment of variceal bleeding Antibiotic prophylaxis (7 d maximum): Norfloxacin 400 mg po bid (ciprofloxacin can be used if IV therapy required) *or* Ceftriaxone 1 g IV daily (if advanced cirrhosis and in center with high quinolone resistance) Vasoactive drugs: Octreotide IV bolus of 50 μg and followed by a continuous infusion of 50 μg/h × 3-5 d *plus* Endoscopic variceal ligation or sclerotherapy	
Secondary prophylaxis of variceal bleeding Nonselective β-blocker (such as propranolol 20 mg po bid or nadolol 40 mg po daily) *plus* Endoscopic variceal ligation	Titrate β-blocker to maximal tolerated dose or 55-60 beats per minute. Combination therapy with nonselective β-blocker plus isosorbide mononitrate can be considered in patients who are unable to undergo endoscopic variceal ligation.

a decrease in cardiac output through β_1-adrenergic blockade and a decrease in splanchnic blood flow through β_2-adrenergic blockade.[12] It has been proven with statistical significance that mortality is lower in cirrhotic patients with esophageal varices that have never bled when those patients are treated with a β-adrenergic blocker.[13] In most studies, the dose of nonselective β-adrenergic blocker was titrated to decrease the heart rate by 25% of baseline.[11] Heart rate does not correlate with reduction in HVPG and direct HVPG measurement is not widely available; therefore, titration of β-blocker therapy to the maximal tolerated dose or a heart rate of 55 to 60 beats per minute is now recommended.[14,15,16] Patients with contraindications to therapy with nonselective β-adrenergic blockers (ie, those with asthma, insulin-dependent diabetes with episodes of hypoglycemia, and peripheral vascular disease) or intolerance to β-adrenergic blockers should be considered for alternative prophylactic therapy with endoscopic variceal ligation (EVL).[11]

In cases of variceal bleeding, vasoactive drug therapy to stop or slow bleeding is routinely used early in patient management in conjunction with EVL.[11,14] Antibiotic therapy to prevent infection, as well as to prevent rebleeding and decrease mortality, should also be implemented. Octreotide is the vasoactive drug most commonly used to manage acute variceal bleeding in the United States and is usually dosed via the IV route. It works as a splanchnic vasoconstrictor thus decreasing portal blood flow and pressure. During octreotide therapy, patients should be monitored for hypo- or hyperglycemia as well as cardiac conduction abnormalities.[11,16] Cirrhotic patients with active bleeding are at high risk of severe bacterial infections.[11] Short-term prophylactic antibiotic therapy to reduce the risk of infection during episodes of bleeding not only reduces the likelihood of development of infections, it also reduces the incidence of rebleeding and increases short-term survival.[17,18,19] Prophylactic antibiotic therapy should be prescribed for all patients with cirrhosis and acute variceal bleeding.[11] A short course (7 days maximum) of oral norfloxacin, or IV ciprofloxacin when the oral route is not available, is recommended. Alternatively, in patients with severe cirrhosis in areas with high quinolone resistance, IV ceftriaxone may be preferable.

The combination of EVL plus pharmacologic therapy to prevent rebleeding is currently considered the most rational therapeutic approach.[11,14,16] Pharmacologic therapy should be initiated with an orally administered nonselective β-blocker such as propranolol or nadolol.[16] β-Blocker therapy should be titrated to achieve a goal heart rate of 55 to 60 beats per minute or the maximal tolerated dose. Patients on nonselective β-blocker therapy should be monitored for evidence of heart failure, bronchospasm, and glucose intolerance, particularly hypoglycemia in patients with insulin-dependent diabetes. EVL should be conducted every 1 to 2 weeks until variceal obliteration, and then the patient should be followed by surveillance endoscopy in 1 to 3 months and then every 6 to 12 months. Combination therapy with orally administered nonselective β-blocker plus isosorbide mononitrate can be considered in patients who are unable to undergo EVL.

Ascites and Spontaneous Bacterial Peritonitis

Ascites is the most common complication of cirrhosis and the development of fluid retention in the setting of cirrhosis is an important landmark in the natural course of liver disease.[20] Physical examination findings of ascites include a full, bulging abdomen and shifting flank dullness. Diagnostic paracentesis is justified in patients admitted with ascites. Spontaneous bacterial peritonitis (SBP) is diagnosed when there is a positive ascitic fluid bacterial culture and an elevated ascitic fluid absolute polymorphonuclear count (greater than or equal to 250 cells/mm^3). SBP is an infection of ascitic fluid which occurs in the absence of any evidence of an intra-abdominal, surgically treatable source of infection. SBP is a common complication which develops in 10% to 20% of patients hospitalized with severe liver disease, cirrhosis, and ascites.[16] The key mechanism behind the development of SBP is thought to be bacterial translocation.[21] Most episodes of SBP are caused by *Escherichia coli, Klebsiella pneumonia,* and *pneumococci.*[12] Drug therapy recommendations for the management of ascites and spontaneous bacterial peritonitis are listed in Table 37-4.[20]

Treatment of ascites includes alcohol avoidance, sodium restriction, and oral diuretic therapy, usually with the combination of spironolactone and furosemide dosed using a ratio of 100:40 mg in order to maintain electrolyte balance. Electrolytes should be monitored in patients on diuretic therapy. Relatively broad-spectrum antibiotic therapy which adequately covers the three most commonly encountered bacteria is warranted in patients with documented or suspected SBP.[16,20,21] Long-term antibiotic therapy for the *prevention* of SBP should be considered in all patients at high risk for this complication including those who have experienced a prior episode of SBP and those with low protein ascites (less than 1.5 g/dL) plus at least one of the following: serum creatinine greater than or equal to 1.2 mg/dL, blood urea nitrogen greater than or equal to 25 mg/dL, serum sodium less than or equal to 130 mEq/L, or Child-Pugh score of greater than or equal to 9 with bilirubin greater than or equal to 3 mg/dL.[20] Long-term prophylaxis may be accomplished with orally administered norfloxacin or a double strength trimethoprim/sulfamethoxazole daily. Daily dosing of antibiotics, rather than intermittent dosing, is recommended in long-term prophylaxis. Albumin infusion may be useful in cases of refractory ascites following large volume paracentesis as well as in certain patients with SBP.

Hepatic Encephalopathy

Hepatic encephalopathy (HE) is a disturbance in central nervous system function because of hepatic dysfunction.[22] Presently, the primary substances thought to be involved in the development of HE are ammonia, glutamate, manganese, and the γ-aminobutyric acid (GABA)-benzodiazepine receptor agonists.[23,24] Treatment approaches for episodic and persistent HE include (1) reducing ammonia blood concentrations by dietary restriction of protein, (2) drug therapy aimed at

TABLE 37-4 **Table of Therapeutic Recommendations: Ascites and Spontaneous Bacterial Peritonitis**[20]

Recommendations	Notes
Ascites	
Initial therapeutic paracentesis should be performed in patients with tense ascites. Sodium restriction of 2000 mg/d should be instituted as well as oral diuretic therapy. Diuretic-sensitive patients should be treated with sodium restriction and diuretics rather than serial paracentesis.	Diuretic therapy: Spironolactone 100 mg po daily with or without furosemide 40 mg po daily. Therapy can be titrated every 3-5 d (maintaining the 100:40 mg ratio) to reach adequate natriuresis and weight loss. Maximal doses are spironolactone 400 mg daily and furosemide 160 mg daily.
Refractory Ascites	
Serial therapeutic paracenteses may be performed. Post-paracentesis albumin infusion of 6-8 g per liter of fluid removed can be considered if large volumes of fluid are removed during paracentesis.	
Treatment of Spontaneous Bacterial Peritonitis	
If ascitic fluid PMN counts are greater than 250 cells/mm3, empiric antibiotic therapy should be instituted. If ascitic fluid PMN counts are less than 250 cells/mm^3, but signs or symptoms of infection exist, empiric antibiotic therapy should be initiated while awaiting culture results. If ascitic fluid PMN counts are greater than 250 cells/mm3, clinical suspicion of spontaneous bacterial peritonitis is present, and the patient has a serum creatinine greater than 1 mg/dL and blood urea nitrogen of greater than 30 mg/dL or total bilirubin greater than 4 mg/dL, 1.5 g/kg albumin should be infused within 6 h of detection and 1 g/kg albumin infusion should also be given on day 3.	Ideal antibiotic choice: cefotaxime 2 g IV every 8 h. Ofloxacin 400 mg po twice daily may be substituted for cefotaxime in patients without prior exposure to quinolones, vomiting, shock, grade II or higher encephalopathy, or serum creatinine greater than 3 mg/dL.
Prophylaxis Against Spontaneous Bacterial Peritonitis	
Patients who survive an episode of spontaneous bacterial peritonitis should receive long-term prophylaxis with either daily norfloxacin 400 mg po daily (or daily trimethoprim/sulfamethoxazole). Long-term prophylaxis may be justified in patients with ascites whose ascitic total protein is less than 1.5 g/dL and at least one of the following is present: serum creatinine greater than or equal to 1.2 mg/dL, blood urea nitrogen is greater than or equal to 25 mg/dL, serum sodium is less than or equal to 130 mg/dL, or Child-Pugh score is greater than or equal to 9 with serum bilirubin greater than or equal to 3 mg/dL.	

Abbreviation: PMN, polymorphonuclear.

inhibiting ammonia production or enhancing its removal and, (3) inhibition of the γ-aminobutyric acid (GABA)-benzodiazepine receptors.[22,25] Additionally, treatment for persistent HE should include avoidance and prevention of precipitating factors (GI hemorrhage, infections, renal and electrolyte disturbances, use of psychoactive medications, constipation, and excessive dietary protein) in an effort to avoid acute decompensation.[22] Therapeutic recommendations for the management of hepatic encephalopathy are listed in Table 37-5.[22,25]

Lactulose administration (via oral route or rectal enema) lowers ammonia levels in the blood in several ways: (1) through creation of a laxative effect which reduces the time period available for ammonia absorption, (2) through leaching of ammonia from the circulation into the colon and increasing bacterial uptake of ammonia by colonic bacteria, and (3) through reducing ammonia production by the small intestine by interfering directly with the uptake of glutamine by the intestinal wall and its subsequent metabolism to ammonia.[25] Patients on lactulose therapy should have their electrolytes monitored periodically, they should be followed for changes in mental status, and lactulose should be titrated to result in two to three stools per day to avoid acute HE.[22] Inhibiting the activity of urease-producing bacteria by using orally administered neomycin or metronidazole can decrease production of ammonia.[26,27] Despite poor absorption, chronic use of neomycin can lead to irreversible ototoxicity, nephrotoxicity, and the possibility of staphylococcal superinfection.[22] As such, neomycin should not be considered first-line therapy for HE. In patients with an inadequate response to lactulose alone, combination therapy with neomycin may be tried. Metronidazole may also produce a favorable clinical response in HE. However, neurotoxicity caused by impaired hepatic clearance of the drug may be problematic. Orally administered rifaximin has been shown to be effective in the treatment of HE and has a favorable side effect profile as compared to other antibiotics in use for HE today.[28] Though studies to date have enrolled

TABLE 37-5 **Table of Therapeutic Recommendations: Hepatic Encephalopathy**[22,25]

Recommendations	Notes
Nutritional Management	
Patients with HE should receive the maximally tolerated amount of protein (goal 1.2 g/kg/d)	Patients with zinc deficiency should receive supplementation.
Zinc sulfate 220 mg po bid	
Reduction of Nitrogenous Load from the Gut	
Lactulose	Lactulose dosing: 45 mL po followed by hourly dosing until evacuation occurs. Then dosing adjusted to achieve 2-3 soft bowel movements per day (typically 15-45 mL every 8-12 h). May also be provided via 1 hour retention enema (250 mL lactulose in 750 mL water).
Antibiotics	
Neomycin	Neomycin dosing: 3-6 g per day for 1-2 weeks then 1-2 g per day. Patients should be monitored for renal function periodically and annually for ototoxicity.
Metronidazole	Metronidazole dosing: 250 mg po bid
Rifaximin	Rifaximin dosing: 400 mg po tid
Inhibition of GABA Receptors	
Flumazenil	Flumazenil dosing: 1 mg IV bolus is indicated for patients in acute HE with possible benzodiazepine intake.
Bromocriptine	Bromocriptine dosing: 30 mg po bid is indicated for chronic HE.

Abbreviation: HE, hepatic encephalopathy.

relatively small numbers of patients and even though it does not carry the indication for HE in the United States, rifaximin is largely considered second-line therapy for patients with HE who fail therapy or have inadequate results with lactulose. Oral zinc supplementation is recommended for long-term management in patients with cirrhosis who are zinc deficient.[22] Flumazenil via intravenous bolus may be considered for short-term therapy in refractory patients with suspected benzodiazepine intake, but cannot be recommended for routine clinical use. Alterations of dopaminergic neurotransmission have also been thought to play a role in the symptoms of HE, particularly the extrapyramidal signs. Improvements of extrapyramidal symptoms have been reported with oral bromocriptine therapy.[29] Bromocriptine is indicated for chronic HE treatment in patient who are unresponsive to other therapies.[22] Prolactin levels may become elevated during bromocriptine treatment and ototoxicity is possible.[22,26] Bromocriptine should be avoided in patients with ascites.[26]

CASE Application

1. Which of the following drugs causes the most cases of hepatic cirrhosis in the western world?
   a. HMG-CoA reductase inhibitors (statins)
   b. Valproic acid
   c. Methotrexate
   d. Ethanol

2. Which of the following is a sign or symptom of hepatic cirrhosis?
   a. Hypoglycemia
   b. Weight gain
   c. Ascites
   d. Pancreatitis

3. Marked elevations (greater than 10 times normal) in AST and ALT are typically associated with which of the following?
   a. Cirrhosis
   b. Acute acetaminophen toxicity
   c. Chronic hepatitis C infection
   d. Chronic hepatitis B infection

4. Which of the following is true?
   a. ALT is more specific for liver damage than AST.
   b. AST is more specific for liver damage than ALT.
   c. An elevation in alk phos is specific for liver disease.
   d. An elevation in prothrombin time is specific for liver disease.

5. BT is a 58-year-old man who has been diagnosed with cirrhosis for the past 2 years. BT is currently having difficulty with overactive bladder and his physician is considering starting him on darifenacin. BT presents with mild ascites and no encephalopathy. His pertinent laboratory values are as follows: total bilirubin 2.1 mg/dL (0.3-1.2), albumin 2.8 g/dL (3.2-4.6), and prothrombin time 20.2 seconds (12.5-15.2). Based on the patient's Child-Pugh score (Table 37-1) and the following information from darifenacin's dosing information, what dose will you recommend for BT?

No liver disease	Mild hepatic insufficiency	Moderate hepatic insufficiency	Severe hepatic insufficiency
15 mg daily	15 mg daily	7.5 mg daily	No clinical experience

   a. BT has grade A cirrhosis and should be started on 15 mg daily.
   b. BT has grade A cirrhosis and should be started on 7.5 mg daily.
   c. BT has grade B cirrhosis and should be started on 7.5 mg daily.
   d. BT has grade C cirrhosis and should not be given darifenacin.

6. Hepatic drug elimination is dependent upon which of the following?
   a. Blood flow, drug binding in blood, and hepatic extraction ratio
   b. Blood flow, drug binding in blood, and bioavailability
   c. Drug binding in blood, bioavailability, and hepatic extraction ratio
   d. Blood flow, drug binding in blood, hepatic intrinsic clearance

7. Which of the following statements is true in liver disease regarding volume of distribution and half-life of drugs normally highly protein bound to albumin in the blood?
   a. Albumin is increased in chronic liver disease leading to increased protein binding, increased volume of distribution, and potentially decreased half-life.
   b. Albumin is decreased in chronic liver disease leading to decreased protein binding, decreased volume of distribution, and potentially decreased half-life.
   c. Albumin is decreased in chronic liver disease leading to decreased protein binding, increased volume of distribution, and potentially increased half-life.
   d. No changes in albumin concentrations normally occur in chronic liver disease, and so no changes in volume of distribution or half-life normally occur.

8. Which of the following drugs would be expected to have a decreased therapeutic effect in cirrhosis due to pharmacodynamic changes associated with chronic liver disease?
   a. Morphine
   b. Furosemide
   c. Lorazepam
   d. Zolpidem

9. Which of the following is true about the oral bioavailability of relatively high hepatic ratio drugs in cirrhosis if portal-systemic shunting has occurred?
   a. Oral bioavailability will be increased and initial dosage should be decreased.
   b. Oral bioavailability will be decreased and initial dosage should be increased.
   c. Oral bioavailability will be increased but no dosage adjustment need be considered.
   d. Oral bioavailability will be unchanged and no initial dosage adjustment need be considered.

10. Pharmacokinetic evaluation of low hepatic extraction and high plasma protein bound drugs should be based on which of the following?
    a. Unbound concentration
    b. Bound concentration
    c. Total drug concentration
    d. Hepatic blood flow

11. Dosage adjustment of low hepatic extraction ratio/low plasma protein bound drugs should be aimed at maintaining which of the following?
    a. Normal unbound plasma concentrations
    b. Normal bound plasma concentrations
    c. Normal total (bound plus unbound) plasma concentrations
    d. No dosage adjustments need be considered

12. Which of the following statements is true?
    a. In liver disease, phase II conjugation metabolism is affected to a greater extent than phase I oxidative reactions.
    b. In liver disease, phase I oxidative metabolism is affected to a greater extent than phase II conjugation reactions.
    c. Chronic liver disease is associated with uniform reductions in metabolism via the different cytochrome P450 pathways.
    d. Serum creatinine is an accurate reflection of renal function in chronic liver disease.

13. Which of the following describes appropriate therapy for primary prevention of variceal bleeding in a patient with portal hypertension who has been found to have varices?
    a. No primary prevention therapy needed; only patients who have experienced an episode of variceal bleeding in the past should receive prophylaxis therapy.
    b. An appropriate prophylaxis therapy would be atenolol 50 mg po daily.
    c. An appropriate prophylaxis therapy would be propranolol 20 mg po daily.
    d. An appropriate prophylaxis therapy would be nadolol 40 mg po daily.

14. RP is a 45-year-old white man with a 20-year history of heavy alcohol use, cirrhosis, and portal hypertension. He presents for emergent care after experiencing hematemesis and is diagnosed with acute esophageal variceal bleeding. Which of the following best describes appropriate therapy for RP at this time?
    a. Pantoprazole IV 40 mg daily plus norfloxacin po 400 mg bid
    b. Octreotide IV 50 μg bolus, then 50 μg/h infusion plus norfloxacin po 400 mg bid
    c. Octreotide IV 50 μg bolus, then 50 μg/h infusion plus pantoprazole IV 40 mg daily
    d. Octreotide IV 50 μg bolus, then 50 μg/h infusion as monotherapy

15. Treatment of ascites includes po diuretic therapy with spironolactone and furosemide. What is the appropriate starting dosing ratio for these two drugs?
    a. Spironolactone 40 mg: furosemide 100 mg
    b. Spironolactone 100 mg: furosemide 40 mg

c. Spironolactone 200 mg: furosemide 40 mg
d. Spironolactone 40 mg: furosemide 200 mg

16. Which of the following therapies is considered first line in addition to dietary protein restriction for patients with hepatic encephalopathy?
    a. Metronidazole po 250 mg bid
    b. Neomycin po 500 mg bid
    c. Lactulose po 15 to 45 mL every 8 to 12 hours
    d. Rifaximin po 400 mg tid

17. Which of the following drugs sometimes used for hepatic encephalopathy is associated with ototoxicity?
    a. Metronidazole
    b. Neomycin
    c. Lactulose
    d. Rifaximin

18. Which of the following drugs increases a cirrhosis patient's risk of developing hepatic encephalopathy?
    a. Alprazolam
    b. Flumazenil
    c. Bromocriptine
    d. Zinc sulfate

19. Which of the following drugs used for the management of hepatic encephalopathy has the possible side effect of neurotoxicity?
    a. Neomycin
    b. Rifaximin
    c. Metronidazole
    d. Cefotaxime

20. PW is a 56-year-old woman with a history of cirrhosis who is admitted with severe ascites and undergoes paracentesis. PW's polymorphonuclear count is found to be 275 cells/mm^3. Which of the following antibiotics is available in IV formulation and is appropriate empiric therapy in PW at this time?
    a. Vancomycin
    b. Cephalexin
    c. Tigecycline
    d. Cefotaxime

TAKEAWAY POINTS ››

- The main causes of cirrhosis in the western world include alcohol abuse and hepatitis C infection. Patients with cirrhosis are strongly encouraged to abstain from alcohol as continued use may speed the onset of complications like ascites.
- Over 1000 drugs have been linked to liver dysfunction. It is important to monitor liver function (through tests such as AST and ALT) during therapy with medications known to cause liver damage.
- Usually acute toxicities or acute damage to the liver causes significant increases in aminotransferase levels. Chronic disease, such as cirrhosis, is more likely to cause only moderate increases in the aminotransferases or they may remain normal.
- The Child-Pugh classification and MELD scoring system can be used to stage the severity of liver disease in a patient with cirrhosis. When available, dosing recommendations for drugs which are metabolized by the liver are usually based on Child-Pugh classification.
- When dosing recommendations are unavailable for a drug in a patient with cirrhosis, some points to consider include:
    - The oral bioavailability of relatively high hepatic extraction ratio drugs can be greatly increased and therefore dosage should be reduced accordingly.
    - Pharmacokinetic evaluation of low hepatic extraction and high plasma protein bound drugs should be based on unbound concentrations and dosage adjustment may be necessary even though total blood/plasma concentrations are within the normal range.
    - Dosage adjustment of low hepatic extraction ratio/low plasma protein bound drugs should be aimed at maintaining normal total plasma concentrations.
    - Elimination of drugs partly excreted unchanged by the kidneys will be impaired in patients with hepatorenal syndrome. Creatinine clearance calculations based on serum creatinine are unreliable in these patients.
    - Volume of distribution of hydrophilic drugs may be increased in patients with cirrhosis and edema or ascites. Loading doses of these drugs may need to be increased if a rapid effect of the drug is required.
    - Extreme caution is recommended when using drugs with a narrow therapeutic index.
- Complications of cirrhosis include portal hypertension, esophageal varices, ascites, spontaneous bacterial peritonitis, encephalopathy, hepatorenal syndrome, hepatopulmonary syndrome, hepatocellular carcinoma, thrombocytopenia, and coagulopathies.
- Patients with portal hypertension found to have medium to large varices should receive primary prophylaxis against variceal bleeding and this can be accomplished with a nonselective β-blocker such

as nadolol or propranolol. Patients with small varices may also be candidates for primary prophylaxis if they have risk factors for variceal hemorrhage (increased risk includes those with Child-Pugh class B or C or the presence of red wale marks on varices). Patients who survive an episode of variceal bleeding should receive secondary prophylaxis against future bleeding with a nonselective β-blocker plus endoscopic variceal ligation (EVL). Combination therapy with nonselective β-blocker and isosorbide mononitrate may be used in patients unable to undergo EVL.

- Octreotide therapy (usually via IV infusion) used in conjunction with EVL is employed in acute variceal hemorrhage to control bleeding. Short-term (7 days) antibiotic prophylaxis which is also recommended in patients with acute variceal bleeding. Oral norfloxacin or IV ciprofloxacin are appropriate.
- Sodium restriction and oral diuretic therapy are used to control ascites in patients with cirrhosis. Oral diuretic therapy often includes spironolactone and furosemide started at doses of 100 mg and 40 mg, respectively and titrated using the ratio of 100:40 in order to maintain electrolyte balance.
- Albumin infusion may be used in patients with ascites who have a large amount of fluid removed during paracentesis and in those with suspected spontaneous bacterial peritonitis.
- Cefotaxime IV is the ideal antibiotic choice for patients with suspected spontaneous bacterial peritonitis.
- Lactulose (via oral or rectal enema administration), along with dietary protein restriction and avoidance of other precipitating factors, is first-line therapy for hepatic encephalopathy. Other options to lower the nitrogenous load from the gut include orally administered neomycin, metronidazole, and rifaximin therapy.
- Patients treated with neomycin should have annual auditory screening and periodic renal function monitoring. Metronidazole can cause neurotoxicity especially in a patient with hepatic dysfunction who is unable to clear the drug adequately.
- Flumazenil IV may be used in a patient with acute hepatic encephalopathy who is thought to have had recent benzodiazepine intake. Oral bromocriptine can be used for chronic hepatic encephalopathy to antagonize GABA receptors.

REFERENCES

1. Schuppan D, Afdhal NH. Liver cirrhosis. *Lancet.* 2008;371(9615):838-851.
2. Heron M, Hoyert DL, Murphy SL, et al. Deaths: Final Data for 2006. *Natl Vital Stat Rep.* 2009;57(14):1-80.
3. Abboud G, Kaplowitz N. Drug-induced liver injury. *Drug Saf.* 2007;30(4):277-294.
4. Giannini EG, Testa R, Savarino V. Liver enzyme alteration: a guide for clinicians. *CMAJ.* 2005;172(3):367-379.
5. Pugh RNH, Murray-Lyon IM, Dawson JL, et al. Transection of the oesophagus for bleeding oesophagus varices. *Br J Surg.* 1973;60:646-649.
6. Malinchoc M, Kamath PS, Gordon FD, et al. A model to predict poor survival in patients undergoing transjugular intrahepatic portosystemic shunts. *Hepatology.* 2000;31:864-871.
7. MELD/PELD Calculator Documentation. Available at: http://www.unos.org/SharedContentDocuments/MELD_PELD_Calculator_Documentation.pdf. Accessed June 29, 2009.
8. Verbeeck RK. Pharmacokinetics and dosage adjustment in patients with hepatic dysfunction. *Eur J Clin Pharmacol.* 2008;64:1147-1161.
9. Wright AS, Rikkers LF. Current management of portal hypertension. *J Gastrointest Surg.* 2005;9(7):992-1005.
10. Abraldes JG, Angermayr B, Bosch J. The management of portal hypertension. *Clin Liv Dis.* 2005;9:685-713.
11. Garcia-Tsao G, Sanyal AJ, Grace ND, et al. Prevention and management of gastroesophageal varices and variceal hemorrhage in cirrhosis. *Hepatology.* 2007;46(3):922-938.
12. Groszmann RJ, Guadalupe G, Bosch J, et al. Beta-blockers to prevent gastroesophageal varices in patients with cirrhosis. *N Engl J Med.* 2005;353:2254-2261.
13. Chen W, Nikolova D, Frederiksen SL, et al. Beta-blockers reduce mortality in cirrhotic patients with oesophageal varices who have never bled (Cocharane review). *J Hepatol.* 2004;40(suppl 1):67 (abstract).
14. de Franchis R. Evolving consensus in portal hypertension: report of the Baveno IV consensus workshop on methodology of diagnosis and therapy in portal hypertension. *J Hepatol.* 2005;43:167-176.
15. Garcia-Tsao G, Grace N, Groszmann RJ, et al. Short term effects of propranolol on portal venous pressure. *Hepatology.* 1986;6:101-106.
16. Garcia-Tsao G, Lim J, and Members of the Veterans Affairs Hepatitis C Resource Center Program. Management and treatment of patients with cirrhosis and portal hypertension: recommendations from the Department of Veterans Affairs hepatitis C resource center program and the national hepatitis C program. *Am J Gastroenterol.* 2009;104:1802-1829.
17. Bernard B, Grange JD, Khac EN, et al. Antibiotic prophylaxis for the prevention of bacterial infections in cirrhotic patients with gastrointestinal bleeding: a meta-analysis. *Hepatology.* 1999;29:1655-1661.
18. Soares-Weiser K, Brezis M, Tur-Kaspa R, et al. Antibiotic prophylaxis for cirrhotic patients with gastrointestinal bleeding (Cochrane Review). The Cochrane Library 2002, Issue 2:CD002907.
19. Hou MC, Lin HC, Liu TT, et al. Antibiotic prophylaxis after endoscopic therapy prevents rebleeding in acute variceal hemorrhage: a randomized trial. *Hepatology.* 2004;39:746-753.
20. Runyon BA. Management of adult patients with ascites due to cirrhosis: an update. *Hepatology.* 2009;49(6):2087-2107.
21. Koulaouzidis A, Bhat S, Saeed AA. Spontaneous bacterial peritonitis. *World J Gastroenterol.* 2009;15(9):1042-1049.

22. Blei AT, Cordoba J. Hepatic encephalopathy. *Am J Gastroenterol.* 2001;96:1968-1976.
23. Stewart CA, Cerhan J. Hepatic encephalopathy: a dynamic or static condition. *Metab Brain Dis.* 2005;20(3):193-204.
24. Mas A. Hepatic encephalopathy: from pathophysiology to treatment. *Digestion.* 2006;73(suppl 1):86-93.
25. Morgan MY, Blei A, Grungreiff K, et al. The treatment of hepatic encephalopathy. *Metab Brain Dis.* 2007;22:389-405.
26. Hawkins RA, Jessy J, Mans AM, et al. Neomycin reduces the intestinal production of ammonia from glutamine. *Adv Exp Med Biol.* 1994;368:125-134.
27. Morgan MH, Read AE, Speller DC. Treatment of hepatic encephalopathy with metronidazole. *Gut.* 1982;23:1-7.
28. Pedretti G, Calzetti C, Missale G, et al. Rifaximin versus neomycin on hyperammonemia in chronic portal systemic encephalopathy in cirrhotics. A double-blind, randomized trial. *Ital J Gastroenterol.* 1991;23:175-178.
29. Uribe M, Farca A, Marquez MA, et al. Treatment of chronic portal systemic encephalopathy with bromocriptine: a double-blind controlled trial. *Gastroenterology.* 1979;76:1347-1351.

CHAPTER

38 Hepatitis

Lisa S. Smith and Joy B. Greene

FOUNDATION OVERVIEW

Hepatitis is the inflammation and damage of hepatocytes in the liver caused by hepatitis A, B, C, D, E viruses, alcohol, and medications. There are 85,000 new cases of acute hepatitis annually and several million people living with chronic hepatitis.[1] Viral hepatitis occurs at any age and is the most common cause of liver disease. The prevalence and incidence may be underreported because patients are often asymptomatic. Acute hepatitis is associated with all five types of viral hepatitis and rarely exceeds 6 months in duration. Chronic viral hepatitis is associated with hepatitis B, C, and D and may lead to the development of ascites, jaundice, hepatic encephalopathy, esophageal varices, cirrhosis, and hepatocellular carcinoma. This chapter focuses on the most common viral forms of hepatitis (hepatitis A, B, and C).

Hepatitis A

Hepatitis A virus (HAV) is an acute viral infection spread via the fecal-oral route that infects 1.4 million people yearly worldwide. In the United States, HAV has declined to 76% since the development of the hepatitis A vaccine, but HAV remains prevalent in underdeveloped countries.[2] HAV is an RNA virus that impacts areas with inadequate sanitation and persons with poor hygienic practices. Other risk factors include IV drug use, exposure to infected individuals, and homosexual activity in men.[3]

Hepatitis B

Hepatitis B virus (HBV) is an acute and chronic viral DNA infection. In the United States, acute HBV is transmitted through exposure to blood and bodily secretions, sexual activity, IV drug use, and occupational exposure. HBV affects more than 2 billion people in the world, with approximately 350 million chronic infections.[4] Deaths related to HBV range from 500,000 to 750,000 annually. Despite having an effective vaccine against HBV, more than 300,000 newly diagnosed infections emerge annually. Approximately 10% to 15% of patients develop chronic HBV disease; therefore, 85% to 90% of acute HBV infections resolve without complications.

Hepatitis C

Approximately 170 million people worldwide are infected with HCV, with more than 4 million in the United States. There are six geographically specific genotypes of HCV.[5] For example, genotype 1 represents 75% of infections within the United States, whereas genotype 4 is common in the Middle East. HCV genotype is used to determine the duration of therapy and the likelihood of therapeutic response.[5]The most common modes of transmission of HCV are IV drug use and blood transfusion prior to 1992.[5] Before 1992 blood banks did not screen for HCV.[6] Other HCV risk factors include tattoos, body piercings, and shared drug paraphernalia. HCV is rarely transmitted through sexual intercourse in heterosexual monogamous relationships. Approximately 10% to 15% of patients with acute HCV resolve without any further sequelae; therefore, 85% to 90% of HCV cases develop into chronic disease.

Clinical Presentation and Diagnosis

Signs and symptoms vary among hepatitis patients and range from asymptomatic to liver failure. Asymptomatic patients may only present with mildly elevated liver enzymes. Common acute symptoms include fatigue, jaundice, nausea and vomiting, weight loss, fever, right upper quadrant pain, and splenomegaly.[7] An overview of HAV, HBC, and HCV can be found in Table 38-1.

Diagnosing viral hepatitis may be difficult because patients may be asymptomatic. Symptoms cannot identify the type of hepatitis; therefore, laboratory serology must be obtained. Viral hepatitis can be diagnosed by the presence of antibodies, antigens, and measured virus. Elevated liver enzymes (eg, AST and ALT) are not specific to viral hepatitis but of hepatocellular injury. In the presence of persistently elevated liver enzymes, lack of antibody production, and continued presence of viral particles in the blood, chronic HBV or HCV can be diagnosed. A liver biopsy is useful for assessing the grade and stage of liver disease in chronic HBV or HCV. The grade reflects the degree of liver inflammation, and the stage reflects extent of fibrosis or presence of cirrhosis.[7]

PREVENTION

Prevention of HAV, HBV, and HCV includes avoiding risk factors for transmission and immunization of children and at-risk adults against HAV and HBV (there is no vaccine for HCV). Screening is recommended for individuals with risk factors for acquiring viral hepatitis. Pregnant females should be screened for HBV to prevent perinatal HBV transmission. Patients acquiring HBV or HCV should be screened for other forms of viral hepatitis because coinfection is common and harder to treat.[7]

TABLE 38-1 **Overview of Hepatitis A, B, and C**

	Hepatitis A	Hepatitis B	Hepatitis C
Route of transmission	Oral-fecal	Blood, bodily secretions	Blood
Risk factors	Geographic areas with poor sanitation, poor hygienic practices, IV drug use, homosexual activity in men	IV drug use, sexual activity, occupational exposure to infected blood or bodily secretions, uterine exposure to infected female	IV drug use, blood transfusion prior to 1992, intranasal drug users who share paraphernalia, tattoos or body piercings if performed without proper infection control practices
Signs and symptoms of acute infection	Elevated liver enzymes, fatigue, jaundice, nausea, vomiting, weight loss, fever, right upper quadrant pain, splenomegaly; may be asymptomatic		
Chronic form (% incidence)	No	Yes (10%); 90% (if acute HBV was perinatally acquired)	Yes (80%-85%)
Screening	Not necessary unless assessing need for vaccine	Patients with above risk factors, pregnant females, patients with HCV or HIV	Recommended for patients who have ever used IV drugs, are on hemodialysis, had a blood transfusion prior to 1992, received blood clotting factors prior to 1987, unexplained elevated liver enzymes, organ transplant, children born to HCV infected mothers, have occupational exposure to HCV infected blood or a needle stick
Prevention for at-risk children and adults	**Havrix** *Adult:* 1440 ELISA units (1 mL) IM with a booster dose of 1440 ELISA units to be given 6-12 mo following primary immunization *Pediatric:* 720 ELISA units (0.5 mL) IM with a booster dose of 720 ELISA units to be given 6-12 mo following primary immunization **Vaqta** *Adult:* 50 units (1 mL) IM with a booster dose of 50 units (1 mL) to be given 6-18 mo after primary immunization *Pediatric:* 25 units (0.5 mL) IM with a booster dose of 25 units (0.5 mL) to be given 6-18 mo after primary immunization **Twinrix** (combination HAV and HBV vaccine) *Adult:* 1 mL IM given on a 0-, 1-, and 6-mo schedule	**Engerix-B** **Recombivax HBA** *Adult (> 19):* 1 mL IM at 0, 1, and 6 mo *Pediatric (0-19 y):* 0.5 mL IM at 0, 1, and 6 mo	None available
Diagnosis	IgM anti-HAV, elevated liver enzyme (nonspecific)	HBsAg, HBcAg, HbeAg, HBV DNA, elevated liver enzymes (nonspecific)	HCV RNA, anti-HCV, elevated liver enzymes (nonspecific)

Abbreviation: IV, intravenous drug.

Hepatitis A Prevention

Good personal hygiene and proper disposal of sanitary waste are required to prevent fecal-oral transmission of HAV. This includes frequent hand washing with soap and water after using the bathroom and prior to eating meals. Drinking bottled water in areas where HAV is most endemic will also minimize the risk of becoming infected with HAV. Individuals at high risk of acquiring HAV should receive either serum immune globulin or HAV vaccine.

Immune Globulin

Immune globulin (IG) contains antibodies from pooled human plasma that provides passive immunization against various infectious diseases, including HAV. Immune globulin is available in intravenous (IVIG) or intramuscular (IGIM) formulations, but only IGIM is used for prevention of HAV. IGIM is effective in providing pre- and postexposure prophylaxis against HAV, but it does not confer lifelong immunity. Adverse effects of IGIM are rare; however, there have been reports of anaphylaxis in individuals who have immunoglobulin A deficiency. IgA deficient patients should not receive IGIM.

HAV Vaccine

HAV vaccine (Havrix, Vaqta) is an inactivated virus administered intramuscularly for adults and children older than 1 year of age. HAV vaccine is recommended for children, persons traveling to countries with endemic HAV, men who have sex with men, chronic liver disease patients, intravenous drug users, patients who receive clotting factors, and people with occupational exposure to primates or HAV. For pretravel vaccination, the HAV vaccine should be administered at least 2 weeks prior to expected exposure.[8,9]

Hepatitis B Prevention

Hepatitis B vaccine (Engerix-B; Recombivax HB) is an inactivated virus administered intramuscularly in multiple doses. Hepatitis B vaccine is indicated for children and adults with occupational exposure to HBV, household and sexual contact of HBV carriers, men who have sex with men, people with multiple heterosexual partners, partners of patients with a newly acquired sexually transmitted disease, patients diagnosed with HIV, intravenous drug users, children born after 1991, infants born to mothers with HBV, patients on hemodialysis, patients with chronic liver disease, and people arriving to the United States from endemic HBV areas.[10,11] Twinrix is a preparation for adults that contains immunizations for HAV and HBV in one vaccine. The preparation contains a trace amount of neomycin and should be used with caution in patients who are allergic to neomycin.[12]

Vaccine Adverse Reactions

Adverse reactions to the HAV and HBV vaccines include soreness, warmth, and erythema at the injection site, drowsiness, headache, and fever. Rare cases (< 1%) of Guillain-Barré syndrome have been reported. The only contraindication to HAV and HBV vaccines includes hypersensitivity to HAV or HBV and yeast (HBV and Twinrix vaccines).[8-12]

HAV and HBV vaccines are pregnancy category C. Pregnancy is not a contraindication for the HAV and HBV vaccines and none of the products contain the preservative thimersol.[8-12]

TREATMENT

The treatment goal of viral hepatitis is supportive in nature and consists of viral suppression and eradication to prevent the long-term complications (eg, cirrhosis and hepatocellular carcinoma).[7] Surrogate endpoints indicating treatment response include normalization of serum liver function tests (ie, ALT), reduced viral load, and histologic improvement. Treatment initiation for HBC and HCV is based upon viral load, liver histology from biopsy, and liver function tests.[7] Table 38-2 summarizes treatment regimens for HBV and HCV.

TABLE 38-2 **Drug Therapy for Chronic HBV and HCV**

	Hepatitis B	Hepatitis C
Treatment	Pegylated-interferon alpha-2a (Pegasys) or one of the following: lamivudine (Epivir), adefovir (Hepsera), entecavir (Baraclude), telbivudine (Tyzeka), tenofovir (Viread)	Pegylated-interferon alpha-2a (Pegasys) or pegylated interferon alpha-2b (PegIntron) weekly plus daily ribavirin
Duration	Pegylated-interferon alpha-2a (Pegasys): 48 wk, NRTIs : 6-12 mo after HBeAg seroconversion if HBeAg positive patient or until loss of HBsAg if HBeAg negative patient	Genotypes 1, 4 (48 wk) Genotypes 2, 3 (24 wk)
Efficacy	Varies per agent and the presence of HBeAg	Genotype 1,4 ~50% Genotype 2,3 ~80%

HBV

Patients with chronic HBV have either e-antigen positive or negative disease. E-antigen negative disease is more difficult to treat and requires longer treatment duration. Chronic HBV can be treated with peg-interferon alpha-2a (Pegasys) or a nucleoside reverse transcriptase inhibitor (NRTI).[4] Peg-interferon alpha-2a and the NRTIs are similar in efficacy for e-antigen positive and negative HBV; however, seroconversion of the e-antigen occurs more often at 1 year for peg-interferon alpha-2a and 2 years for NRTIs. Viral resistance does not develop to peg-interferon alpha-2a, but is associated with NRTIs.[4]

The most common interferon adverse effects are flu-like symptoms (fever, headache, nausea, musculoskeletal pain, myalgia, and weakness), thrombocytopenia, neutropenia, depression, alopecia, fatigue, anxiety, and insomnia. Severe adverse effects include hepatic decompensation, bone marrow suppression, gastrointestinal hemorrhage or ischemic colitis, hemorrhagic or ischemic stroke, pulmonary disease including respiratory failure, and severe psychiatric side effects (depression, suicidal ideation, and suicide attempt). There are black box warnings for caution in patients with neuropsychiatric disorders, autoimmune disease, persistent severe infections, and ischemic disorders. Contraindications to interferon therapy include hypersensitivity to the drug, autoimmune hepatitis, and decompensated cirrhosis.[13-15]

The NRTIs, including lamivudine (Epivir), adefovir (Hepsera), entecavir (Baraclude), telbivudine (Tyzeka), and tenofovir (Viread), inhibit HBV polymerase. Administered orally, they are well tolerated with few adverse effects. Headache and gastrointestinal problems are the most commonly reported side effects. Rare, but serious side effects include lactic acidosis, hepatomegaly with steatosis, and HBV exacerbation upon discontinuation of the NRTI (black box warning).[16-20] Adefovir and tenofovir can cause nephrotoxicity; therefore serum creatinine should be monitored closely. Telbivudine may cause peripheral neuropathy and increased creatine kinase.

Lamivudine was the first NRTI used to treat chronic HBV, but it is plagued with a high incidence of viral resistance and cross-resistance. Newer NRTIs display less resistance and cross-resistance.[4] Studies involving combination therapy with NRTIs have not shown improved results compared to monotherapy; therefore, combination therapy is not warranted in most patients.

HCV

HCV patients treated with a nonpegylated interferon display a low sustained virologic response (SVR). Combination therapy of interferon and oral ribavirin improves SVR and the development of peg-interferon allows for weekly dosing and improved response over nonpegylated interferon. Oral ribavirin administered daily with weekly peg-interferon alpha-2a (Pegasys) or peg-interferon alpha-2b (PegIntron) has a 50% SVR for genotypes 1and 4 and 80% SVR for genotypes 2 and 3.[21] Interferon alfacon-1 (Infergen), a nonpegylated interferon, is reserved for patients who are nonresponders or partial responders to peg-interferon and ribavirin.[4] All interferon products are contraindicated in patients with decompensated cirrhosis.

Ribavirin is a weak antiviral drug indicated for treatment of HCV when used in combination with peg-interferon alpha.[21] Ribavirin requires dosage modifications in renal dysfunction and is contraindicated for patients with CrCl less than 50 mL/min. Other contraindications include pregnancy, male partners of pregnant females, autoimmune hepatitis, decompensated cirrhosis, and sickle cell anemia.

Adverse effects to ribavirin include rash, dry skin, nausea, anorexia, decreased weight, alopecia, and dose-related hemolytic anemia. There are black box warnings for hemolytic anemia, pregnancy, and warnings against ribavirin monotherapy.[22]

SPECIAL CONSIDERATIONS

Pregnant females with chronic HBV should be treated with an NRTI during the third trimester to prevent perinatal transmission. Approximately 90% of children whose mothers were not treated with antiviral therapy during the third trimester will develop HBV within 6 months of birth. Most of the safety data in pregnancy has been collected with lamivudine and tenofovir.[23]

Peg-interferon is pregnancy category C, but severe birth defects have occurred in fetuses exposed to ribavirin (pregnancy category X) either directly from the pregnant female or indirectly from the male sexual partner. All men and women of childbearing age should use two forms of contraception during ribavirin therapy and for 6 months following discontinuation of ribavirin.[22] A Ribavirin Registry is required by the FDA to collect and evaluate in utero exposure to ribavirin during gestation and up to 6 months preconception. Both health care providers and patients can provide information to this important registry.

HBV or HCV coinfection with HIV is common and presents a treatment challenge secondary to drug interactions and side effects from complex drug regimens. NRTI monotherapy should be avoided in coinfection because HIV may develop resistance to the NRTIs used to treat HBV (exception—telbivudine). Therefore, unless telbivudine is used, combination NRTI therapy is warranted. Continued long-term therapy with the NRTIs is common because the HBV poorly responds to treatment in the HBV/HIV coinfected patient population.

HCV treatment in HCV/HIV coinfected patients should not begin until the patient's HIV is well controlled on medications. If the HIV regimen contains didanosine, either an alternative HIV medication should be chosen or ribavirin should be excluded from the HCV treatment regimen. The only peg-interferon treatment indicated for HCV/HIV coinfection is peg-interferon alpha-2a (Pegasys).

HBV/HCV coinfection leads to more severe liver disease and an increased risk of hepatocellular carcinoma. There are no treatment guidelines for treating HBV/HCV coinfected patients, treatment should be individualized to the patient.[24-25]

POSTEXPOSURE PROPHYLAXIS

Postexposure prophylaxis for HAV and HBV includes vaccination and immune globulin within 14 days of exposure to the virus.[23] Immune globulin (GamaSTAN) and hepatitis B immune globulin (HepaGam B; HyperHEP B S/D; Nabi-HB) provide protection by imparting passive immunity for patients exposed to HBV and HAV respectively.[26]

Adverse reactions to intramuscular immune globulin and HBIG include pain and swelling at the injection site, headache, muscle pain, nausea and vomiting. Because immune globulins are prepared from human plasma, a risk exists for acquiring HIV or viral hepatitis. The only contraindications to immune globulin and HBIG are hypersensitivity to the products. Immune globulin and HBIG are pregnancy category C.[27-28]

CASE Application

1. Select the most common mode of transmission for the hepatitis A virus (HAV).
   a. Blood
   b. Fecal-oral route
   c. Perinatal exposure
   d. Semen

2. Which of the following forms of viral hepatitis can be cured?
   a. Chronic hepatitis A
   b. Chronic hepatitis B
   c. Chronic hepatitis C
   d. Viral hepatitis can never be cured

3. A rare side effect associated with Twinrix (hepatitis A/B vaccine) is
   a. Stevens-Johnson syndrome
   b. Neuroleptic syndrome
   c. Guillain-Barré syndrome
   d. Red-man syndrome

4. Peg-interferon alpha-2a and ribavirin cotherapy is pregnancy category
   a. B
   b. C
   c. D
   d. X

5. CR is a 58-year-old man diagnosed with chronic hepatitis C (HCV) genotype 1. Today he will begin peg-interferon alpha-2b and ribavirin therapy. Which of the following counseling topics is appropriate?
   a. CR should use two forms of birth control.
   b. CR's therapy will last 24 weeks.
   c. CR likely developed HCV from a contaminated food source.
   d. CR likely acquired HCV from perinatal transmission.

6. LO is a 28-year-old woman who discovered her boyfriend has chronic hepatitis B (HBV). They are sexually active and plan to marry in 6 months. Which of the following is the appropriate plan for LO?
   a. Administer HBIG and begin the HBV vaccine series.
   b. Administer HBIG.
   c. Begin the HBV vaccine series.
   d. Begin treating her for HBV.

7. Which of the following signs and symptoms may LO experience if she develops HBV?
   a. Jaundice
   b. Nausea
   c. Elevated liver enzymes
   d. She may experience no physical symptoms
   e. All of the above

8. MO is a 19-year-old Asian man diagnosed with chronic HBV acquired from perinatal exposure. He will begin therapy with entecavir today. Entecavir will likely:
   a. Be combined with ribavirin
   b. Be ineffective
   c. Develop resistance
   d. Cause minimal side effects

9. Which of the following medications for HCV is administered subcutaneously three times per week?
   a. Interferon alfacon-1
   b. Peg-interferon alpha-1a
   c. Peg-interferon alpha-2b
   d. Ribavirin

10. Immune globulin (GamaSTAN) is indicated for postexposure prophylaxis of
    a. Autoimmune hepatitis
    b. Hepatitis A virus
    c. Hepatitis B virus
    d. Hepatitis C virus

11. Which of the following drugs has the highest incidence of hemolytic anemia?
    a. Ribavirin
    b. Peg-interferon alpha-2a
    c. Lamivudine
    d. Tenofovir

12. DP is a 42-year-old woman who has developed chronic HBV from occupational exposure as a nurse. Her physician asks you to recommend a NRTI that has both high potency and low viral resistance. The best choice is
    a. Entecavir
    b. Tenofovir
    c. Lamivudine
    d. Both a and b
    e. All of the above

13. Chronic HCV genotype 2 should be treated with peg-interferon and ribavirin for
    a. 24 weeks
    b. 48 weeks
    c. 1 year
    d. 5 years

14. RM is a man who has just learned he is coinfected with HIV/HCV. When should RM's chronic HCV be treated?
    a. Immediately.
    b. As soon as his HIV is well controlled with medication.
    c. Never. His HCV is not treatable.
    d. After he develops decompensated cirrhosis.

15. DA has been diagnosed with chronic HCV genotype 1. His past medical and social histories include a history of intravenous drug abuse, alcoholism, a wife (married 30 years) with chronic HCV and a blood transfusion in 2002. During your patient counseling session, DA asks you how he most likely acquired HCV. You correctly tell him
    a. Blood transfusion in 2002
    b. Sexually transmitted from his wife
    c. Intravenous drug abuse
    d. Alcoholism

16. BR is a 47-year-old woman coinfected with HBV and HIV. The physician wants to prescribe a nucleoside reverse transcriptase inhibitor (NRTI) monotherapy to treat BR's chronic HBV. Which of the following NRTIs should you recommend?
    a. Lamivudine
    b. Entecavir
    c. Telbivudine
    d. Tenofovir

17. Which of the following drugs has been given a black box warning by the FDA for the risk of severe depression and suicidal risk?
    a. Ribavirin
    b. Peg-interferons
    c. Nucleoside reverse transcriptase inhibitors
    d. Hepatitis B immune globulin (HBIG)

18. Which of the following products should not be given concomitantly with live vaccines?
    a. Engerix-B
    b. Recombivax HB
    c. Twinrix
    d. GamaSTAN

19. When is it appropriate to treat chronic viral hepatitis with peg-interferon alpha-2a monotherapy?
    a. When the patient has renal dysfunction (CrCl <50 mL/min).
    b. When the patient has chronic HCV genotype 1.
    c. When the patient has chronic HBV.
    d. Both a and c.
    e. None of the above.

20. MM, a 21-year-old woman, has been exposed to hepatitis C. Which of the following is the most appropriate course of action?
    a. Do nothing unless MM acquires hepatitis C.
    b. Administer immune globulin.
    c. Begin peg-interferon and ribavirin.
    d. Begin lamivudine.

TAKEAWAY POINTS ››

- The most common forms of viral hepatitis are HAV, HBV, and HCV.
- HAV is an acute disease; while HBV and HCV are acute and chronic diseases.
- Viral hepatitis is spread via the following route(s): HAV (fecal-oral route), HBV (blood and bodily secretions), and HCV (blood).
- Acute and chronic viral hepatitis patients are often asymptomatic with elevated liver enzymes being the first indicator of disease.
- Prevention vaccines are available for HAV and HBV, but there is no vaccine for HCV.
- The duration of chronic HBV treatment is 1 year for peg-interferon alpha-2a, but is usually greater than 1 year for monotherapy with nucleoside reverse transcriptase inhibitors (NRTIs).
- The NRTIs drugs have few side effects, but viral resistance and cross-resistance are common.
- Pregnant females with HBV should be treated with NRTIs in the third trimester to reduce the transmission of HBV to the fetus.
- NRTI monotherapy should be avoided in patients with HIV/HBV coinfection because HIV can develop resistance to all of the NRTIs used to treat HBV with the exception of telbivudine. Therefore, unless telbivudine is used, combination NRTI therapy is warranted.
- Chronic HCV treatment should include cotherapy with daily oral ribavirin and weekly subcutaneous peg-interferon for 48 weeks in genotype 1 or 4 and for 24 weeks in genotype 2 or 3.
- Interferon products are associated with serious adverse effects including hepatic decompensation, bone marrow suppression, gastrointestinal hemorrhage or ischemic colitis, hemorrhagic or ischemic stroke, pulmonary disease including respiratory failure, and severe psychiatric side effects (depression, suicidal ideation, and suicide attempt).
- Ribavirin is pregnancy category X. Pregnant women should forgo treatment for chronic HCV until after delivery. All men and women of childbearing age should use two forms of contraception during therapy and for 6 months following discontinuation of ribavirin. A Ribavirin Registry is required by the FDA to collect and evaluate in utero exposure to ribavirin during gestation and up to 6 months preconception.
- Patients coinfected with HIV/HCV should not be treated for chronic HCV unless HIV is well controlled with medication.
- Postexposure prophylaxis for HAV and HBV involves the provision of passive immunity with an immune globulin and the HAV and HBV vaccines. There is no postexposure prophylaxis for HCV.

REFERENCES

1. Centers for Disease Control and Prevention. Statistics and surveillance. Available at: http://www.cdc.gov/hepatitis/statistics.htm. Accessed August 25, 2009.
2. Wasley A, Samandari T, Bell B. Incidence of hepatitis A in the United States in the era of vaccination. *JAMA*. 2005;294:194-201.
3. Alter MJ, Mast EE. The epidemiology of viral hepatitis in the United States. *Gastroenerol Clin North Am*. 1994;23(3):437-455.
4. Dienstag JL. Hepatitis B viral infection. *N Engl J Med*. 2008;359:1486-1500.
5. Memon MI, Memon M. Hepatitis C: an epidemiological review. *J Viral Hepat*. 2002; 9(2):84-100.
6. Roth WK, Weber M, Seifried E. Feasibility and efficacy of routine PCR screening of blood donations for hepatitis C virus, hepatitis B virus, and HIV-1 in a blood-bank setting. *Lancet*. 1999;353:359-363.
7. Nguyen Tung T, Lingappa Vishwanath R. Liver disease. In: Stephen J. McPhee, William F. Ganong. *Pathophysiology of Disease: An Introduction to Clinical Medicine*. 5th ed. Available at: http://www.accesspharmacy.com/content.aspx?aID=2089114. Accessed November 11, 2009.
8. Havrix [package insert]. Rixensart, Belgium: GlaxoSmith-Kline Biologicals; 2009.
9. Vaqta [package insert]. Whitehouse Station, NJ: Merck & Co., Inc.; 2007.
10. Engerix-B [package insert]. Rixensart, Belgium: GlaxoSmithKline Biologicals; 2009.
11. Recombivax HB [package insert]. Whitehouse Station, NJ: Merck & Co., Inc.; 2007.
12. Twinrix [package insert]. Rixensart, Belgium: GlaxoSmithKline Biologicals; 2009.
13. Pegasys [package insert]. Nutley, NJ: Hoffman-La Roche Inc.; 2008.
14. PegIntron [package insert]. Kenilworth, NJ: Schering Corporation; 2009.
15. Infergen [package insert]. Costa Mesa, CA: Valeant Pharmaceuticals North America; 2006.
16. Epivir [package insert]. Research Triangle Park, NC: GlaxoSmithKline; 2009.
17. Hepsera [package insert]. East Melbourne, Victoria: Gilead Sciences Pty Limited; 2006.
18. Baraclude [package insert]. Princeton, NJ: Bristol-Myers Squibb Company; 2009.
19. Tyzeka [package insert]. East Hanover, NJ: Novartis Pharmaceuticals Corporation; 2009.
20. Viread [package insert]. Foster City, CA: Gilead Sciences, Inc.; 2008.
21. American Gastroenterological Association Technical Review on the Management of Hepatitis C. *Gastroenterology*. 2006;130:231-264.
22. Ribavirin monograph. Lexi-Comp Online™. Lexi-Comp Inc. Hudson, OH. Available at: http://www.crlonline.com/crlonline. Accessed September 12, 2009.
23. Tran TT. Management of hepatitis B in pregnancy: weighing the options. *Cleve Clin J Med*. 2009;76(3):S25-S29.
24. Crockett SD, Keeffe EB. Natural history and treatment of hepatitis B virus and hepatitis C virus coinfection. *Ann Clin Microbiol Antimicrob*. 2005;4:13.
25. Dienstag Jules L. Acute viral hepatitis. In: Dennis L. Kasper, Eugene Braunwald, Anthony S. Fauci, et al. *Harrison's Principles of Internal Medicine*. 17th ed. Available at: http://www.accesspharmacy.com/content.aspx?aID=2873725. Accessed November 11, 2009.
26. GamaSTAN [package insert]. Research Triangle Park, NC: Talecris Biotherapeutics, Inc.; 2008.
27. Immune globulin monograph. Lexi-Comp Online™. Lexi-Comp Inc. Hudson, OH. Available at: http://www.crlonline.com/crlonline. Accessed September 12, 2009.
28. Hepatitis B immune globulin monograph. Lexi-Comp Online™. Lexi-Comp Inc. Hudson, OH. Available at: http://www.crlonline.com/crlonline. Accessed September 12, 2009.

CHAPTER

39 Upper Gastrointestinal Disorders

Bryan L. Love and Lisa T. Meade

FOUNDATION OVERVIEW: PEPTIC ULCER DISEASE

Approximately 10% of Americans develop chronic peptic ulcer disease (PUD) during their lifetime.[1] An estimated 60% to 100% of ulcers recur within 1 year of healing with conventional treatment.[1] In the United States roughly 30% to 40% of the population is infected with *Helicobacter pylori (H. pylori)*, but not all will develop PUD.[2] Most people acquire the infection during childhood.

Peptic ulcers are lesions in the stomach or duodenum that extend deeper into the gastrointestinal (GI) tract than other acid related disorders. These lesions develop in response to damage by gastric acid and pepsin. Gastric ulcers can occur anywhere in the stomach, but most are located on the lesser curvature. In contrast, duodenal ulcers occur in the first part of the duodenum. PUD is commonly divided into three forms: *H. pylori* induced, nonsteroidal anti-inflammatory drug (NSAID) induced, and stress related mucosal damage (SRMD). *Helicobacter pylori* is a spiral shaped, gram-negative bacteria that resides in the gastric epithelium and produces urease. The exact mechanism of gastric injury is unknown, but some possibilities include: the production of a cytotoxin, an increase gastric acid production and alterations in the host immune response.[3]

Damage from NSAIDs can occur by two mechanisms: direct irritation of the gastric epithelium and systemic inhibition of prostaglandin (cyclooxygenase-1 [COX-1] and cyclooxygenase-2 [COX-2]) synthesis. Up to 25% of chronic NSAID users will develop ulcer disease.[4]

Stress ulcers are superficial lesions that form in the mucosal layer of the stomach within hours of major stressful event (trauma, burns, surgery, organ failure, or sepsis). The most common cause of gastrointestinal bleeding in the intensive care unit is stress ulcers and the presence of a GI bleed is associated with a fivefold increase in mortality. The incidence of stress related mucosal bleeding (SRMB) is 1% to 6%. SRMB can increase hospital stays and health care cost.[5]

Signs and Symptoms

The clinical presentation of PUD can vary but may include nonlocalized epigastric pain. Other symptoms of PUD include heartburn, belching, bloating, nausea, and anorexia. Pain due to a duodenal ulcer may be worse with an empty stomach (at night or between meals) and may be relieved by food. *Helicobacter pylori* infection is more commonly associated with duodenal ulcers, but can occur with gastric ulcers. Gastric ulcer pain may occur at any time or may be worsened with eating. NSAID use is associated with gastric ulcers. Both types of ulcers can occur in the absence of symptoms and this is especially true with gastric ulcers in the elderly.[4] Patients can present with similar symptoms, therefore no one symptom can differentiate between *H. pylori* and NSAID-induced ulcers.

Diagnosis

Upper GI radiography and upper endoscopy can be used to visualize the ulcer and diagnose PUD.[6] Testing for *H. pylori* is recommended for patients with active ulcer disease, a past history of peptic ulcer disease and gastric mucosa associated lymphoid tissue (MALT) lymphoma.[7]

There is no single test that is considered the gold standard for diagnosing *H. pylori*. Endoscopic tests are more expensive, uncomfortable, and invasive. Rapid urease testing, histology, and culture are endoscopic tests for *H. pylori*. Nonendoscopic tests are more convenient, less expensive, and noninvasive. The urea breath test (UBT) and fecal antigen are more reliable than antibody testing for identifying active *H. pylori* before treatment.[7] Testing for *H. pylori* is only recommended if eradication therapy will be offered. The UBT is the most reliable test to document eradication.[7] Testing to confirm eradication is recommended for any patient with a *H. pylori*-associated ulcer, persistent dyspeptic symptoms despite treatment, *H. pylori* associated MALT lymphoma, and resection of early gastric cancer.[7] The term eradication or cure is only used when the organism is not detected 4 weeks after the end treatment.

PREVENTION

Primary prevention of NSAID-induced ulcers should include the use of a NSAID with the least gastrointestinal (GI) toxicity, and at the lowest effective dose. Partially selective and nonacetylated products may be associated with lower GI toxicity.[8-10] See Table 39-1 for a list of nonselective and selective NSAIDs.

The selection of an agent to use with an NSAID for prevention of GI toxicity depends on risk factors and the use of low-dose aspirin therapy. Risk factors that can cause NSAID GI complications include prior history of gastrointestinal event

TABLE 39-1 NSAIDs and COX-2 Inhibitors[6,8-10]

Salicylates		Risk of GI Toxicity
Acetylated	Aspirin	Intermediate
Nonacetylated	Salsalate (Disalcid) Trisalicylate (Trilisate)	Low Low
Nonsalicylates		
Partially selective	Etodolac (Lodine) Nabumetone (Relafen) Meloxicam (Mobic)	Low Low Low
COX-2 selective	Celecoxib (Celebrex)	Low
Nonselective	Ibuprofen (Motrin) Diclofenac (Voltaren) Indomethacin (Indocin) Naproxen (Naprosyn) Flurbiprofen (Ansaid) Ketoprofen (Orudis) Piroxicam (Feldene) Sulindac (Clinoril)	Low Intermediate Intermediate Intermediate High High High High

(ulcer, hemorrhage), age > 65, high-dose NSAID, and concurrent use of corticosteroids, low-dose aspirin, clopidogrel or anticoagulants.[10] See Table 39-2 for risk factors for GI toxicity from NSAIDs and prevention of ulcer complications. Patients in the high-risk category should be treated with a COX-2 inhibitor and either misoprostol or a proton pump inhibitor (PPI). Treatment for the moderate-risk patient should be a COX-2 inhibitor alone or a NSAID plus either misoprostol or PPI. To minimize the risk of cardiovascular events in patients treated with celecoxib the total daily dose should not exceed 400 mg per day. Patients with low or no risk of NSAID-induced ulcers do not require any protective measures.

Compared to traditional NSAIDs, COX-2 inhibitors have a lower incidence of duodenal and gastric ulcers. However, the gastroprotective effect of COX-2 inhibitors is lost in patients taking low-dose aspirin.[9,10] The FDA requires all COX-2 inhibitors and NSAIDs to include a boxed warning to highlight the increased risk of cardiovascular events.[11] Results from two meta-analyses suggest that naproxen has a neutral effect on the cardiovascular system.[12,13] This remains controversial, but recent guidelines recommend naproxen combined with misoprostol or PPI for patients on low-dose aspirin therapy and at low or moderate risk of GI toxicity from a NSAID.[10]

See Table 39-2 for recommended prevention of NSAID induced ulcers in patients taking low-dose aspirin. Patients requiring low-dose aspirin to prevent cardiovascular events and other risk factors (recent ulcer or two or more risk factors) for GI bleeding are considered high risk and should not be treated with NSAIDs or COX-2 inhibitors.

Ibuprofen reduces the antiplatelet effect of low-dose aspirin. The American Heart Association recommends patients take aspirin 30 minutes before the ibuprofen or at least 8 hours after to avoid this interaction and maintain the cardioprotective effects.[14] The FDA has concluded that all NSAIDs, including COX-2 inhibitors, are contraindicated for pain management in patients immediately after coronary artery bypass grafting (CABG) surgery due to the increased risk of myocardial infarction (MI) and stroke.[15]

Misoprostol

Misoprostol, the prostaglandin E1 analog, is indicated to prevent NSAID-induced gastric ulcers. Diarrhea occurs in 10% to 30% of patients and other side effects include nausea, abdominal cramping, headache, and flatulence. Taking misoprostol with food can minimize the diarrhea. Misoprostol is category X in pregnancy and should be avoided in women of childbearing age unless the patient is at high risk of complications from gastric ulcers. Patients should receive both written and oral

TABLE 39-2 Risk Factors for GI Toxicity and Recommended Prevention of NSAID Ulcer Complications[10]

	Treatment Recommendations	
Risk Category	**With Low-Dose Aspirin**	**Without Low-Dose Aspirin**
Very High Risk		
History of recent complicated ulcer	Avoid NSAIDs or COX-2	Avoid NSAIDs if possible or COX-2 plus either misoprostol or PPI
High Risk		
Prior history of ulcer disease plus low-dose aspirin, clopidogrel, warfarin or corticosteroid or multiple (> 2) risk factors	Avoid NSAIDs or COX-2	COX-2 plus either misoprostol or PPI
Moderate Risk (1-2 risk factors)		
Age > 65 High-dose NSAID Prior history of uncomplicated ulcer Concurrent use of corticosteroids, low-dose aspirin or anticoagulants	Naproxen plus misoprostol or PPI	COX-2 alone or NSAID plus either misoprostol or PPI
Low Risk		
No risk factors	Naproxen plus misoprostol or PPI	NSAID

warnings of the dangers of misoprostol and should be capable of complying with effective contraceptive measures. A negative serum pregnancy test within 2 weeks prior to starting therapy is required and female patients should start misoprostol on the second or third day of their next normal menstrual cycle.[16] Arthrotec is a combination product containing diclofenac and misoprostol.

Stress Ulcers

Two independent risk factors for SRMB include patients with respiratory failure (mechanical ventilation for longer than 48 hours) or coagulopathy defined as a platelet count < 50,000 mm^3, an international normalized ratio of > 1.5 or a partial thromboplastin time of > 2 times normal.[17] Patients with these risk factors should receive prophylaxis for stress ulcers. Other risk factors include severe burns (> 35% of body surface area), multiple trauma, sepsis, surgery, or organ failure.[17] It is not cost effective to use prophylaxis for all patients, therefore, prophylaxis should be reserved for those patients at high risk of SRMB. Adverse effects, drug interactions and frequent dosing make antacids and sucralfate less favorable than H2-receptor antagonists (H2RAs) and PPIs for the prevention of SRMB.[18] Clinical trials demonstrate that H2RAs significantly reduce the risk of GI bleeding in critically ill patients. However, tolerance can develop within 42 hours and the pH control can deteriorate with the use of H2RAs. PPIs provide more consistent acid suppression and unlike H2RAs tolerance does not develop. There are fewer studies that review the use of PPIs for SRMD. Both H2RAs and PPIs may be given by mouth, nasogastric tube, or intravenously.

TREATMENT

The four goals of treatment for PUD are: relief of symptoms, ulcer healing, prevention of ulcer recurrence, and reduction of complications.[1,2]

NSAID-Induced Ulcers

In regards to therapy, two issues that most often need to be addressed are prevention of NSAID-induced ulcers and treatment of the ulcers once they occur. When the NSAID is stopped most uncomplicated ulcers will heal. If the NSAID must be continued as in the case of arthritis a PPI is the agent of choice. Treatment for *H. pylori* is recommended for patients on NSAIDs if they test positive for the organism.

Sucralfate

Sucralfate is indicated for the management of duodenal ulcers, but is also used in the treatment of gastric ulcers, GERD, and esophagitis.[19] Adding sucralfate to NSAID therapy is not effective in preventing gastric or duodenal ulcers.[9] Sucralfate does not effect acid secretion, but forms a physical barrier over ulcerated tissue. The most common side effect with sucralfate is constipation. Other side effects include dry mouth, nausea, rash, and metallic taste. Elderly patients who have difficulty swallowing the large tablets may tolerate the suspension. Sucralfate may reduce the absorption of other drugs (digoxin, fluoroquinolones, ketoconazole, levothyroxine, phenytoin, quinidine, tetracycline, theophylline, and warfarin) and should be administered 2 hours after the interacting medication(s).[19] In order to prevent a delay in onset and reduced efficacy, sucralfate should be dosed 30 minutes after a PPI.

H2-Receptor Antagonists

H2RAs reversibly inhibit H2 receptors on the parietal cell, which results in a decrease of basal and food stimulated acid secretion. After 30 days of therapy some patients develop a tolerance to H2RA. H2RAs are not very effective for healing or preventing gastric ulcers, but do prevent duodenal ulcers.[9] The overall incidence of side effects is less than 3% but can include headache, dizziness, fatigue, somnolence, and either diarrhea or constipation. Adverse effects are more likely in elderly patients and those with reduced renal function. Cimetidine has numerous drug interactions (warfarin, phenytoin, theophylline, and lidocaine) due to the inhibition of several CYP450 isoenzymes.[20] Famotidine, ranitidine, and nizatidine are excreted renally and require dose reduction or extension of the dosing interval in renal insufficiency.

Proton Pump Inhibitors

PPIs are effective for healing both duodenal and gastric ulcers, and they also have a protective effect against NSAID-related mucosal injury. PPIs irreversibly inhibit the final step in gastric acid secretion. These agents inhibit greater than 90% of gastric acid secreted in 24 hours. All PPIs provide similar ulcer healing rates and relief of symptoms. Compared to H2RAs, PPIs relieve symptoms and heal more quickly, but are more expensive. Patients should take PPIs 30 to 60 minutes before eating. Elimination of PPIs is almost entirely hepatic and dosage adjustment is required in severe liver disease. Dosage adjustment for hepatic impairment varies between PPIs and is not always correlated to a Child-Pugh score. Pantoprazole requires no dosage adjustment for hepatic impairment, but esomeprazole, omeprazole, and dexlansoprazole recommends a maximum dose of 20 to 30 mg per day. Omeprazole and esomeprazole decrease the elimination of phenytoin, diazepam, and warfarin by inhibiting the CYP2C19.[21,22] Currently there is some data to suggest PPIs may decrease the effectiveness of clopidogrel, increasing the risk of MI or death.[23,24] Clopidogrel is a prodrug requiring hepatic conversion by the CYP2C19 to its active metabolite. One theory suggests some PPIs inhibit the CYP2C19, which would decrease the antiplatelet effect of clopidogrel.[24] In general, PPIs are well tolerated and the side effects are similar to H2RAs which include headache, nausea, dizziness, somnolence, diarrhea, constipation, and vitamin B_{12} deficiency.

TABLE 39-3 **Drug Regimens to Eradicate *H. pylori*[7]**

	PPI or H2RA	Antibiotic 1	Antibiotic 2	Bismuth	Duration
Clarithromycin-based triple therapy	PPI bid or esomeprazole once daily	Clarithromycin 500 mg bid	Amoxicillin 1000 mg bid or metronidazole 500 mg bid		14 d
Bismuth quadruple therapy	H2RA or PPI bid or esomeprazole once daily	Metronidazole 250 mg qid	Tetracycline 500 mg qid or amoxicillin 500 mg qid	Bismuth subsalicylate 525 mg qid	10-14 d
Prepackaged Products					
Prevpac	Lansoprazole 30 mg bid	Clarithromycin 500 mg bid	Amoxicillin 1000 mg bid		10-14 d
Helidac (metronidazole, tetracycline and bismuth)	PPI or H2RA	Metronidazole 250 mg qid	Tetracycline 500 mg qid	Bismuth subsalicylate 525 mg qid	14 d
Pylera (metronidazole, tetracycline and bismuth)	Omeprazole 20 mg bid for 10 d	Metronidazole 125 mg qid	Tetracycline 125 mg qid	Bismuth subcitrate 140 mg qid	10 d

H. pylori-Induced Ulcers

Primary treatment for confirmed *H. pylori* should be triple therapy (PPI, clarithromycin, and amoxicillin or metronidazole) for 14 days or quadruple therapy (PPI or H2RA, bismuth, metronidazole, and tetracycline) for 10 to 14 days.[7] Fourteen day regimens are preferred, since eradication rates are lower with 7 day regimens.[7,25] Metronidazole may be substituted for amoxicillin in penicillin allergic patients. Treatment with a PPI prior to starting one of the treatment regimen has no effect on outcomes. If initial treatment is unsuccessful, then the second course of therapy (salvage therapy) should avoid antibiotics that were previously used. See Table 39-3 for treatment regimens to eradicate *H. pylori.*

Amoxicillin and clarithromycin can cause gastrointestinal upset and diarrhea. Altered taste may also occur with clarithromycin. Metronidazole can cause metallic taste, dyspepsia, and disulfiram-like reaction with alcohol consumption. Finally, bismuth may darken tongue and stool in addition to some nausea.[25]

GI bleeding, perforation, and obstruction can occur with *H. pylori* or NSAID-induced ulcer disease. Symptoms of bleeding include vomiting blood or black colored stools.

Perforation may begin as a sharp sudden pain, but then the pain spreads to the abdomen area. Obstruction tends to occur over time and may present with bloating, nausea and vomiting. Upper GI bleeding and perforation occur more often in patients taking NSAIDs.[9]

SPECIAL CONSIDERATIONS

The incidence of *H. pylori* infection, peptic ulcer disease, and gastric malignancy is uncommon in children in the United States. Even though the same agents used to treat *H. pylori* in adults appears to be effective in children there are no standard guidelines.[3] Gastric ulcers generally do not develop before age 40 and the incidence of duodenal ulcers increases with age up to 60 years of age. H2RAs and PPIs are pregnancy category B or C and both are excreted in breast milk.

FOUNDATION OVERVIEW: GASTROESOPHAGEAL REFLUX DISEASE

Gastroesophageal reflux disease (GERD) is a commonly encountered disorder caused by abnormal reflux of gastric contents into the esophagus. An exact incidence of GERD is difficult to quantify since many patients never seek treatment or self-medicate with over-the-counter products. Considering these limitations, it is estimated that between 10% to 20% of people in Western countries have symptoms of GERD on a weekly basis, and it represents the most common gastrointestinal diagnosis reported during outpatient visits.[26]

Abnormal reflux of gastric contents into the esophagus is the underlying cause of GERD and in many cases results from a defect in lower esophageal sphincter (LES) function. Additionally, abnormal defense mechanisms may promote the development of gastroesophageal reflux: anatomic factors (hiatal hernia), reduced esophageal clearance, delayed gastric emptying, inadequate mucus secretion, and decreased salivary buffering all are believed to contribute to GERD pathophysiology. The composition, volume, and duration of exposure of refluxate are important aggravating factors.[27] The classic symptom of GERD is heartburn usually described as substernal warmth or burning starting in the epigastric area often radiating to the neck. Warning signs and symptoms of complicated GERD include dysphagia, early satiety, gastrointestinal bleeding, iron deficiency anemia, odynophagia, vomiting, or weight loss.[27,28] There is no widely accepted standard method for diagnosing the disease; rather diagnosis is usually made based upon symptoms. Endoscopy, manometry, and other diagnostic testing should be reserved for patients with complicated GERD or those refractory to initial therapy.[29-31]

Excessive reflux of acid and pepsin resulting in mucosal damage and inflammation is termed reflux esophagitis. Less commonly, reflux can even lead to erosion of squamous epithelium lining the esophagus or erosive esophagitis. Long-term

TABLE 39-4 Therapeutic Lifestyle Changes Recommended for the Treatment of Gastroesophageal Reflux Disease[28,29,33]

Dietary and Medication Aggravating Factors		Lifestyle Changes
Directly irritating foods: Citrus fruits Carbonated beverages Onions Spicy foods Tomatoes	Directly irritating medications: Bisphosphonates Aspirin/NSAIDs Iron Potassium	General: Smoking cessation Weight reduction if overweight Reduction of alcohol consumption Avoid aggravating factors
Foods which lower esophageal sphincter tone: Caffeinated beverages Chocolate Fried or fatty foods Mint	Medications which lower esophageal sphincter tone: Anticholinergics Estrogen/progesterone Nicotine Nitrates Tetracyclines Theophylline	Nighttime symptoms: Avoid eating within 3 h before bedtime Elevate head of bed Postprandial symptoms: Eat smaller and more frequent meals Avoid lying down after meals

complications of reflux include development of strictures, Barrett esophagus, and esophageal adenocarcinoma.[27,28,32] Additionally, chronic reflux may cause extraesophageal syndromes such as chronic cough, laryngitis, asthma, and erosion of dental enamel.[29]

PREVENTION

Lifestyle modification and dietary avoidance are commonly recommended therapies initiated and continued throughout the course of therapy for GERD. Generally, these measures include avoiding foods that may precipitate reflux, acidic foods that are directly irritating and may precipitate heartburn, and instituting behaviors to minimize heartburn or reflux (Table 39-4). Evidence supporting lifestyle modifications is contradictory, although elevating the head of bed, lying on the left side while sleeping, and weight loss have the best supporting evidence.[33] Other lifestyle recommendations may be effective for individual patients when considering their specific symptoms. For example, patients who experience GERD symptoms following ingestion of alcohol or caffeinated beverages will benefit from avoidance of these triggers.

TREATMENT

The four goals of treatment for GERD include relieving symptoms, reducing the frequency of recurrent symptoms, promoting healing of mucosal injury, and preventing complications.[28] Reducing the gastric acidity decreases reflux symptoms and allows esophagitis to heal. An empiric trial of acid suppression therapy for 4 to 8 weeks is indicated for patients with typical symptoms and the absence of atypical manifestations or symptoms suggesting complicated disease.[27-29] Either a step-up or step-down approach to therapy can be used for the empirical trial. Step-up involves starting with twice daily H2-receptor antagonists (H2RA) for 8 weeks and changing to standard-dose proton pump inhibitor (PPI) if symptoms persist. Step-down therapy begins with PPI for 8 weeks, and treatment intensity is reduced to the lowest effective dose of acid suppressive therapy that provides symptom relief.[28,29] Improvements in heartburn are less predictable than with esophagitis; however, similar to esophagitis greater improvements are seen with more potent acid suppression (ie, proton pump inhibitors > H2-receptor antagonists > placebo). GERD is considered a chronic disease requiring maintenance therapy to ameliorate reflux symptoms. Clinical trials demonstrate that maintenance therapy with acid suppressive medications maintained relief of symptoms and prevented the recurrence of esophagitis.[34,35] The most common treatment strategy is continued use of either a PPI or H2RA as needed to maintain symptom control. See Table 39-5 for a list of medications used in the treatment of GERD.

Antacids

Over-the-counter antacid and antacid-alginic acid preparations are generally considered effective and are considered appropriate therapy for GERD. Antacids may be effective alone for mild heartburn. Antacids are beneficial for immediate symptomatic relief and may be used in conjunction with other acid-suppression regimens; however, they are not recommended as sole treatment for erosive esophagitis.[29] Gastrointestinal adverse effects are commonly encountered (diarrhea or constipation) and vary depending on the product used. Electrolyte disturbances and drug interactions are important considerations when selecting a product.

Sucralfate

Sucralfate (Carafate) is a prescription product which acts by creating a barrier to acid penetration in the esophagus.[19] Clinical studies of sucralfate have demonstrated little or no efficacy in patients with GERD; thus, it is not routinely recommended.[28]

H2-Receptor Antagonists

Cimetidine (Tagamet), famotidine (Pepcid), nizatidine (Axid), and ranitidine (Zantac) are all approved for use as over-the-counter products for heartburn with the dose of each medication half of the lowest prescription dosage. Higher doses taken more frequently are usually needed for mild to moderate GERD symptoms. Esophageal healing rates and heartburn symptoms are improved with H2RA when compared with placebo; however, they are less effective when compared with PPIs.

TABLE 39-5 Treatment Options for GERD[27,28]

Therapeutic Category	Generic Name	Brand Name	Standard Dose	Pregnancy Category
Antacids	Combination of aluminum hydroxide, magnesium hydroxide, and simethicone	Maalox or Mylanta	30 mL with meals and at bedtime	C
Proton pump inhibitors	Omeprazole Lansoprazole Rabeprazole Pantoprazole Esomeprazole	Prilosec Prevacid Aciphex Protonix Nexium	20-40 mg daily 15-30 mg daily 20 mg daily 40 mg daily 20-40 mg daily	C B B B B
H2-receptor antagonists	Cimetidine Famotidine Nizatidine Rantidine	Tagamet Pepcid Axid Zantac	400 mg bid 20 mg bid 150 mg bid 150 mg bid	B B B B
Gastric protectants	Sucralfate	Carafate	1 g four times per day	B
Promotility agents	Metoclopramide Bethanechol Baclofen	Reglan Urecholine Lioresal	10 mg four times per day 25 mg four times per day 5-10 mg tid	B C C

Esophageal healing rates are approximately 50% with standard doses of H2RA. Available H2RAs have similar efficacy and are generally considered interchangeable, although cimetidine is generally avoided due to an increased risk of drug interactions resulting from inhibition of multiple cytochrome P-450 enzymes.[27-29,36]

Proton Pump Inhibitors

Proton pump inhibitors (PPIs) inhibit gastric H^+/K^+-adenosine triphosphatase in gastric parietal cells thereby blocking gastric acid secretion. While some physiologic studies suggest modest benefits when comparing individual agents, all PPIs are superior to H2RA in treating patients with moderate to severe GERD symptoms, including patients with erosive esophagitis.[31,36,37] Approximately 80% of patients achieve symptomatic relief and endoscopic healing following 8 weeks of prescription-strength therapy.[29] Although the incidence is similar to placebo, the most common adverse effects of PPIs are abdominal pain, constipation, diarrhea, and headache.[37] In general long-term use of PPIs is considered safe; however, there are both potential and confirmed risks associated with continuous acid suppression. In theory, potent acid suppression with PPIs poses additional risks with long-term use including malabsorption, excessive gastrin secretion (hypergastrinemia) leading to gastric carcinomas, and hypochlorhydria resulting in bacterial overgrowth. More recently, large studies have revealed a 40% increase in hip fractures in patients over 50 years of age thought to be related to calcium malabsorption.[38]Additionally, PPIs increase the risk of infectious gastroenteritis by a 50% and double the risk of *Clostridium difficile* colitis.[39,40]

Promotility Therapy

Diminished esophageal sphincter tone, esophageal clearance, and delayed gastric emptying contribute to the pathogenesis of GERD. Several agents including metoclopramide, bethanechol, and baclofen have been used to improve these factors; however, central nervous system side effects including drowsiness, confusion, and dystonia limit their usefulness in large numbers of patients. Side effects typically occur in a dose-dependent manner, and are more commonly encountered in elderly patients or patients with renal insufficiency. Although these agents may provide symptomatic improvement in some patients with GERD, they are generally considered last-line therapy and should always be used in conjunction with acid suppressive therapy.[28,29]

Surgery

Surgery is considered an alternative approach to management for patients with chronic GERD symptoms particularly patients who are refractory to typical pharmacotherapy. The most common procedure is the Nissen fundoplication where the proximal portion of the stomach is wrapped around the distal esophagus to create an antireflux barrier. Surgery results in a similar rate of recurrent esophagitis when compared with maintenance PPI therapy. Surgical treatments possess inherent risks not associated with medical therapy, including need for repeat surgery, increased flatulence, inability to belch, severe dysphagia, and changes in bowel habits (diarrhea, bloating, abdominal pain, or constipation).[29,31]

SPECIAL CONSIDERATIONS

Gastroesophageal reflux occurs in about 18% of pediatric patients. Although rare, similar complications as seen in adult patients are possible. Dietary adjustments and postural changes during and after feedings are usually effective. Additionally, smaller and more frequent feedings may also be beneficial.[41] A similar approach to medical management is useful in pediatric patients, although combined use of a promotility agent and an acid suppressant provides quicker relief of symptoms. H2RAs and PPIs are considered safe and used in pediatric and neonatal patients, although most PPIs are only indicated for patients over 1 year of age. Available H2RA and PPIs are classified as either pregnancy category B or C, and both classes of agents are passed into breast milk.[41-46]

CASE Application

1. Patients with NSAID induced ulcers are more likely to have which of the following?
   a. Superficial ulcer depth
   b. A duodenal ulcer
   c. Stress related mucosal bleeding
   d. Damage to the gastric mucosa

2. JD is a 62-year-old man with a documented NSAID-induced ulcer, who is *H. pylori* negative. He must continue the NSAID for osteoarthritis. Which is the preferred medication for treating NSAID-induced ulcer?
   a. Lansoprazole
   b. Misoprostol
   c. Ranitidine
   d. Sucralfate

3. CT is a 40-year-old man with epigastric pain and recently diagnosed with a duodenal ulcer. A urea breath test confirmed *H. pylori*. The patient denies any allergies to medications. What is recommended as primary therapy for *H. pylori*?
   a. PPI + metronidazole + levofloxacin
   b. PPI + metronidazole + clarithromycin
   c. PPI + amoxicillin + clarithromycin
   d. PPI + metronidazole + bismuth + tetracycline

4. Which of the following is a nonendoscopic test used to diagnose *H. pylori*?
   a. Urea breath test
   b. Mucosal biopsy
   c. Culture
   d. Antibody detection

5. A patient calls the pharmacy to complain about her tongue turning black after starting a new regimen for peptic ulcer disease. Which medication is causing the side effect?
   a. Amoxicillin
   b. Metronidazole
   c. Bismuth subsalicylate
   d. Clarithromycin

6. If a patient was treated initially with PPI, amoxicillin, and clarithromycin, which regimen is recommended for salvage therapy?
   a. PPI + amoxicillin
   b. PPI + tetracycline + metronidazole + bismuth
   c. PPI + metronidazole + clarithromycin
   d. PPI + amoxicillin + levofloxacin

7. What is the recommended duration of treatment for *H. pylori* using clarithromycin-based triple therapy?
   a. 5 days
   b. 7 days
   c. 10 days
   d. 14 days

8. SL is a 62-year-old woman with rheumatoid arthritis and atrial fibrillation (AF). She controls her arthritis pain with high-dose nabumetone and takes warfarin for AF. Which medication regimen(s) is recommended for prevention of NSAID ulcer complications?
   a. Change to celecoxib plus PPI
   b. Add PPI to current NSAID
   c. Change to celecoxib
   d. b and c
   e. All of the above

9. A patient heard on Good Morning America that indomethacin can cause ulcers. She calls the pharmacy to find out if there is a better alternative to treat her arthritis. The patient is age 58 and does not have any other significant medical problems. What recommendation would be most appropriate?
   a. Sulindac
   b. Etodolac
   c. Piroxicam
   d. Naproxen

10. TC is a 55-year-old woman with hyperlipidemia, post-MI, HTN. Medications include atorvastatin 20 mg once daily, ASA 81 mg once daily, and metoprolol 100 mg bid. If the patient needs chronic NSAID therapy what is recommended to prevent ulcers?
    a. COX-2 inhibitor
    b. Naproxen
    c. COX-2 inhibitor plus PPI
    d. Naproxen plus PPI

11. Which of the following describes the clinical presentation of duodenal ulcers?
    a. Pain may be accompanied by coughing up blood.
    b. Pain is worse at night or between meals.
    c. Pain is worse with food.
    d. Pain is caused by damage from NSAIDs.

12. Which of the following requires a negative pregnancy test prior to starting therapy?
    a. Celecoxib
    b. Misoprostol
    c. PPIs
    d. Amoxicillin

13. A patient is admitted to the intensive care unit after a car accident. The patient has been on mechanical ventilation for 72 hours and has a head injury. Which of the

following is recommended for this patient for stress ulcer prophylaxis?

a. Ranitidine by mouth
b. Intravenous pantoprazole
c. Sucralfate by nasogastric tube
d. Patient does not require stress ulcer prophylaxis

Use the following case to answer questions 14 and 15.

AM is a 45-year-old obese woman with HTN and diabetes who presents with complaints of "severe" heartburn after meals and occasionally at night. She admits to smoking and occasional alcohol consumption. She consumes 4 to 5 caffeinated beverages daily. Medications include: hydrochlorothiazide (HCTZ) 12.5 mg daily and metformin 850 mg twice daily.

14. Which of the following factors may worsen GERD symptoms in this patient?
    a. Alcohol consumption
    b. Caffeine consumption
    c. Obesity
    d. Smoking
    e. All of the above

15. Which of the following represents the best initial treatment option with the highest probability of symptom control?
    a. Famotidine
    b. Metoclopramide
    c. Pantoprazole
    d. Sucralfate

16. HG is a 65-year-old woman with osteoporosis, GERD, and HTN. Medications include: alendronate 70 mg weekly, calcium carbonate 600 mg + vitamin D 400 units, omeprazole 20 mg daily, and enalapril 10 mg bid. Which of the following are possible consequences of this regimen?
    a. Alendronate may worsen GERD symptoms.
    b. Enalapril may worsen GERD symptoms.
    c. Omeprazole may reduce calcium absorption.
    d. a and c.

17. Which of the following is a typical sign or symptom of patients with GERD?
    a. Iron deficiency anemia
    b. Dysphagia
    c. Regurgitation
    d. Weight loss

18. Which of the following acts by competitively inhibiting histamine at the H2 receptor of gastric parietal cells?
    a. Omeprazole
    b. Pantoprazole
    c. Rabeprazole
    d. Ranitidine

19. NJ, a 50-year-old woman, presented to her physician approximately 8 weeks ago with complaints of heartburn, regurgitation, and dysphagia which resulted in an endoscopy. At that time her physician diagnosed GERD with erosive esophagitis and prescribed 2 months of lansoprazole 30 mg daily. Today at her follow-up visit, she reports improvement in her symptoms. What would you recommend as maintenance therapy for NJ?
    a. Lansoprazole 15 mg daily
    b. Lansoprazole 30 mg daily
    c. No further therapy required
    d. Either a or b

20. Select the trade name for pantoprazole.
    a. Axid
    b. Aciphex
    c. Prevacid
    d. Protonix
    e. Tagamet

21. Which of the following would be appropriate health information to discuss with a patient presenting to your pharmacy with GERD symptoms?
    a. Eating smaller meals more often
    b. Elevating the head of the bed 6 to 8 in
    c. Weight reduction for patients who are overweight
    d. Smoking cessation
    e. All of the above

TAKEAWAY POINTS ››

- PUD is commonly divided into three forms: *H. pylori* induced, NSAID induced and stress related mucosal damage.
- The clinical presentation of PUD can vary but may include nonlocalized epigastric pain.
- Symptoms cannot differentiate between *H. pylori* and NSAID-induced ulcer.
- The urea breath test (UBT) and fecal antigen are reliable for identifying active *H. pylori* before treatment.
- Testing for *H. pylori* is only recommended if eradication therapy will be offered.
- Misoprostol, a prostaglandin analog is indicated to prevent NSAID-induced gastric ulcers. Diarrhea and other gastrointestinal side effects limit the use of this agent.

- Misoprostol is pregnancy category X.
- Respiratory failure (mechanical ventilation for longer than 48 hours) or coagulopathy are two risk factors for stress related mucosal bleeding (SRMB).
- The preferred treatment options for prophylaxis of SRMB are H2RAs and PPIs.
- For the treatment of NSAID-induced ulcer disease, if the NSAID must be continued, a proton pump inhibitor (PPI) is the agent of choice.
- Sucralfate is indicated for the management of duodenal ulcers, but constipation and frequent dosing limit the use of this agent.
- H2RAs are not very effective for healing or preventing gastric ulcers, but do prevent duodenal ulcers.
- All PPIs provide similar ulcer healing rates and relief of symptoms for gastric and duodenal ulcers.
- Compared to H2RAs, PPIs relieve symptoms and heal more quickly, but are more expensive.
- PPIs may decrease the effectiveness of clopidogrel.
- Primary treatment for *H. pylori* should be triple therapy (PPI, clarithromycin, and amoxicillin or metronidazole) for 14 days or quadruple therapy (PPI or H2RA, bismuth, metronidazole, and tetracycline) for 10 to 14 days.
- If initial treatment is unsuccessful, then the second course of therapy should avoid antibiotics that were previously used.
- GI bleeding, perforation, and obstruction are complications of PUD.
- Lifestyle modifications may be beneficial in patients with GERD, although additional pharmacologic therapy is required for symptom control in most patients.
- Patients with typical symptoms may be treated empirically if no signs or symptoms suggesting complicated GERD are present.
- Endoscopy, manometry, and other diagnostic testing should be reserved for patients with complicated GERD or those refractory to initial therapy.
- The goals of GERD treatment include relieving symptoms, reducing the frequency of recurrent symptoms, promoting healing of mucosal injury, and preventing complications.
- Acid suppression is the foundation of GERD treatment, and either a step-up or step-down approach to therapy may be used for the 8-week empirical trial.
- Although less effective overall when compared to PPIs, H2RA in divided doses may be beneficial in mild to moderate GERD.
- PPIs typically provide the greatest symptomatic relief and have the highest healing rates in patients with reflux esophagitis.
- Antacids and OTC acid suppressants are options for patient-directed therapy for heartburn and regurgitation.
- Promotility agents (eg, metoclopramide) may be useful in selected patients when used as an adjunct to acid suppression.
- Since GERD is a chronic condition, maintenance therapy is appropriate to control symptoms and prevent complications.
- A PPI is the drug of choice for maintenance therapy in patients with moderate-to-severe GERD. The lowest effective dose of acid suppressive therapy should be used.
- Antireflux surgery is an option for patients with GERD intolerant of or refractory to standard acid suppressive therapy.

REFERENCES

1. Del Valle J, Chey WD, Scheiman JM, et al. Acid peptic disorders. In: Yamada T, Aplers DH, Kaplowitz N, et al. ed. *Textbook of Gastroenterology*. 4th ed. Philadelphia, PA: Lippincott Williams & Wilkins; 2003:1321-1376.
2. Peterson WL, Fendrick AM, Cave DR, Peura DA, Garabedian-Ruffalo SM, Laine L. Helicobacter pylori-related disease: guidelines for testing and treatment. *Arch Intern Med.* 2000;160(9):1285-1291.
3. Solnick JV, Siddiqui J. *Helicobacter pylori*. In: Wilson WR, Sande MA, eds. *Current Diagnosis and Treatment in Infectious Disease.* New York, NY: Lange Medical Books/McGraw-Hill; 2001.
4. Larkai EN, Smith JL, Lidsky MD, Graham DY. Gastroduodenal mucosa and dyspeptic symptoms in arthritic patients during chronic nonsteroidal anti-inflammatory drug use. *Am J Gastroenterol.* 1987;82(11):1153-1158.
5. Stollman N, Metz DC. Pathophysiology and prophylaxis of stress ulcer in intensive care unit patients. *J Critical Care.* 2005;20(1):35-45.
6. Berardi RR, Welage LS. Peptic ulcer disease. In: Dipiro JT, Talbert RL, Yee G, Matzke G, Wells B, Posey L, eds. *Pharmacotherapy: A Pathophysiologic Approach*. 7th ed. New York, NY: McGraw-Hill; 2008:569-587.
7. Chey WD, Wong BC. American College of Gastroenterology guideline on the management of Helicobacter pylori infection. *Am J Gastroenterol.* 2007;102(8):1808-1825.
8. Laine L. Gastrointestinal effects of NSAIDs and coxibs. *J Pain Sympt Manage.* 2003;25(2 suppl):S32-S40.
9. Lanza FL. A guideline for the treatment and prevention of NSAID-induced ulcers. Members of the Ad Hoc Committee on Practice Parameters of the American College of Gastroenterology. *Am J Gastroenterol.* 1998;93(11):2037-2046.
10. Lanza FL, Chan FK, Quigley EM. Guidelines for prevention of NSAID-related ulcer complications. *Am J Gastroenterol.* 2009;104(3):728-738.
11. Antman EM, Bennett JS, Daugherty A, et al. Use of nonsteroidal antiinflammatory drugs: an update for clinicians: a scientific statement from the American Heart Association. *Circulation.* 2007;115:1634-1642.
12. Kearney PM, Baigent C, Godwin J, et al. Do selective cyclo-oxygenase-2 inhibitors and traditional non-steroidal

anti-inflammatory drugs increase the risk of atherothrombosis? Meta-analysis of randomized trials. *BMJ*. 2006;332:1302-1308.

13. McGettigan P, Henry D. Cardiovascular risk and inhibition of cyclooxygenase: a systematic review of observational studies of selective and nonselective inhibitors of cyclooxygenase 2. *JAMA*. 2006;296:1633-1644.
14. US Food and Drug Administration: New Information for Health care Professionals Concomitant Use of Ibuprofen and Aspirin. US Food and Drug Administration, Rockville, Maryland, Sept. 8, 2006. Available at: http://www.fda.gov/cder/drug/InfoSheets/HCP/ibuprofen_aspirinHCP.htm. Accessed October 23, 2009.
15. US Food and Drug Administration: Medication Guide for Non-Steroidal Anti-Inflammatory Drugs (NSAIDs). Available at: http://www.fda.gov/downloads/Drugs/DrugSafety/ucm088567.pdf. Accessed October 23, 2009.
16. Cytotec [package insert]. G.D. Searle & Co.
17. ASHP Therapeutic Guidelines on Stress Ulcer Prophylaxis. ASHP Commission on Therapeutics and approved by the ASHP Board of Directors on November 14, 1998. *Am J Health Syst Pharm*. 1999;56(4):347-379.
18. Brett S. Science review: the use of proton pump inhibitors for gastric acid suppression in critical illness. *Critical care* (London, England). 2005;9(1):45-50.
19. Carafate [package insert]. Birmingham, AL: Axcan Pharma US, Inc; 2008.
20. Tagamet [package insert]. Research Triangle Park, NC: GlaxoSmithKline, Inc.; 2006.
21. Prilosec [package insert]. Wilmington, DE: AstraZeneca LP; 2008.
22. Nexium [package insert]. Wilmington, DE: AstraZeneca LP; 2008.
23. Gilard M, Arnaud B, Cornily JC, et al. Influence of omeprazole on the antiplatelet action of clopidogrel associated with aspirin: the randomized, double-blind OCLA (Omeprazole CLopidogrel Aspirin) study. *J Am Coll Cardiol*. 2008;51(3):256-260.
24. Pezalla E, Day D, Pulliadath I. Initial assessment of clinical impact of a drug interaction between clopidogrel and proton pump inhibitors. *J Am Coll Cardiol*. 2008;52(12):1038-1039.
25. Howden CW, Hunt RH. Guidelines for the management of Helicobacter pylori infection. Ad Hoc Committee on Practice Parameters of the American College of Gastroenterology. *Am J Gastroenterol*. 1998;93(12):2330-2338.
26. Camilleri M, Dubois D, Coulie B, et al. Prevalence and socioeconomic impact of upper gastrointestinal disorders in the United States: results of the US Upper Gastrointestinal Study. *Clin Gastroenterol Hepatol*. Jun 2005;3(6):543-552.
27. Kahrilas PJ. Clinical practice. Gastroesophageal reflux disease. *N Engl J Med*. 2008;359(16):1700-1707.
28. Heidelbaugh JJ, Nostrant TT, Kim C, Van Harrison R. Management of gastroesophageal reflux disease. *Am Fam Physician*. 2003;68(7):1311-1318.
29. DeVault KR, Castell DO. Updated guidelines for the diagnosis and treatment of gastroesophageal reflux disease. *Am J Gastroenterol*. 2005;100(1):190-200.
30. DeVault KR, Castell DO. Updated guidelines for the diagnosis and treatment of gastroesophageal reflux disease. The Practice Parameters Committee of the American College of Gastroenterology. *Am J Gastroenterol*. 1999;94(6):1434-1442.
31. Kahrilas PJ, Shaheen NJ, Vaezi MF. American Gastroenterological Association Institute technical review on the management of gastroesophageal reflux disease. *Gastroenterology*. 2008;135(4):1392-1413, :1392-1413, 1413.e1-5.
32. Spechler SJ. Clinical practice. Barrett's esophagus. *N Engl J Med*. 2002;346(11):836-842.
33. Kaltenbach T, Crockett S, Gerson LB. Are lifestyle measures effective in patients with gastroesophageal reflux disease? An evidence-based approach. *Arch Intern Med*. 2006;166(9):965-971.
34. Johnson DA, Benjamin SB, Vakil NB, et al. Esomeprazole once daily for 6 months is effective therapy for maintaining healed erosive esophagitis and for controlling gastroesophageal reflux disease symptoms: a randomized, double-blind, placebo-controlled study of efficacy and safety. *Am J Gastroenterol*. 2001;96:27-34.
35. Klinkenberg-Knol EC, Nelis F, Dent J, et al. Long-term omeprazole treatment in resistant gastroesophageal reflux disease: efficacy, safety, and influence on gastric mucosa. *Gastroenterology*. 2000;118:661-669.
36. Khan M, Santana J, Donnellan C, Preston C, Moayyedi P. Medical treatments in the short-term management of reflux oesophagitis. *Cochrane Database Syst Rev*. 2007(2):CD003244.
37. Horn J. The proton-pump inhibitors: similarities and differences. *Clin Ther*. 2000;22(3):266-280.
38. Yang YX, Lewis JD, Epstein S, Metz DC. Long-term proton pump inhibitor therapy and risk of hip fracture. *JAMA*. 2006;296(24):2947-2953.
39. Garcia Rodriguez LA, Ruigomez A. Gastric acid, acid-suppressing drugs, and bacterial gastroenteritis: how much of a risk? *Epidemiology*. 1997;8(5):571-574.
40. Dial S, Alrasadi K, Manoukian C, Huang A, Menzies D. Risk of Clostridium difficile diarrhea among hospital inpatients prescribed proton pump inhibitors: cohort and case-control studies. *CMAJ*. 2004;171(1):33-38.
41. Gold BD. Review article: epidemiology and management of gastro-oesophageal reflux in children. *Aliment Pharmacol Ther*. 2004;19 (suppl 1):22-27.
42. Barron JJ, Tan H, Spalding J, Bakst AW, Singer J. Proton pump inhibitor utilization patterns in infants. *J Pediatr Gastroenterol Nutr*. 2007;45(4):421-427.
43. Canani RB, Cirillo P, Roggero P, et al. Therapy with gastric acidity inhibitors increases the risk of acute gastroenteritis and community-acquired pneumonia in children. *Pediatrics*. 2006;117(5):e817-820.
44. Colletti RB, Di Lorenzo C. Overview of pediatric gastroesophageal reflux disease and proton pump inhibitor therapy. *J Pediatr Gastroenterol Nutr*. 2003;37 (suppl 1):S7-S11.
45. Gibbons TE, Gold BD. The use of proton pump inhibitors in children: a comprehensive review. *Paediatr Drugs*. 2003;5(1):25-40.
46. Gold BD. Gastroesophageal reflux disease: could intervention in childhood reduce the risk of later complications? *Am J Med*. 2004;117 (suppl 5A):23S-29S.

CHAPTER

40 Nausea and Vomiting

Kelly K. Nystrom and Amy M. Pick

FOUNDATION OVERVIEW

Nausea and vomiting are two of the most common side effects experienced by patients receiving chemotherapy.[1] If not appropriately controlled, nausea and vomiting can lead to serious complications such as electrolyte imbalances and esophageal tears.[2] It is much easier to prevent nausea and vomiting than to try to treat it once it has started. Although significant progress has been made in drug therapy for nausea and vomiting, these side effects continue to be some of the most worrisome and undesirable effects reported by patients receiving chemotherapy.

The etiology of nausea and vomiting is quite complex. The chemoreceptor trigger zone (CTZ), located outside of the blood-brain barrier, is activated by chemotherapy and other irritants. The CTZ is triggered by various neurotransmitters including dopamine, serotonin, histamine, and neurokinin-1 (substance P)[3,4] (Figure 40-1). The activation of the CTZ stimulates the vomiting center. This process is common in chemotherapy-induced nausea and vomiting (CINV). In addition to the CTZ, the gastrointestinal tract (GI) tract releases serotonin in response to chemotherapy, which can also cause CINV.[5] Our current antiemetic medications block these neurotransmitters to stop the initiation of CINV.

There are several risk factors that increase the possibility of experiencing CINV. The emetogenic potential of the chemotherapy agent or agents is probably the most important factor.[5] Agents are classified into high, moderate, low, or minimal risk for causing CINV. These risk categories were developed based on the percentage of patients experiencing CINV when receiving a particular chemotherapy agent without an antiemetic medication[5-11] (Table 40-1). Dose and rate of infusion of the agent can also affect risk. Generally, the higher the dose of chemotherapy, the higher the risk of CINV. Bolus infusions also tend to have higher risk of CINV than extended infusions. Younger patients (< 50 years old), women, patients with a history of motion sickness or nausea with pregnancy and patients with a history of poorly controlled CINV are at increased risk of developing problems despite adequate antiemetic treatment. Interestingly, a history of alcoholism can decrease a patient's risk of CINV.[5,8,9,12,13] One theory is that this occurs because the patient's body has become desensitized to toxins and irritants.[14]

There are several types of CINV: acute, delayed, anticipatory, breakthrough, and refractory.[4,5,11] Acute CINV is defined as nausea and vomiting that occurs within the first 24 hours following the administration of chemotherapy, but most commonly occurs within 5 to 6 hours of the dose. Delayed CINV develops more than 24 hours after chemotherapy is administered and can persist up to 7 days.[11] Chemotherapeutic agents that commonly cause delayed CINV include cisplatin, carboplatin, cyclophosphamide, and doxorubicin[11] (Table 40-2). Anticipatory CINV occurs after a negative experience with chemotherapy, and thus can only occur if chemotherapy has been previously received. The incidence of this type of nausea or vomiting ranges from 18% to 57%.[11] Breakthrough CINV occurs when preventative antiemetic therapy fails and patients have at least one episode of nausea and/or vomiting that may require antiemetic treatment despite preventative antiemetic premedication. The last type is refractory CINV. This occurs when premedications and breakthrough therapy fail to prevent CINV from occurring after chemotherapy administration.

CHEMOTHERAPY-INDUCED NAUSEA AND VOMITING

Antiemetics

Serotonin (5-HT3) Receptor Antagonists

Serotonin is one of the most common neurotransmitters involved in CINV. The serotonin (5-HT3) receptor antagonists block serotonin in the GI tract and the CTZ to prevent CINV.[14] There are four 5-HT3 receptor antagonists on the market in the United States[4,8,9,14,15] (Table 40-3). These agents are effective in the prevention of acute CINV and have a limited role in delayed CINV (with the exception of palonosetron). Palonosetron has a longer half-life and is the only one in the class FDA-approved for both acute and delayed CINV in moderately emetogenic chemotherapy. There is currently no data to support superiority of one agent over another in the prevention of acute CINV.[14] Choice of agent should be based on availability and cost. The oral route has been shown to be just as effective as the IV route and, therefore, the oral route is preferred for prevention of CINV because of ease of administration and decreased cost.[11,14] Another option available is topical granisetron. This is applied 24 to 48 hours prior to chemotherapy and can remain on the skin for up to 7 days. The most common toxicities are headache and constipation.[14,15] An infrequent, but more serious, toxicity is the ability of the 5-HT3 receptor antagonists to cause QT prolongation, although this has not been shown to be clinically significant to date.[14]

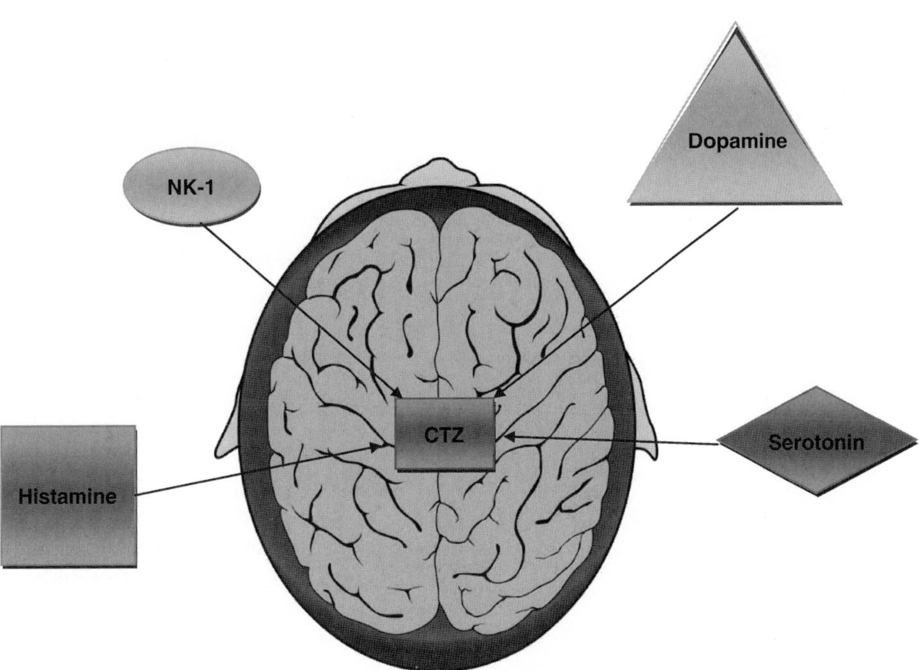

FIGURE 40-1 Chemoreceptor trigger zone (CTZ) and activating neurotransmitters. NK-1, neurokinin-1.

Corticosteroids

Corticosteroids can be used alone for the prevention of CINV with low-risk chemotherapy agents. Dexamethasone is the most commonly used corticosteroid, although one corticosteroid has not been proven superior to another[4,14] (see Table 40-3). Corticosteroids are commonly used in conjunction with a 5-HT3 receptor antagonist with or without aprepitant for the prevention of CINV with moderate or high emetogenic chemotherapy agents or regimens to improve the efficacy of these agents.[7,8,14,16] The mechanism of action is not well understood, but one theory is that they prevent serotonin release in the GI tract and block the 5-HT3 receptors in the GI tract as well.[7] Oral and IV routes are considered equivalent.[14] Since the use of corticosteroids for CINV is only short-term, the most common toxicities are generally limited to GI upset, insomnia, fluid retention, increased appetite, and increased blood sugars.[14,15]

Neurokinin-1 Receptor Antagonists

The neurokinin-1 (NK-1) receptor antagonists are a new class of antiemetics. Aprepitant and the IV prodrug, fosaprepitant dimeglumine, are the only two agents from this class currently approved in the United States. They are approved for prevention of acute and delayed CINV with highly emetogenic agents and with the cyclophosphamide/doxorubicin combination (see Table 40-3). The NCCN guidelines also recommend use with certain moderate emetic risk agents that have the potential for delayed CINV[11] (see Table 40-2). Substance P exerts its effect on the NK-1 receptors causing nausea and vomiting. Aprepitant and fosaprepitant dimeglumine block substance P, thus preventing nausea and vomiting.[4,14] The oral route is preferred unless the patient is having difficulty taking oral medications; the IV route is approved on day 1 only before chemotherapy. The most common side effects are headache, abdominal pain, and mild transaminase elevations.[14,15] In addition, aprepitant is metabolized by CYP 3A4, and is a substrate and moderate inhibitor of CYP 3A4 so drug interactions should be considered. Important drug interactions include oral contraceptives, warfarin, and dexamethasone.[17,18] This is why the dexamethasone dose should be decreased by 50% when given with aprepitant.

Dopamine Receptor Antagonists

Dopamine is a common neurotransmitter affecting the CTZ resulting in CINV[4,5] (see Figure 40-1). Common dopamine receptor antagonists are the phenothiazines (prochlorperazine, promethazine), the butyrophenones (droperidol, haloperidol), and metoclopramide (Table 40-4). These agents are used for breakthrough nausea and vomiting. Toxicities include sedation and extrapyramidal side effects.[4,5,15] A black box warning has been added to the package insert for metoclopramide warning of tardive dyskinesia with high doses or long-term use of metoclopramide. These dyskinesias may continue after the metoclopramide is discontinued.[19]

Cannabinoids

Cannabinoids produce their antiemetic activities through various effects on the CNS and GI tract, including activity at the cannabinoid receptor[5,14] (see Table 40-4). The cannabinoid

TABLE 40-1 Emetic Risk of Commonly Administered Chemotherapy Agents

Emetic Risk	Incidence Without Antiemetics	Agent
High	> 90%	Cisplatin
High	> 90%	Cyclophosphamide (≥ 1500 mg/m^2)
High	> 90%	Cyclophosphamide/doxorubicin combination
High	> 90%	Cyclophosphamide/epirubicin combination
Moderate	30%-90%	Carboplatin
Moderate	30%-90%	Cytarabine (> 1 gm/m^2)
Moderate	30%-90%	Doxorubicin
Moderate	30%-90%	Ifosfamide
Moderate	30%-90%	Imatinib (po)
Moderate	30%-90%	Irinotecan
Moderate	30%-90%	Oxaliplatin
Low	10%-30%	Capecitabine (po)
Low	10%-30%	Docetaxel
Low	10%-30%	Etoposide
Low	10%-30%	Fluorouracil
Low	10%-30%	Gemcitabine
Low	10%-30%	Methotrexate
Low	10%-30%	Paclitaxel
Minimal	< 10%	Bevacizumab
Minimal	< 10%	Dasatinib
Minimal	< 10%	Erlotinib (po)
Minimal	< 10%	Rituximab
Minimal	< 10%	Sorafenib (po)
Minimal	< 10%	Vincristine

Abbreviation: po, oral.

dronabinol is a Schedule III controlled substance that is particularly helpful for patients with refractory nausea and vomiting. Side effects include sedation, dysphoria, dizziness and dry mouth, and elderly patients may be more sensitive to these side effects.[5,8,15] These agents may also increase appetite, which may be beneficial in patients with refractory nausea and vomiting resulting in weight loss.

Prevention of Acute Chemotherapy-Induced Nausea and Vomiting

Guidelines exist from several organizations on the treatment and prevention of CINV. The most commonly used guidelines are the National Comprehensive Cancer Network (NCCN) guidelines, which are updated at least annually, the American Society of Clinical Oncology (ASCO) guidelines updated in

TABLE 40-2 Chemotherapy Agents With Increased Risk of Delayed Nausea and Vomiting

Chemotherapy Agents Requiring Treatment for Prevention of Delayed Nausea and Vomiting	
Cisplatin	Doxorubicin
Cyclophosphamide (≥ 1500 mg/m^2)	Epirubicin
Cyclophosphamide/doxorubicin combination	Ifosfamide
Cyclophosphamide/epirubicin combination	Irinotecan
Carboplatin	Methotrexate

2006 and the Multinational Association of Supportive Care in Cancer (MASCC) guidelines updated in 2008.[10,11,17]

For highly emetogenic chemotherapy or for the combination of cyclophosphamide/doxorubicin, the recommendation is to give a 5-HT3 receptor antagonist, dexamethasone and aprepitant prior to the chemotherapy[10,11,17] (see Table 40-3). An agent for breakthrough nausea and vomiting should be prescribed for use on an as needed basis[1,4,5,10,11,14,15,17] (see Table 40-4).

For moderately emetogenic chemotherapy, a 5-HT3 receptor antagonist with dexamethasone should be used[10,11,17] (see Table 40-3). The NCCN guidelines recommend adding aprepitant for regimens containing drugs known to cause delayed CINV such as carboplatin and ifosfamide. An agent for breakthrough nausea and vomiting should be prescribed for use on an as needed basis[1,4,5,10,11,14,15,17] (see Table 40-4).

For low emetogenic risk agents, the recommendation is a single-agent antiemetic such as dexamethasone given 30 to 60 minutes prior to chemotherapy administration.[10,11,17] An agent for breakthrough nausea and vomiting should be prescribed for use on an as needed basis. For minimal risk agents, scheduled antiemetics should be avoided, and antiemetics should only be used on an as needed basis.[1,4,5,10,11,14,15,17] (see Table 40-4).

Treatment of Acute Chemotherapy-Induced Nausea and Vomiting

Even with adequate prevention for CINV, patients may experience breakthrough CINV within the first 24 hours after chemotherapy. There are many drugs available for treatment of breakthrough CINV with a variety of factors to consider when choosing an agent[1,4,5,10,11,14,15,17] (see Table 40-4). When choosing an agent, it is important to remember to use an agent with a different mechanism of action than was prescribed for prevention of acute CINV. In order to get the CINV controlled, it may be helpful to schedule the breakthrough antiemetic around the clock until the CINV subsides.

Prevention of Delayed Chemotherapy-Induced Nausea and Vomiting

For highly emetogenic agents and moderately emetogenic agents with a high risk of delayed CINV as identified by the NCCN guidelines, if aprepitant was given on day 1 of chemotherapy, then

TABLE 40-3 **Antiemetics Used for Prevention of Chemotherapy-Induced Nausea and Vomiting**

Antiemetic	Trade Name	Dose	Route	Frequency
5-HT3 Receptor Antagonists				
Ondansetron	Zofran	8-12 mg 16-24 mg	IV po	30-60 min before chemotherapy
Granisetron	Kytril	2 mg 1 mg bid 1 mg 0.01 mg/kg	po po IV IV	30-60 min before chemotherapy
	Sancuso	Delivers 3.1 mg/24 h	Topical	24-48 h before chemotherapy
Dolasetron	Anzemet	100 mg 100 mg	po IV	30-60 min before chemotherapy
Palonosetron	Aloxi	0.25 mg	IV	30 min before chemotherapy
Corticosteroid				
Dexamethasone	Decadron	12-20 mg 12 mg 8 mg	IV po po	30-60 min before chemotherapy Daily with aprepitant or bid alone for 2-3 d after chemotherapy
Neurokinin-1 Receptor Antagonists				
Aprepitant	Emend	125 mg 80 mg	po po	30-60 min before chemotherapy On days 2 and 3
Fosaprepitant dimeglumine	Emend	115 mg	IV	30 min before chemotherapy

Abbreviations: IV, intravenous; po, oral.

it should be continued on days 2 and 3 at 80 mg orally daily. Dexamethasone 8 mg orally daily should also be continued for two to three more days after chemotherapy to prevent delayed CINV.[5,11]

For moderately emetogenic agents when aprepitant is not used, dexamethasone 8 mg orally twice daily should be used for 2 to 4 days following chemotherapy.[5] As previously stated, palonosetron is FDA-approved for prevention of both acute and delayed nausea and vomiting for moderately emetogenic agents and may provide added protection against delayed nausea and vomiting when used as a component of the acute prophylaxis regimen.

TABLE 40-4 **Select Antiemetics Used for Breakthrough Chemotherapy-Induced Nausea and Vomiting**

Drug	Trade Name	Dose	Route	Frequency	Special Notes
Dopamine Antagonists					
Droperidol	Inapsine	0.625-1.25 mg	IV	Every 4-6 h prn	Black box warning for risk of QT prolongation
Haloperidol	Haldol	0.5-2 mg	IV/IM/po	Every 4-6 h prn	
Metoclopramide	Reglan	20-40 mg 1-2 mg/kg	IV/po IV	Every 4-6 h prn Every 4-6 h prn	Black box warning for permanent EPSE
Prochlorperazine	Compazine	5-10 mg 25 mg	IV/IM/po PR	Every 4-6 h prn Every 12 h prn	
Promethazine	Phenergan	12.5-25 mg	IV/IM/po/PR	Every 4-6 h prn	Concentrated solution may cause tissue damage if extravasated; dilute before administration
Benzodiazepines					
Lorazepam	Ativan	0.5-2 mg	IV/IM/po/ SL	Every 4-6 h prn	Works well for anticipatory CINV
Miscellaneous					
Dronabinol	Marinol	5-10 mg	po	Every 3-6 h prn	Works well to increase appetite; use with caution in elderly as may see increased side effects; schedule II medication
Olanzapine	Zyprexa	2.5-5 mg	po	bid prn	May be used for acute and refractory, although it is not FDA-approved for this indication

Abbreviations: IV, intravenous; po, oral; IM, intramuscular; EPSE, extrapyramidal side effects; CINV, chemotherapy-induced nausea and vomiting.

Treatment of Delayed Chemotherapy-Induced Nausea and Vomiting

Treatment would include the same breakthrough medications used in the treatment of acute CINV, keeping in mind that it is much harder to treat delayed CINV than acute CINV[1,4,5,10,11,14,15,17] (see Table 40-4).

Anticipatory Nausea and Vomiting

Anticipatory nausea is more common than anticipatory vomiting, but both are conditioned responses, so they occur only after a poor experience with chemotherapy.[11] Benzodiazepines can help control this type of nausea and vomiting. Lorazepam is the most commonly used benzodiazepine for this purpose, and is usually given in combination with other antiemetics for CINV[5,8,11] (see Table 40-4). The most common toxicities are sedation, dizziness, and amnesia.[5]

POSTOPERATIVE NAUSEA AND VOMITING

Postoperative nausea and vomiting (PONV) are two of the most common problems following surgery and anesthesia and can result in unanticipated hospital admissions.[20-22] The Society for Ambulatory Anesthesia published guidelines for the management of PONV in 2007. Patients at increased risk of PONV include female sex, nonsmokers, history of PONV or motion sickness, and postoperative opioid use.[20,21,23] The addition of each risk factor increases the risk of PONV by 20%. The type of anesthetic used, the duration of surgery, and the type of surgery also play a role in the risk of PONV.[20,21]

Prevention of Postoperative Nausea and Vomiting

Strategies such as avoiding certain anesthetics, minimizing intraoperative and postoperative opioids, and use of regional anesthetics are used to decrease the risk of PONV.[20,21] Patients with low risk of PONV will probably not benefit from prophylaxis and should not receive this treatment unless they are at risk of medical adverse effects from vomiting including patients with wired jaws and increased intracranial pressure. Patients with moderate to high risk of PONV should receive prophylactic antiemetic therapy (Table 40-5). For patients with moderate risk, prophylaxis with one or more agents is recommended; whereas for patients with high risk, combination prophylaxis with two to three agents from different classes is recommended.

Treatment of Postoperative Nausea and Vomiting

Patients who experience PONV and who have not received prophylaxis should be treated with a low-dose 5-HT3 receptor antagonist (dolasetron 12.5 mg, ondansetron 1 mg, granisetron 0.1 mg).[20,21,23] If a patient has received dexamethasone prior to the procedure and experiences PONV, then a low-dose 5-HT3 receptor antagonist can be tried.[20,21,23] When a 5-HT3 receptor antagonist is used, if PONV is experienced within 6 hours of initial administration, then a drug with a different mechanism of action should be used and the 5-HT3 antagonist dose should not be repeated.[20,21] If a patient is still in post-anesthesia care, propofol, 20 mg as needed, can be used for PONV when a 5-HT3 receptor antagonist is given as initial prophylaxis.

TABLE 40-5 **Antiemetics Used for Prevention of Postoperative Nausea and Vomiting**

Antiemetic	Trade Name	Dose	Route	Frequency
5-HT3 Receptor Antagonists				
Granisetron	Kytril	0.35-1 mg	IV	End of surgery
Dolasetron	Anzemet	12.5 mg	IV	End of surgery
Ondansetron	Zofran	4-8 mg	IV	End of surgery
Palonosetron	Aloxi	0.075 mg	IV	End of surgery
Corticosteroid				
Dexamethasone	Decadron	2.5-10 mg	IV	Before induction
Neurokinin-1 Receptor Antagonist				
Aprepitant	Emend	40 mg	po	Within 3 h prior to induction
Dopamine Antagonists				
Droperidol	Inapsine	0.625-1.25 mg	IV	End of surgery
Prochlorperazine	Compazine	5-10 mg	IV	End of surgery
Promethazine	Phenergan	12.5-25 mg	IV	End of surgery
Miscellaneous				
Scopolamine transdermal patch	Trans Scop	1 patch	Topical	Applied prior evening or 4 h before end of surgery

Abbreviations: IV, intravenous; po, oral.

Propofol may also be needed if initial triple antiemetic therapy fails. When PONV occurs more than 6 hours after the initial agent was given, any of these drugs can be used again for treatment of PONV.

CASE Application

1. Select the correct statement. Patients more susceptible to nausea and vomiting include:
   a. Chronic alcoholics
   b. Female patients
   c. Patients older than 50 years of age
   d. Patients with a smoking history
2. Select the correct statement. Delayed nausea and vomiting:
   a. Is easier to prevent than acute nausea and vomiting
   b. Occurs within the first 24 hours following drug administration
   c. Occurs more commonly with cisplatin and cyclophosphamide
   d. Commonly resolves within 72 hours of chemotherapy administration
3. Which neurotransmitter has no involvement in CINV?
   a. Dopamine
   b. Neurokinin-1
   c. Norepinephrine
   d. Serotonin
4. DS is a 35-year-old woman undergoing surgery for a hysterectomy. She has a history of PONV and motion sickness. Which drug should be administered during or following surgery for the prevention of PONV?
   a. Haloperidol
   b. Ondansetron
   c. Prochlorperazine
   d. Scopolamine
5. Select the correct dose and route of aprepitant for prevention of PONV.
   a. 40 mg orally
   b. 80 mg IV injection
   c. 115 mg IV injection
   d. 125 mg orally
6. Select the serotonin (5-HT3) receptor antagonist that has a prolonged half-life and is given as a single-dose injection prior to the start of chemotherapy for the prevention of acute and delayed CINV.
   a. Aloxi
   b. Anzemet
   c. Kytril
   d. Zofran
7. Which serotonin (5-HT3) receptor antagonist is available as a transdermal patch?
   a. Dolasetron
   b. Granisetron
   c. Ondansetron
   d. Palonosetron
8. DH is undergoing chemotherapy for breast cancer with doxorubicin and cyclophosphamide. Select which antiemetic combination will give her optimal prevention for CINV?
   a. Aprepitant, dolasetron, and prochlorperazine
   b. Aprepitant, prochlorperazine, and dexamethasone
   c. Aprepitant, haloperidol, and promethazine
   d. Aprepitant, ondansetron, and dexamethasone
9. Select the correct statement.
   a. Dolasetron has similar efficacy to ondansetron when used at equipotent doses.
   b. Granisetron is the only 5-HT3 antagonist approved for prevention of delayed CINV with highly emetogenic chemotherapy.
   c. Palonosetron is superior to prochlorperazine for the treatment of breakthrough nausea and vomiting.
   d. The IV route of administration of ondansetron is superior to oral administration.
10. Select the correct dose of IV ondansetron when used in the prevention of PONV.
    a. 4 mg
    b. 12 mg
    c. 20 mg
    d. 32 mg
11. Which is the preferred antiemetic for breakthrough nausea and vomiting?
    a. Aprepitant
    b. Dronabinol
    c. Ondansetron
    d. Prochlorperazine
12. Significant drug interactions with aprepitant include:
    a. Dexamethasone
    b. Oral contraceptive pills (OCP)
    c. Warfarin
    d. All of the above
13. Which antiemetic should be diluted when given intravenously to minimize extravasation potential?
    a. Droperidol
    b. Fosaprepitant
    c. Palonosetron
    d. Promethazine

14. Select which antiemetic has a black box warning associated with irreversible extrapyramidal side effects.
    a. Aprepitant
    b. Dexamethasone
    c. Dolasetron
    d. Metoclopramide
15. Which antiemetic should be avoided in patients with the potential for a prolonged QT-interval?
    a. Aprepitant
    b. Droperidol
    c. Metoclopramide
    d. Scopolamine
16. Of the agents listed, select the chemotherapy agent with the highest emetic risk.
    a. Cisplatin
    b. Etoposide
    c. Paclitaxel
    d. Vincristine
17. Anticipatory nausea and vomiting may be prevented with:
    a. Dexamethasone
    b. Dronabinol
    c. Lorazepam
    d. Palonosetron
18. Sancuso transdermal patch delivers antiemetic activity for:
    a. 24 hours
    b. 72 hours
    c. 5 days
    d. 7 days
19. Which statement is correct?
    a. Dronabinol is a Schedule II substance.
    b. Dronabinol is reserved for the treatment of CINV in patients with anorexia or HIV.
    c. Dronabinol is associated with sedation, euphoria, and dizziness.
    d. All of the above.
20. Factors that increase the risk of PONV include:
    a. Duration of surgery
    b. Type of anesthetic used
    c. Type of surgery
    d. All of the above

TAKEAWAY POINTS ››

- Nausea and vomiting are two of the most common side effects experienced by patients receiving chemotherapy.
- Various neurotransmitters are involved in the pathogenesis of nausea and vomiting, including dopamine, serotonin, histamine, and neurokinin-1.
- Risk factors for developing CINV include rate of infusion, dose of drug, younger patients, female patients, and those with a history of motion sickness or nausea with pregnancy.
- Acute and delayed CINV are easier to prevent than to treat. Antiemetic drug therapy should be directed toward the prevention of acute and delayed CINV.
- Serotonin (5-HT3) antagonists and dexamethasone should be used in the prevention, not treatment, of acute CINV.
- Aprepitant is useful in the prevention, not the treatment, of acute and delayed nausea and vomiting and should be used in highly emetogenic regimens, regimens at risk for delayed nausea, or for the combination of cyclophosphamide/doxorubicin.
- Dopamine antagonists such as promethazine are used in the treatment of breakthrough nausea and vomiting.
- When treating breakthrough CINV, a drug with a different mechanism of action than prescribed previously should be used.
- Benzodiazepines such as lorazepam are useful in the prevention of anticipatory CINV.
- Risk factors for developing PONV include type of anesthetic used, duration of surgery, type of surgery, female patients, nonsmokers, and history of PONV.
- Serotonin antagonists are the antiemetic class most often given for patients at high risk for PONV.

REFERENCES

1. Baribeault D, Erb CH. New directions in the treatment of chemotherapy-induced nausea and vomiting. A Supplement to *The Oncology Pharmacist.* 2009;2:1-12.
2. Kloth DD. New Pharmacologic findings for the treatment of PONV and PDNV. *Am J Health Syst Pharm.* 2009;66 (suppl 1): S11-S18.
3. Berger AM, Clark-Snow RA. Adverse effects of treatment: nausea and vomiting. In: DeVita Jr. VT, Hellman S, Rosenberg SA (eds). *Cancer: Principles and Practice of Oncology.* 7th ed. Philadelphia, PA: Lippincott Williams and Wilkins; 2005:2515-2523.
4. Navari RM. Pharmacological management of chemotherapy-induced nausea and vomiting. *Drugs.* 2009;69:515-533.

5. Lohr L. Chemotherapy-induced nausea and vomiting. *Cancer J.* 2008;14:85-93.
6. Grunberg SM, Osoba D, Hesketh PJ, et al. Evaluation of new antiemetic agents and definition of antineoplastic agent emetogenicity—an update. *Support Care Cancer.* 2005;15:80-84.
7. Grunberg SM. Antiemetic activity of corticosteroids in patients receiving cancer chemotherapy: dosing, efficacy, and tolerability analysis. *Ann Oncol.* 2007;18:233-240.
8. Jordan K, Sippel C, Schmoll HJ. Guidelines for antiemetic treatment of chemotherapy-induced nausea and vomiting: past, present and future recommendations. *Oncologist.* 2007;12:1143-1150.
9. Hesketh PJ. Chemotherapy-induced nausea and vomiting. *N Engl J Med.* 2008;358:2482-2494.
10. Kris MG, Hesketh PJ, Somerfield MR, et al. American Society of Clinical Oncology guideline for antiemetics in oncology: Update 2006. *J Clin Oncol.* 2006;24:2932-2947.
11. The NCCN Clinical Practice Guidelines in Oncology™ Antiemesis (Version 3.2009). © 2009 National Comprehensive Cancer Network, Inc. Available at: NCCN.org. Accessed [August 2, 2009]. To view the most recent and complete version of the NCCN Guidelines, go online to NCCN.org.
12. Osoba D, Zee B, Pater J, et al. Determinants of postchemotherapy nausea and vomiting in patients with cancer. *J Clin Onocol.* 1997;15:116-123.
13. Sullivan JR, Leyden MJ, Bell R. Decreased cisplatin-induced nausea and vomiting with chronic alcohol ingestion. *N Engl J Med.* 1983;309:796.
14. Jordan K, Schmoll HJ, Aapro MS. Comparative activity of antiemetic drugs. *Crit Rev Oncol Hematol.* 2006;61:162-175.
15. Klasco RK (ed). DRUGDEX® System (electronic version). Thomson Micromedex, Greenwood Village, Colorado, USA. Available at: http://www-thomsonhc-com.cuhsl.creighton.edu. Accessed August 24, 2009.
16. Ioannidis JPA, Hesketh PJ, Lau J. Contribution of dexamethasone to control of chemotherapy-induced nausea and vomiting: a meta-analysis of randomized evidence. *J Clin Oncol.* 2000;19:3409-3422.
17. Herrstedt J. Antiemetics: an update and the MASCC guidelines applied in clinical practice. *Nat Clin Pract Oncol.* 2008:5:32-43.
18. Shadle CR, Lee Y, Majumdar AK, et al. Evaluation of potential inductive effects of aprepitant on cytochrome P450 3A4 and 2C9 activity. *J Clin Pharmacol.* 2004;44:215-223.
19. FDA requires boxed warning and risk mitigation strategy for metoclopramide-containing drugs. FDA News Release, Feb 26, 2009. Available at: http://www.fda.gov/Safety/MedWatch/SafetyInformation/SafetyAlertsforHumanMedicalProducts/ucm106942.htm . Accessed October 27, 2009.
20. Gan TJ, Meyer T, Apfel CC, et al. Consensus guidelines for managing postoperative nausea and vomiting. *Anesth Analg.* 2003;97:62-71.
21. Gan TJ, Meyer TA, Apfel CC, et al. Society for ambulatory anesthesia guidelines for the management of postoperative nausea and vomiting. *Anesth Analg.* 2007;105:1615-1628.
22. Wender RH. Do current antiemetic practices result in positive patient outcomes? Results of a new study. *Am J Health Syst Pharm.* 2009;66(suppl 1):S3-S10.
23. DiPiro CV. Nausea and vomiting. In: DiPiro JT, Talbert RL, Yee GC, et al, eds. *Pharmacotherapy: A Pathophysiologic Approach.* 7th ed. New York, NY: McGraw-Hill Medical; 2008:607-616.

CHAPTER

41 Inflammatory Bowel Disease

Brian A. Hemstreet

FOUNDATION OVERVIEW

Inflammatory bowel disease (IBD) is a chronic inflammatory condition that affects mainly the gastrointestinal (GI) tract and consists of two major subtypes, ulcerative colitis (UC) and Crohn disease (CD). The incidence of UC in the United States is estimated to be 2 to 7 cases per 100,000 population per year, while CD is reported as approximately 5 cases per 100,000 population per year.[1,2] While the underlying pathophysiology of IBD involves an abnormal response directed against the intestinal tract, the true cause of IBD has not been identified.[2,3] Both genetic and environmental factors have been implicated as contributors to the development of IBD.[4] Inflammatory bowel disease has been observed to occur more commonly in patients who report a positive family history of IBD.[5] Another leading theory is that the inflammatory response is induced by the local bacterial flora that inhabit the human GI tract.[3-6] Ultimately, the inflammatory response results in injury to the GI tract that may vary in location, depth, severity, and duration.

While both forms of IBD involve inflammation of the GI tract, there are some key differences between UC and CD. Ulcerative colitis is localized to the colon and is characterized by diffuse continuous mucosal inflammation with the absence of granulomatous changes.[1,5] The rectal area is involved in 95% of patients with UC.[1] In contrast, CD may affect any area of the GI tract, but most frequently involves the ileum or colon.[2,4] The inflammation is often observed to be discontinuous in nature, resulting in "skip lesions," and often penetrates much deeper into the intestinal wall compared to UC.[5] Inflammation confined to the intestinal wall is referred to as luminal CD, and may progress to fibrostenotic disease with development of strictures and luminal obstruction. Likewise, severe inflammation resulting in fistula formation occurs in 20% to 40% of patients with CD, while patients with UC do not develop fistulae.[2]

Due to the location and inflammatory nature of the disease, most patients with UC will present with bloody diarrhea, urgency, and tenesmus as their main symptoms.[1,4] Patients with CD may exhibit similar symptoms, but most commonly present with diarrhea, abdominal pain, weight loss, fever, perianal lesions, and signs of malnutrition.[2] Interestingly, patients with IBD may also develop inflammation in various other organ systems, referred to as extraintestinal symptoms. Examples include arthritis, erythema nodosum, pyoderma gangrenosum, uveitis, episcleritis, and primary sclerosing cholangitis, among others.[7]

The diagnosis of IBD is based collectively on presenting signs and symptoms, along with radiographic and endoscopic findings. Endoscopy is particularly helpful in characterizing the extent and location of the disease, as well as ruling out other potential causes of intestinal inflammation. Determining where the disease is located also directly impacts selection of drug therapy. Patients with UC can be classified as having "extensive" disease if inflammation extends proximal to the splenic flexure.[1] The terms "distal" or "left-sided" disease is used if inflammation is distal to the splenic flexure.[1,8] Lastly, ulcerative proctitis denotes inflammation localized to the rectum, while proctosigmoiditis involves both the rectum and sigmoid colon.[8] While these terms are used for denoting the subtype of UC based on extent and location of inflammation, the extent and location of CD is also determined via endoscopy in a similar manner.[2,6]

Disease severity in UC is classified based on various parameters, such as the number and characteristics of stools per day, presence of systemic signs of inflammation, such as fever or elevated erythrocyte sedimentation rate, among others. The designations used for UC are mild, moderate, moderate severe, and fulminant.[1] While a validated scoring system, the Crohn Disease Activity Index, may be used to classify disease severity, a similar designation to UC also exists and includes classifications of mild-moderate, moderate-severe, and severe/fulminant disease.[2]

TREATMENT

Once disease extent, location, and severity have been determined, pharmacologic therapies may be instituted to address the underlying inflammation. Major goals of drug therapy are to suppress acute inflammation, improve patient symptoms and quality of life, avoid or minimize toxicities, and prevent complications of the disease. Drug therapies should aim to induce disease remission, and then maintain long-term remission if possible. Extraintestinal manifestations of IBD also need to be managed in conjunction with the GI aspects of the disease. In some instances, patients who are refractory to medical therapy or develop severe complications may require surgical intervention.

An important aspect of drug therapy for IBD is that the choice of drug therapy depends on the disease subtype, as well as the severity and location of the disease. More severe

or extensive forms of IBD may require administration of systemic medications, either in oral or parenteral forms. Alternatively, disease that is mild or moderate in nature and is located in areas distal to the splenic flexure may be treated with rectal dosage forms, also referred to as "topical" therapies.[1,2,8] Suppositories can be used to treat up to 20 cm of the rectal area and are preferred for patients with proctitis.[1,8] Enemas may reach inflammation that extends to the splenic flexure and thus may be used for patients with left-sided disease.[8] Oral formulations of some drugs used in the management of IBD are designed to release in specific areas of the small or large intestine and should be chosen based on the target area of inflammation. Systemic and topical therapies may be combined for maximal effectiveness. As many drug therapies for IBD may have serious adverse effects or complicated dosing regimens, counseling to promote patient adherence is key to obtain the optimal outcome.[9]

Aminosalicylates

The aminosalicylate drug class consists of the prototypical agent sulfasalazine and other agents formulated to deliver mesalamine, also known as 5-aminosalicylate or 5-ASA, the active component of sulfasalazine, to various locations within the GI tract (Table 41-1). Sulfasalazine consists of mesalamine bound to sulfapyridine via a diazo bond.[10,11] When administered orally, bacteria located in the colon cleave the diazo bond and release mesalamine which acts locally in the colon. The sulfapyridine component is systemically absorbed. Patients with allergies to sulfonamides should avoid sulfasalazine, as the sulfapyridine component may lead to hypersensitivity reactions. Adverse effects from sulfasalazine are mostly related to the sulfapyridine component and may be dose related or idiosyncratic. Common adverse effects are nausea, diarrhea, headache, and abdominal pain.[12]

Newer formulations of mesalamine lack the sulfapyridine component and deliver the drug to the GI through various delayed release mechanisms.[13] All of these formulations are safe to use in patients with allergies to sulfonamides. Some products use inert carrier molecules in place of sulfapyridine, such as balsalazide (Colazal), while others, such as olsalazine (Dipentum), use two molecules of mesalamine linked via a diazo bond to deliver the drug to the colon. Other formulations use pH-dependent coated tablets (Asacol) or microgranules (Pentasa). The newest formulations of mesalamine use pH-dependent multimatrix tablets (Lialda) or granules with a polymer matrix (Apriso) to allow for once daily dosing and improved patient adherence. Lastly, mesalamine is also available as a suppository or an enema, which are preferred formulations for patients with distal disease.[8,14] The nonsulfa-containing aminosalicylates are better tolerated than sulfasalazine and thus are used more often.

The choice of an aminosalicylate is based on the type of disease, as well as the location and severity. The formulation of drug chosen should release or deliver mesalamine to the site of inflammation. The aminosalicylates can be used in UC for both induction and maintenance of remission in patients with both distal or extensive mild to moderate disease.[1,8] The aminosalicylates can be also be used in mild to moderate CD, but appear to be less efficacious than in UC. Patients should be instructed to take the appropriate number of tablets or capsules and not to crush or break them. Likewise, proper instruction on use of suppositories and enemas will ensure maximal effectiveness.

Corticosteroids

Corticosteroids have potent anti-inflammatory effects and do have specific roles in the management of IBD. The main role for corticosteroids in IBD is to rapidly suppress inflammation

TABLE 41-1 **Aminosalicylate Products Used in the Treatment of IBD**

Brand Name(s)	Formulation	Site of Action
	Topical Mesalamine Therapies	
Rowasa	Enema	Rectum, distal colon
Canasa	Suppository	Rectum
	Oral Products	
Sulfasalazine		
Azulfidine Azulfidine Entabs	Immediate release or enteric-coated tablets	Colon
Mesalamine		
Asacol Asacol HD	Table coated with Eudragit-S (delayed-release acrylic resin)	Terminal ileum and colon
Pentasa	Encapsulated ethylcellulose microgranules (capsule)	Small bowel and colon
Dipentum	Dimer of mesalamine (capsule)	Colon
Colazal	Mesalamine bound to inert carrier molecule (capsule)	Colon
Lialda	Once daily tablet with pH-dependent coating and MMX mutimatrix core	Terminal ileum and colon
Apriso	Once daily pH-dependent tablet with mesalamine granules in a Intellicor polymer matrix	Colon

in patients with moderate to severe symptoms or in those patients unresponsive to aminosalicylates.[15] There are many different formulations of corticosteroids available including oral, parenteral, and topical agents. In general, short courses (7-10 days) of oral prednisone at doses of 40-60 mg daily are used for moderate to severe UC and CD.[1,2] Parenteral hydrocortisone or methylprednisolone can be used for hospitalized patients with severe disease. Budesonide (Entocort), a corticosteroid with limited systemic bioavailability, is formulated to release in the ileum and ascending colon and can be considered a first-line agent in the management of mild-moderate CD in place of an aminosalicylate.[2,16] Topical hydrocortisone products, available as enemas or suppositories, can be used for patients with distal disease who do not initially respond to aminosalicylates.[8] Corticosteroids are generally ineffective for treatment of fistulae associated with CD.[15]

Despite their ability to rapidly suppress inflammation, corticosteroids are ineffective as long-term treatments and have no role in the maintenance of remission of IBD.[1,2,15,16] The potential for serious adverse effects precludes the long-term use of these agents. Patients who become corticosteroid dependent may develop hypertension, osteoporosis, glucose intolerance, and psychiatric disturbances among others.[12] Thus, efforts should be made to limit corticosteroid exposure and to utilize other agents that may have steroid-sparing effects should patients become dependent on steroids for controlling their disease.

Immunomodulators

Immunomodulators, such as azathioprine, 6-mercaptopurine (6-MP), and methotrexate, have potent immunosuppressive effects and are used mostly as maintenance therapy in IBD, particularly for patients who are resistant to or dependent on corticosteroids[2,15] (Table 41-2).

Azathioprine is the pro-drug of 6-MP, and requires hepatic activation to 6-MP following absorption. 6-MP is then taken up into the cell and further metabolized by various enzymes, including xanthine oxidase and thiopurine methyltransferase (TPMT).[17] Genetic polymorphisms in the TPMT enzyme may predispose patients to toxicity from azathioprine and 6-MP, so patients should have TPMT activity or genotype evaluated prior to initiating therapy.[2,17,18]

Oral azathioprine 2 to 3 mg/kg/d or 6-MP 1 to 1.5 mg/kg/d are recommended as maintenance therapy, following steroid-induced remission, in patients with moderate to severe IBD or in those who have failed corticosteroids or aminosalicylates.[1,2,15,16] Recent data also suggest that azathioprine in combination with infliximab is better than either drug alone in biologic or immunomodulator naïve patients with CD.[19] Both azathioprine and 6-MP have delayed effects and often take >3 to 4 months to work.[15,17] Toxicities associated with azathioprine and 6-MP include bone marrow suppression, hepatitis, pancreatitis, rash, fever, arthralgia, lymphoma, and diarrhea.[12] Patients should have complete blood cell counts and liver transaminases monitored regularly during treatment.[2]

Methotrexate is a folate antagonist that is used mostly in CD as a maintenance therapy. Like azathioprine and 6-MP, methotrexate has a slow onset of action and thus is not used as an induction therapy in patients with active disease. Methotrexate has steroid sparing effects in patients with steroid dependence and can be also used in patients who are steroid refractory.[2,15,16] Weekly intramuscular or subcutaneous doses of 15 to 25 mg are recommended for patients with CD.[2] Potential toxicities associated with methotrexate therapy include nausea, abdominal pain, diarrhea, bone marrow suppression, pneumonitis, and hepatotoxicity.[12] Methotrexate is teratogenic and should be avoided in women of child-bearing age. If therapy is deemed necessary, then reliable forms of contraception should be used.[20]

TABLE 41-2 Immunomodulator and Biologic Therapies Used in the Treatment of IBD

Drug	Brand Name(s)	Formulation
Immunomodulator Therapies		
Azathioprine	Imuran, Azasan	Tablet
6-Mercaptopurine	Purinethol	Tablet
Methotrexate	Trexall	Tablet, injection (IM,SC)
Biologic Therapies		
Infliximab	Remicade	Injection (IV)
Adalimumab	Humira	Injection (SC)
Certolizumab	Cimzia	Injection (SC)
Natalizumab	Tysabri	Injection (IV)

Abbreviations: IM, intramuscular; SC subcutaneous; IV intravenous.

Biologic Therapies

Several biologic agents have now been approved for both the treatment of acute, active IBD and for maintaining remission (Table 41-2). The most widely used biologic agents are designed to antagonize the effects of tumor necrosis factor alpha (TNF-α) and include infliximab, adalimumab, and certolizumab.[21] These agents are typically indicated for patients with moderate to severe disease as an alternative to corticosteroids, for patients who are steroid dependent, or those that have failed other therapies. The TNF-α antagonists are the drugs of choice for patients with fistulizing CD.[22] All of the TNF-α antagonists require parenteral administration and are very costly compared to the available oral therapies.

Infliximab is a chimeric antibody that is given intravenously and is indicated in both moderate to severe UC and CD, with specific indications in pediatric and fistulizing CD. Doses of 5 mg/kg intravenously given at 0, 2, and 6 weeks, followed by 5 mg/kg every 8 weeks are typically used.[2,15] Due to it chimeric structure, antibodies to infliximab may develop over time, which may lead to subsequent loss of efficacy.[23] Adalimumab is a fully humanized antibody to TNF-α that is approved only for moderate to severe CD. Adalimumab is given subcutaneously at dose of 160 mg on day 1, then 80 mg on day 15 of therapy, followed by 40 mg subcutaneously every

other week starting on day 29 of therapy. Since it is a humanized molecule, it may be used in patients who develop loss of efficacy to infliximab due to antibody development or as a first line biologic agent.[23] Certolizumab is a pegylated, humanized, antigen-binding fragment with complementary determining regions derived from a murine source.[21] Certolizumab is given subcutaneously at a dose of 400 mg initially, and then at 2 and 4 weeks followed by 400 mg subcutaneously every 4 weeks if an initial response is achieved.[24] Patients with initial C-reactive protein concentrations >10 mg/dL tend to respond better to certolizumab compared to those with concentrations <10 mg/dL.[23,24]

All of the TNF-α antagonists carry a risk of serious potential adverse effects, particularly predisposition to infections. Prior to initiating therapy with a TNF-α antagonist, patients should be evaluated for latent tuberculosis.[25] Patients being evaluated for possible TNF-α therapy should not have a current serious infection or sepsis. Heart failure may be precipitated or worsened, so use should be avoided in patients with advanced heart failure. Infliximab may cause infusion-related reactions, such as urticaria, erythema, dizziness, and nausea, which can be managed by slowing the infusion or premedicating with acetaminophen and diphenhydramine.[2,12,15] Delayed infusion reactions may also occur, ranging from 3 to 14 days after the injection, and may consist of myalgia, fever, rash, urticaria, and pruritis.[2] Due to their administration as subcutaneous injections, adalimumab and certolizumab carry a lower risk of injection-related adverse effects. Other less common adverse effects of TNF-α antagonists include a lupus-like syndrome, lymphoma, and nerve demyelination.[15]

In addition to the TNF-α antagonists, natalizumab is the only other biologic agent approved for IBD. Natalizumab is a humanized monoclonal antibody that prevents leukocyte α-4 mediated adhesion, preventing transmigration across endothelial cells.[23] It is indicated for the induction and maintenance of remission of moderate to severely active CD in patients who have failed other therapies, including TNF-α antagonists. It is administered intravenously at a dose of 300 mg initially, and then 300 mg intravenously every 4 weeks. An important aspects of natalizumab therapy is that patients who do not respond within 12 weeks of treatment have little chance of experiencing efficacy and should have therapy discontinued.[23,26] Natalizumab also carries a risk of progressive multifocal leukoencephalopathy and is only available by registering through the manufacturer's prescribing program. Patients should be monitored for any signs of neurologic abnormality while receiving natalizumab. Infusion-related reactions and hepatotoxicity have also been reported.[12]

Antibiotics

Given that bacteria may play a role in the pathogenesis of IBD, antibiotics have been observed to have some roles in IBD treatment. Metronidazole and ciprofloxacin are the two most-studied antimicrobial agents used in IBD therapy.[27] These two agents are recommended in patients with UC who develop pouchitis following ileoanal pouch anastamosis.[1] In patients with CD, metronidazole alone or in combination with ciprofloxacin has the most favorable effects as short-term adjunctive therapy in patients with colonic, perianal, or fistulizing disease.[2,22,25,27] Common adverse effects of metronidazole include nausea, diarrhea, and metallic taste. Long-term use is associated with the development of peripheral neuropathy and should be avoided if possible.[2,12,22] Ciprofloxacin may be associated with diarrhea, particularly overgrowth of *Clostridium difficile*, and may also precipitate tendon rupture in rare instances.[12]

Special Considerations

Patients with active IBD may be at risk for development of acute colonic dilation, also known as toxic megacolon, particularly if medications are used that decrease intestinal motility. Patients with active disease should have drugs such as loperamide, narcotics, and anticholinergic agents discontinued.[28] Patients who receive prolonged courses of corticosteroids may require calcium and vitamin D supplementation for prevention of bone loss and possible use of a bisphosphonate as preventative therapy.[1,29] Patients who smoke have a higher risk of steroid dependence, so efforts should be made to institute smoking cessation techniques or therapies, particularly in patients with CD.[2] Nicotine replacement therapy, typically with a patch, is a viable adjunctive treatment option in UC, and appears to be most efficacious in ex-smokers.[1,8] Lastly, patients who undergo multiple surgeries for IBD may require long-term parenteral or enteral nutrition, particularly if they develop short bowel syndrome.[1,2,25]

CASE Application

1. Select the characteristic that is a feature of Crohn disease, but not of ulcerative colitis.
   a. Disease distribution limited to the colon
   b. Presence of extraintestinal manifestations
   c. Inflammation affecting only the mucosal layer
   d. Inflammation penetrating below the mucosal layer

2. Which drug formulation of mesalamine is most effective as initial therapy for patients with mild to moderate ulcerative proctitis?
   a. Suppository
   b. Enema
   c. Tablet
   d. Intravenous injection

3. Which enzyme involved in the metabolism of azathioprine is subject to genetic polymorphism?
   a. Rasburicase
   b. Dihydrofolate reductase
   c. Thiopurine methyltransferase
   d. Hyaluronidase

4. BD is a 27-year-old white man who is newly diagnosed with moderate extensive ulcerative colitis. He reports a drug allergy to sulfonamide-containing medications, which manifests as a rash. Which product would be most appropriate as initial therapy for this patient?
   a. Canasa
   b. Azulfidine
   c. Colazal
   d. Entocort

5. Which product is available only as an intravenous solution for injection?
   a. Purinethol
   b. Colazal
   c. Flagyl
   d. Remicade

6. Which laboratory parameter(s) should be monitored closely in patients who are initiated on methotrexate therapy?
   a. Complete blood count
   b. Serum potassium
   c. Serum calcium
   d. Lipase

7. Which condition is considered a contraindication to receiving a TNF-α antagonist?
   a. Migraine headache
   b. Previous myocardial infarction
   c. Asthma
   d. Sepsis

8. JJ is a 37-year-old woman who has been receiving Asacol for treatment of ulcerative colitis. She is receiving maximal doses of Asacol, but continues to have daily moderate symptoms including urgency, abdominal pain, and rectal bleeding. Which therapy would be best for treatment of her symptoms at this time?
   a. Entocort
   b. Trexall
   c. Remicade
   d. Apriso

9. A 48-year-old male patient with Crohn disease is prescribed Humira for treatment of severe symptoms. Which counseling point should you provide to this patient prior to starting this therapy?
   a. Correct number of tablets to take on a daily basis
   b. Proper injection technique
   c. Monitor for development of diarrhea.
   d. The next dose should be given in 8 weeks

10. Which medication would be most efficacious in a patient with fistulizing Crohn disease?
    a. Ciprofloxacin
    b. Mesalamine
    c. Prednisone
    d. Certolizumab

11. Which drug may be most commonly associated with the development of pancreatitis as a potential adverse effect?
    a. Methotrexate
    b. Azathioprine
    c. Adalimumab
    d. Natalizumab

12. What is the role of oral prednisone in the treatment of inflammatory bowel disease (IBD)?
    a. Preferred treatment for maintenance of remission
    b. First line for treatment of mild disease
    c. No role in the management of IBD
    d. Short-term use in patients unresponsive to aminosalicylates

13. Which product has the ability to be administered on a once daily basis?
    a. Asacol
    b. Lialda
    c. Azulfidine
    d. Dipentum

14. A patient receiving long-term therapy with metronidazole should be monitored for the development of which adverse effect?
    a. Peripheral neuropathy
    b. Hepatitis
    c. Pulmonary fibrosis
    d. Anemia

15. What is the mechanism of action of natalizumab in the treatment of IBD?
    a. Antagonism of TNF-α
    b. Inhibition of arachidonic acid formation
    c. Down regulation of interleukin-1 production
    d. Inhibition of leukocyte adhesion

16. A patient who presents with left-sided ulcerative colitis has inflammation extending from the rectum to which area within the GI tract?
    a. Sigmoid colon
    b. Hepatic flexure
    c. Splenic flexure
    d. Terminal ileum

17. What is the generic drug name for Entocort?
    a. Prednisone
    b. Hydrocortisone
    c. Methylprednisolone
    d. Budesonide

18. Which medication requires that the prescriber registers with the manufacturer's prescribing program?
    a. Humira
    b. Cimzia
    c. Tysabri
    d. Remicade

19. How does sulfasalazine differ from mesalamine?
    a. Sulfasalazine is the active component of mesalamine.
    b. Sulfasalazine contains the carrier molecule sulfapyridine while mesalamine does not.
    c. Sulfasalazine can be used in patients with sulfa allergies, while mesalamine cannot.
    d. Sulfasalazine is available in enema form, while mesalamine is not.

20. A patient receiving Tysabri for Crohn disease develops mental status changes after 24 weeks of therapy. This may indicate development of which adverse effect?
    a. Meningitis
    b. Progressive multifocal leukoencephalopathy
    c. Central pontine myelinolysis
    d. Multi-infarct dementia

TAKEAWAY POINTS ››

- IBD consists of both UC and CD and is considered an inflammatory disorder with no known definitive cause.
- Differences exist between UC and CD in regards to disease location, depth and pattern of inflammation, and presenting signs and symptoms.
- Patients may also manifest extraintestinal symptoms of IBD, such as arthritis.
- Choice of drug therapy for active IBD should be based on the subtype of IBD, the disease location and severity, and considerations of potential contraindications to therapy.
- Aminosalicylates are generally first-line agents for UC and CD and should be chosen based on the formulation that will deliver the active component, mesalamine, to the site of inflammation.
- Topical mesalamine products are preferred for patients with distal disease.
- Corticosteroids are used short-term in the setting of active IBD and should not be used as maintenance therapy.
- Immunomodulators, such as azathioprine and methotrexate, are used for long-term maintenance therapy, particularly for patients who are steroid dependent.
- Biologic agents that antagonize TNF-α can be used as first-line therapies for moderate to severe IBD and are the drugs of choice for fistulizing CD.
- TNF-α antagonist use predisposes patients to the development of serious infections.
- Antibiotics are considered adjunctive therapies in patients with fistulizing or perianal CD.

REFERENCES

1. Kornbluth A, Sachar DB. Ulcerative colitis practice guidelines in adults: American Collecge of Gastroenterology, Practice Parameters Committee. *Am J Gastroenterol.* 2010;105:501-523.
2. Lichtenstein GR, Hanauer SB, Sandborn WJ; The Practice Parameters Committee of the American College of Gastroenterology. Management of Crohn's disease in adults. *Am J Gastroenterol.* 2009;104:465-483.
3. Kocaman O, Sahin T, Aygun C, Senturk O, Hulagu S. Endothelial dysfunction in patients with ulcerative colitis. *Inflamm Bowel Dis.* 2006;12:166-171.
4. Podolsky DK. Inflammatory bowel disease. *N Engl J Med.* 2002;347:417–429.
5. Lakatos PL, Fischer S, Lakatos L, Gal I, Papp J. Current concept on the pathogenesis of inflammatory bowel disease—crosstalk between genetic and microbial factors: pathogenic bacteria and altered bacterial sensing or changes in mucosal integrity take "toll". *World J Gastroenterol.* 2006;12(12):1829-1841.
6. Viscido A, Aratari A, Maccioni F, Signore A, Caprilli R. Inflammatory bowel diseases: clinical update of practical guidelines. *Nucl Med Comm.* 2005;26:649-655.
7. Kethu SR. Extraintestinal manifestations of inflammatory bowel diseases. *J Clin Gastroenterol.* 2006;40(6):467-475.
8. Regueiro M, Loftus EV, Steinhart AH, Cohen RD. Clinical guidelines for the medical management of left-sided ulcerative colitis and ulcerative proctitis: summary statement. *Inflamm Bowel Dis.* 2006;12:972-978.
9. Kane SV. Systematic review: adherence issues in the treatment of ulcerative colitis. *Aliment Pharmacol Ther.* 2006;23:577-585.
10. Hanauer SB. Review article: high dose aminosalicylates to induce and maintain remission in ulcerative colitis. *Aliment Pharmacol Ther.* 2006;24(suppl 3):37-40.
11. Cohen HD, Das KM. The metabolism of mesalamine and its possible use in colonic diverticulitis as an anti-inflammatory agent. *J Clin Gastroenterol.* 2006;40(supp 3):S150-S154.
12. Juillerat P, Pittet V, Felley C, et al. Drug safety in Crohn's disease therapy. *Digestion.* 2007;76:161-168.
13. Tindall WN. New approaches to adherence issues when dosing oral aminosalicylates in ulcerative colitis. *Am J Health-Syst Pharm.* 2009;66:451-457.
14. Gionchetti P, Rizzello F, Morselli C, et al. Review article: aminosalicylates for distal colitis. *Aliment Pharmacol Ther.* 2006;24(suppl 3):41-44.
15. Lichtenstein GR, Abreu MT, Cohen R, Tremaine W. American Gastroenterological Association Institute technical review on

corticosteroids, immunomodulators, and infliximab in inflammatory bowel disease. *Gastroenterology*. 2006;130:940-987.
16. Sandborn WJ, Feagan BG, Lichtenstein GR. Medical management of mild to moderate Crohn's disease: evidence-based treatment algorithms for induction and maintenance of remission. *Aliment Pharmacol Ther*. 2007;26:987-1003.
17. Derijks LJJ, Gilissen LPL, Hooymans PM, et al. Review article: thiopurines in inflammatory bowel disease. *Aliment Pharmcol Ther*. 2006;24:715-729.
18. Dubinsky MC, Sandborn WJ. Optimizing thiopurine response in IBD: the clinical utility of TMPT testing and metabolite monitoring. *Gastroenterol Hepatol*. 2006;2(8, supp 6):3-8.
19. Sandborn J, Rutgeerts P, Reinisch W, et al. "SONIC: a randomized, double-blind, controlled trial comparing infliximab and infliximab and azathioprine to azathioprine in patients with Crohn's disease naïve to immunomodulators and biologic therapy." *Am J Gastroenterol*. 2008;103(S1):S436.
20. Ferrero S, Ragni N. Inflammatory bowel disease: management issues during pregnancy. *Arch Gynecol Obstet*. 2004;270:79-85.
21. Tracey D, Klareskog L, Sasso EH, Salfeld JG, Tak PP. Tumor necrosis factor antagonist mechanisms of action: a comprehensive review. *Pharmacol Ther*. 2008;117:244-279.
22. Bressler B, Sands BE. Review article: medical therapy for fistulizing Crohn's disease. *Aliment Pharmacol Ther*. 2006;24:1283-1293.
23. Jones J, Panaccione R. Biologic therapy in Crohn's disease: state of the art. *Curr Opin Gastroenterol*. 2008;24:475-481.
24. Sandborn WJ, Feagan BG, Stoinov S, et al. Certolizumab pegol for the treatment of Crohn's disease. *N Engl J Med*. 2007;357:228-238.
25. Cummings JR, Keshav S, Travis SP. Medical management of Crohn's disease. *BMJ*. 2008;336:1062-1066.
26. Sandborn WJ, Colombel JF, Enns R, et al. Natalizumab induction and maintenance therapy in Crohn's disease. *N Engl J Med*. 2005;353:1912-1925.
27. Guslandi M. Antibiotics for inflammatory bowel disease: do they work? *Eur J Gastroenterol Hepatol*. 2005;17:145-147.
28. Gan SI, Beck PL. A new look at toxic megacolon: an update and review of incidence, etiology, pathogenesis, and management. *Am J Gastroenterol*. 2003;98:2363-2371.
29. American Gastroenterological Association Medical Position Statement. Guidelines on osteoporosis in gastrointestinal diseases. *Gastroenterol*. 2003;124:791-794.

PART

6

Respiratory Disorders

CHAPTER

42 Chronic Obstructive Pulmonary Disease

Miranda R. Andrus and S. Scott Sutton

FOUNDATION OVERVIEW

The prevalence, morbidity, and mortality of chronic obstructive pulmonary disease (COPD) are directly linked to cigarette smoking and air pollution.[1] COPD cases are expected to continue to increase, due to the continued exposure to risk factors (cigarette smoke and air pollution) and individuals living longer.[1] According to the 2007 United States National Health Interview Survey, approximately 11 million Americans over the age of 18 years have COPD.[2] It is projected that worldwide, COPD will become the third leading cause of death by the year 2020.[1]

COPD is a preventable chronic disease of the airways that is characterized by gradual, progressive loss of lung function. It is characterized by airflow limitation that is not fully reversible.[1] The airflow limitation is associated with an abnormal inflammatory response of the lung to noxious particles or gases.[1] Emphysema and chronic bronchitis are often present in COPD, but patients must also have abnormal spirometry to be formally diagnosed with COPD. Emphysema is an abnormal permanent enlargement of the airspaces distal to the terminal bronchioles, accompanied by destruction of their walls and without obvious fibrosis. Chronic bronchitis is inflammation of the bronchioles with mucus hypersecretion and chronic productive cough when all other causes of cough have been ruled out.

The most common risk factor for COPD is cigarette smoking, however, not all smokers develop COPD, which suggests a possible genetic factor or predisposition.[3] A rare genetic disorder called alpha 1 antitrypsin (AAT) deficiency is a risk factor for COPD.[4] This hereditary deficiency is a recessive trait most commonly seen in individuals of Northern European descent.[5] Patients with AAT deficiency develop COPD at an early age (20-50 years). Patients presenting with COPD at an early age or a strong family history should be screened for this disorder.[4] Inhalation exposure risk factors include occupational dusts and chemicals (chemical agents and fumes), indoor air pollution (wood, animal dung, crop residues, and coal burned in open fires), and outdoor air pollution.[6-9] Another potential risk factor is impaired lung growth during gestation, birth, and childhood. A positive association has been found between birth weight and forced expiratory volume in 1 second (FEV_1) in adulthood.[10] Oxidative stress, or a depletion of antioxidants in the lungs plays a role in the development of COPD and can initiate lung inflammation and injury.[11] Respiratory infections, both viral and bacterial, may contribute to the pathogenesis of COPD and are considered a risk factor.[12]

COPD is caused by amplification of the normal inflammatory response to chronic irritants such as cigarette smoke. Inflammatory mediators increased in COPD patients include neutrophils, macrophages, and lymphocytes. Oxidative stress generated by oxidants released by cigarette smoke and other inhaled substances and a reduction in endogenous antioxidants also contribute to lung inflammation. An imbalance between the proteases that break down connective tissue in the lung and the antiproteases that protect against this is also seen in COPD. These characteristics lead to airflow limitation and air trapping, resulting in hyperinflation of the lungs. This reduces the capacity of the lungs to fill during inspiration, resulting in dyspnea, particularly during exertion. Gas exchange abnormalities also result, with hypoxemia and hypercapnia common in COPD. Finally, mucus hypersecretion and chronic productive cough are often present due to chronic irritation of the airway.[1,13]

The clinical presentation of COPD includes dyspnea, chronic cough, sputum production, and exposure to risk factors.[1] Dyspnea is usually present every day, worsened by exertion, and progressively worsens over time. Patients may describe an increased effort to breathe or gasping. Patients with symptoms of COPD and exposure to risk factors should be tested with spirometry to confirm a diagnosis. The Global Initiative for Chronic Obstructive Lung Disease (GOLD) guidelines define COPD as a post-bronchodilator forced expiratory volume in 1 second (FEV_1) to forced vital capacity (FVC) ratio as less than 0.7 and FEV_1 less than 80% predicted.[1] This demonstrates airflow limitation that is not fully reversible. The GOLD guidelines also define specific stages of COPD which are described in Table 42-1.

COPD is a progressive disease, and even with the best treatment, will worsen over time. There is no cure, with most treatment directed at managing symptoms. The most common complication of COPD is exacerbations of symptoms. A COPD exacerbation is defined as an acute change from baseline in cough and/or sputum production that is beyond day-to-day variations.[1] Exacerbations affect the prognosis of COPD, and lead to poor long-term outcomes and increased hospital mortality.[14] Late in the disease, pulmonary hypertension may develop due to hypoxic vasoconstriction of the pulmonary arteries.[15] This may eventually lead to the development

TABLE 42-1 **Classification of COPD per GOLD Guidelines[1]**

Stage	Description	FEV_1/FVC	FEV_1
I	Mild	< 0.7	≥ 80% predicted with or without symptoms
II	Moderate	< 0.7	< 80% and ≥ 50% predicted with or without symptoms
III	Severe	< 0.7	< 50% and ≥ 30% predicted with or without symptoms
IV	Very severe	< 0.7	< 30% predicted or < 50% predicted + chronic respiratory failure or right heart failure

of cor pulmonale. Patients with severe COPD also can develop several systemic features which can worsen morbidity and mortality. These include cachexia, skeletal muscle wasting, osteoporosis, depression, anemia, and increased risk of cardiovascular disease.[16]

TREATMENT

The GOLD guidelines emphasize that a COPD management plan should include four components, which are summarized in Table 42-2. In stages I and II of COPD, treatment will concentrate on avoiding risk factors and treating symptoms as needed with medications. In stages III and IV, treatment will require multiple disciplines and treatment approaches. The ultimate goal would be to prevent development of COPD altogether, but once it is diagnosed the goal is effective management.[1] The goals of management are listed in Table 42-3.

Nonpharmacologic Treatment

Smoking cessation is the single most effective treatment for reducing the progression of COPD.[1] Tobacco dependence is a chronic condition that warrants intensive and repeated treatment with both counseling and pharmacotherapy until continued abstinence is achieved.[17]

Pulmonary rehabilitation should be considered for patients with COPD, and it has been shown to have numerous benefits including improved exercise capacity, improved health-related quality of life, reduced number of hospitalizations, reduced anxiety and depression, and improved survival.[1] A comprehensive pulmonary rehabilitation program will include exercise training, nutrition counseling, and education.

TABLE 42-2 **Components of a COPD Management Plan[1]**

1	Assess and monitor disease
2	Reduce risk factors
3	Manage stable COPD
4	Manage exacerbations

TABLE 42-3 **Goals of Treatment for COPD[1]**

Relieve symptoms
Prevent disease progression
Improve exercise tolerance
Improve health status
Prevent and treat complications
Prevent and treat exacerbations
Reduce mortality

Oxygen therapy is often necessary for patients with stage IV COPD. Oxygen therapy for patients with chronic respiratory therapy has been shown to increase survival.[18,19] Other benefits include improvement in exercise capacity, lung mechanics, and mental state.[20] Oxygen therapy can also prevent the progression of pulmonary hypertension.[21,22]

All patients with COPD should receive the influenza vaccine annually.[1] The 2008 GOLD guidelines only recommend the pneumococcal polysaccharide vaccination in COPD patients over the age of 65 and for patients less than 65 years of age with an FEV_1 less than 40%.[1] However, the more updated 2009 CDC recommendations state that all patients with chronic lung disease or who are chronic smokers should receive the pneumococcal vaccine.[23]

Pharmacologic Treatment

The medications available for COPD are effective for reducing or relieving symptoms, improving exercise tolerance, reducing the number and severity of exacerbations, and improving the quality of life. No medications presently available have been shown to slow the rate of decline in lung function.[1]

Bronchodilators

Bronchodilators are the mainstay of treatment for symptomatic COPD. They reduce symptoms and improve exercise tolerance and quality of life.[1] Bronchodilator medications commonly utilized for COPD include β_2-agonists, anticholinergics, and theophylline (theophylline would be considered a last-line agent because of potential adverse reactions). The inhaled route is the preferred route for β_2-agonists and anticholinergics, but attention must be paid to proper inhaler technique.[1] Clinicians should advise, counsel, and observe patient technique with the devices frequently and consistently. Combining different bronchodilator therapies improves efficacy and is preferred over increasing the dose of a single agent, due to increased risk of adverse drug reactions. Additionally, the dose-response relationship using FEV_1 is relatively flat for single-agent therapy.[1,24-31] Bronchodilators work by reducing the tone of airway smooth muscle (relaxation), thus minimizing airflow limitation.[1,24] In patients with COPD, the clinical benefits of bronchodilators include increased exercise capacity, decreased air trapping in the lungs, and relief of symptoms. However, the use of bronchodilators may not be associated with significant improvements in pulmonary function measurements such as FEV_1.[1] The initial therapy for COPD patients who experience symptoms intermittently are short-acting bronchodilators. Among these agents, the choices are short-acting β_2-agonists or an anticholinergic. Either class of agents has a rapid onset of action, relieves symptoms, and improves lung function. For patients with moderate to severe COPD who experience symptoms on a regular and consistent basis, or in whom short-acting therapies do not provide relief, long-acting bronchodilator therapies are recommended.[1,24,32-33] Long-acting therapy may be administered as a β_2-agonist or anticholinergic.

β_2-Agonists β_2-Agonists cause airway smooth muscle relaxation by stimulating adenyl cyclase to increase the formation of cyclic adenosine monophosphate (cAMP).[24-28] cAMP is responsible for mediating relaxation of bronchial smooth muscle, leading to bronchodilation. β_2-Agonists are available in inhalation, oral, and parenteral dosage forms; the inhalation route is preferred because of fewer adverse reactions. β_2-Agonists are available in short-acting, long-acting, and selective/nonselective formulations (Table 42-4). Short-acting β_2-agonists are used for acute symptom relief and maintenance therapy. Short-acting β_2-agonists require frequent dosing (albuterol 2 puffs every 6 hours when prescribed on a scheduled basis) and often lose effectiveness when used regularly for more than 3 months (tachyphylaxis). Long-acting β_2-agonists (see Table 42-4)

TABLE 42-4 β_2-Agonists for COPD[a]

Generic Name	Brand Name	Selectivity	Formulations	Indication	Special Considerations
Short-Acting β_2-Agonists					
Albuterol	Proventil; Ventolin	$\beta_1 < \beta_2$	Inhalation, nebulization, oral	Rescue and maintenance for COPD	Tachyphylaxis; requires frequent dosing for maintenance therapy. Adverse reactions: tachycardia, heart palpitations, tremor; use with caution in patients with cardiovascular disease, diabetes, hyperthyroidism, or hypokalemia.
Levalbuterol	Xopenex	$\beta_1 < \beta_2$	Inhalation, nebulization	Rescue and maintenance for COPD	Tachyphylaxis; requires frequent dosing for maintenance therapy. Adverse reactions (less than albuterol): tachycardia, heart palpitations, tremor; use with caution in patients with cardiovascular disease, diabetes, hyperthyroidism, or hypokalemia.
Isoproterenol	Isuprel	β_1 and β_2	Injection, solution	Ventricular and brady arrhythmias	Sympathomimetic with significant stimulatory effect on β_1 receptor (therefore no role in COPD). Adverse effects: cardiovascular—tachycardia, arrhythmias, hyper-/hypotension
Pirbuterol	Maxair	$\beta_1 < \beta_2$	Inhalation	Rescue or maintenance for COPD	Same as albuterol
Epinephrine	Adrenalin; EpiPen; Epifrin; Primatene Mist	β_1 and β_2	Inhalation; injection; solution; ophthalmic solution	Cardiac arrest; open-angle glaucoma; acute treatment of bronchospasm	Same as isoproterenol
Long-Acting β_2-Agonists					
Formoterol	Foradil	$\beta_1 < \beta_2$	Powder for oral inhalation	Maintenance for COPD	Should not be used as rescue inhaler. β_2 (short- and long-acting) may increase risk of arrhythmias, decrease serum potassium, prolong QTc interval, or increase serum glucose. Use with caution in patients with cardiovascular disease, diabetes, hyperthyroidism, or hypokalemia. β-Agonists may cause elevation in blood pressure, heart rate, and result in CNS stimulation/excitation.
Salmeterol	Serevent	$\beta_1 < \beta_2$	Powder for oral inhalation	Maintenance for COPD	Same as formoterol

[a]Albuterol, levalbuterol, salmeterol, and formoterol are used in the management of COPD. Other β_2-agonists listed are not commonly used in COPD, but are listed for you to be able to compare and contrast the different types of β_2-agonists.

last at least 12 hours, allowing for twice daily dosing and have not been shown to lose effectiveness with regular use. Long-acting β_2-agonists are more effective and convenient than short-acting β_2-agonists for maintenance therapy, but more expensive. If a patient has a prescription for a long-acting β_2-agonist, patients should also have a short-acting β_2-agonists available for as-needed use (rescue). Less-selective β_2-agonists (eg, metaproterenol, isoproterenol, and epinephrine) should not be used because of short duration of action and increased cardiostimulatory effects. Short-acting, selective β_2-agonists (albuterol, levalbuterol, and pirbuterol) are preferred for therapy. Adverse effects of β_2-agonists are dose-related and include palpitations, tachycardia, and tremor. Sleep disturbances may also occur and appear to be worse with higher doses of inhaled long-acting β_2-agonists.[24-28] Increasing doses beyond those clinically recommended is without benefit and could be associated with increased adverse effects.

Anticholinergics Ipratropium and tiotropium are inhaled anticholinergic medications commonly used for COPD. The anticholinergics produce bronchodilation by competitively blocking muscarinic receptors in bronchial smooth muscle.[32-33] This activity blocks acetylcholine, with the net effect of a reduction in cyclic guanosine monophosphate. Cyclic guanosine monophosphate normally causes bronchial smooth muscle constriction. They may also decrease mucus secretion, although this effect is variable. Tiotropium dissociates from receptors extremely slowly resulting in a half-life longer than 36 hours, allowing for once-daily dosing.[33] Ipratropium has an elimination half-life of about 2 hours, necessitating dosing every 6 to 8 hours.[32] Inhaled anticholinergics are well-tolerated with the most common adverse effect being dry mouth. Occasional metallic taste has also been reported with ipratropium. Other anticholinergic adverse effects include constipation, tachycardia, blurred vision, urinary retention, and precipitation of narrow-angle glaucoma symptoms.[32-33] Atropine is an anticholinergic available in oral and inhalation formulations. Atropine has a tertiary structure and is absorbed across the oral and respiratory mucosa, whereas ipratropium and tiotropium have quaternary structures that are poorly absorbed. The lack of systemic absorption of ipratropium and tiotropium greatly diminishes the anticholinergic side effects compared to atropine. Table 42-5 compares the inhaled anticholinergics.

Methylxanthines Methylxanthines, including theophylline and aminophylline, have been available for the treatment of COPD for decades and at one time was considered a first-line agent. Currently the role of methylxanthines has been limited to a patient not responding to β_2-agonists, anticholinergics, or corticosteroids.[1] Although theophylline is available in a variety of oral dosage forms, sustained relief preparations are most appropriate for the long-term management of COPD.[1,34] These products have the advantage of improving patient compliance and achieving more consistent serum concentrations over rapid release theophylline and aminophylline preparations. However, caution must be used when switching from one sustained release preparation to another because there are considerable variations in sustained-release characteristics. Aside from IV aminophylline, there is no need to use any of the various salt forms of theophylline. Methylxanthines are nonspecific phosphodiesterase inhibitors that increase intracellular cAMP within airway smooth muscle resulting in bronchodilation.[34] It has a modest bronchodilator effect and its use is limited due to a narrow therapeutic index, multiple-drug interactions, and adverse effects. Theophylline's bronchodilator effects are dependent upon achieving adequate serum concentrations, and therapeutic drug monitoring is needed to optimize therapy because of wide interpatient variability.[34] If theophylline is used, serum concentrations in the range of 5 to 15 mg/L (28 to 83 μmol/L) provide adequate clinical response with a greater margin of safety than the traditionally recommended range of 10 to 20 mg/L (55 t o110 μmol/L).[1] The most common adverse effects include heartburn, restlessness, insomnia, irritability, tachycardia, and tremor.[34] Dose-related adverse effects include nausea and vomiting, seizures, and arrhythmias.[34] Tobacco smoke contains a chemical that induce the cytochrome P-450 isoenzymes 1A1, 1A2, and 2E1.[34] Theophylline is metabolized by 1A2 and 2E1, and therefore, smoking leads to increased clearance of theophylline.

Corticosteroids

Symptomatic patients with severe COPD (FEV_1 less than 50% predicted) and frequent exacerbations should be considered for treatment with inhaled corticosteroids. Regular treatment with *inhaled* corticosteroids decreases the number of exacerbations per year and improves health status; however, corticosteroids therapy does not slow the long-term decline in

TABLE 42-5 **Inhaled Anticholinergics for COPD**

Generic Name	Brand Name	Formulation	Duration	Indication for COPD	Special Considerations
Ipratropium	Atrovent	Oral inhalation; nasal spray	Short	Maintenance therapy for COPD	Paradoxical bronchospasm may occur; not indicated for initial treatment of acute episodes of bronchospasm; use with caution in patients with myasthenia gravis, narrow-angle glaucoma, and benign prostatic hyperplasia
Tiotropium	Spiriva	Powder for oral inhalation	Long	Maintenance therapy for COPD	Same as ipratropium

TABLE 42-6 Inhaled Corticosteroids[a,b] for COPD

Generic Name	Brand Name	Formulations
Beclomethasone	Beconase AQ	Aerosol for inhalation; suspension (nasal)
Budesonide	Pulmicort	Powder for oral inhalation; suspension (nasal)
Ciclesonide	Alvesco	Aerosol for oral inhalation; suspension (nasal)
Flunisolide	AeroBid	Aerosol for oral inhalation; suspension (nasal)
Fluticasone	Flovent	Aerosol for oral inhalation; cream; lotion; ointment; powder for oral inhalation; suspension (nasal)
Mometasone	Asmanex	Powder for oral inhalation; suspension (nasal); cream; lotion; ointment
Triamcinolone	Azmacort	Aerosol for oral inhalation; cream; injection; lotion; paste; powder; suspension (nasal)

[a]Special considerations: Rinse mouth and throat after use to prevent *Candida* infection. Not for use for the relief of acute bronchospasm (oral systemic corticosteroids may be utilized for COPD exacerbations). Monitoring parameters—growth (adolescents and children[b]), signs and symptoms of adrenal suppression.

[b]Orally inhaled and intranasal corticosteroids may cause a reduction in growth velocity in pediatric patients. COPD patients are often 50 years of age or greater and therefore growth reduction would not be an issue; however, these inhalers may be utilized in younger patients diagnosed with asthma.

pulmonary function.[1] The anti-inflammatory mechanisms of corticosteroids include: (1) reduction in capillary permeability to decrease mucus, (2) inhibition of release of proteolytic enzymes from leukocytes, and (3) inhibition of prostaglandins.[1,35-41] Currently, the appropriate situations to consider corticosteroids in COPD include (1) short-term systemic use for acute exacerbations and (2) inhalation therapy for chronic COPD.[1] Long-term systemic corticosteroid use should be avoided due to an unfavorable risk/benefit ratio. The steroid myopathy that can result from long-term use of oral corticosteroids weakens muscles, further decreasing the respiratory drive in patients with advanced disease.[1] Other long-term adverse effects of systemic corticosteroid therapy include osteoporosis, thinning of the skin, development of cataracts, and adrenal suppression and insufficiency.[35-41] The use of chronic inhaled corticosteroid therapy has been of interest for the past decade. Their use has been common despite the lack of firm evidence about significant clinical benefit until recently. Inhaled corticosteroids have an improved risk-to-benefit ratio compared to systemic corticosteroid therapy. Upon discontinuation of inhaled corticosteroids, some patients experience deterioration in lung function and an increase in dyspnea and mild exacerbations; it is reasonable to reinstitute the medication in these patients. The most common adverse effects from inhaled corticosteroid therapy include oropharyngeal candidiasis and hoarse voice.[35-41] These can be minimized by rinsing the mouth after use and by using a spacer device with metered-dose inhalers (MDI). Table 42-6 lists the inhaled corticosteroids and Table 42-7 lists formulations and doses for commonly used COPD medications.

SPECIAL CONSIDERATIONS

Other Pharmacologic Therapies

The American Thoracic Society and the European Respiratory Society have published standards for the diagnosis and management of patients with Alpha1-antitrypsin (AAT) deficiency. They recommend augmentation therapy for individuals with AAT deficiency and moderate airflow obstruction (FEV_1 35%-60% predicted).[1,42] Augmentation therapy consists of weekly transfusions of pooled human AAT with the goal of maintaining adequate plasma levels of the enzyme. Augmentation therapy is not recommended for individuals with AAT deficiency who do not demonstrate lung disease.

Leukotriene modifiers (zafirlukast and montelukast) have not been adequately evaluated in COPD patients and are not recommended for routine use. Nedocromil, a mast cell stabilizer, has not been adequately tested in COPD patients and is not included in the GOLD recommendations. *N*-acetylcysteine has antioxidant and mucolytic activity, which makes it a promising agent for COPD treatment, but current evidence have produced conflicting results. Routine use of *N*-acetylcysteine cannot be recommended at this time. Prophylactic antibiotics have no effect on the frequency of COPD exacerbations and should only be used for treating infectious exacerbations. Antitussives are contraindicated in COPD because cough has an important protective role.[1]

Pharmacologic Therapy of COPD Exacerbations

An exacerbation is a sustained worsening of the patient's symptoms from his or her usual stable state that is beyond normal day to day variations. Commonly reported symptoms are worsening of dyspnea, increased sputum production, and change in sputum color. The most common causes of an exacerbation are respiratory infection and air pollution, but the cause cannot be identified in about one-third of severe exacerbations. Treatment depends upon the symptoms and severity of the exacerbation. Mild exacerbations can often be treated at home with an increase in bronchodilator therapy with or without oral corticosteroids. Antibiotics are indicated only if there are clinical signs of airway infection (eg, increased volume and change in color of sputum and/or fever). Moderate to severe exacerbations require management in the emergency department or hospital. Management should consist of controlled oxygen therapy, bronchodilators, oral or IV corticosteroids, antibiotics if indicated, and consideration of mechanical ventilation.

TABLE 42-7 Formulations and Doses for Commonly Used COPD Medications

Generic/Brand Name	Formulation	Onset	Usual Dose
Short-Acting β_2-Agonists			
Albuterol	Nebulization	5-15 min	2.5 mg every 6-8 h (max: 30 mg/d)
	Inhalation	5-15 min	MDI (90 μg/puff) 1-2 puffs every 4-6 h (max: 1080 μg/d)
	Oral	7-30 min	2-4 mg three to four times per d; extended release: 4-8 mg every 12 h (max:32 mg/d)
Levalbuterol (Xopenex)	Nebulization	10-20 min	0.63-1.25 mg tid, 6-8 h apart (max: 3.75 mg/d)
	Inhalation	5-10 min	MDI (45 μg/puff) 1-2 puffs every 4-6 h (max: 540 μg/d)
Long Acting β_2-Agonists			
Salmeterol (Serevent)	Inhalation	10 min-2 h	Powder (50 μg/inhalation) one inhalation every 12 h (max: 100 μg/d)
Formoterol (Foradil)	Inhalation	1-3 min	Powder 912 μg/inhalation) one inhalation every 12 h (max: 24 μg/d)
Inhaled Corticosteroids			
Beclomethasone	Inhalation	1-7 d	MDI (40, 80 μg/puff) 40-160 μg bid (max:640 μg/d)
Budesonide	Inhalation	1-7 d	Powder (200 μg/inhalation) one to two inhalations twice a d
Fluticasone	Inhalation	1-7 d	MDI (44, 110, 220 μg/puff) 88-440 μg twice a d (max: 1760 μg/d)
Triamcinolone	Inhalation	1-7 d	MDI (100 μg/puff) two puffs three to four times per d or four puffs twice a d (max: 1600 μg/d)
Methylxanthines			
Theophylline	Oral	0.2-2 h	400-600 μg/d divided every 6-24 h based upon the formulation. Doses vary widely and should be based upon pharmacokinetic considerations and plasma theophylline concentrations. Aminophylline is the most widely used salt of theophylline. Aminophylline is usually administered by slow IV injection. The bronchodilation effects of theophylline are proportional to the log of the theophylline concentration. This means that as the theophylline concentration increases, there will be a less than proportional increase in bronchodilation. Patients should always be maintained at the lowest possible theophylline-plasma concentration that produces a satisfactory response. There are numerous factors or disease states that impact theophylline clearance (smoking, cirrhosis, heart failure, drug interactions). The formulation Theo-24 has been associated with dose-dumping when combined with a high-fat meal, other formulations have not been associated with dose dumping.

Outcome Evaluation

COPD patients should be monitored for improvement or worsening of symptoms (dyspnea, cough, sputum production, and fatigue). Changes in the FEV_1 should not be the main outcome that is monitored. FEV_1 changes are weakly related to symptoms, exacerbations, and health related quality of life.

CASE Application

1. A patient presents with symptoms of shortness of breath, nonproductive cough and the following spirometry results: prebronchodilator FEV_1: 69% predicted; post-bronchodilator FEV_1: 70% predicted; FEV_1/FVC ratio: 0.64. How would you interpret these findings?
   a. This patient has COPD with reversible airway obstruction
   b. This patient has COPD with irreversible airway obstruction
   c. This patient has asthma with reversible airway obstruction
   d. This patient has asthma with irreversible airway obstruction
   e. This patient does not have COPD or asthma

2. Which of the following characterized alpha1 antitrypsin (AAT) deficiency?
   a. Onset at a late age (> 50 years)
   b. Disease caused by environmental factors
   c. Disease caused by genetic factors
   d. Prominent in African American populations
   e. Disease caused by oxidative stress

3. Which of the following is first-line treatment for a patient diagnosed with COPD (stage I)?
   a. Short-acting bronchodilator
   b. Long-acting anticholinergic
   c. Long-acting β-agonist
   d. Inhaled corticosteroid
   e. Oral theophylline

4. A patient with COPD complains of developing a tremor since starting one of his medications. Which medication is the most likely cause?

   a. Ipratropium
   b. Tiotropium
   c. Fluticasone
   d. Prednisone
   e. Albuterol

5. Which of the following is the most likely side effect to be caused by inhaled corticosteroids?

   a. Oral candidiasis
   b. Glucose intolerance
   c. Tachycardia
   d. Immunosuppression
   e. Weight gain

6. Which of the following are advantages of using a spacer device with a metered-dose inhaler?

   a. Decreased oropharyngeal deposition
   b. Enhanced lung delivery
   c. Less hand-lung coordination needed
   d. Reduced side effects from inhaled corticosteroids
   e. All of the above

7. SS is a 68-year-old woman who smokes and has recently been diagnosed with mild COPD. In addition to a short-acting bronchodilator, what would you recommend for her treatment?

   i. Smoking cessation
   ii. Influenza vaccine yearly
   iii. Pneumococcal vaccine
   iv. Oxygen therapy

   a. i only
   b. i and ii
   c. i, ii, and iii
   d. i and iii
   e. All of the above

8. The clinical presentation of COPD can include which of the following?

   a. Dyspnea
   b. Chronic cough
   c. Sputum production
   d. Exposure to risk factors
   e. All of the above

9. When should a trial of inhaled corticosteroids be considered for a patient with COPD?

   a. Stage I with a short-acting β-agonist
   b. Stage II with a long-acting β-agonist
   c. Stage II with a long-acting anticholinergic
   d. Stage III with at least two other medications
   e. Stage III with repeated exacerbations

10. PL is a 75-year-old man who has been experiencing increased dyspnea for the last month. He was diagnosed with COPD 3 years ago and has been taking albuterol metered-dose inhaler on an as needed (prn) basis. His most recent spirometry results are: FEV_1/FVC ratio of 0.65 and FEV_1 65% of predicted. Which of the following is the best choice for changing his medication regimen?

    a. Add scheduled tiotropium and continue prn albuterol
    b. Add scheduled fluticasone and continue prn albuterol
    c. Add prn salmeterol and continue prn albuterol
    d. Add scheduled theophylline and continue prn albuterol
    e. No changes are necessary at this time.

11. Select the COPD medications that can be used concurrently in a maintenance regimen for a patient with stage III COPD.

    a. Levalbuterol and albuterol
    b. Albuterol and formoterol
    c. Formoterol and salmeterol
    d. Fluticasone and flunisolide
    e. Theophylline and aminophylline

12. Select the disease state or factor that can affect the clearance of theophylline.

    a. Smoking history
    b. Hepatic cirrhosis
    c. Drug interactions (cytochrome P-450 inhibitors especially 1A2, 2E1, 3A4)
    d. a and b
    e. a, b, and c

13. Select the formulation of the corticosteroid that should be utilized in maintenance therapy for COPD.

    a. IV/injection (methylprednisolone)
    b. Oral (prednisone)
    c. Inhalation (fluticasone)
    d. Nasal (fluticasone)

14. Select the central nervous system side effect of aminophylline when levels exceed 20 μg/mL.

    a. Hypotension
    b. Arrhythmias
    c. Nausea and vomiting
    d. Seizures

15. Albuterol is a short-acting bronchodilator recommended for treatment of COPD by treatment guidelines. Select the dose(s) of albuterol that may be utilized/preferred in the treatment of COPD.

    a. Albuterol inhalation (metered-dose inhaler—90 μg/puff) —two puffs every 6 hours
    b. Albuterol inhalation (metered-dose inhaler—90 μg/puff)— as needed "rescue" (prn)
    c. Albuterol oral—4 mg tid.
    d. a and b
    e. a, b, and c

16. A patient is receiving 32 mg/h of aminophylline. The patient is ready to be changed to oral theophylline. What would the daily dose of theophylline be that would equal 32 mg/h of aminophylline? Aminophylline's salt factor is 0.8.
    a. 614 mg
    b. 768 mg
    c. 300 mg
    d. 900 mg
17. Select the generic name of Symbicort.
    a. Fluticasone + salmeterol
    b. Albuterol + ipratropium
    c. Budesonide + formoterol
18. KT is a patient that presents to your clinic on Theo-24 (a sustained release/once a day theophylline product). She has experienced the dose-dumping effect when the agent is taken with a high-fat meal. She would like to be changed to another sustained release theophylline product that does not have the dose-dumping effect. Select the product that Theo-24 could be changed to:
    a. Theo-Dur twice daily
    b. Slo-Bid twice daily
    c. Uniphyl once daily
    d. All of the above
19. Select the COPD bronchodilator that is a phosphodiesterase inhibitor.
    a. Albuterol
    b. Salmeterol
    c. Ipratropium
    d. Fluticasone
    e. Theophylline
20. Select the albuterol formulation with the fastest onset.
    a. Nebulization
    b. Inhalation
    c. Oral
    d. a and c
    e. a and b

TAKEAWAY POINTS ››

- The prevalence, morbidity, and mortality trends of chronic obstructive pulmonary disease (COPD) are directly linked to the prevalence of cigarette smoking and air pollution.
- COPD is a preventable chronic disease of the airways that is characterized by gradual, progressive loss of lung function. It is characterized by airflow limitation that is not fully reversible.
- COPD is a progressive disease, and even with the best treatment, will worsen over time. There is no cure, with most treatment directed at managing symptoms. The most common complication of COPD is exacerbation of symptoms. A COPD exacerbation is defined as an acute change from baseline in cough and/or sputum production that is beyond day-to-day variations.
- Smoking cessation is the single most effective treatment for reducing the progression of COPD.
- All patients with COPD should receive the influenza vaccine annually. The CDC guidelines recommend the pneumococcal polysaccharide vaccination in all patients with chronic lung disease and in chronic smokers.
- Bronchodilators are the mainstay of treatment for symptomatic COPD. They reduce symptoms and improve exercise tolerance and quality of life. Bronchodilator medications commonly utilized for COPD include β_2-agonists and anticholinergics.
- In symptomatic patients with severe COPD (FEV_1 less than 50% predicted) and frequent exacerbations, regular treatment with *inhaled* corticosteroids decreases the number of exacerbations per year and improves health status; however, corticosteroid therapy does not slow the long-term decline in pulmonary function.
- COPD patients should be monitored for improvement or worsening of symptoms (dyspnea, cough, sputum production, and fatigue).

REFERENCES

1. Global Initiative for the Chronic Obstructive Lung Disease. Global strategy for the diagnosis, management, and prevention of chronic obstructive pulmonary disease. Available at: www.goldcopd.com. Updated 2008. Accessed August 11, 2009.
2. Pleis JR, Lucas JW. Summary health statistics for U.S. adults: National Health Interview Survey, 2007. National Center for Health Statistics. *Vital Health Stat.* 2009;10(240):1-159.
3. Smith CA, Harrison DJ. Association between polymorphism in gene for microsomal epoxide hydrolase and susceptibility to emphysema. *Lancet.* 1997;350(9078):630-633.
4. Stoller JK, Aboussouan LS. Alpha 1 antitrypsin deficiency. *Lancet.* 2005;365(9478):2225-2236.
5. Blanco I, de Serres FJ, Fernandez-Bustillo E, et al. Estimated numbers and prevalence of PI*S and PI*Z alleles of alpha 1 antitrypsin deficiency in European countries. *Eur Respir J.* 2006;27(1):77-84.
6. Hnizdo E, Sullivan PA, Bang KM, et al. Association between chronic obstructive pulmonary disease and employment by industry and occupation in the US population: a study of data from the Third National Health and Nutrition Examination Survey. *Am J Epidemiol.* 2002;156(8):738-746.

7. Balmes J, Becklake M, Blanc P, et al. American Thoracic Society Statement: occupational contribution to the burden of airway disease. *Am J Respir Crit Care Med.* 2003;167(5):787-797.
8. Ezzati M. Indoor air pollution and health in developing countries. *Lancet.* 2005;366(9480):104-106.
9. Abbey DE, Burchette RJ, Knutsen SF, et al. Long-term particulate and other air pollutants and lung function in nonsmokers. *Am J Respir Crit Care Med.* 1998;158(1):289-298.
10. Lawlor DA, Ebrahim S, Davey Smith G. Association of birth weight with adult lung function: findings from the British Women's Heart and Health Study and a meta-analysis. *Thorax.* 2005;60(10):851-858.
11. MacNee W. Pulmonary and systemic oxidant/antioxidant imbalance in chronic obstructive pulmonary disease. *Proc Am Thorac Soc.* 2005;2(1):50-60.
12. Seemungal T, Harper-Owen R, Bhowmik A, et al. Respiratory viruses, symptoms and inflammatory markers in acute exacerbations and stable chronic obstructive pulmonary diseases. *Am J Respir Crit Care Med.* 2001;164(9):1618-1623.
13. Hogg JC. Pathophysiology of airflow limitation in chronic obstructive pulmonary disease. *Lancet.* 2004;364(9435):709-721.
14. Conners AF, Jr., Dawson NV, Thomas C, et al. Outcomes following acute exacerbation of sever chronic obstructive lung disease. The SUPPORT investigators (Study to Understand Prognoses and Preferences for Outcomes and Risks of Treatments). *Am J Respir Crit Care Med.* 1996;154(4 Pt 1):959-967.
15. Barbera JA, Peinado VI, Santos, S. Pulmonary hypertension in chronic obstructive pulmonary disease. *Eur Respir J.* 2003;21(5):892-905.
16. Agusti AG, Noguera A, Sauleda J, et al. Systemic effects of chronic obstructive pulmonary disease. *Eur Respir J.* 2003;21(2):347-360.
17. Fiore MC, Jaen CR, Baker TB, et al. Treating tobacco use and dependence: 2008 Update. *Clinical Practice Guideline.* Rockville, MD: U.S. Department of Health and Human Services. Public Health Service; May 2008.
18. Nocturnal Oxygen Therapy Trial Group. Continuous or nocturnal oxygen therapy in hypoxemic chronic obstructive lung disease: a clinical trial. *Ann Intern Med.* 1980;93(3):391-398.
19. Report of the Medical Research Council Working Party. Long-term domiciliary oxygen therapy in chronic hypoxic cor pulmonale complicating chronic bronchitis and emphysema. *Lancet.* 1981;1(8222):681-686.
20. Targpy SP, Celli BR. Long-term oxygen therapy. *N Engl J Med.* 1995;333(11):710-714.
21. Weitzenblum E, Sautegeau A, Ehrhart M, Mammosser M, Pelletier A. Long-term oxygen therapy can reserve the progression of pulmonary hypertension in patients with chronic obstructive pulmonary disease. *Am Rev Respir Dis.* 1985;131(4):493-498.
22. Zielinski J, Tobiasz M, Hawrylkiewicz I, et al. Effects of long-term oxygen therapy on pulmonary hemodynamics in COPD patients: a 6-year prospective study. *Chest.* 1998;113(1):65-70.
23. Centers for Disease Control and Prevention. Recommended adult immunization schedule—United States, 2009. *MMWR.* 2008;57(53).
24. Proventil [package insert]. Kenilworth, NJ: Schering Corporation; 2009.
25. Ventolin [package insert]. Research Triangle Park, NC: GlaxoSmithKline; 2009.
26. Xopenex [package insert]. Marlborough, MA: Sepracor Inc.; 2009.
27. Isuprel [package insert]. Chicago, IL: Abbott Laboratories; 2006
28. Maxair [package insert]. Northridge, CA: 3M Pharmaceuticals; 2006
29. Epinephrine injection [package insert]. North Chicago, IL: Abbott Laboratories; 2009.
30. Foradil [package insert]. Kenilworth, NJ: Schering Corporation; 2010.
31. Serevent [package insert]. Research Triangle Park, NC: GlaxoSmithKline; 2010.
32. Atrovent [package insert]. Ridgefield, CT: Boehringer Ingelheim Pharmaceuticals; 2010.
33. Spiriva [package insert]. Ridgefield, CT: Boehringer Ingelheim Pharmaceuticals; 2006.
34. Uniphyl [package insert]. Stamford, CT: The Purdue Frederick Company; 2010.
35. Beconase AQ [package insert]. Research Triangle Park, NC: GlaxoSmithKline; 2009.
36. Pulmicort [package insert]. Wilmington, DE: AztraZeneca; 2010.
37. Alvesco [package insert]. Florham, NJ: Nycomed; 2007.
38. AeroBid [package insert]. St Louis, MO: Forest Laboratories; 2002.
39. Flovent [package insert]. Research Triangle Park, NC. GlaxoSmithKline; 2008.
40. Asmanex [package insert]. Kenilworth, NJ: Schering Corporation: UCB Inc.; 2010.
41. Azmacort [package insert]. Cranbury, NJ: KOS Pharmaceuticals; 2007.
42. Juvelekian GS, Stroller JK. Augmentation therapy for alpha 1 antitrypsin deficiency. *Drugs.* 2004;64(16):1743-1756.

CHAPTER

43 Asthma

Wendy Brown

FOUNDATION OVERVIEW

According to the National Health Interview Survey (NHIS), asthma prevalence rates in the United States are 7.3% in adults and 9.3% in children. This equates to $16.1 billon in indirect and direct expenses associated with asthma according to the American Lung Association Epidemiology and Statistics Unit Research Program. In the pediatric population males are more likely to report current asthma symptoms and in the adult population females are more likely to report the presence of asthma.[1] Evaluation of national surveillance data within a 3 year time period revealed 12.3 million physician visits, 1.3 million outpatient department visits within hospital systems, 1.8 million emergency department visits, and 4210 deaths attributed to asthma.[2] The rate of a health care encounter for asthma does not differ by race. When evaluating race in regard to health care settings, whites tend to utilize physician offices, whereas blacks have higher rates for hospital-based sites for asthma management.

Pathophysiology

The major characteristics of asthma are airway inflammation and bronchial hyper-responsiveness which cause variable degree of airflow obstruction.[3] In the asthmatic response, a genetically predisposed or atopic individual is exposed to a specific reactive stimuli or trigger. The most common asthma triggers are to molds, pollen, animal dander, and dust mites. Minutes after repeated exposure, the immediate asthmatic response occurs causing bronchoconstriction which resolves spontaneously or easily by β_2-agonist use. Within 4 to 12 hours after the immediate asthmatic response, the late asthmatic response, caused by influx of inflammatory cells primarily eosinophils, Th2 lymphocytes, mast cells, macrophages, and mediators such as leukotrienes, histamine, and prostaglandin infiltrate the airway. The reaction is often more severe and prolonged and is referred to as an asthma exacerbation. This chronic inflammation is postulated to cause hypertrophy and hyperplasia of the bronchial smooth muscle and mucus glands which may lead to permanent, irreversible obstruction termed airway remodeling.[4] The combination of airway obstruction and inflammation leads to the common symptoms of asthma which are cough, wheezing, chest tightness, and dyspnea.[5] Among children, nighttime cough may be the only symptom present.[6]

Diagnosis and Assessment of Control

Diagnosis is based on a thorough history with special focus on symptoms and genetic predisposition. The definitive diagnosis is made through the use of spirometry. This is a diagnostic test where a person exhales forcefully into a machine to determine if airflow obstruction is present. To determine if obstruction is present the ratio of the forced expiratory volume in 1 second (FEV_1) over forced vital capacity (FVC) is reviewed. (Table 43-1) To determine reversibility, as in asthma, a short-acting β-agonist (albuterol) is given and the post-bronchodilator FEV_1 is evaluated. If the FEV_1 improves greater or equal to 12% and 200 mL when compared to prebronchodilator value the person is diagnosed with asthma.[7] Once diagnosis is made, further age-specific evaluation based on impairment and risk is determined in order to classify severity and control of asthma. (Tables 43-1 and 43-2) A person is always assigned to the highest step based on the most severe symptom and then once control has been maintained for at least 3 months, therapy maybe stepped down.

TREATMENT

Asthma medications are classified into two broad categories of quick relief and long-term control. Independent of severity, all persons with asthma should have a quick relief medication readily available. The class of medication most commonly used as quick relievers are short-acting β_2-selective adrenergic agonists. (Table 43-3) Their mechanism of action is to stimulate β_2-receptor on bronchial smooth muscle to cause relaxation. All are equally effective, have an onset of action within 5 minutes, a peak at 30 to 60 minutes and duration of 4 to 6 hours.[8] The most common side effects associated with short-acting β_2-agonists are tremor, anxiety, and tachycardia. Small dose dependent decreases in serum potassium and magnesium have been observed. Overuse of short-acting β_2-agonists is defined as need for medication use for symptoms of asthma more than 2 days per week or more than twice in a month for nighttime awakenings.[7] Long-term controller medication should be evaluated for patients who overuse short-acting β_2-agonists. Of the long-term controller medications, "Inhaled corticosteroids constitute the drug class that has the greatest effect in helping patients achieve well-controlled asthma."[5] Through their broad effects on gene transcription, they suppress but do not cure,

TABLE 43-1 **Asthma Severity Classification**

	Age	Intermittent[a]— Step 1	Mild Persistent[a]—Step 2	Moderate Persistent[a]—Step 3	Severe Persistent[a]— Steps 4-6
FEV_1/FVC Normal **8-19 y = 85%** **20-39 y = 80%** **40-59 y = 75%** **60-80 y = 70%**	0-4 y	≤2 d/wk symptoms 0 (zero) HS awakenings ≤ 2 d/wk SABA use No limit on normal activity Exacerbation 0-1 × y	>2d/wk symptoms 1-2 × mo HS awakenings > 2 d/wk SABA use; not qd SABA Minor limit on normal activity Exacerbation ≥2 × 6 mo; >4 wheezing episodes 1 y lasting >1 d	Daily symptoms 3-4 × mo HS awakenings Daily SABA use Some limit on normal activity Exacerbation ≥2 × 6 mo; >4 wheezing episodes 1 y lasting > 1 d	Symptoms throughout the day >1 ×/wk HS awakenings Several times qd SABA use Extremely limits normal activity Exacerbation ≥2 × 6 mo; >4 wheezing episodes 1 y lasting >1 d
	5-11 y	Symptoms, HS awakenings SABA use, activity, and exacerbation same 12+ FEV_1>80%, Normal FEV_1/FVC	Symptoms, HS awakenings SABA use, activity, and exacerbation same 12+ FEV_1 = 80%, FEV_1/FVC>80%	Symptoms, HS awakenings SABA use, activity, and exacerbation same 12+ FEV_1 60%-80% FEV_1/FVC 75%-80%	Symptoms, HS awakenings SABA use, activity, and exacerbation same 12+ FEV_1<60%, FEV_1/FVC <75%
	12 + y	≤2 d/wk symptoms ≤2 × mo HS awakenings ≤ 2 d/wk SABA No limit on normal activity FEV_1 >80%, Normal FEV_1/FVC Exacerbation 0-1 × y	>2d/wk symptoms 3-4 × mo HS awakenings > 2 d/wk; not qd; not >1 ×/d SABA Minor limit on normal activity FEV_1 >80%, Normal FEV_1/FVC Exacerbation ≥2 × y	Daily symptoms >1 ×/wk not every HS awakenings Daily SABA Some limit on normal activity FEV_1>60% and < 80%, FEV_1/FVC decreased ≤5% Exacerbation ≥ 2 × y	Symptoms throughout the day 7 ×/wk HS awakenings Several times qd SABA use Extremely limits normal activity FEV_1<60%, FEV_1/FVC decreased >5% Exacerbation ≥2 × y
			Treatment[d]		
	0-4 y	SABA prn	Low ICS Alternatives: Cromolyn/Montelukast	Medium ICS	Step 4: Medium ICS + LABA or montelukast Step 5: High ICS+ LABA or montelukast Step 6: High ICS+ LABA or montelukast + po steroid
	5-11 y	SABA prn	Low ICS Alternatives: Cromolyn/LTRA/Theophylline	Low ICS + LABA, LTRA, or theophylline or Medium ICS	Step 4: Medium ICS + LABA[b] Step 5: High ICS+ LABA[b] Step 6: High ICS+ LABA+ po steroid[b]
	12 + y	SABA prn	Low ICS Alternatives: Cromolyn/LTRA/Theophylline	Low ICS + LABA or Medium ICS Alternative: Low ICS + LTRA/Theophylline or zileuton	Step 4: Medium ICS + LABA[c] Step 5: High ICS+ LABA consider omalizumab Step 6: High ICS+ LABA+ po steroid consider omalizumab

[a]Require a SABA prn regardless of need for controller therapy.

[b]Alternatives: ICS + LTRA or theophylline

[c]Alternatives: ICS + LTRA, theophylline, or zileuton

[d]Patient is reassessed in 2-6 wk for effectiveness of therapy. When patient is controlled for 3 mo, therapy is step down.

Abbreviation: HS, at bedtime.

Reproduced with permission from Expert Panel Report 3-Diagnosis and Management of Asthma. NIH Publication Number 09-6147

TABLE 43-2 **Asthma Control Classification**

Age	Well-controlled	Not well-controlled	Very poorly controlled
0-4 y	≤2 d/wk symptoms ≤1 ×/mo HS awakenings ≤ 2 d/wk SABA No limit on normal activity 0-1 × y Exacerbation requires po steroids	>2d/wk symptoms >1 ×/ mo HS awakenings > 2 d/wk SABA Some limit on normal activity 2-3/y exacerbation requires po steroids	Daily symptoms > 1 × wk HS awakenings Several times per day SABA Extreme limit on normal activity > 3/y exacerbation requires po steroids
5-11 y	≤2 d/wk not more than once qd symptoms ≤1 ×/mo HS awakenings ≤ 2 d/wk SABA No limit on normal activity 0-1 × y exacerbation requires po steroids FEV_1or PEF>80%, FEV_1/FVC>80%	>2 d/wk or multiple times qd ≤2 d/wk symptoms ≥2 ×/mo HS awakenings > 2 d/wk SABA Some limit on normal activity ≥2 × y exacerbation requires po steroids FEV_1 or PEF 60%-80%, FEV_1/FVC 75%-80%	Throughout the day ≥2 ×/wk HS awakenings Several times per day SABA Extreme limit on normal activity ≥2 × y exacerbation requires po steroids FEV_1 or PEF <60%, FEV_1/FVC <75%
12 + y	≤2 d/wk symptoms ≤2 × mo HS awakenings ≤ 2 d/wk SABA No limit on normal activity FEV_1 or PEF >80% ATAQ = 0, ACQ ≤0.75, ACT ≥20 Exacerbation 0-1 × y	>2d/wk symptoms 1-3 ×/wk HS awakenings >2 d/wk SABA Some limit on normal activity FEV_1 or PEF 60%-80% ATAQ = 1-2, ACQ ≥1.5, ACT = 16-19 Exacerbation ≥2 × y	Throughout the day ≥4 ×/wk HS awakenings Several times per day SABA Extreme limit on normal activity FEV_1 or PEF>60% ATAQ = 3-4, ACQ = N/A, ACT ≤15 Exacerbation ≥ 2 × y
		Treatment[a]	
0-4 y	Continue current treatment Follow up 1-6 mo Step down when controlled for 3 mo	Step up one step Follow up 2-6 wk if no improvement consider alternative dx or adjusting therapy for SE consider alternative tx	Burst po corticosteroid Step up 1-2 steps Follow up 2 wk if no improvement consider alternative dx or adjusting therapy for SE consider alternative tx
5-11 y	Continue current treatmentFollow up 1-6 mo	Step up one step Follow up 2-6 wk	Burst po corticosteroid
12 + y	Step down when controlled for 3 mo	SE consider alternative treatment options	Step up 1-2 steps SE consider alternative treatment options

[a]Before step up on therapy review medication adherence, inhaler technique, environmental control

Abbreviations: ACT, asthma control test; ACQ, asthma control questionnaire; ATAQ, asthma therapy assessment questionnaire; dx, diagnosis; FEV_1,forced expiratory volume in one second; FVC, forced vital capacity; ICS, inhaled corticosteroid; HS, at bedtime; LABA, long-acting β-agonist; LTRA, leukotriene receptor antagonist; SABA, short-acting β-agonist; SE, side effects; tx, treatment.

Reproduced with permission from Expert Panel Report 3-Diagnosis and Management of Asthma. NIH Publication Number 09-6147

multiple mediators of airway inflammation.[9] All are equally effective at controlling bronchial inflammation and decreasing airway hyperresponsiveness, however, they are not equivalent on a microgram per microgram or puff per puff basis.[7] In order to achieve maximum benefit they must be used on a daily basis and education must be provided that it will take at least 2 weeks to 1 month for full effect. The most common side effects of low to medium dose-inhaled corticosteroids are thrush and dysphonia.[10] To minimize and prevent these side effects, persons with asthma should be encouraged to rinse and spit with water after inhaler use. At high doses over prolonged periods, patient's risk of developing adrenal suppression, osteoporosis, skin thinning, and cataract formation increases.[1] To maintain a low to medium steroid dose, additional long-term medications such as long-acting β_2-agonists, leukotriene modifiers, cromolyn, theophylline, and/or omalizumab (Xolair) are added based on patient's asthma severity. Current long-acting β_2-agonists (LABA) have a duration of action of approximately 12 hours. Due to the SMART trial and subsequent black box warning in regard to increased risk of death, these medications should never be used alone for control of asthma.[11] Subsequently, there are three formulations available: Fluticasone/salmeterol (Advair), budesonide/formoterol (Symbicort), and Mometasone/formoterol (Dulera). Leukotriene modifiers are divided into two categories to target inflammation. Two antagonize the leukotriene receptor where as the original drug, Zileuton, within this class acts as a 5-lipoxygenase inhibitor (Table 43-3). Common side effects are related to the gastrointestinal tract and most recently a caution has been added to monitor for behavior and mood changes. Zafirlukast absorption is affected by food and zileuton may elevate liver enzymes. Theophylline is currently considered as an adjunct option due to its long-acting bronchial dilatory properties, however, it is not used as often due to its narrow therapeutic range, dose-related

TABLE 43-3 **Medications**

Mechanism of Action	Drugs
Short-acting β_2-selective adrenergic agonists	Albuterol (ProAir, Provental, Ventolin), levalbuterol (Xopenex), and pirbuterol (Maxair)
Long-acting β_2-selective adrenergic agonists	Salmeterol (Serevent) and formoterol (Foradil)
Inhaled corticosteroids	Beclomethasone (QVAR), budesonide (Pulmicort) [only pregnancy category B corticosteroid], ciclesonide (Alvesco) [a pro-drug that activates via enzymes in respiratory tract], flunisolide (AeroBid, Aerospan), fluticasone (Flovent), and mometasone (Asmanex)
Leukotriene receptor antagonists	Montelukast (Singulair) and zafirlukast (Accolate)
5-Lipoxygenase inhibitor	Zileuton (Zyflo CR)
Methylxanthine	Theophylline (Theo-Dur, Theo-24, Uniphyl)
Mast cell stabilizer	Cromolyn (Intal, Nalcrom)
Monoclonal antibody	Omalizumab (Xolair)

side effects, and significant drug-drug interactions due to its metabolism via the CYP-450 enzyme system. An additional alternative is the use of the mast cell stabilizer cromolyn. It has an extensive safety profile with minimal side effects. However due to its short duration of activity requiring three to four times a day dosing and decreased efficacy compared to inhaled corticosteroids, it is considered an alternative for patients with mild persistent asthma. For patients who are not well-controlled despite high-dose inhaler corticosteroids, have a significant allergic component and meet weight criteria, omalizumab (Xolair) may be prescribed. Omalizumab is a monoclonal antibody that attaches to free circulating IgE to prevent it from binding to mast cells, thus inhibiting part of the inflammatory response. It is given as a subcutaneous injection every 2 to 4 weeks. The most common side effect is injection site reaction. The clinically significant side effect that prompted a black box warning was related to anaphylaxis that may occur at any time during treatment.

Assessment of proper inhalation technique is important for maximal deposition of medication into the respiratory tract. With meter-dose inhaler formulations, a slow deep inhalation with the aid of a spacer or holding chamber is preferred. Dry powder formulation such as the Diskus, Twisthaler, Flexhaler, Aerolizer require a more forceful and deep inhalation. Prior to any adjustment of medication inhaler technique, adherence to medications via asthma action plan and environmental triggers should be evaluated.

For acute exacerbation of asthma, a 7- to 10-day course of oral corticosteroid may be required for quick relief of significant lung inflammation.

SPECIAL POPULATIONS

β-Blocker Use

In patients with asthma who have experienced a myocardial infarction and require a β-blocker, cardioselective β-blockers may be used. They have twenty times more affinity for the β_1 receptor versus β_2; thus at therapeutic doses (less than 50 mg/day for atenolol and 75 mg/day for metoprolol) their β_2-blocking effect is negligible.[12]

Pregnancy

In pregnancy, asthma may get better, stay the same, or get worse. When a person is well controlled on current therapy, continue therapy. The majority of asthma medications are category C and maintaining oxygenation is of greatest benefit to prevent preterm labor, low birth weight, and increased risk for caesarian section deliveries. When initiating inhaled corticosteroid therapy, budesonide (Pulmicort) has shown to be safe to use in pregnancy and has a category B designation.[13]

Children

The use of inhaled corticosteroids in children to control asthma is safe and effective with the greatest side effect of decrease in growth, velocity of 1 cm within the first year. Children are able to catch up in growth thus not affecting overall height.[14]

Exercise-Induced Bronchospasm

Exercise-induced asthma is diagnosed when there is a drop in FEV_1 by 15% after completion of physical activity. For prevention of bronchospasm, encourage a 10 minute warm up and cool down. One of the following medications may be given: short-acting β_2-agonist (albuterol, pirbuterol, or levalbuterol) or mast cell stabilizer at least 10 minutes before exercise (duration 2-3 hours or 1-2 hours, respectively), long-acting β2-agonist at least a half an hour before exercise (last 10-12 hours) or leukotriene receptor antagonist (LTRA) montelukast ≥ 2 hours before exercise.[15]

Comorbid Conditions

In persons with asthma who despite proper severity classification and medication management display poor control, additional comorbid conditions such as gastroesophageal reflux disease (GERD), obstructive sleep apnea, allergic rhinitis, and obesity should be evaluated.

Immunizations

All persons with asthma should receive an annual influenza vaccination. Pneumococcal polysaccharide (PPSV) is to be administered to all adults with asthma and a booster given after age 65.[16]

CASE Application

1. Select the statement that most accurately characterizes asthma.
   a. Airway inflammation and bronchial hyperresponsiveness
   b. Airway inflammation and esophageal hyperresponsiveness
   c. Adrenal inflammation and bronchial hyperresponsiveness
   d. Adrenal inflammation and esophageal hyperresponsiveness

2. Select the mechanism(s) for development of asthma.
   a. Ectopy and exposure to environmental triggers
   b. Ectopy and activation of neutrophils
   c. Atopy and exposure to environmental triggers
   d. Atopy and activation of neutrophils

3. The late asthmatic response is caused by influx of which primary inflammatory cell?
   a. Natural killer cells
   b. Eosinophils
   c. Monocytes
   d. Immunoglobulin A

4. Irreversible obstruction or airway remodeling may occur in susceptible persons with asthma due to uncontrolled inflammation within which structure?
   a. Bronchial smooth muscle
   b. Esophageal smooth muscle
   c. Pharynx
   d. Alveoli

5. Among children this may be the only nighttime symptom to consider a diagnostic work up for asthma.
   a. Dyspnea
   b. Cough
   c. Reflux
   d. Enuresis

6. What is the preferred treatment for an 18-year-old man with off and on chest tightness that occurred 4 days this past week with no nocturnal awakening, FEV_1/FVC = 70%, and FEV_1 = 75%?
   a. Low-dose inhaled corticosteroid
   b. Medium-dose inhaled corticosteroid
   c. High-dose inhaled corticosteroid
   d. Leukotriene modifier

7. You are providing follow up education for a 3-year-old child with asthma who in the last month is scheduling their AccuNeb 1.25 mg tid for symptoms. The child and his parents have completed the following questionnaire:

Have your child complete these questions.

1. How is your asthma today?				
0: Very bad	1: Bad	2: Good	3: Very good	**Score: 2**
2. How much of a problem is your asthma when you run, exercise, or play sports?				
0: It is a big problem. I cannot do what I want to do.	1: It is a problem and I do not like it.	2: It is a little problem but it is okay.	3: It is not a problem.	**Score: 2**
3. Do you cough because of your asthma?				
0: Yes, all the time.	1: Yes, most of the time.	2: Yes, sometimes.	3: No, never.	**Score: 2**
4. Do you wake up during the night because of your asthma?				
0: Yes, all the time.	1: Yes, most of the time.	2: Yes, sometimes	3: No, never.	**Score: 2**

Please complete the following questions on your own.

5. During the *last 4 weeks,* how many days did your child have any daytime asthma symptoms?						
5: Not at all	4: 1-3 days	3: 4-10 days	2: 11-18 days	1: 19-24 days	0: Everyday	**Score: 2**
6. During the *last 4 weeks,* how many days did your child wheeze during the day because of asthma?						
5: Not at all	4: 1-3 days	3: 4-10 days	2: 11-18 days	1: 19-24 days	0: Everyday	**Score: 3**
7. During the *last 4 weeks,* how many days did your child wake up during the night because of asthma?						
5: Not at all	4: 1-3 days	3: 4-10 days	2: 11-18 days	1: 19-24 days	0: Everyday	**Score: 2**

What is the best treatment option given the patients current asthma control?
   a. Continue current treatment
   b. Step up one step
   c. Step down one step
   d. Oral steroid burst

8. After assessing environmental control and medication adherence what additional factor should be addressed prior to stepping up asthma therapy?
   a. Inhaler technique
   b. IgE level
   c. Serum glucose
   d. pH monitoring

9. Independent of asthma severity all persons with asthma should have this class of medication readily available.
   a. Short-acting β_2-agonist
   b. Short-acting β_2-antagonist

c. Long-acting β_2-agonist
d. Long-acting β_2-antagonist

10. Select the brand name for levalbuterol.

 a. Serevent
 b. Flovent
 c. Xolair
 d. Xopenex

11. Which is the best medication for control of inflammation in persistent asthma?

 a. Formoterol
 b. Zileuton
 c. Budesonide
 d. Cromolyn

12. Which medication would be an absolute contraindication when given alone for the treatment of persistent asthma?

 a. Mometasone
 b. Zafirlukast
 c. Theophylline
 d. Salmeterol

13. What is the mechanism of action of montelukast?

 a. Antagonist to leukotriene receptors
 b. Agonist to leukotriene receptors
 c. Antagonist to muscarinic receptors
 d. Agonist to muscarinic receptors

14. Select the agent that is administered as a subcutaneous injection in patients with allergic asthma not controlled with high-dose inhaled corticosteroids.

 a. Pirbuterol
 b. Omalizumab
 c. Ciclesonide
 d. Adalimumab

15. What is the preferred treatment option for a 46-year-old man with the diagnosis of asthma? Current complaints are wheezing in morning that gets better as day progresses. One episode of cough in last month required three courses of oral steroids within the last year with an FEV_1 of 55%.

 a. Medium-dose inhaled corticosteroid (ICS)
 b. Low-dose ICS and LABA
 c. Medium-dose ICS and LABA
 d. Theophylline

16. Select the brand name for ciclesonide.

 a. AeroBid
 b. Asmanex
 c. Azmacort
 d. Alvesco

17. What is the follow-up treatment recommendation for a 16-year-old girl currently on QVAR 80 µg 2 puffs bid who is experiencing no limitation on activity and has not used her SABA in over 3 months?

 a. Step up therapy
 b. Step down therapy
 c. Continue current treatment
 d. Discontinue SABA

18. What is the most common adverse reaction of short-acting β-agonists?

 a. Hypernatremia
 b. Tremor
 c. Anaphylaxis
 d. Thrush

19. You are counseling the parents of a 2-year-old child who will be released from the hospital with a new prescription for a medium-dose inhaled corticosteroid. What side effect should you educate the parents about?

 a. Reduced glucose production
 b. Permanente growth suppression
 c. Intermitted expiratory wheezing
 d. Reduced growth velocity

20. You are counseling a 25-year-old woman with asthma who is well-controlled with Advair 250/50 µg 1 puff bid and albuterol 2 puffs every 4 to 6 hours prn. She presents a prescription for prenatal vitamin from her initial obstetric appointment. What is the safest medication to recommend for *control* of her asthma?

 a. Albuterol 2 puffs qid
 b. Advair 250/50 1 puffs bid
 c. Alvesco 160 µg 1 puff daily
 d. Pulmicort 90 mg 1 puff bid

TAKEAWAY POINTS ››

- The major characteristics of asthma are airway inflammation and bronchial hyperresponsiveness which cause variable degrees of airflow obstruction.
- Uncontrolled inflammation causes hypertrophy and hyperplasia of the bronchial smooth muscle and mucus glands which in susceptible individuals leads to permanent, irreversible obstruction termed airway remodeling.
- The definitive diagnosis of asthma is made through the use of spirometry when the post-bronchodilator FEV_1 improves greater or equal to 12% and 200 mL when compared to the prebronchodilator value.

- Persons with asthma should have a quick relief medication (albuterol) readily available.
- Inhaled corticosteroids are the preferred treatment for controlling inflammation in persons with persistent asthma.
- Monotherapy with long-acting β_2-agonists is absolutely contraindicated in treatment of asthma due to increased risk of asthma-related death (black box warning). Long acting β_2 -agonists should only be used as adjuvant therapy in patients not adequately controlled on inhaled corticosteroids or whose disease requires two maintenance therapies.
- Patients with asthma who have had a myocardial infarction and require β-blocker use may use cardioselective β-blockers without adversely affecting their asthma control.
- Children with asthma who are treated with inhaled corticosteroids will have a transient decrease in growth velocity but will not affect overall height.

REFERENCES

1. United States: National Health Interview Survey, 2006.Current asthma prevalence percents by age. Available at: http://www.cdc.gov/asthma/nhis/06/table4-1.htm. Accessed August 16, 2009.
2. Moorman J, Rudd R, Johnson CA, et al. National surveillance for asthma—United States, 1980-2004. *MMWR.* 2007;56(SS08):1-14,18-54.
3. Busse WW, Lemanske RF Jr. Asthma. *N Engl J Med.* Feb 1 2001;344 (5):350-362.
4. Ten Hacken NH, Postma DS, Timens W. Airway remodeling and long-term decline in lung function in asthma. *Curr Opin Pulm Med.* Jan 2003;9(1):9-14.
5. Fanta C. Asthma. *N Engl J Med.* 2009; 360:1002-1014.
6. Antoniu SA, Mihaescu T, Donner CF. Pharmacotherapy of cough-variant asthma. *Expert Opin Pharmacother.* 2007;8(17):3021-3028.
7. Expert Panel Report 3 (EPR-3): Guidelines for the Diagnosis and Management of Asthma-Summary Report 2007. National Asthma Education and Prevention Program. *J Allergy Clin Immunol.* Nov 2007;120(5 suppl):S94-S138
8. Nelson H. β-Adrenergic bronchodilators. *N Engl J Med.* 1995;333:499-506.
9. Colice G. Comparing inhaled corticosteroids. *Respir Care.* 2000;45(7):846-853
10. Lipworth BJ. Systemic adverse effects of inhaled corticosteroid therapy: a systematic review and meta-analysis. *Arch Intern Med.* 1999;159(9):941-955.
11. Nelson H, Weiss S, Bleecker E, Yancey S, Dorinsky P, et al. The Salmeterol Multicenter Asthma Research Trial—a comparison of usual pharmacotherapy for asthma or usual pharmacotherapy plus salmeterol. *Chest.* 2006;129(1):15-26.
12. Salpetr S, Ormistron T, Salpeter E. Cardioselective β-blockers in patients with reactive airway disease: a meta-analysis. *Annals of Internal Medicine.* 2002; 137(9):715-725.
13. Quick Reference summarizes the findings of the NAEPP Working Group Report on Managing Asthma During Pregnancy: Recommendations for Pharmacologic Treatment—Update 2004 (NIH Publication No. 05-3279). Available at: http://www.nhlbi.nih.gov/health/prof/lung/asthma/astpreg.htm. Accessed October 30, 2009.
14. The Childhood Asthma Management Program (CAMP) Research Group. Long-term effects of budesonide or nedocromil in children with asthma. *N Engl J Med.* 2000;343(15): 1054-1063.
15. Randolph C. Exercise-induced bronchospasm in children. *Clin Rev Allergy Immunol.* 2008;34:205-216.
16. Summary of recommendations for adult immunizations. Available at: www.immunize.org/catg.d/p2011.pdf. Accessed October 30, 2009.

CHAPTER

44 Cystic Fibrosis

Holly J. Watson

FOUNDATION OVERVIEW

Cystic fibrosis (CF) is the most common lethal, genetic disease in the white population. CF occurs in about 1 of every 2000 live births in the United States and 5% of the general population are gene carriers.[1] CF is a disease of the epithelial cells in the body; especially those lining the intestinal tract and airways of the lungs. Normally, epithelial cells transport chloride through the cystic fibrosis transmembrane regulator (CFTR) with sodium and water following the ion flux. CF is the loss of the function of the CFTR with defective movement of Cl and water in the body. Thus, the composition of fluid secreted by the pancreas, hepatobiliary tree, reproductive tract, sweat glands, and the airways is thick and leads to obstruction with malfunction. This malfunction eventually leads to widespread organ system disease (Table 44-1).

Clinical presentation of CF patients can be divided into early disease and disease later in life. Early disease is usually milder while later disease is more advanced and severe. Early obstruction in the gastrointestinal system manifests as abdominal distention, pain, vomiting, and change in stool output. Early maldigestion, due to lipase deficiency, produces stools with high fat content known as steatorrhea. Symptoms of steatorrhea in the patient are stools with foul odor, bulkiness, greasiness, and more frequent in number. Late maldigestion leads to varying degrees of malnutrition. Late pancreatic disease leads to a relative insulin deficiency known as cystic fibrosis-related diabetes (CFRD) which can be symptomatic or can present as untreated diabetes mellitus type 2. Late disease in the biliary tract leads to obstruction and liver failure (Table 44-2).

Pulmonary disease can also be divided into early and late disease. Early obstruction in the pulmonary system leads to coughing, sputum production, wheezing, retractions, tachypnea, dyspnea, and cyanosis. Early pulmonary infection begins with a slow cycling pattern with well-being alternating with pulmonary deterioration known as exacerbations. These early exacerbations are commonly caused by *Staphylococcus aureus, Haemophilus influenzae,* and *Pseudomonas aeruginosa* with later infections caused by more resistant organisms such as *Stenotrophomonas maltophilia* and *Burkholderia cepacia*. Late pulmonary disease leads to increasing oxygen requirements, digital clubbing, increased anterior-posterior chest diameter, and flattened diaphragm. The destruction of lung tissue due to the chronic infection and inflammation leads to permanent decrease in pulmonary function tests (PFTs) (see Table 44-2). Symptoms of chronic sinusitis may include nasal obstruction, pain, and anosmia.

The diagnosis of CF is made based on elevated sweat chloride concentrations. Two samples of sweat are collected with the use of pilocarpine iontophoresis with a positive test having chloride concentrations of 60 mEq/L or more. The presence of respiratory obstruction, exocrine pancreatic dysfunction, and a positive family history provide additional support for the diagnosis of CF. CFTR mutation analysis may be necessary for 2% of the population with an inconclusive sweat test.

PREVENTION

The cystic fibrosis gene was identified and cloned in 1989.[2] Prevention of CF is based on family genetic counseling and understanding autosomal recessive inheritance. Ninety-five percent of males with CF are sterile due to obstruction of the epididymis, vas deferens, and seminal vesicles. Females with CF have reduced fertility due to abnormal cervical mucous. CF carriers who marry can produce a CF child and the incidence of the carrier state is 5% in the white population. CFTR mutation analysis can detect heterozygotes (carriers) who have no signs or symptoms of CF. For a couple where each parent is a carrier, a child has a 1:4 chance of having the disease, 1:2 chance of being a carrier, and a 1:4 chance of being normal (neither the disease nor carrier state). Gene therapy may be a preventative treatment in the future but current results have been disappointing.

TREATMENT

Treatment outcomes for CF are divided into short-term and long-term outcomes. The short-term goals for the intestinal disease are normal bowel habits, weight gain, and normal vitamin levels. The long-term goal for the intestinal disease is optimal nutrition. The short-term goals for the pulmonary treatment are to reduce the airway infection, inflammation, and obstruction. The goal of an acute exacerbation is to return pulmonary function to the preexacerbation status. The long-term goal of pulmonary treatment is to arrest the persistent decline in forced vital capacity (FVC), forced expiratory volume at 1 s (FEV_1), and increase in residual volume (RV).

TABLE 44-1 Organ System Effects of Cystic Fibrosis

Organ Obstruction	Malfunction	Clinical Effect
Pancreatic duct	Duct obstruction	Enzyme deficiency, maldigestion
Biliary duct	Duct obstruction	Cirrhosis, portal hypertension, esophageal varices
Intestines	Viscous secretions	Distal intestinal obstructive syndrome (DIOS)
Pulmonary	Viscous secretions	Obstruction, infection
Sweat glands	Fail to reabsorb Na ("salty taste of skin")	Hyponatremia
Reproductive	♂ Obstruction epididymis, vas deferens, seminal vesicles	Aspermia
	♀ Obstruction cervix	Decreased fertility
Bone, joint	Unknown	Arthritis, osteopenia

TABLE 44-2 Early Versus Late Disease in CF Patients

Organ Malfunction	Early Disease	Late Disease
	Gastrointestinal	
Obstruction	Distention, pain, nausea and vomiting	DIOS, liver failure, CFRD
Maldigestion	Steatorrhea, malnutrition	Severe malnutrition
	Pulmonary	
Obstruction	Cough, ↑sputum	COPD, cor pulmonale
Infection	Acute exacerbations	Permanent ↓PFTs

Gastrointestinal Disease

Pancreatic Enzyme Replacement Therapy

Gastrointestinal treatment is primarily accomplished with pancreatic enzyme replacement therapy. The preferred products are the microencapsulated pancreatic enzymes (Table 44-3). The enteric-coated spheres inside these capsules are protected from destruction by gastric acid and therefore can be given in much lower doses than the older noncoated products. These products are dosed based on the lipase component at an initial dose of 1000 lipase units/kg/meal; one-half of this amount is administered with snacks.[3] For patients unable to swallow capsules, the contents may be opened and sprinkled over applesauce, jelly, or some nonalkaline soft food. Side effects are associated with high doses of the enzyme products. Hyperuricosuria has been reported due to the high purine content of the products. Proximal colonic stricture is associated with doses in excess of 24,000 units/kg/d. Histamine H2-receptor antagonists and proton pump inhibitors have been used to decrease the enzyme dose in patients who are hypersecretors of acid. Constant acid in the colon prevents the enteric coating from dissolving.

Vitamin Replacement Therapy

Vitamins are required in CF patients who pass fat in their stools; especially the fat-soluble vitamins. These deficiencies become clinically evident as neurologic dysfunction (vitamin E); demineralization of the bone (vitamin D); bleeding problems (vitamin K); and dermatitis, vision difficulties (vitamin A). Vitamin K, at a dose of 5 mg twice weekly, should be given to patients with a prolonged international ratio (INR).[3] Recommended daily allowance (RDA) of the fat-soluble vitamins are administered in water-miscible products, such as ADEK, that are better absorbed in the CF patient but more expensive. Higher doses of the older fat-soluble vitamin products overcome this poor bioavailability and are much less expensive. These products can be administered starting at twice the RDA and adjusted as needed.

Choleretic Therapy

The older CF patient can benefit from ursodeoxycholic acid (UDCA), a bile acid with choleretic properties. This medication has been shown to produce morphologic and functional improvement in patients with liver disease. Doses range from 15 to 20 mg/kg/d in combination with taurine supplementation.[3] This agent is recommended to be given prophylactically to prevent end-stage liver failure.

Pulmonary Disease

Pulmonary treatment is focused on three areas: anti-obstruction, anti-inflammation, and anti-infective therapy.

Anti-Obstructive Therapy

The main treatment for removal of mucous and secretions from the airways is percussion and postural drainage. Vibrations loosen mucous and secretions (eg, percussion) and placing

TABLE 44-3 Enteric Coated Pancreatic Enzyme Products

Product	Lipase	Protease	Amylase
Pancrease	4,000	25,000	20,000
Pancrease MT 4	4,000	12,000	12,000
Pancrease MT 10	10,000	30,000	30,000
Pancrease MT 16	16,000	48,000	48,000
Pancrelipase	4,000	25,000	20,000
Ultrase MT 12	12,000	39,000	39,000
Ultrase MT 20	20,000	65,000	65,000
Ultrase MT 18	24,000	78,000	78,000

the head lower than the body (eg, postural drainage) facilitates removal of the mucous and secretions. Nebulized mucolytics, such as sterile sodium chloride or *N*-acetylcysteine (eg, Mucomyst), can increase the results of the percussion; and nebulized bronchodilators, such as albuterol, can increase the results of postural drainage. Two new nebulized products have been studied for long-term chronic use to prevent the accumulation of mucous and secretions in the lungs of CF patients. The first is recombinant human DNAse to be given by inhalation (2.5 mg once or twice daily) to reduce the viscosity of pulmonary secretions. This medication has been shown to increase the time between pulmonary exacerbations in CF patients. The second nebulized product for chronic use is hypertonic saline in a 7% sterile solution. It is thought that this product will slow the progression of lung damage in CF patients.[4,5]

Anti-Inflammatory Therapy

Anti-inflammatory treatments for CF patients can be accomplished with three groups of medications: oral corticosteroids, inhaled corticosteroids, and ibuprofen. Oral corticosteroids have shown improvements in pulmonary function tests but detrimental effects on linear growth and glucose metabolism.[6] Inhaled corticosteroids have not been studied sufficiently in this population. High-dose ibuprofen slowed the rate of progression of pulmonary disease but serum concentration monitoring is needed and is very costly. Low-dose ibuprofen has been shown to increase inflammation.[7]

Antibiotic Therapy

Antibiotic therapy for CF results in clinical improvement without eradicating all bacteria from the sputum (ie, suppressive therapy). The primary bacteria in the lungs of the CF patient is *P. aeruginosa* which secretes an extracellular matrix known as a biofilm that protects it from local host defenses and most antibiotics. Also, the bacteria is colonizing the airway surface, rather than penetrating the tissue as a pathogen and this is another way the bacteria is protected from host defenses and antibiotics (ie, endobronchial infection). Suppressive antibiotic therapy is aimed at *P. aeruginosa* and *S. aureus* and is accomplished with an aminoglycoside *plus* an extended-spectrum penicillin. Double antibiotic therapy is recommended to take advantage of synergy with the antibiotic combination and to prevent the emergence of resistance.[8] Since most of the *S. aureus* encountered are β-lactamase producers, the use of an extended-spectrum penicillin plus a β-lactamase inhibitor combination (eg, ticarcillin-clavulanate) will avoid triple antibiotic therapy. Double-drug therapy has shown superiority over treatment with single drugs[9-12] and decreases the development of resistance.[12] Unlike other lower respiratory tract infections, CF sputum cultures correlate well with lower tract organisms and should guide therapy. Older CF patients will usually have resistant organisms such as MRSA (ie, methicillin-resistant *S. aureus*), *B. cepacia,* and *S. maltophilia*. These organisms are generally resistant to most antibiotics and treatment should be guided by the culture and sensitivity report. Older antibiotics with unique mechanisms of action (eg, colistin, polymyxin B) may exhibit susceptibility in patients with resistant organisms. Patients with resistant organisms should wear a respirator mask when with other CF patients as they have been shown to pass these organisms to other CF patients. Because of this observation, CF camps have been discontinued.

Oral antibiotics have been prescribed in symptomatic outpatients with susceptible organisms. This "prophylactic practice" is discouraged because the beneficial effect does not outweigh the risk of the development of resistant organisms.[13] The fluoroquinolone antibiotic ciprofloxacin has activity against all the CF pathogens and has been evaluated in adults undergoing CF exacerbation. Studies are inconclusive due to flaws in design but suggest this oral therapy is as effective as IV therapy.[14] This agent appears to be safe but should be used with caution in those younger than 18 years due to the possibility of joint or cartilage toxicity.[15]

Once-daily dosing of aminoglycosides has been attempted in this population to achieve higher pulmonary concentrations of antibiotic. More studies are needed to determine the efficacy and safety of this method of administration.[16]

The inhaled route of antibiotic delivery has also been tried in the CF population. Topical delivery via inhalation ensures delivery of the drug in high concentrations to the site of infection while avoiding systemic toxicity. Original studies with small doses reported a high incidence of resistant organisms during inhalation treatment. A more recent placebo-controlled, multicenter trial of tobramycin 600 mg administered by aerosol three times daily produced a statistically significant improvement in FEV_1, FVC, FEV 25% to 75%, *P. aeruginosa* density in the sputum, and peripheral WBC count.[17] Appropriate clinical use of this therapy (prophylaxis, treatment, length of therapy, frequency of therapy) remains to be determined. More studies are needed and preservative-free antibiotic preparations should be used with these larger doses.

SPECIAL CONSIDERATIONS

CF patients have increased clearance of many antibiotics including aminoglycosides, some β-lactams, and trimethoprim-sulfamethoxazole. Increased clearance means higher doses in most patients. A CF dosing chart such as Table 44-4 should be consulted for dosing in this population and subsequent pharmacokinetic calculations performed to further individualize the dose.

TABLE 44-4 Antibiotic Doses in Cystic Fibrosis

Antibiotic	Dose[a]	Max Dose[b]	Regimen	Serum Level[c]
Tobra/Gent	6-9	NA	Every 8 h	Peak >8, trough <2
Amikacin	20-30	NA	Every 8 h	Peak >24, trough <9
Aztreonam	200	8	Every 6 h	NA
Ceftazidime	150	6	Every 8 h	NA
Colistin	2.5-6	NA	Every 6-8 h	NA
Imipenem	45-100	4	Every 6 h	NA
Nafcillin	100	6	Every 4-6 h	NA
Ticarcillin	400	18	Every 4-6 h	NA
Ticarcillin + clavulanate	400	18	Every 4-6 h	NA
Piperacillin	400	18	Every 4-6 h	NA
		Oral		
Amoxicillin	20	NA	Every 8 h	NA
Amoxicillin + clavulanate	20	NA	Every 6 h	NA
Ciprofloxacin	1.5 g/d	1.5	Every 12 h	NA
Cephalexin	50-100	6	Every 6-8 h	NA
Dicloxacillin	80-100	6	Every 6 h	NA
Trim/Sulfa	10-15	0.64	Every 12 h	NA
		Inhaled		
Tobra/Gent	0.6-1.8 g/d	NA	Every 12 h	NA
Colistin	150 mg/d	NA	Every 6-12 h	NA
Polymyxin B	250 mg/d	NA	Every 6-12 h	NA

[a]mg/kg/d, [b]g/d, [c]µg/mL.

CASE Application

1. JN is a 2-year-old (8 kg) with repeat visits to her physician for pneumonia. There is a positive family history for CF. What test should be ordered in this patient to diagnose CF?
   a. Chest x-ray
   b. Sputum culture
   c. Sweat test
   d. DNA test

2. JN is diagnosed with CF and treatment for her pneumonia needs to be initiated. Which test should be ordered to guide the antibiotic selection?
   a. Sputum culture and sensitivity
   b. Chest x-ray
   c. Chest MRI
   d. Chest CAT scan

3. Which organism would you empirically treat for in this patient with CF?
   a. *Burkholderia cepacia*
   b. *Pseudomonas aeruginosa*
   c. *Stenotrophomonas maltophilia*
   d. *Haemophilus influenzae*

4. Which combination of antibiotics would be appropriate to treat JN's pneumonia?
   a. Aminoglycoside and amoxicillin
   b. Aminoglycoside and ticarcillin
   c. Aminoglycoside and Timentin (ticarcillin plus clavulanate)
   d. Ciprofloxacin

5. High serum peaks are needed to penetrate and adequately treat gram-negative pulmonary infections. Low troughs are needed to ensure low toxicity. What are the appropriate serum levels you would aim for with JN's aminoglycoside therapy?
   a. Peak > 8 and trough > 2
   b. Peak > 8 and trough < 2
   c. Peak < 8 and trough > 2
   d. Peak < 8 and trough < 2

6. What general statement can you make regarding the initial dose of antibiotics in CF patients?

   a. Higher antibiotic doses are needed in CF patients.
   b. The same doses are needed in CF patients as other patients with pneumonia.
   c. Doses vary with each patient and should be individualized.
   d. a and c.
   e. All of the above.

7. How long should the IV antibiotics be continued for JN's pulmonary exacerbation?

   a. 7 days
   b. 10 days
   c. 21 days
   d. Until her PFTs return to baseline for a 2 year old

8. Give two reasons why double IV antibiotic therapy should be used to treat JN's pulmonary exacerbation.

   a. Antibiotic synergy and decreased bacterial resistance
   b. Antibiotic synergy and increased bacterial resistance
   c. Broader antibacterial coverage and antibiotic synergy
   d. Narrower antibacterial coverage and antibiotic synergy

9. What other therapy should be initiated along with antibiotics for JN's pneumonia?

   a. Percussion and drainage
   b. Pancreatic enzyme replacement therapy
   c. Vitamin replacement therapy
   d. Hormone replacement therapy

10. JN is ready to go home from the hospital and needs to be started on pancreatic enzyme replacement therapy. She eats three meals each day and has three snacks. She weighs 21 kg. Calculate her beginning enzyme dose per meal.

    a. 15,000 units/meal
    b. 21,000 units/meal
    c. 22,000 units/meal
    d. 23,000 units/meal

11. Which product would you select for JN to receive with each meal?

    a. Pancrease MT 4 (2 with meals)
    b. Pancrease MT 10 (1 with meals)
    c. Pancrease MT 16 (1 with meals)
    d. Pancrease MT 20 (1 with meals)

12. What is the dose of pancreatic enzyme replacement for JN to take with her three snacks each day?

    a. Pancreatic MT 4 (1 with snacks)
    b. Pancreatic MT 10 (1 with snacks)
    c. Pancreatic MT 16 (1 with snacks)
    d. Pancreatic MT 20 (1 with snacks)

13. How would you instruct JN's mother to administer her pancreatic enzyme replacement therapy?

    a. Administer the capsule whole with water.
    b. Administer the capsule whole with juice.
    c. Open the capsule and sprinkle over soft, nonalkaline food. Do not chew the beads.
    d. Open the capsule and sprinkle over soft, alkaline food. Do not chew the beads.

14. How would you instruct JN's mother to monitor the effectiveness of her child's pancreatic enzyme replacement therapy?

    a. ↓ Steatorrhea, ↑ weight
    b. ↓ Steatorrhea, ↓ weight
    c. ↑ Steatorrhea, ↑ weight
    d. ↑ Steatorrhea, ↓ weight

15. What side effects would you instruct JN's mother to monitor with the pancreatic enzyme replacement therapy?

    a. Sore mouth and diaper rash
    b. Sore mouth and sunburn
    c. Diaper rash
    d. Sore mouth

16. JN's mother has heard CF patients are deficient in vitamins. She wants to know which ones.

    a. Fat-soluble vitamins
    b. Water-soluble vitamins
    c. None
    d. All vitamins

17. The child down the hall with CF is older and has liver failure. Her mother wants to know if there is a drug to prevent this awful disease.

    a. Pancreatic supplements
    b. Vitamin supplements
    c. Antibiotics
    d. Ursodeoxycholic acid

18. When JN goes home, the doctors would like to give a medicine shown to increase the time between pulmonary exacerbations. What would you recommend?

    a. Inhaled corticosteroids
    b. Inhaled albuterol
    c. Inhaled DNAse
    d. Inhaled *N*-acetylcysteine (Mucomyst)

19. What other therapy can be given to JN to help prevent pulmonary infections?

    a. Influenza vaccine
    b. Meningococcal vaccine
    c. MMR vaccine
    d. Hepatitis vaccine

20. As JN's mother leaves the hospital with JN, she wants to know the likelihood of development of CF in other children she may have. Neither of JN's parents has been diagnosed with CF.
    a. 25%
    b. 50%
    c. 75%
    d. 100%

TAKEAWAY POINTS ››

- Cystic fibrosis is the most common lethal genetic disease in the white population. It is inherited in an autosomal recessive manner with carriers being completely asymptomatic.
- Cystic fibrosis is a disorder of chloride transport in all body epithelial cells. The majority of problems occur in the gastrointestinal and pulmonary systems.
- The pathology of CF results in the abnormal movement of sodium (Na) and water in the body. This results in thick secretions that obstruct systems, block exocrine gland ducts, and constantly produce infections with inflammation.
- Thick secretions in the gastrointestinal system lead to obstruction in the tract, the pancreatic duct, and the biliary duct. This leads to deficiency in digestive enzymes with malabsorption of food which leads to malnutrition.
- Treatment of the gastrointestinal system involves replacement of pancreatic enzymes and vitamins.
- Thick secretions in the pulmonary system lead to obstruction in the lungs, bacterial colonization, and chronic inflammation.
- Treatment of the pulmonary system is aimed at reducing the infection and the inflammation.
- Treatment of the pulmonary infection involves IV antibiotic therapy for CF exacerbations and prophylactic antibiotics to reduce the progression of the disease. Antibiotic therapy is aimed at *P. aeruginosa* that is the most common pathogen in the CF lung.
- Treatment of the pulmonary inflammation is aimed at decreasing the lung destruction that occurs over time.
- The overall goal of CF therapy is to slow the progression of the disease, prevent malnutrition, and help the patient to have as normal a lifestyle as possible.

REFERENCES

1. Steinberg AG, Brown DC. On the incidence of cystic fibrosis of the pancreas. *Am J Hum Genet.* 1960;12:416-424.
2. Wright SE, Morton NE. Genetic studies on cystic fibrosis in Hawaii. *Am J Hum Genet.* 1968;20:157-169.
3. Bosso JA, Milavetz G. Cystic fibrosis. In: DiPiro JT, Talbert RL, Yee GC, et al, eds. *Pharmacotherapy: A Pathophysiologic Approach.* 7th ed. New York, NY: McGraw Hill; 2008:563-574.
4. Riordan JR, Rommens JM, Kerem B, et al. Identification of the cystic fibrosis gene: cloning and characterization of complementary DNA. *Science.* 1989;245:1066-1073.
5. Donaldson SH, Bennett WE, Zeman KL, et al. Mucus clearance and lung function in cystic fibrosis with hypertonic saline. *N Engl J Med.* 2006;354:241-250.
6. Rosenstein BJ, Eigen H. Risks of alternate-day prednisone in patients with cystic fibrosis. *Pediatrics.* 1991;87:245-246.
7. Konstan MW, Byard PJ, Hoppel CL, et al. Effect of high-dose ibuprofen in patients with cystic fibrosis. *N Engl J Med.* 1995;332:848-854.
8. Parry MF, Neu HC, Merlino M, et al. Treatment of pulmonary infections in patients with cystic fibrosis: a comparative study of ticarcillin and gentamicin. *J Pediatr.* 1977;90:144-148.
9. Moller NE, Hoiby N. Antibiotic treatment of chronic *Pseudomonas aeruginosa* infection in cystic fibrosis patients. *Scand J Infect Dis.* 1981;24(suppl):87-91.
10. Friis B. Chemotherapy of chronic infections with mucoid *Pseudomonas aeruginosa* in lower airways of patients with cystic fibrosis. *Scand J Infect Dis.* 1979;11:211-217.
11. Krause PJ, Young LS, Cherry JD, et al. The treatment of exacerbations of pulmonary disease in cystic fibrosis: Netilmicin compared with netilmicin and carbenicillin. *Curr Ther Res.* 1979;25:609-617.
12. Bosso JA, Allen JE, Matsen JM. Changing susceptibility of *Pseudomonas aeruginosa* isolates from cystic fibrosis patients with the clinical use of newer antibiotics. *Antimicrob Agents Chemother.* 1989;33:526-528.
13. Beardsmore CS, Thompson JR, Williams A, et al. Pulmonary function in infants with cystic fibrosis. *Arch Dis Child.* 1994;71:133-137.
14. Bosso JA. Use of ciprofloxacin in cystic fibrosis patients. *Am J Med.* 1989;87(suppl 5A):123S-127S.
15. Hoiby N, Pedersen SS, Jensen T, et al. Fluoroquinolones in the treatment of cystic fibrosis. *Drugs.* 1993;45:(suppl 3):98-101.
16. Tackett KL, Watson HJ, Stallworth JR. Efficacy of once-daily aminoglycosides as compared to traditional thrice daily dosing in children with cystic fibrosis pulmonary exacerbation. *eJourn SC Med Assoc.* 2003;99:274-279.
17. Ramsey BW, Dorkin HL, Eisenberg JD, et al. Efficacy of aerosolized tobramycin in patients with cystic fibrosis. *N Engl J Med.* 1993;328:1740-1746.
18. Moore RD, Smith CR, Lietman PS. Association of aminoglycoside plasma levels with therapeutic outcome in gram-negative pneumonia. *Am J Med.* 1984;77:657-662.

PART

7

Bone and Joint Disorders

CHAPTER

45 Gout

Michelle M. Bottenberg, Karly A. Hegge, Kristin K. Horning, and Sheryl L. Compton

FOUNDATIONAL OVERVIEW

Gout is a chronic metabolic disease which is frequently encountered in primary care and hospital practice settings.[1] Although awareness of this condition dates back many years, the understanding of gout has improved significantly, and a correlation has been established between the risk of developing gout and maintaining a diet high in red meats or seafood.[2] Men are at a substantially higher risk, with diagnosis occurring about seven to nine times more often in men compared to women.[3] Serum uric acid (SUA) measurement remains an important assessment parameter for gout. SUA concentrations tend to be higher with increasing age, blood pressure, body weight, and alcohol intake.[4] However, gout flares can occur in individuals with normal SUA levels, while many patients with elevated SUA concentrations do not develop gout.

Gouty arthritis is the most common inflammatory arthritis in men over age 40.[5] In the United States, an estimated 6.1 million adults have experienced an acute flare of gout.[6] Recently, a renewed interest has highlighted the potential implications of this disease, including the relationship to common comorbidities such as obesity, type 2 diabetes, dyslipidemia, hypertension, and heart disease.[7] The economic burden of this increasingly prevalent condition is substantial, with new gout cases in the United States costing an estimated 27 million dollars annually.[8]

Pathophysiology

Gout is characterized by acute and often recurrent arthritis mediated by the formation of monosodium urate (MSU) crystals within the joints and surrounding tissues, resulting in pain, erythema, and inflammation. Hyperuricemia, or elevated SUA concentrations, can be a result of various causes, including a defect in purine metabolism, a decrease in uric acid excretion, increased nucleic acid turnover, or increased purine production. Uric acid is a metabolic by-product of purine compounds, which are derived from either dietary sources or the breakdown of DNA material within the body's cells. Uric acid is primarily excreted by the kidneys, but it can accumulate if its production exceeds excretion. A vast majority of patients with gout accumulate excessive uric acid due to underexcretion of the compound, although some cases of gout are caused by overproduction. Regardless of the cause, excessive intake of foods high in purine can contribute to hyperuricemia and thereby exacerbate gout, including red meats, seafood, and beer (Table 45-1).

Clinical Presentation

The classic presentation for gout is an acute monoarthritis which is typically self-limited and often involves a joint of the lower extremity, such as the first metatarsophalangeal joint or knee (Table 45-2). At some point, up to 90% of patients experience podagra, or acute attacks of gouty arthritis in the great toe.[8] Symptoms usually develop rapidly and include excruciating pain, erythema, warmth, and swelling near the affected joint. Although acute attacks often occur spontaneously, they can be precipitated by stress, infection, surgery, or ingestion of alcohol or medications which can affect SUA concentrations. Exacerbations may initially occur infrequently; however, gout is a chronic disease with recurrent flare-ups which often increase in frequency over time. If untreated, an acute gouty attack may last 1 to 2 weeks, followed by an asymptomatic period.

In addition to traditional gout symptoms, patients may experience other complications such as tophi, or urate crystal deposits that can damage surrounding soft tissue and cause significant pain and joint destruction. Finally, elevated urinary uric acid levels may contribute to the formation of uric acid stones in the kidney (uric acid nephrolithiasis).

Diagnosis

Hyperuricemia is defined as a SUA level of > 7 mg/dL in men or > 6 mg/dL in women.[9] Although asymptomatic hyperuricemia is common, it rarely requires medical treatment. Therefore, other clinical features of gout must also be considered when evaluating patients with elevated SUA concentrations. According to recommendations from the European League Against Rheumatism (EULAR) and criteria from the American College of Rheumatology (ACR), the presence of MSU crystals on synovial fluid analysis is the gold standard in diagnosing gout.[9,10] However, in the absence of a needle aspiration, clinicians frequently diagnose gout based on certain patient criteria, including physical examination, patient and family history, and current medications. Radiographs of affected joints may reveal damage consistent with gout but should not be used alone for diagnosis.

TABLE 45-1 Dietary Components Which May Affect SUA Levels

Increased SUA
▪ Red and organ meat (liver, kidney), seafood (shellfish, anchovies), beer, and spirits[24,25]
▪ Sugar-sweetened soft drinks and fructose[26,27]
Decreased SUA
▪ Vitamin C[28]
▪ Coffee[29]
▪ Dairy products[30]

TREATMENT—ACUTE GOUT EPISODES

Early, appropriate therapy is associated with less pain, less disability, and decreased duration of the gout attack. Current available pharmacologic options for acute episodes of gout include nonsteroidal anti-inflammatory drugs (NSAIDs), colchicine, and corticosteroids (Table 45-3). Goals of therapy include quickly alleviating symptoms, preventing recurrent attacks, and preventing complications. First-line treatment should include either oral colchicine or NSAIDs to relieve pain and inflammation.[9,11,12] Additionally, the affected joints should be rested and treated with cold packs, while application of heat should be avoided.[13,14]

NSAIDs

Although indomethacin (Indocin) is classically described as the drug of choice in gout, any short-acting NSAID at equipotent, anti-inflammatory doses should be efficacious. NSAIDs exert anti-inflammatory, analgesic, and antipyretic effects by inhibiting prostaglandin synthesis.[15] Adverse effects include gastropathy, fluid retention, and a risk of renal dysfunction. Proton pump inhibitors or cyclooxygenase-2 (COX-2) selective inhibitors may have a role in limiting gastrointestinal (GI) toxicity, although cost and potential cardiovascular risk of COX-2 inhibitors must be considered.[16] Caution should be used in patients with renal or hepatic dysfunction, ulcers, heart failure, or bleeding risk. Monitoring parameters include signs and symptoms of bleeding, as well as effects on pain, serum creatinine, blood pressure, and electrolytes.

TABLE 45-2 Clinical Signs and Symptoms of Gout

Signs
▪ Affected joint(s) are swollen, erythematous, and warm
▪ Mild fever
▪ Tophi may be present in chronic, severe disease (usually on ears, hands, wrists, elbows, or knees)
Symptoms
▪ Severe pain, swelling, and warmth in the affected joint(s)
▪ Attack is usually monoarticular; most common sites are metatarsophalangeal and knee joints
▪ Elderly patients may exhibit atypical presentation, such as insidious onset of symptoms and polyarticular joint involvement, often involving the hand or wrist joints

Colchicine

Oral colchicine is effective for acute gout attacks, but its use may be limited by its narrow therapeutic index and poor tolerability. Colchicine exerts its anti-inflammatory effects by reducing phagocytosis and lactic acid production in joints thereby reducing deposition of urate crystals. It is most effective when given in the first 24 to 48 hours of the attack. Colchicine commonly causes significant GI intolerance (eg, nausea, vomiting, diarrhea, abdominal pain), as well as less common effects such as myopathy and bone marrow suppression. The risk of toxicity is greater in patients with arrhythmias or with renal or hepatic impairment.[17] Other drawbacks to colchicine include its slow onset of action and potential to interact with multiple drugs, including cyclosporine and HMG-CoA reductase inhibitors.

Therefore, oral colchicine should be reserved for patients who are at risk for NSAID-induced gastropathy or who have failed NSAID therapy. Intravenous colchicine is not recommended due to the increased risk of serious adverse effects, including leukopenia, extravasation, and even death.[18] Consequently, as of 2008, intravenous colchicine is no longer being manufactured.[19]

Corticosteroids

Corticosteroids are recommended as an alternative treatment option for patients who are unable to take NSAIDs or colchicine, such as those with renal insufficiency or a history of gastrointestinal bleeding. Corticosteroids may be administered either orally or via intra-articular injection, depending on the number and location of affected joint(s). Prior to intra-articular injections, the joint fluid obtained by arthrocentesis should be examined to rule out infection. Systemic administration is most commonly recommended for patients with severe oligoarticular or polyarticular attacks and for attacks in sites which are not readily available to aspiration (eg, the midfoot). Patients taking systemic corticosteroids should be monitored for adverse effects, including hyperglycemia, central nervous system stimulation, fluid retention, weight gain, and increased risk of infection. Although corticotropin (adrenocorticotropic hormone, ACTH) has been used for acute gouty flares, it is not a preferred agent.

PREVENTION—CHRONIC MANAGEMENT OF GOUT

The primary goal of urate-lowering therapy is to prevent further manifestations of urate crystal formation and deposition, as well as to enhance dissolution of these crystals. Prevention of gouty flares includes both nonpharmacologic and pharmacologic approaches, although the most effective method involves a combination of these measures.[9] Patients should be

TABLE 45-3 **Pharmacologic Options for Patients With Acute Gout**

Drug Class	Examples	Typical Dose	Comments
NSAIDs	Indomethacin (Indocin) Naproxen (Naprosyn) Sulindac (Clinoril)	50 mg po tid, then taper and discontinue once response is achieved 750 mg po initially, then 250 mg po tid until attack has subsided 200 mg bid × 7 d	Any NSAID at anti-inflammatory dosing is effective Caution in patients with renal or hepatic insufficiency Caution in patients with a history of GI bleeding or ulcers
Colchicine	Colcrys	1.2 mg at first sign of flare, then 0.6 mg every hour; maximum 1.8 mg po over a 1 h period	Best used if within 24 h of the attack Avoid intravenous use; intravenous formulation no longer manufactured Most common adverse effects—nausea, vomiting, diarrhea Rare but serious adverse effects: myelosuppression, neuromyopathy Caution in patients with renal or hepatic insufficiency Potential drug interactions with erythromycin, simvastatin, and cyclosporine can increase risk of colchicine-induced toxic effects
Corticosteroids	Prednisone Triamcinolone acetonide (Kenalog) Methylprednisolone (Depo-Medrol)	40-60 mg po daily × 3 d, then decrease by 10 mg every 3 d until discontinuation 60 mg IM × 1 dose 10-40 mg × 1 dose by intra-articular injection	Useful for patients in whom NSAIDs and colchicine are contraindicated or in polyarticular flares Caution in patients subject to hyperglycemia Intra-articular therapy may be treatment of choice if only one or two accessible joints are involved

encouraged to decrease dietary intake of purine-rich foods, maintain a healthy weight, and avoid medications which may increase SUA concentrations. Certain pharmacologic agents can increase uric acid levels and increase the risk of gout attacks, including thiazide diuretics, levodopa, niacin, low-dose aspirin, cytotoxic agents, cyclosporine, ethambutol, or pyrazinamide.

Several pharmacologic agents are approved for the prevention of future gout attacks (Table 45-4). Based on whether they are classified as overproducers or underexcretors of uric acid, patients should be treated with urate-lowering therapy such as xanthine oxidase inhibitors or uricosuric agents.[20] Urate-lowering therapy is recommended for patients who experience ≥ 2 attacks per year or who have tophi or radiographic evidence of joint damage. The target SUA level should be ≤ 6, with patients typically requiring 3 to 12 months of continued therapy.

Xanthine Oxidase Inhibitors

Allopurinol (Zyloprim) is a purine analogue inhibitor that blocks the conversion of xanthine to uric acid.[15] It is effective in both overproducers and underexcretors of uric acid and is

TABLE 45-4 **Pharmacologic Options for Urate-Lowering Therapy in Patients with Chronic Gout**

Generic Name (Trade Name)	Typical Dose	Comments
Allopurinol (Zyloprim)	100-300 mg po daily	Adjust dose for renal insufficiency May precipitate acute gout attack Adjust dose based on SUA levels Can cause rare life-threatening hypersensitivity reaction Can be used to treat both urate overproduction and renal urate underexcretion
Febuxostat (Uloric)	40-80 mg po daily	Avoid in patients with severe hepatic impairment
Probenecid (Benemid)	250-500 mg po bid	Adjust dose based on SUA levels May precipitate acute gout attack Modifies renal excretion of other drugs; monitor for drug interactions Maintain adequate hydration
Colchicine (Colcrys)	CrCl ≥ 50 mL/min: 0.6 mg po bid; CrCl 35-49 mL/min:0.6 mg po daily; CrCl 10-34 mL/min: 0.6 mg po every 2-3 d; CrCl < 10 mL/min: Avoid use	Avoid IV use; IV formulation no longer manufactured Most common adverse effects—nausea, vomiting, diarrhea Rare but serious adverse effects: myelosuppression, neuromyopathy Caution in patients with renal or hepatic insufficiency Potential drug interactions with erythromycin, simvastatin, and cyclosporine can increase risk of colchicine-induced toxic effects

typically dosed at 100 to 300 mg daily. When initiating therapy, the patient's SUA level should be considered. In addition, renal function should be evaluated as the dose of allopurinol must be reduced in renal insufficiency. Furthermore, allopurinol should not be started during an acute gout attack as it can worsen arthritis. The most commonly reported side effects are GI intolerance and skin rash.

Febuxostat (Uloric) is a nonpurine analogue inhibitor recently approved for the management of chronic hyperuricemia in symptomatic gout patients.[15] Febuxostat is metabolized by the liver, so no dosage adjustments are required for renal insufficiency. The most common side effects reported are liver enzyme abnormalities, nausea, and rash.

Colchicine

Recently, colchicine (Colcrys) was approved for prophylaxis of gout in addition to treatment of gout flares, although limited clinical evidence exists for this indication. When used for prophylaxis, the maximum daily dose is 1.2 mg, with lower doses recommended for patients with renal insufficiency. Please refer to the acute treatment and special considerations sections for more specific information regarding side effects and monitoring of colchicine.

Uricosuric Agents

Probenecid (Benemid) is the preferred uricosuric agent for patients with either refractory hyperuricemia or intolerance to xanthine oxidase inhibitors.[21] Probenecid is indicated for underexcretors of uric acid as it blocks reuptake at the proximal tubule in the kidney. The recommended dose is 250 to 500 mg twice daily; however, doses of up to 3 g per day may be required. It is not recommended in patients with a history of kidney stones or reduced renal function (estimated creatinine clearance [CrCl] < 50 mL/min). As with xanthine oxidase inhibitors, probenecid should not be initiated during an acute gout attack. Additionally, if patients have other comorbidities, such as hypertension and hyperlipidemia, consider use of losartan (Cozaar) and fenofibrate (Tricor, Trilipix) as both have modest uricosuric effects.[15]

SPECIAL CONSIDERATIONS

Renal and Hepatic Impairment

Selecting therapy for patients with gout can be challenging since many medications used for this condition require monitoring and dose adjustment in renal insufficiency. NSAIDs should be avoided in patients with either renal or hepatic impairment.[15] SUA concentrations should be monitored with allopurinol and probenecid. Both of these medications require renal dosage adjustment, while colchicine should be avoided altogether in severe renal dysfunction (CrCl < 10 mL/min).[21-22] In addition, probenecid is not effective in patients with reduced kidney function (CrCl < 50 mL/min).[21] Therefore, patients with renal dysfunction are typically candidates for either corticosteroids or febuxostat. Although febuxostat is metabolized in the liver, no dosage adjustment is needed for mild or moderate hepatic impairment (Child-Pugh Class A or B). Caution should be used in severe hepatic impairment, as no studies have been conducted in these patients.[21,23]

History of Gastrointestinal Bleeding/ Ulcers

Patients who are at increased bleeding risk or who have a history of GI bleeding or ulcers should avoid NSAIDs due to increased risk for gastropathy. Corticosteroids may provide a safer treatment option for these populations, although GI adverse events are still possible.[15] Moreover, patients on anticoagulation therapy are also at risk for bleeding, so NSAIDs should be used with caution.

Drug Interactions

Drug interactions should be carefully considered when selecting therapy for gout, since many medications can interact with treatment options for this condition. Concurrent use of erythromycin, simvastatin, and cyclosporine may alter the elimination of colchicine, resulting in an increased risk for adverse effects. Furthermore, concurrent use of warfarin and allopurinol can increase warfarin concentrations, so careful monitoring of INR values with possible subsequent dosage adjustments are warranted.[15] Allopurinol can also increase serum concentrations of theophylline, azathioprine, 6-mercaptopurine, so close monitoring and dosage adjustments may be needed.[15]

Major drug interactions of febuxostat include azathioprine, 6-mercaptopurine, and theophylline, all of which are xanthine oxidase substrates. Since coadministration can increase concentrations of these agents and potentially result in toxicity, febuxostat is contraindicated with these medications.

Since the uricosuric effect of probenecid is diminished by low-dose aspirin, this treatment combination may not be appropriate for patients taking aspirin for primary or secondary cardiovascular protection. Furthermore, probenecid inhibits renal tubular secretion of some medications, including penicillins, most cephalosporins, rifampin, and methotrexate, thereby increasing plasma concentrations and possibly leading to increased incidence of adverse effects.

CASE Application

1. Which of the following is *not* a risk factor for increased SUA levels?
   a. Increased age
   b. Female sex
   c. Increased body weight
   d. Increased alcohol intake

2. Which of the following foods is most likely to have the highest purine content?

   a. Liver
   b. Apple
   c. Popcorn
   d. Potatoes

3. Which of the following is *not* consistent with the typical clinical presentation of gout?

   a. Commonly affects the great toe
   b. Bilateral joint involvement
   c. Rapid onset of symptoms
   d. Self-limiting pain and erythema

4. A 76-year-old woman with a 10-year history of gout presents to the clinic with recently developed painful MSU crystal deposits in her hand tissues. Which of the following terms most accurately describes this complication of gout?

   a. Atheromas
   b. Podagra
   c. Tophi
   d. Uric acid nephrolithiasis

5. A 60-year-old man presents to the pharmacy with a past medical history of hypertension and gout. After reviewing his medication profile, which of the following medications is *most* likely to cause elevated SUA levels?

   a. Hydrochlorothiazide
   b. Lisinopril
   c. Metoprolol
   d. Indomethacin

6. Which of the following is the brand name for allopurinol?

   a. Uloric
   b. Zyloprim
   c. Zebeta
   d. Benemid

7. Which of the following is a *true* statement?

   a. Use of allopurinol increases warfarin levels and increases theophylline levels.
   b. Use of allopurinol increases warfarin levels and decreases theophylline levels.
   c. Use of allopurinol decreases warfarin levels and decreases theophylline levels.
   d. Use of allopurinol decreases warfarin levels and increases theophylline levels.

8. A resident approaches you about a patient who was just admitted for an acute gout flare. He wants to start the patient on corticosteroid therapy. Which of the following would be important to communicate to the resident regarding monitoring parameters?

   a. Recommend to monitor serum creatinine for renal dysfunction.
   b. Recommend to monitor blood glucose levels.
   c. Recommend to monitor for diarrhea.
   d. Recommend to monitor for presence of skin rash.

9. A 63-year-old man presents to your clinic complaining of excruciating pain in his left big toe. After being diagnosed with an acute gout flare, his physician wants to start him on therapy. His medical history is positive for hypertension, hyperlipidemia, peptic ulcer disease, and glaucoma. Which of the following is the most appropriate therapy for this patient?

   a. Ibuprofen
   b. Indomethacin
   c. Allopurinol
   d. Prednisone

10. In a patient with a creatinine clearance of less than 10 mL/min, which acute gout medication is most appropriate?

    a. Prednisone
    b. Ibuprofen
    c. Nabumetone
    d. Colchicine

11. A patient is picking up a new prescription for colchicine. Which of the following are the appropriate counseling points to discuss with the patient?

    a. The patient should be counseled on gastrointestinal side effects of nausea, vomiting, diarrhea, and abdominal pain.
    b. The patient should be counseled on possibility of a rash.
    c. The patient should be counseled on signs and symptoms of bleeding.
    d. The patient should be counseled on close monitoring of blood glucose levels.

12. Which of the following statements most accurately describes how NSAIDs work in the treatment of gout?

    a. NSAIDs work by reducing phagocytosis and lactic acid production in joints, thereby reducing deposition of urate crystals.
    b. NSAIDs work by blocking the conversion of xanthine to uric acid.
    c. NSAIDs work by exerting anti-inflammatory, analgesic, and antipyretic effects by inhibiting the synthesis of prostaglandin.
    d. NSAIDs work by inhibiting proximal renal tubule reabsorption of uric acid to decrease serum levels.

13. Which of the following statements is *true* regarding febuxostat?

    a. Febuxostat is a good choice for patients with liver failure.
    b. Febuxostat is the drug of choice for acute gout.

c. Febuxostat is an option for patients with renal insufficiency.
d. Febuxostat has no drug interactions.

14. Intravenous colchicine is not recommended due to the possibility of which adverse effect?

a. Leukopenia
b. Diarrhea
c. Hyperglycemia
d. Abdominal pain

15. Which of the following is a *true* statement regarding the use of NSAIDs in the treatment of gout?

a. Indomethacin is the NSAID of choice for treating gout.
b. Short-acting NSAIDs at equipotent, anti-inflammatory doses are the drugs of choice for acute gout in the absence of contraindications.
c. Intravenous administration of NSAID is the preferred route of administration for the treatment of gout.
d. NSAIDs are second-line treatment behind colchicine for the treatment of gout.

16. A 68-year-old man presents to the clinic with a history of three acute episodes of gout in the past year. He is classified as an overproducer of uric acid. He has liver impairment but no renal insufficiency. Which of the following medications is *most* appropriate for chronic prophylaxis of gout?

a. Allopurinol
b. Febuxostat
c. Probenecid
d. Sulfinpyrazone

17. What is the mechanism of action by which probenecid produces its effect?

a. Inhibition of xanthine oxidase
b. Blocks excretion of uric acid
c. Blocks reuptake of uric acid at the proximal tubule
d. Inhibits prostaglandin synthesis

Please use the following case to answer questions 18 and 19.

A 75-year-old man is started on allopurinol for gout prevention. His baseline serum uric acid level is 11.6 mg/dL. He is overweight (BMI 30 mg/m^2) and drinks 1 to 2 cans of beer a day.

18. Which of the following statements *best* describes the role of allopurinol for gout prevention?

a. Allopurinol is most effective when initiated within 24 to 48 hours of an acute attack.
b. The usual starting dose is 300 mg po daily.
c. Treatment with allopurinol should be continued for 3 to 12 months.
d. Serous side effects include myopathy and bone marrow suppression.

19. Regarding nonpharmacologic treatment of gout, which of the following measures should be avoided?

a. Weight loss
b. Reduction of alcohol consumption
c. Application of cold packs
d. Application of heat

20. The target serum uric acid level when treating gout is typically:

a. $\le$ 6 mg/dL
b. $\le$7 mg/dL
c. $\le$8 mg/dL
d. $\le$9 mg/dL

TAKEAWAY POINTS ››

- Gout is an acute and often recurrent monoarthritis caused by formation of MSU crystals in the joints and surrounding tissues.
- Hyperuricemia is defined as SUA concentrations > 7 mg/dL in men or > 6 mg/dL in women.
- Individuals with hyperuricemia do not always develop gout, while gouty attacks can occur with normal SUA concentrations.
- Definitive diagnosis of gout requires the observation of MSU crystals on needle aspirate, although many clinicians make the diagnosis based on clinical presentation.
- Signs and symptoms of hyperuricemia include pain, erythema, warmth, and swelling near the affected joint.
- Potential complications of gout include tophi, which can cause joint damage, and uric acid nephrolithiasis.
- Treatment of gout involves a combination of nonpharmacologic and pharmacologic approaches.
- Drugs of choice for acute gouty arthritis include NSAIDs and colchicine, which help to relieve pain and inflammation.
- Urate lowering therapy can be used for the chronic gout management to prevent flare-ups. Xanthine oxidase inhibitors, particularly allopurinol, are most commonly prescribed, but an alternative choice is a uricosuric agent such as probenecid.

REFERENCES

1. Mikuls TR, Farrar JT, Bilker WB, et al. Gout epidemiology: results from the UK General Practice Research Database, 1990-1999. *Ann Rheum Dis.* 2005;64:267-272.
2. Choi HK, Atkinson K, Karlson EW, et al. Purine-rich foods, dairy and protein intake, and the risk of gout in men. *N Engl J Med.* 2004;350:1093-1103.
3. Kramer HM, Curhan G. The association between gout and nephrolithiasis: The National Health and Nutrition Examination Survey III, 1988-1994. *Am J Kidney Dis.* 2002;40:37-42.
4. Chang HY, Pan WH, Yeh WT, et al. Hyperuricemia and gout in Taiwan: results of the nutritional and health survey in Taiwan (1993-1996). *J Rheumatol.* 2001;28:1640-1646.
5. Roubenoff R, Klag MJ, Mead LA, et al. Incidence and risk factors for gout in white men. *JAMA.* 1991;266:3004-3007.
6. Lawrence RC, Felson DT, Helmick CG, et al. Estimates of the prevalence of arthritis and other rheumatic conditions in the United States: Part II. *Arthritis Rheum.* 2008;58:26-35.
7. Johnson RJ, Rideout BA. Uric acid and diet—insights into the epidemic of cardiovascular disease. *N Engl J Med.* 2004;350:1071-1073.
8. Kim KY, Ralph Schumacher H, Hunsche E, et al. A literature review of the epidemiology and treatment of acute gout. *Clin Ther.* 2003;25:1593-1617.
9. Zhang W, Doherty M, Bardin T, et al. EULAR evidence based recommendations for gout. Part II: Management. Report of a task force of the EULAR Standing Committee for International Clinical Studies Including Therapeutics (ESCISIT). *Ann Rheum Dis.* 2006;65:1312-1324.
10. Wallace SL, Robinson H, Masi AT, et al. Preliminary criteria for the classification of the acute arthritis of primary gout. *Arthritis Rheum.* 1997;20:895-500.
11. Mikuls TR, MacLean CH, Olivieri J, et al. Quality of care indicators for gout management. *Arthritis Rheum.* 2004;50:937-943.
12. Jordan KM, Cameron JS, Snaith M, et al. British Society for Rheumatology and British Health Professionals in Rheumatology guideline for the management of gout. *Rheumatology.* (Oxford) 2007;46:1372-1374.
13. Schlesinger N, Baker DK, Beutler AM, et al. Local ice therapy during bouts of acute gouty arthritis. *J Rheumatol.* 2002;29:331-334.
14. Schlesinger N. Management of acute and chronic gouty arthritis. *Drugs.* 2004;64:2399-2416.
15. Keith MP, Gilliland WR. Updates in the management of gout. *Am J Med.* 2007;120:221-224.
16. Wall GC, Cooper SA. Gout and hyperuricemia: new guidelines and treatments. *J Pharm Prac.* 2009;22:104-115.
17. Singh H, Torralba KD. Therapeutic challenges in the management of gout in the elderly. *Geriatrics* 2008;6:13-20.
18. Bonnel RA, Villalba ML, Karwoski CB, et al. Deaths associated with inappropriate intravenous colchicine administration. *J Emerg Med.* 2002;22:385-387.
19. FDA News Release, 6 February 2008. Available at: http://www.fda.gov/NewsEvents/Newsroom/PressAnnouncements/2008/ucm116853.htm. Accessed October 30, 2009.
20. Keith MP, Gilliland WR. Updates in the management of gout. *Am J Med.* 2007;120:221-224.
21. Eggebeen AT. Gout: an update. *Am Fam Physician.* 2007;76:801-808.
22. Colchicine. In DRUGDEX System [Internet database]. Greenwood Village, Colo: Thomson Reuters (Healthcare) Inc. Updated periodically.
23. Uloric [package insert]. Available at: http://www.uloric.com/hcp/coming-soon.aspx. Accessed October 26, 2009.
24. Rimm EB, Giovannucci EL, Stampfer MJ, Colditz GA, Litin LB, Willett WC. Reproducibility and validity of an expanded self-administered semiquantitative food frequency questionnaire among male health professionals. *Am J Epidemiol.* 1992;135:1114-1126.
25. Willett WC, Sampson L, Stampfer MJ, et al. Reproducibility and validity of a semi-quantitative food frequency questionnaire. *Am J Epidemiol.* 1985;122:51-65.
26. Feskanich D, Rimm EB, Giovannucci EL, et al. Reproducibility and validity of food intake measurements from a semiquantitative food frequency questionnaire. *J Am Diet Associ.* 1993;93:790-796.
27. Wallace SL, Robinson H, Masi AT, Decker JL, McCarty DJ, Yu TF. Preliminary criteria for the classification of the acute arthritis of primary gout. *Arthritis Rheum.* 1997;20:895-900.
28. Choi HK, Gao X, Curhan G. Vitamin C intake and the risk of gout in men: a prospective study. *Arch Intern Med.* 2009;169;5:502-507.
29. Willett W. *Nutritional Epidemiology.* 2nd ed. New York, NY: Oxford University Press, 1998.
30. Garrel DR, Verdy M, PetitClerc C, Martin C, Brule D, Hamet P. Milk- and soy-protein ingestion: acute effect on serum uric acid concentration. *Am J Clin Nutr.* 1991;53:665-669.

CHAPTER

46 Osteoporosis

Thomas F. Oppelt

FOUNDATION OVERVIEW

Osteoporosis is a disease of the skeleton marked by low bone mass and microarchitectural degeneration of bone tissue, with a subsequent increase in fracture risk.[1,2] In the United States, 10 million people are estimated to have osteoporosis and almost 34 million more are believed to have osteopenia (low bone mass), placing them at risk of developing osteoporosis.[3] Studies suggest that over 2 million osteoporosis-related fractures occur in the United States annually, with an estimated cost of $17 billion.[4,5] Some speculate that the prevalence of these bone metabolism disorders may be on the rise, in part, due to a decrease in the overall routine utilization of hormone replacement therapy (HRT) for most postmenopausal women. In 2002, the Women's Health Initiative (WHI) was published suggesting that the risks of long-term estrogen plus progestin supplementation outweighed any benefits (namely, the FDA-approved prevention of osteoporosis).[5] Also, while osteoporosis is less prevalent in men than women, men account for almost 30% of low bone mass related (fragility) fractures.[4]

The human adult skeleton is essentially comprised of two types of bone: cortical (80%) and trabecular (20%). Cortical bone forms the exterior portion, while trabecular bone forms the porous interior, as well as at the ends of long bones, vertebrae and distal forearms. Throughout life, bone undergoes remodeling, a process where old, damaged bone is routinely removed and replaced by new bone.[6] The resorption (removal) phase is conducted by osteoclasts utilizing proteolytic enzymes to dissolve a targeted area. This is closely followed by the formation (replacement) phase, as osteoblasts utilize calcium and phosphorous, among other ions, to lay down newly formed bone tissue. This process normally tends to favor bone formation over resorption until the age of 30 years, when bone reaches its peak mass and formation and resorption become balanced.[7] Osteopenia, and ultimately osteoporosis, is the result of an uncoupling of this balance in favor of osteoclast-driven resorption.[6,8,9] Modalities of prevention and treatment of osteoporosis typically target osteoblastic or osteoclastic function, either directly or indirectly.

Osteoporosis is routinely asymptomatic. In some cases, osteoporosis may present as shortened stature (kyphosis, or humpbacked; lordosis, or bent backward), bone pain or most frequently as a fracture of the vertebra, hip, or forearm.[5] Therefore, it is critical to provide screening to those patients at risk (Table 46-1).[8,9] The diagnosis of osteoporosis is characteristically made by evaluating bone mineral density (BMD) via dual energy x-ray absorptiometry (DXA). A BMD is recorded as a T-score, which is the difference between a patient's bone mineral density (g/cm^2) and the expected BMD of a sex-matched young healthy adult.[1] The World Health Organization (WHO) uses specific T-score ranges to assist in the diagnosis of osteopenia and osteoporosis (Table 46-2).[1]

The National Osteoporosis Foundation (NOF) recommends patients should have a BMD measured every 2 years (though some clinicians may assess annually with higher risk patients).[2] In general, a BMD should be considered for postmenopausal women under age 65 with one or more risk factors, all women over the age of 65, men between age 50 to 70 with one or more risk factors and all men over 70 years old (see Table 46-1).[2] It is important to note that BMD is specific but not sensitive for fracture risk. Over 50% of patients with a hip fracture, for example, have a T-score > -2.5.[9] The WHO has provided an online risk assessment tool known as FRAX (www.shef.ac.uk/FRAX), which accounts for 12 risk factors and BMD, to account for this disparity.[10] The WHO recommends considering pharmacologic therapy for those with a 10-year fracture probability $\geq 3\%$ for the hip or $\geq 20\%$ for any major fracture.

PREVENTION

Preventing osteoporosis and reaching maximum bone mass usually begins with a healthy lifestyle, including a proper diet and weight bearing exercise. In addition, patients should be advised to avoid the use of tobacco and the excessive consumption of alcoholic beverages.[9] These basic steps are followed by ensuring the adequate intake of calcium and vitamin D (Vit D). The NOF recommends the following for adult women and men:[11]

- 19 through 49 years old—Calcium 1000 mg qd and vitamin D 400 to 800 IU qd
- 50+ years old—Calcium 1200 mg qd and vitamin D 800 to 1000 IU qd

Calcium is most commonly available as two salt forms: calcium carbonate and calcium citrate. A patient experiences peak

Disclosure: Thomas Oppelt is a Regional Account Scientific Director (RASD) with US Medical Affairs for Novartis Pharmaceutical Corporation. Novartis manufactures/markets zoledronic acid and calcitonin.

TABLE 46-1 **Common Risk Factors for Osteoporosis**

- Estrogen deficiency (a result of menopause)
- Amenorrhea (absence of menstrual periods)
- Advanced age
- Caucasian/Asian/Latino race
- Family history of osteoporosis
- Low weight and body mass index (BMI < 21 kg/m^2)
- History of prior fracture (after age 50)
- Current smoking
- Alcoholism
- Calcium and/or vitamin D deficiency
- Cushing syndrome
- Hypogonadism (low testosterone in men)
- Anorexia/eating disorders
- Celiac sprue
- Inflammatory bowel disease (IBD)
- Hyperparathyroidism
- Hyperthyroidism
- Rheumatoid arthritis (RA)

absorption when the carbonate form is taken with food, while the citrate form can be taken with or without food (but often costs more).[11] It should be noted that vitamin D deficiency (25(OH)D serum concentration < 20 ng/mL) is very common throughout the United States in children and adults.[12] One predicted cause of this may be the increased use of sunscreen. Sunscreen lowers the risk of certain skin cancers, but also affects the body's ability to absorb vitamin D from sunlight.[12] The lower the baseline vitamin D serum concentration, the more difficult it is to get to an appropriate level (> 30+ ng/mL) and often requires a loading dose (given orally or intramuscularly).[12,13] A general rule of thumb is to ensure a patient has adequate and sustained calcium and vitamin D levels prior to initiating pharmacologic therapy.

Antiresorptive Agents

Bisphosphonates

Bisphosphonates (BPs) are within a class of medications known as antiresorptive agents, because they target the effects of osteoclasts. Specifically, BPs selectively adhere to and incorporate with bone (leading to long terminal half-lives often measured in years) and cause osteoclast apoptosis during the bone remodeling process.[14,15] This results in a prevention of bone loss, as observed by a stabilization or improvement in BMD, as well as a reduction in fractures. As of September 2009, the US Food and Drug Administration (FDA) has approved the following BPs for the prevention of osteoporosis: alendronate, risedronate, ibandronate and zoledronic acid (Table 46-3). Initially, BPs were given as a daily pill. However, it became evident that the appropriate use of these medications was plagued with poor patient compliance. Therefore, the oral BPs were reexamined utilizing different dosing strategies to allow weekly and monthly dosing and a subsequent improvement in adherence.[16,17] More recently, intravenous (IV) zoledronic acid became available for osteoporosis prevention and is dosed every 2 years.[18] The most recognized side effects of oral BPs include abdominal pain, esophageal irritation, and nausea.[19,20,21] To minimize these gastrointestinal (GI) side effects and maximize absorption, patients are directed to take their oral BP first thing in the morning, with a full glass of water, and remain upright without eating or drinking for 30 to 60 minutes.[19,20,21] It is noteworthy to remember that ions, including calcium, can decrease the bioavailability of oral BPs and patients may need to consider using water that has a low mineral content as opposed to tap or well water (ie, certain bottled water may need to be considered).[22] The IV BPs, which do have some GI side effects (albeit lower than the oral BPs), are associated with post-dose flu-like symptoms, musculoskeletal pain, and mild to moderate injection site reactions.[23,24] Osteonecrosis of the jaw (ONJ), defined as an area of exposed bone in the maxillofacial region that does not heal within 8 weeks, has been reported in patients taking BPs (oral or IV).[25] However, a causal relationship has not been determined.[25] In general, BPs are contraindicated in patients with hypocalcemia and patients with renal dysfunction (creatinine clearance≤ 30-35 mL/min, based on individual product labeling).

Estrogen and Selective Estrogen Receptor Modulators

As previously mentioned, estrogen is FDA approved for the prevention of postmenopausal osteoporosis, though not routinely used because of the increased risk of cardiovascular disease, blood clotting, and breast cancer (Table 46-4).[4] Raloxifene is a selective estrogen receptor modulator (SERM) that activates estrogen pathways in some tissues, while blocking those same pathways in others. In general, both estrogen and raloxifene inhibit osteoclast formation and recruitment (by osteoblasts).[26,27] Clinically, this results in raloxifene increasing BMD, decreasing vertebral fractures, and lowering serum total cholesterol and low-density lipoprotein cholesterol much like estrogen, but does not stimulate activity at the endometrium or breast tissue.[26,27] The side effect profile of raloxifene includes leg cramps, hot flushes, and venous thromboembolism.[26,27]

TABLE 46-2 **World Health Organization (WHO) Definitions**

BMD	Definition
T-score < −1.0 to > −2.5	Osteopenia
T-score ≤ −2.5	Osteoporosis

TREATMENT

Antiresorptive Agents

Several bisphosphonates are FDA approved for the treatment of postmenopausal osteoporosis, as discussed previously

TABLE 46-3 FDA-Approved Bisphosphonates for the Management of Osteoporosis

Generic (Brand[a])	Indication(s)/Dose(s)
Alendronate (Fosamax) *Also available as Fosamax Plus D*	Prevention: ▪ 35 mg po every week ▪ 5 mg po qd Treatment: ▪ 70 mg po every week ▪ 10 mg po qd Treatment in men: ▪ 70 mg po every week ▪ 10 mg po qd Treatment of glucocorticoid-induced osteoporosis: ▪ 5-10 mg po qd
Risedronate (Actonel) *Also available as Actonel with Calcium*	Prevention and treatment: ▪ 35 mg po every week ▪ 75 mg po every 2 consecutive days monthly ▪ 150 mg po every month ▪ 5 mg po qd Treatment in men: ▪ 35 mg po every week Prevention and treatment of glucocorticoid-induced osteoporosis: ▪ 5 mg po qd
Ibandronate (Boniva)	Prevention and treatment: ▪ 150 mg po every month ▪ 2.5 mg po qd Treatment: ▪ 3 mg IV every 3 months
Zoledronic acid (Reclast)	Prevention: ▪ 5 mg IV once every 2 years Treatment: ▪ 5 mg IV once a year Treatment in men: ▪ 5 mg IV once a year Prevention and treatment of glucocorticoid-induced osteoporosis: ▪ 5 mg IV once a year

[a]US trade name:
Fosamax and Fosamax Plus D are registered trademarks of Merck & Co, Inc.
Actonel and Actonel with Calcium are registered trademarks of Procter & Gamble Pharmaceuticals.
Boniva is a registered trademark of Roche Therapeutics Inc.
Reclast is a registered trademark of Novartis Pharmaceuticals Corp.

(see Table 46-3). In addition, there are a number of BPs available for the treatment of men with low bone mass, as well as the prevention and treatment of glucocorticoid-induced osteoporosis. Raloxifene is also indicated for postmenopausal osteoporosis treatment. The side effect profiles of BPs and raloxifene are as previously discussed.

Calcitonin

Calcitonin is a synthetic hormone that inhibits bone resorption through a decrease in osteoclast formation and its attachment to bone during the remodeling process.[28] Subsequently, nasal calcitonin has been shown to reduce the risk of new vertebral fractures in postmenopausal women, as well as increase lumbar spine BMD.[29] Nasal calcitonin is generally well tolerated but has been known to cause nasal congestion/discharge, sneezing, dry mouth, and nausea.[29] Due to the lack of compelling data showing prevention in hip fracture, nasal calcitonin is generally reserved for those who cannot tolerate other agents. Injectable salmon calcitonin is approved for the treatment of osteoporosis as well, but is rarely used due to its cost (compared to the nasal form) and route of administration.

Anabolic Agents

Teriparatide

Teriparatide is a recombinant form of parathyroid hormone (PTH^{1-34}) that has an anabolic effect, in that it stimulates bone formation.[30] Unlike antiresorptive agents that target osteoclasts, PTH^{1-34} increases osteoblastic formation while inhibiting osteoblast apoptosis.[30,31] The clinical response to this agent includes increases in BMD and a decrease in the risk of vertebral and nonvertebral fractures.[32] Despite its novel mechanism of action,

TABLE 46-4 **FDA-Approved Medications for the Management of Osteoporosis (Other Than Bisphosphonates)**

Medication Class	Generic (Brand[a])	Indication(s)/Dose(s)
Antiresorptive agents	Estrogen (multiple brands)	Prevention: ▪ Multiple forms and formulations
	Raloxifene (Evista)	Prevention and treatment: ▪ 60 mg po qd [a]Indicated for reduction in the risk of invasive breast cancer in postmenopausal women
	Salmon calcitonin (Miacalcin nasal spray or injectable)	Treatment—Nasal: ▪ One spray (200 IU) in the nose qd, alternating nostrils Treatment—Injectable: ▪ Half cc (100 IU) SQ or IM qd
Anabolic agents	Teriparatide (Forteo)	Treatment: ▪ 20 μg SQ qd Treatment in men: ▪ 20 μg SQ qd Treatment of glucocorticoid-induced osteoporosis: ▪ 20 μg SQ qd

[a]US trade name:
Evista is a registered trademark of Eli Lilly and Company.
Miacalcin is a registered trademark of Novartis Pharmaceuticals Corp.
Forteo is a registered trademark of Eli Lilly and Company.

PTH^{1-34} is generally reserved for men or women at "high risk" of fracture or "severe" osteoporosis, as well as those who develop glucocorticoid-induced osteoporosis.[31,33] This is essentially due to its high cost, coupled with the fact that it is indicated as a daily injection.[31] PTH^{1-34} has side effects including dizziness and leg cramps, and hypercalcemia and hypercalciuria should be monitored.[31,32] Of note, teriparatide was associated with osteosarcoma in rats, though this has not been routinely seen with human use.[31,32] Nevertheless, PTH^{1-34} should not be used in patients at risk for osteosarcoma, including patients with Paget disease or bone metastases/malignancies. PTH^{1-34} should not be used in patients for more than 2 years and clinicians often follow therapy with an antiresorptive agent to preserve the improvements in BMD.[34]

CASE Application

1. Which of the following are correct?
   a. While osteoporosis is more prominent in women, osteopenia is equally common in men and women.
   b. Due to the availability of many medications, the prevalence of osteoporosis has been declining in the United States.
   c. Osteoporosis is most commonly associated with musculoskeletal pain.
   d. The most common sites for osteoporotic fractures include the spine and hip.
   e. Low bone mass is common in patients under the age of 30, but improves in time under normal physiologic conditions.

2. SD is a 45-year-old woman. She does not have any significant past-medical history and currently smokes one-half pack a day and drinks alcohol socially. She attends a health fair and learns her T-score is −1.5. Which is the best course of action?
   a. SD has osteopenia and should be started on alendronate 70 mg po every week.
   b. SD has no physical signs or symptoms of osteoporosis and should be advised to quit smoking and to have her BMD checked again in 6 months.
   c. SD is young and should be started on teriparatide 20 μg SQ qd to rebuild her bone mass to more normal levels.
   d. SD should be started on calcium 1000 mg and vitamin D 800 IU qd.

3. Which of the following is true?
   a. Osteoclasts are primarily responsible for the formation phase of bone remodeling and are stimulated by calcium and vitamin D.
   b. Bone remodeling is generally reserved for areas of bone that suffer acute damage.
   c. Osteoblastic function is stimulated by bisphosphonates.
   d. None of the above is true.

4. Select the risk factors for osteoporosis.
   a. HRT therapy that is prescribed at a slightly higher dose than recommended by the FDA
   b. Low body mass index (BMI < 21 kg/m^2)
   c. Being African American
   d. All of the above

5. JR is a 58-year-old white man who presents to the emergency department (ED) with a hip fracture after rolling out of his bed in his home. His vitals and laboratory values are generally unremarkable. He is 5 ft 8 in and weighs 133 lb. His medical history includes mild asthma and rheumatoid

arthritis. His current medications include albuterol inhaler every 4 to 6 hours prn, prednisone 10 mg qd, and a multivitamin. After discharge from the hospital, he is sent to your clinic about 3 weeks later for further evaluation. Which of the following is the best answer?

a. JR should have a BMD checked immediately to determine if he has osteoporosis.
b. JR is a candidate for zoledronic acid 5 mg IV with repeat dosing every other year.
c. JR is a candidate for raloxifene 60 mg po qd.
d. JR is a candidate for teriparatide 20 μg SQ qd.
e. JR should start taking calcium and vitamin D and follow-up in 6 months.

6. Select the agent that can be administered monthly for osteoporosis treatment.

a. Risedronate
b. Raloxifene
c. Zoledronic acid
d. Alendronate
e. None of the above

7. RS is a 67-year-old Asian woman with a T-score −2.7. She is 5 ft 6 in and 127 lb. She was admitted to the hospital with leg swelling that was diagnosed as deep vein thrombosis (DVT) and was ultimately referred to your clinic upon resolution and discharge. Her medical history includes hypertension, osteoarthritis, and diabetes. She currently takes furosemide, Accupril, celecoxib, metformin, and aspirin. Which of the following is the best answer?

a. RS should begin taking calcium 1000 mg qd and vitamin D 400 IU qd.
b. RS is a candidate for estrogen 0.625 mg po qd.
c. RS is a candidate for ibandronate 3 mg IV every 3 months.
d. RS is a candidate for raloxifene 60 mg po qd.

8. Which of the following condition(s) would suggest caution for receiving a bisphosphonate?

a. Creatinine clearance CrCl < 30 mL/min
b. Peanut allergy
c. History of stroke
d. History of Paget disease
e. All of the above

9. Which of the following is true regarding teriparatide?

a. It may be associated with hypercalcemia.
b. It is contraindicated in a patient with Paget disease.
c. It is available as a monthly IM injection.
d. It should only be used for a maximum of 3 years.
e. More than one of the above is true.

10. Which of the following is true regarding bisphosphonates?

a. Ibandronate po should be taken with food to minimize any GI side effects.
b. Risedronate should be taken at bedtime to minimize any CNS side effects, including dizziness.
c. A patient receiving zoledronic acid should avoid drinking high-mineral water (ie, well water).
d. A patient taking alendronate should also routinely be taking calcium and vitamin D.

11. Select the brand name for raloxifene.

a. Evista
b. Fosamax
c. Premarin
d. Reclast
e. Actonel

12. Select the osteoporosis medication that is available as a nasal spray.

a. Ibandronate
b. Teriparatide
c. Calcitonin
d. Zoledronic acid
e. None of the above

13. KG is a 59-year-old postmenopausal woman who is sent to you on referral. She recently had her BMD checked and had a T-score of −2.3. Her past medical history is unremarkable, and she only takes a multivitamin with additional calcium and vitamin D. Her family history is remarkable for a mother who had osteoporosis and died of breast cancer and a father who has diabetes. Which of the following is the best answer?

a. KG has osteopenia but is taking appropriate calcium and vitamin D.
b. KG is a good candidate for risedronate 5 mg po qd.
c. KG is a good candidate for alendronate 70 mg IV every week.
d. KG is a good candidate for raloxifene 60 mg po qd.
e. KG is a good candidate for calcitonin 100 IU IM qd.

14. MF is a 63-year-old postmenopausal woman who recently learned her T-score is −2.9 (it was −2.8 a year ago) despite being on an oral bisphosphonate, calcium, and vitamin D. She is not on any additional medications. Which of the following should her pharmacist do first?

a. Explain to her that at 63 years and being postmenopausal, such a small change in BMD is not surprising.
b. Suggest she talk to her doctor about taking a different bisphosphonate.
c. Recommend to her physician that raloxifene should be added to the current regimen.
d. Counsel the patient to see how she is taking her medications and review her refill records to see if she is filling the bisphosphonate as expected.

15. Which of the following is true regarding vitamin D?

a. Low serum vitamin D levels are common throughout the United States.
b. For postmenopausal patients, vitamin D 400 IU qd is typically adequate.

c. If a patient has significantly low serum vitamin D levels, vitamin D 800 IU qd will usually correct this over time.
d. All of the above are true.

16. Which of the following is true?

a. FRAX is an online tool for patients to use when learning about bisphosphonates.
b. FRAX helps determine who might be the best candidates for osteoporosis therapy.
c. FRAX is generally not useful for patients with a T-score > −1.4.
d. All of the above.

17. Which of the following matches the medication with a commonly associated side effect.

a. Alendronate—Nasal congestion
b. Ibandronate—Gout
c. Raloxifene—Hot flushes
d. Teriparatide—Memory loss
e. Zoledronic acid—Dry mouth

18. SM is a 65-year-old postmenopausal woman with a T-score of −3.0. Her past medical history is notable for osteoarthritis. She currently takes naproxen, as well as calcium 1200 mg and vitamin D 1000 IU qd. Which of the following is correct?

a. SM is on the appropriate doses of calcium and vitamin D according to WHO guidelines.
b. SM is a candidate for risedronate 150 mg po every month, despite the fact she is on naproxen.
c. SM should have her vitamin D level checked, despite the high dose of vitamin D she is currently taking.
d. SM is a candidate for zoledronic acid 5 mg IV once a year, but normal renal function should be observed prior to receiving each dose.
e. All of the above.

19. Which of the following is true?

a. The human skeleton is comprised of two types of bone: subcortical and trochanter.
b. BMD is specific but not sensitive for fracture risk.
c. A radiographic x-ray cannot determine osteoporosis.
d. ONJ is an area of exposed bone in the maxillofacial region that does not heal within 2 weeks of its occurrence.

20. Which of the following are risk factors for osteoporosis?

a. History of fracture while in college playing rugby
b. Amenorrhea starting at age 45
c. Occasionally drinking a glass of wine with dinner
d. b and c

TAKEAWAY POINTS ››

- Osteoporosis is a common disease that is often asymptomatic and ultimately preventable and treatable.
- The process of bone remodeling is driven by osteoclasts, which cause resorption, and osteoblasts, which lead to formation of bone. Osteopenia and osteoporosis are the result of this process favoring resorption.
- The WHO defines osteoporosis as having a BMD T-score ≤ −2.5 as determined by DXA, though fractures are somewhat common in patients above this threshold.
- FRAX is an online tool that combines a T-score with 12 risk factors to determine a patient's risk of fracture. This risk allows clinicians to determine who is a potential candidate for therapy.
- The target of antiresorptive agents, including bisphosphonates, estrogen, and SERMs, as well as calcitonin, is to inhibit osteoclastic function.
- The target of anabolic agents, namely teriparatide (PTH^{1-34}), is to stimulate osteoblastic function.
- Calcium and vitamin D are essential to the prevention and treatment of osteoporosis.
- Bisphosphonates, which improve/stabilize BMD and prevent fractures, are available in numerous formulations and dosing schedules to attempt to offset the risks of poor compliance.
- Therapies including bisphosphonates, estrogen (to some degree), SERMs, calcitonin, and teriparatide all have unique properties that can be used to customize therapy based on individual patient needs.

REFERENCES

1. World Health Organization. Prevention and management of osteoporosis. *World Health Organ Tech Rep Ser*. 2003; 921:1-164.
2. National Osteoporosis Foundation. Osteoporosis: Review of the evidence for prevention, diagnosis and treatment and cost-effectiveness analysis. *Osteoporosis Int*. 1998;8(suppl 4):1-88.
3. Looker AC, Orwoll ES, Johnston CC Jr, et al. Prevalence of low femoral bone density in older U.S. adults from NHANES III. *J Bone Miner Res*. 1997;12:1761-1768.
4. Burge R, Dawson-Hughes B, Solomon DH, et al. Incidence and economic burden of osteoporosis-related fracture in the United States, 2005-2025. *J Bone Miner Res*. 2007;22(3):465-475.

5. Writing group for the Women's Health Initiative Investigators. Risks and benefits of estrogen plus progestin in healthy postmenopausal women: principal results from the Women's Health Initiative randomized control trial. *JAMA*. 2002;288:321-333.
6. Raisz LG. Local and systemic factors in the pathogenesis of osteoporosis. *N Engl J Med*. 1988;318(13):818-828.
7. Bonjour JP, Theintz G, Law F, et al. Peak bone mass. *Osteoporos Int*. 1994;4(suppl 1):7-13.
8. Kanis JA. Diagnosis of osteoporosis and assessment of fracture risk. *Lancet*. 2002;359:1929-1936.
9. Nanes MS, Kallen CB. Clinical assessment of fracture risk and novel therapeutic strategies to combat osteoporosis. *Fertil Steril*. 2009;92(2):403-412.
10. World Health Organization Collaborating Centre for Metabolic Bone Diseases. WHO Fracture Risk Assessment Tool (FRAX®). University of Sheffield, UK. WHO; 2009. Available at: http://www.shef.ac.uk/FRAX/. Accessed September 3, 2009.
11. National Osteoporosis Foundation. *What you should know about calcium*. Washington, DC: National Osteoporosis Foundation; 2008. Available at: http://www.nof.org/prevention/calcium2.htm. Accessed September 4, 2009.
12. Holick MF. Vitamin D deficiency. *N Engl J Med*. 2007;357(3):266-281. Available at: http://www.nof.org/prevention/calcium2.htm. Accessed September 4, 2009.
13. Roux C, Bischoff-Ferrari HA, Papoulos SE, et al. New insights into the role of vitamin D and calcium in osteoporosis management: an expert roundtable discussion. *Curr Med Res Opin*. 2008;24(5):1363-1370.
14. Drake MT, Clarke BL, Khosla A. Bisphosphonates: mechanism of action and role in clinical practice. *Mayo Clin Proc*. 2008;83(9):1032-1045.
15. Khan SA, Kanis JA, Vasikaran S, et al. Elimination and biochemical responses to intravenous alendronate in postmenopausal osteoporosis. *J Bone Miner Res*. 1997;12:1700-1707.
16. Recker RR, Gallagher R, Maccosbe PE. Effects of dosing frequency on bisphosphonate medication adherence in a large longitudinal cohort of women. *Mayo Clin Proc*. 2005;80:856-861.
17. Cooper A, Drake J, Brankin E. Treatment persistence with once-monthly ibandronate and patient support vs. once-weekly alendronate: results from the PERSIST study. *Int J Clin Pract*. 2006;60:896-905.
18. Biennial IV zoledronic acid (Reclast) for prevention of osteoporosis. *Med Lett Drugs Ther*. 2009;51:49.
19. Black DM, Cummings SR, Karpf DB, et al. Randomised trial of effect of alendronate on risk of fracture in women with existing vertebral fractures. *Lancet*. 1996;348:1535-1541.
20. Harris ST, Watts NB, Genant HK, et al. Effects of risedronate treatment on vertebral and nonvertebral fractures in women with postmenopausal osteoporosis: a randomized controlled trial. Vertebral Efficacy With Risedronate Therapy (VERT) Study Group. *JAMA*. 1999;282(14):1344-1352.
21. Chestnut CH, Skag A, Christiansen C, et al. Oral Ibandronate Osteoporosis Vertebral Fracture Trial in North America and Europe (BONE). Effects of oral ibandronate administered daily or intermittently on fracture risk in postmenopausal osteoporosis. *J Bone Miner Res*. 2004;19(8):1241-1249.
22. Morr S, Cuartas E, Alwattar B, et al. How much calcium is in your drinking water? A survey of calcium concentrations in bottled and tap water and their significance for medical treatment and drug administration. *HSS Journal*. 2006;2(2):130-135.
23. Eisman JA, Civitelli R, Adami S, et al. Efficacy and tolerability of intravenous ibandronate injections in postmenopausal osteoporosis: 2-year results from the DIVA study. *J Rheum*. 2008;35:488-497.
24. Black DM, Delmas PD, Eastell R, et al. Once-yearly zoledronic acid for treatment of postmenopausal osteoporosis. *N Engl J Med*. 2007;356:1809-1822.
25. Khosla S, Burr D, Cauley J, et al. American Society for Bone and Mineral Research. Bisphosphonate-associated osteonecrosis of the jaw: report of a task force of the American Society for Bone and Mineral Research. *J Bone Miner Res*. 2007;22(10):1479-1491.
26. Delmas PD, Bjarnason NH, Mitlak BH, et al. Effects of raloxifene on bone mineral density, serum cholesterol concentrations, and uterine endometrium in postmenopausal women. *N Engl J Med*. 1997;337(23):1641-1647.
27. Ettinger B, Black DM, Mitlak BH, et al. Reduction of vertebral fracture risk in postmenopausal women with osteoporosis treated with raloxifene: results from a 3-year randomized clinical trial. Multiple Outcomes of Raloxifene Evaluation (MORE) Investigators. *JAMA*. 1999;282:637-645.
28. Baron B, Vignery A. Behavior of osteoclasts during a rapid change in their number induced by high doses of parathyroid hormone or Calcitonin in intact rats. *Metab Bone Dis Relat Res*. 1981;2:339-346.
29. Chestnut CH, Silverman S, Andriano K, et al. A randomized trial of nasal spray salmon calcitonin in postmenopausal women with established osteoporosis: the prevent recurrence of osteoporotic fractures study. PROOF Study Group. *Am J Med*. 2000;109:267-276.
30. Dempster DW, Cosman F, Parisien M, et al. Anabolic actions of parathyroid hormone on bone. *Endocr Rev*. 1993;14:690-709.
31. Hodsman AB, Bauer DC, Dempster DW, et al. Parathyroid hormone and teriparatide for the treatment of osteoporosis: a review of the evidence and suggested guidelines for its use. *Endocr Rev*. 2005;26(5):688-703.
32. Neer RM, Arnaud CD, Zanchetta JR, et al. Effect of parathyroid hormone (1-34) on fractures and bone mineral density in postmenopausal women with osteoporosis. *N Engl J Med*. 2001;344:1434-1441.
33. Saag KG, Shane E, Boonen S, et al. Teriparatide or alendronate in glucocorticoid-induced osteoporosis. *N Engl J Med*. 2007;357:2028-2039.
34. Black DM, Bilezikian JP, Ensrud KE, et al. One year of alendronate after one year of parathyroid hormone (1-84) for osteoporosis. *N Engl J Med*. 2005;353(6):555-565.

CHAPTER

47 Rheumatoid Arthritis

Alison M. Reta, Rory E. O'Callaghan, Steven W. Chen

FOUNDATION OVERVIEW

Rheumatoid arthritis (RA) is a chronic systemic disorder that strikes approximately 1% of the world's population.[1,2] The onset is usually at a young age (15-45 years), and occurs more frequently in women than in men.[3] The exact etiology of RA is not well understood, and the factors that initiate the inflammatory process are unknown, but it is clearly an autoimmune disease involving T-lymphocytes, B-lymphocytes, macrophages, and cytokines.[3] The body's immune cells are unable to differentiate between self and nonself, and begin to target the joint tissue. T-lymphocytes produce proinflammatory cytokines and produce cytotoxic substances that lead to the erosion of bone and cartilage. Activated B-lymphocytes produce plasma cells, which form antibodies that attack joint tissues. Macrophages begin to release prostaglandins and cytotoxins to cause further injury and inflammation.[3]

RA is classically characterized by the presence of chronic inflammation and symmetric erosive synovitis, leading to joint deterioration and deformity. Early in the disease course, patients may develop vague, generalized symptoms such as fatigue, malaise, diffuse musculoskeletal pain, and morning stiffness in joints that lasts for longer than 30 minutes.[4] In the majority of cases, these symptoms develop insidiously over weeks to months.[4] The small joints of the hands, wrists, and feet are most likely to be involved and may appear swollen and feel warm to the touch. At later stages, joints of the fingers may become deformed because of the erosive effect of the disease on bones, tendons, and ligaments. RA patients occasionally have extra-articular involvement associated with their disease such as vasculitis, Sjögren, rheumatoid nodules, and pulmonary or cardiac complications.[3]

There are no specific laboratory tests that establish a diagnosis of RA, but several tests suggest the diagnosis.[4] About 60% to 70% of RA patients will test positive for rheumatoid factor (RF), and approximately 25% of patients will test positive for antinuclear antibody (ANA). Erythrocyte sedimentation rates and C-reactive protein (CRP) levels may also be elevated, although these are nonspecific markers of inflammation. A complete blood count (CBC) may reveal anemia of chronic disease or thrombocytopenia.[3]

According to the American College of Rheumatology, a diagnosis of RA is made when patients meet four of the following seven criteria for at least 6 weeks: morning stiffness (lasting more than 1 hour), swelling in three or more joint areas, swelling in the hand or wrist joints, symmetrical arthritis, rheumatoid nodules, positive RF, and radiological changes (joint erosions or decalcifications).[5]

With time, RA can vary in activity and severity among individuals and within the same patient. For this reason is it important to assess disease duration, activity level, and prognostic factors for each patient. Disease duration is classified as "early" if it has persisted for <6 months, "intermediate" if for 6 to 24 months, and "long" if for >24 months. Several validated instruments (the RA Disease Activity Score and Simplified Disease Activity Index, to name two) are available to measure RA disease activity more objectively and consistently; these instruments generally provide a disease activity score used to classify disease activity as low, moderate, or high, which is then considered when making further treatment decisions.[6,7] Poor prognostic factors include active disease with high (>20) tender and swollen joint counts, increased RF level, extra-articular involvement, radiographic erosions, increased anticyclic citrullinated peptide antibodies, and functional limitation (as assessed by the Health Assessment Questionnaire disability index).[1,4,8]

TREATMENT

The five goals of therapy for RA are to minimize symptoms, alleviate pain, maintain joint function and range of motion, prevent disease progression, and create a drug treatment plan that maximizes medication efficacy, safety, and tolerance.[5,8] Current RA treatment guidelines recommend the initiation of disease-modifying antirheumatic drugs (DMARDs) soon after RA diagnosis, but nonsteroidal and other analgesic medications may be used as concurrent initial therapy while waiting for the therapeutic onset of DMARD agents.[1] Biologic DMARDs can be used, but typically only after a patient has experienced treatment failure with nonbiologics, particularly methotrexate. Generally speaking, patients early in the disease course presenting with low disease activity are not candidates for biologic therapy.[5]

Nondrug Therapy

In addition to medication therapy, all RA patients should receive self-management education and training. Education and emotional support for both patient and his or her family is

TABLE 47-1 Use of Nonbiologic DMARD Agents Relative to Disease Status

Nonbiologic DMARDs	Disease Duration[a]	Disease Activity[b]	Poor Prognostic Factors[c]
	Monotherapy		
Methotrexate	All	All	+/–
Leflunomide	All	All	+/–
Hydroxychloroquine	Early/intermediate	Low	–
	Combination		
MTX + hydroxychloroquine	Long All All	Low Moderate High	+/– +/– +/–
MTX + leflunomide	Intermediate/long	High	+/–
MTX + sulfasalazine	All	High	+
Hydroxychloroquine + leflunomide	Intermediate	High	–
MTX + hydroxychloroquine + sulfasalazine	All	Moderate/high	+

[a]Disease duration: early <6 months, intermediate 6-24 months, long >24 months.

[b]Disease activity: low, moderate, high.

[c]Poor prognostic factors: positive, poor prognostic factors present; negative, without poor prognostic factors; positive/negative, recommendation independent of prognostic factors.

Adapted from Saag KG, Teng GG, Patkar NM, et al. Recommendations for the use of nonbiologic and biologic disease-modifying antirheumatic drugs in rheumatoid arthritis. *Am Coll Rheumat.* 2008;59:762-784.

important.[1,4] Local application of heat or cold therapy and rest of acutely inflamed joints is advisable. Patients should avoid physical stressors that worsen their condition, eat a healthy diet, and perform regular exercise (as tolerated) to maintain muscle strength and joint range-of-motion.[5] Physical therapy or occupational therapy may be beneficial.[1] Surgery is usually considered a last resort for conditions that cannot be adequately managed by drug therapy, such as correction of joint deformities or relief of intractable pain.[1,9]

Non-DMARD Therapy

Non-DMARD therapies used in the treatment of RA do not alter the course of the disease.[1,10] As a result, these drugs must be used concomitantly with DMARDs or only temporarily during initiation of disease-modifying RA drug therapy.[4]

Aspirin, nonsteroidal anti-inflammatory drugs (NSAIDs), and selective COX-2 inhibitors reduce inflammation and pain by inhibiting prostaglandin synthesis. Higher doses of these agents are necessary to reduce inflammation as opposed to reducing pain, and anti-inflammatory benefits can require several weeks of continuous therapy to manifest. Oral corticosteroid agents such as prednisone also provide relief from inflammation and have demonstrated disease-modifying properties in RA.[4] However, because of major undesirable long-term adverse effects such as osteoporosis and adrenal suppression, corticosteroids are usually prescribed temporarily for acute RA flares or short term during "bridge therapy" as a patient awaits the onset of DMARD therapy. On occasion, long-term corticosteroid therapy at low doses may be required for patients refractory to NSAID or DMARD therapy, but this is not preferred.[8]

Patients must take NSAIDs or corticosteroids with food to minimize the risk of gastric mucosa damage. For patients requiring long-term NSAID use, concurrent proton pump inhibitor or misoprostol therapy should be considered to reduce the risk of NSAID-induced peptic ulcer disease.[1]

DMARD Therapy

DMARDs have proven to reduce or prevent joint damage and preserve joint function and integrity.[1,10] All RA patients, except those with very limited disease status or with very severe disease when little reversibility is expected, are candidates for DMARD therapy.[1,4]

DMARD therapy should be initiated early after RA diagnosis, typically within 3 months of diagnosis if more conservative measures are inadequate.[1] These agents generally have a slow onset of effect (1-6 months), and as a result, bridge therapy with an NSAID or corticosteroid is often recommended until DMARD efficacy is demonstrated.[1,8] Patients have variable responses to different DMARD agents. If a first-choice DMARD is not effective, a second agent should be tried.

Several principles can be used to guide DMARD therapy: DMARDs should be given at the maximum-tolerated dose, they should not be stopped unless there is toxicity or disease remission, they should be added to current therapy and not replace it, and medication regimens that provide <50% improvement ought to be modified.[8] Because single-agent therapy often fails to control disease progression or clinical symptoms, multidrug therapy is often prescribed.[1,10] Nonbiologic DMARDs may be given alone or together with other nonbiologic or biologic DMARDs. See Tables 47-1 and 47-2 for recommended DMARD combinations based on disease duration, disease activity, and presence of poor prognostic features. Refer to Table 47-3 for nonbiologic DMARD dosing information.

Nonbiologic DMARDs

Methotrexate Methotrexate is the gold standard for DMARD therapy. Its mechanism of action is not fully understood, but it

TABLE 47-2 **Use of Biologic DMARD Agents Relative to Disease Status**

Biologic-DMARDS	Disease Duration[a]	Disease Activity[b]	Poor Prognostic Factors[c]	Previous or Concurrent Therapies
TNF-α inhibitors	Early Intermediate/long Intermediate/long Intermediate/long	High Moderate High Moderate/high	+ + +/− +/−	With methotrexate Must have failed MTX monotherapy Must have failed MTX monotherapy Must have failed MTX + nonbiologic DMARD
Abatacept	Not specified	Moderate/high	+	Must have failed MTX + nonbiologic DMARD
Rituximab	Not specified	High	+	Must have failed MTX + nonbiologic DMARD
Biologic combination	Not recommended in any patients based on data indicating increased risk of adverse events and/or lack of additive efficacy			

[a]Disease duration: early <6 months, intermediate 6-24 months, long >24 months.

[b]Disease activity: low, moderate, high.

[c]Poor prognostic factors: positive, poor prognostic factors present; negative, without poor prognostic factors; positive/negative, recommendation independent of prognostic factors.

Adapted from Saag KG, Teng GG, Patkar NM, et al. Recommendations for the use of nonbiologic and biologic disease-modifying antirheumatic drugs in rheumatoid arthritis. *Am Coll Rheumat.* 2008;59;762-784.

appears to exert its anti-inflammatory effect through immunosuppression. Methotrexate is dosed on a weekly basis. Common side effects include nausea, vomiting, diarrhea, alopecia, and general malaise.[1,10] Elevation of liver transaminases, renal toxicity, and thrombocytopenia or bone marrow suppression may occur in some patients.[1] Methotrexate should not be used in patients with transaminases more than twice the upper limit of normal, in patients with very poor renal function (ClCr < 30 mL/min), or in patients with a white blood cell count $<3000/mm^3$ or with a platelet count of $<50 \times 10^9/L$.[5,8] In addition, methotrexate should not be initiated or resumed in patients with active tuberculosis, bacterial infection, herpes zoster, or life-threatening fungal infection.[5] Liver transaminases (alanine transaminase and aspartate transaminase), serum creatinine (SCr), and a

TABLE 47-3 **Nonbiologic DMARD Dosing Information**

Generic Name	Trade Name	Dosage Range	Administration Schedule	Routes of Administration
Methotrexate	Rheumatrex, Trexall	Initial: 7.5 mg Maximum: 20 mg	Once weekly	po, IM, SQ, IV
Leflunomide	Arava	Dose (load): 100 mg/d × 3 d Maintenance: 20 mg/d[a]	1-2 doses/d	po
Hydroxychloroquine	Plaquenil	Initial: 400-600 mg × 4-12 wk Maintenance: 200-400 mg	Once daily	po
Sulfasalazine	Azulfidine	Initial: 0.5-1 g Maintenance: 2-3 g Maximum: 3 g/d	2-3 divided doses/d	po
Gold sodium thiomalate	Myochrysine	25-50 mg	Every 2-4 wk	IM
Auranofin	Ridaura	3-6 mg Maximum: 9 mg/d	1-2 doses/d	po
D-Penicillamine	Cuprimine	Initial: 125-250 mg/d[b] Maintenance: 500-1500 mg	2-3 doses/d	po
Cyclophosphamide[c]	Cytoxan	1-2 mg/kg	Once daily	po, IV
Azathioprine	Imuran	Initial: 1 mg/kg Maintenance: 1-2.5 mg/kg[d]	1-2 doses/d	po, IV
Cyclosporine[c]	Neoral	2.5-5 mg/kg	Once daily	po, IV
Minocycline[c]	Minocin	100-200 mg	2 doses daily	po

[a]May decrease to 10 mg/d if unable to tolerate 20 mg daily.

[b]Increase dose at 1 to 3 month intervals by 125 or 250 mg/d, as patient response and tolerance indicate; if no improvement and no serious toxicity after 2 to 3 months, increases of 250 mg/d at 2 to 3 month intervals may be continued until remission or toxicity.

[c]Not FDA approved for rheumatoid arthritis.

[d]May titrate from initial dose by 0.5 mg/kg/d after 6 to 8 weeks and every 4 weeks thereafter, maximum dose is 2.5 mg/kg/d. May decrease maintenance dose by lowering dose to 0.5 mg/kg/d every 4 weeks until lowest effective dose is reached.

Abbreviations: IM, intramuscular; IV, intravenous; po, oral; SQ, subcutaneous.

CBC should be measured at baseline, every 2 to 4 weeks after initiation of therapy for 3 months, and then periodically (every 6 months) thereafter.[5] Routine liver biopsies for RA patients receiving methotrexate are no longer recommended. Liver biopsy does not appear to be cost-effective when liver transaminases are normal. However, persistently elevated liver transaminases are an indication for liver biopsy.

The risk of stomach upset, which occurs as a result of gastrointestinal endothelial damage caused by methotrexate, can be reduced by administering folic acid 1 mg daily (except the day of the methotrexate dose). Methotrexate is pregnancy category X. Based on strong evidence of efficacy, relatively low toxicity, and rapid response, methotrexate is the preferred first-line DMARD for RA.[1]

Leflunomide Methotrexate or leflunomide are currently recommended as first-line monotherapy agents for all levels of RA disease activity.[5] Leflunomide hinders the body's immune response by interfering with the proliferation of T-cells. Common side effects include diarrhea, rash, alopecia, headache, weight loss, and elevated liver transaminase.[2] Leflunomide should not be used in patients with transaminase levels greater than twice the upper limit of normal, in patients with active tuberculosis, bacterial, herpes zoster, or life-threatening fungal infection, or in patients who have a white blood cell count $<3000/mm^3$ or a platelet count of $<50 \times 10^9/L$.[5,8] It is pregnancy category X and is teratogenic in both female and male patients; both women and men should avoid leflunomide if attempting conception. Following discontinuation, it may take 2 years for leflunomide to clear fully from the body due to its long half-life.[1] If a patient decides to become pregnant, leflunomide should be discontinued 3 months prior to conception and the patient must undergo a drug elimination procedure with cholestyramine. Similar to methotrexate, key laboratory tests (liver transaminases, SCr, CBC) should be measured at baseline, every 2 to 4 weeks for the first 3 months of therapy, and then every 6 months thereafter.[5]

Hydroxychloroquine Hydroxychloroquine may be appropriate for patients with a less active, milder form of RA.[1,8] It is an antimalarial agent that has both anti-inflammatory and immunomodulatory effects. Its mechanism of action in RA disease processes is unknown. Following a loading dose, hydroxychloroquine is dosed daily. It is generally a well-tolerated drug, though some patients may experience gastrointestinal upset, diarrhea, abdominal cramping, rash, or headache. Hydroxychloroquine is not associated with hepatic or renal toxicities or with bone marrow suppression. Patients receiving hydroxychloroquine should have an ophthalmological examination within 1 year of treatment initiation due to the risk of macular damage and retinal toxicity. High-risk patients should have the opthalmological examination repeated every 6 to 12 months, while low-risk patients may repeat the examination every 5 years.[5]

Sulfasalazine Sulfasalazine exerts anti-inflammatory effect by inhibiting prostaglandin synthesis. Nausea, vomiting, and anorexia are common side effects as well as bone marrow suppression, rash, photosensitivity, and elevated liver transaminases. Sulfasalazine should not be used in patients with transaminases more than twice the upper limit of normal, or in patients with established sulfa allergies.[1,3]

Other agents Many other DMARD agents are available for use (some lacking Federal Drug Administration approval), but are not commonly utilized in clinical practice because of limited efficacy and/or high risk of major toxicity. These include gold compounds, penicillamine, cyclophosphamide, azathioprine, cyclosporine, and minocycline.[1,5,8]

Biologic DMARDs

Biologic DMARDs, also referred to as biologic agents, are effective in reducing disease activity and improving function and quality of life in RA patients for whom nonbiological treatment is unsuccessful. Biologic agents can be separated into two groups—those that attack tumor necrosis factor alpha (TNF-α) and those that target other immune mediators. Biologic agents should not be used in combination with one another because of greater risk of major adverse effects, particularly infections. It is recommended that patients initiating biologic DMARD therapy receive baseline liver transaminase, SCr, and CBC laboratory tests.[5] They should also be screened for tuberculosis and have a negative tuberculin-purified protein derivative skin test before starting therapy with a biologic agent.[5,8] Patients on any biologic DMARD agent should continually be monitored for signs of infection, since these drugs decrease immune response.[1,2,10] Biologic agents should not be initiated or resumed in any patient with active infections including bacterial, tuberculosis infection, herpes zoster, life-threatening fungal, or acute Hepatitis B or C disease.[1,2,5,10] Prescribers should exercise caution when using these medications in patients with severe active upper respiratory tract infections or open skin wounds. Anti-TNF-α agents are contraindicated in patients with New York Heart Association Class III or IV heart failure. Refer to Table 47-4 for dosing information for the biologic DMARDs.

Infliximab Infliximab is an IgG anti-TNF-α human-murine chimeric antibody that binds to TNF, preventing it from binding to its receptor target. It is given as an intravenous infusion and should be taken concurrently with oral methotrexate to reduce the risk of human antichimeric antibody formation. Side effects include increased risk of infection, headache, and rash. Patients may be pretreated with diphenhydramine to prevent an infusion-related reaction.[1,3]

Etanercept Etanercept competitively binds to TNF, preventing it from binding to the surfaces of inflammatory cells. It is given as a weekly or biweekly subcutaneous injection. Etanercept is not associated with dose-related toxicities, but can increase the risk of infection. There is no recommended laboratory monitoring for this drug.[1,3]

Adalimumab Adalimumab is a recombinant human monoclonal antibody that binds to TNF-α receptor sites, inhibiting

TABLE 47-4 **Biologic DMARD Dosing Information**

Generic	Brand	Dosage Range	Administration Schedule	Routes of Administration
Infliximab	Remicade	3 mg/kg[a]	Weeks 0, 2, and 6, and then every 8 wk	IV
Etanercept	Enbrel	25 mg twice weekly or 50 mg once weekly	1-2 doses/wk	SQ
Adalimumab	Humira	40 mg	Every 14 d	SQ
Abatacept	Orencia	Weight based: <60 kg = 500 mg 60-100 kg = 750 mg >100 kg = 1000 mg	Weeks 0, 2, and 4, and then every 4 wk	IV
Rituximab	Rituxan	1000 mg IV infusion: Initial: 50 mg/h, may increase every 30 min to max 400 mg/h Subsequent: 100 mg/h, may increase every 30 min to max 400 mg/h[b]	Repeat in 14 d, then discontinue	IV
Anakinra	Kineret	100 mg	Once daily	SQ

[a]For incomplete response: may increase dose to 10 mg/kg or decrease dosing interval to every 4 weeks.

[b]Maximum: total of two doses, safety data unknown past two doses. Premedicate with corticosteroid, acetaminophen, and an antihistamine prior to each dose.

Abbreviations: IV, intravenous; SQ, subcutaneous.

the binding of endogenous TNF-α to those targets. Adalimumab is given on a weekly or biweekly basis depending on whether the patient is taking concurrent methotrexate. Side effects include headache, rash, and injection site reactions as well as increased risk of infection.[1,3]

Abatacept Abatacept is an immunoglobulin protein agent that inhibits T-lymphocyte activation through blockade of its stimulation by antigen-presenting cells. It is given by IV infusion and can be used as monotherapy in some patients. Patients refractory to nonbiologic DMARDs and anti-TNF biologic agents have been successfully treated with abatacept. Common side effects include nausea, headache, and infusion-related reactions.[1,3] Because of risk of major infections (even greater than anti-TNF biologic agents), abatacept is reserved for patients with at least moderate RA disease activity and poor prognostic manifestations who have experienced an inadequate response to methotrexate in combination with DMARDs or to sequential use of other nonbiologic DMARDs.[5]

Rituximab Rituximab is a monoclonal antibody that targets the CD20 antigen on B-lymphocytes. It is given as two IV infusions 2 weeks apart. The most common side effect is infusion-related reactions.[1,3] Similar to abatacept, patients refractory to nonbiologic DMARDs and anti-TNF biologic agents have been successfully treated with rituximab. Because of the risk of serious adverse effects including several black box warnings (eg, fatal infusion reactions, tumor lysis syndrome, severe mucocutaneous reactions, progressive, multifocal leukoencephalopathy), rituximab is reserved for patients with high RA disease activity and poor prognostic manifestations, who have experienced an inadequate response to methotrexate in combination with DMARDs or sequential use of other nonbiologic DMARDs.[5]

Anakinra Anakinra is a recombinant human interleukin-1 (IL-1) receptor antagonist. It inhibits the binding of cytokines IL-1a and IL-1b to their IL-1 receptor. Anakinra is available as a daily, subcutaneous injection. Noted side effects are injection site reactions and neutropenia.[2] Anakinra is generally less effective than anti-TNF agents and, therefore, is not considered a first-line biologic agent.

SPECIAL CONSIDERATIONS

RA patients should receive an influenza vaccine prior to starting DMARD therapy, and should be revaccinated on a yearly basis as long as treatment continues.[5] They should also receive the pneumococcal vaccine if starting methotrexate, leflunomide, sulfasalazine, or any biologic DMARD. If risk factors for Hepatitis B are present, patients on a biologic DMARD should receive the vaccine series.[5] Because of their lowered threshold for infection, patients on biologic agents should not receive live vaccines and should avoid their scheduled doses for the week before and after undergoing surgical procedures.[5] Patients should also be screened for tuberculosis infection prior to starting therapy with a biologic agent.[5,8]

CASE Application

1. Select the classic signs and symptoms of rheumatoid arthritis.
   a. Morning stiffness that lasts more than 1 hour
   b. Swelling in the small joints of the hands, wrists, and feet
   c. Positive rheumatoid factor
   d. All of the above

2. Which of the following DMARDs would be contraindicated in a patient with a history of a sulfa allergy?
   a. Neoral
   b. Arava
   c. Rheumatrex
   d. Azulfidine
   e. Cytoxan

3. JJ was diagnosed with RA with moderate disease activity and has been exhibiting symptoms for about 2 months. His physician is seeking your advice in designing an initial medication regimen for him. Which of the following medications would you include for the most appropriate recommendation?

   i. Ibuprofen
   ii. Prednisone
   iii. Leflunomide
   iv. Etanercept

   a. i only
   b. i and ii
   c. i, ii, and iii
   d. All of the above

4. Corticosteroids may be used

   a. During acute RA flares
   b. During "bridge therapy" while awaiting the onset of DMARD therapy
   c. At low doses in patients who are refractive to traditional NSAID or DMARD therapy
   d. All of the above

5. Which of the following nondrug therapies would be recommended for a patient with RA?

   a. Heat or cold therapy.
   b. Physical therapy.
   c. Weight reduction.
   d. All of the above.
   e. Nonpharmacologic therapy is not effective for RA.

6. Which of the following is the correct mechanism of action for Enbrel?

   a. Monoclonal antibody which targets the CD20 antigen on B-lymphocytes
   b. TNF-α inhibitor
   c. Immunoglobulin protein which inhibits T-lymphocytes
   d. Dihydrofolate reductase inhibitor

7. DMARDs are preferred over non-DMARD therapy because

   a. DMARD agents have fewer adverse reactions than non-DMARDs.
   b. Non-DMARD agents are less cost-effective than DMARDs.
   c. DMARD agents may reduce or prevent joint damage and preserve joint function.
   d. Non-DMARD agents require close laboratory monitoring.

8. Which brand/generic name is correctly matched?

   a. Adalimumab/Enbrel
   b. Entanercept/Orencia
   c. Abatacept/Humira
   d. Infliximab/Remicade

9. Which of the following agents is dosed weekly?

   a. Methotrexate
   b. Leflunomide
   c. Hydroxychloroquine
   d. Sulfasalazine

10. Choose the correct mechanism of action for leflunomide.

    a. Inhibits prostaglandin synthesis
    b. Interferes with the proliferation of T cells
    c. Prevents activation of inflammatory cells by binding to tumor necrosis factor
    d. Prevents tumor necrosis factor from binding to its receptor site

11. A serious adverse reaction of hydroxychloroquine is

    a. Bone marrow suppression
    b. Hepatic toxicity
    c. Renal impairment
    d. Retinal damage

12. The adverse reaction common to all biological DMARD agents is

    a. Bone marrow suppression
    b. Heart failure exacerbation
    c. Increased susceptibility to infection
    d. Teratogenicity

13. All of the following biological agents work by interfering with the actions of tumor necrosis factor *except*:

    a. Adalimumab
    b. Etanercept
    c. Infliximab
    d. Rituximab

14. Which of the following conditions would be a contraindication for receiving methotrexate?

    a. Slight renal impairment (ClCr = 50 mL/min)
    b. Mild thrombocytopenia (platelets = 100×10^9/L)
    c. Pregnancy
    d. Latent tuberculosis infection

15. Which of the following is true about DMARD therapy?

    a. DMARDs reduce or prevent joint damage in RA.
    b. Onset of action is usually 1 to 2 weeks.
    c. Reserved for use in severe long-term RA.
    d. If a patient fails one DMARD, they will likely fail all DMARDs.
    e. All of the above are true.

16. AA is a 34-year-old woman who regularly picks up her Arava and Ortho Tri-Cyclen refills at your pharmacy. Today she arrives to pick up her Arava and states she will no longer need her Ortho Tri-Cyclen as she and her husband have decided to start trying to have a baby. Which of the following would be the most appropriate response to this information?

a. Continue Arava at a lower dose when she becomes pregnant, as rheumatoid arthritis typically improves during pregnancy.
b. Change Arava to methotrexate during pregnancy.
c. Discontinue Arava 2 to 3 weeks prior to trying to get pregnant.
d. Undergo drug-elimination with cholestyramine prior to trying to get pregnant.

17. Folic acid supplementation is recommended for patients taking methotrexate because

a. Folic acid can prevent renal toxicity.
b. Folic acid can prevent gastrointestinal toxicity.
c. Most people with rheumatoid arthritis have folic acid deficiencies.
d. Folic acid will enhance the efficacy of methotrexate.

18. Which of the following agents is available as an SQ injection?

a. Abatacept
b. Cytoxan
c. Etanercept
d. Remicade
e. Rituxan

19. Select the brand name for hydroxychloroquine.

a. Arava
b. Cytoxan
c. Humira
d. Plaquenil
e. Rituxan

20. Which of the following is true about Rituximab?

i. It is available for administration IV or SQ.
ii. Premedication with corticosteroid, APAP, and antihistamine should be done prior to each dose.
iii. Dosing may be repeated every 7 days.
iv. Recommended infusion dose is 1000 mg.

a. i only
b. ii and iv
c. i, ii, and iv
d. All of the above

TAKEAWAY POINTS ››

- Rheumatoid arthritis (RA) is a chronic autoimmune disorder that affects approximately 1% of the world's population.
- RA is typically characterized by the presence of chronic inflammation and symmetric erosive synovitis that may eventually lead to joint deterioration and deformity.
- There are no specific laboratory tests available to establish a diagnosis of RA, but patients may test positive for rheumatoid factor (RF) or antinuclear antibody. Erythrocyte sedimentation rates and C-reactive protein levels may also be elevated.
- Diagnosis of RA is made when patients meet four of the following seven criteria: morning stiffness that lasts more than 1 hour, swelling in three or more joint areas, swelling in the hand or wrist joints, symmetrical arthritis, rheumatoid nodules, positive RF, and radiological changes (joint erosions or decalcifications).
- All RA patients should receive self-management education and training, including use of local heat or cold therapy, joint rest, proper exercise to maintain joint range of motion and muscle strength, healthy eating, and physical and occupational therapy as needed.
- Disease activity levels can be measured with validated instruments and be used to help guide the treatment approach for a given RA patient.
- Treatment guidelines recommend the initiation of disease-modifying antirheumatic drugs (DMARDs) soon after RA diagnosis, but other options such as nonsteroidal anti-inflammatory drugs and corticosteroids may be used in the beginning of treatment while awaiting the therapeutic onset of DMARD agents.
- DMARDs have been proven to reduce or prevent joint damage and preserve joint function and integrity.
- A variety of DMARDs (nonbiologic and biologic) are available for RA. The nonbiologic methotrexate or leflunomide are recommended as first-line monotherapy agents for all levels of disease activity.
- Biological DMARDs are used typically after a patient has experienced treatment failure with nonbiologics, particularly methotrexate.
- Combinations of biological DMARDs are not recommended because of increased risk of serious adverse events (eg, infection) and/or lack of additive benefit.
- Abatacept and rituximab have demonstrated efficacy in RA patients refractory to nonbiologic DMARDs and anti-TNF biologic agents.

REFERENCES

1. Kwoh CK, Anderson LG, Greene JM, et al. Guidelines for the management of rheumatoid arthritis. *Arthritis Rheum.* 2002;46:328-46.
2. Olsen NJ, Stein CM. New drugs for rheumatoid arthritis. *N Eng J Med.* 2004;21:2167-79.
3. Schuna AA. Rheumatoid arthritis. In: Dipiro JT, Talbert RL, Yee GC, et al, eds. *Pharmacotherapy: A Pathophysiologic Approach.* 7th ed. New York: McGraw-Hill; 2008:1505-1517.
4. Rindfleisch JA, Muller D. Diagnosis and management of rheumatoid arthritis. *Am Fam Physician.* 2005;72:1037-1047.

5. Saag KG, Teng GG, Patkar NM, et al. Recommendations for the use of nonbiologic and biologic disease-modifying antirheumatic drugs in rheumatoid arthritis. *Am Coll Rheum.* 2008;59;762-784.
6. Felson DT, Anderson JJ, Boers M, et al. The American College of Rheumatology preliminary core set of disease activity measures for rheumatoid arthritis clinical trials. *Arthritis Rheum.* 1993;36:729-740.
7. Smolen JS, Breedveld1 FC, Schiff MH, et al. A simplified disease activity index for rheumatoid arthritis for use in clinical practice. *Rheumatology.* 2003;42:244-257.
8. Zvaifler NJ. The evaluation and treatment of rheumatoid arthritis. In: Koopman WJ, Moreland LW, eds. *Arthritis and Allied Conditions.* 15th ed. Philadelphia, PA: Lippincott Williams & Wilkins; 2005.
9. Chung KC, Burns PB, Wilgis EF, et al. A multicenter clinical trial in rheumatoid arthritis comparing silicone metacarpophalangeal joint arthroplasty with medical treatment. *J Hand Surg Am.* 2009;34:815-823.
10. Vaz A, Lisse J, Rizzo W, et al. DMARDs and biologic therapies in the management of inflammatory joint diseases. *Expert Rev Clin Immunol.* 2009;5(3):261-269.

CHAPTER

48 Osteoarthritis

Cynthia M. Phillips and Amy D. Grant

FOUNDATION OVERVIEW

Osteoarthritis is a disorder arising from different pathophysiological causes with manifestations of joint damage, mechanical stress, and loss of articular cartilage resulting in functional and mechanical joint failure.[1-3]

As the most common degenerative joint disease, it affects 12% of the population between the ages of 25 to 74, and up to 85% of those over the age of 75.[4-6] Women over 50 years experience increased hand, knee, and foot osteoarthritis while older men are more affected with hip pain. Risk factors associated with osteoarthritis include advanced age, female gender, genetics, obesity, history of joint trauma, repetitive movement, malalignment, and quadriceps weakness.[4-8]

A normal joint is composed of subchondral bone covered by a thin layer of articular cartilage on one end.[7,9,10] The interarticular space separates the adjoining subchondral bone and is cushioned with synovial fluid.[7,9,10] Articular cartilage allows frictionless movement and uniform load distribution.[7,9,10] Muscles, ligaments, and tendons surround the joint providing strength, maintaining stability, and absorbing load.[7,9,10] Weight-bearing joints such as the knee and hip are mainly affected in osteoarthritis; however, joints of the hand, foot, lumbar and cervical spine may also be involved.[7,9,10] Certain features, common to joint degeneration, lead to development of pain and decreased mobility.[7,9,10] Changes within the articular cartilage cells or chondrocytes result from increased synthesis of proteoglycans and the collagen matrix accompanied by increased destruction from metalloproteinases (MMPs) secondary to inflammation from release of cytokines within the synovium and bone.[7,9,10] Chondrocyte destruction exceeds formation resulting in interarticular joint space narrowing and development of fibrillations (cartilage clefts). Subchondral bone sclerosis occurs when cartilage is destroyed.[7,9,10] Bone remodeling results in osteophyte development and cyst formation (cavities within the bone).[9,10] The result is a weakened joint susceptible to instability with loss of dexterity.[7,9,10]

Patients with osteoarthritis may present clinically with history of pain and tenderness of the joint, limited joint mobility, joint instability, and crepitus with joint movement.[3,11] First signs of osteoarthritis may occur on radiographs with absence of clinical symptoms. Symptoms may progress from absence of pain, to joint pain upon movement relieved by rest, to ultimately pain with rest. Loss of functional ability displays as stiffness with inactivity, limited range of motion, and gait instability. Bony or cartilaginous enlargement of the joint, such as the Heberden (located on distal interphalangeal joint) and Bouchard (present on proximal interphalangeal joint) nodes, is an outward physical sign of osteoarthritis. Advanced disease will manifest with joint space narrowing, formation of new bone at joint margins (osteophytosis), and subchondral sclerosis on radiographs.

Diagnosis of osteoarthritis is commonly based on patient history and physical examination. Radiographic evidence and laboratory testing may be useful in diagnostic confirmation and elimination of other disease.[3] The American College of Rheumatology criteria for classification of osteoarthritis of the knee and hip share common elements including: age >50 years, joint-specific pain, and joint stiffness. Diagnosis of knee or hip osteoarthritis also includes bone tenderness and enlargement with radiographic evidence of osteophytes. Pain with internal rotation of the hip joint further validates osteoarthritis diagnosis. Laboratory testing with normal erythrocyte sedimentation rate eliminates alternate etiology.[11-13] Hard tissue enlargement, swollen joints, and deformity in addition to hand pain with aching or stiffness, are criteria used to diagnose osteoarthritis of the hand.[13] Assessment of how the pain affects activities of daily living, measures taken to cope with pain, and psychological distress are useful to determine treatment modalities.[3,14]

PREVENTION

Addressing local biomechanical risk factors such as obesity with weight loss, potential joint injury with joint protection, and muscle weakness with exercise are strategies for prevention of osteoarthritis.[7,15,16] Increased body mass is associated with muscle weakness, altered gait, decreased function, and fall risk.[15] Weight loss reduces the probability of developing osteoarthritis.[17] Weight loss should be a primary strategy for overweight adults with knee osteoarthritis.[18] Joint injury predisposes patients for osteoarthritis later in life.[19,20] Current treatment of injury in those without osteoarthritis may include surgery, joint rehabilitation, muscle strengthening, and maintaining a healthy weight to prevent development of osteoarthritis later in life.[16,20-22] Regular physical activity and muscle strengthening through resistance exercise in those without osteoarthritis may be a preventative strategy.[16,23] Because muscles provide movement, absorb load, and stabilize the joint, strengthening can improve muscle function.[16]

TREATMENT

Disease state awareness, relieving pain, and improving musculoskeletal movement and function are the focal points for osteoarthritis. These goals can be accomplished by lifestyle changes, orthotics, physical rehabilitation, and pharmacologic therapy.[24-29] Surgical modalities should be considered after all other options are exhausted.[24-29] Regular contact should be established with the patient through office visits or telephone contact to discuss pain status, compliance with pharmacologic and nonpharmacologic treatment, adverse effects of medications, and barriers to any therapy[28,29] (Figure 48-1).

Nonpharmacologic

Obesity is a preventable risk factor of osteoarthritis. Obese patients should lose weight to reduce strain on joints.[24-29] A fitness program focusing on improving muscle strength, mobility, and coordination should be developed for every patient. Physical and/or occupational therapy should be used to maintain or regain range of motion and strengthen muscles. Patients should wear appropriate footwear that supports and cushions the joints. Heat can be applied topically or through hydrotherapy during noninflammatory situations, such as immediately prior to exercise.[24-29] Assistive devices such as canes, crutches, joint supports, and insoles can be used to protect joints from overuse.[24-29]

Pharmacologic

A stepwise approach should be used in order to determine the most effective patient-specific therapy.

Analgesics

Relief of pain and inflammation is the primary objective of pharmacologic treatment.[24-29] Therefore, first-line therapy for osteoarthritis is acetaminophen, which should be maximized at 4 g/24 h before attempting a different agent[24-31] (Table 48-1). Acetaminophen blocks the action of central cyclooxygenase, which prevents prostaglandin (agents that enhance pain sensations) synthesis. Though effective for pain relief, acetaminophen does not eliminate inflammation, as it is a centrally acting drug. Acetaminophen affects the hepatic, renal, and hematologic systems. Monitoring of bilirubin,

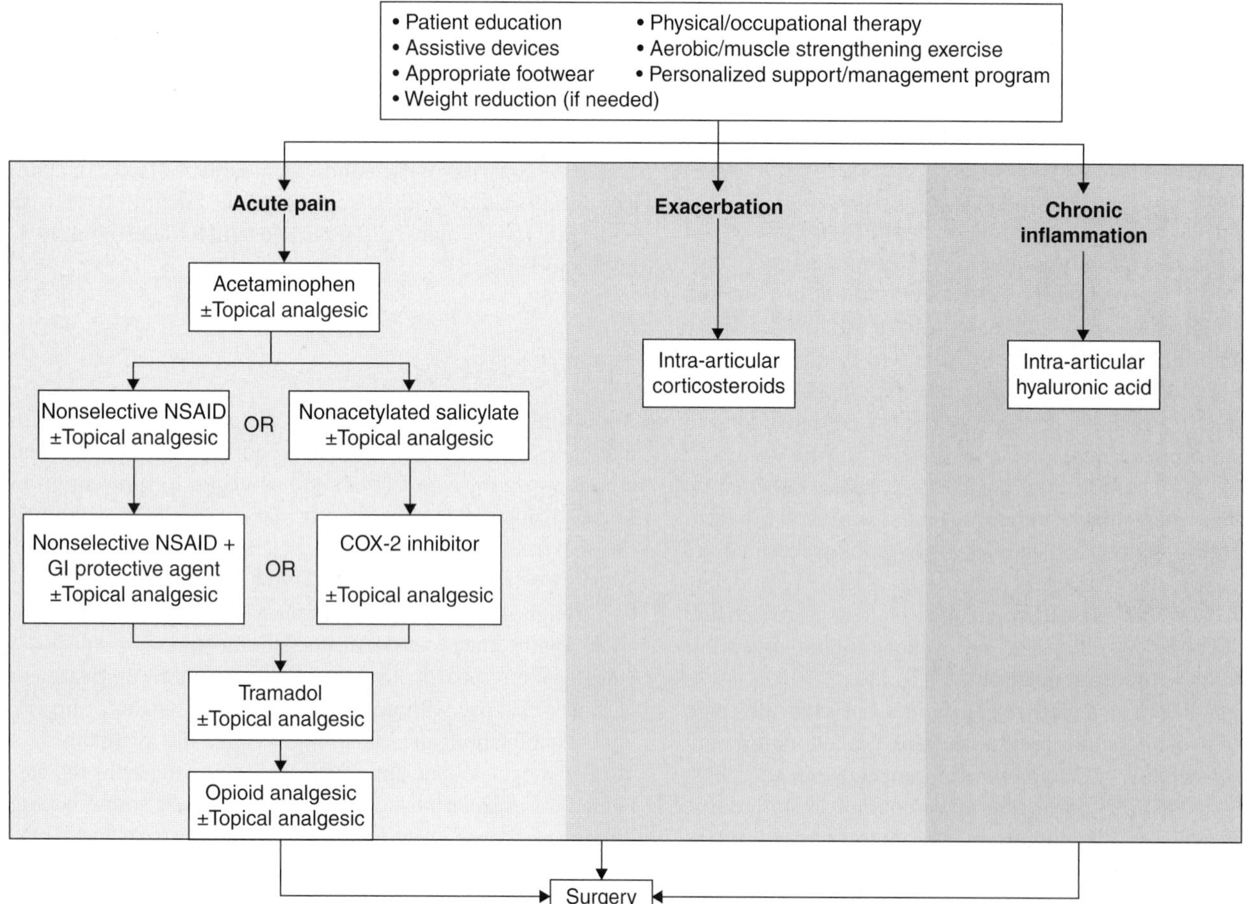

FIGURE 48-1 Osteoarthritis treatment algorithm.[24-31, 33]

TABLE 48-1 **Comparison of Medications Commonly Used in Osteoarthritis[24-29]**

Drug	Dose/Frequency	Maximum Daily Dose
	Oral Analgesics	
Acetaminophen[a]	325-650 mg every 4-6 h	4000 mg
Tramadol[a]	50-100 mg every 4-6 h	300-400 mg
	Topical Analgesics	
Capsaicin 0.025% or 0.075%	Apply 3-4 times daily	
Methylsalicylate	Apply 3-4 times daily	
	Nutritional Supplements	
Glucosamine HCl	500 mg 3-4 times daily	
Chondroitin sulfate	200 mg 2-3 times daily	1200 mg
	Salicylates	
Acetylated Salicylates		
Aspirin	325-650 mg every 4-6	4000 mg
Nonacetylated Salicylates		
Choline magnesium trisalicylate[a]	500-1500 mg 2-3 times daily	4500 mg
	NSAIDS	
Salicylic Acid Derivative		
Salsalate[a]	1500 mg bid or 1000 mg tid	3000 mg
Diflunisal[a]	500-1000 mg daily in two divided doses	1500 mg
Acetic Acids		
Etodolac	400 mg bid or 300 mg tid or 500 mg bid	1000 mg
Diclofenac	100-150 mg daily in 2-3 divided doses	
Indomethacin	25-50 mg 2-3 times daily	200 mg
Ketorolac	10 mg every 4-6 h	40 mg
Sulindac	150 mg bid	400 mg
Tolmetin	400 mg tid	1800 mg
Propionic Acids		
Fenoprofen	300-600 mg 3-4 times daily	3200 mg
Flurbiprofen	200-300 mg daily in 2-4 divided doses	300 mg
Ibuprofen	400-800 mg 3-4 times daily	3200 mg
Ketoprofen[a]	50 mg qid or 75 mg tid	300 mg
Naproxen	500-1000 mg daily in two divided doses	
Oxaprozin[a]	600-1200 mg daily	>50 kg: 1800 mg <50 kg: 1200 mg
Fenamates		
Meclofenamate	50 mg every 4-6 h up to 100 mg every 6 h	400 mg
Nonacidic		
Nabumetone	1000 mg daily	2000 mg
Oxicams		
Piroxicam	10-20 mg daily	20 mg
Meloxicam	7.5-15 mg daily	15 mg
Coxibs		
Celecoxib	200 mg daily	800 mg

(*Continued*)

TABLE 48-1 **Comparison of Medications Commonly Used in Osteoarthritis[24-29] (*Continued*)**

Drug	Dose/Frequency	Maximum Daily Dose
Corticosteroids		
Betamethasone	0.25-2 mL (6 mg/mL)	
Dexamethasone	0.4-6 mg	
Methylprednisolone	4-80 mg every 1-5 wk	
Triamcinolone	Acetonide: 2.5-40 mg every 3-4 wk Hexacetonide: 2-20 mg every 3-4 wk	80 mg total each time
Miscellaneous Antirheumatic		
Hyaluronate	16-30 mg every week for 3-5 wk	
Opioids		
Acetaminophen/codeine[a]	30-60 mg codeine every 4-6 h	4000 mg APAP
Acetaminophen/hydrocodone[a]	5-10 mg hydrocodone every 6 h	4000 mg APAP
Acetaminophen/oxycodone[a]	2.5-30 mg oxycodone every 4-6 h	4000 mg APAP

[a]Adjust in renal dysfunction. Most NSAIDs have warnings not to administer drug in severe renal dysfunction though no specific dosing guidelines are given.

alkaline phosphatase, serum creatinine, bruising, and signs and symptoms of bleeding should occur for all patients receiving chronic acetaminophen doses.[24-29]

If an acetaminophen trial of 1 to 2 weeks is ineffective, a low-dose nonselective nonsteroidal anti-inflammatory drug (NSAID) or nonacetylated salicylate may be used.[24-29,30] Nonselective NSAIDs inhibit cyclooxygenase enzymes (COX-1 and COX-2), which block prostaglandin synthesis.[24-29] The most common adverse drug reactions occurring in 10% to 60% of patients using nonselective NSAIDs are gastrointestinal effects, including nausea, diarrhea, cramping, and dyspepsia. More serious reactions are perforation, ulceration, obstruction, and gastrointestinal bleeding.[24-29] Nonselective NSAIDs can also cause renal insufficiency. Monitoring should include serum creatinine, blood urea nitrogen, serum potassium, blood pressure, edema, weight gain, and colored or bloody urine or stool.[24-29] If pain persists on a low-dose nonselective NSAID, then a full-dose nonselective NSAID or COX-2 inhibitor (selective NSAID) should be prescribed.[24-29,30] Sulfonamide allergy is a contraindication to COX-2 inhibitor use. While COX-2 inhibitors are considered to have a lesser side effect profile than nonselective NSAIDs, a controversy exists over the causal relationship of COX-2 inhibitors and increased cardiovascular risk. Data is also inconclusive regarding the decreased risk of gastrointestinal adverse events in the use of COX-2 inhibitors compared to nonselective NSAIDs.[24-29]

Tramadol is a centrally acting analgesic that inhibits the reuptake of serotonin and norepinephrine and should be used for patients with contraindications to NSAIDs or have failed previous drug trials. Tramadol has an adverse effect profile including nausea, dizziness, headache, vomiting, constipation, and somnolence.[24-29] Use of tramadol has been associated with decrease of the seizure threshold necessitating appropriate precautions and patient monitoring.[25-27]

Opiates bind to opiate receptors in the central nervous system (CNS) causing an altered perception and response to pain. Opiates are reserved as a last resort to eliminate pain.[24-29] As with tramadol, use of opiates can cause central nervous system depression calling for appropriate precautions.[25-27] Common adverse effects associated with opioid use are constipation, nausea, somnolence, and dizziness.[24-29]

Topical analgesic creams, capsaicin, and methylsalicylate are options for patients who do not wish to take systemic treatment or as adjunctive therapy to oral medications.' Topical agents deplete and prevent the reaccumulation of the CNS neurons of substance P, a mediator of pain. Limited adverse effects exist with topical treatment, including burning, stinging, and erythema.[24-29]

Corticosteroids

Intra-articular corticosteroids are an option for patients experiencing an exacerbation or are not candidates for NSAIDs.[24-29] The mechanism of action for pain relief and inflammation reduction is currently undefined, but several theories exist, including reduction in antibodies and cytokines, reduction in macrophage movement, and changes in synovial membrane permeability.[32] A local anesthetic is often coadminstered with the corticosteroid as well as arthrocentesis (joint aspiration) prior to the injection.[31] Improvement in pain occurs 2 to 3 days following injection and lasts between 4 and 8 weeks.[24,32,33] More efficacy data exists for knee and hand osteoarthritis, but corticosteroids can be used for any osteoarthritis-affected joint.[32] Adverse effects seen with intra-articular administration include facial flushing, skin depigmentation, glucose intolerance exacerbation, adrenal insufficiency, hypercorticism, sodium and fluid retention, and joint infections.[24,32] Injections are limited to three times per year and 20 in a lifetime for one joint.[27,32]

Hyaluronic Acid

Hyaluronic acid (HA) treatment can be considered for exacerbations or as alternate therapy for patients unable to tolerate other pharmacologic options.[24,28,33,34] Hyaluronic acid is most effective in knee osteoarthritis.[24,34] It is a component of synovial fluid; therefore, exogenous drug stimulates HA synthesis by synoviocytes in arthritic joints.[24,34] It has a slower onset of action than corticosteroids.[33] Data is inconclusive as to whether hyaluronic acid or glucocorticoids have a longer duration of pain relief.[33] Patients treated with hyaluronic acid may have less joint aspirations and injections.[33] The downfall to this treatment is the requirement of a weekly injection for 3 to 5 weeks.[34] It is well tolerated but should not be given to patients with allergies to avian products.[34]

Glucosamine and Chondroitin

Glucosamine and chondroitin are two dietary supplements often used in combination as therapy or adjunct therapy.[24,31-35] Glucosamine presumably maintains elasticity, strength, and resiliency in joint cartilage and may also be anti-inflammatory in nature.[27,35,36] It should be avoided in patients with shellfish allergy and those taking medications that increase risk of bleeding and is contraindicated in active bleeding.[25-27] Side effects are mild; gastrointestinal discomfort and upset are most common.[25-27] Chondroitin is a compound in connective tissue and cartilage that absorbs water, increasing cartilage thickness.[35,36] Chondroitin should be used with caution in patients with hemostatic problems or a history of bleeding.[25-27] It should also be avoided in those taking medications that increase bleeding risk.[25-27] Glucosamine is synergistic with chondroitin.[35] Numerous studies compare these agents to traditional therapies.[35-36] Some studies show improvement in pain and stiffness; however, most do not show a statistically significant difference from traditional treatment.[35-36]

SPECIAL CONSIDERATIONS

Patients at risk for gastrointestinal bleeding (concomitant aspirin and NSAID therapy, prior history of GI bleeds) should use the lowest-possible dosage of NSAIDs if an alternative drug class is not a viable option.[24,28-29] A gastroprotective agent such as misoprostol should be added.[24,27-29,31] Histamine H_2 antagonists (H_2 antagonists) and proton pump inhibitors (PPI) demonstrate some gastroprotective properties, yet are not as effective as misoprostol.[24,27-29] Pregnancy is a contraindication for misoprostol use.[24,27-29]

More than one NSAID at a time should not be used in any population, though concomitant low-dose aspirin used for cardioprotection is acceptable.[24-25,29,36] NSAID use should be considered carefully in patients with hypertension, congestive heart failure, or renal insufficiency as NSAIDs promote sodium and water retention.[24-25,29,36] Patients with a history of or at high risk for cardiovascular disease should be very cautious using NSAIDs (nonselective and COX-2 inhibitors).[24,36] Selective NSAIDs and diclofenac have demonstrated increased risk of myocardial infarction, stroke, heart failure, and hypertension, but some studies show this may be a drug class effect.[28-29,36]

CASE Application

1. EM is a 63-year-old obese man with a history of increasing pain in his left knee. He presently cares for his 85-year-old mother who has had bilateral knee replacements secondary to osteoarthritis. During his college years, he played on the university team and suffered several knee injuries. During his career as a radio announcer for sports, he maintained a sedentary lifestyle and does not presently exercise. Which of the following are risk factors for the development of osteoarthritis in EM?
   a. Age
   b. Genetics
   c. Joint injury
   d. Obesity
   e. All of the above

2. Which of the following pathophysiological changes occur in a patient with osteoarthritis?
   a. Interarticular narrowing
   b. Bone remodeling
   c. Cytokine release
   d. Chondrocyte destruction
   e. All of the above

3. Which of the following is a sign or symptom of a patient with clinical presentation of osteoarthritis?
   a. Joint stiffness with rest
   b. Normal range of motion with joint
   c. Joint stability
   d. Joint pain with movement
   e. Frictionless joint movement

4. Diagnosis of a patient with osteoarthritis of the hip could be made with which of the following?
   a. Pain with external rotation of the hip
   b. Age >40
   c. Osteophyte development
   d. Joint pain with osteophytes on radiograph and normal laboratory values
   e. Abnormal erythrocyte sedimentation rate

5. Preventative measures in patients without osteoarthritis but who have joint injury include:
   a. Resistance exercise
   b. Maintaining a healthy weight
   c. Surgery
   d. Regular exercise
   e. All of the above

6. SL is a 62-year-old obese man with a history of degenerative joint disease in his entire left knee. Past medical history is significant for dyslipidemia treated with gemfibrozil and diabetes with NPH 10 U at bedtime and glipizide 10 mg bid. Blood sugar readings are not at goal with HgA1c

of 8.5%. Current blood pressure is 130/80 mm Hg. He receives his second injection of 40 mg of Kenalog in his left knee today. Which side effect could cause a drug–disease state interaction in this patient?

a. Skin depigmentation
b. Adrenal insufficiency
c. Joint infection
d. Hyperglycemia
e. All of the above

7. What is the primary objective of medication therapy for osteoarthritis?

a. Improve mobility
b. Weight loss
c. Pain relief
d. Improve muscle and joint strength
e. All of the above

8. What is the most preventable risk factor for developing osteoarthritis?

a. Genetics
b. Joint trauma history
c. Repetitive movement
d. Obesity
e. All of the above

9. Select the first-line pharmacologic agent for treating osteoarthritis?

a. Acetaminophen
b. Intra-articular corticosteroids
c. Tramadol
d. Ibuprofen
e. All of the above

10. Which of the following help to reduce NSAID-induced GI toxicity?

a. Nonacetylated salicylates
b. COX-2 inhibitors
c. Addition of misoprostol
d. Addition of PPI
e. All of the above

11. Which of the following is *not* a goal of osteoarthritis treatment?

a. Teaching patient about the disease state
b. Curing osteoarthritis
c. Providing pain relief
d. Improving musculoskeletal movement
e. Maintaining ability to perform activities of daily living

12. Which of the following is the *correct* order in which treatment options should be trialed?

a. Acetaminophen → COX-2 inhibitor → nonselective NSAID → opioid → joint replacement
b. Acetaminophen → nonselective NSAID → opioid → COX-2 inhibitor → intra-articular corticosteroid
c. Nonselective NSAID → COX-2 inhibitor → opioid → intra-articular hyaluronic acid → joint replacement
d. Nonselective NSAID → COX-2 inhibitor → opioid analgesic → intra-articular corticosteroid → Ultram
e. Acetaminophen → nonselective NSAID → COX-2 inhibitor → opioid analgesic → joint replacement

13. AZ is a 72-year-old woman with a history of atrial fibrillation treated with warfarin. Her height is 5 ft 2 in, weight is 198 lb, blood pressure is 116/76 mm Hg, and SCr is 1.1. AZ is now complaining of pain and stiffness in her left knee. X-ray shows joint space narrowing and osteophytes at the joint. Which treatment should be initiated at this point?

a. Weight reduction
b. Tylenol
c. Celebrex
d. Both a and b
e. Both a and c

14. BY is a 65-year-old man with confirmed osteoarthritis. He has been pain free on his current regimen of acetaminophen 1000 mg every 6 hours for 2 years. Past medical history is significant for gastrointestinal bleed 4 years ago and hypertension. He now presents to your clinic with pain in his left hip. BY's medication regimen also consists of lisinopril 40 mg daily and hydrochlorothiazide 25 mg daily. What recommendation will you present to the physician?

a. Increase acetaminophen to 1000 mg every 4 hours, reinforce fitness program.
b. Add pantoprazole 40 mg daily to his regimen, reinforce fitness program.
c. Stop acetaminophen, begin ibuprofen 400 mg tid, reinforce fitness program.
d. Stop acetaminophen, begin Anaprox 250 mg bid, Protonix 40 mg daily, reinforce fitness program.
e. Add celecoxib 200 mg daily, reinforce fitness program.

15. CK is a 58-year-old woman who presents to your pharmacotherapy clinic today with an INR of 4.2 (she was previously stable for 6 months). She has a PMH of diabetes, atrial fibrillation, and hypertension. The list of medications that she gives you from her pharmacy are as follows: metformin 1000 mg and glipizide 10 mg bid; warfarin 5 mg on Monday, Wednesday, and Friday and 2.5 mg on Sunday, Tuesday, Thursday, and Saturday; amlodipine 10 mg daily; potassium chloride 10 mEq daily; and hydrochlorothiazide 25 mg daily. CK has not had a warfarin dosage change in over 1 year. She tells you her right knee has been bothering her much more frequently than usual. Which of the following is the most likely reason for her INR fluctuation?

a. CK took 5 mg warfarin tablets every day in the past week.
b. After questioning CK about OTC use, she tells you she has been using Capsaicin- HP on her knee for the past week.

c. After questioning CK about OTC use, she tells you she has been taking acetaminophen 650 mg every 6 hours to relieve her from knee pain for the past week.
d. CK is not telling you about an herbal product she has begun taking.
e. All of the above.

16. DP is a 55-year-old man who has hypertension and a positive family history of early cardiovascular disease. His medications include aspirin 81 mg daily and metoprolol 25 mg bid. DP's osteoarthritis is no longer controlled with acetaminophen 1000 mg q 6 h. The physician wants to begin DP on a regimen including an NSAID. Which treatment do you recommend?

a. Naproxen 250 mg bid
b. Naproxen 500 mg tid
c. Celebrex 200 mg daily
d. Celebrex 400 mg daily
e. None of the above

17. The physician does not take your advice for DP in Question 16. She prescribes ibuprofen 800 mg tid. Which of the following do you need to counsel DP concerning?

a. Do not take this medication, it might cause you harm.
b. Take ibuprofen at least 30 minutes after aspirin or aspirin 8 hours after ibuprofen. Monitor your BP more often.
c. Stop taking your aspirin. Do not take ibuprofen on an empty stomach.
d. Stop taking your aspirin. Monitor your BP more often.
e. None of the above.

18. A 44-year-old woman with a history of GI bleed presents to your community pharmacy. She tells you her pregnancy test from last night was positive. She presents refill bottles for her prescription of ibuprofen 400 mg every 8 hours and Cytotec 200 μg bid and asks if these are okay for her to keep taking. You respond:

a. Stop taking Cytotec. It is ok to continue ibuprofen.
b. Stop taking ibuprofen. It is ok to continue Cytotec.
c. Continue taking both medications. Call your physician as soon as you can.
d. Continue taking both medications. Your pregnancy test may not be accurate.
e. Stop taking both prescriptions. Let's call your physician together to discuss your situation.

19. Which of the following medications is contraindicated in patients with documented sulfa allergy?

a. Ultram
b. Toradol
c. Celebrex
d. Aspirin
e. Glucosamine

20. AM is a 52-year-old woman whose medications include acetaminophen 500 mg qid, gabapentin 300 mg tid, gemfibrozil 600 mg bid, and fluoxetine 20 mg daily. At the direction of her physician, AM added ibuprofen 800 mg bid and capsaicin cream 0.025% tid prn to her regimen. While putting on her contacts this morning, she experienced an immediate burning pain in her eyes. She immediately takes out her contacts, flushes her eyes, and calls you, her pharmacist. Which of the following is most likely causing her eye pain?

a. Capsaicin cream
b. Acetaminophen
c. Drug interaction between acetaminophen and gemfibrozil
d. Drug interaction between acetaminophen and gabapentin
e. None of the above

21. KT is a 73-year-old woman with osteoarthritis of the hand. Her medication list includes: salsalate 500 mg bid, Lantus 10 U at bedtime, hydrochlorothiazide 25 mg daily, and ibuprofen 400 mg prn that was recently increased to 800 mg bid prn because of pain. What recommendation(s) do you give to the physician during rounds?

a. KT should not be on more than one NSAID at a time.
b. Ibuprofen should not be given prn for osteoarthritis.
c. Ibuprofen should be dosed 3 to 4 times daily
d. Both a and b
e. All of the above

22. GM is an 81-year-old woman with history of bilateral knee osteoarthritis for 25 years. She has contraindications to surgery and has received one injection of hyaluronic acid (Hyalgan) weekly for the last 2 weeks. She complains that she has not felt any pain relief. You explain:

a. She will not experience pain relief at this point.
b. She may need to complete the series of five injections before improvement.
c. She may need concomitant administration of intra-articular glucocorticoid.
d. She should take glucosamine and chondroitin in addition to the use of hyaluronic acid.
e. She should stop NSAID therapy while Hyalgan is administered.

23. A 59-year-old man with history of 2 months of joint pain in his knees with movement decides to treat with glucosamine chondroitin. He reports an allergy to shellfish. He asks for your recommendation. You tell him:

a. No significant benefit is seen with use of glucosamine chondroitin as monotherapy.
b. Glucosamine chondroitin demonstrates benefit when used in combination with NSAIDS.
c. Glucosamine chondroitin is contraindicated in those with shellfish allergies.

d. Gastrointestinal symptoms of gas, bloating, and cramps may occur with use of glucosamine chondroitin.
e. All of the above.

24. Corticosteroids work to provide pain relief in osteoarthritis by:

a. Reduction of interarticular space narrowing
b. Reduction of cytokine production
c. Depletion of substance P
d. Prostaglandin synthesis inhibition
e. Inhibition of serotonin and norepinephrine

25. Your technician brings you an IV bag to check. The label states "Cerebyx 1200 mg IV daily for pain." You check the patient's profile as your hospital does not have Cerebyx on formulary and find the patient has a history of osteoarthritis and hypertension with hospitalization for an acute gout episode. Identify the errors in this drug order.

a. Indication
b. Dose
c. Route of administration
d. Drug
e. All of the above

TAKEAWAY POINTS ››

- Osteoarthritis, a common degenerative joint disease in those over age 50, commonly affects joints in the knee, hip, and hand.
- Risk factors associated with osteoarthritis include advanced age, female gender, genetics, obesity, history of joint trauma, repetitive movement, malalignment, and quadriceps weakness.
- Joint changes associated with osteoarthritis include articular cartilage destruction, release of inflammatory cytokines, subchondral bone remodeling, and interarticular space narrowing.
- Signs and symptoms of osteoarthritis are specific joint pain and tenderness, stiffness and pain with inactivity, swollen joints, and limited range of motion.
- Diagnosis of osteoarthritis is made on patient history, physical examination, and evidence of radiographic changes such as presence of osteophytes, subchondral sclerosis, and joint space narrowing.
- Preventative strategies for osteoarthritis include weight loss, joint protection, muscle strengthening with exercise, and rehabilitation.
- Osteoarthritis treatment goals are disease state awareness, pain relief, and musculoskeletal movement and function improvement.
- Nonpharmacologic osteoarthritis treatment therapies include: weight reduction for overweight individuals, physical/occupational therapy, muscle-strengthening exercises, use of appropriate footwear and assistive devices, heat application to affected joints, and regular patient contact with a provider.
- Pharmacologic agents include: oral and topical analgesics, NSAIDs, nutritional supplements, intra-articular corticosteroids and hyaluronic acid, and opioids.
- First-line therapy for osteoarthritis is acetaminophen. The maximum daily dose is 4000 mg/d.
- Nonselective NSAIDs and nonacetylated salicylates are used when acetaminophen is contraindicated or ineffective.
- Selective NSAIDs (COX-2 inhibitors) can be used in place of nonselective NSAIDs. The only available drug in the United States is celecoxib, which contains a sulfa component.
- If other analgesics are ineffective, tramadol can be trialed for pain relief. Opiates should be a final alternative due to their addictive and respiratory depression effects.
- Patients at risk for gastrointestinal bleeding should avoid nonselective NSAIDs if possible. If unavoidable, a gastroprotective agent should be added.
- NSAID (nonselective and selective) should be used cautiously in patients with hypertension, congestive heart failure, or renal insufficiency.
- Topical analgesic creams are an option for patients who do not wish to take systemic treatment or as an adjunct to drug therapy.
- Intra-articular corticosteroids are an option during osteoarthritis exacerbations or in those who are not NSAID candidates. Side effects include facial flushing, skin depigmentation, glucose intolerance exacerbation, adrenal insufficiency, hypercorticism, sodium and fluid retention, and joint infections.
- Intra-articular hyaluronic acid can be used in place of intra-articular corticosteroids for chronic inflammation.
- Glucosamine and chondroitin are dietary supplements used solely or as an adjunct in osteoarthritis. Studies do not show a statistically significant difference in pain improvement.

REFERENCES

1. Sharma L, Kapoor D. Epidemiology of osteoarthritis. In: Moscowitz RW, Altman RD, Hochberg MC, Buckwlater JA, Goldberg VM, eds. *Osteoarthritis: Diagnosis and Medical/Surgical Management*. 4th ed. Philadelphia, PA: Lippincott, Williams and Wilkins; 2007:3-26.
2. Brandt KD, Dieppe P, Radin E. Etiopathogenesis of osteoarthritis. *Med Clin North Am*. 2009;93:1-24.
3. Hunter DJ, McDougall JJ, Keefe FJ. The symptoms of osteoarthritis and the genesis of pain. *Rheum Dis Clinic North Am*. 2008;34:623-643.

4. ACR Subcommittee on Osteoarthritis Guidelines. Recommendations for the medical management of osteoarthritis of the hip and knee: 2000 update. *Arthritis Rheum.* 2000;43:1905-1915.
5. Lawrence RC, Helmick CG, Arnett FC, et al. Estimates of the prevalence of arthritis and selected musculoskeletal disorders in the United States. *Arthritis Rheum.* 1998;41:778-799.
6. Dillon CF, Rasch EK, Gu Q, Hirsch R. Prevalence of knee osteoarthritis in the United States: arthritis data from the Third National Health Nutrition Examination Survey 1991-91. *J Rheumatol.* 2006;33:2271-2279.
7. Felson DT, Lawrence RC, Dieppe PA, et al. Osteoarthritis: new insights. Part 1: the disease and its risk factors. *Ann Intern Med.* 2000:133:635-646.
8. Zhang Y, Jordan JM. Epidemiology of osteoarthritis. *Rheum Dis Clin N Am.* 2008;34:515-529.
9. Dieppe PA, Lomander LS. Pathogenesis and management of pain in osteoarthritis. *Lancet.* 2005;325:965-973.
10. Aspden RM. Osteoarthritis: a problem of growth not decay? *Rheumatology.* 2008;47:1452-1460.
11. Altman R, Asch E, Bloch D et al. The American College of Rheumatology criteria for classification and reporting of osteoarthritis of the knee. *Arthritis Rheum.* 1986;29:1039-1049.
12. Altman R, Alarcon G, Appelrouth D, et al. The American College of Rheumatology criteria for the classification and reporting of osteoarthritis of the hip. *Arthritis Rheum.* 1991;34:505-514.
13. Altman R, Alarcon G, Appelrouth D, et al. The American College of Rheumatology criteria for the classification and reporting of osteoarthritis of the hand. *Arthritis Rheum.* 1990;33:1601-1608.
14. Penninx BW, Messier SP, Rejeski WJ, et al. Physical exercise and the prevention of disability in activities of daily living in older persons with osteoarthritis. *Arch Intern Med.* 2001;161:2309-2316.
15. Messier SP. Obesity and osteoarthritis: disease genesis and nonpharmacologic weight management. *Med Clin North Am.* 2009;93:149-159.
16. Bennell KL, Hunt MA, Wrigley TV, et al. Muscle and exercise in the prevention and management of knee osteoarthritis: an internal medicine specialist's guide. *Med Clin North Am.* 2009;93:161-177.
17. Felson DT, Zhang Y, Anthony JM, Naimark A, Anderson JJ. Weight loss reduces the risk for symptomatic knee osteoarthritis in women. The Framingham Study. *Ann Intern Med.* 1992;116:535-539.
18. Christensen R, Bartels EM, Astrup A, Bliddal H. Effect of weight reduction in obese patients diagnosed with knee osteoarthritis: a systematic review and meta analysis. *Ann Rheum Dis.* 2007;66:433-439.
19. Gelber AC, Hochberg MC, Mead LA, Wang NY, Wigley FM, Klag MJ. Joint injury in young adults and risk for subsequent knee and hip osteoarthritis. *Ann Intern Med.* 2000;133:321-328.
20. Roos EM. Joint injury causes knee osteoarthritis in young adults. *Curr Opin Rheumatol.* 2005;17:195-200.
21. Lomander LS, Englund PM, Dahl LL, Roos EM. The long-term consequence of anterior cruciate ligament and meniscus injuries: osteoarthritis. *Am J Sports Med.* 2007;35:1756-1769.
22. Nicholson S, Dickman K, Maradiegue A. Reducing premature osteoarthritis in the adolescent through appropriate screening. *J Pediatr Nurs.* 2009;24:69-74.
23. Teichtahl AJ, Wluka AE, Forbes A, et al. Longitudinal effect of vigorous physical activity on patella cartilage morphology in people without clinical knee disease. *Arthritis Rheum.* 2009:61:1095-1102.
24. Buys LM, Elliott E. Osteoarthritis. In: DiPiro JT, Talbert RL, Yee GC, et al, eds. *Pharmacotherapy: A Pathophysiologic Approach.* 7th ed. New York, NY: McGraw-Hill; 2008:1519.
25. Micromedex® Healthcare Series. n.d. Greenwood Village, CO: Thompson Reuters (Healthcare) Inc. Available at: http://www.thomsonhc.com. Accessed September 2, 2009.
26. Wolters Kluwer Health, Inc. Drug Facts and Comparisons 4.0 online. 2009. Available at: www.xyzal.com. Accessed September 2, 2009.
27. Lexi-comp ONLINE Web site. http://crlonline.com. Copyright 1978-2009. Accessed September 2, 2009.
28. Altman RD, Hochberg MC, Moskowitz RW, Schnitzer TJ. Recommendations for the medical management of osteoarthritis of the hip and knee. *Arthritis Rheum.* 2000;43(9):1905.
29. Zhang W, Moskowitz RW, Nuki G, et al. OARSI recommendations for the management of hip and knee osteoarthritis. Part II: OARSI evidence-based, expert consensus guidelines. *Osteoarthritis Cartilage.* 2008;16(2):137.
30. American Academy of Orthopaedic Surgeons. *Clinical Practice Guideline on the Treatment of Osteoarthritis of the Knee (Non-Arthroplasty).* Rosemont, IL: American Academy of Orthopaedic Surgeons (AAOS); 2008.
31. Stitik TP, Kumar A, Foye PM. Corticosteroid injections for osteoarthritis. *Am J Phys Med Rehabil.* 2006;85(suppl):S51.
32. Bahadur C, Onal B, Dayan VY, et al. Comparison of therapeutic effects of sodium hyaluronate and corticosteroid injections on trapeziometacarpal joint osteoarthritis. *Clin Rheumatol.* 2009;28:529.
33. Hochberg MC. Role of intra-articular hyaluronic acid preparations in medical management of osteoarthritis of the knee. *Semin Arthritis Rheum.* 2000;30(2 suppl 1):2.
34. Clegg DO, Domenic RJ, Harris CL, et al. Glucosamine, chondroitin sulfate, and the two in combination for painful knee osteoarthritis. *New Engl J Med.* 2006;354:795.
35. Sawitzke AD, Shi H, Finco MF, et al. The effect of glucosamine and/or chondroitin sulfate on the progression of knee osteoarthritis. *Arthritis Rheum.* 2008;58(10):3183.
36. Farkouh ME, Greenberg BP. An evidence-based review of the cardiovascular risks of nonsteroidal anti-inflammatory drugs. *Am J Cardiol.* 2009;103:1227.

PART

8

Neurologic Disorders

CHAPTER

49 Epilepsy

S. Scott Sutton and Holly J. Watson

FOUNDATION OVERVIEW

Epilepsy is a chronic disease of disturbed electrical activity in the brain, resulting in recurrent seizures with or without convulsions. The age-adjusted prevalence of epilepsy is 4 to 7 cases per 1,000 persons, with approximately 125,000 new cases of epilepsy annually. Developing countries have higher rates of epilepsy related to poor health care and prenatal care, increased risk of neurologic trauma, and increased rates of infection.

Epilepsy is a disorder with profound impact on lifestyle and patients are often dependent upon caregivers to assist with medications and transportation. All states impose limitations on driving for individuals who have recently had a seizure with impaired consciousness.[1]

The pathophysiology of a seizure is due to an unstable cell membrane in the gray matter of the brain. The cause of the unstable cell membrane has been linked to three causes: an abnormality in potassium conductance, an abnormality in voltage-sensitive ion channels, or a deficiency in membrane ATPases linked to ion transport. Excitatory neurotransmitters (glutamate, aspartate, acetylcholine, norepinephrine) enhance the propagation of seizures while inhibitory neurotransmitters (GABA, dopamine) decrease the propagation of seizure activity in the brain. The spread can be local (partial seizure) or throughout the entire brain (generalized seizure). The different types of epilepsies are due to the different pathophysiologic abnormalities.[1]

Epilepsy is classified by the seizure presentation (Table 49-1).[2-3] The classification system is based on how the seizure begins; therefore, obtaining an adequate description from a third party is important. The classifications of epilepsy are:

- Absence seizures (petit mal)—sudden interruption of activities and a blank stare.
- Myoclonic seizures—brief shock-like contraction of a muscle group.
- Clonic seizures—jerking motion while tonic seizures involve a sustained muscle contraction.
- Tonic-clonic seizures (grand mal)—alternating muscle contraction and jerking.
- Atonic seizures involve a sudden loss of muscle tone known as "drop attacks."

Epilepsy syndromes are another classification system of epilepsies based on seizure type and etiology. The syndrome approach provides a tool to aid clinical management and provide prognosis.[3]

- *Idiopathic* epilepsy—no underlying etiology and is presumed genetic.
- *Symptomatic* epilepsy—an underlying cause which is usually brain damage.
- *Cryptogenic* epilepsy—presumed to have an underlying etiology that cannot be identified.

Epilepsy is a clinical diagnosis made when the patient has recurrent seizures. An isolated seizure does not justify the diagnosis of epilepsy. Laboratory tests are evaluated to rule out treatable causes of seizures such as hypoglycemia, altered electrolytes, and infections. A seizure produced by treatable causes does not represent epilepsy. Electroencephalogram (EEG) can be useful to confirm a seizure and identify seizure types based on the spike and wave pattern generated; however, the EEG may be normal in some patients.[4]

The underlying etiology of epilepsy is unknown in 80% of patients. The most common recognized causes of epilepsy are head trauma and stroke. Developmental and genetic defects represent 5% of epilepsy cases. Central nervous system tumors, infections, metabolic disturbances (hyponatremia and hypoglycemia), neurodegenerative diseases, and medications represent other causes. Medications associated with causing seizures include tramadol, bupropion, theophylline, some antidepressants, some antipsychotics, amphetamines, cocaine, imipenem, lithium, excessive doses of penicillins or cephalosporins, sympathomimetics, and stimulants.

PREVENTION

Epilepsy cannot be prevented, but the seizures experienced by the patient can be minimized in both number and duration. There is a positive association between early initiation of antiepileptic drug (AED) therapy and seizure control. The inability to control seizures early can lead to increased frequency in seizure activity and the generation of other seizure types. External factors known to precipitate seizures in patients with epilepsy include hyperventilation, sleep deprivation, sensory stimuli, emotional stress, and hormonal fluctuations during pregnancy/menses/puberty. These external factors should be minimized in the epilepsy population.

TABLE 49-1 International Classification of Epileptic Seizures

I. Partial seizures (seizures begin locally)
   A. Simple (without impairment of consciousness)
      1. With motor symptoms
      2. With special sensory or somatosensory symptoms
      3. With psychic symptoms
   B. Complex (with impairment of consciousness)
      1. Simple partial onset followed by impairment of consciousness, with or without automatisms
      2. Impaired consciousness at onset, with or without automatisms
   C. Secondarily generalized (partial onset evolving to generalized tonic-clonic seizures)
II. Generalized seizures (bilaterally symmetrical and without local onset)
   A. Absence
   B. Myoclonic
   C. Clonic
   D. Tonic
   E. Tonic-clonic
   F. Atonic
   G. Infantile spasms
III. Unclassified seizures
IV. Status epilepticus

TREATMENT

The goal of epilepsy treatment is complete elimination of seizures with no drug side effects. This is not always possible and the patient should be involved in deciding the balance between frequency of seizures and occurrence of side effects. In certain situations, some seizure control may be sacrificed to improve the patient's day to day functioning. Optimal quality of life requires balancing seizures, side effects, and addressing life issues (eg, driving, safety, relationships, and social stigma). Epilepsy patients may have neuropsychiatric diseases such as depression, anxiety, and sleep disturbances which require treatment to optimize quality of life.[5-7]

Initial therapy is initiated with one AED and up to 70% of patients are controlled on monotherapy. Initial management of seizure disorders depends upon the type of seizure (Table 49-2). Combination AED therapy is required in 30% of patients in order to achieve seizure control; however, combination therapy increases the chance of side effects and drug interactions. Combination AED therapy is achieved by combining seizure medications with different mechanisms of action.[5-7] Table 49-3 lists key AED properties that impact medication selection, dosing, and adverse reactions.

SPECIAL CONSIDERATIONS

Complications of Therapy

Adverse effects of AEDs are often dose limiting or cause a drug to be discontinued. AED adverse reactions are classified as dose related or idiosyncratic (see Table 49-3). Dose-related adverse reactions are associated with the dose or concentration. Dose-related adverse effects include sedation, ataxia, and diplopia. Idiosyncratic adverse reactions are not related to the dose of the AED and often lead to discontinuation of the AED. Examples of idiosyncratic reactions include rash, hepatotoxicity, and hematologic toxicities. Because idiosyncratic reactions may be life threatening, the AED should be discontinued. Idiosyncratic reactions are associated with an immunologic reaction; therefore cross-reactivity among AEDs is possible.[6-7]

Switching AEDs

Switching AEDs requires a titration process, because abrupt discontinuation of an AED may lead to breakthrough seizures. The process requires starting the new AED at a low dose and titrating up to the minimal effective dose. Once the minimal effective dose is reached, the drug to be discontinued is gradually tapered, while the dose of the new AED continues to be increased to the target dose.

Discontinuing AEDs

Epilepsy is considered a lifelong disorder; however, patients who are seizure-free may desire to discontinue their medication. Factors favoring successful withdrawal of AEDs include a seizure-free period of 2 to 4 years, complete seizure control within 1 year of onset, an onset of seizures after age 2 but before age 35, and a normal neurologic examination and EEG. Withdrawal of AEDs is done slowly with a dose tapered over at least 3 months.[8]

Drug Interactions

AEDs are associated with numerous drug interactions related to absorption, metabolism, and protein binding. Tube feedings and antacids reduce the absorption of phenytoin and carbamazepine. Phenytoin, carbamazepine, and phenobarbital are potent inducers of the cytochrome P-450 (CYP-450) isoenzyme system and valproic acid is an inhibitor of the P-450 isoenzyme system (Table 49-4).[9]

Special Populations

Children require prompt control of seizures to avoid interference with development of the brain and cognition. AED doses are increased rapidly and frequent changes in the regimen are made to maximize control of seizures. Due to high metabolic rates in children, doses of AEDs are higher on a milligram per kilogram basis compared to adults.

Women of child-bearing potential or who are pregnant have recommendations for AED management (Table 49-5). Several AEDs have been implicated in minor and serious birth defects. Valproic acid and carbamazepine are associated with neural tube defects (eg, spina bifida). The majority of pregnant epileptic patients receiving AEDs produce a normal infant, but special recommendations must be followed. AEDs induce hepatic CYP-450 isoenzymes and decrease the effectiveness of hormonal contraceptives. Epileptic women taking AEDs and hormonal contraceptives are recommended to use other forms of birth control.[10]

TABLE 49-2 **Evidence-Based Guidelines for Initial Monotherapy Treatment of Epilepsy**

Seizure Type	American Academy of Neurology	Scottish Intercollegiate Guidelines Network	United Kingdom National Institute for Clinical Excellence
Primary generalized tonic-clonic	Carbamazepine[a] Lamotrigine[a] Oxcarbazepine[a] Phenobarbital[a] Phenytoin[a] Topiramate[a] Valproate[a]	Lamotrigine Valproate	Carbamazepine Lamotrigine Topiramate Valproate *Second line:* Clobazam[b] Levetiracetam Oxcarbazepine
Absence	Lamotrigine (children)	Ethosuximide Lamotrigine Valproate	Ethosuximide Lamotrigine Valproate *Second line:* Clobazam[b] Clonazepam Topiramate
Myoclonic	Not mentioned	Lamotrigine Valproate	Valproate Topiramate (children with severe myoclonic epilepsy of infancy) *Second line:* Clobazam[b] Clonazepam Lamotrigine Levetiracetam Piracetam[b] Topiramate
Tonic	Not mentioned	Not mentioned	Lamotrigine Valproate *Second line:* Clobazam[b] Clonazepam Levetiracetam Topiramate
Atonic	Not mentioned	Not mentioned	Lamotrigine Valproate *Second line:* Clobazam[b] Clonazepam Levetiracetam Topiramate
Partial with or without secondary generalization	Carbamazepine Gabapentin Lamotrigine Oxcarbazepine Phenobarbital Phenytoin Topiramate Valproate	Phenytoin Carbamazepine Valproate Lamotrigine Oxcarbazepine	Carbamazepine Lamotrigine Oxcarbazepine Valproate Topiramate *Secondl ine:* Clobazam[b] Gabapentin Levetiracetam Phenytoin Tiagabine

[a]Based upon data from newly diagnosed epilepsy patients of multiple seizure types.

[b]Not currently available in the United States.

Reproduced with permission from: Welty TE, Faught E. In: Chisholm-Burns MA, Wells BG, Schwinghammer TL, et al, eds. *Pharmacotherapy Principles & Practice.* New York, NY: McGraw-Hill; 2008: 443-460.

TABLE 49-3 Characteristics of Common Antiepileptic Drugs

Drug	Mechanism of Action	Dose	Pharmacokinetic Parameters	Usual Serum Concentration Range	Dose-Related Adverse Effects	Idiosyncratic Adverse Effects
Carbamazepine	Modulate sodium channels	*Loading dose:* Not recommended due to excessive dose-related toxicity *Maintenance dose:* Titrate dosage to target over 3-4 wk Adults: 10-20 mg/kg/d as a divided dose Children: 20-30 mg/kg/d as a divided dose	*Half-life:* 10-25 h with chronic dosing *Apparent volume of distribution:* 0.8-1.9 L/kg *Protein binding:* 67%-81% *Primary elimination route:* Hepatic	4-12 μg/mL (17-51 μmol/L)	Diplopia, drowsiness, nausea, sedation	Aplastic anemia, hyponatremia, leukopenia, osteoporosis, rash
Clonazepam	Enhance GABA activity	*Loading dose:* Not recommended due to increased adverse effects *Maintenance dose:* Initiate at 0.5 mg one to three times daily, titrate dose to effectiveness usually 3-5 mg daily in 2-3 divided doses	*Half-life:* 30-40 h *Apparent volume of distribution:* 3.2 L/kg *Protein binding:* 47%-80% *Primary elimination route:* Hepatic	Not established	Ataxia, memory impairment, sedation, slowed thinking	
Ethosuximide	Modulate calcium channels	*Loading dose:* Not recommended due to increased adverse effects *Maintenance dose:* Initiate at 250 mg twice daily and titrate to 500-1000 mg twice daily	*Half-life:* 60 h *Apparent volume of distribution:* 0.6-0.7 L/kg *Protein binding:* None *Primary elimination route:* Hepatic	40-100 μg/mL (283-708 μmol/L)	Ataxia, sedation	Hepatotoxicity, neutropenia, rash
Felbamate	Inhibit glutamate activity	*Loading dose:* Not recommended due to increased adverse effects *Maintenance dose:* 1200-3600 mg/d in 3-4 divided doses	*Half-life:* Monotherapy: 20 h Concurrent enzyme inducers: 11-16 h *Apparent volume of distribution:* 0.7-0.8 L/kg *Protein binding:* 25%-35% *Primary elimination route:* Hepatic	Not established	Anxiety, insomnia, nausea	Anorexia, aplastic anemia, headache, hepatotoxicity, weight loss

Gabapentin	Modulate calcium channels and enhance GABA activity	*Loading dose:* Not recommended due to short half-life *Maintenance dose:* 900-3600 mg/d in 3-4 divided doses (doses up to 10,000 mg/d have been tolerated)	*Half-life:* 5-7 h (proportional to creatinine clearance) *Apparent volume of distribution:* 0.6-0.8 L/kg *Protein binding:* >10% *Primary elimination route:* Renal	Not established	Drowsiness, sedation	Peripheral edema, weight gain
Lamotrigine	Modulate sodium channels	*Loading dose:* Not recommended due to increased risk of rash *Maintenance dose:* 150-800 mg/d in 2-3 divided doses. Doses should be initiated and titrated according to the manufacturer's recommendations to reduce the risk of rash	*Half-life:* Monotherapy: 24 h Concurrent enzyme inducers: 12-15 h Concurrent enzyme inhibitors: 55-60 h *Apparent volume of distribution:* 1.1 L/kg *Protein binding:* 55% *Primary elimination route:* Hepatic	Not established	Ataxia, drowsiness, headache, insomnia, sedation	Rash
Levetiracetam	Unknown	*Loading dose:* Not recommended due to excessive adverse effects *Maintenance dose:* 1000-3000 mg/d Start at 1000 mg/d and titrate upward as indicated by response	*Half-life:* 6-8 h *Apparent volume of distribution:* 0.5-0.7 L/kg *Protein binding:* >10% *Primary elimination route:* 70% renal 30% hepatic	Not established	Somnolence, dizziness	Depression
Oxcarbazepine	Modulate sodium channels	*Loading dose:* Not recommended due to excessive adverse effects *Maintenance dose:* 600–1200 mg/d Start at 300 mg twice daily and titrate upward as indicated by response	*Half-life:* Parent drug ~2 h 10-monohydroxy metabolite ~9 h *Apparent volume of distribution:* 0.5–0.7 L/kg *Protein binding:* 40% *Primary elimination route:* Hepatic	Not established	Diplopia, dizziness, somnolence	Hyponatremia, 25%-30% cross sensitivity in patients with hypersensitivity to carbamazepine
Phenobarbital	Modulate sodium channels	*Loading dose:* 10-20 mg/kg as single or divided intravenous infusions or orally in divided doses over 24-48 h *Maintenance dose:* Adults: 1-4 mg/kg/d as a single or divided dose Children: 3-6 mg/kg/d as divided dose Neonates: 1-3 mg/kg/d as divided dose	*Half–life:* Adults: 49-120 h Children: 37-73 h Neonates: ~115 h *Volume of distribution:* 0.7-1 L/kg *Protein binding:* ~50% *Primary elimination route:* Hepatic	15-40 μg/mL (65-172 μmol/L)	Ataxia, drowsiness, sedation	Attention deficit, cognitive impairment, hyperactivity, osteoporosis, passive-aggressive behavior

(Continued)

TABLE 49-3 **Characteristics of Common Antiepileptic Drugs (*Continued*)**

Drug	Mechanism of Action	Dose	Pharmacokinetic Parameters	Usual Serum Concentration Range	Dose-Related Adverse Effects	Idiosyncratic Adverse Effects
Phenytoin	Modulate sodium channels	*Loading dose:* Adults: 15-20 mg/kg single intravenous dose or divided oral dose Infants > 3 mo: 10-15 mg/kg single intravenous dose Neonates: 15-20 mg/kg single intravenous dose *Maintenance dose:* Adults: 5-7 mg/kg/d as single or divided dose Children: 6-15 mg/kg/d as divided dose Neonates: 3-8 mg/kg/d as divided dose	*Half-life:* Follows capacity-limited or Michaelis-Menten pharmacokinetics Half-life increases as the dose and serum concentration increases *Volume of distribution:* Adults: 0.7 L/kg Children: 0.8 L/kg Neonates: 1.2 L/kg *Protein binding:* Adults, children: 88%-92% Neonates: 65% *Primary elimination route:* Hepatic	10-20 μg/mL (40-79 μmol/L) total concentration 1-2 μg/mL (4-8 μmol/L) unbound concentration	Ataxia, diplopia, drowsiness, sedation	Anemia, gingival hyperplasia, hirsutism, lymphadenopathy, osteoporosis, rash
Pregabalin	Modulate calcium channels	*Loading dose:* Not recommended due to increased adverse effects *Maintenance dose:* Initiate at 150 mg/d in 2-3 divided doses and titrate to a maximum dose of 600 mg/d	*Half-life:* 6.3 h, proportional to creatinine clearance *Apparent volume of distribution:* 0.5 L/kg *Protein binding:* Negligible *Primary elimination route:* Renal	Not established	Ataxia, blurred vision, dizziness, dry mouth, somnolence	Edema, weight gain
Tiagabine	Enhance GABA activity	*Loading dose:* Not recommended due to excessive adverse effects *Maintenance dose:* 32-56 mg/d in four divided doses Doses should be titrated upward over 6 wk, starting at 4 mg/d	*Half-life:* Monotherapy: 7-9 h Concurrent enzyme inducers: 2.5-4.5 h *Apparent volume of distribution:* 0.6-0.8 L/kg *Protein binding:* 96% *Primary elimination route:* Hepatic	Not established	Dizziness, somnolence, irritability, slowed thinking	

Topiramate	Modulate sodium channels; inhibit glutamate activity; enhance GABA activity	*Loading dose:* Not recommended due to excessive adverse effects *Maintenance dose:* 100-400 mg/d in 2-3 divided doses Doses should be started at 25-50 mg/d and gradually titrated upward over 3-6 wk to avoid excessive adverse effects	*Half-life:* Monotherapy: 21 h Concurrent enzyme inducers: 11-16 h *Apparent volume of distribution:* 0.55-0.8 L/kg *Protein binding:* 13%-17% *Primary elimination route:* 60% renal 40% hepatic	Not established	Ataxia, dizziness, drowsiness, slowed thinking	Acute glaucoma, metabolic acidosis, oligohidrosis, paresthesias, renal calculi, weight loss
Valproic acid/ divalproex sodium	Modulate sodium channels	*Loading dose:* 20-40 mg/kg *Maintenance dose:* Adults: 15-45 mg/kg/d in 2-4 divided doses Children: 5-60 mg/kg/d in 2-4 divided doses	*Half-life:* Adults: 8-15 h Children: 4-15 h Infants > 2 mo: 65 h *Volume of distribution:* 0.1-0.5 L/kg *Protein binding:* 90% (decreases with increasing serum concentrations) *Primary elimination route:* Hepatic	50-100 μg/mL (346-693 μmol/L); children may require concentrations up to 150 μg/mL (1040 μmol/L)	Drowsiness, nausea, sedation, tremor	Hepatotoxicity, osteoporosis, pancreatitis, weight gain
Zonisamide	Modulate sodium and calcium channels	*Loading dose:* Not recommended due to excessive adverse effects *Maintenance dose:* 100-600 mg/d; start at 100 mg/d and titrate upward as indicated by response	*Half-life:* ~63 h *Apparent volume of distribution:* 1.45 L/kg *Protein binding:* 40% *Primary elimination route:* Hepatic	Not established	Dizziness, somnolence	Metabolic acidosis, oligohidrosis, paresthesias, renal calculi

Abbreviation: GABA, γ-aminobutyric acid.

Reproduced with permission from: Welty TE, Faught E. In: Chisholm-Burns MA, Wells BG, Schwinghammer TL, et al, eds. *Pharmacotherapy Principles & Practice*. New York, NY: McGraw-Hill; 2008: 443-460.

TABLE 49-4 **Drug Interaction Properties with Antiepileptic Drugs**

Enzyme	Substrate	Inducers	Inhibitors
CYP 1A2	Carbamazepine	Carbamazepine Phneytoin Phenobarbital	
CYP 2C9	Phenobarbital Phenytoin Carbamazepine Valproic acid	Carbamazepine Phenytoin Phenobarbital	Valproic acid
CYP 2C19	Phenobarbital Phenytoin Valproic acid		Felbamate Topiramate Zonisamide
CYP 2D6	Zonisamide	Carbamazepine	
CYP 3A4	Carbamazepine	Carbamazepine Phenytoin Phenobarbital	
Uridine diphosphate glucuronyl-transferase	Lamotrigine Carbamazepine	Lamotrigine Phenobarbital Phenytoin	Valproic acid

Michaelis-Menten Metabolism

Phenytoin exhibits dose-dependent capacity-limited (Michaelis-Menten) pharmacokinetics, meaning the maximum capacity of hepatic enzymes to metabolize the drug is reached within the normal dosage range. Therefore, small changes in doses result in disproportionate and large changes in serum concentrations. Due to individual differences in metabolism, each patient follows a different curve in the relationship between dose and serum concentrations.[4,6]

Protein Binding

Phenytoin and valproic acid are highly protein bound and only unbound medication is able to produce clinical and adverse effects. When interpreting serum concentrations for highly protein-bound AEDs, it is important to remember that the value represents the total concentration (bound and unbound). Patients with decreased protein (albumin) will have the same total concentration of AEDs, but the unbound concentration (active component) will be increased. Also, certain diseases states and medications may displace AEDs from protein, thereby increasing the unbound concentration. Examples of patients with low protein or disease states/medications that increase the unbound concentration of AEDs include:

- Patients with renal failure
- Patients with hypoalbuminemia
- Neonates
- Pregnant women
- Patients taking other highly protein bound medications
- Critical care patients

Alterations in protein binding of phenytoin will result in increased dose-related side effects. In patients with suspected changes in protein binding, it is useful to measure or calculate unbound (free) phenytoin concentrations.[6]

TABLE 49-5 **Management of Antiepileptic Drugs During Pregnancy**

▪ Give supplemental folic acid 1-4 mg daily to all women of child-bearing potential
▪ Use monotherapy when possible
▪ Use lowest dose possible to control seizures
▪ Monitor AED serum concentrations at the start of pregnancy and monthly thereafter
▪ Administer supplemental vitamin K during the eighth month of pregnancy to women receiving enzyme-inducing AEDs

Autoinduction

Carbamazepine is a potent inducer of the CYP-450 isoenzyme system, leading to increased clearance of many medicines and itself. Carbamazepine displays autoinduction of its own metabolism.

Serum Concentration Monitoring

A therapeutic range should be established for each patient and this range should define concentrations that result in minimal side effects and optimal seizure control. Table 49-3 lists usual serum concentrations for the AEDs.

Status Epilepticus

Status epilepticus (SE) is a neurologic emergency that can lead to permanent brain damage or death. SE is defined as any seizure lasting more than 30 minutes, with or without a loss of

TABLE 49-6 Parenteral Medications Used in Status Epilepticus in Adults

Drug Name (Brand Name)	Loading Dose	Administration Rate	Therapeutic Level	Side Effects	Comments
Diazepam (Valium)	0.15 mg/kg	5 mg/min (IVP)	N/A	Hypotension, respiratory depression	Rapid redistribution rate; can be given rectally
Lorazepam (Ativan)	0.1 mg/kg	2 mg/min (IVP)	N/A	Hypotension, respiratory depression	May be longer-acting than diazepam
Midazolam (Versed)	0.2 mg/kg	2 mg/min (IVP)	N/A	Sedation	Can also be given IM, buccally, intranasally; expensive
Phenytoin (Dilantin)	15-20 mg/kg	Up to 50 mg/min	10-20 μg/mL (39.6-79.2 μmol/L)	Arrhythmias, hypotension,	Hypotension, especially in elderly
Fosphenytoin (Cerebyx)	15-20 mg PE/kg	Up to 150 mg PE/min	10-20 μg/mL	Paresthesias, hypotension	Can be given IM; less CV side effects than phenytoin; expensive
Phenobarbital (Luminal)	20 mg/kg	50-100 mg/min	15-40 μg/mL (64.7-172.4 μmol/L)	Hypotension, sedation, respiratory depression	Long-acting
Valproate sodium (Depacon)	15-20 mg/kg (up to 40 mg/kg)	3-6 mg/kg/min	50-150 mcg/mL (346.5-1039.5 μmol/L)		Less CV side effects than phenytoin
Propofol (Diprivan)	1-2 mg/kg	~ 40 mg/10 s	N/A (typically titrated to EEG)	Hypotension, respiratory depression	Requires mechanical intubation; high lipid load (increased calories); propofol infusion syndrome
Pentobarbital (Nembutal)	10-15 mg/kg	Up to 50 mg/min	10-20 μg/mL (typically titrated to EEG)	Hypotension, respiratory depression, cardiac depression, infection, ileus	Requires mechanical intubation, pressors, hemodynamic monitoring

Abbreviations: CV, cardiovascular; EEG, electroencephalogram; IM, intramuscular; IVP, intravenous push; N/A, not applicable; PE, phenytoin equivalents.

Reproduced with permission from Brophy GM, Tesoro EP. Status epileptieus. In: Chisholm-Burns MA, Wells BG, Schwinghammer TL, et al, eds. *Pharmacotherapy Principles and Practice.* New York, NY: McGraw-Hill, 2008;461-471.

consciousness; or having recurrent seizures without regaining consciousness between seizure episodes.[11] The goals for treatment of SE include the cessation of any seizure activity and the prevention of further seizures. Ideally, this is accomplished through directed pharmacotherapy with minimization of adverse reactions. Treatment of SE includes benzodiazepines and anticonvulsants (Table 49-6).

Phenytoin and Fosphenytoin in Status Epilepticus

Phenytoin is administered intravenously as a loading dose (for patients not previously on phenytoin) of 15 to 20 mg/kg. The loading dose is infused no faster than 50 mg/min due to risks of hypotension and arrhythmias. Continuous monitoring of ECG and blood pressure is recommended. Maintenance dosing can be started in 12 hours after the loading dose. Phenytoin should not be administered via the intramuscular route due to alkaline nature. Extravasation of the drug can cause local discoloration, edema, pain, and sometimes necrosis.

Fosphenytoin is a water-soluble, prodrug of phenytoin that is rapidly converted to phenytoin in the body. Unlike phenytoin, fosphenytoin is compatible with most intravenous solutions and is tolerated as an intramuscular injection. Fosphenytoin is dosed on phenytoin equivalents (PE), and it can be infused up to 150 mg PE/min. The loading dose for patients not taking phenytoin is 15 to 20 mg PE/kg. Although fosphenytoin has fewer cardiovascular side effects compared to phenytoin, blood pressure and ECG should still be monitored.[12]

AED Brand Names and Formulations

Table 49-7 lists brand/generic names and formulations of antiepileptic drugs.

TABLE 49-7 **Brand/Generic Names and Formulations of AEDs**

Generic	Brand	Formulations
Sodium Channel Modulators		
Carbamazepine	Tegretol, Tegretol XR Epitol Equitro	Tablet Chewable tablet Extended release tablet Extended release capsule Suspension
Lamotrigine	Lamictal	Tablet Chewable tablet Disintegrating tablet
Oxcarbazepine	Trileptal	Tablet Suspension
Valproic acid	Depacon Depakene Stavzor	Softgel capsule Solution
Divalproex	Depakote Depakote ER	Delayed release capsule Extended release tablet Delayed release/enteric coated tablet
Phenytoin	Dilantin Phenytek	Capsule Extended release capsule Chewable tablet Suspension IV solution for injection
Fosphenytoin	Cerebyx	IV/IM solution for injection
Phenobarbital	Luminal	Tablet Elixir IV solution for injection
Calcium Channel Modulators		
Ethosuximide	Zarontin	Liquid-filled capsule Syrup
Pregabalin	Lyrica	Capsule
GABA Modulators		
Clonazepam	Klonopin Klonopin Wafers	Tablet Disintegrating tablet
Glutamate Modulators		
Felbamate	Felbatol	Tablet Suspension
Combination Modulators		
Gabapentin	Neurontin	Capsule Tablet Solution
Topiramate	Topamax	Capsule/sprinkles Tablet
Zonisamide	Zonegran	Capsule
Unknown Mechanism of Action		
Levetiracetam	Keppra Keppra XR	Tablet Extended release tablet IV solution for injection Solution

CASE Application

1. Select the type of epilepsy that results in a sudden interruption of activities and a blank stare.
   a. Absence seizures
   b. Tonic-clonic
   c. Myoclonic
   d. Atonic

2. Select the treatable cause of seizures.
   i. Hypoglycemia
   ii. Altered electrolytes
   iii. Infections
   iv. Cryptogenic
   a. i and ii
   b. i and iii
   c. i, ii, and iii
   d. iii and iv

3. Select the drug-induced cause of seizures.
   i. Bupropion
   ii. Tramadol
   iii. Amoxicillin
   a. i
   b. iii
   c. i and iii
   d. ii and iii
   e. i, ii, and iii

4. Select the dose-related adverse reaction of AEDs.
   a. Neutropenia
   b. Sedation
   c. Thrombocytopenia
   d. All of the above
   e. a and c

5. Select the patient population or condition that often leads to fast titration of AEDs.
   a. Switching AEDs
   b. Discontinuing AEDs
   c. Children
   d. Women of child-bearing potential

6. Select the medication that exhibits dose-dependent, capacity-limited pharmacokinetics.
   i. Dilantin
   ii. Cerebyx
   iii. Keppra
   iv. Neurontin
   a. i and ii
   b. i and iii
   c. i and iv
   d. i, ii, iii, and iv

7. Select the AED that has CYP-450 3A4 isoenzyme induction and autoinduction.
   a. Topiramate
   b. Carbamazepine
   c. Phenytoin
   d. Phenobarbital

8. Select the example of partial seizures.
   i. Complex
   ii. Simple
   iii. Tonic-clonic
   iv. Myoclonic
   a. i
   b. iii
   c. i and iv
   d. i and ii
   e. ii and iv

9. Select the AED that modulates sodium channels.
   a. Clonazepam
   b. Ethosuximide
   c. Gabapentin
   d. Carbamazepine

10. Select the AED which is primarily eliminated through renal route.
   a. Clonazepam
   b. Ethosuximide
   c. Gabapentin
   d. Carbamazepine

11. Select the idiosyncratic adverse reaction of carbamazepine.
   a. Aplastic anemia
   b. Hyponatremia
   c. Rash
   d. All of the above

12. Select the AED that modulates sodium channels.
   i. Phenytoin
   ii. Phenobarbital
   iii. Oxcarbazepine
   iv. Lamotrigine
   a. i and ii
   b. i and iii
   c. i, ii, iii, and iv
   d. ii, iii, and iv

13. Select the AED that is associated with the idiosyncratic adverse effect of gingival hyperplasia.
   a. Phenobarbital
   b. Primidone
   c. Tiagabine
   d. Phenytoin

14. Select the AED that has a usual serum concentration of 50 to 100 μg/mL.
   a. Phenytoin
   b. Carbamazepine
   c. Valproic acid
   d. Oxcarbazepine

15. Select the AED that has an unbound (free) concentration of 1 to 2 μg/mL.
   a. Phenytoin
   b. Carbamazepine
   c. Valproic acid
   d. Oxcarbazepine

16. Select the AED that has a primary route of elimination (substrate) of CYP-450 3A4.
   i. Carbamazepine
   ii. Zonisamide
   ii. Levetiracetam
   a. i and iii
   b. i and ii
   c. ii and iii
   d. i, ii, and iii

17. Select the AED that is a substrate and inducer of the CYP-450 2C9.
   a. Phenytoin
   b. Phenobarbital
   c. Gabapentin
   d. All of the above
   e. a and b

18. Select the water-soluble prodrug of phenytoin that is rapidly converted to phenytoin in the body.
   a. Trileptal
   b. Tegretol
   c. Keppra
   d. Cerebyx
   e. Dilantin

19. Intravenous dosing of phenytoin cannot be infused faster than 50 mg/min. Select the adverse reactions that are associated with infusions faster than 50 mg/min.
   a. Hypotension
   b. Gingival hyperplasia
   c. Anemia
   d. Rash

20. Select the AED that is available in oral and parenteral formulations.
   a. Neurontin
   b. Dilantin
   c. Keppra
   d. Trileptal

TAKEAWAY POINTS ››

- Epilepsy is a chronic disease of disturbed electrical activity in the brain resulting in recurrent seizures with or without convulsions.
- The pathophysiology of a seizure is due to an unstable cell membrane in the gray matter of the brain.
- The classifications of epilepsy are: absence seizures (petit mal)—sudden interruption of activities and a blank stare; myoclonic seizures—brief shock-like contraction of a muscle group; clonic seizures—jerking motion while tonic seizures involve a sustained muscle contraction; tonic-clonic seizures (grand mal)—alternating muscle contraction and jerking; atonic seizures involve a sudden loss of muscle tone know as "drop attacks."
- Laboratory tests are evaluated to rule out treatable causes of seizures, such as hypoglycemia, altered electrolytes, and infections. A seizure produced by treatable causes does not represent epilepsy.
- Medications associated with causing seizures include tramadol, bupropion, theophylline, some antidepressants, some antipsychotics, amphetamines, cocaine, imipenem, lithium, excessive doses of penicillins or cephalosporins, sympathomimetics, and stimulants.
- The goal of epilepsy treatment is complete elimination of seizures with no drug side effects. This is not always possible and the patient should be involved in deciding the balance between frequency of seizures and occurrence of side effects.
- Initial therapy is initiated with one AED and up to 70% of patients are controlled on monotherapy.
- Adverse effects of AEDs are often dose limiting or cause a drug to be discontinued. AED adverse reactions are classified as dose related or idiosyncratic.
- Dose-related adverse effects include sedation, ataxia, and diplopia. Idiosyncratic adverse reactions are not related to the dose of the AED and often lead to discontinuation of the AED.
- AEDs are associated with numerous drug interactions related to absorption, metabolism, and protein binding.
- Phenytoin exhibits dose-dependent capacity-limited (Michaelis-Menten) pharmacokinetics, meaning the maximum capacity of hepatic enzymes to metabolize the drug is reached within the normal dosage range.
- Phenytoin and valproic acid are highly protein bound and only unbound medication is able to produce clinical and adverse effects.
- A therapeutic range should be established for each patient and this range should define concentrations that result in minimal side effects and optimal seizure control.
- Status epilepticus (SE) is a neurologic emergency that can lead to permanent brain damage or death.

REFERENCES

1. Armijo JA, Shushtarian M, Valdizan EM, Cuadrado A, de las Cuevas I, Adín J. Ion channels and epilepsy. *Curr Pharm Des.* 2005;11:1975-2003.
2. Commission on Classification and Terminology of the International League Against Epilepsy. Proposal for revised clinical and electroencephalographic classification of epileptic seizures. *Epilepsia.* 1981;22:489-501.
3. Commission on Classification and Terminology of the International League Against Epilepsy. Proposal for revised classification of epilepsies and epileptic syndromes. *Epilepsia.* 1989;30:389-399.
4. Karceski S, Morrell MJ, Carpenter D. Treatment of epilepsy in adults: expert opinion. *Epilepsy Behav.* 2005; 7:S1-S64.
5. Perruca E. An introduction to antiepileptic drugs. *Epilepsia.* 2005;46(suppl 4):31-37.
6. French JA, Kanner AM, Bautista J, et al. Efficacy and tolerability of the new antiepileptic drugs I: treatment of new onset epilepsy, report of the Therapeutics and Technology Assessment Subcommittee and Quality Standards Subcommittee of the American Academy of Neurology and the American Epilepsy Society. *Neurology.* 2005;62:1252-1260.
7. French JA, Kanner AM, Bautista J, et al. Efficacy and tolerability of the new antiepileptic drugs II: treatment of new onset epilepsy, report of the Therapeutics and Technology Assessment Subcommittee and Quality Standards Subcommittee of the American Academy of Neurology and the American Epilepsy Society. *Neurology.* 2005;62:1261-1273.
8. Quality Standards Subcommittee of the American Academy of Neurology. Practice parameter: a guideline for discontinuing antiepileptic drugs in seizure free patients [summary statement]. *Neurology.* 1996;47:600-602.
9. Patsalos PN, Froscher W, Pisani F, van Rijn CM. The importance of drug interactions in epilepsy therapy. *Epilepsia.* 2002;43: 365-385.
10. Crawford P. Best practice guidelines for the management of women with epilepsy. *Epilepsia.* 2005;46(suppl 9):117-124.
11. Commission on Classification of Terminology, International League Against Epilepsy. Proposal for revised clinical and electroencephalographic classification of epileptic seizures. *Epilepsia.* 1981;22;489-501.
12. Pryor FM, Gidal B, Ramsay RE, DeToledo J, Morgan RO. Fosphenytoin: pharmacokinetics and tolerance of intramuscular loading doses. *Epilepsia.* 2001:42(2):245-250.

CHAPTER

50 Parkinson Disease

Michele A. Faulkner

FOUNDATION OVERVIEW

Parkinson disease (PD) is a highly prevalent neurodegenerative disorder secondary in prevalence only to Alzheimer disease.[1] Approximately 2% of the geriatric population is affected, though younger persons can also develop the disease.[2] The mean age of onset is 65 years, and men are affected more often than women. Associated morbidity is substantial, and results in increased hospitalizations, increased prescription drug utilization and more frequent placement in long-term care facilities as compared to the general population.[3] Though in most cases persons with PD can expect to live into old age, their life expectancy is somewhat shorter than average.[4,5] The disease is progressive, and no cure has been identified to date.

The underlying mechanism of PD development is not well understood, but genetic predisposition, environmental toxins, and the sequelae of infection have all been implicated.[6] Loss of nigrostriatal neurons in the substantia nigra pars compacta and Lewy body formation (misfolded proteins) are the pathological hallmarks of the disease. By the time symptoms emerge and a diagnosis is made, it is estimated that 80% of nigrostriatal neurons have been lost.[7] Due to a resultant deficiency in the neurotransmitter dopamine, there is less inhibitory output from the basal ganglia.[8] The neurotransmitter imbalance allows for relative overactivity of acetylcholine, and is responsible for the abnormalities of motor function that characterize the disease. The cardinal features of PD include tremor, bradykinesia, rigidity, and postural instability (though this symptom is rare in the early stages of the disease). PD symptoms typically begin unilaterally in the extremities, and spread to the opposite side as the disease progresses. Presentation varies among individuals and can differ substantially from person to person.

Tremor is the most common PD symptom, however not all patients have one.[9] Some may complain of feeling an internal vibration that is not outwardly apparent. In mild disease, the tremor (often described by the term "pill rolling" as the fingers and thumb move in opposite directions), disappears with purposeful movement and during sleep. In some cases tremor may also be present in the lips, chin, and jaw.

Bradykinesia, or slow movement, may result in difficulty with tasks requiring repetitive movements and fine motor control (such as teeth brushing). Arm-swing when walking may be diminished or absent, and spontaneous gesturing and facial expression are often blunted. A shuffling gait may become apparent, and difficulty turning in bed or rising from a chair may affect the PD patient's ability to function. Handwriting frequently becomes smaller (micrographia) and difficult to read. Bradykinesia is the symptom that most PD patients consider most distressing. Eventually, all voluntary movements will be affected to some degree.

Rigidity is more common in older patients upon initial presentation.[6] This symptom will be observed as resistance in the muscles upon initiation of passive movement. The rigidity of PD is often described as "jerky" or "cogwheeling" in nature.[10] Vague muscle aches, especially in the back, shoulder, or arm on the side where symptoms eventually appear, may be the first sign of rigidity. Some patients experience painful dystonias and cramping in the feet.[9]

Postural instability (or postural reflex impairment) typically appears later in the disease process. As impairment progresses, patients may be observed in a stooped position with flexion at the knees, hips, and waist. Patients may also be observed walking on the balls of their feet. Impairment of posture contributes substantially to the risk of injury secondary to falling.[11]

PD remains a diagnosis of exclusion. Because many neurological disorders share common features, the diagnosis is sometimes made in error as evidenced by examination of the brain postmortem.[5] There are no biological or laboratory tests that can confirm the diagnosis of PD. In general, if two of the cardinal features of the disease are present, and characteristics suggestive of another disorder are absent, the diagnosis is made. A positive response to administration of the drug levodopa (which will temporarily increase dopamine levels in the central nervous system) may be used as a confirmatory test. Medication-induced parkinsonism, associated most often with phenothiazine antiemetics, metoclopramide, and neuroleptic medications, should be ruled out.[12,13]

TREATMENT

The primary goal of PD treatment is to maintain the patient's functional ability by controlling motor symptoms. Recent studies suggest that one or more medications may have a role in slowing the progression of the disease, but symptom control remains the principal focus at this time. Therapy should be tailored to the individual needs of the patient (Figure 50-1).

Carbidopa/Levodopa

No treatment has been shown to be better at controlling the motor symptoms of PD than levodopa.[13] Conversion of

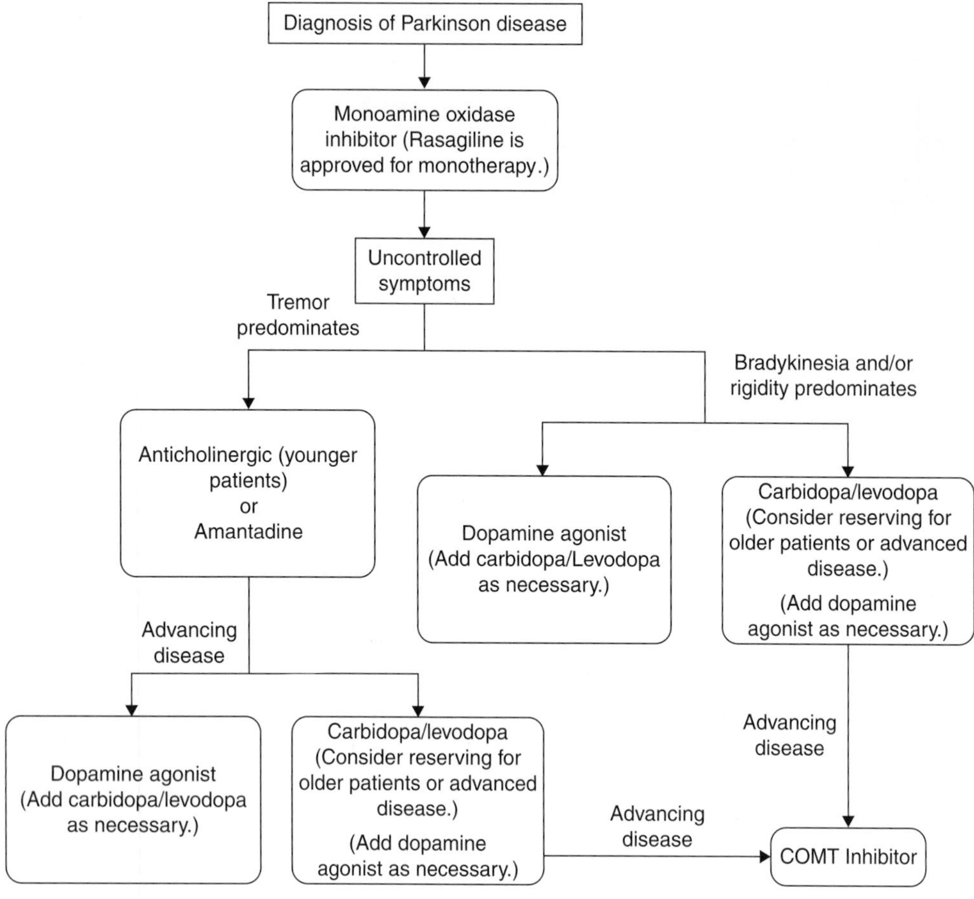

FIGURE 50-1 General approach to pharmacologic management of Parkinson disease.[a]

levodopa to dopamine results in direct replacement of the neurotransmitter in the brain. The carbidopa component inhibits the activity of the enzyme dopa decarboxylase, thus preventing the conversion of levodopa to dopamine in the periphery. Without this inhibition, levels of dopamine in the CNS would be diminished, and the patient would be subject to profound nausea and orthostatic hypotension. A minimum daily dose of 75 to 100 mg of carbidopa is recommended to prevent peripheral conversion, and carbidopa supplementation may be given without an increase in the levodopa dose if necessary.[13] The typical starting dose of carbidopa/levodopa is 25/100 mg orally given tid (Table 50-1). The drug is best taken on an empty stomach, but if side-effects necessitate that it be taken with food, a low protein meal is preferred as amino acids compete with levodopa for transport into the CNS.[5] An immediate-release formulation and a controlled-release formulation of carbidopa/levodopa are available, as is an orally dissolving tablet that may be taken without liquid. The controlled-release formulation is not absorbed as well, and may require a 30% increase in daily dose if a conversion from the immediate-release form is desired.[5]

Carbidopa/levodopa works well for the entire range of motor symptoms, and most patients can be maintained on 600 mg of levodopa or less for the first several years. However, the efficacy of levodopa will eventually begin to decrease secondary to a decline in the ability of the brain to store dopamine. The result is a return of symptoms prior to the next administration time known as "wearing off." In contrast, "on-off" phenomena also begins to appear after extended use of levodopa, but the return of symptoms occurs in an unpredictable manner and typically lasts only seconds to minutes.[14] This unpredictability can be distressing for patients, particularly as symptom breakthrough begins to occur with increasing frequency.

Dyskinesias, primarily dystonia and chorea, are involuntary movements that may occur in a patient taking levodopa.[8] These movements often appear when the motor symptoms of PD are under optimal control, and for this reason they are sometimes referred to as "peak dose" dyskinesias. Previously, dopamine receptor overstimulation was thought to be responsible, but there is now evidence that therapies resulting in fluctuating receptor stimulation play a role. Some practitioners elect

TABLE 50-1 Dosing of Medications Used in the Treatment of Parkinson Disease

Drug	Dosing	Renal adjustment
Carbidopa/levodopa (Sinemet, Parcopa)	Initial dose—25/100 mg po tid Initial dose (CR formulation)—50/200 mg po bid Usual maximum dose (levodopa)—6000 mg	
Bromocriptine (Parlodel)	Initial dose 1.25 mg po bid Maximum dose—100 mg qd	
Pramipexole (Mirapex)	Initial dose—0.125 mg po tid Initial dose (ER formulation)—0.375 mg po qd Maximum dose—4.5 mg qd	Cl_{cr} 35-59 mL/min—0.125mg po bid Cl_{cr} 15-34 mL/min—0.125mg po qd Cl_{cr}<15 mL/min—not recommended
Ropinirole (Requip)	Initial dose—0.25 mg po tid Initial dose (XR formulation)—2 mg po qd Maximum dose—24 mg qd	
Selegiline (Eldepryl, Zelapar)	Initial/maximum dose—5 mg po bid or 10 mg po qd Initial dose (disintegrating tab)—1.25 mg po qd Maximum dose (disintegrating tab)—2.5 mg po qd	
Rasagiline (Azilect)	Initial dose (with levodopa)—0.5 mg po qd levodopa) Maximum dose (with levodopa)—1 mg po qd Initial/maximum dose (monotherapy)—1 mg po qd	
Amantadine (Symmetrel)	Initial dose—100 mg po bid Maximum dose—400 mg qd	Cl_{cr} 30-50 mL/min—100 mg qd Cl_{cr} 15-29 mL/min—100 mg po qd Cl_{cr}<15 mL/min or dialysis—200 mg po every wk
Anticholinergics	Dosing varies by agent	
Entacapone (Comtan)	200 mg po with each dose of levodopa Maximum dose—800 mg qd	
Tolcapone (Tasmar)	Initial dose—100 mg po tid Maximum dose—200 mg po tid	

to delay the use of levodopa, especially in younger patients, in an effort to delay the onset of these motor fluctuations.

Common adverse effects associated with carbidopa/levodopa include confusion, changes in bowel habits, CNS depression, dizziness, and nausea. The drug should be tapered when discontinued to avoid neuroleptic malignant syndrome which may result in delirium, fevers, muscular rigidity, and a general instability of the CNS.

Dopamine Agonists

Four dopamine agonists (DA) are currently indicated for the treatment of PD as initial therapy or as add-on therapy. Three of them, rotigotine, pramipexole, and ropinirole, are nonergolines and bind to D_2 and D_3 receptors, both of which are inhibitory. (Rotigotine, the only transdermal DA, is currently unavailable in the United States due to manufacturing issues). Pramipexole is typically initiated at a dose of 0.375 mg daily divided every 8 hours or once daily for the extended-release formulation, though adjustment for renal dysfunction is recommended. The dose may be increased every 5 to 7 days as needed up to maximum of 4.5 mg daily. The immediate-release formulation of ropinirole is initiated at a dose of 0.25 mg tid, and is increased weekly to effect, while the extended-release formulation is initiated at a dose of 2 mg daily with an additional 2 mg added to the daily dose no more often than every 7 days. The maximum daily dose of either formulation is 24 mg. Bromocriptine is an ergot derivative which binds to D_2 receptors, but also to excitatory D_1 receptors.[7] Usual dosing is 1.25 mg twice daily with dose increases occurring every 2 to 4 weeks. Doses as high as 100 mg daily have been employed. The oldest of the DAs, apomorphine, is not used to treat the cardinal symptoms of PD, but does have a place in the treatment of severe off periods.

The DAs work by bypassing nigrostriatal neurons and directly stimulating postsynaptic dopamine receptors.[15] The efficacy of the DAs is slightly less than levodopa; however, they are less likely to cause dyskinesias. Most patients on DA monotherapy experience good symptom control for several years. If a DA is added to levodopa therapy when wearing off has begun to occur, the dose of the latter should initially be decreased by one-fourth to one-third to help avoid dyskinesias.

Many DA side-effects are similar to those associated with levodopa including nausea, somnolence, and hypotension. DAs cause psychiatric side-effects (delusions, hallucinations) three times more often than levodopa.[16] Edema of the lower extremities has been noted with the DAs, as has impulsive behavior leading to gambling, excessive shopping, and hypersexuality. Some users claim to have experienced sleep attacks described as being similar to narcolepsy. The ergot derivatives have been associated with pulmonary and retroperitoneal fibrosis which has decreased use. Like levodopa, DA doses should be slowly tapered when therapy is being discontinued.

Monoamine Oxidase Inhibitors

The older of the two monoamine oxidase (MAO) inhibitors used for the treatment of PD, selegiline, is approved for add-on therapy. Traditional dosing is 5 mg orally given twice daily, but a single 10 mg daily dose may be given. An orally disintegrating selegiline tablet with a quicker onset of action is now available, and is initiated at a dose of 1.25 mg daily. After 6 weeks of therapy, the dose may be increased to a maximum of 2.5 mg daily if necessary. A second agent, rasagiline, is approved as both monotherapy and as add-on therapy. When given alone, the dose is 1 mg daily. However if the drug is being added to levodopa, the starting dose is 0.5 mg daily. These drugs work by hindering dopamine breakdown by MAO in the brain. At normal doses, the inhibitors used in the treatment of PD are selective for MAO type B, the primary type present in the basal ganglia.[17] As MOA inhibition by these agents is irreversible, it may take weeks before levels of MAO are back to normal after an inhibitor is discontinued. Of note, there is some recent evidence that rasagiline may slow the advancement of PD, and as such, consideration should be given to using an MAO inhibitor as initial therapy.[18]

Side-effects associated with MAO inhibitors include nausea, headache, and dizziness. Selegiline in particular is associated with insomnia due to its amphetamine metabolite. Doses of selegiline should be given no later than early afternoon in order to avoid sleep disturbances. The orally disintegrating tablet is less likely to cause insomnia because it avoids first pass metabolism. Due to their selectivity, selegiline and rasagiline are less likely to lead to serotonin toxicity when given in conjunction with other drugs; however caution should be used when administering them in conjunction with other medications including selective serotonin and norepinephrine reuptake inhibiting antidepressants, sympathomimetics, dextromethorphan, meperidine, and tramadol.[17,19] Similarly, tyramine interactions that increase levels of norepinephrine leading to sympathomimetic effects such as hypertension and tachycardia are unlikely when selegiline and rasagiline are used at normal doses. There have however been rare reports of this interaction (sometimes referred to as the "cheese effect") occurring with selegiline when users have ingested foods such as aged cheese, and pickled or fermented foods and drinks.

Amantadine

Amantadine is an antiviral drug that was serendipitously found useful for the treatment of PD. Because its effects are mild and transient, its place in therapy is limited.[5] The drug is typically employed near the time of diagnosis, and is best used when tremor is a predominant symptom. However, the drug has recently found a new place in therapy as an agent used to control dyskinesias. When used early in the treatment of PD, amantadine's effectiveness typically wanes after several months. The usual dose is 100 mg twice daily, and adjustment for renal disease is recommended. Amantadine's mechanism of action is not well understood, but the drug is an NMDA receptor antagonist, and may decrease the activity of the excitatory neurotransmitter glutamate. It also has anticholinergic properties. Constipation and leg edema have been associated with amantadine use. Nightmares, hallucinations, and confusion have also been reported.[5] Amantadine should be slowly tapered when discontinuing use as rebound symptoms have occurred.

Anticholinergics

Multiple anticholinergic agents have been used in the treatment of PD, but the most common are benztropine, diphenhydramine, and trihexyphenidyl. These drugs act primarily to correct the relative overactivity of acetylcholine that occurs due to diminished levels of dopamine. Like amantadine, anticholinergics are used primarily to control tremor. Use in older patients is limited due to frequent side-effects which include dry mucous membranes, tachycardia, memory impairment, and orthostatic hypotension.[5] Anticholinergic drugs should be tapered to avoid rebound PD symptoms.

Catechol-*O*-Methyltransferase Inhibitors

Two catechol-*o*-methyltransferase (COMT) inhibitors are currently available for PD treatment. These enzyme-inhibiting drugs help prevent the breakdown of both levodopa and dopamine by COMT. Though it is normally a secondary enzymatic pathway, COMT predominates when dopa decarboxylase activity is being inhibited by carbidopa.[20] COMT inhibitors should only be used as an adjunct to levodopa therapy. They are particularly useful for PD patients who are experiencing "off time."

The two available COMT inhibitors are tolcapone and entacapone. Tolcapone, the older drug, is the more potent of the two. It works in both the periphery and the brain. However, due to several cases of liver failure associated with the drug, it is now used infrequently, and is best reserved for patients who do not respond adequately to other agents. The normal dose for therapy initiation is 100 mg tid. Liver function tests are recommended every 2 to 4 weeks for 6 months, and then periodically thereafter when tolcapone is used.[21] The drug may be given independent of the timing of levodopa administration. In contrast, entacapone is administered simultaneously with levodopa, usually at a dose of 200 mg. It exerts its action in the periphery only. A combination drug containing carbidopa/levodopa and entacapone is available for use when appropriate doses of the individual ingredients have been established.

Dyskinesias are possible when COMT inhibitors are used, but decreasing the levodopa dose when the drugs are initially added (typically by ~25%) can help avoid this problem. Patient counseling should include a discussion regarding diarrhea, the onset of which might not occur until weeks after the drug has been started. In some cases, the problem is significant enough that the drug must be discontinued. Patients may also experience orange discoloration of body fluids.

SPECIAL CONSIDERATIONS

Though the primary neurotransmitter derangement associated with PD is dopamine deficiency, serotonergic, adrenergic, and cholinergic pathways may also be affected. As such, there are several comorbid conditions that frequently exist with PD. Several of these conditions are neuropsychiatric in nature. Depression is estimated to occur in up to 60% of patients, and may even be part of the disease.[22] No class of antidepressant is preferred over another, but other comorbidities (insomnia, hypersomnia, and sexual dysfunction) must be taken into consideration when choosing a therapeutic agent. Some antidepressant classes have been associated with drug-induced tremor, and these drugs should be evaluated as a possible cause if symptoms worsen. Additionally, caution is warranted when using some antidepressants in conjunction with medications used to treat PD (such as the MAO inhibitors). Psychosis and dementia also commonly exist in the PD population. If antipsychotic therapy is warranted, more antidopaminergic drugs should be avoided. Preferred agents include quetiapine and clozapine. Rivastigmine is indicated for PD dementia, but because it inhibits cholinesterase, it has the potential to make PD symptoms worse by potentiating the relative overactivity of acetylcholine. Bladder dysfunction, constipation, hypotension (both medication-induced and disease-related), and falls predisposing patients to fracture are also common in the PD patient and frequently warrant intervention with drug therapy.

CASE Application

1. What is the primary neurotransmitter deficiency in Parkinson disease?
   a. Acetylcholine
   b. Dopamine
   c. Norepinephrine
   d. Serotonin

2. Which of the cardinal features of Parkinson disease is least likely to be present upon diagnosis?
   a. Bradykinesia
   b. Postural instability
   c. Rigidity
   d. Tremor

3. What is the primary goal of Parkinson disease treatment?
   a. Cessation of disease progression
   b. Facilitate an increase in the storage capacity of dopamine
   c. Maintenance of functional ability
   d. Reversal of neuronal loss

4. What is the role of carbidopa in the treatment of Parkinson disease?
   a. It inhibits acetylcholine.
   b. It inhibits dopa decarboxylase.
   c. It inhibits catechol-*o*-methyltransferase.
   d. It inhibits monoamine oxidase.

5. Which of the following describes off-time associated with "on-off" phenomena?
   a. It lasts for several hours.
   b. It typically happens at the end of a dosing interval.
   c. It is associated with receptor overstimulation.
   d. It is unpredictable.

6. What is the maximum recommended daily dose of pramipexole?
   a. 0.375 mg
   b. 4.5 mg
   c. 24 mg
   d. 100 mg

7. Which of the following medications has been implicated in causing impulsive behavior?
   a. Amantadine
   b. Entacapone
   c. Rasagiline
   d. Ropinirole

8. Which drug is frequently associated with insomnia due to the action of its metabolite?
   a. Amantadine
   b. Benztropine
   c. Pramipexole
   d. Selegiline

9. Anticholinergics are primarily used to control which cardinal Parkinson disease symptom?
   a. Bradykinesia
   b. Postural instability
   c. Rigidity
   d. Tremor

10. The use of which of the following medication requires monitoring of liver function tests?
    a. Levodopa
    b. Rasagiline
    c. Ropinirole
    d. Tolcapone

11. Which drug should be dosed simultaneously with levodopa?
    a. Amantadine
    b. Entacapone
    c. Pramipexole
    d. Rasagiline

12. Parkinsonian symptoms have been noted in patients exposed to which of the following medications?
    a. Haloperidol
    b. Metoclopramide
    c. Prochlorperazine
    d. All of the above

13. What is the mechanism of action of ropinirole?
    a. Direct replacement of dopamine in the central nervous system
    b. Direct stimulation of postsynaptic dopamine receptors
    c. Inhibition of the enzymatic breakdown of dopamine in the central nervous system
    d. Inhibition of the enzymatic breakdown of dopamine in the periphery

14. Which antipsychotic is preferred when treatment of psychosis is necessary in the Parkinson patient?
    a. Chlorpromazine
    b. Haloperidol
    c. Quetiapine
    d. Risperidone

15. Which medication is available as an orally disintegrating tablet that may be taken without liquid?
    a. Carbidopa/levodopa
    b. Pramipexole
    c. Selegiline
    d. Both a and c are correct

16. Which medication can cause rebound Parkinson symptoms if stopped abruptly?
    a. Amantadine
    b. Carbidopa/levodopa
    c. Pramipexole
    d. Rasagiline

17. GR was recently diagnosed with Parkinson disease. His family practitioner initiated therapy with carbidopa/levodopa 10/100 mg tid. He has been taking the medication with meals, but he is experiencing significant nausea. GR has noticed very little difference in his symptoms. What is the most probable reason GR is experiencing such significant nausea?
    a. Carbidopa/levodopa should be taken on an empty stomach.
    b. Carbidopa/levodopa should be taken with a meal high in protein.
    c. The levodopa component is being converted to dopamine in the periphery.
    d. Carbidopa/levodopa always causes nausea.

18. Comorbid conditions frequently present in persons with Parkinson disease include which of the following?
    a. Depression
    b. Constipation
    c. Hypotension
    d. All of the above

19. Which dopamine agonist is most likely to be associated with fibrotic complications?
    a. Bromocriptine
    b. Pramipexole
    c. Ropinirole
    d. Rotigotine

20. Which of the following is/are true of dyskinesias in a person with Parkinson disease?
    a. They often appear when the cardinal symptoms are under good control.
    b. Intermittent dopamine receptor stimulation is believed to contribute to dyskinesia development.
    c. They are associated with extended use of levodopa.
    d. All of the above.

TAKEAWAY POINTS ››

- Parkinson disease is the second most common neurological disease.
- There are currently no medications that halt or reverse disease progression.
- The pathological hallmarks of Parkinson disease are loss of nigrostriatal neurons in the substantia nigra which leads to dopamine deficiency and the formation of Lewy bodies.
- The decrease in dopamine concentration in the brain causes a relative overactivity of acetylcholine. It is this neurotransmitter imbalance that is responsible for the movement derangements that are the primary symptoms of Parkinson disease.
- The cardinal features of the disease are bradykinesia, rigidity, tremor, and postural instability.
- Carbidopa/levodopa administration results in the direct replacement of dopamine. The carbidopa component prevents peripheral conversion of levodopa to dopamine prior to its entrance into the brain.
- Carbidopa/levodopa efficacy wanes after several years of use resulting in periods of off-time. Dyskinesias, particularly dystonia and chorea, often appear after several years as well.
- The dopamine agonists bypass the nigrostriatal neurons directly stimulating postsynaptic dopamine receptors.
- The MAO inhibitors used for the treatment of Parkinson disease are selective for MAO type B. At normal doses they are much less likely to interact with tyramine or contribute to serotonin toxicity than nonselective agents.
- Amantadine is an antiviral agent that is helpful for the control of tremor in Parkinson disease. Its effects are mild and typically wane after several months of use. Amantadine has recently been employed to treat dyskinesias associated with levodopa use.

- The anticholinergic medications are used primarily for tremor. They serve to offset the imbalance between dopamine and acetylcholine activity. Use is limited in older patients due to the high frequency of side-effects.
- The COMT inhibitors prevent the breakdown of both levodopa and carbidopa in the periphery allowing levodopa to cross the blood–brain barrier for conversion.
- The COMT inhibitor tolcapone has been associated with liver failure and its use requires monitoring of liver function tests.
- The COMT inhibitor entacapone should be dosed simultaneously with levodopa, while tolcapone may be dosed independently.
- Multiple comorbidities are associated with Parkinson disease. The selection of medications used to treat them must be done with care so as to avoid significant drug interactions or exacerbation of parkinsonian symptoms.

REFERENCES

1. Schapira AHV. Progress in neuroprotection in Parkinson's disease. *Eur J Neurol.* 2008;15(suppl 1):5-13.
2. Clarke C, Morroe AP. Parkinson's disease. *Clin Evid.* 2005;13:1658-1677.
3. Huse DM, Schulman K, Orsini L, et al. Burden of illness in Parkinson's disease. *Mov Disord.* 2005;20:1449-1454.
4. Nutt JF, Wooten GF. Clinical practice. Diagnosis and initial management of Parkinson's disease. *N Engl J Med.* 2005;353: 1021-1027.
5. Tarsy D. Initial treatment of Parkinson's disease. *Curr Treat Options Neurol.* 2006;8:224-235.
6. Gancher ST. Parkinson disease in young adults. Available at: http://emedicine.medscape.com/article/1154474-overview. Accessed September 6, 2009.
7. Bonuccelli U, Pavese N. Dopamine agonists in the treatment of Parkinson's disease. *Expert Rev Neurother.* 2006;8:81-89.
8. Brotchie JA, Lee J, Venderova K. Levodopa-induced dyskinesia in Parkinson's disease. *J Neural Transm.* 2005;112:359-391.
9. Bhat V, Weiner WJ. Parkinson's disease. Diagnosis and the initiation of therapy. *Minerva Med.* 2005;96:145-154.
10. Jankovic J. Parkinson's disease: clinical features and diagnosis. *J Neurol Neurosurg Psychiat.* 2008;79:368-376.
11. Scott L. Identifying poor symptom control in Parkinson's disease. *Nursing Times.* 2006;102:30-32.
12. Gershanik OS. Drug-induced parkinsonism in the aged: recognition and prevention. *Drug Aging.* 1994;5:127-132.
13. Lang AE, Miyasaki J, Olanow CW, et al. A forum on the early management of Parkinson's disease. *Can J Neurol Sci.* 2005;32(3):277-286.
14. Schapira AH, Obeso J. Timing of treatment initiation in Parkinson's disease: a need for reappraisal? *Ann Neurol.* 2006;59:559-562.
15. Montastruc JL, Rascol O, Senared JM. Treatment of Parkinson's disease should begin with a dopamine agonist. *Mov Disord.* 1999;14:725-730.
16. Bonuccelli U, Pavese N. Role of dopamine agonists in Parkinson's disease: an update. *Expert Rev Neurother.* 2007;7:1391-1399.
17. Henchcliffe C, Schumacher HC, Burgut F. Recent advances in Parkinson's disease therapy: use of monoamine oxidase inhibitors. *Expert Rev Neurother.* 2005;5:811-821.
18. Olanow CW. Early rasagiline treatment slows UPDRS decline in the ADAGIO delayed start study. *Ann Neurol.* 2008; 64(suppl 12):S68.Abstract.
19. Chen JJ, Swoope DM, Dashtipour K. Comprehensive review of rasagiline, a second-generation monoamine oxidase inhibitor, for the treatment of Parkinson's disease. *Clin Ther.* 2007;29:1825-1849.
20. Hermanowicz N. Drug therapy for Parkinson's disease. *Semin Neurol.* 2007;27:97-105.
21. Borges N. Tolcapone in Parkinson's disease: liver toxicity and clinical efficacy. *Expert Opin Drug Saf.* 2005;4:69-73.
22. Lagopoulos J, Malhi GS, Ivanovski B, et al. A matter of motion or an emotional matter? Management of depression in Parkinson's disease. *Exp Rev Neurother.* 2005;5:803-810

CHAPTER

51 Headache

Carrie Foust Koenigsfeld, Darla Klug Eastman, and Anisa Fornoff

FOUNDATION OVERVIEW

Headaches are a common chief complaint of patients seeking advice from a pharmacist. It is estimated that 18% of women and 6% of men experience migraine headache.[1] Prevalence is highest between the ages of 25 and 45 in both males and females.[2] Migraines are considered to be one of the top 20 most disabling diseases worldwide by the World Health Organization.[3] Tension headaches are the most common type of primary headaches with an estimated prevalence of 86% in women and 63% in men with the rates occurring highest between the ages of 20 and 50.[4] Cluster headaches may be relatively uncommon, with the prevalence estimated to be 56 to 401 per 100,000 with onset typically occurring over the age of 20.[5]

The pathophysiologic and etiologic mechanisms of migraine are not completely known at this time. The sensory sensitivity may be due to a dysfunction of monoaminergic sensory control systems of the brainstem and thalamus. It is speculated that the trigeminovascular input from the meningeal vessels is a pathway for pain recognized in migraine headaches. There is a release of vasoactive neuropeptides, specifically calcitonin gene-related peptide (CGRP), when the cells in the trigeminal nucleus are activated. There is a deficiency of serotonin levels in the plasma during a migraine attack. The use of serotonin agonists, triptans, in migraine therapy has demonstrated the role of serotonin in treatment, being potent agonists of 5-HT_{1B}, 5-HT_{1D}, and 5-HT_{1F}. Dopamine may also play a role in migraine headaches as dopamine receptor antagonists are effective treatments administered as monotherapy or with other antimigraine medications; however, there is a lack of clinical data to support this theory.[6]

The pathophysiology behind tension headache also remains unknown, but one hypothesis is that stress may be an important stimulus. Cluster headaches may be precipitated by hypothalamic-related changes in cortisol, prolactin, testosterone, growth hormone, luteinizing hormone, endorphins, or melatonin.[7]

When considering the diagnosis of headaches, a comprehensive history of present illness and physical examination are critical. A thorough history will include time of onset, attack frequency, duration, aggravating and relieving factors, characteristics of pain, associated signs and symptoms, family history, social history, treatment history, and impact on daily living. Some history and physical examination findings that may be suggestive of a secondary headache disorder include, but are not limited to, the worst headache ever, increase in frequency or severity of usual headaches, head pain with exercise, increased head pain with sneezing or coughing, headache that wakes patient from sleep, signs of infection, ataxia or uncoordinated limbs, new headaches in a person ≥ age 40, history of head trauma, and changes in mental status.[8] Headaches beginning after the age of 50 may suggest underlying issues such as a mass lesion or cerebrovascular disease. Any of these findings are considered "red flags" that warrant a referral to the physician.

The three main categories of primary headache disorder according to the International Headache Society are migraine headaches, tension-type headaches, and cluster headaches. Headaches are differentiated from each other based upon duration, location, frequency, severity, and quality of pain. Tension headaches last from 30 minutes to 7 days and are located in the occipital or frontal region of the head with a band-like tightness. Pain associated with cluster headaches is unilateral and the headaches are more vascular in nature producing pain around the eye, temple, or forehead. Cluster headaches resolve within 3 hours with the pain being accompanied with one or more symptoms, such as nasal congestion, watering of the eyes, eyelid edema, or ptosis. There is clinical variability among migraine headaches. Onset of migraine pain is usually gradual with the peak of pain happening in minutes to hours. In adults, pain may last 4 to 72 hours and is most often located in the frontal or temporal region of the head. Patients often describe the headache as moderate to severe, pulsating in nature, and aggravated by physical activity. A combination of nausea, vomiting, photophobia and phonophobia accompany the headache.[3] More than 10% of patients experience a migraine both with and without aura and 60% or more of patients with migraines have headaches without aura.[9] An aura refers to the neurologic symptoms that can precede an attack. These symptoms may occur as diplopia, scotomas, blurry vision, ataxia, and vertigo.

PREVENTION

Headaches may be triggered by a variety of patient-specific factors. Possible triggers include emotional stress; changes in sleeping habits; physical activity; environmental factors such as flickering lights and loud noises; ingestion of chocolate, red wine, caffeine, alcohol, nitrates, aspartame, and medications including oral contraceptives.[10] Patients should avoid possible triggers. Encouraging patients to keep a headache diary can be helpful in tracking the duration and frequency of symptoms, possible triggers, and responses to treatment interventions.

Nonpharmacologic treatment may be considered for prevention and for adjunctive treatment for alleviating headaches. Headache sufferers may find relief by reducing activity and sensory input and by sleep. Some patients have used relaxation therapy, including biofeedback, hypnosis, or acupuncture to alleviate the pain.[10] Patients should avoid identified triggers and consider a wellness program focused on a consistent sleep pattern, exercise, healthy diet, and limited caffeine and nicotine intake.[10]

TREATMENT

Migraine Headache

Acute Therapy

The goals for treatment of an acute migraine headache are to treat attacks quickly and consistently while avoiding recurrence, restore the patient's ability to function, optimize self-care, minimize adverse effects, and be cost-effective.[11,12] Several medications may be used during an acute migraine attack, including nonsteroidal antiinflammatory drugs (NSAIDs), analgesic combination products, ergot derivatives, serotonin agonists (triptans), and opiates. (Table 51-1) A stratified approach to treatment of an acute migraine attack is typically employed although a step-wise approach may be used at times.[13] The stratified approach tailors initial therapy to the severity and disability of the headache using a migraine-specific medication. A patient would have multiple medications available to select appropriate drug therapy based on headache severity.

A step-wise approach initiates a safe, effective, and inexpensive medication as first-line therapy. Examples of initial pharmacotherapy in a step-wise approach would be NSAIDs or analgesic combination products. If the first agent does not work, a second agent which is more specific for migraine, such as a triptan or ergot derivative, is selected.[11]

Many factors must be taken into consideration when choosing an appropriate abortive agent for acute headache therapy. The severity of headache and its effect on patient function should be taken into account. Past response of headaches to treatment is also an important factor in selecting an option. Route of administration should be considered due to patient preference, necessity of a certain route, and differences in the onset of action. Duration of action of medications is also important as medications with longer half-lives may require less frequent dosing and may limit headache recurrence. Medical history, adverse effect profile, and cost should also be considered.

NSAIDs and analgesic combination products may be appropriate for mild to moderate migraine headaches. Acetaminophen monotherapy has not been shown to provide adequate relief and should not be recommended.[14] Caution should

TABLE 51-1 **Medication Therapy for Headache**

Class	Generic (Brand)	Route	Mechanism of Action	Adverse Reactions	Contraindications
NSAID	Ibuprofen	po	Inhibit prostaglandin synthesis, which may prevent inflammation in the trigeminovascular system	GI upset, somnolence, dizziness	Caution with peptic ulcer disease, renal dysfunction, hypersensitivity to aspirin or NSAIDs
	Aspirin	po			
	Naproxen (Naprosyn)	po			
	Ketorolac (Toradol)	IV			
	Diclofenac (Voltaren)	po			
Analgesic	Acetaminophen	po, PR	Inhibition of prostaglandins	Rash, increased LFTs or bilirubin	Cautious use along with alcohol or other products containing acetaminophen
Combination product	Acetaminophen/ aspirin/caffeine (Excedrin Extra Strength, Excedrin Migraine, Excedrin Tension Headache)	po	Inhibition of prostaglandins	Overuse, medication-overuse headache, withdrawal	Cautious use along with alcohol or other products containing acetaminophen
	Butalbital/caffeine + aspirin (Fiorinal) or acetaminophen (Fioricet)	po			
	Isometheptene/ dichloralphenazone/ acetaminophen (Midrin)	po			

(*Continued*)

TABLE 51-1 **Medication Therapy for Headache *(Continued)***

Class	Generic (Brand)	Route	Mechanism of Action	Adverse Reactions	Contraindications
Opioid	Meperidine (Demerol)	IV, po	Binds to opiate receptors altering perception and response to pain	Dependence, medication-overuse headache, constipation, nausea/vomiting	
	Butorphanol (Stadol)	IV, intranasal			
	Oxycodone	IV, po			
	Hydromorphone	IV, po			
Serotonin agonist (Triptan)	Sumatriptan (Imitrex)—t1/2 2-2.5 h Sumatriptan/naproxen (Treximet)	po, SQ, intranasal	Vasoconstriction of dilated intracranial arteries	Parasthesias, fatigue, dizziness, flushing warmth, somnolence, chest tightness, pain in the chest or neck	Ischemic heart disease, uncontrolled hypertension, cerebrovascular disease, hemiplegic or basilar migraine, use of ergot derivative within 24 h, use of SSRI or SNRI
	Rizatriptan (Maxalt, Maxalt MLT)—t1/2 2-3 h	po, oral disintegrating			
	Zolmitriptan (Zomig, Zomig ZMT)—t1/2-3 h	po, oral disintegrating			
	Naratriptan (Amerge)—t1/2-6 h	po			
	Frovatriptan (Frova)—t1/2-26 h	po			
	Eletriptan (Relpax)—t1/2-4 h	po			
	Almotriptan (Axert)—t1/2-3 h	po			
Ergot derivative	Ergotamine (Ergomar)	Sublingual	Constriction of intracranial blood vessels that decreases neurogenic inflammation in the trigeminovascular system	Nausea/vomiting, vasoconstriction, retroperitoneal fibrosis, ergotism or intense vasoconstriction resulting in peripheral vascular ischemia or gangrene	Peripheral vascular disease, hepatic or renal failure, coronary artery disease, sepsis, uncontrolled hypertension, concomitant use of strong inhibitors of CYP 3A4, pregnancy, triptan use within 24 h
	Dihydroergotamine (Migranal)	IM, SQ, intranasal			
Antiemetic	Metoclopramide (Reglan)	IV	Blocks dopamine and serotonin receptors in the CNS, enhances acetylcholine in the GI tract	Drowsiness, fatigue, EPS	Seizure history
	Prochlorperazine (Compro)	IV, IM, PR	Blocks dopamine receptors in the CNS	Sedation, hypotension, anticholinergic effects	Reye syndrome, children less than 2 y old
Miscellaneous	100% oxygen	IH	Unknown but likely vasoconstriction	None	Caution in COPD and smokers
	Lidocaine	Intranasal	Blocks pain impulses	Local irritation	

Abbreviations: CNS, central nervous system, COPD, chronic obstructive pulmonary disease; EPS, extrapyramidal syndrome; IH, inhalation; PR, per rectum; SSRI, selective serotonin reuptake inhibitor; SNRI, serotonin-norepinephrine reuptake inhibitor.

be taken to avoid medication overuse when these drugs are employed. Many of these medications are available over the counter, which makes them convenient, less expensive choices for some patients.

Ergot derivatives, including ergotamine tartrate and dihydroergotamine, are migraine-specific medications that should be used for moderate to severe migraine headaches. Individual dosage forms carry specific guidelines for repeating doses if some, but not full, benefit is realized from the initial dose. Dihydroergotamine nasal spray (Migranal) once assembled must be used within 8 hours and the remaining solution must be discarded. Also noteworthy is the risk of ergotism. Ergotism is severe peripheral ischemia that may present as cold and painful extremities, paresthesias, decreased peripheral pulses, and claudication that may ultimately result in gangrene.[13] There are several contraindications to use of ergot derivatives including peripheral vascular disease, coronary artery disease, uncontrolled hypertension, hepatic or renal failure, sepsis, pregnancy or lactation, and use of a triptan within 24 hours.

Triptans are also migraine-specific and should be used for moderate to severe migraines. Triptan medications carry specific guidelines related to repeating doses as needed for full effect. Two important considerations about triptans are the risk of serotonin syndrome when combined with other agents affecting serotonin and the fact that triptans and ergot derivatives should never be used within 24 hours of each other due to their vasoconstrictive effects. Finally, patients who have ischemic heart disease, uncontrolled hypertension, cerebrovascular disease, or hemiplegic or basilar migraine should not receive a triptan as these are contraindications to therapy.

Due to the risk of causing medication-overuse headaches, opioid use is generally limited to patients who require rescue therapy when an initial agent has failed to achieve the goals of therapy. Its use may also be considered in patients who have contraindications to take other agents.[11,14] Patients should be counseled on medication-overuse headache potential These are headaches that occur as the acute treatment wears off, resulting in additional medication use to provide relief for the new headache pain.[3] This may result in a cycle of further increased headaches and use of acute therapy.[3]

In addition to abortive therapy, some patients may require adjuvant therapy with antiemetic medications such as metoclopramide or prochlorperazine. Antiemetics given 15 to 30 minutes prior to an oral abortive medication may limit nausea and vomiting and improve absorption. These medications have also shown benefit in monotherapy, though the exact mechanism is unknown.[14]

Preventative Therapy

Appropriateness of preventative therapy should be evaluated in patients treated for acute migraine attacks. Considerations for prophylactic therapy include frequency of attacks, impact on activities of daily living, ability to use abortive medications, and complexity of medical condition.[11]

Agents that may be used for preventative therapy include beta blockers, antidepressants, anticonvulsants, NSAIDs, calcium-channel blockers, and serotonergic agents, including the ergot derivatives. (Tables 51-1 and 51-2)

When selecting an agent for preventative therapy, it is important to consider a patient's medical history. Although the data are limited for herbal or vitamin alternatives, the American Academy of Neurology recognizes feverfew, riboflavin, and magnesium as possible preventative treatment options.

It is preferable to select an agent that is indicated for a comorbid condition whenever possible. For example, a beta blocker or calcium-channel blocker would be preferred in a patient with hypertension.

Cluster Headache

The goal for treatment of an acute cluster headache is to abort an attack as quickly as possible.[15] It is important for treatment to have a very fast onset of action due to the rapid and short-lived nature of cluster headaches. As a result, oral medications have a limited role in the treatment of an acute attack, while subcutaneous injections, intranasal, or inhaled products are more useful.[15]

Subcutaneous sumatriptan or inhaled 100% oxygen via a nonrebreather mask are currently the treatments of choice for acute cluster headaches.[15,16] Other triptans or ergotamine derivatives may also be considered.

Preventative therapy may be considered for cluster headache patients when individuals suffer more than two attacks daily or when acute treatment is ineffective or is limited by adverse effects.[16]

The prophylactic medication should be started early in the cluster headache cycle and continued through the cycle until the patient is headache free for at least 2 weeks.[13] The calcium-channel blocker verapamil, ergot derivative ergotamine, lithium, corticosteroids, or anticonvulsant valproic acid may be considered. Comorbid conditions, adverse effects, and drug interaction potential should guide agent selection.

Tension Headache

The goal of treatment for tension headache is to alleviate symptoms while avoiding recurrence. Most tension headaches can be treated with medications available over the counter, including NSAIDs or combination simple analgesic products with aspirin, acetaminophen, and/or caffeine.[17] Failure of these agents to provide adequate relief may warrant prescription therapy. Preventative therapy may be considered in patients who have more than two headaches weekly, duration of headaches exceed 3 to 4 hours, or severity of headache results in medication overuse or significant disability.[13] Tricyclic antidepressants or botulinum toxin injections may be considered.

TABLE 51-2 **Medication Therapy for Headache Prevention**[a]

Class	Generic (Brand)	Mechanism of Action	Adverse Reactions	Contraindications
Beta antagonist	Atenolol Metoprolol (Toprol) Nadolol Propranolol Timolol	Unknown but may raise the migraine threshold by modulating adrenergic or serotonergic neurotransmission	Fatigue, depression, nausea, dizziness, insomnia, bradycardia, impotence	Caution in CHF, PVD, atrioventricular conduction disturbances, asthma, depression, and diabetes
Antidepressant	Amitriptyline Doxepin Imipramine Nortriptyline Protriptyline	Unknown but may cause downregulation of central serotonin and adrenergic receptors	Sedation, urinary retention, dry eyes, increased appetite	Concurrent use of MAOI Caution with BPH, glaucoma, hypotension
	Fluoxetine (Prozac)		Fewer side effects than TCAs but increased risk of serotonin syndrome	Concurrent use of MAOI Caution with triptan use and risk for serotonin syndrome
Anticonvulsant	Gabapentin (Neurontin)	Inhibition of GABA, glutamate modulation, inhibition of sodium and calcium ion channels	Somnolence, dizziness, asthenia	Avoid abrupt withdrawal
	Topiramate (Topamax)		Paresthesia, fatigue, anorexia, diarrhea, weight loss, nausea	
	Valproic acid (Depakote/ Depakote ER)		Nausea/vomiting, alopecia, tremor, asthenia, somnolence, weight gain	Pregnancy
Calcium channel antagonist	Verapamil	Inhibition of calcium ions from entering areas of the vascular smooth muscle	Gingival hyperplasia, constipation, edema, hypotension, dizziness, nausea	Left ventricular dysfunction, hypotension
Other	Lithium	Alters cation transport in nerve and muscle cells; influences reuptake of serotonin	Tremor, lethargy, nausea, diarrhea, GI upset	Use with severe renal or cardiovascular disease, dehydration, pregnancy, or concomitant diuretic use

[a]Please note that NSAIDs and ergot derivatives may also be used for preventative therapy, see Table 51-1.

Abbreviations: BPH, benign prostatic hypertrophy; CHF, congestive heart failure; GABA, gamma-aminobutyric acid; GI, gastrointestinal; MAOI, monoamine oxidase inhibitor; PVD, peripheral vascular disease; TCA, tricyclic antidepressant.

CASE Application

1. Which of the following is most likely to play a role in migraine pathogenesis?
   a. Norepinephrine
   b. Serotonin
   c. Dopamine

2. A patient presents to your community pharmacy complaining of a headache. She rates the headache as a 7 on a scale of 1 to 10, and the pulsating worsens as the headache progresses. She experiences nausea and sensitivity to light until the headache dissipates after about 12 hours. She is unable to function during the headache. Which of the following headache types is this patient likely experiencing?

a. Migraine
b. Tension
c. Cluster

3. Which of the following signs/symptoms are classified as "red flags," indicating need for physician referral and diagnostic evaluation?

   a. "Worst headache of my life"
   b. Acute headache that occurs after coughing/sneezing
   c. Headache onset age ≥40 years
   d. All of the above

4. LK suffers from chronic migraines and is currently experiencing an acute attack. Which of the following situations within the past few days could have triggered her migraine?

   a. The wine and cheese party she attended last night.
   b. She recently stopped drinking regular coffee.
   c. She started a triphasic oral contraceptive 10 days ago.
   d. All of the above.

5. Which of the following would be an absolute contraindication for receiving a selective 5-HT_1 receptor agonist (triptan)?

   a. Diabetes
   b. Ischemic heart disease
   c. Anemia
   d. Controlled hypertension

6. Which of the following is the brand name for rizatriptan?

   a. Imitrex
   b. Maxalt
   c. Amerge
   d. Frova

7. A patient is taking Zomig ZMT. Which of the following is true regarding this medication?

   i. It is a subcutaneous injection
   ii. Liquid is not required for administration
   iii. It is an orally disintegrating tablet

   a. i and ii
   b. i and iii
   c. ii and iii
   d. i, ii, and iii

8. A patient who currently takes oral sumatriptan often experiences headache recurrence, where the headache comes back within 24 hours after a positive response to the medication. Her physician would like a recommendation of a selective 5-HT_1 receptor agonist (triptan) with a longer half-life. Which of the following would you recommend?

   a. Frovatriptan
   b. Rizatriptan
   c. Zolmitriptan
   d. Almotriptan

9. Which of the following are correct repeat dose instructions for the migraine medication?

   a. Zomig tablets: take one tablet now; may repeat in 2 hours
   b. Imitrex subcutaneous injection: use one injection now; may repeat in 2 hours
   c. Amerge tablets: take one tablet now; may repeat in 2 hours
   d. All of the above are correct

10. Treximet is a combination headache medication made up of which of the following?

    a. Sumatriptan and naproxen
    b. Acetaminophen, aspirin, and caffeine
    c. Acetaminophen, isometheptene mucate, and dichloralphenazone
    d. Acetaminophen, butalbital, and caffeine

11. CJ is a 30-year-old patient admitted to the hospital with an unremitting migraine headache. She has tried two doses of naratriptan in the past 12 hours. She also takes lisinopril 10 mg once daily for her blood pressure and terbinafine for her onychomycosis. Her vital signs are BP 132/88 mm Hg, HR 70 bpm, Ht 5 ft 5 in and Wt: 130 lb. The physician plans to administer dihydroergotamine. Which of the following contraindications present to her receiving this treatment?

    a. Uncontrolled hypertension
    b. Elevated heart rate
    c. Terbinafine
    d. Naratriptan

12. A severe adverse effect that may result from taking ergotamine tartrate is:

    a. Purple toe syndrome
    b. Ergotism
    c. Pruritus
    d. Nausea

13. JB is a 55-year-old woman who has suffered from migraines for many years. Her zolmitriptan 5 mg works well to abort her headaches when they occur. Over the past few months, her headaches have increased in frequency to one every 2 weeks. She also complains of difficulty sleeping. Her vital signs today upon physical examination are Ht 5 ft 6 in, Wt 140 lb, BP 120/80 mm Hg, and HR 60 bpm. Her physician would like to start her on prophylactic drug therapy. Which of the following drug therapy options is the best option for prophylaxis for this patient?

    a. Propranolol
    b. Botulinum toxin type A
    c. Amitriptyline
    d. Phenelzine

14. Which of the following are prophylactic treatment options for migraine headache?

    i. Verapamil
    ii. Topiramate
    iii. Valproic acid

    a. i and ii
    b. i and iii
    c. ii and iii
    d. i, ii, and iii

15. JJ is a 49-year-old man who experiences headache cycles two times a year, usually in the spring and fall. The headaches occur for about 3 to 4 weeks. Each day during the headache series he may have up to 5 headaches. He describes the headaches as an unbearable type of pain that comes suddenly, located in his left eye, and goes within 1 to 2 hours. He experiences severe ocular and nasal symptoms, such as nasal stuffiness or rhinorrhea, ocular lacrimation, and ptosis. He tells you that in order to attempt to stop the pain, he sometimes rubs the areas of pain or even beats his head against objects. Which of the following are appropriate abortive treatment options for this patient's headache?

    a. Oxygen
    b. Imitrex (sumatriptan) tablets
    c. Amitriptyline
    d. a and c

16. AB is a 25-year-old college student who has been having headaches 3 to 4 times a month that last for 12 to 24 hours for the past couple of months. He describes them as having a gripping quality with pressure on both sides of his head, as if someone is squeezing his head with a rubber band. He does not experience nausea or vomiting. His headaches do not stop him from going to class, but sometimes he finds himself having to turn off his radio when studying since he just can't handle any noise. Light does not bother him during his headaches. Which of the following abortive treatment options would be appropriate recommendations for AB's headache?

    i. NSAIDS
    ii. Imitrex (sumatriptan)
    iii. Amitriptyline

    a. i only
    b. i and iii
    c. ii and iii
    d. i, ii, and iii

17. DT is a 31-year-old woman who is 36 weeks pregnant. She currently has a headache with presentation most like a tension-type headache. She is requesting a recommendation for treatment. Which of the following is the best recommendation?

    a. NSAIDs
    b. Ergotamine
    c. Acetaminophen

18. MM presents to the emergency room (ER) with a severe migraine headache and nausea and vomiting. He has taken one dose of zolmitriptan 5 mg po within the past 6 hours, but vomited within 10 minutes. Which of the following would be the most appropriate next step for treatment?

    a. Metoclopramide 10 mg IV
    b. Biofeedback
    c. Three days of inpatient dihydroergotamine IV
    d. Acetaminophen 650 mg PR

19. A physician calls your pharmacy asking which serotonin receptor agonist migraine medications are available as a nasal spray. You respond:

    i. Sumatriptan
    ii. Rizatriptan
    iii. Zolmitriptan

    a. i and ii
    b. i and iii
    c. ii and iii
    d. i, ii, and iii

20. A patient is picking up a prescription for Migranal (dihydroergotamine). Which of the following is an important counseling point to provide?

    a. Remove the foil wrapper before inserting PR
    b. Once prepared, use within 8 hours
    c. Wear latex-free gloves to apply
    d. Take with a full glass of water

21. Select the brand name for eletriptan.

    a. Maxalt
    b. Zomig
    c. Ergomar
    d. Relpax

22. Which of the following herbal medications has evidence of support for the treatment of migraine?

    a. Glucosamine
    b. Black cohosh
    c. Feverfew

23. A patient presents to pick up a new prescription for sumatriptan tablets. When verifying the prescription, the computer alerts you of a contraindication with a current prescription: Paxil 20 mg. Which of the following is the reason for this contraindication?

    a. Stevens-Johnson syndrome
    b. Serotonin syndrome
    c. Neuroleptic malignant syndrome
    d. Computer error—there is no contraindication

TAKEAWAY POINTS »

- Headaches are a common, disabling disorder that pharmacists encounter.
- A thorough history and physical examination may be useful in determining the types of headache and appropriate therapy.
- "Worst headache ever," increased frequency or severity of headache, head pain with exercise, new headaches after age 40, history of head trauma, and changes in mental status are "red flags" that should prompt referral to a physician.
- Migraine headaches typically have gradual onset of pain in the frontal or temporal region of the head, last 4 to 72 hours, and may or may not present with an aura.
- Tension headaches are often described as a band-like pressure in the occipital or frontal region of the head lasting 30 minutes to 1 week.
- Cluster headaches present as unilateral pain around the eye, temple, or forehead lasting for less than 3 hours.
- A headache diary may help patients identify and avoid headache triggers.
- Acute therapy for a mild to moderate migraine headache may include NSAIDs or analgesics.
- Ergot derivatives may be used for a moderate to severe acute migraine attack but use should be avoided in patients with peripheral vascular disease, coronary artery disease, uncontrolled hypertension, or within 24 hours of triptan use.
- Triptans, or serotonin agonists, may be used for moderate to severe migraine headaches. Triptans should not be used in patients with coronary artery disease, uncontrolled hypertension, or within 24 hours of ergot administration.
- Beta blockers, antidepressants, anticonvulsants, NSAIDs, calcium-channel blockers, or serotonergic agents may be considered as preventative therapy for migraine sufferers.
- Subcutaneous sumatriptan or inhaled 100% oxygen are first-line options for cluster headaches.
- Tension headaches can typically be treated with NSAIDs or simple analgesics.

REFERENCES

1. Lipton RB, Stewart WF, Diamond S, et al. Prevalence and burden of migraine in the United States: Data from the American Migraine Study II. *Headache.* 2001;41:646.
2. Lipton RB, Bigal ME. The epidemiology of migraine. *American Journal of Medicine.* 2005;18(suppl 1):S3.
3. Headache Classification Committee of the International Headache Society. The international classification of headache disorders, 2nd ed. *Cephalalgia.* 2004;24(suppl1):1.
4. Mueller L. Tension-type, the forgotten headache. *Postgraduate Medicine.* 2002;111:25.
5. Russell MB. Epidemiology, genetics and cluster headaches. *Lancet Neurology.* 2004;3:279.
6. Goadsby PJ, Raskin NH. Headache. Kasper DL, Braunwald E, Fauci AS, et al, eds. *Harrison's Principles of Internal Medicine,* 17th ed. New York, NY: McGraw-Hill; 2008. http://www.accesspharmacy.com/content.aspx?aID=2890365. Accessed 09/30/2009.
7. McGeeney BE. Cluster headache pharmacotherapy. *American Journal of Therapeutics.* 2005;12(4):351-358.
8. Lawrence, EC. Diagnosis and management of migraine headaches. *Southern Medical Journal.* 2004;97:1069.
9. Launer LJ, Terwindt GM , Ferrari MD. The prevalence and characteristics of migraine in a population based cohort: the GEM study. *Neurology.* 1999;53:537.
10. Pryse-Phillips WEM, Dodick DW, Edmeads JG, et al. Guidelines for the nonpharmacologic management of migraine in clinical practice. *Canadian Medical Association Journal.* 1998;159:47.
11. Snow V, Weiss K, Wall EM, et al. Pharmacologic management of acute attacks of migraine and prevention of migraine headache. *Ann Intern Med.* 2002;137:840.
12. Silberstein SD. Practice parameter: evidence-based guidelines for migraine headache (an evidence-based review). *Neurology.* 2000;55:754.
13. Minor DS, Wofford MR. Headache disorders. In: Dipiro JT, Talbert RL, Yee GC, et al, eds. *Pharmacotherapy: A Pathophysiologic Approach.* 7th ed. McGraw-Hill; 2008.
14. Matchar DB, Young WB, Rosenberg JA, et al. Evidence-based guidelines for migraine headache in the primary care setting: Pharmacological management of acute attacks. The U.S. Headache Consortium, 2000. www.americanheadachesociety.org/professionalresources/USHeadacheConsortiumGuidelines.asp. Accessed 8/10/09.
15. Leone M, Franzini A, Cecchini AP, et al.: Cluster headache: pharmacologic treatment and neurostimulation. *Nature Clinical Practice* 5(3):153, 2009.
16. Ekbom K, Hardebo JE.: Cluster headache: aetiology, diagnosis and management. *Drugs.* 2002;62(1):61.
17. Jensen R, Olesen J. Tension-type headache: an update on mechanisms and treatment. *Curr Opin Neurol.* 2000; 13:285.

CHAPTER

52 Pain Management

Peter J. S. Koo

FOUNDATION OVERVIEW

Pain is an unpleasant sensation that can negatively affect all areas of a person's life, including comfort, thought, sleep, emotion, and normal daily activity.[1] Pain, as defined by the International Association for the Study of Pain, is, "An unpleasant sensory and emotional experience associated with actual or potential tissue damage or described in terms of such damage. Pain is always subjective." Because pain is a variable and personal experience, it is difficult to completely describe and measure objectively. The clinician must therefore guard against personal biases, which can interfere with treatment. One must also rely on tools such as pain scales to communicate with patients and understand the extent of their pain.

Types of Pain

Pain is categorized according to its cause, location, duration, and clinical features. The most simplistic categorization involves differentiating brief-duration (acute) pain from long-lasting (chronic) pain.[1-2] Other types of pain include visceral, somatic, and neuropathic.

Acute Pain

Acute pain results from injury or surgery. Acute pain is limited in duration and associated with objective features, such as increased heart rate, pulse pressure, anxiety, and/or sweating. Acute pain is intense at the beginning and will decrease in intensity over time or become intermittent depending on the individual's activities.

Chronic Pain

Chronic pain is a long-term experience, and sometimes subjective. A chronic disease that is characteristically painful for which there is no cure may lead to chronic pain, examples include: arthritis, cancer, migraine headaches, fibromyalgia, and diabetic neuropathy. Psychological conditions such as depression may exacerbate or cause chronic pain.

Visceral Pain

Visceral pain results from stimulation of internal organ pain receptors. Examples are pancreatic cancer pain or cancer metastases. The painful stimuli from the internal organ receptors enter the spinal cord at multiple levels along with somatic fibers, and therefore patients may describe the sensation as pressure-like, deep squeezing, and usually not very well localized or defined. In general, the patients often cannot pinpoint the source of the pain.

Somatic Pain

Somatic pain originates from irritation of pain fibers in the body surface or deep tissues. Examples are surgical incisional pain or surgical bone pain. Painful stimuli enter spinal cord at a single level, and the painful stimuli can be mapped on parietal cortex. The patient may describe the pain as sharp, piercing from body surface or dull aching from deep tissues, and the individual can usually pinpoint the precise location of the painful origin.

Neuropathic Pain

Neuropathic pain can be initiated or caused by a primary lesion, dysfunction, or transitory alteration in the peripheral or central nervous system resulting in sensations of burning, tingling, or electric shock-like quality. These sensations can be triggered by very slightest touches that are normally tolerated, and result in an exaggerated painful sensation.

TREATMENT

Effective treatment considers the cause, duration, and intensity of pain and matches the appropriate intervention to the situation. The goal of therapy is to eliminate or reduce the pain to the lowest tolerable intensity and prevent it from recurring. The clinical situation must be considered when selecting analgesics; for example:

- It would be irrational to treat severe abdominal cramping pain caused by constipation with morphine, which may worsen the constipation.
- Elimination and prevention of chronic pain is best accomplished by using analgesics at fixed time intervals rather than on an as-needed basis.
- Patients with severe acute or malignant pain may require additional analgesics for breakthrough pain, as the scheduled analgesics alone may not be adequate.

Drug selection, doses, routes of administration, and dosing frequency should be adjusted as needed until the goals of therapy are met. Until the dosage is stabilized, all patients who are receiving analgesics should be monitored for efficacy of analgesia as well as untoward side effects. Successful pain management may also include the use of nonpharmacological

TABLE 52-1 **Mechanism of Action of Analgesics (Drugs That Modify the Source of Pain)**

Effect	Agents
↓ Pain stimulus	NSAIDs, antihistamines, sympatholytics
↓ Pain transmission	Membrane stabilizers, antidepressants
Alter central perception	Opioids, antidepressants

measures, such as ensuring that the patient receives adequate rest and emotional support. Table 52-1 is a summary of the mechanism of action of analgesics.

Opioids remain the standard for management of acute, traumatic, and many types of chronic painful conditions, while NSAIDs are useful for musculoskeletal pain syndromes.[3-5] However, some painful conditions, particularly those associated with chronic or neuropathic pain, are poorly responsive to opioids and NSAIDs.[6] In addition, opioids may have limited benefits in chronic neuropathic pain syndromes due to dose-limiting side effects. Adjunct medications are often synergistic with other analgesics. Tricyclic antidepressants, anticonvulsants, and other membrane stabilizers have demonstrated utility in managing neuropathic pain as well as other conditions such as migraine headache. The practicing pharmacist should be familiar with "nontraditional" drugs for pain management, including their utility, adverse effects, and dose regimens, and advantages over other analgesic classes.

Nonsteroidal Anti-Inflammatory Agents (NSAIDs)

NSAIDs are valuable in the management of postprocedural, acute, and chronic pain. They are also used for the therapy of autoimmune inflammatory disorders (eg, rheumatoid arthritis). NSAIDs exhibit highly individual responses with respect to efficacy and side effects experienced. NSAIDs have two key pharmacologic properties and they are:

1. Anti-inflammatory: peripheral prostaglandin inhibition
2. Analgesia: central inhibition of prostaglandins/other neuroactive chemicals

The anti-inflammatory duration (but not analgesic duration of action) correlates to serum half-life. The advantages of NSAIDs include: minimal central nervous system (CNS) side-effects, they do not slow intestinal motility (eg, not constipating), and they provide synergism with opioid analgesics. The disadvantages of NSAIDs include:

- They have a ceiling analgesic effect (eg, higher doses do not provide better pain relief, but do provide a slightly longer duration of analgesic action).
- Analgesic duration is shorter than predicted by half-life of drug.
- Gastrointestinal irritation and bleeding.
- Antiplatelet effects: irreversible with aspirin and lasts 5 to 10 days. For nonaspirin NSAIDs, duration approximates analgesic duration, although antiplatelet activity increases with chronic dosing.
- Decreased renal function: Decreased glomerular filtration rate (GFR), analgesic nephropathy, acute tubular necrosis (ATN). Patients with hypovolemia, compromised circulation, or dehydration are at greater risk.
- Other effects: Fluid retention; agranulocytosis; dermatologic/photosensitivity; asthma exacerbation; tinnitus, headache, cognitive dysfunction; mild reversible hepatic enzyme elevation.
- Increase cardiovascular events with chronic use or immediately after cardiovascular bypass surgery.

NSAID drug interactions reduce or increase the effect of certain medications. NSAIDs reduce the effects of ACE inhibitors, beta-blockers, loop diuretics, and thiazide diuretics, and increase the effects of anticoagulants, cyclosporine (nephrotoxicity), digoxin, phenytoin, lithium, methotrexate, and probenecid.

Acetaminophen

Acetaminophen has central (spinal cord) prostaglandin inhibition similar to NSAIDs. The dosing of acetaminophen is similar to aspirin (eg, 325-650 mg q 4-6 hours as needed for pain), and should not exceed 4 g per day. Acetaminophen is used as monotherapy for pain associated with degenerative joint disease and in combination with opioid for moderate pain (eg, acetaminophen 325 mg/oxycodone 5 mg every 4 hours). Caution should be used in patients with hepatic or renal disease and patients receiving chronic fixed-ratio opioid combinations (eg, Percocet). Unlike NSAIDs, acetaminophen has no anti-inflammatory properties.

Adjunct Analgesics/Neuropathic Pain

Tricyclic Antidepressants

Tricyclic antidepressants (TCAs) exert analgesic effects by working in the spinal cord to reduce trafficking of pain signals by enhancing serotonin and/or norepinephrine. TCAs also potentiate opioid analgesia. The starting dose usually is 10 to 25 mg at bedtime and the dose is titrated to pain relief. The dose should be titrated slowly in elderly patients (ie, every 7-14 days). In general, tricyclic antidepressants should be avoided in the elderly patient population. Side effects associated with TCAs include:

- Anticholinergic (eg, dry mouth, blurred vision, constipation)
- Cardiovascular (eg, tachycardia, heart blockade, orthostasis)
- Central nervous system (eg, dizziness, drowsiness, confusion, tremor, seizure)
- Dermatological (eg, photosensitivity)

Anticonvulsants

Anticonvulsants prolong the depolarization of nerves causing reduced neuronal excitability and decrease in pain signaling. Examples of anticonvulsants used in pain include:

- Carbamazepine—Used for trigeminal neuralgia and neuropathies.
    - Side effects: Sedation, ataxia, rare blood dyscrasias (anemia, neutropenia, thrombocytopenia).
    - CYP-450 drug interactions and auto-induces own metabolism initially.
- Valproate—Used for migraine headaches and neuropathic pain. GABA-enhancing mechanism that reduces nerve firing in the transmission of pain signals.
    - Side effects: Ataxia, dizziness, rash, weight gain, GI distress.
- Gabapentin—Used for chronic neuropathic pain and postherpetic neuralgia.
    - Side effects: Somnolence, ataxia, dizziness, fatigue, nystagmus, tremor, diplopia, rhinitis.
- Pregabalin—Used for fibromyalgia.
- Topiramate, lamotrigine, and newer anticonvulsants—Used to treat diabetic neuropathy and other neuropathic pain syndromes.

Systemic Local Anesthetics

Systemic local anesthetics prolong nerve depolarization via sodium channels in the nerve membranes. Examples include lidocaine and mexiletine.

- Lidocaine—Regional nerve blocks and local anesthesia applications. May need to be repeated or infused via a regional nerve catheter.
- Mexiletine—Oral congener of lidocaine used for neuropathy, neuralgia, and sympathetic pain syndromes.

Side effects associated with systemic use include nausea, vomiting, dyspepsia, anorexia, tremor, ataxia, nystagmus, confusion, diplopia, hypotension, torsades de pointes, bradycardia, arrhythmia, and photosensitivity.

Other Agents

- Capsaicin—Topical 0.025% and 0.075% used for diabetic and other neuropathies. Alters function of pain-sensitive nerve endings (nociceptors) through substance-P depletion as well as alter the activities of the nociceptors.
- Lidocaine 5% patches (Lidoderm)—Approved for the treatment of postherpetic neuralgia. Analgesic effect due to decrease in sensory activities of the pain receptors through local anesthetic effects. Tachyphylaxis can occur with continuous use; therefore, patients require a 12-hour break between the patch changes daily.
- Skeletal muscle relaxants—Cyclobenzaprine has tricyclic structure and is primarily used for musculoskeletal spasms. Baclofen and benzodiazepines are GABA agonists. Tizanidine, a congener of clonidine, has antinociceptive (pain relieving) properties. These agents are used for spasms from spinal origin such as nerve root impingement or spinal cord compression and irritation.

Opioid Analgesics

Opioids are more potent than nonopioid analgesics such as NSAIDs, although the range of potencies is wide with this class of medicines. They are generally recommended for moderate to severe pain intensity and are used in acute and chronic pain syndromes that are refractory to other classes of agents. The administration of opioid analgesics is frequently complicated by the need to convert between different routes of administration or different opioid formulations. The approximate equianalgesic doses of parenteral and oral opioid analgesics are listed in Table 52-2. Rational use of opioid analgesics must start with patient and technology assessment. Opioid dosing has to be based on the patient's history of opioid analgesic used, the specific patient's needs, and on the delivery system being utilized. In order for the pharmacist to make the appropriate assessment of the dose and frequency of an opioid analgesic ordered, the pharmacist must have a basic understanding of the delivery system, in addition to the pharmacology of the opioid analgesic. Depending on the delivery system and the route, the dose of opioid can vary by a factor of 10 to 100. Therefore, changes in the route of opiate delivery can result in significant changes in the patient's clinical response or toxicity. Often, the concept of equianalgesic dosing is the source of confusion and misunderstanding. Key properties of opioid analgesics are listed below.

1. Morphine
    a. Rectal absorption better than oral. At large doses, metabolite can cause CNS excitability and results in increased anxiety or restlessness.
    b. Morphine is a smooth muscle relaxant, which can cause vasodilatation and hypotension which is often associated with intravenous administration.
2. Meperidine (*Not recommended without good justification*)
    a. Active metabolite (Normeperidine) is renally excreted and can accumulate and cause CNS irritability and myoclonic seizures if the dose of meperidine is pushed too high or if the patient's renal function is decreased.
    b. Widely variable intramuscular absorption from injection site after repeated injections.
3. Levorphanol
    a. 16-hour half-life, drug can accumulate with frequent repetitive dosing.

TABLE 52-2 **Equianalgesic Adult Opioid Doses**

Drug	IM/SQ	Oral	Rectal
Fentanyl	150-200 μg	400 μg	NA
Hydrocodone	NA	20 mg	NA
Hydromorphone	1.5-2 mg	6 mg	3 mg
Methadone	2.5 mg	2.5 mg	NA
Morphine	8-10 mg	30 mg	20 mg
Oxycodone	NA	20 mg	NA

b. May need to reduce dose after one day of therapy to prevent drug accumulation.
c. Analgesic half-life is shorter than the serum half-life of drug, and therefore frequent dosing can lead to drug accumulation, especially at the beginning of therapy.

4. Hydromorphone
   a. It may have less cognitive impairment in the elderly than morphine at equianalgesic doses.
   b. Pharmacologically it is similar to morphine, except it is more potent than morphine on milligram per milligram basis.
5. Methadone
   a. 24-hour average half-life, dosage must be carefully adjusted because as with levorphanol frequent dosing can lead to drug accumulation. Avoid rapid dose escalation when initiating methadone therapy, especially in opiate naïve patients.
   b. Good oral bioavailability due to low first pass effect and extraction ratio.
   c. Metabolism by CYP-450 3A4, and CYP inducers can increase metabolism significantly to decrease effectiveness.
6. Oxymorphone
   a. Less emesis and sedation than equianalgesic morphine doses.
   b. Rapid onset with IV administration because it is highly lipophilic.
7. Fentanyl
   a. Passive diffusion fentanyl patch has a slow onset, but has a long 72-hour duration of action. Patches are most often used in chronic pain. In acute pain patients with rapidly changing needs, the patches are not responsive or sensitive enough to be useful. In patients with rapidly changing analgesic needs, IV, transmucosal, or iontophoresis active transdermal routes might be more appropriate.
   b. Less hypotensive effect than morphine or hydromorphone at equianalgesic doses, especially when it is administered intravenously.
   c. Transdermal patches need to be disposed and discarded carefully to prevent accidental poisoning of animals or children. It is only recommended for use in opiate tolerant patients. Tolerance is defined by taking more than 60 mg or oral morphine daily for more than 2 weeks.
8. Codeine
   a. Requires metabolic conversion by CYP 2D6 to active metabolite, morphine.
   b. CYP-450 2D6 inhibition can reduce efficacy.
9. Hydrocodone
   a. Requires metabolic conversion to active metabolite, hydromorphone.
   b. Only available in combination with acetaminophen for pain.
   c. Causes less emesis than codeine, and no cross sensitivity in nausea, vomiting, or itching with codeine.
   d. CYP-450 2D6 inhibition can reduce efficacy.
10. Tramadol
    a. It is a mu_1-specific agonist and mild opiate analgesic.
    b. Should start with lower doses in elderly.
    c. Tramadol also has SSRI properties.
    d. Tramadol can produce either CNS excitation or sedation depending on the specific patient during initiation of therapy.
    e. Most effective when used for the management of mild neuropathic pain.

Adverse effects of opioid analgesics associated with opioid analgesics include:

- Slowed mentation—Most often associated with morphine in elderly patients. Effect may be reduced with an alternative opioid analgesic.
- Urinary retention—May be managed with bethanechol or terazosin.
- Constipation—Should always be therapeutically prevented while receiving opioid analgesics. Treat with stimulant laxatives such as senna, cascara, or bisacodyl in addition to stool softeners. In severe cases, oral naloxone, metoclopramide or polyethylene glycol or magnesium citrate may be used.
- Unavoidable sedation—Can be managed with amphetamine 5 mg at 8 AM and 12 noon for chronic malignant pain.
- CNS irritability—Frequently associated with meperidine due to its metabolite normeperidine, but can also occur with high doses of morphine analogs secondary to the 6-glucuronide metabolites, which is centrally active.
- Hypotension—Most pronounced immediately following general anesthesia or in volume-depleted patients. Most frequently associated with intravenous opiate boluses. Fentanyl is frequently used in critical care situations because it has the least amount of hypotensive effect.
- Respiratory depression—Occurs only occasionally at therapeutic doses, most often is associated with rapid IV boluses, and can be reversed easily with naloxone if it is identified early. The patients are especially at risk when opiates are given together with other CNS depressants.
- Opioid abstinence symptoms—This may occur after patient is abruptly discontinued of chronic opioids. Opiate abstinence may occur in opiate dependent patients whose pain is managed with spinal analgesia alone. These abstinence symptoms may be relieved by systemic opioids or clonidine.

Dosing regimens and delivery systems for opioid analgesics include:

1. Intermittent on demand dosing (prn)—The preferred regimen for patients who are neurologically or hemodynamically unstable.

2. Scheduled dosing (round-the-clock)—The preferred method for controlling severe pain or chronic pain. This method should also be used for the oral regimen when transitioning a patient from PCA to the oral route.
3. Continuous infusion—Used only for patients when other routes of analgesic administration is either unavailable or impractical. Not recommended outside of the critical care or monitored environment. May be used for managing cancer pain.
4. Patient-controlled IV analgesia (PCA)—The preferred method for controlling postoperative pain. It allows the patient to control the pain on their own.
5. Spinal analgesia (epidural or intrathecal)—Duration of analgesia depends on the lipophilicity of the opioid used. Less lipophilic opioids have a longer duration of action. More lipophilic opioids have a shorter duration of analgesia. The analgesic effect of epidural or intrathecal morphine may last 12 to 24 hours. The epidural morphine dose is between 1 to 5 mg, and the intrathecal morphine dose is between 0.5 to 2 mg. *(Use of low molecular weight heparins are* ***contraindicated*** *within 12 hours before spinal analgesia administration or spinal catheter insertion or within 2 hours after spinal analgesia administration or spinal catheter removal.)*
6. Regional analgesia (nerve plexus blocks or nerve blocks)—This is different from spinal analgesia, because local anesthetic and opiate are administered around the peripheral nerve outside the spine. *(Low molecular weight heparin* ***is also contraindicated within 12 hours of catheter placement or 2 hours after removal.****)*
7. Sustained release opioids—Used for controlling chronic pain after the patient is stabilized by the immediate release preparation. It has a slower onset, but a long lasting duration of action of 8 to 24 hours. The use of sustained release opioid is not appropriate for the management of acute pain immediately after surgery or trauma, because the delayed onset and exceptionally long duration of opiate effect can lead to delay in pain control or unforeseen toxicity.
8. Transdermal fentanyl—Should only be used for constant but stable persistent pain where the patient cannot take oral medications. It should not be used in patients with rapidly escalating or unstable pain because of delayed maximum effects of at least 8 hours. Fentanyl transdermal use should be limited to patients who are opiate tolerant. Transdermal fentanyl is not recommended in opiate-naive patients. One should always treat the patient with other short-acting opioid analgesics during the first 8 hours after patch application. Must tell the patient to discard the used patch carefully to prevent accidental poisoning of either children or pets. It is primarily used for the management of persistent chronic pain. Usually, oral sustained release opioids can be just as effective. *(Opiate tolerance is defined by taking equivalent to 60 mg of oral morphine daily for 2 weeks.)*

CASE Application

MAG is a 58-year-old woman with a chief complaint of left arm, shoulder, and axillary pain. Patient underwent a left subtotal mastectomy and chemotherapy for breast cancer 6 years ago and received radiation therapy and bone marrow transplant at that time. Patient is currently free of cancer, but complains of burning and stinging pain down her left arm and nothing has worked well for her. She is also complaining of severe constipation. Her current medications are Bupropion (Wellbutrin) 150 mg po bid, Ibuprofen 600 mg po one tablet tid, Morphine sulfate extended release (ER) 30 mg bid, Atenolol 50 mg po every morning, and Tamoxifen 10 mg po bid.

1. What is best therapeutic plan of this patient's analgesic regimen?
   a. Analgesic regimen should be discontinued, because long-acting opiate is not appropriate for this patient's pain.
   b. Increase morphine ER to 30 mg po every 4 hours since it is not providing adequate analgesia.
   c. Increase morphine ER to 60 mg po tid since it is not optimally controlling patient's pain.
   d. Add pain medication to focus on neuropathic symptoms.

2. What is the best approach for the burning pain in this patient?
   a. Add amitriptyline 50 mg po at bedtime.
   b. Add duloxetine 20 mg po at bedtime because it has less side effects.
   c. Add nortriptyline 50 mg po at bedtime.
   d. Add gabapentin 300 mg po every bedtime, and titrate to 300 mg po tid over next 7 to 10 days for patient's neuropathic pain.

3. Select the pain medication that has a ceiling effect (eg, higher doses do not provide better pain relief).
   a. Oxycodone
   b. Gabapentin
   c. Ibuprofen
   d. Morphine

4. NSAIDs are commonly used to treat pain. Select the potential disadvantage(s) of using NSAIDs for pain management.
   a. Gastrointestinal bleeding
   b. Antiplatelet effects
   c. Decreased renal function
   d. Fluid retention
   e. All of the above

5. Select the medication(s) that may have reduced effectiveness when used with NSAIDs.
   a. ACE inhibitors
   b. Beta-blockers
   c. Thiazide diuretics
   d. All of the above

6. QP is a 44-year-old patient diagnosed with severe diabetic neuropathy. He is currently being treated with an alpha-blocker (terazosin) for an enlarged prostate. Terazosin has significantly improved the symptoms of the enlarged prostate, but the patient is having orthostatic hypotension episodes. Select the medication that would be most appropriate for QP's diabetic neuropathy.
   a. Naproxen
   b. Morphine
   c. Nortriptyline
   d. Gabapentin

7. Select the side effect(s) associated with tricyclic antidepressants.
   a. Gastrointestinal bleeding
   b. Heart blockade
   c. Respiratory depression
   d. Anemia

8. Select the medication(s) that may cause central nervous system side effects.
   a. Gabapentin
   b. Opioids
   c. TCAs
   d. All of the above

9. Select the medication that is used for trigeminal neuralgia and neuropathies and is associated with significant CYP-450 drug interactions.
   a. Valproate
   b. Gabapentin
   c. Topiramate
   d. Carbamazepine

10. Select the medication that alters function of pain-sensitive nerve endings through substance-P depletion.
    a. Capsaicin
    b. Amitriptyline
    c. Carbamazepine
    d. Topiramate

11. Select the side effect associated with the active metabolite of meperidine when the dose is too high or the patient has renal dysfunction.
    a. Seizures
    b. Gastrointestinal bleeding
    c. Respiratory depression
    d. a and c
    e. All of the above

12. Select the opioid that is available in multiple formulations, including a transdermal patch.
    a. Morphine
    b. Oxycodone
    c. Meperidine
    d. Fentanyl

13. IT is a 74-year-old man with severe chronic pain. He has been previously treated with nonopioid analgesics, but is prescribed morphine today. The patient will be receiving morphine chronically. Select the medication that IT should receive in addition to morphine.
    a. Ibuprofen
    b. Gabapentin
    c. Capsaicin
    d. Bisacodyl

14. Select the medication that can reverse respiratory depression caused by opioids.
    a. Flumazenil
    b. Naloxone
    c. Acetylcysteine
    d. All of the above

15. Select the dosing method that should be employed when treating acute severe pain.
    a. Intermittent
    b. Scheduled dosing
    c. Directly observed therapy
    d. b and c

16. Select the medication that decreases pain transmission.
    a. Naproxen
    b. Carbamazepine
    c. Oxycodone
    d. Capsaicin

17. Select the opioid that is available in oral, parenteral, and rectal formulations.
    a. Fentanyl
    b. Hydrocodone
    c. Hydromorphone
    d. Morphine

18. Select the opioid that has the same dose when administered intramuscularly and orally.
    a. Fentanyl
    b. Oxycodone
    c. Methadone
    d. Hydrocodone

19. Select the nonopioid analgesic that is minimally associated with central nervous system side effects and does not slow intestinal motility.
    a. Naproxen
    b. Hydrocodone
    c. Carbamazepine
    d. Amitriptyline

20. Select the analgesic that affects pain by enhancing neurotransmitters serotonin and norepinephrine.
    a. Ibuprofen
    b. Amitriptyline
    c. Carbamazepine
    d. Tramadol
    e. b and c

TAKEAWAY POINTS ››

- Pain is an unpleasant sensation that can negatively affect all areas of a person's life, including comfort, thought, sleep, emotion, and normal daily activity.
- Pain is categorized according to its cause, location, duration, and clinical features. The most simplistic categorization involves differentiating brief-duration (acute) pain from long-lasting (chronic) pain.
- Effective treatment considers the cause, duration, and intensity of pain and matches the appropriate intervention to the situation. The goal of therapy is to eliminate or reduce the pain to the lowest tolerable intensity and prevent it from recurring. The clinical situation must be considered when selecting analgesics.
- Drug selection, doses, routes of administration, and dosing frequency should be adjusted as needed until the goals of therapy are met. Until the dosage is stabilized, all patients who are receiving analgesics should be monitored for efficacy of analgesia as well as untoward side effects.
- Opioids remain the standard for management of acute, traumatic, and many types of chronic painful conditions, while NSAIDs are useful for musculoskeletal pain syndromes.
- Some painful conditions, particularly those associated with chronic or neuropathic pain, are poorly responsive to opioids and NSAIDs.
- Tricyclic antidepressants, anticonvulsants, and other membrane stabilizers have demonstrated utility in managing neuropathic pain as well as other conditions such as migraine headache.
- The advantages of NSAIDs include: minimal central nervous system (CNS) side-effects, they do not slow intestinal motility (eg, not constipating), and they provide synergism with opioid analgesics.
- Side effects associated with TCAs include anticholinergic, cardiovascular, central nervous system, and dermatological.
- Anticonvulsants prolong the depolarization of nerves causing reduced neuronal excitability and decrease in pain signaling.
- Opioids are more potent than nonopioid analgesics such as NSAIDs, although the range of potencies is wide with this class of medicines.
- Opioids are recommended for moderate to severe pain intensity and are used in acute and chronic pain syndromes that are refractory to other classes of agents.

REFERENCES

1. AGS Panel on Persistent Pain in Older Persons. The management of persistent pain in older persons. *JAGS*. 2002;50:S205-S224.
2. Argoff CE. Pharmacologic management of chronic pain. *J Am Osteopath Assoc*. 2002 September;102(9 suppl 3):S21-S27.
3. Dellemijn P. Are opioids effective in relieving neuropathic pain? *Pain*. 1999 April; 80(3):453-462.
4. Freedman GM. Chronic pain. Clinical management of common causes of geriatric pain. *Geriatrics*. 2002 May;57(5):36-42.
5. Goldstein FJ. Adjuncts to opioid therapy. *J Am Osteopath Assoc*. 2002 September;102(9 suppl 3):S15-S21.
6. Guay DR. Adjunctive agents in the management of chronic pain. *Pharmacotherapy*. 2001 September;21(9):1070-1081.
7. Lucas LK, Lipman AG. Recent advances in pharmacotherapy for cancer pain management. *Cancer Pract*. 2002 May-June; 10(suppl 1):S14-S20.
8. Portenoy RK. Current pharmacotherapy of chronic pain. *J Pain Symptom Manage*. 2000 Jan;19(1 suppl):S16-S20.
9. Moore RA, Straube S, Wiffen PJ, Derry S, McQuay HJ. Pregabalin for acute and chronic pain in adults. *Cochrane Database Syst Rev*. 2009(3):CD007076.
10. Jensen TS, Madsen CS, Finnerup NB. Pharmacology and treatment of neuropathic pains. *Curr Opin Neurol*. 2009;22(5):467-474.
11. Goodyear-Smith F, Halliwell J. Anticonvulsants for neuropathic pain: gaps in the evidence. *Clin J Pain*. 2009;25(6):528-536.
12. Freynhagen R, Bennett MI. Diagnosis and management of neuropathic pain. *BMJ*. 2009;339:b3002.
13. Moulin DE, Clark AJ, Gilron I, et al. Pharmacological management of chronic neuropathic pain—consensus statement and guidelines from the Canadian Pain Society. *Pain Res Manag*. 2007;12(1):13-21.
14. Goodyear-Smith F, Halliwell J. Anticonvulsants for neuropathic pain: gaps in the evidence. *Clin J Pain*. 2009;25(6): 528-536.

PART

9 Psychiatric Disorders

CHAPTER

53 Depression

S. Scott Sutton and John C. Voris

FOUNDATION OVERVIEW

Major depressive disorder (MDD) is diagnosed when an individual experiences one or more major depressive episodes without a history of manic, mixed, or hypomanic episodes. An MDD episode is defined by the criteria listed in the *Diagnostic and Statistical Manual of Mental Disorders*, fourth edition, text revision (DSM-IV-TR).[1] Depression is associated with significant functional disability, morbidity, and mortality. Individuals with MDD experience significant and pervasive symptoms that can affect mood, thinking, physical health, work, and relationships. Unfortunately, suicide may be a result of MDD that has not been diagnosed and treated adequately.

The true prevalence of MDD in the United States is unknown. The National Comorbidity Survey Replication found that 16.2% of the population studied had a history of MDD in their lifetime, and more than 6.6% had an episode within the past 12 months.[2] Women are twice as likely as men to experience MDD. Although MDD may begin at any age, the average age of onset is the mid-20s.[1] MDD patients may also suffer from anxiety disorders and substance-use disorders.[2]

Pathophysiology

The exact cause of MDD is unknown, but appears to be multifactorial. There are biologic, psychological, and social theories that attempt to explain depressive disorders, however, none of them do so completely.

Genetics: The occurrence of MDD exhibits a genetic pattern. First-degree relatives of MDD patients are more likely to develop MDD compared to first-degree relatives of control individuals.

Stress: Depression can occur in the absence or presence of major life stressors. However, there is an association between life stressors and depression. In addition, when a genetic predisposition accompanies significant life stress chances for depression increase.

Neurotransmitter and receptor: Classic views for the cause of MDD focus on the neurotransmitters such as norepinephrine (NE), serotonin (5-HT), and dopamine (DA). The neurotransmitter hypothesis asserts that depression is due to a deficiency of neurotransmitters. The supporting evidence for this hypothesis is that existing antidepressants increase neurotransmitters concentrations.[3-4] The neurotransmitter receptor hypothesis suggests that depression is related to abnormal functioning of neurotransmitter receptors. In this model, antidepressants exert therapeutic effects by altering receptor sensitivity. Chronic administration of antidepressants causes desensitization (down regulation) of beta adrenergic receptors and various 5-HT receptors. Importantly, the time required for changes in receptor sensitivity corresponds to the onset of action of antidepressant therapy.[3-4]

While such models of depression are useful in conceptualizing the mechanisms behind antidepressant activity, they most likely represent an oversimplification of the actual pathophysiology process of the disorder. Depression likely involves a complex dysregulation of neurotransmitter systems, and these systems modulate or are modulated by other biologic systems. Thus, the underlying cause of depression may extend beyond dysfunction of the neurotransmitter system.[5]

Clinical Presentation and Diagnosis

MDD patients typically present with a combination of emotional, physical, and cognitive systems. Table 53-1 lists the clinical presentation for patients with depression. Symptoms of a major depressive episode usually develop over days to weeks, but mild depressive and anxiety symptoms may be present for weeks to months prior to the onset of the full syndrome. Left untreated, major depressive episodes typically last 6 months or more. A minority of patients experience chronic episodes that can last for at least 2 years. Approximately two-thirds of patients will recover fully from major depressive episodes and return to usual mood and functioning, whereas the other third will have partial remission and may continue to experience various degrees of symptoms.[1]

The diagnosis of MDD requires the presence of at least five depressive symptoms present every day that cause clinically significant effects and the symptoms must last for a minimum of 2 weeks. Examples of the symptoms are: depressed mood, diminished interest in usual activities, change in appetite or weight, change in psychomotor activity, change in amount of sleep, loss of energy, feelings of worthlessness or guilt, diminished ability to think or concentrate, or recurrent thought of death or suicide.[1]

When a patient presents with depressive symptoms, it is necessary to investigate the possibility of a contributing medical or drug-induced condition. For example:

- Up to 40% of patients with neurological disorders (eg, stroke, Alzheimer disease) develop depressive symptoms.[1]
- Individuals experiencing withdrawal from substances of abuse (eg, cocaine) can present with depressive symptoms.[6]

TABLE 53-1 **Clinical Presentation of Depression**[a]

- Emotional
  - Sadness
  - Anhedonia
  - Irritability
  - Anxiety
  - Worthlessness
  - Suicidal ideation (SI)
- Physical
  - Disturbed sleep
  - Change in weight/appetite
  - Psychomotor changes
  - Decreased energy
  - Body aches and pains
- Cognitive
  - Impaired concentration
  - Indecisiveness
  - Poor memory

[a]Severely depressed patients may also present with psychotic symptoms (hallucinations or delusions).

Depressed patients should have a complete physical examination, mental status examination, and basic laboratory workup, including a complete blood count, thyroid function tests, and electrolyte determinations to identify any potential medical problems. A complete medication review should be performed because several medications can contribute to depressive symptoms. Once a medical condition or concomitant medication has been ruled out as the cause of depressive symptoms, the patient should be evaluated for a major depressive disorder. Table 53-2 lists conditions and medications associated with depressive symptoms.

TREATMENT

The goals of treatment are to reduce the symptoms of acute depression, facilitate the patient's return to a level of functioning before the onset of illness, and prevent further episodes of depression. An extremely important outcome in the treatment of MDD is the prevention of suicide attempts.

Antidepressants can be classified in several ways, including classification by chemical structure and the mechanism of antidepressant activity. Although the link between the mechanism of action and antidepressant response is tenuous, the classification has the advantage of being based on established pharmacology and explains some of the common, but expected adverse effects. Historically, studies have found that antidepressants are of equivalent efficacy in groups of patients when administered in comparable doses. However, a meta-analysis shows a potential hierarchy within the antidepressant group regarding efficacy and acceptability.[7] Because one cannot predict which antidepressant will be the most effective in an individual patient, the initial choice is often made empirically. Factors that influence the choice of an antidepressant include the patient's history of response, pharmacogenetics (history of familial antidepressant response), patient's concurrent medical history, presenting symptoms, potential for drug–drug interactions, adverse events profile, patient preference, and drug cost.

TABLE 53-2 **Medical Conditions, Substance Use Disorders, and Medications Associated with Depressive Symptoms**

- Medical conditions
  - Endocrine diseases (hypothyroidism, Addison, Cushing)
  - Deficiency states (severe anemia, Wernicke encephalopathy)
  - Infections (encephalitis, human immunodeficiency virus, tuberculosis, mononucleosis)
  - Collagen disorder (systemic lupus erythematous)
  - Metabolic disorders (hypo/hyperkalemia)
  - Cardiovascular disease (coronary artery disease, heart failure, myocardial infarction)
  - Neurologic disorders (Alzheimer disease, epilepsy, Parkinson disease, multiple sclerosis, Huntington disease)
  - Malignant disease
- Substance use disorders (intoxication or withdrawal)
  - Alcoholism
  - Marijuana abuse and dependence
  - Nicotine dependence
  - Opiate abuse and dependence
  - Psychostimulant abuse and dependence (eg, cocaine)
- Drug therapy
  - Antihypertensives (clonidine, diuretics, guanethidine, hydralazine, methyldopa, propranolol, reserpine)
  - Hormonal therapy (oral contraceptives, steroids)
  - Acne therapy (isotretinoin)
  - Interferon

Tricyclic Antidepressants

Tricyclic antidepressants (TCAs) are effective in treating all depressive subtypes, but their use has diminished greatly because of the availability of equally effective therapies that are much safer in overdose and better tolerated. TCAs potentiate the activity of NE and 5-HT by blocking their reuptake into presynaptic terminals. The potency and selectivity of TCAs for the reuptake inhibition varies greatly within in the class.[8] Because TCAs affect other receptor systems (cholinergic, neurologic, and cardiovascular) adverse events are reported frequently during therapy. TCAs produce a wide range of pharmacologic actions, including unwanted adverse effects. The most common side effects are dose related and are associated with blockade of cholinergic receptors (anticholinergic effects) and their affinity to adrenergic receptors (orthostatic hypotension). TCAs may cause cardiac conduction delays and can induce heart block and produce arrhythmias (in overdose). Abrupt withdrawal of TCAs is associated with symptoms of cholinergic rebound (eg, dizziness, nausea, diarrhea, insomnia, and restlessness). Therefore, the dose should be tapered over several days. The TCAs are often used in low doses to treat neuropathic pain and their sedative profile usually requires the dose to be administered at bedtime. Table 53-3 lists key parameters for TCAs.

TABLE 53-3 **Antidepressants Medications**

Antidepressant	Mechanism of Action	Contraindications (C)/ Warnings (W)	Adverse Reactions	General Information
Tricyclic antidepressants[a]	Inhibits reuptake of NE and 5-HT	C: Hypersensitivity to TCA; use of MAOI inhibitor within 14 d; acute recovery of myocardial infarction W: Closely monitor for clinical worsening, suicidal tendencies, or unusual changes in behavior	Anticholinergic, sedation, orthostatic hypotension, seizures (high doses), conduction abnormalities (high doses), weight gain, sexual dysfunction	Withdrawal symptoms with abrupt withdrawal; pregnancy category C; substrate and inhibitor of cytochrome P-450
Serotonin and norepinephrine reuptake inhibitors[b]	Inhibits reuptake of NE and 5-HT; weak inhibitor of dopamine reuptake	C: Concomitant use or within 2 wk of MAO inhibitors; uncontrolled narrow angle glaucoma W: Closely monitor for clinical worsening, suicidal tendencies, or unusual changes in behavior	Gastrointestinal effects (nausea and diarrhea), insomnia, sexual dysfunction, increased blood pressure	Pregnancy category C; substrate and inhibitor of cytochrome P-450
Triazolopyridines[c]	Inhibits 5-HT reuptake; 5-HT_2 receptor antagonist; blocks alpha_1 adrenergic and histaminergic receptors	C: Hypersensitivity to trazodone/nefazodone W: closely monitor for clinical worsening, suicidal tendencies, or unusual changes in behavior; priapism (trazodone); hepatic injury (nefazodone)	Dizziness, orthostatic hypotension, sedation, cognitive slowing, somnolence, dry mouth, gastrointestinal effects (nausea and diarrhea)	Pregnancy category C; substrate and inhibitor of CYP450
SSRIs[d]	Inhibits reuptake of 5-HT	C: Hypersensitivity to SSRI; use of MAO inhibitor within 14 d W: Closely monitor for clinical worsening, suicidal tendencies, or unusual changes in behavior	Gastrointestinal effects (nausea and diarrhea), sexual dysfunction, headache, insomnia	Pregnancy risk factor C; substrate and inhibitor of CYP450; abrupt discontinuation may produce withdrawal syndrome
Aminoketone[e]	Inhibits reuptake of dopamine (and possibly NE)	C: Hypersensitivity to bupropion or any component of the formulation; seizure disorder; anorexia or bulimia; patients receiving another dosage form of bupropion W: Closely monitor for clinical worsening, suicidal tendencies, or unusual changes in behavior	Gastrointestinal effects (nausea and diarrhea), tachycardia, tremor, insomnia, dry mouth	Pregnancy category C; substrate and inhibitor of CYP450; should not be taken in patients with eating disorders as they are prone to electrolyte disorders and are therefore at higher risk of seizures
Tetracyclics[f]	Central presynaptic alpha_2-adrenergic antagonist effects, which results in increased release of NE and 5-HT Additionally potent antagonist of $5\text{-HT}_{2\&3}$ serotonin receptors and H1 receptors and moderate peripheral alpha_1-adrenergic and muscarinic antagonist	C: Hypersensitivity to mirtazipine; use of MAO inhibitor within 14 d W: Closely monitor for clinical worsening, suicidal tendencies, or unusual changes in behavior	Somnolence, weight gain, dry mouth, constipation	Pregnancy category C; may increase appetite/weight; substrate and inhibitor of CYP450

(Continued)

TABLE 53-3 Antidepressants Medications (*Continued*)

Antidepressant	Mechanism of Action	Contraindications (C)/ Warnings (W)	Adverse Reactions	General Information
Monoamine oxidase inhibitors[g]	Increases endogenous concentrations of NE, 5-HT, and DA through inhibition of the enzyme monoamine oxidase	C: Hypersensitivity to MAOI; heart failure, abnormal liver function tests, renal disease, concurrent use of sympathomimetics, foods high in tyramine content W: Closely monitor for clinical worsening, suicidal tendencies, or unusual changes in behavior	Orthostatic hypotension, weight gain, sexual dysfunction, hypertensive crisis	Pregnancy category C; 2 wk should elapse between discontinuation of MAOI and initiation of another antidepressant; 5 wk should elapse before start of fluoxetine

[a]Tertiary amines, amitriptyline, clomipramine, doxepin, imipramine; secondary amines, desipramine, nortriptyline.

[b]Venlafaxine, desvenlafaxine, and dulexetine.

[c]Trazodone and nefazodone.

[d]Fluoxetine, citalopram, sertraline, paroxetine, escitalopram, and fluvoxamine.

[e]Bupropion.

[f]Mirtazapine.

[g]Phenelzine, tranylcypromine.

Serotonin/Norepinephrine Reuptake Inhibitors

Venlafaxine (Effexor), desvenlafaxine (Pristiq), and duloxetine (Cymbalta) are serotonin/norepinephrine reuptake inhibitors (SNRIs). Venlafaxine inhibits 5-HT reuptake at low doses, with additional NE reuptake inhibition at higher doses. Duloxetine inhibits 5-HT and NE across all doses. The most commonly reported adverse effects associated with venlafaxine are dose related and include gastrointestinal problems (nausea and diarrhea), sexual dysfunction, and activation. Venlafaxine can also cause a dose-related increase in diastolic blood pressure.[9] Blood pressure should be monitored regularly during therapy. Duloxetine is associated with gastrointestinal effects (nausea and diarrhea), dry mouth, decreased appetite, insomnia, and sweating.[10] Table 53-3 lists key parameters for SNRIs.

Triazolopyridines

Trazodone (Desyrel) and nefazodone are effective in treating depression; however, they both carry risks that limit their use as antidepressants. Trazodone and nefazodone have dual actions on serotonergic neurons, acting as 5-HT_2 receptor antagonists and 5-HT reuptake inhibitors. Trazodone blocks alpha$_1$ adrenergic and histaminergic receptors leading to increased side effects (eg, dizziness and sedation) that limit its use as an antidepressant. Nefazodone's use as an antidepressant has declined after reports of hepatoxicity. The FDA-approved nefazodone labeling includes a black box warning describing rare cases of liver failure.[11] Because of the potential for hepatic injury associated with nefazodone use, treatment should not be initiated in individuals with active liver disease or with elevated baseline serum transaminases. A rare but potentially serious adverse effect of trazodone is priapism, which is reported to occur in 1 in 6,000 male patients. Table 53-3 lists key parameters for triazolopyridines.

Sedation, cognitive slowing, and dizziness are the most frequent dose-limiting side effects associated with trazodone. It is the expected side effect of sedation that leads to trazodone's major use as a soporific. Common adverse effects associated with nefazodone include light-headedness, dizziness, orthostatic hypotension, somnolence, dry mouth, nausea, and weakness.

Selective Serotonin Reuptake Inhibitors

The efficacy of selective serotonin reuptake inhibitors (SSRIs) is superior to placebo and comparable to other classes of antidepressants. SSRIs are generally chosen as first-line antidepressants because of their safety in overdose and improved tolerability.[12] The SSRIs have a low affinity for histaminergic, alpha$_1$ adrenergic, and muscarinic receptors; therefore, they produce fewer anticholinergic and cardiovascular side effects. Side effects associated with SSRIs are mild, but prevalent and include gastrointestinal effects (nausea and diarrhea), sexual dysfunction, headache, and insomnia.[13] To mitigate the potential insomnia, SSRIs (with the exception of paroxetine) are most frequently administered in the morning. Paroxetine is the most sedating of the SSRIs and thus usually requires dosing at bedtime. A withdrawal syndrome can occur if the

SSRIs are abruptly discontinued (particularly short-acting paroxetine). Table 53-3 lists key parameters for SSRIs.

Aminoketone

Bupropion (Wellbutrin) is a dopamine reuptake inhibitor (thus a stimulant) used in the treatment of MDD. Adverse effects associated with bupropion include gastrointestinal issues, tremor, insomnia, dry mouth, and skin reactions. Sexual side effects are minimal with this drug. The occurrence of seizures with bupropion is dose related and may be increased by head trauma.[14] Due to its stimulant properties, bupropion should be dosed either in the morning or in the morning and early afternoon to avoid disrupting sleep.

Tetracyclics

Mirtazapine (Remeron) enhances noradrenergic and serotonergic activity through the antagonism of central presynaptic alpha$_2$ adrenergic autoreceptors and heteroreceptors. Mirtazapine also antagonizes 5-HT$_2$ and 5-HT$_3$ leading to lower gastrointestinal and anxiety side effects and histamine receptors leading to sedative properties.[15] The most common adverse effects of mirtazapine are somnolence, weight gain, dry mouth, and constipation. Certain side effects of mirtazapine are dose dependent, for example, weight gain and sedation are decreased with larger mirtazapine doses because of different mechanisms of action at different doses (such as increased noradrenergic transmission as the dose is increased).[16]

Monoamine Oxidase Inhibitors

Monoamine oxidase inhibitors (MAOIs) increase the concentration of NE, 5-HT, and DA within the neuronal synapse through inhibition of the MAO enzyme. The most common MAOI side effect is orthostatic hypotension. Other common adverse effects include weight gain and sexual side effects. Hypertensive crisis is a serious, life-threatening, rare reaction that may occur when MAOIs are taken concurrently with certain foods, especially those high in tyramine or medications. Ten milligrams of tyramine can cause a marked pressor effect, and 25 mg can result in serious hypertensive crisis. These incidents can culminate in cerebrovascular accidents and death. Symptoms of hypertensive crisis include headache, stiff neck, gastrointestinal effects (nausea and diarrhea), sweating, and sharply elevated blood pressure.

SPECIAL CONSIDERATIONS

Drug Interactions

Antidepressants cause pharmacodynamic (eg, additive pharmacologic effects) and pharmacokinetic (eg, changes in drug levels) interactions with other medications. The pharmacodynamic interactions involve receptor blockade by the antidepressants. For example:

- TCAs can cause significant additive effects with other medications that cause sedation, hypotension, or anticholinergic effects.
- Nefazodone and mirtazapine can interact with other drugs that cause hypotension and sedation effects, respectively.

The most concerning pharmacodynamic interactions are hypertensive crisis and serotonin syndrome. Hypertensive crisis is characterized by sharply elevated blood pressure, headache, stiff/sore neck, nausea, vomiting, and sweating. It may result during MAOI therapy if the patient takes a sympathomimetic (eg, ephedrine, pseudoephedrine, phenylephrine) or if the patient consumes foods rich in tyramine (eg, tap beers, aged cheese, fava beans, yeast extracts, liver, sauerkraut, or tofu). Since many over-the-counter products contain sympathomimetics, patients should always be told to consult their pharmacist prior to using any drugs. Serotonin syndrome is characterized by confusion, restlessness, fever, abnormal muscle movements, hyperreflexia, sweating, diarrhea, and shivering.[16] It may result when a serotonergic agent is added to any serotonergic antidepressant. The MAOIs are associated with severe cases of serotonin syndrome. Certain medications may complicate the serotonin syndrome diagnosis because they are not obvious serotonergic agents (eg, dextromethorphan, meperidine, tramadol).

Several antidepressants are known to inhibit various cytochrome P-450 isoenzymes, thereby elevating plasma levels of substrates for those isoenzymes and thus potentially leading to increased adverse effects or toxicity of those drugs.[17-18] The propensity to cause these interactions varies with the antidepressant. Table 53-4 lists select antidepressant interactions.

Efficacy

Antidepressants, when dosed properly, have a response rate of 60% to 80%. Various factors must be taken into account when selecting antidepressant activity to optimize efficacy. Examples include: patient's past history of response, family history of antidepressant response, side effects, drug interactions, and cost.

Time Course of Response

Antidepressants do not produce a clinical response immediately. Improvement in physical symptoms (sleep, appetite, energy) can occur within the first week of treatment. Improvement of emotional symptoms of depression will take at least 2 to 4 weeks and up to 6 to 8 weeks for full effects.

TABLE 53-4 Select Drug Interactions of Antidepressants[a]

Antidepressant	Type of Interaction	Examples of Interacting Drugs
TCAs Trazodone Mirtazapine	Pharmacodynamic–additive sedation	Benzodiazepines Alcohol Antihistamines
TCAs Trazodone	Pharmacodynamic—additive hypotensive effects	Prazosin (alpha blockers) Antipsychotics
TCAs	Pharmacodynamic—additive anticholinergic effects	Phenothiazines Benzotropine Antipsychotics
TCAs	Pharmacodynamic—additive cardiac toxicity	Thioridazine Quinidine
TCAs	Pharmacodynamic—decreased antihypertensive effect	Guanethidine Clonidine Methyldopa
Bupropion	Pharmacodynamic—increased seizure risk	TCAs Phenothiazines
MAOIs	Pharmacodynamic—hypertensive crisis	Tyramine-rich foods Sympathomimetics
MAOIs TCAs SSRIs SNRIs	Pharmacodynamic—serotonin syndrome	Serotonergic antidepressants Meperidine Dextromethorphan Tramadol
Fluvoxamine	Pharmacokinetic—CYP1A2 inhibition	TCAs Clozapine Theophylline
Fluoxetine Fluvoxamine Sertraline	Pharmacokinetic—CYP2C inhibition	TCAs Phenytoin Warfarin
Fluoxetine Paroxetine Duloxetine Sertraline	Pharmacokinetic—CYP2D6 inhibition	TCAs Haloperidol Risperidone Codeine Propranolol
Nefazodone Fluoxetine Fluvoxamine	Pharmacokinetic—CYP3A4 inhibition	TCAs Alprazolam Verapamil Carbamazepine Lovastatin

[a]Not an all-inclusive list.

Abbreviations: MAOI, monoamine oxidase inhibitor; SNRI, serotonin norepinephrine reuptake inhibitor; SSRI, selective serotonin reuptake inhibitor; TCAs, tricyclic antidepressant.

CASE Application

1. The pathophysiology of major depressive disorder (MDD) is associated with:
   a. Genetic factors
   b. Stress factors
   c. Neurotransmitter factors
   d. All of the above
2. Select the neurotransmitter(s) that is involved in the pathophysiology of depression.
   a. Norepinephrine
   b. Serotonin
   c. Dopamine
   d. All of the above
3. Select the symptom(s) of major depressive disorder.
   a. Depressed mood
   b. Diminished interest in usual activities
   c. Change in appetite or weight
   d. All of the above
4. Select the antidepressant that inhibits the reuptake of NE and 5-HT.
   a. Tricyclics (TCAs)
   b. Serotonin norepinephrine reuptake inhibitors (SNRIs)
   c. Selective serotonin reuptake inhibitors (SSRIs)
   d. a and b
   e. All of the above
5. Select the mechanism of action of trazodone that leads to the side effect of dizziness and sedation.
   a. 5-HT receptor antagonist
   b. 5-HT reuptake inhibitor
   c. Alpha$_1$ adrenergic and histaminergic antagonism
   d. All of the above
6. Select the antidepressant that has a black box warning for rare cases of liver failure.
   a. Duloxetine
   b. Bupropion
   c. Amitriptyline
   d. Nefazodone
7. Select the aminoketone that is a dopamine reuptake inhibitor.
   a. Wellbutrin
   b. Elavil
   c. Prozac
   d. Cymbalta
8. Select the answer that would represent the highest chance of developing the side effect of hypertensive crisis.
   a. Utilization of phenelzine
   b. Utilization of imipramine

c. Utilization of phenelzine plus pseudoephedrine
d. Utilization of imipramine plus benzodiazepine

9. Select the medication that is associated with causing depression.

a. Propranolol
b. Clonidine
c. Reserpine
d. a and c
e. All of the above

10. UW is a 49-year-old patient who suffered a myocardial infarction 5 days ago. Upon discharge, it was noted that UW appeared depressed. After a complete evaluation, UW met the criteria for diagnosis. Other past medical histories include: hypertension, diabetes, and severe uncontrolled narrow angle glaucoma. Select the antidepressant that would be the most effective and safest pharmacotherapy option for UW.

a. Elavil
b. Effexor
c. Zoloft
d. a and b
e. All of the above

11. UW has fully recovered from his myocardial infarction and is feeling much better since initiation of his antidepressant 4 weeks ago. UW presents for a follow-up today and states that while he is happy with the results of antidepressant, he is concerned about his acquired sexual dysfunction. Select the antidepressant that would be *least* likely to cause sexual dysfunction.

a. Wellbutrin
b. Pamelor
c. Prozac
d. Cymbalta

12. Select the medication property(ies) that is associated with tricyclic antidepressants.

a. Pregnancy category B
b. Causes orthostatic hypotension
c. Inhibits reuptake of dopamine
d. a and c
e. All of the above

13. TM is a 49-year-old patient diagnosed with major depression disorder. His past medical history is significant for alcohol-induced liver damage (patient has increased liver function tests), hypertension, and hyperlipidemia. Select the antidepressant that would be appropriate for TM.

i. Nefazodone
ii. Sertraline
iii. Mirtazapine

a. i and ii
b. ii and iii
c. i and iii
d. i, ii, and iii

14. KG is a 44-year-old patient with a history of anorexia who has had several hospitalizations for anorexia because of severe weakness and electrolyte abnormalities. KG has been diagnosed with major depressive disorder. Select the antidepressant that may be utilized for KG.

i. Wellbutrin
ii. Paxil
iii. Cymbalta

a. i and ii
b. ii and iii
c. i and iii
d. All of the above

15. Select the drug interaction(s) associated with TCA antidepressants.

i. Alcohol
ii. Antipsychotics
iii. Meperidine

a. i and ii
b. ii and iii
c. i and iii
d. All of the above

16. BC is a 54-year-old patient diagnosed with major depressive disorder. BC is currently receiving the following medications: lisinopril for hypertension and warfarin for a recent deep venous thrombosis. BC currently has an INR within range (INR = 2.5); however, the patient has had a difficult time achieving a goal INR level and has had elevated INRs in the past (most recent 14 days ago INR was 5.9). Select the antidepressant that would have the least impact on the activity of warfarin.

a. Fluvoxamine
b. Sertraline
c. Fluoxetine
d. Venlafaxine

17. BN is a patient with major depressive disorder currently taking a monoamine oxidase inhibitor. She has been experiencing major sinus pressure, headaches, and congestion. She approaches your pharmacy and asks if she can take a decongestant for the congestion. You inform her that she cannot take the decongestant with the MAOI because of a high incidence of what side effect.

a. Serotonin syndrome
b. Hypertensive crisis
c. Orthostatic hypotension
d. Sexual dysfunction

18. Select the drug interaction(s) associated with fluvoxamine.

i. Verapamil
ii. Carbamazepine
iii. Lovastatin

a. i and ii
b. ii and iii
c. i and iii
d. All of the above

19. Select the brand name of paroxetine.

a. Paxil
b. Zoloft
c. Prozac
d. Effexor

20. Select the generic name of Remeron.

a. Duloxetine
b. Amitriptyline
c. Mirtazapine
d. Trazodone

TAKEAWAY POINTS ››

- Major depressive disorder (MDD) is diagnosed when an individual experiences one or more major depressive episodes without a history of manic, mixed, or hypomanic episodes.
- An MDD episode is defined by the criteria listed in the *Diagnostic and Statistical Manual of Mental Disorders*, Fourth Edition, Text Revision (DSM-IV-TR).
- Depression is associated with significant functional disability, morbidity, and mortality. Individuals with MDD experience significant and pervasive symptoms that can affect mood, thinking, physical health, work, and relationships.
- The exact cause of MDD is unknown, but appears to be multifactorial. Biologic, psychological, and social theories appear to work together or precipitate depressive disorders.
- Classic views for the cause of MDD focus on the neurotransmitters norepinephrine (NE), serotonin (5-HT), and dopamine (DA).
- The diagnosis of MDD requires the presence of at least five depressive symptoms that cause clinically significant effects and the symptoms must last for a minimum of 2 weeks.
- The goals of treatment are to reduce the symptoms of acute depression, facilitate the patient's return to a level of functioning before the onset of illness, and prevent further episodes of depression. An extremely important outcome in the treatment of MDD is the prevention of suicide attempts.
- Tricyclic antidepressants (TCAs) are effective in treating all depressive subtypes, but their use has diminished greatly because of the availability of equally effective therapies that are much safer in overdose and better tolerated. TCAs potentiate the activity of NE and 5-HT by blocking their reuptake; however, the potency and selectivity of TCAs for the reuptake inhibition varies greatly within in the class.
- Venlafaxine (Effexor), desvenlafaxine (Pristiq), and duloxetine (Cymbalta) are serotonin/norepinephrine reuptake inhibitors (SNRIs).
- Trazodone (Desyrel) and nefazodone are effective in treating depression; however, they both carry risks that limit their usefulness as antidepressants. Trazodone and nefazodone have dual actions on serotonergic neurons, acting as 5-HT_2 receptor antagonists and 5-HT reuptake inhibitors. Trazodone's primary use is as a sedative/hypnotic.
- The efficacy of selective serotonin reuptake inhibitors (SSRIs) is superior to placebo and comparable to other classes of antidepressants. SSRIs are generally chosen as first-line antidepressants because of their safety in overdose and improved tolerability.
- Bupropion (Wellbutrin) is a dopamine reuptake inhibitor and stimulant used in the treatment of MDD.
- Mirtazapine (Remeron) enhances noradrenergic and serotonergic activity through the antagonism of central presynaptic $alpha_2$ adrenergic autoreceptors and heteroreceptors. Mirtazapine also antagonizes 5-HT_2 and 5-HT_3 leading to gastrointestinal effects and antianxiety side effects. The antagonism of histamine receptors leads to sedative properties.
- Monoamine oxidase inhibitors (MAOIs) increase the concentration of NE, 5-HT, and DA within the neuronal synapse through inhibition of the MAO enzyme. The most common MAOI side effect is postural hypotension.
- Hypertensive crisis is a serious, life-threatening, rare reaction that may occur when MAOIs are taken concurrently with certain foods, especially those high in tyramine or sympathomimetic medications.
- Antidepressants cause pharmacodynamic (eg, additive pharmacologic effects) and pharmacokinetic (eg, changes in drug levels) interactions with other medications.
- When dosed properly for an appropriate time, antidepressants have a response rate of 60% to 80%.
- Antidepressants do not produce a clinical response immediately. Improvement in physical symptoms (sleep, appetite, energy) can occur within the first week of treatment. Improvement of emotional symptoms of depression will take at least 2 to 4 weeks and up to 6 to 8 weeks for full effects.

REFERENCES

1. American Psychiatric Association. *Diagnostic and Statistical Manual of Mental Disorders*. 4th ed. Text Revision. Washington, DC: American Psychiatric Association; 2000.
2. Kessler RC, Berglund P, Demler O. The epidemiology of major depressive disorders: results from the National Comorbidity Survey Replication (NCS-R). *JAMA*. 2003;289:3095-3105.

3. Boland RJ, Keller MB. Antidepressants. In: Tasman A, Kay J, Lieberman JA, eds. *Psychiatry Therapeutics*. 2nd ed. Hoboken, NJ: Wiley; 2003:292-334.
4. Stahl SM. *Essential Psychopharmacology: Neuroscientific Basis and Practical Applications*. 2nd ed. New York, NY: Cambridge University Press; 2000:135-295.
5. Ressler KJ, Nemeroff CB. Role of serotonergic and noradrenergic systems in the pathophysiology of depression and anxiety disorders. *Depress Anxiety*. 2000;12(suppl 1):2-19.
6. Sofuoglu M, Dudish-Poulsen S, Poling J, Mooney M, Hatsukami DK. The effect of individual cocaine withdrawal symptoms on outcomes in cocaine users. *Addict Behav*. 2005;30:1125-1134.
7. Cipriani A, Furukawa TA, Salanti G, et al. Comparative efficacy and acceptability of 12 new-generation antidepressants: a multiple-treatment meta-analysis. *Lancet*. 2009;373:746-758.
8. Baldessarini RJ. Drugs and the treatment of psychiatric disorders: depression and anxiety disorders. In: Hardman JG, Limbrid LE, Goodman A, et al, eds. *Goodman and Gilman's The Pharmacological Basis of Therapeutics*. 10th ed. New York, NY: McGraw Hill, 2000:447-484.
9. Feighner JP. Cardiovascular safety in depressed patients: focus on venlafaxine. *J Clin Psychiatry*. 1995;56:574-579.
10. Stahl SM, Grady MM, Moret C, Briley M. SNRIs: their pharmacology, clinical efficacy, and tolerability in comparison with older classes of antidepressants. *CNS Spectr*. 2005;10:732-747.
11. Ables AZ, Baughman III OL. Antidepressants: update on new agents and indications. *Am Fam Physician*. 2003;67:547-554.
12. Mann JJ. The medical management of depression. *N Engl J Med*. 2005;353:1819-1834.
13. Masand PS, Gupta S. Long term side effects of newer generation antidepressants: SSRIs, venlafaxine, nefazodone, bupropion, and mirtazapine. *Ann Clin Psychiatry*. 2002;14:175-182.
14. Johnston JA, Lineberry CG, Ascher JA. A 102-center prospective study of seizures in association with buproprion. *J Clin Psychiatry*. 1991;52:450-456.
15. Gorman JM. Mirtazapine: clinical overview. *J Clin Psychiatry*. 1999;60(suppl 17):9-13.
16. Boyer EW, Shannon M. The serotonin syndrome. *N Engl J Med*. 2005;352:1112-1120.
17. Michalets EL. Update: clinically significant cytochrome P-450 drug interactions. *Pharmacotherapy*. 1998;18:84-112.
18. Spina E, Scordo MG. Clinically significant drug interactions with antidepressants in the elderly. *Drug Aging*. 2002;19:299-320.

CHAPTER

54 Bipolar Disorders

Susie H. Park

FOUNDATION OVERVIEW

Bipolar disorder, formerly known as manic depressive disorder, is a recurrent psychiatric illness characterized by recurring episodes of mania and depression. There can be extreme shifts in mood, energy level, thinking, and daily functioning and activities. Bipolar patients require lifelong treatment to control their symptoms. Bipolar disorder affects 2.6% of the US population over the age of 18 and has a lifetime prevalence of 1%.[1-2] Bipolar disorders are more common in women.[2] The mean age of onset for bipolar disorder is 21 and often begins in adolescence or early adulthood.[2] There is a high comorbidity of substance use disorders in bipolar disorders.

Pathophysiology

The exact cause of bipolar disorder is unknown; however, there is evidence that a chemical imbalance with several neurotransmitters is involved in its pathophysiology. It is thought that there may be an excess of norepinephrine and dopamine in mania, whereas there may be a deficiency of serotonin, norepinephrine, and dopamine in depression. Medications used to manage the symptoms of bipolar disorder alter the transmission of serotonin, dopamine, norepinephrine, as well as gamma-aminobutyric acid (GABA), glutamate, and aspartate.

Family, twin, and adoptions studies provide strong evidence for a major genetic contribution to the risk of developing bipolar disorder. Identifying that bipolar disorders tend to run in families has led to the identification of candidate genes interacting to play a role in determining illness susceptibility.

Clinical Presentation and Diagnosis

Discrete types of mood episodes are classified as manic, hypomanic, depressive, or mixed type. Mania is the unique hallmark of bipolar disorder. The signs and symptoms of *mania* include an elated, euphoric, expansive, or irritable mood; increased self-esteem or grandiosity; a decreased need for sleep; more talkative or pressured speech; racing thoughts or flight of ideas; distractibility; increased goal-directed activities; and psychomotor agitation. The patient may also report an increase in risk-taking behaviors or excessive involvement in pleasurable activities without thinking about the consequences of engaging in such activities (ie, sexual promiscuity, unrestrained buying sprees). Three or more of these associated symptoms must be present in a given patient if his/her mood is euphoric or expansive; four or more if the mood is irritable.[3] These symptoms must last at least 1 week or can be of any duration if hospitalization was required. During a manic episode, people with bipolar disorder engage in unsafe behaviors that may result in hospitalization and incarceration. Psychosis may sometimes accompany a manic episode. *Hypomania* is a less severe form of mania, lasting at least 4 days and not requiring hospitalization. These patients may describe that they feel more creative, important, and productive and do not think that they need any kind of medical treatment. A *depressive* episode may alternate with manic episodes, and the patient would be said to have bipolar depression (as opposed to unipolar depression, otherwise known as major depressive disorder; see Chapter 53, Depression). One example of the episodic course of bipolar disorder includes one manic episode followed by three depressive episodes over the course of many years, possibly with or without a return to mania. Another example may include an initial depressive episode lasting a few months followed by a manic episode, then a return to a depressive episode several months to years later. *Mixed* (or dysphoric) type includes episodes of both mania and major depression occurring at the same time for at least 1 week. Agitation, psychosis, and suicidality are symptoms associated with mixed episodes. Rapid cycling is a term to describe when a patient experiences four or more episodes of depression or mania within a 12-month period.

There are four different types of bipolar disorders that can be diagnosed in an individual. *Bipolar I disorder* includes manic or mixed episodes usually accompanied by major depressive episodes. *Bipolar II* is major depressive episodes plus hypomanic episodes. *Cyclothymic disorder* is recurring hypomania plus depressive symptoms that recur for a minimum of 2 years. *Bipolar disorder not otherwise specified* (NOS) describes bipolar features that do not meet criteria for a specific bipolar disorder.

TREATMENT

The goal of treating an acute manic episode is to control the patient's agitation, reduce any risk of self-harm or harm to others, and to generally slow the patient down to allow a return of normal functioning. This may take the form of sedating the patient and inducing sleep, especially if the patient has not slept for several days due to a decreased need for sleep and increased energy. A mood stabilizer such as lithium or divalproex sodium with or without an antipsychotic or a benzodiazepine is used

for the treatment of acute manic episodes. Benzodiazepines such as clonazepam or lorazepam can be used as an adjunctive treatment to promote sleep in agitated and overactive patients.[4] The goal of maintenance treatment is to prevent or minimize future episodes, prevent rehospitalizations, and maximize the patient's functioning ability and quality of life. Maintenance treatment involves the use of lithium, divalproex sodium, carbamazepine, lamotrigine, with or without atypical antipsychotics and antidepressants. The precise mechanism of action of mood stabilizers is not well known. Table 54-1 lists the medications used for treating bipolar disorder. Multiple medication combinations may be used at one time to manage the symptoms. In the case of treating bipolar depression, the goal is to relieve the depression without inducing a manic episode. This requires treatment using an antidepressant agent with a concomitant mood stabilizer or an antipsychotic. Antidepressants should not be used as monotherapy, even when treating the depressive episode in bipolar disorder due to their ability to precipitate a rapid mood switch from depression to mania.

Lithium

Lithium is an effective antimanic agent and is used as one option for first-line treatment in acute manic or mixed episodes, as well as for ongoing maintenance treatment.[5,6] Lithium confers a therapeutic advantage by decreasing suicidality in bipolar patients, however, it has a slow onset of action which may limit its use in acute manic episodes. It is a cation eliminated primarily through the kidneys and is most known for its narrow therapeutic effect. Serum concentration monitoring is required and correlates with treatment response: 0.5 to 1.2 mEq/L for acute manic episodes and 0.6 to 0.8 mEq/L for maintenance treatment. Lithium serum concentrations >1.5mEq/L can lead to lithium toxicity. Lithium toxicity may manifest as coarse hand tremor, persistent diarrhea, uncoordinated motor movements (ataxia), slurred speech, and confusion. Levels >2.5 mEq/L may result in renal failure, seizure, and coma. Table 54-2 lists the required monitoring parameters associated with lithium and Table 54-3 lists some common drug interactions with lithium. The recommended starting dose is 300 mg tid or less, depending on patient's age and weight[5] with a maximum recommended dose of 2,400 mg/d. Common adverse effects of lithium include nausea, vomiting, diarrhea, hand tremor, polyuria, polydipsia, sedation, weight gain, acne, and hypothyroidism.[7] Patients should be counseled about maintaining adequate water intake (dehydration increases lithium concentrations), maintaining consistent sodium quantities in their diets (low sodium can increase lithium), and the effect of caffeine decreasing lithium concentrations via increased diuresis. Lithium should not be used in people with renal failure and women who are pregnant in their first trimester. It is pregnancy category D and has been associated with causing Ebstein anomaly, a cardiac abnormality.[8]

Valproic Acid/Divalproex Sodium

Valproate (divalproex sodium, Depakote or Depakote ER and valproic acid, Depakene; VPA) is another first-line agent for acute manic episodes and is sometimes preferred over lithium due to its wider margin of safety and its faster onset. It is the preferred agent for mixed episodes of bipolar.[9] The therapeutic range of VPA is 50 to 125 μg/mL. The recommended starting dose is 250 mg tid with a maximum daily dose of 60 mg/kg.[5] During an acute episode, VPA can be given as a loading dose of 20 to 30 mg/kg in divided doses. Baseline laboratory monitoring tests should be performed: CBC with differential including platelets, liver function tests, and a pregnancy test in women of childbearing age. Adverse effects include nausea, vomiting, dyspepsia, sedation, tremor, alopecia, weight gain, elevated liver enzymes, and thrombocytopenia. VPA has also been associated with causing polycystic ovary syndrome (PCOS) in women, hyperammonemia, and pancreatitis. Patients should be counseled to take VPA with food to minimize GI adverse effects. Patients may take selenium and zinc to treat hair loss, however, the dose of VPA should be separated by at least 4 hours. VPA is involved in multiple cytochrome P450 isoenzyme 2C9 drug-drug interactions and is highly protein bound. VPA is pregnancy category D, but unlike lithium, its teratogenic effect is spina bifida.[10] If used during pregnancy, folic acid 5 mg/d is recommended for the pregnant patient taking VPA or other anticonvulsants.[11]

Carbamazepine

Carbamazepine (Tegretol, Equetro; CBZ) is effective in manic and mixed episodes (FDA-approved indication) and maintenance treatment in bipolar disorder, although it is not a first-line agent.[5] It may be used as an alternative agent when lithium, VPA, or atypical antipsychotics fail. The recommended starting dose is 200 mg bid, up to 1,600 mg/d if needed. CBZ is a cytochrome P450 enzyme inducer, potentially lowering the blood concentrations of concomitantly administered medications, such as oral contraceptives. Other P4503A4 substrates include haloperidol, midazolam, valproate, and warfarin. Dosage adjustments would be required of these agents when used with CBZ. Also an autoinducer, CBZ induces its own metabolism. Blood concentration monitoring is required of CBZ: 4 to 12 μg/mL; levels >12 μg/mL are associated with toxicity. CBZ is associated with causing Stevens-Johnson syndrome (SJS) and toxic epidermal necrolysis (TEN), two potentially fatal dermatologic reactions. The allelic variation of the *HLA-B* gene, *HLA-B*1502*, has been linked to these two adverse drug reactions. Genotyping susceptible patients is advised prior to starting CBZ. Adverse effects of CBZ include sedation, dizziness, weight gain, nausea, diplopia, elevated liver enzymes, and hyponatremia. It has rare adverse effects of causing agranulocytosis and aplastic anemia. CBZ is also pregnancy category D, associated with causing spina bifida.

Lamotrigine

Lamotrigine (Lamictal) is FDA approved for maintenance treatment of bipolar I disorder and may be used as an alternative to lithium for bipolar depressive episodes.[5] It is an effective treatment for bipolar depressive episodes[12] but does not

TABLE 54-1 **Medications Used for the Treatment of Bipolar Disorder**

Agent	Dosage Forms and Strengths	Brand Name	Daily Dosing Range (mg)	Comments
Lithium carbonate	150 mg, 600 mg capsules 300 mg tablets 300 mg capsules 450 mg ER tablets 300 mg ER tablets	 Eskalith Eskalith CR Lithobid slow-release	600-2400	Therapeutic range Acute: 0.5-1.2 mEq/L Maintenance : 0.6-0.8 mEq/L
Lithium citrate	300 mg/5 mL oral solution	Cibalith-S		
Valproic acid	250 mg capsules 250 mg/5mL	Depakene	750-3500	Therapeutic range: 50-125 μg/mL Loading dose in acute manic or mixed episodes: 20-30 mg/kg/day
Divalproex sodium	125, 250, 500 mg tabs	Depakote		
Divalproex sodium ER	250, 500 mg tablets	Depakote ER		
Carbamazepine[a]	100 mg chewable tablets 200 mg tablets 100 mg/5mL oral suspension 100, 200, 400 mg ER tablets 100, 200, 300 mg ER caps	Tegretol Tegretol XR Equetro	200-1600	Therapeutic range: 4-12 μg/mL to avoid toxicity
Oxcarbazepine	150, 300, 600 mg tablets 300 mg/5 mL oral suspension	Trileptal	600-2400	Not FDA-approved for BPD
Lamotrigine	25, 100, 150, 200 mg tablets 25, 50, 100, 200 mg ODT 2, 5, 25 mg chewable dispersible tablets	Lamictal	100-400	Indicated for maintenance treatment of BDI Dosing is based on concomitant medications
Olanzapine/Fluoxetine	3/25, 6/25, 6/50, 12/25, 12/50 mg capsules	Symbyax	6/25-12/50	Bipolar depression
Quetiapine	25, 50, 100, 200, 300, 400 mg tablets	Seroquel	200-800	Bipolar depression Acute mania Maintenance
Quetiapine XR	50, 150, 200, 300, 400 mg ER tablets	Seroquel XR		
Olanzapine[b]	2.5, 5, 7.5, 10, 15, 20 mg tablets 5, 10, 15, 20 mg ODT	Zyprexa Zydis	5-20	Acute mania Maintenance
Aripiprazole[b]	2, 5, 10, 15, 20, 30 mg tablets 1 mg/mL oral solution 10, 15 mg ODT	Abilify Discmelt	15-30	Acute mania Maintenance
Risperidone long-acting injection	12.5, 25, 37.5, 50 mg vial kits for IM injection	Consta	25-50	Maintenance
Risperidone	0.25, 0.5, 1, 2, 3, 4 mg tablets 1 mg/mL oral solution 0.5, 1, ,2, 3, 4 mg ODT	Risperdal M-Tab	2-6	Acute mania
Ziprasidone	20, 40, 60, 80 mg caps	Geodon	40-160	Acute mania Maintenance
Asenapine	5, 10 mg sublingual tablets	Saphris	10-20	Acute mania
Paliperidone	1.5, 3, 6, 9 mg tabs	Invega	3-12	Acute treatment of schizoaffective disorder

[a]Other brand name products of carbamazepine include Carbatrol and Epitol. Equetro is the only FDA-approved brand for BPD treatment.

[b]Olanzapine and aripiprazole are available in IM formulations and FDA approved for acute agitation associated with bipolar I mania in adults.

Abbreviations: BPD, bipolar disorder; BDI: bipolar I disorder; ER & XR, extended-release; ODT, orally disintegrating tablet; to be placed on top of the tongue with dry hands.

TABLE 54-2 **Lithium Monitoring**

Baseline Laboratory/ Ongoing Monitoring	Explanation
SCr, BUN	Renal excretion of lithium
Urine-specific gravity	Polyuria caused by lithium Lithium decreases the kidney's ability to concentrate the urine
Electrolytes	Hyponatremia and dehydration can lead to ↑ renal reabsorption of lithium: ↑ lithium levels: lithium toxicity Hypokalemia may ↑ the risk of lithium-induced cardiac toxicity
CBC with differential	Lithium can ↑ WBC (except basophils) Lithium can ↑ platelets
TSH; T_4	Hyperthyroidism can mimic mania Lithium can induce hypothyroidism with long-term treatment
ECG (in patients with cardiovascular disease risk; age >40)	Lithium can worsen cardiac disease Lithium can cause cardiac conduction abnormalities
Weight	Lithium causes weight gain
Pregnancy test	Lithium is pregnancy category D Lithium can cause teratogenicity: Ebstein anomaly
Lithium levels	Lithium is a narrow-therapeutic index drug; avoid toxicity Levels assist in determining therapeutic response

TABLE 54-3 **Lithium Drug Interactions**

Drugs that Increase (↑) Lithium
ACE inhibitors result in volume depletion and a reduction in glomerular filtration rate → reduced Li^+ excretion → increased Li^+ levels
▪ Reports of angiotensin II receptor blockers (ARBs; eg, losartan) also increase Li^+
Diuretics, especially thiazide diuretics cause the greatest ↑ in Li^+; all diuretics can cause sodium depletion → Na^+ depletion causes an ↑ in proximal tubular reabsorption of both Na^+ and Li^+
▪ Loop diuretics and potassium-sparing diuretics appear less interacting
NSAIDs can increase Li^+ by up to 50%; most likely due to enhanced reabsorption of sodium and lithium secondary to inhibition of prostaglandin synthesis
▪ Not likely to occur with aspirin or sulindac (Clinoril)
Drugs that Decrease (↓) Lithium
Acetazolamide may impair the proximal tubular reabsorption of Li^+
Sodium promotes the renal clearance of lithium
Theophylline and *caffeine* will ↑ the renal clearance of lithium and can ↓ Li^+ by 20%
Drugs that Increase Lithium Toxicity
Carbamazepine can cause an increase in neurotoxicity
▪ No change in lithium levels
Calcium channel blockers cause an increase in neurotoxicity; mostly caused by nondihydropyridine CCBs (eg, diltiazem, verapamil)
▪ No change in lithium levels
Methyldopa may increase neurotoxicity
Phenytoin may increase neurotoxicity

appear to be effective for treating manic episodes. The starting dose of lamotrigine depends on concomitant medications taken by the patient. For patients taking lamotrigine without concomitant cytochrome P450 enzyme inhibitors or inducers, the dose starts at 25 mg/d for weeks 1 to 2, followed by 50 mg/d for weeks 3 to 4, 100 mg/d for week 5, and then is increased to 200 mg/d beginning week 6. If lamotrigine is taken with valproate, the starting dose is 25 mg every other day (qod) with a target dose of 100 mg at week 6. If lamotrigine is taken with carbamazepine, an enzyme inducer, start 50 mg/d with a target dose of 400 mg/d by week 6. Higher doses are usually given in bid dosing and doses are titrated slowly in order to avoid potentially life-threatening rashes. Factors that may increase the risk of rash include coadministration with valproate, exceeding recommended initial doses of lamotrigine, or exceeding the recommended dose escalation schedule.[13] It is also recommended that lamotrigine be discontinued at the first sign of rash, unless the rash does not appear to be drug related.[13] Other adverse drug reactions of lamotrigine include headache, dizziness, sedation, blurred vision, and GI distress.

Other Anticonvulsants

Oxcarbazepine (Trileptal),[14] topiramate (Topamax),[15,16] gabapentin (Neurontin),[17] phenytoin (Dilantin),[18] zonisamide (Zonegran),[19] and levetiracetam (Keppra)[20] have been studied for use in bipolar disorders with some evidence of efficacy and safety. However, these agents are not standard treatments and are not FDA approved for treatment of bipolar disorders. They are used as adjunctive treatment or in refractory treatment cases.

Atypical Antipsychotics

The role of atypical antipsychotics (AAPs; ie, second-generation antipsychotics) in the treatment of bipolar disorder is growing. These agents are indicated for use as monotherapy or as adjunct therapy with lithium or divalproex. Olanzapine (Zyprexa), aripiprazole (Abilify), quetiapine (Seroquel), quetiapine XR (Seroquel XR for once-daily dosing), and ziprasidone (Geodon) are atypical antipsychotic agents FDA approved for the treatment of both acute manic or mixed episodes as well as maintenance treatment in bipolar I disorder. Risperidone

(Risperdal) and asenapine (Saphris) are currently approved only for the treatment of acute manic or mixed episodes. Ziprasidone should be taken consistently with food to increase its absorption up to two-fold. Moreover, quetiapine and its XR formulation are approved for bipolar depression, specifically. The olanzapine plus fluoxetine combination product (Symbyax) is also indicated for bipolar depression. Risperidone long-acting injection is approved for maintenance treatment of bipolar I disorder. This agent is administered intramuscularly (IM) every 2 weeks. Oral risperidone or other antipsychotic should be given with the first IM injection for the first 3 weeks in order to ensure an adequate therapeutic plasma concentration.[21] Paliperidone (Invega), the active metabolite of risperidone, is uniquely indicated for the acute treatment of schizoaffective disorder. The presence of psychosis (ie, hallucinations, delusions) accompanying the manic or depressive episode warrants the use of an antipsychotic medication until the mood episode is well-controlled. In schizoaffective disorder, however, the antipsychotic may be used as long as the psychotic symptoms persist concurrent to the depressive, manic, or mixed episode. A major limitation to the use of AAPs is the metabolic side effects associated with their long-term use. These include weight gain and glucose intolerance, requiring regular monitoring during treatment.

Antidepressants

Antidepressants are used to treat the depressive episode in bipolar disorder; however, they should be used in combination treatment with a mood stabilizer at all times. This is because all antidepressants can potentially precipitate a manic episode especially if used as monotherapy in a patient with bipolar disorder. Therefore, antidepressants should generally not be used in the absence of a concomitant mood stabilizer that can help prevent treatment-emergent mania. SSRIs such as fluoxetine (Prozac), paroxetine (Paxil), and sertraline (Zoloft) and the dopamine/norepinephrine reuptake inhibitor, bupropion (Wellbutrin) are less likely to cause a conversion into mania compared to TCAs.[22,23] Other SSRIs safe to use are citalopram (Celexa) and escitalopram (Lexapro).

Other Treatments for Bipolar Disorder

Calcium channel blockers, such as verapamil,[24] have been used for treating bipolar mania. There are conflicting results regarding the efficacy of this class of agents.[5] There is growing interest and research in omega-3 fatty acid for the treatment of bipolar disorder[25] and has been shown to be efficacious in patients with bipolar disorder.[26]

Special Populations

Bipolar disorder is challenging to treat during pregnancy. Since the classic agents like lithium, valproic acid, and carbamazepine are all pregnancy category D, these agents are often avoided. Typical, high-potency antipsychotics, such as haloperidol, have been used to manage acute mania. Patients taking lithium or an anticonvulsant may switch to a first-generation antipsychotic either for the first trimester or the entire pregnancy.[27] There is growing evidence for the use of atypical, second-generation antipsychotics during pregnancy. Electroconvulsive therapy (ECT) is also very effective and safe in managing bipolar disorder in pregnancy.

CASE Application

1. Which of the following is *not* a sign and symptom of a manic episode?

   a. Irritable mood
   b. Anhedonia
   c. Racing thoughts
   d. Psychomotor agitation
   e. Decreased need for sleep

2. Hypomania is characterized by:

   a. Multiple hospitalizations
   b. Psychotic episodes
   c. Impairment in social functioning
   d. Impairment in occupational functioning
   e. An inflated self-esteem

3. Rapid cycling describes when a bipolar patient has ____ or more manic or depressive episodes within a __________ period.

   a. 2; 6-month
   b. 2; 1-year
   c. 3; 2-year
   d. 4; 1-year
   e. 4; 2-year

4. In treating patients with bipolar disorder, which medications are used either as monotherapy or in combination with other agents?

   i. Lithium
   ii. Aripiprazole
   iii. Lamotrigine
   iv. Citalopram

   a. i only
   b. i and iii only
   c. i and iv only
   d. i, iii, and iv only
   e. i, ii, iii, and iv

5. Which of the following is a common adverse drug reaction of lithium?

   a. Alopecia
   b. Increased urination
   c. Hyperammonemia
   d. Hyperthyroidism
   e. Diplopia

6. What is the recommended starting dose of lithium?
   a. 300 mg tid
   b. 15 mg qhs
   c. 200 mg bid
   d. 500 mg bid
   e. 50 mg qd

7. The teratogenicity associated with lithium use in the first trimester of pregnancy is:
   a. Cardiovascular
   b. Renal
   c. Hepatic
   d. Neuromuscular
   e. Dermatological

8. Which of the following is *not* something you would counsel to your lithium-user patient?
   a. "You should avoid dehydration, so maintain your water intake."
   b. "Stop your medication if you experience persistent diarrhea."
   c. "Use caution while operating machinery or driving a car."
   d. "Ask your pharmacist before starting any new pain medications."
   e. "You should reduce your sodium intake while taking lithium."

9. What is the target therapeutic concentration of a patient taking lithium for 3 years?
   a. 4 to 12 μg/mL
   b. 4 to 12 mEq/L
   c. 50 to 125 μg/mL
   d. 0.6 to 0.8 mEq/L
   e. 1 to 1.8 mEq/L

10. Your 42-year-old patient is on several medications and reports the following:

    Aleve (naproxen sodium) 1 tablet twice daily for back pain when working. Motrin (ibuprofen) 400 mg 1 tablet every 8 hours as need for headache occurring three times per month, Cozaar (losartan) 50 mg 1 tablet bid, Glucophage (metformin) 850 mg 1 tablet bid. Patient smokes six to seven cigarettes per day, drinks alcohol occasionally, and has one to two cups of coffee every morning except Fridays and Saturdays.

    Which of the following factors can affect the level of lithium when he draws his blood at the next clinic visit?

    i. Aleve
    ii. Cozaar
    iii. Glucophage
    iv. Smoking
    v. Alcohol
    vi. Coffee

    a. ii and vi only
    b. ii and iii only
    c. i, ii, and vi only
    d. i and v only
    e. iv, v, and vi only

11. The physician wants to know what extended-release preparations of lithium are available, if any. You advise that the prescription be written for:
    a. Lithium citrate
    b. Lithium carbonate tablets
    c. Lithium carbonate capsules
    d. Eskalith
    e. Lithobid

12. Which of the following is *not* a required laboratory monitoring parameter for patients taking lithium?
    a. Serum creatinine
    b. Electrocardiogram
    c. Thyroid function tests
    d. Liver enzyme tests
    e. Electrolytes

13. Polycystic ovary syndrome (PCOS) has been associated with which of the following medications?
    a. Aripiprazole
    b. Divalproex sodium
    c. Lithium
    d. Lamotrigine
    e. Olanzapine

14. What is the recommended loading dose of Depakote (in kg/d) for a patient who has just been admitted into the psychiatry emergency department for an acute manic episode?
    a. 5 mg
    b. 10 to 15 mg
    c. 20 to 30 mg
    d. 40 mg
    e. 50 to 55 mg

15. Your bipolar patient is concerned about using certain medications for her psychiatric condition. She heard that there are some medications associated with causing a neural tube defect if taken during pregnancy. You confirm her suspicion and tell her that there are some agents associated with causing this condition in the newborn when used by the mother during pregnancy. You list the following agent(s):

    i. Lithium
    ii. Divalproex sodium
    iii. Carbamazepine
    iv. Olanzapine
    v. Risperidone

a. i only
b. i and ii only
c. ii and iii only
d. ii and iv only
e. iv and v only

16. It is recommended that the human leukocyte antigen type B, *HLA-B*1502*, allele is genotyped in Asian patients prior to taking:

a. Lithium
b. Carbamazepine
c. Lorazepam
d. Haloperidol
e. Quetiapine

17. You discover that your bipolar patient in the hospital ward is "cheeking" his medication for the past 4 days. You decide to recommend the same medication in an orally disintegrating tablet (ODT) formulation. Which of the following medications is available in this dosage form?

a. Carbamazepine
b. Haloperidol
c. Lithium
d. Quetiapine
e. Risperidone

18. Which of the following factors is *not* likely to increase the risk of lamotrigine-related rash?

a. Coadministration with another anticonvulsant, valproate
b. Coadministration with another anticonvulsant, carbamazepine
c. Exceeding the recommended initial dose of lamotrigine
d. Exceeding the recommended maximum dose of lamotrigine
e. Exceeding the recommended dose escalation schedule of lamotrigine

19. The psychiatric treatment team decides to start Risperdal Consta on a patient who has a history of nonadherence to his mood stabilizer for bipolar disorder for the past 6 years. They ask you, the clinical pharmacist, for the recommended starting dose and directions for administration. You reply with the following:

a. 2 mg tablet, 1 tab po bid
b. 3 mg ODT, 1 tab on top of the tongue everyday
c. 25 mg SQ every 2 weeks
d. 25 mg IM every 2 weeks
e. 50 mg IM every 2 weeks

20. Which agent is the safest option for treating a pregnant female with acute bipolar mania?

a. Carbamazepine
b. Chlorpromazine
c. Haloperidol
d. Lithium
e. Valproic acid

21. Symbyax is a product that contains the following agents for treating bipolar depression:

a. Lithium + divalproex sodium
b. Risperidone + fluoxetine
c. Olanzapine + fluoxetine
d. Risperidone + sertraline
e. Olanzapine + sertraline

22. Which antidepressant is most likely to cause a switch to mania?

a. Amitriptyline
b. Bupropion
c. Citalopram
d. Escitalopram
e. Sertraline

23. Which of the following medication classes have *not* been used to stabilize a patient's mood in bipolar disorder?

a. ACE-inhibitors
b. Anticonvulsants
c. Antidepressants
d. Antipsychotics
e. Calcium channel blockers

24. Which agent is effective for the treatment of bipolar I disorder, and may be more effective than lithium for bipolar depression?

a. Dilantin
b. Lamictal
c. Lamisil
d. Neurontin
e. Trileptal

TAKEAWAY POINTS ››

- Bipolar disorders are classified as follows: bipolar I, bipolar II, cyclothymia, and bipolar disorder not otherwise specified.
- The clinical presentation of bipolar disorder may include: mania, hypomania, mixed (or dysphoric) mania, major depression, and rapid cycling.

- The difference between mania and hypomania is that there is not necessarily a loss of social or occupational functioning, or hospitalization seen during hypomanic episodes.
- Mood stabilizers such as lithium and divalproex sodium (valproate) are commonly used as monotherapy or in combination treatment for treating bipolar disorder.
- Atypical antipsychotics, monotherapy or in combination with mood stabilizers, are used in the treatment of bipolar disorder.
- Antidepressant monotherapy should be avoided in bipolar disorder treatment.
- Lithium has a narrow therapeutic window that requires careful monitoring before and during treatment.
- Lithium is implicated in numerous drug interactions.
- Valproate may be more effective than lithium for mixed episodes.
- Lamotrigine is effective for treating bipolar depression but not for acute manic episodes.
- Lithium, valproate, and carbamazepine should be avoided during the first trimester of pregnancy.
- Treatment adherence is important in preventing relapse, suicidal behavior, and rehospitalization.
- Lifelong pharmacotherapy may be required for many bipolar disorder patients.

REFERENCES

1. Kessler RC, Chiu WT, Demler O, Walters EE. Prevalence, severity, and comorbidity of 12-month DSM-IV disorders in the National Comorbidity Survey Replication (NCS-R). *Arch Gen Psychiatry* 2005;62:617-627.
2. Merikangas KR, Akiskal HS, Angst J, Greenberg PE, Hirschfeld RMA. Lifetime and 12-month prevalence of bipolar spectrum disorder in the national comorbidity survey replication. *Arch Gen Psychiatry.* 2007;64:543-552.
3. American Psychiatric Association. Mood disorders. In: *Diagnostic and Statistical Manual of Mental Disorder.* 4th ed. Text Revision. Washington, DC: American Psychiatric Association;2000:382.
4. Goodwin GM. Evidence-based guidelines for treating bipolar disorder: revised second edition—recommendations from the British Association for Psychopharmacology. *J Psychopharmacol.* 2009;23:346-388.
5. Hirschfeld RMA, Bowden CL, Gitlin MJ, et al. Practice guideline for the treatment of patient with bipolar disorder (revision). *Am J Psychiatry.* 2002;159:1-50.
6. Suppes T, Dennehy EB, Hirschfeld RMA, et al. The Texas implementation of medication algorithms: update to the algorithms for treatment of bipolar I disorder. *J Clin Psychiatry.* 2005;66:870-886.
7. Peet M, Pratt JP. Lithium: current status in psychiatric disorders. *Drugs.* 1993;46:7-17.
8. Ernst CL, Goldberg JF. The reproductive safety profile of mood stabilizers, atypical antipsychotics, and broad-spectrum psychotropics. *J Clin Psychiatry.* 2002;63(suppl 4):42-55.
9. Freeman TW, Clothier JL, Pazzaglia P, Lesem MD, Swann AC. A double-blind comparison of valproate and lithium in the treatment of acute mania. *Am J Psychiatry.* 1992;149: 108-111.
10. Lindhout D, Meinardi H. Spina bifida and in-utero-exposure to valproate (letter). *Lancet.* 1984;2:396.
11. Crawford P, Appleton R, Betts T, Duncan J, Guthrie E, Morrow J for The Women With Epilepsy Guidelines Development Group. Best practice guidelines for the management of women with epilepsy. *Seizure.* 1999;8:201-17.
12. Goodwin GM, Bowden CL, Calabrese JR, et al. A pooled analysis of 2 placebo-controlled 18 month trials of lamotrigine and lithium maintenance in bipolar I disorder. *J Clin Psychiatry.* 2004;65:432-441.
13. Lamictal [package insert]. Research Triangle Park, NC: GlaxoSmithKline; 2009.
14. Pratoomsri W, Yatham LN, Bond DJ, Lam RW, Sohn CH. Oxcarbazepine in the treatment of bipolar disorder: a review. *Can J Psychiatry.* 2006;51:540-545.
15. Marcotte D. Use of topiramate, a new anti-epileptic as a mood stabilizer. *J Affect Disord.* 1998;50:245-251.
16. Chengappa KNR, Gershon S, Levine J. The evolving role of topiramate among other mood stabilizers in the management of bipolar disorder. *Bipolar Disord.* 2001;3:215-232.
17. Pande AC, Crockatt JG, Janney CA, Werth JL, Tsaroucha G for Gabapentin Bipolar Disorder Study Group. Gabapentin in bipolar disorder: a placebo-controlled trial of adjunctive therapy. *Bipolar Disord.* 2000;2:249-255.
18. Mishory A, Yaroslavsky Y, Bersudsky Y, Belmaker RH. Phenytoin as an antimanic anticonvulsant: a controlled study. *Am J Psychiatry.* 2000;157:463-465.
19. McElroy SL, Suppes T, Keck PE, et al. Open-label adjunctive zonisamide in the treatment of bipolar disorders: a prospective trial. *J Clin Psychiatry.* 2005;66:617-624.
20. Post RM, Altshuler LL, Frye MA, et al. Preliminary observation on the effectiveness of levetiracetam in the open adjunctive treatment of refractory bipolar disorder. *J Clin Psychiatry.* 2005;66:370-374.
21. Risperdal Consta [package insert]. Titusville, NJ: Janssen; 2009.

22. Peet M. Induction of mania with selective serotonin re-uptake inhibitors and tricyclic antidepressants. *Br J Psychiatry*. 1994; 164:549-550.
23. Sachs GS, Lafer B, Stoll AL, et al. A double-blind trial of bupropion versus desipramine for bipolar depression. *J Clin Psychiatry*. 1994;55:391-393.
24. Barton BM, Gitlin MJ. Verapamil in treatment-resistant mania: an open trial. *J Clin Psychopharmacol*. 1987;7:101-103.
25. Freeman MP, Hibbeln JR, Wisner KL, et al. Omega-3 fatty acids: evidence basis for treatment and future research in psychiatry. *J Clin Psychiatry*. 2006;67:1954-1967.
26. Stoll AL, Severus E, Freeman MP, et al. Omega-3 fatty acids in bipolar disorder: a preliminary double-blind, placebo-controlled trial. *Arch Gen Psychiatry*. 1999;56:407-412.
27. Yonkers KA, Wisner LK, Stowe Z, et al. Management of bipolar disorder during pregnancy and the postpartum period. *Am J Psychiatry*. 2004;161:608-620.

CHAPTER

55 Anxiety Disorders

Kelly C. Lee

FOUNDATION OVERVIEW

Anxiety disorders, as a group, are the most common psychiatric disorders in the United States with the exception of substance abuse disorders.[1] Anxiety disorders are divided into six different disorders with different clinical presentations, prevalence/incidence, pathophysiology, treatments, and prognosis. These include panic disorder (PD), generalized anxiety disorder (GAD), obsessive-compulsive disorder (OCD), post-traumatic stress disorder (PTSD), social anxiety disorder (SAD), and specific phobic disorders. Specific phobia refers to an individual's phobia or fear of certain objects or situations and is rarely treated with medications.[2] Specific phobia will not be addressed in this chapter. It should also be noted that for patients to be diagnosed with any of the anxiety disorders discussed below, the symptoms must not be due to a general medical condition or substance and the symptoms must cause significant impairment in social or occupational functioning.[2]

Panic Disorder

The lifetime prevalence of PD is 1.6% to 2.2%, although 10% to 15% of the population may experience a single panic attack during their lifetime.[3] Panic disorder is characterized by at least two unexpected panic attacks with associated anticipatory anxiety for at least 1 month.[2] Those with PD may have associated agoraphobia or the fear of being in a place or situation where escape may be difficult. Panic attack is characterized by somatic or cognitive symptoms such as chest pain, palpitations, sweating, shortness of breath, fear of dying, dizziness, or hot flashes. These symptoms appear suddenly and last about 10 minutes. While patients can have multiple panic attacks in their lifetime, they may not necessarily have a PD. Patients with PD have approximately 40% lifetime prevalence of comorbid major depressive disorder (MDD).[4]

Generalized Anxiety Disorder

Generalized anxiety disorder is experienced by 5% of individuals during their lifetime and lasts for at least 6 months. It is characterized by chronic excessive worry and anxiety about life events.[2] Additional symptoms may include feeling restless, difficulty concentrating, muscle tension or sleep disturbance, and easy fatigueability. Generalized anxiety disorder is more common among women and usually has a long course of illness. There does not appear to be a genetic link to development of GAD and there is a high incidence of comorbidity with MDD.

Obsessive-Compulsive Disorder

The lifetime prevalence of OCD is 1.6% and men tend to have an earlier onset of symptoms than women.[5] There is a strong genetic link for OCD, as well as an association with antistreptococcal antibodies in a subgroup of children with OCD or tic disorders.[6] Patients with OCD have either obsessions, compulsions, or both obsessions and compulsions. Obsessions are marked by recurrent and persistent thoughts that are inappropriate and cause significant anxiety in the person.[2] Compulsions are characterized by repetitive behaviors that a person feels driven to perform. Adults who have either obsessions or compulsions recognize that these feelings are excessive, but they are unable to control these thoughts or actions. These behaviors generally take more than 1 h/d.

Post-Traumatic Stress Disorder

Post-traumatic stress disorder is characterized by a collection of symptoms that occur after exposure to a traumatic event such as military combat or violent personal attack. Symptoms must be present for 1 month and must include the following types of symptoms: reexperiencing (flashbacks, dreams), avoidance (of activities or people associated with the trauma), and increased arousal (sleep disturbance, exaggerated startle response).[2] There is a wide range for prevalence rates depending on groups that are studied but community-based studies estimate about 8% lifetime prevalence.[7] Comorbidity with another psychiatric illness such as MDD is common in patients with PTSD, and duration and severity of the trauma are the most significant predictors for development of PTSD. Most symptoms of PTSD occur within 3 months of exposure to the trauma but they can appear at any time during a patient's lifetime.

Social Anxiety Disorder

Patients with SAD have a persistent fear of at least one or more social or performance situations that make them embarrassed or fearful of being scrutinized or humiliated.[2] They may have a fear of performing tasks in public, such as speaking, eating, or writing. The social exposure produces significant anxiety to the point that they may lead to panic attacks or avoidance of public situations. The lifetime prevalence of SAD is 3% to 13% and patients have an increased risk of developing SAD if the condition is present in a relative.[8] Patients may have SAD during the entire lifetime although the severity may fluctuate with stressors. Social anxiety disorder is commonly comorbid with alcohol abuse disorders.

TREATMENT

The goals of treatment for anxiety disorders are to reduce symptoms and prevent recurrence of symptoms or episodes. Anxiety disorders are often difficult to treat because of the chronic course of illness. Medications need to be titrated to an effective dose and they are most effective when combined with psychotherapy. Patients should be educated on the importance of medication adherence with panic disorders. Nonpharmacologic treatment of anxiety disorders usually involves cognitive-behavioral therapy (CBT), which is a form of psychotherapy. Cognitive-behavioral therapy is considered first line for treating all anxiety disorders either as monotherapy or in combination with pharmacologic treatment, depending on the severity and duration of illness.

There are three major classes of medications that are used to treat most anxiety disorders: antidepressants, benzodiazepines, and buspirone. Antidepressants include selective serotonin reuptake inhibitors (SSRIs), atypical antidepressants (venlafaxine, duloxetine), and tricyclic antidepressants (TCAs). While other antidepressants such as bupropion, mirtazapine, nefazodone, and monoamine oxidase inhibitors (MAOIs) may be used in some anxiety disorders, their limited effectiveness and tolerability place them as third- or fourth-line agents. These agents will not be discussed in this section. Table 55-1 lists the medications that have been approved for use in different anxiety disorders. Antidepressants may increase anxiety or restlessness at the initiation of therapy in patients with anxiety disorders; therefore, lowest effective dose should be used and doses should be titrated slowly.

Selective Serotonin Reuptake Inhibitors

Selective serotonin reuptake inhibitors are generally effective for most anxiety disorders regardless of their FDA-approved indications. The SSRIs work by preventing the reuptake of serotonin by the presynaptic neuron, thereby leaving more serotonin in the synaptic cleft. The mechanism of how these agents work in anxiety disorders is generally unknown. They are considered first line for treating all of the anxiety disorders due to their tolerability, safety, and decreased risk for dependence and/or withdrawal. All of the SSRIs are available orally in tablet/capsule and all of them are available in liquid formulation except for fluvoxamine.

The most common adverse effects of SSRIs include sleep disturbances, gastrointestinal upset, headache, and sexual dysfunction.[9] With the exception of sexual dysfunction, most of the adverse effects are limited to the first 2 weeks of therapy. All of the SSRIs are metabolized by the liver, so caution should be exercised in patients with significant liver function impairment. The use of SSRIs is contraindicated in patients who are also receiving MAOIs and caution should be used in those who are also receiving other agents that increase serotonin, such as TCAs, venlafaxine, duloxetine, and nefazodone. Upon discontinuation of SSRIs, patients must wait 2 weeks before starting therapy with MAOIs. Selective serotonin reuptake inhibitors may also interact with nonpsychiatric medications such as linezolid and serotonin 1A agonists such as sumatriptan and

TABLE 55-1 FDA-Indicated Antidepressants for Treatment of Anxiety Disorders

Anxiety Disorder	Fluoxetine	Paroxetine	Fluvoxamine	Sertraline	Escitalopram	Venlafaxine XR	Duloxetine	Buspirone	Clomipramine
Panic disorder	X	X		X		X			
Generalized anxiety disorder		X			X	X	X	X	
Obsessive-compulsive disorder	X	X	X	X					X
Post-traumatic stress disorder		X		X					
Social anxiety disorder		X	X[a]	X		X			

[a]Luvox CR only.

increase the risk of serotonin syndrome. Pharmacokinetic drug interactions are common and many SSRIs inhibit the cytochrome P450 enzymes. Most notably, fluoxetine inhibits CYP2C9/2C19, CYP2D6, and CYP3A4 enzymes, fluvoxamine inhibits CYP1A2 enzyme, and paroxetine is a potent inhibitor of CYP2D6 enzyme. Drugs that undergo metabolism by these enzymes may have elevated concentrations if they are given concomitantly with these antidepressants. Withdrawal symptoms may also occur upon abrupt discontinuation of SSRIs with short half-lives such as paroxetine. Dosing should be individualized per patient and the specific anxiety disorder that is being treated. In general, treatment of OCD requires higher doses than those used for depression.[10]

Selective serotonin reuptake inhibitors and serotonin norepinephrine reuptake inhibitors are considered superior to other classes of agents for use in PTSD. While many adjunctive agents may be used to treat specific symptoms of PTSD, antidepressants should be the treatment of choice for long-term management of PTSD.

Atypical Antidepressants

Venlafaxine is a serotonin and norepinephrine reuptake inhibitor that is used for multiple anxiety disorders (see Table 55-1).[9] It does not have anticholinergic, alpha-adrenergic blocking or antihistaminic properties. The most common adverse effects of venlafaxine include gastrointestinal upset, sedation, sexual dysfunction, and dose-related hypertension (at doses >150 mg/d). Dosing in anxiety disorders is similar to that used for depression. Venlafaxine also has a short half-life which may predispose a patient to withdrawal symptoms if the medication is discontinued abruptly. Withdrawal symptoms may include agitation, dizziness, sensory disturbances, sweating, and tremor. Duloxetine is another serotonin and norepinephrine reuptake inhibitor and is approved for use in GAD. Duloxetine is most often associated with nausea, dry mouth, constipation, and sexual dysfunction. Venlafaxine and duloxetine should not be used in combination with MAOIs. Both drugs are available orally either in tablet or capsule forms.

Tricyclic Antidepressants

Tricyclic antidepressants, while efficacious for anxiety disorders, have been designated as second line to SSRIs because of their adverse effect profile and toxicity in overdose situations. These agents block the reuptake of serotonin and norepinephrine but they also inhibit muscarinic, histaminic, and alpha-adrenergic receptors. These additional receptors are responsible for the myriad of adverse effects such as sedation, dry mouth, weight gain, and orthostasis that are common with TCAs. Tricyclic antidepressants also have the potential to lower seizure threshold, cause sexual dysfunction, and induce cardiac arrhythmias in overdose situations. Of the TCAs, imipramine and clomipramine have been widely studied in PD.[11] Clomipramine has been shown to be the most efficacious TCA for OCD and is often used in patients who are refractory to SSRIs. Tricyclic antidepressants have minimal or conflicting evidence for use in PTSD and SAD. One of the advantages of TCAs is that levels of the drugs can be measured—levels may be useful in situations of overdose, nonadherence, and toxicity. Liver function test should also be monitored during TCA treatment. Most of the TCAs undergo metabolism by CYP2D6 enzyme; therefore, concomitant drugs that inhibit or induce this enzyme may elevate or lower the TCA concentration, respectively.[9] The use of TCAs with MAOIs is contraindicated. Alcohol and other CNS depressants should also be avoided.

Benzodiazepines

Benzodiazepines act at the GABA-A receptors and act to increase the frequency of opening of chloride channels in the presence of GABA.[9] Benzodiazepines may be used on a short-term basis during the initial period when an antidepressant is initiated. They may also be used on scheduled basis in lieu of antidepressant when a patient cannot tolerate an antidepressant. Finally, some patients may use benzodiazepines on an as needed basis in combination with antidepressants. Benzodiazepines are widely used as monotherapy or adjunctive agents in PD. The utility of benzodiazepines in other anxiety disorders are often as second- or third-line agents due to the potential for physical dependence and abuse. Benzodiazepines are sometimes preferred by patients due to their rapid onset of effect compared to antidepressants. The most common adverse effects of benzodiazepines are sedation, cognitive impairment, anterograde amnesia, respiratory depression, and dependence. Paradoxical effects such as excitation and disinhibition, especially in elderly and younger patients, may also occur. Abrupt discontinuation of long-term benzodiazepine treatment should be avoided to minimize the risk of withdrawal symptoms and seizures. Benzodiazepines differ in pharmacokinetic properties (Table 55-2). Benzodiazepines that have short durations of action have the highest potential for withdrawal symptoms and risk for physical dependence. Benzodiazepines that undergo

TABLE 55-2 **Pharmacokinetic Properties of Benzodiazepines**

Benzodiazepine	Onset	Duration	Metabolism
Alprazolam	Intermediate	Short	Oxidation
Clonazepam	Intermediate	Long	Nitroreduction
Diazepam	Very fast	Short (single dose) Long (chronic dose)	Oxidation
Lorazepam	Intermediate (single dose)	Short	Conjugation
Oxazepam	Slow	Intermediate	Conjugation
Temazepam	Slow	Intermediate	Conjugation

conjugative metabolism are preferred in patients who have liver dysfunction, are elderly, or on concomitant medications that may induce or inhibit cytochrome P450 enzymes.[9] Triazolobenzodiazepines (alprazolam, triazolam, and midazolam) are significantly affected by CYP3A4 inhibitors and inducers; caution should be used when these drugs are combined. Benzodiazepines are available in oral formulation as well as IM and IV formulations. Lorazepam administered as IM injections produce more reliable absorption and concentration compared to diazepam.

Buspirone

While the exact mechanism of buspirone is unclear, the primary pharmacologic activity is theorized as a serotonin 1A partial agonist.[9] Buspirone is primarily indicated for use in GAD. It does not have any benzodiazepine-like or antidepressant properties, but it is used commonly with SSRI for antidepressant augmentation. Similar to antidepressants, the onset of effect is at least 2 weeks and full effect may not be observed until 4 to 6 weeks. Buspirone is an option in those who have not responded to or cannot tolerate antidepressants. In addition, buspirone may be desired in those patients with a substance abuse history when benzodiazepines should be avoided. The most common adverse effects of buspirone are nausea, headache, and jitteriness. The drug is metabolized by CYP3A4 and caution is advised when combining other serotonergic agents. Buspirone is also contraindicated for use with MAOIs. Buspirone is available in tablet formulation.

Special Populations

General

All antidepressants have the potential to exacerbate anxiety symptoms when initiated in patients with anxiety disorders. In patients with PD, antidepressants such as SSRIs can precipitate panic attacks. Caution should be used when initiating these agents and the lowest dose should be used with slow titration. Tricyclic antidepressants should be avoided in patients with active suicidality due to its potential for death in an overdose situation. These agents have narrow therapeutic windows and can cause life-threatening arrhythmias with relatively low doses.

Benzodiazepines should be avoided in patients with active substance abuse/dependence or histories of abuse/dependence. Patients should be cautioned against combining CNS depressants like alcohol with benzodiazepines. Benzodiazepines should be avoided in elderly patients due to the increased risk for impaired cognition, falls, and hip fractures.

Pregnancy

The decision to use psychotropic agents during pregnancy should be based upon the risks and benefits to both the mother and fetus. While some women may want to avoid any medications during pregnancy, the severity of the anxiety disorder and the potential risks of not treating the illness should be considered.

The safety of SSRIs during pregnancy has been studied extensively and has led to labeling changes by the manufacturer. Paroxetine, when taken during the first trimester, has been associated with fetal heart defects and has a pregnancy category D.[12] The other SSRIs have pregnancy category C and risks must be balanced against the benefit of use during pregnancy. In the second trimester, SSRIs have been associated with persistent pulmonary hypertension (PPHN) in newborns. Based upon this data, the American College of Obstetricians and Gynecologists recommend that paroxetine be avoided if possible during the first trimester.[13]

Poor neonatal adaptation syndrome (or neonatal withdrawal syndrome) has been reported in 15% to 30% of women with major depression who took SSRIs in late pregnancy.[14-15] Symptoms may include hypoglycemia, irritability, temperature instability, and seizures in the infant. Symptoms are usually transient and usually resolve by 2 weeks after delivery.

Benzodiazepines have been associated with the risk of cleft lip/palate and other defects and should be avoided during first trimester of pregnancy. When used in the third trimester, they can cause sedation and withdrawal symptoms in the newborn. Benzodiazepines have a pregnancy category D. Buspirone has a pregnancy category B and is considered generally safe for use in pregnancy.

Lactation

Benzodiazepines should be avoided during lactation as they pass into the breast milk and can cause lethargy and temperature dysregulation in the infant. All SSRIs pass into the breast milk and have been rarely associated with various symptoms in the infant such as irritability, crying, poor feeding, and colic-like symptoms.[9]

Children and Adolescents

The use of antidepressants in children and adolescents is controversial in many anxiety disorders. Fluoxetine is FDA-indicated for use in children with OCD and sertraline is FDA-indicated for OCD in children and adolescents. All of the SSRIs and atypical antidepressants are labeled with a black box warning for suicidality in children and young adults (up to age 24 years old). A medication guide should be dispensed with all prescriptions for these medications. Patients should be monitored for signs and symptoms of increased agitation, anxiety, or changes in mood/behavior especially at the initiation of therapy or dose changes.

CASE Application

1. Buspirone is most likely used in the treatment of which anxiety disorder?
    a. Generalized anxiety disorder
    b. Obsessive-compulsive disorder
    c. Panic disorder
    d. Post-traumatic stress disorder
    e. Social anxiety disorder

2. Which of the following benzodiazepines has the longest duration of action at steady state?
   a. Alprazolam
   b. Clonazepam
   c. Diazepam
   d. Triazolam
   e. Lorazepam

3. Which of the following antidepressants is the most appropriate initial treatment for social anxiety disorder?
   a. Fluvoxamine
   b. Mirtazapine
   c. Nefazodone
   d. Trazodone
   e. Venlafaxine

4. The most significant concern for patients with panic disorder starting an antidepressant is:
   a. Anxiety
   b. Bruxism
   c. Gastrointestinal upset
   d. Headache
   e. Sexual dysfunction

5. The generic name for Cymbalta is:
   a. Duloxetine
   b. Escitalopram
   c. Nefazodone
   d. Trazodone
   e. Venlafaxine

6. Which of the following medications is most effective for obsessive-compulsive disorder?
   a. Buspirone
   b. Clomipramine
   c. Clonazepam
   d. Nefazodone
   e. Venlafaxine

7. For the treatment of anxiety disorders, which of the following is an advantage of an SSRI compared to a tricyclic antidepressant?
   a. Safer in overdose
   b. Less likely to cause sedation
   c. Can treat comorbid depression
   d. Less likely to cause gastrointestinal upset
   e. Less likely to cause insomnia

8. The SSRIs are effective for treating which of the following anxiety disorders?
   a. Generalized anxiety disorder
   b. Obsessive-compulsive disorder
   c. Post-traumatic stress disorder
   d. Panic disorder
   e. All of the above

9. Patients with significant impairment in liver function may receive which of the following benzodiazepines to minimize risk of adverse effects?
   a. Alprazolam, clonazepam, estazolam
   b. Chlordiazepoxide, clorazepate, diazepam
   c. Lorazepam, oxazepam, temazepam
   d. Lorazepam, clonazepam, triazolam
   e. Diazepam, clonazepam, lorazepam

10. The most significant dose-related adverse effect of venlafaxine is:
    a. Sedation
    b. Seizures
    c. Hypertension
    d. Hepatotoxicity
    e. Renal dysfunction

11. Valproic acid is used to treat irritability and impulse control in patients with which anxiety disorder?
    a. Panic disorder
    b. Generalized anxiety disorder
    c. Social anxiety disorder
    d. Obsessive-compulsive disorder
    e. Post-traumatic stress disorder

12. Alprazolam is most likely to have a significant drug–drug interaction with which of the following medications?
    a. Citalopram
    b. Carbamazepine
    c. Paroxetine
    d. Phenytoin
    e. Warfarin

13. Which of the following medications has the highest risk for withdrawal symptoms?
    a. Clonazepam
    b. Diazepam
    c. Lorazepam
    d. Midazolam
    e. Triazolam

14. The mechanism of action of buspirone is:
    a. Selective serotonin reuptake inhibitor
    b. Serotonin and norepinephrine reuptake inhibitor
    c. Dopamine 2A partial agonist
    d. Serotonin 1A partial agonist
    e. Serotonin and dopamine antagonist

15. JK is a 38-year-old man with panic disorder who needs treatment. He has also recently completed an alcohol detoxification program. Which of the following treatment is most appropriate for JK?
    a. Alprazolam
    b. Diazepam
    c. Imipramine

d. Phenelzine
e. Sertraline

16. Which of the following nonpharmacologic treatments are effective for treating most anxiety disorders?
    a. Cognitive-behavioral therapy
    b. Dialectical behavior therapy
    c. Exposure therapy
    d. Hypnotic therapy
    e. Interpersonal therapy

17. A 32-year-old pregnant woman in her first trimester presents with worsening of her OCD symptoms. Due to the potential risk of her compulsive behaviors on her fetus, she has agreed to start pharmacologic treatment. Which of the following agents should be avoided?
    a. Citalopram
    b. Fluoxetine
    c. Fluvoxamine
    d. Paroxetine
    e. Sertraline

18. Which of the following medications has the lowest risk of causing serotonin syndrome when combined with sertraline?
    a. Clonazepam
    b. Fluoxetine
    c. Imipramine
    d. Phenelzine
    e. Venlafaxine

19. The brand name for escitalopram is:
    a. Celexa
    b. Effexor
    c. Lexapro
    d. Paxil
    e. Zoloft

20. Benzodiazepines should be avoided in pregnant women during the first trimester due to the risk of:
    a. Cleft palate
    b. Heart defects
    c. Limb abnormalities
    d. Pulmonary hypertension
    e. Renal defects

TAKEAWAY POINTS ››

- Anxiety disorders are the most common psychiatric disorders and include panic disorder, generalized anxiety disorder, obsessive-compulsive disorder, post-traumatic stress disorder, and social anxiety disorder.
- Selective serotonin reuptake inhibitors are first-line agents to treat anxiety disorders and can treat acute symptoms as well as prevent recurrent symptoms.
- Selective serotonin reuptake inhibitors should be recommended during pregnancy if benefits outweigh the risks to the fetus; paroxetine should be avoided if possible.
- Atypical antidepressants such as venlafaxine and duloxetine are effective for selected anxiety disorders and are preferred over TCAs and benzodiazepines.
- Tricyclic antidepressants are reserved as third- or fourth-line agents to treat anxiety disorders due to their tolerability and safety profiles.
- Benzodiazepines may be used as sole treatment or as adjunctive agents to treat anxiety disorders; however, caution should be used in high-risk populations such as patients with substance abuse problems, elderly patients, and patients who are pregnant.
- Buspirone is reserved for use in generalized anxiety disorder and does not have any risk for physical dependence or abuse.

REFERENCES

1. Kessler RC, McGonagle KA, Zhao S, et al. Lifetime and 12-month prevalence of DSM-III-R psychiatric disorders in the United States. Results from the National Comorbidity Survey. *Arch Gen Psychiatry*. 1994;51:8-19.
2. American Psychiatric Association. Task Force on DSM-IV. *Diagnostic and Statistical Manual of Mental Disorders: DSM-IV-TR*. 4th ed. Text Revision. Washington, DC: American Psychiatric Association; 2000.
3. Weissman MM, Bland RC, Canino GJ, et al. The cross-national epidemiology of panic disorder. *Arch Gen Psychiatry*. 1997;54:305-309.
4. Kessler RC, Chiu WT, Jin R, Ruscio AM, Shear K, Walters EE. The epidemiology of panic attacks, panic disorder, and agoraphobia in the National Comorbidity Survey Replication. *Arch Gen Psychiatry*. 2006;63:415-424.
5. Torres AR, Prince MJ, Bebbington PE, et al. Obsessive-compulsive disorder: prevalence, comorbidity, impact, and help-seeking in the British National Psychiatric Morbidity Survey of 2000. *Am J Psychiatry*. 2006;163:1978-1985.
6. Mell LK, Davis RL, Owens D. Association between streptococcal infection and obsessive-compulsive disorder, Tourette's syndrome, and tic disorder. *Pediatrics*. 2005; 116:56-60.
7. Kessler RC, Sonnega A, Bromet E, Hughes M, Nelson CB. Post-traumatic stress disorder in the National Comorbidity Survey. *Arch Gen Psychiatry*. 1995;52:1048-1060.

d. Phenelzine
e. Sertraline

16. Which of the following nonpharmacologic treatments are effective for treating most anxiety disorders?

a. Cognitive-behavioral therapy
b. Dialectical behavior therapy
c. Exposure therapy
d. Hypnotic therapy
e. Interpersonal therapy

17. A 32-year-old pregnant woman in her first trimester presents with worsening of her OCD symptoms. Due to the potential risk of her compulsive behaviors on her fetus, she has agreed to start pharmacologic treatment. Which of the following agents should be avoided?

a. Citalopram
b. Fluoxetine
c. Fluvoxamine
d. Paroxetine
e. Sertraline

18. Which of the following medications has the lowest risk of causing serotonin syndrome when combined with sertraline?

a. Clonazepam
b. Fluoxetine
c. Imipramine
d. Phenelzine
e. Venlafaxine

19. The brand name for escitalopram is:

a. Celexa
b. Effexor
c. Lexapro
d. Paxil
e. Zoloft

20. Benzodiazepines should be avoided in pregnant women during the first trimester due to the risk of:

a. Cleft palate
b. Heart defects
c. Limb abnormalities
d. Pulmonary hypertension
e. Renal defects

TAKEAWAY POINTS ››

- Anxiety disorders are the most common psychiatric disorders and include panic disorder, generalized anxiety disorder, obsessive-compulsive disorder, post-traumatic stress disorder, and social anxiety disorder.
- Selective serotonin reuptake inhibitors are first-line agents to treat anxiety disorders and can treat acute symptoms as well as prevent recurrent symptoms.
- Selective serotonin reuptake inhibitors should be recommended during pregnancy if benefits outweigh the risks to the fetus; paroxetine should be avoided if possible.
- Atypical antidepressants such as venlafaxine and duloxetine are effective for selected anxiety disorders and are preferred over TCAs and benzodiazepines.
- Tricyclic antidepressants are reserved as third- or fourth-line agents to treat anxiety disorders due to their tolerability and safety profiles.
- Benzodiazepines may be used as sole treatment or as adjunctive agents to treat anxiety disorders; however, caution should be used in high-risk populations such as patients with substance abuse problems, elderly patients, and patients who are pregnant.
- Buspirone is reserved for use in generalized anxiety disorder and does not have any risk for physical dependence or abuse.

REFERENCES

1. Kessler RC, McGonagle KA, Zhao S, et al. Lifetime and 12-month prevalence of DSM-III-R psychiatric disorders in the United States. Results from the National Comorbidity Survey. *Arch Gen Psychiatry*. 1994;51:8-19.
2. American Psychiatric Association. Task Force on DSM-IV. *Diagnostic and Statistical Manual of Mental Disorders: DSM-IV-TR*. 4th ed. Text Revision. Washington, DC: American Psychiatric Association; 2000.
3. Weissman MM, Bland RC, Canino GJ, et al. The cross-national epidemiology of panic disorder. *Arch Gen Psychiatry*. 1997;54:305-309.
4. Kessler RC, Chiu WT, Jin R, Ruscio AM, Shear K, Walters EE. The epidemiology of panic attacks, panic disorder, and agoraphobia in the National Comorbidity Survey Replication. *Arch Gen Psychiatry*. 2006;63:415-424.
5. Torres AR, Prince MJ, Bebbington PE, et al. Obsessive-compulsive disorder: prevalence, comorbidity, impact, and help-seeking in the British National Psychiatric Morbidity Survey of 2000. *Am J Psychiatry*. 2006;163:1978-1985.
6. Mell LK, Davis RL, Owens D. Association between streptococcal infection and obsessive-compulsive disorder, Tourette's syndrome, and tic disorder. *Pediatrics*. 2005; 116:56-60.
7. Kessler RC, Sonnega A, Bromet E, Hughes M, Nelson CB. Post-traumatic stress disorder in the National Comorbidity Survey. *Arch Gen Psychiatry*. 1995;52:1048-1060.

2. Which of the following benzodiazepines has the longest duration of action at steady state?

   a. Alprazolam
   b. Clonazepam
   c. Diazepam
   d. Triazolam
   e. Lorazepam

3. Which of the following antidepressants is the most appropriate initial treatment for social anxiety disorder?

   a. Fluvoxamine
   b. Mirtazapine
   c. Nefazodone
   d. Trazodone
   e. Venlafaxine

4. The most significant concern for patients with panic disorder starting an antidepressant is:

   a. Anxiety
   b. Bruxism
   c. Gastrointestinal upset
   d. Headache
   e. Sexual dysfunction

5. The generic name for Cymbalta is:

   a. Duloxetine
   b. Escitalopram
   c. Nefazodone
   d. Trazodone
   e. Venlafaxine

6. Which of the following medications is most effective for obsessive-compulsive disorder?

   a. Buspirone
   b. Clomipramine
   c. Clonazepam
   d. Nefazodone
   e. Venlafaxine

7. For the treatment of anxiety disorders, which of the following is an advantage of an SSRI compared to a tricyclic antidepressant?

   a. Safer in overdose
   b. Less likely to cause sedation
   c. Can treat comorbid depression
   d. Less likely to cause gastrointestinal upset
   e. Less likely to cause insomnia

8. The SSRIs are effective for treating which of the following anxiety disorders?

   a. Generalized anxiety disorder
   b. Obsessive-compulsive disorder
   c. Post-traumatic stress disorder
   d. Panic disorder
   e. All of the above

9. Patients with significant impairment in liver function may receive which of the following benzodiazepines to minimize risk of adverse effects?

   a. Alprazolam, clonazepam, estazolam
   b. Chlordiazepoxide, clorazepate, diazepam
   c. Lorazepam, oxazepam, temazepam
   d. Lorazepam, clonazepam, triazolam
   e. Diazepam, clonazepam, lorazepam

10. The most significant dose-related adverse effect of venlafaxine is:

    a. Sedation
    b. Seizures
    c. Hypertension
    d. Hepatotoxicity
    e. Renal dysfunction

11. Valproic acid is used to treat irritability and impulse control in patients with which anxiety disorder?

    a. Panic disorder
    b. Generalized anxiety disorder
    c. Social anxiety disorder
    d. Obsessive-compulsive disorder
    e. Post-traumatic stress disorder

12. Alprazolam is most likely to have a significant drug–drug interaction with which of the following medications?

    a. Citalopram
    b. Carbamazepine
    c. Paroxetine
    d. Phenytoin
    e. Warfarin

13. Which of the following medications has the highest risk for withdrawal symptoms?

    a. Clonazepam
    b. Diazepam
    c. Lorazepam
    d. Midazolam
    e. Triazolam

14. The mechanism of action of buspirone is:

    a. Selective serotonin reuptake inhibitor
    b. Serotonin and norepinephrine reuptake inhibitor
    c. Dopamine 2A partial agonist
    d. Serotonin 1A partial agonist
    e. Serotonin and dopamine antagonist

15. JK is a 38-year-old man with panic disorder who needs treatment. He has also recently completed an alcohol detoxification program. Which of the following treatment is most appropriate for JK?

    a. Alprazolam
    b. Diazepam
    c. Imipramine

8. Kessler RC, Chiu WT, Demler O, Merikangas KR, Walters EE. Prevalence, severity, and comorbidity of 12-month DSM-IV disorders in the National Comorbidity Survey Replication. *Arch Gen Psychiatry*. 2005;62:617-627.
9. Selective serotonin reuptake inhibitors. Drug Facts and Comparisons. Facts & Comparisons® eAnswers [online]. 2010. Available from Wolters Kluwer Health, Inc. Accessed October 6, 2010.
10. Koran LM, Hanna GL, Hollander E, Nestadt G, Simpson HB. Practice guideline for the treatment of patients with obsessive-compulsive disorder. *Am J Psychiatry*. 2007;164:5-53.
11. Work Group on Panic Disorder. Practice guideline for the treatment of patients with panic disorder. American Psychiatric Association. *Am J Psychiatry*. 1998;155:1-34.
12. Use of Paxil CR Tablets or Paxil Tablets During Pregnancy. Avialble at http://www.gsk.com/media/paroxetine/mi_letter_paroxetine_pregnancy.pdf. Accessed on August 28, 2009.
13. ACOG Practice Bulletin. Clinical management guidelines for obstetrician-gynecologists number 92, April 2008 (Replaces practice bulletin number 87, November 2007). Use of psychiatric medications during pregnancy and lactation. *Obstet Gynecol*. 2008;111:1001-1020.
14. Chambers CD, Hernandez-Diaz S, Van Marter LJ, et al. Selective serotonin-reuptake inhibitors and risk of persistent pulmonary hypertension of the newborn. *N Engl J Med*. 2006; 354:579-587.
15. Chambers CD, Johnson KA, Dick LM, Felix RJ. Birth outcomes in pregnant women taking fluoxetine. *N Engl J Med*. 1996; 335:1010-1015.
16. Oberlander T, Warburton W, Misri S, Aghajanian J, Hertzman C. Effects of timing and duration of gestational exposure to serotonin reuptake inhibitors: population based study. *Br J Psychiatry*. 2008;192:338-343.

CHAPTER

56 Schizophrenia

Krina H. Patel

FOUNDATION OVERVIEW

Schizophrenia is a disabling and challenging psychiatric illness. The lifetime prevalence of schizophrenia is approximately 1%.[1,2] This illness affects males and females equally and the onset occurs in the late teens to mid-thirties. The exact etiology of schizophrenia is unknown but research indicates that genetics and alteration of neurotransmitters, such as dopamine, has a significant role in the development of schizophrenia.[3]

Symptoms

One common misconception is that schizophrenia means "split personalities" or "multiple personalities." Schizophrenia, in fact, is an illness that is associated with various types of symptoms and is not a "split personality" disorder. Positive symptoms, negative symptoms, and cognitive symptoms are the different types of symptoms associated with schizophrenia.[1,4,5] Positive symptoms are symptoms that are considered an "excess" of normal functions or "added" to normal functions.[1] Delusion and hallucinations are common examples of positive symptoms. Negative symptoms are "loss" of normal functions or qualities that "subtracted" from an individual's personality.[1] Examples of common negative symptoms include alogia, avolition, and anhedonia. Negative symptoms, at times, may be more difficult to assess compared to positive symptoms since negative symptoms are also associated with other psychiatric disorders. Finally, cognitive symptoms such as impaired attention or memory may be present.[5] In addition to these symptoms, individuals with schizophrenia will likely present with social and occupational dysfunction.[1] For example, patients may have difficulty with self-care, maintaining employment or maintaining interpersonal relationships.

Diagnosis

Currently, there are no objective measures to confirm the diagnosis of schizophrenia. At present, the accepted method of diagnosing schizophrenia can be carried out by evaluating the patient's symptoms and assessing the patient to determine if he meets the criteria for schizophrenia. The Diagnostic and Statistical Manual of Mental Disorders, fourth edition, Text Revision (DSM-IV-TR) is a diagnostic reference which provides the criteria for schizophrenia diagnosis.[1] Characteristic symptoms, social and occupational dysfunction, duration and ruling out other disorders are the key components of the DSM-IV criteria for schizophrenia.

TREATMENT

The goal, when treating a patient with schizophrenia, is to develop a treatment plan that decreases symptoms, improves quality of life, and improves patient functioning while minimizing adverse effects.[4,6] The current treatment options for schizophrenia include nonpharmacolgic therapy and pharmacologic therapy. Both nonpharmacologic and pharmacologic therapy are beneficial for the treatment of schizophrenia. Nonpharmacologic therapy such as psychosocial support groups and programs generally focus on enhancing patient functioning. The use of nonpharmacologic treatment is beneficial in combination with pharmacologic treatment.[4] Antipsychotics are a mainstay for the treatment of schizophrenia. Currently the two classes of antipsychotics which are used for schizophrenia are the first-generation antipsychotics (FGAs) and the second-generation antipsychotics (SGAs). Table 56-1 provides a list of current antipsychotics. Antipsychotics are an effective class of agents that will help control the symptoms associated with schizophrenia. Both antipsychotic classes are quite effective for improving positive symptoms. However, one significant difference is that SGAs are more likely to improve negative symptoms when compared to FGAs.[5]

Pharmacologic Treatment

The FGAs, also known as the typical or conventional antipsychotics, were introduced to the market in the 1950s. The FGAs are high-affinity dopamine-2 (D_2) receptor antagonists. Currently there are several FGAs available. Although the FGAs are effective for the treatment of schizophrenia, this class is usually not considered as first-line therapy for schizophrenia due to the safety and tolerability concerns associated with this class. FGAs can induce extrapyramidal symptoms (EPS) which are movement disorders such as dystonia, akathisia, pseudoparkinsonism, and tardive dyskinesia (TD) (Table 56-2).[7] Tardive dyskinesia is an especially concerning adverse effect because in some cases it can be irreversible. The risk of EPS associated with FGAs is often why this class is not used as first-line treatment of schizophrenia. Overall, the FGAs may be further classified as high, medium, and low-potency agents; however, these agents are equally effective in equipotent doses. These agents may however differ by the adverse effect profiles. For example, low-potency agents are more likely to cause anticholinergic adverse effects, while high-potency agents are more likely to cause extrapyramidal symptoms.

TABLE 56-1 **Antipsychotics**

First-Generation Antipsychotics (FGAs)	Second-Generation Antipsychotics (SGAs)
[a]Haloperidol	Clozapine
[b]Chlorpromazine	Risperidone
[a]Fluphenazine	Olanzapine
Loxapine	Quetiapine
Molindone	Ziprasidone
Perphenazine	Aripiprazole
[a]Pimozide	Paliperidone
[b]Thioridazine	Iloperidone
[a]Thiothixene	Asenapine
Trifluoperazine	

[a]High-potency agents.
[b]Low-potency agents.

The SGAs are also referred to as atypical antipsychotics. This class of antipsychotics was introduced to the market in the 1990s and currently there are nine SGAs available. The SGAs are also D_2 receptor antagonists, however the affinity for the D_2 receptor is less when compared to FGAs.[8] The SGAs generally exhibit greater affinity toward serotonin 5-HT_2 compared to D_2 receptor affinity. Each SGA differs in their D_2 and 5HT_2 activity along with variable affinity for histamine, muscarinic and alpha receptors. This variation in mechanism of action among each SGA is one of the reasons why each displays a slightly different adverse effect profile.[8] SGAs, with the exception of clozapine, are considered as first-line treatment.[9] The use of SGAs may be advantageous due to the decreased risk EPS associated with this class. Clozapine is the only SGA with proven superior efficacy in the management of treatment-resistant patients; however, is not considered as first-line treatment due to its safety profile. Risperidone was introduced to the market after clozapine. Risperidone at higher doses (>6mg) tends to lose its atypical profile and tends to resemble a FGA. Olanzapine, quetiapine, and ziprasidone are also other SGAs which are available. Aripiprazole displays a unique mechanism different than the other SGAs. Aripiprazole exhibits both D_2 antagonist and agonist activities depending on the current dopaminergic status. Paliperidone is an extended-release formulation which is actually the active metabolite of risperidone. Iloperidone and asenapine are the two newest additions to this class of antipsychotics. Although the SGAs are within the same class, each SGA exhibits a unique mechanism and a different adverse effect profile.[8]

TABLE 56-2 **Extrapyramidal Symptoms**

Type of EPS	Common Characteristics
Dystonia	Muscle spasms (generally head and neck)
Akathisia	Restlessness, inability to sit still
Pseudoparkinsonism	Bradykinesia, rigidity, akinesia, tremor
Tardive dyskinesia	Abnormal orofacial movements, choreiform, and athetoid movements

Adverse Effects

Antipsychotics are useful and effective for the treatment of schizophrenia, however, the adverse effects associated with the class of medications may be a disadvantage for patients. Antipsychotics in general may cause adverse effects such as anticholinergic effects, sedation, EPS, metabolic abnormalities, orthostasis, QTc prolongation, and prolactin elevation. The likelihood of antipsychotics causing these adverse effects varies based on the class of antipsychotic and many times varies among each agent. For example, patients treated with FGAs are at higher risk for developing EPS, prolactin elevation, and neuroleptic malignant syndrome (NMS). A few common signs and symptoms associated with NMS include autonomic instability, altered level of consciousness, muscle rigidity, and an elevated creatine kinase.

Patients treated with SGAs are at higher risk for metabolic abnormalities. SGAs may cause metabolic abnormalities such as glucose dysregulation, lipid abnormalities, and weight gain. Clozapine and olanzapine are most likely to induce metabolic abnormalities, while aripiprazole and ziprasidone are least likely.[10] It is believed that quetiapine and risperidone have a moderate potential for metabolic abnormalities.[10] Prolactin elevation is generally associated with FGAs, however, risperidone may also cause elevated prolactin levels. Additionally, although there is a decreased risk of EPS with SGAs use compared to FGAs, the potential for EPS with SGAs is still a possibility. Risperidone at high doses (>6 mg) is more likely to cause EPS compared to lower doses. Quetiapine, on the other hand generally has a very low potential of inducing EPS. Finally, clozapine is also associated with a couple of serious adverse effects. Increased risk of seizures and the occurrence of agranulocytosis may occur with clozapine use.

Monitoring

There are several monitoring recommendations associated with antipsychotics. Patients receiving SGA treatment should have parameters such as weight, fasting lipids, fasting glucose, and blood pressure monitored.[10] Frequent monitoring of these parameters will allow detection of metabolic abnormalities which may arise. Patients receiving clozapine treatment should have their white blood cell (WBC) and absolute neutrophil count (ANC) strictly monitored (Table 56-3). If

TABLE 56-3 Clozapine Monitoring

Therapy	Frequency of Monitoring	WBC and ANC Values
First 6 mo of clozapine treatment	Weekly	WBC >3500/mm^3 ANC >2000/mm^3
6-12 mo of clozapine treatment	Every 2 wk	WBC >3500/mm^3 ANC >2000/mm^3
After 12 mo of clozapine treatment	Every 4 wk	WBC >3500/mm^3 ANC >2000/mm^3

WBC and ANC fall below the recommended values additional monitoring along with clozapine discontinuation may be necessary. Monitoring other parameters such as prolactin levels or electrocardiac abnormalities may also be recommended depending on the prescribed agent. For example, QTc monitoring is recommended with ziprasidone treatment. Also, patients receiving treatment with FGAs or risperidone should have their prolactin levels monitored. All patients should also be monitored for any signs of EPS, especially those receiving FGAs. If EPS is suspected, benzodiazepines, dopamine agonists, and anticholinergic agents such as diphenhydramine and benztropine may be utilized.

Treatment Algorithm

The treatment algorithm provides guidance for making pharmacotherapeutic recommendations for the treatment of schizophrenia (Figure 56-1).[9] The algorithm indicates that SGAs are first-line treatment and FGAs are generally initiated after the treatment failure with a SGA. The algorithm also indicates that clozapine may be used if a patient has no response with SGAs and FGAs. Combination therapy may also be utilized in later stages if no response to monotherapy is observed, however, the data supporting combination therapy are inconsistent and limited.[9] Therefore, based on the guidelines monotherapy is the mainstay of antipsychotic treatment.[9] Selection of a specific antipsychotic agent should be based on guidelines and other factors, such as cost, adverse effect profile, monitoring parameters, patient response, and adherence to treatment may also need consideration.

Treatment Adherence

Schizophrenia is a chronic disorder that requires maintenance treatment. Treatment adherence among this population may be a challenge. Some reasons for nonadherence may include presence of paranoid symptoms, medication adverse effects, and lack of insight.[11,12] Factors such as these may contribute to medication nonadherence and it may be difficult to encourage patients to continue treatment. Providing patient education as well as using long-acting formulations may be options for patients who tend to have problems with treatment adherence.[13,14]

Special Populations

The use of antipsychotics during pregnancy is a complex issue. Risks and benefits of continuing antipsychotics during pregnancy should be evaluated for each individual patient.[15,16] Discontinuing antipsychotics may put the female at risk for relapse which may lead to complications during pregnancy. Currently the association of teratogenicity with the antipsychotics is not clear. Most antipsychotics are classified as pregnancy category C and are excreted in breast milk.[16,17] In most cases a discussion with the patient to determine a treatment plan during pregnancy is the best option.

The use of antipsychotics in elderly patients with dementia-related psychosis must also be used with extreme caution. Recently a box warning was assigned to all antipsychotics indicating an increased risk of death associated with the use of antipsychotics for the treatment of dementia-related psychosis.[18] Nonpharmacologic treatment may be an option for certain patients, however, those who are nonresponsive to nonpharmacologic treatment or present with severe symptoms may require antipsychotic treatment. A careful assessment of the risks and benefits of antipsychotic treatment in this population should be considered prior to the treatment. In cases when antipsychotic treatment is a must, using lower doses and careful monitoring of adverse effects is essential.

CASE Application

1. Which of the following symptoms are associated with schizophrenia?
   a. Tangentiality and disorganized speech
   b. Flat affect and alogia
   c. Impaired memory and attention
   d. All of the above

2. Which of the following is an accepted and reliable method of diagnosing a patient with schizophrenia?
   a. Diagnosis can be confirmed by laboratory measure such as a blood test.
   b. Diagnosis can be confirmed if the patient meets the Diagnostic and Statistical Manual-IV (DSM-IV) criteria for schizophrenia.
   c. Diagnosis can be confirmed by conducting a brain imaging study on the patient.
   d. All of the above.

3. The best way to reduce the risk of relapse is:
   a. Acute treatment with antipsychotic therapy
   b. Acute treatment with nonpharmacologic therapy
   c. Maintenance treatment with nonpharmacologic therapy
   d. Maintenance treatment with antipsychotic therapy

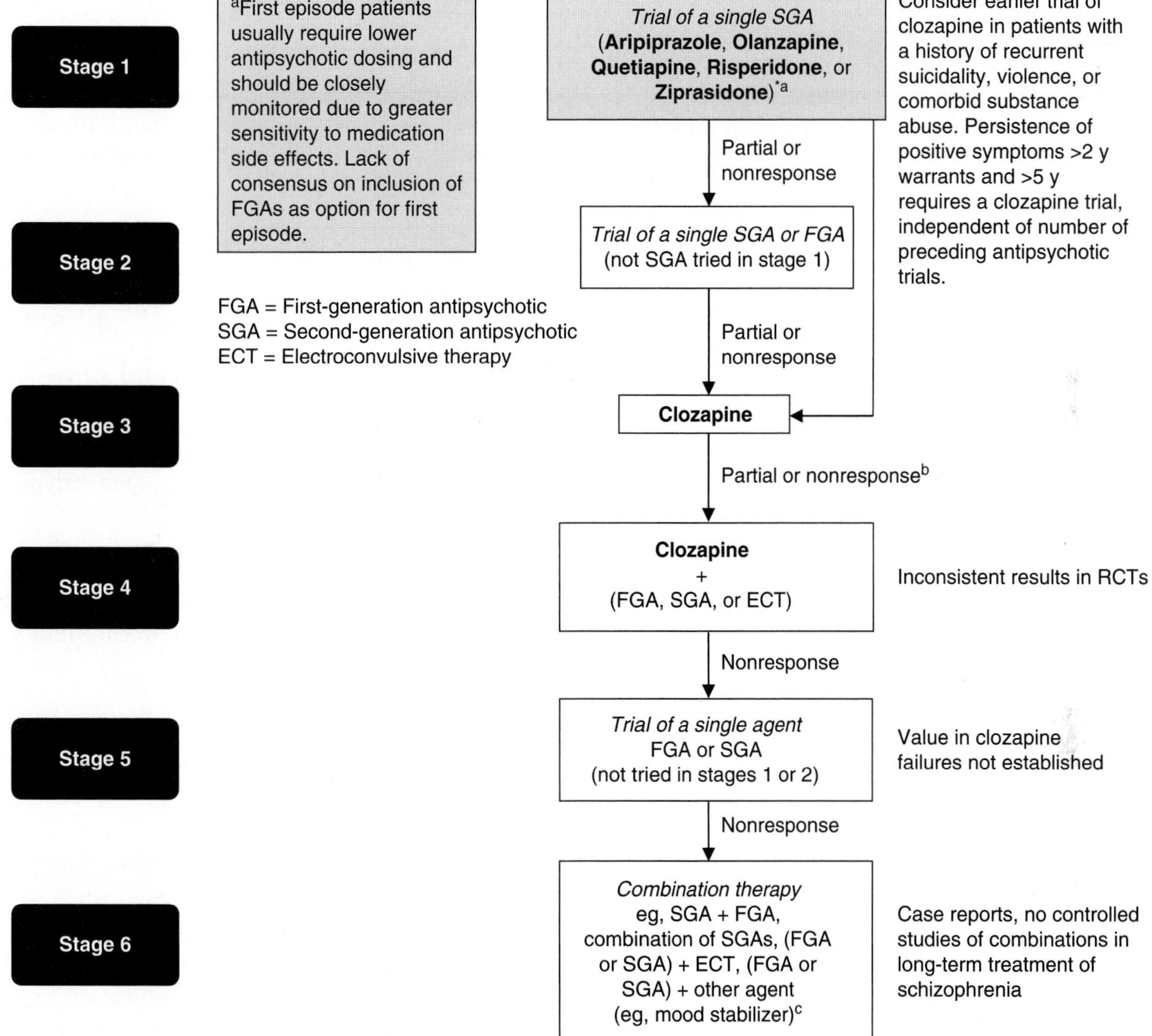

[a]If patient is inadequately adherent at any stage, the clinician should assess and consider a long-acting antipsychotic preparation, such as risperidone microspheres, haloperidol decanoate, or fluphenazine decanoate.

[b]A treatment refractory evaluation should be performed to reexamine diagnosis, substance abuse, medication adherence, and psychosocial stressors. Cognitive Behavioral Therapy (CBT) or Psychosocial augmentation should be considered.

[c]Whenever a second medication is added to an antipsychotic (other than clozapine) for the purpose of improving **psychotic** symptoms, the patient is considered to be in stage 6.

FIGURE 56-1 Algorithm for the treatment of schizophrenia.

4. Which of the following antipsychotics is most likely to improve positive symptoms, negative symptoms, and cognitive symptoms?
   a. Haloperidol
   b. Chlorpromazine
   c. Perphenazine
   d. Quetiapine

5. Which of the following antipsychotics exhibits a mechanism of action with greater affinity for D_2 receptors compared to serotonin receptors?
   a. Paliperidone
   b. Ziprasidone
   c. Haloperidol
   d. Olanzapine

6. Which of the following is *not* a SGA?
   a. Ziprasidone
   b. Fluphenazine
   c. Paliperidone
   d. Clozapine

7. MT is a 30-year-old man who is admitted to the hospital for his first psychotic episode. He is diagnosed with schizophrenia. He is not taking any medications and does not have any other medical conditions. What is the best treatment for MT?
   a. Aripiprazole
   b. Clozapine
   c. Haloperidol
   d. Chlorpromazine

8. Which of the following is an adverse effect that can occur with antipsychotic use?
   a. Anticholinergic effects
   b. Orthostasis
   c. Sedation
   d. All of the above

9. Which of the following is *not* a true statement regarding clozapine?
   a. Clozapine may cause agranulocytosis.
   b. Frequent WBC and ANC monitoring is required with clozapine.
   c. Clozapine is associated with the risk of seizures.
   d. Clozapine is not an effective agent for the treatment of schizophrenia.

10. Which of the following is a movement disorder that may occur with antipsychotic use?
    a. Akathisia
    b. Dystonia
    c. Pseudoparkinsonism
    d. Tardive dyskinesia
    e. All of the above

11. Which of the following adverse effects are most commonly associated with FGAs?
    a. Prolactin elevation and EPS
    b. Metabolic abnormalities and weight gain
    c. Pancreatitis and Stevens-Johnson syndrome
    d. Depression and mood swings

12. RT is a 35-year-old man with a recent diagnosis of schizophrenia. He is refusing to take any antipsychotics because he has read on the internet that these types of medications can cause weight gain and diabetes. After much encouragement from the psychiatrist he has agreed to try an antipsychotic. The attending psychiatrist would like to initiate RT on an antipsychotic that is least likely to cause weight gain and metabolic disturbances. Which of the following is the best option for RT?
    a. Clozapine
    b. Olanzapine
    c. Aripiprazole
    d. Any of the above agents is appropriate

13. YM is a 55-year-old man with a 20-year history of schizophrenia. He has a significant history of stopping his medications. Which of the following is the best option for YM given his history of not adhering to his medication regimen?
    a. Haloperidol decanoate
    b. Thioridazine
    c. Ziprasidone
    d. Pimozide

14. Which of the following is true regarding paliperidone?
    a. Paliperidone is a FGA.
    b. Paliperidone is a metabolite of risperidone.
    c. ANC and WBC monitoring is required with paliperidone treatment.
    d. Paliperidone is considered third-line treatment.

15. Which of the following is a recommended monitoring parameter for patients receiving treatment with a SGA?
    a. Fasting glucose
    b. Blood pressure
    c. Fasting plasma lipids
    d. Weight
    e. All of the above

16. The recommended WBC and ANC values during clozapine treatment should be:
    a. WBC $<3000/\text{mm}^3$ and ANC $<2000/\text{mm}^3$
    b. WBC $>2000/\text{mm}^3$ and ANC $>1000/\text{mm}^3$
    c. WBC $>3000/\text{mm}^3$ and ANC $>1500/\text{mm}^3$
    d. WBC $>3500/\text{mm}^3$ and ANC $>2000/\text{mm}^3$

17. SW is a 45-year-old woman with a 15-year history of schizophrenia. She was started on haloperidol a few days ago. She presents today with a stiff neck and muscle spasms. Her psychiatrist has identified this reaction as dystonia. Which of the following agents may be used to treat SW's EPS?
    a. Cyclobenzaprine
    b. Quetiapine
    c. Benztropine
    d. Clozapine

18. MJ was recently started on fluphenazine for the treatment of schizophrenia. He has been taking the fluphenazine for 3 days now and is not feeling well on this treatment. MJ is experiencing muscle rigidity, hyperthermia, hypertension, and presents with an altered

level of consciousness. Which of the following is MJ experiencing?

a. Tardive dyskinesia
b. Dystonia
c. Neuroleptic malignant syndrome
d. Serotonin syndrome
e. Hypertensive crisis

19. Which of the following may be associated with QTc prolongation?

a. Aripiprazole
b. Olanzapine
c. Ziprasidone
d. Quetiapine

20. The blockade of which of the following receptors is responsible for inducing EPS?

a. Serotonin
b. Dopamine-2 (D_2)
c. Norepinephrine
d. All of the above

21. RT is a 35-year-old man who is being switched to a FGA. He states that he does not like being on antipsychotics because he gets unwanted side effects such as extreme dry mouth, constipation, and urinary incontinence. Which of the following is the best option for RT?

a. Haloperidol
b. Chlorpromazine
c. Loxapine
d. Thioridazine

22. TS is a 30-year-old woman with a 2-year history of schizophrenia. She has been on a few FGAs in the past which have caused her prolactin levels to rise. The psychiatrist treating TS would like to avoid any agents which are likely to elevate prolactin levels. Which of the following agents should be avoided when treating TS?

a. Aripiprazole
b. Risperidone
c. Ziprasidone
d. Quetiapine

TAKEAWAY POINTS ››

- Schizophrenia is a chronic and complex disorder of thought and effect.
- Patients with schizophrenia may present with positive, negative, and cognitive symptoms.
- The Diagnostic and Statistical Manual of Mental Disorders (DSM-IV) provides the criteria for schizophrenia.
- The goal of treatment is to decrease symptoms, improve quality of life, improve patient functioning, and minimize adverse effects.
- FGAs and SGAs are the two classes of antipsychotics that are used for the treatment of schizophrenia.
- SGAs, with the exception of clozapine, are considered first-line therapy for the treatment of schizophrenia.
- FGAs and SGAs are effective for the treatment of schizophrenia; however, adverse effects and monitoring parameters vary among the two classes. FGAs are likely to cause EPS and prolactin elevation while SGAs are likely to cause metabolic effects. Other common adverse effects associated with antipsychotics in general include sedation, anticholinergic effects, and orthostasis.
- Patients receiving clozapine treatment should have their ANC and WBC monitored on a regular basis due to the risk of agranulocytosis which may occur with clozapine treatment.
- When making pharmacotherapeutic recommendations, adverse effects, monitoring parameters, cost, patient response, and adherence to treatment are all factors which should be considered.

REFERNCES

1. American Psychiatric Association. Schizophrenia and other psychotic disorders. In: *Diagnostic and Statistical Manual of Mental Disorders.* 4th ed., Text Revision. Washington, D.C.: American Psychiatric Association; 2000:297-319.
2. National Institute of Mental Health. *Schizophrenia.* Available at: www.nimh.nih.gov/health/topics/schizophrenia/index.html. Accessed June 3, 2009.
3. Meisenzahl EM, Schmitt GJ, Scheuerecker J, et al. The role of dopamine for the pathophysiology of schizophrenia. *Int Rev Psychiatry.* 2007;19:337-345.
4. Lehman AF, Lieberman JA, Dixon LB, et al. Practice guidelines for the treatment of patients with schizophrenia, second edition. *Am J Psychiatry.* 2004;161:1-56.
5. Burton S. Symptom domains of schizophrenia: the role of atypical antipsychotic agents. *J Psychopharmacol.* 2006;20:6-19.
6. Juckel G, Morosini PL. The new approach: psychosocial functioning as a necessary outcome criterion for therapeutic success in schizophrenia. *Curr Opin Psychiatry.* 2008;21:630-639.
7. Wirshing WC. Movement disorders associated with neuroleptic treatment. *J Clin Psych.* 2001;62:15-21.
8. Collaborative Working Group on Clinical Trial Evaluations. Measuring outcome in schizophrenia: differences among atypical antipsychotics. *J Clin Psych.* 1998;59:3-9.
9. Moore TA, Buchanan RW, Buckley PF, et al. The Texas Medication Algorithm Project antipsychotic algorithm for schizophrenia: 2006 update. *J Clin Psych.* 2007;68:1751-1762.

10. American Diabetes Association, American Psychiatric Association, American Association of Clinical Endocrinologists, North American Association for the Study of Obesity. Consensus development conference on antipsychotic drugs and obesity and diabetes. *Diabetes Care.* 2004;27:596-601.
11. Perkins DO. Predictors of noncompliance in patients with schizophrenia. *J Clin Psych.* 2002;63:1121-1128.
12. Hudson TJ, Owen RR, Thrush CR, et al. A pilot study of barriers to medication adherence in schizophrenia. *J Clin Psych.* 2004;65:211-216.
13. Toprac MG, Dennehy EB, Cormody TJ, et al. The Texas Medication Algorithm Project patient and family education program. *J Clin Psych.* 2006;67:1362-1372.
14. McEvoy JP. Risks versus benefits of different types of long-acting injectable antipsychotics. *J Clin Psych.* 2006;67:15-18.
15. American Academy of Pediatrics. Use of psychoactive medication during pregnancy and possible effects on fetus and newborn. *Pediatrics.* 2000;105:880-887.
16. American College of Obstetricians and Gynecologists Committee on Practice Bulletins. Clinical management guidelines for obstetrician-gynecologists: use of psychiatric medications during pregnancy and lactation. *Obstet Gynecol.* 2008;111:1001-1020.
17. Gentile S. Infant safety with antipsychotic therapy in breast-feeding: a systematic review. *J Clin Psych.* 2008;69:666-673.
18. Gill SS, Bronskill SE, Normand ST, et al. Antipsychotic drug use and mortality in older adults with dementia. *Ann Intern Med.* 2007;146:775-786.

CHAPTER

57 Post-Traumatic Stress Disorder

Joshua Caballero and Jehan Marino

FOUNDATION OVERVIEW

Post-traumatic stress disorder (PTSD) is an anxiety disorder that develops as a result of emotional or psychological trauma, or physical harm (eg, unwanted sexual act, physical injury). PTSD usually occurs after a tragic event that results in feeling fear, stress, or helplessness.[1] PTSD may also develop after experiencing or learning about a life-threatening event such as a war or hurricane.

Prevalence

PTSD accounts for approximately 4% of US mental disorders with women being twice as likely to experience PTSD as compared with men.[2,3] The occurrence of PTSD in victims of interpersonal violence and combat veterans is about 25%, and the lifetime prevalence rate ranges from 5% to 10% with a 12 month rate ranging from 2% to 5%.[4,5]

Risk Factors

Intense or repeated traumatic events increase the risk of PTSD. Genetic factors may predispose a person's susceptibility to experience an episode.[6] Neurobiologic changes, such as decreased hippocampus size, hypocortisolism, or a hyperactive amygdala, increases the risk.[6-8] Additionally, preexisting mental disorders (eg, depression, anxiety), poor socioeconomic or educational status, and substance abuse also enhance the risk of developing PTSD.[9,10]

Pathophysiology

The development of PTSD may be due to a dysregulation of the hypothalamus-pituitary-adrenal (HPA) axis.[6] The HPA axis is responsible for regulating responses to stress. Dysregulation of the HPA axis causes elevated glucocorticoid negative feedback sensitivity of the HPA axis which results in hypocortisolism. Since cortisol is a glucocorticoid that reduces stress, below normal concentrations cause an elevated stress response.[6,11]

Several neurotransmitters play a role in the pathophysiology of PTSD. The two most common neurotransmitters are serotonin (5-HT) and norepinephrine (NE). Gamma aminobutyric acid (GABA) and dopamine (DA) may indirectly play a role as well. The primary neurotransmitters (ie, 5-HT, NE) are implicated in PTSD in the following way:

1. Serotonin affects sleep, motor function, impulsivity, and aggression. Patients with PTSD have decreased 5-HT concentrations and neurotransmission which may result in insomnia, abnormal motor function, and aggressive behavior.[12,13]
2. Norepinephrine may be involved in regulating fear, arousal, emotional memories, and vigilance. Alpha receptors are auto-receptors which inhibit NE release. Therefore, in PTSD a down regulation of alpha-2 receptors results in increased NE concentrations and overactivity in the noradrenergic system.[13]

Clinical Presentation

PTSD typically occurs within 3 months after a traumatic event, yet may be deferred until after 6 months or more[1] (Table 57-1). After the initial onset, patients may experience three core symptom clusters. The three clusters include reexperiencing the traumatic event, avoidance or numbing symptoms, and hyperarousal symptoms.[1,5] Patients with PTSD may suffer from sleep disturbances such as insomnia.[14] Additionally, patients may present with general psychiatric distress, poor physical health, and social dysfunctioning.[5,15]

Diagnosis

According to the Diagnostic and Statistical Manual of Mental Disorders (DSM-IV-TR) criteria, a patient with a diagnosis of PTSD must have all of the following symptoms lasting for ≥1 month:[1]

1. Exposure to traumatic event:
   - Had an intense feeling of fear or vulnerability at an event experienced or heard about
2. Traumatic event is persistently reexperienced:
   - May appear as a recurrent dream, thought, or feeling
3. Persistence of three or more avoidance or numbing symptoms including:
   - Avoids activities linked to the trauma, such as thoughts, conversations, or emotions
   - Avoids people, places, and has decreased interests in events that will stimulate thoughts of the trauma
   - Inability to recall an important aspect of the trauma
   - Feelings of decreased view on life with minimal feelings expressed toward people

TABLE 57-1 Categories of PTSD Based on Symptom Onset[1]

Type of PTSD	Time of Onset of Symptoms
Acute	<3 mo
Chronic	3-6 mo
Delayed onset	≥6 mo after trauma

4. Persistence of two or more hyperarousal symptoms including:
   - Exaggerated startle response
   - Irritability or anger
   - Hypervigilance
   - Difficulty falling or staying asleep
5. All symptoms cause distress and impair social or occupational functioning

PREVENTION

One technique used to prevent PTSD from developing is cognitive behavioral therapy (CBT).[16,17] This includes an emphasis on return to normalcy and normal daily routine with trauma focused anxiety management. Additionally, medications have been studied for the prevention of PTSD. One example includes the use of propranolol, administered within 3 months of trauma given for a 10 day course to block memory consolidation. However, the use of propranolol remains controversial since other studies have shown no effectiveness in this population.[18,19]

TREATMENT

The primary short-term goal of PTSD treatment is reduction in symptom severity.[20] The long-term goals carry more emphasis on quality of life improvement, including adaptive functioning improvement and overall remission, as well as preventing trauma-based comorbid conditions and relapse.[20] The ultimate outcome of the various methods of intervention is to return the patient to the pretraumatic state. The goal for duration of treatment for acute PTSD is between 6 to 12 months; however, a minimum of 12 months is highly recommended for chronic PTSD.[21] It is important to discuss idealistic treatment goals with the patient, since complete resolution of symptoms is very difficult to accomplish. Also, because of black box warnings regarding a possible increase in suicidality or worsening of symptoms, all patients should be closely monitored (eg, early follow-up, phone communication) when beginning antidepressant therapy.

Nonpharmacologic Treatment

Nonpharmacologic treatment includes CBT, exposure desensitization, stress training, communication therapy, coping skills, and relaxation training.[21-23] However, most of the published data support the use of CBT.

Pharmacologic Treatment

First-Line Agents

Consensus guidelines state that selective serotonin reuptake inhibitors (SSRIs) should be recommended as first-line treatment since they have been found to be effective and provide a safer adverse event profile compared to other agents.[21] Overall, SSRIs are effective in reducing numbing symptoms. Among the SSRIs, paroxetine and sertraline are FDA approved and most commonly used (Table 57-2). Paroxetine has shown efficacy in several trials lasting almost 3 months in doses between 20 and 60 mg/d. However, paroxetine is among the highest anticholinergic SSRIs, with excessive sedation and weight gain being the most common adverse effects. Other SSRIs such as fluoxetine, citalopram, escitalopram, and fluvoxamine have also shown benefits.[24-31] There are some data that suggest sertraline may be better than citalopram in reducing numbing symptoms.[30] Finally, long-term studies have shown efficacy for fluoxetine (9 months) and sertraline (16 months).[28, 32] All SSRIs should be initiated at low doses and titrated over several weeks to average dosing ranges (see Table 57-2). It is important to note that clinical response may not be evident until 8 to 12 weeks of treatment. Some of the common adverse events associated with SSRIs include diarrhea and sexual dysfunction. Similar to use in other anxiety disorders, SSRIs may cause initial insomnia and agitation; however, the use of paroxetine may minimize these symptoms, since it is considered the most sedating SSRI. All SSRIs are considered pregnancy category C, except for paroxetine (category D).[33] Tapering for all SSRIs (possible exception may be fluoxetine) is highly recommended since withdrawal symptoms (eg, nausea/vomiting, sweating, dizziness) may occur with abrupt discontinuation.

Second-Line Agents

Second-line agents include another SSRI not previously used or venlafaxine. Venlafaxine, which works as a 5-HT/NE reuptake inhibitor (SNRI) and may provide increased concentrations in 5-HT and NE. As mentioned previously, 5-HT and NE are the two most commonly implicated neurotransmitters in PTSD. Venlafaxine extended release (mean dose: 221 mg/d) has shown benefits lasting for 6 months.[34] Another study showed venlafaxine extended release (mean dose: 225 mg/d) had similar efficacy to sertraline (mean dose: 151 mg/d) over 12 weeks.[35]

Third-Line Agents

Third-line agents include mirtazapine or the use of tricyclic antidepressants (TCAs). Mirtazapine enhances serotonergic activity, while TCAs increase both 5-HT and NE. In two small studies, mirtazapine demonstrated efficacy in doses up to 45 mg/d over 8 to 12 weeks.[36,37] Due to its pharmacologic profile, mirtazapine exhibits greater sedation and weight gain at lower doses; however, as the dose is increased the

TABLE 57-2 **Pharmacologic Treatments for PTSD**[21,24-31,33-43]

Drug (Brand)	FDA Approved[a]	Initial Dose (mg/d)	Dosage Range (mg/d)	Schedule[b]	Formulations[c]	Comments/ Class Side Effects
				SSRIs		
Citalopram (Celexa)	N	20	20-60	qd	S, T	SSRIs are first line Need 8-12 wk for improvement Sertraline and paroxetine are FDA approved for PTSD Paroxetine is most sedating CYP-450 interactions with fluoxetine (3A4, 2D6), paroxetine (2D6), and fluvoxamine (2D6, 1A2, 2C19) Paroxetine is pregnancy category D. All other SSRIs are pregnancy category C Nausea/vomiting Sexual dysfunction Diarrhea/constipation
Escitalopram (Lexapro)	N	10	10-20	qd	S, T	
Fluoxetine (Prozac)	N	10-20	10-80	qd	C, S, SY, T	
Fluvoxamine (Luvox)	N	50	100-250	qd, bid	EC, T	
Paroxetine (Paxil)	Y	10-20	20-50	qd	ET, OS, T	
Sertraline (Zoloft)	Y	25-50	50-200	qd	S, T	
				Other Agents		
Venlafaxine extended-release (Effexor XR)	N	37.5	37.5-225	qd, bid, tid	EC, ET, T	Second line Increased blood pressure at high doses Nausea/vomiting Sexual dysfunction
Amitriptyline (Elavil)	N	25-50	50-300	qd, bid, tid	T	Third line due to intolerable adverse events
Imipramine (Tofranil)	N	25-50	50-300	qd, bid, tid	T	Anticholinergic symptoms (eg, constipation, blurred vision, dry mouth) Sedation Sexual dysfunction
Mirtazapine (Remeron)	N	15	15-45	qhs	D, T	Third line due to limited evidence and adverse events Increased appetite/weight gain Sedation
Phenelzine (Nardil)	N	15	15-90	tid, qid	T	Last line due to drug-food interactions and adverse events Avoid eating foods high in tyramine Orthostatic hypotension Sedation Edema, weight gain Sexual dysfunction
Prazosin (Minipress)	N	1	1-14	qd, bid, tid	C	Mostly used adjunctively Preferably for nightmares High doses may be necessary Orthostatic hypotension Angina, tachycardia

[a]N, No; Y, Yes.

[b]bid, twice daily; qd, daily; qid, four times daily; qhs, at bedtime; tid, three times daily.

[c]C, capsule; D, (oral tablet) disintegrating; EC, extended-release capsule; ET, extended-release tablet; OS, oral suspension; S, oral solution; SY, oral syrup; T, tablet.

medication becomes less sedating. Among TCAs, imipramine and amitriptyline may be used, as they have demonstrated effectiveness over 8 weeks.[38-40] However, TCAs are reserved as third-line agents since they may carry more adverse events compared to SSRIs or venlafaxine. Phenelzine, a monoamine oxidase inhibitor (MAOI), may also be used, and data suggest greater efficacy compared to imipramine.[39] However, phenelzine should be reserved as a last-line treatment option due to unfavorable drug-food interactions and adverse events. Additionally, TCAs and MAOIs may be lethal in overdose, which may be an issue in those who have suicidal ideations.

Other Agents

Prazosin may also play a role in the treatment of PTSD. This alpha-1 adrenergic antagonist has demonstrated some benefits especially in patients with nighttime complications (eg, nightmares) with high doses in two small trials lasting for 8 to 20 weeks.[41-43] Prazosin should be considered in patients with PTSD who present with primary complaints of nightmares and sleep disturbances; however, caution is warranted in patients with cardiac disease.

Second-generation antipsychotics (SGAs) may be recommended as adjunctive therapy to antidepressants or those experiencing psychotic symptoms (eg, aggressiveness, hallucinations). Risperidone, olanzapine, and quetiapine have been used with favorable results in small studies. Ziprasidone has shown effectiveness in one case report.[44] Metabolic syndrome is one of the major complications with SGAs, especially with olanzapine. Proper monitoring (eg, weight, body mass index, fasting blood glucose) should be done in patients receiving these agents.

Benzodiazepines, commonly used in other anxiety disorders, are not effective in PTSD. Additionally, bupropion and duloxetine do not currently have any supporting evidence for use. Bupropion showed no efficacy in a trial lasting for 8 weeks.[45] Duloxetine showed some benefits in one case report, but exacerbated symptoms in another.[46] However, these case reports are confounded by comorbid illnesses and concomitant psychotropic agents. Mood stabilizers (eg, topiramate, divalproex, tiagabine) have been studied but have shown very limited or no efficacy.[22]

SPECIAL POPULATIONS

Children and adolescents can be treated with nonpharmacologic and pharmacologic treatments. Some examples of nonpharmacologic treatment includes CBT, psychotherapy, debriefing, and supportive therapy.[47-49] However, CBT is the most studied and may be the preferred treatment.

Medications for children and adolescents are focused on the use of antidepressants primarily with SSRIs. However, there is a black box warning for suicide in this population (as well as young adults up to the age of 25) and caution is warranted.[50] First-line pharmacologic treatment for elderly patients includes SSRIs due to a safer side effect profile compared to TCAs.

RELAPSE PREVENTION

Long-term treatment has been studied with fluoxetine and sertraline.[28,32] One trial demonstrated efficacy of fluoxetine (mean dose: 53 mg/d) over an additional 24 weeks of treatment after patients had initially completed 12 weeks of therapy.[28] Another study showed benefits with sertraline (mean dose: 137 mg/d) over an additional 28 weeks of treatment after patients had initially completed 36 weeks of therapy.[32]

CASE Application

1. Which of the following is *not* a core symptom of PTSD?
   a. Recurrent, intrusive, distressing memories of the trauma
   b. Ability to recall an important aspect of the trauma
   c. Avoidance of conversations about the trauma
   d. Hypervigilance
2. Which agent would be used as a first-line treatment for PTSD?
   a. Phenelzine
   b. Paroxetine
   c. Amitriptyline
   d. Bupropion
3. Which of the following nonpharmacologic treatment for PTSD has the most evidence supporting its use?
   a. Group counseling
   b. Stress inoculation treatment
   c. Psychoeducation
   d. Cognitive behavioral treatment
4. Which of the following SSRIs is/are approved by FDA for the acute treatment of PTSD?
   a. Sertraline
   b. Fluoxetine
   c. Paroxetine
   d. Both a and c
5. Which of the following agents is *not* effective for the treatment of PTSD?
   a. Alprazolam
   b. Imipramine
   c. Mirtazapine
   d. Phenelzine
6. Which agent is *not* effective in patients with chronic PTSD?
   a. Risperidone
   b. Venlafaxine
   c. Bupropion
   d. Prazosin
7. What is the *correct* dosing range for sertraline recommended for the treatment of PTSD?
   a. 2 to 8 mg/d
   b. 20 to 60 mg/d

c. 50 to 200 mg/d
d. 200 to 800 mg/d

8. Which of the following generic-brand name matches is *incorrect*?

a. Sertraline—Zoloft
b. Paroxetine—Prozac
c. Citalopram—Celexa
d. Imipramine—Tofranil

9. AB is a 32-year-old woman diagnosed with chronic PTSD. She asks the pharmacist how long she needs to take the medication for the prevention of symptom recurrence. What is the goal for duration of treatment for chronic PTSD?

a. 1 month
b. 6 months
c. 12 months
d. 5 years

10. CR is a 42-year-old man who was diagnosed with acute PTSD. He was prescribed citalopram 20 mg daily. He returns for a refill 1 month later and states, "I feel somewhat better, but still have flashbacks." How would you counsel this patient?

a. Call the MD to change the medication to another SSRI, such as paroxetine.
b. Call the MD to change the medication to venlafaxine.
c. Remind the patient, it may take 8 to 12 weeks for the medication to show full benefits.
d. Advise the patient that according to Federal laws, it is not your responsibility to counsel.

11. MN is a 23-year-old obese female who was diagnosed with PTSD after a car accident several years ago. Although MN has been treated with a SSRI and other agents, she still has recurrent, disturbing dreams of the event with minor daytime hallucinations. Her psychiatrist wants to prescribe an atypical antipsychotic for augmentation therapy. Which agent are you *least* likely to recommend as a clinical pharmacist?

a. Risperidone
b. Quetiapine
c. Olanzapine
d. None of the above

12. Which agent has pregnancy category D?

a. Paroxetine
b. Fluoxetine
c. Citalopram
d. Sertraline

13. For which of the following medication would you counsel a patient regarding drug-food interactions, especially avoiding tyramine containing foods?

a. Prazosin
b. Phenelzine
c. Venlafaxine
d. Zoloft

14. AS is a 49-year-old woman diagnosed with PTSD. She is taking warfarin 5 mg daily. The MD decides to initiate a SSRI. Which of the following medications would you *avoid* due to CYP-450 drug interactions?

a. Luvox
b. Sertraline
c. Celexa
d. Both b and c

15. Which are the two most important neurotransmitters implicated in PTSD?

a. 5-HT and GABA
b. GABA and NE
c. 5-HT and NE
d. NE and DA

16. Which medication class has a black box warning for increased risk of suicidal ideations in pediatrics?

a. Antipsychotics
b. Benzodiazepines
c. SSRIs
d. None of the above

17. Which of the following are environmental triggers which can cause PTSD?

a. War
b. Rape
c. Natural disaster
d. All of the above

18. SB is a 23-year-old woman who has PTSD and presents to the outpatient clinic with complaints of nightmares and difficulty sleeping. She is currently on paroxetine 40 mg daily and cannot tolerate higher dosages. Which of the following medications would you consider using as adjunctive therapy?

a. Olanzapine
b. Prazosin
c. Bupropion
d. Alprazolam

19. SSRIs have demonstrated overall effectiveness in which of the following core symptoms?

a. Reexperiencing
b. Numbing
c. Avoidance
d. All of the above

20. Which two agents are available in extended-release formulations?

a. Citalopram—escitalopram
b. Venlafaxine—paroxetine
c. Phenelzine—sertraline
d. Fluoxetine—venlafaxine

TAKEAWAY POINTS ››

- CBT may be the preferred nonpharmacologic treatment used in PTSD.
- SSRIs remain first-line treatment for PTSD in any population.
- Response may not be observed until 8 to 12 weeks of treatment.
- Sertraline and paroxetine are the only SSRIs that are FDA approved for PTSD.
- Paroxetine may carry more sedative properties and weight gain among the SSRIs.
- Venlafaxine may be used as a second-line agent if patient fails to respond to SSRIs.
- Mirtazapine or TCAs (eg, imipramine, amitriptyline) may be used as third-line agents.
- Prazosin may play a role in reducing nightmare severity in this population.
- Second-generation atypical antipsychotics may be used as adjunctive therapy to antidepressants if partial response or psychotic features are present.
- Benzodiazepines, bupropion, and duloxetine have not demonstrated any effectiveness in PTSD.
- Mood stabilizers have very limited evidence in treating PTSD.

REFERENCES

1. American Psychiatric Association. *Diagnostic and Statistical Manual of Mental Health Disorders.* 4th ed, Text revision (DSM-IV-TR). Arlington, VA: American Psychiatric Association, 2000.
2. Narrow WE, Rae DS, Robins LN, et al. Revised prevalence estimates of mental disorders in the United States: using a clinical significance criterion to reconcile 2 surveys' estimates. *Arch Gen Psychiatry.* 2002;59:115-123.
3. Stein MB, Walker JR, Hazen AL, et al. Full and partial posttraumatic stress disorder: findings from a community survey. *Am J Psychiatry.* 1997;154:1114-1119.
4. Alonso J, Angermeyer MC, Bernert S, et al. Prevalence of mental disorders in Europe: results from the European Study of the Epidemiology of Mental Disorders (ESEMeD) project. *Acta Psychiatr Scand.* 2004;420:21-27.
5. Germain A, Hall M, Krakow B, et al. A brief sleep scale for posttraumatic stress disorder: Pittsburgh Sleep Quality Index Addendum for PTSD. *J Anxiety Disord.* 2005;19:233-244.
6. Yehuda R. Advances in understanding neuroendocrine alterations in PTSD and their therapeutic implications. *Ann NY Acad Sci.* 2006;1071:137-166.
7. Bremner JD, Elzinga B, Schmahl C, et al. Structural and functional plasticity of the human brain in posttraumatic stress disorder. *Prog Brain Res.* 2008;167:171-186.
8. Shin LM, Rauch SL, Pitman RK. Amygdala, medial prefrontal cortex, and hippocampal function in PTSD. *Ann NY Acad Sci.* 2006;1071:67-79.
9. Costello EJ, Erkanli A, Fairbank JA, et al. The prevalence of potentially traumatic events in childhood and adolescence. *J Trauma Stress.* 2002;15:99-112.
10. Stein MB, Hofler M, Perkonigg A, et al. Patterns of incidence and psychiatric risk factors for traumatic events. *Int J Methods Psychiatr Res.* 2002;11:143-153.
11. Heim C, Ehlert U, Hellhammer DH. The potential role of hypocortisolism in the pathophysiology of stress-related bodily disorders. *Psychoneuroendocrinology.* 2000;25:1-35.
12. Ressler KJ, Nemeroff CB. Role of serotonergic and noradrenergic systems in the pathophysiology of depression and anxiety disorders. *Depress Anxiety.* 2000;12:2-19.
13. Heim C, Nemeroff CB. Neurobiology of posttraumatic stress disorder. *CNS Spectr.* 2009;14:13-24.
14. Krakow B, Melendrez D, Pedersen B, et al. Complex insomnia: insomnia and sleep-disordered breathing in a consecutive series of crime victims with nightmares and PTSD. *Biol Psychiatry.* 2001;49:948-953.
15. Krakow B, Melendrez D, Johnston L, et al. Sleep-disordered breathing, psychiatric distress, and quality of life impairment in sexual assault survivors. *J Nerv Ment Dis.* 2002;190:442-452.
16. Foa EB, Cahill SP, Boscarino JA, et al. Social, psychological, and psychiatric interventions following terrorist attacks: recommendations for practice and research. *Neuropsychopharmacol.* 2005;30:1806-1817.
17. Foa EB, Hearst-Ikeda D, Perry KJ. Evaluation of a brief cognitive-behavioral program for the prevention of chronic PTSD in recent assault victims. *J Consult Clin Psychol.* 1995;63:948-955.
18. Pitman RK, Sanders KM, Zusman RM, et al. Pilot study of secondary prevention of posttraumatic stress disorder with propranolol. *Biol Psychiatry.* 2002;51:189-192.
19. Stein MB, Kerridge C, Dimsdale JE, et al. Pharmacotherapy to prevent PTSD: results from a randomized controlled proof-of-concept trial in physically injured patients. *J Trauma Stress.* 2007;20:923-932.
20. Stein DJ, Ipser JC, Seedat S. Pharmacotherapy for posttraumatic stress disorder (PTSD). Cochrane database of systematic reviews (online) 2006:CD002795. Available at: http://www2.cochrane.org/reviews/en/ab002795.html. Accessed August 28, 2009.
21. Bandelow B, Zohar J, Hollander E, et al. World Federation of Societies of Biological Psychiatry (WFSBP) guidelines for the pharmacological treatment of anxiety, obsessive-compulsive and posttraumatic stress disorders—first revision. *World J Biol Psychiatry.* 2008;9:248-312.
22. Benedek DM, Friedman MJ, Zatzick D, et al. Guideline watch (March 2009): practice guidelines for the treatment of patients with acute stress disorder and posttaumatic stress disorder. *APA Guidelines.* 2009.
23. Cloitre M. Effective psychotherapies for posttraumatic stress disorder: a review and critique. *CNS Spectr.* 2009;14:32-43.
24. Stein DJ, Van der Kolk BA, Austin C, et al. Efficacy of sertraline in posttraumatic stress disorder secondary to interpersonal trauma or childhood abuse. *Ann Clin Psychiatry.* 2006;18:243-249.
25. Neylan TC, Metzler TJ, Schoenfeld FB, et al. Fluvoxamine and sleep disturbances in posttraumatic stress disorder. *J Trauma Stress.* 2001;14:461-467.

26. Marshall RD, Beebe KL, Oldham M, et al. Efficacy and safety of paroxetine treatment for chronic PTSD: a fixed-dose, placebo-controlled study. *Am J Psychiatry*. 2001;158:1982-1988.
27. Tucker P, Zaninelli R, Yehuda R, et al. Paroxetine in the treatment of chronic posttraumatic stress disorder: results of a placebo-controlled, flexible-dosage trial. *J Clin Psychiatry*. 2001;62:860-868.
28. Martenyi F, Brown EB, Zhang H, et al. Fluoxetine v. placebo in prevention of relapse in post-traumatic stress disorder. *Br J Psychiatry*. 2002;181:315-320.
29. Tucker P, Smith KL, Marx B, et al. Fluvoxamine reduces physiologic reactivity to trauma scripts in posttraumatic stress disorder. *J Clin Psychopharmacol*. 2000;20:367-372.
30. Tucker P, Potter-Kimball R, Wyatt DB, et al. Can physiologic assessment and side effects tease out differences in PTSD trials? A double-blind comparison of citalopram, sertraline, and placebo. *Psychopharmacol Bull*. 2003;37:135-149.
31. Robert S, Hamner MB, Ulmer HG, et al. Open-label trial of escitalopram in the treatment of posttraumatic stress disorder. *J Clin Psychiatry*. 2006;67:1522-1526.
32. Davidson J, Pearlstein T, Londborg P, et al. Efficacy of sertraline in preventing relapse of posttraumatic stress disorder: results of a 28-week double-blind, placebo-controlled study. *Am J Psychiatry*. 2001;158:1974-1981.
33. Tuccori M, Testi A, Antonioli L, et al. Safety concerns associated with the use of serotonin reuptake inhibitors and other serotonergic/noradrenergic antidepressants during pregnancy: a review. *Clin Ther*. 2009;31:1426-1453.
34. Davidson J, Baldwin D, Stein DJ, et al. Treatment of post-traumatic stress disorder with venlafaxine extended release: a 6-month randomized controlled trial. *Arch Gen Psychiatry*. 2006;63:1158-1165.
35. Davidson J, Rothbaum BO, Tucker P, et al. Venlafaxine extended release in posttraumatic stress disorder: a sertraline- and placebo-controlled study. *J Clin Psychopharmacol*. 2006;26:259-267.
36. Davidson JR, Weisler RH, Butterfield MI, et al. Mirtazapine vs. placebo in posttraumatic stress disorder: a pilot trial. *Biol Psychiatry*. 2003;53:188-191.
37. Alderman CP, Condon JT, Gilbert AL. An open-label study of mirtazapine as treatment for combat-related PTSD. *Ann Pharmacother*. 2009;43:1220-1226.
38. Frank JB, Kosten TR, Giller EL, Jr., et al. A randomized clinical trial of phenelzine and imipramine for posttraumatic stress disorder. *Am J Psychiatry*. 1988;145:1289-1291.
39. Kosten TR, Frank JB, Dan E, et al. Pharmacotherapy for posttraumatic stress disorder using phenelzine or imipramine. *J Nerv Ment Dis*. 1991;179:366-370.
40. Davidson J, Kudler H, Smith R, et al. Treatment of posttraumatic stress disorder with amitriptyline and placebo. *Arch Gen Psychiatry*. 1990;47:259-266.
41. Raskind MA, Peskind ER, Kanter ED, et al. Reduction of nightmares and other PTSD symptoms in combat veterans by prazosin: a placebo-controlled study. *Am J Psychiatry*. 2003;160:371-373.
42. Raskind MA, Peskind ER, Hoff DJ, et al. A parallel group placebo controlled study of prazosin for trauma nightmares and sleep disturbance in combat veterans with post-traumatic stress disorder. *Biol Psychiatry*. 2007;61:928-934.
43. Taylor FB, Martin P, Thompson C, et al. Prazosin effects on objective sleep measures and clinical symptoms in civilian trauma posttraumatic stress disorder: a placebo-controlled study. *Biol Psychiatry*. 2008;63:629-632.
44. Siddiqui Z, Marcil WA, Bhatia SC, et al. Ziprasidone therapy for post-traumatic stress disorder. *J Psychiatry Neurosci*. 2005;30:430-431.
45. Becker ME, Hertzberg MA, Moore SD, et al. A placebo-controlled trial of bupropion SR in the treatment of chronic posttraumatic stress disorder. *J Clin Psychopharmacol*. 2007;27:193-197.
46. De Berardis D, Serroni N, Carano A, et al. The role of duloxetine in the treatment of anxiety disorders. *Neuropsychiatr Dis Treat*. 2008;4:929-935.
47. Donnelly CL. Pharmacologic treatment approaches for children and adolescents with posttraumatic stress disorder. *Child Adolesc Psychiatr Clin N Am*. 2003;12:251-269.
48. Scott RW, Mughelli K, Deas D. An overview of controlled studies of anxiety disorders treatment in children and adolescents. *J Natl Med Assoc*. 2005;97:13-24.
49. National Institute for Clinical Excellence. Post traumatic stress disorder: the management of PTSD in adults and children in primary and secondary care. *Clinical Guideline*. 2005.
50. Caballero J, Nahata MC. Selective serotonin-reuptake inhibitors and suicidal ideation and behavior in children. *Am J Health Syst Pharm*. 2005;62:864-867.

PART

10 Endocrinologic Disorders

CHAPTER

58 Diabetes Mellitus

Jessica L. Kerr

FOUNDATION OVERVIEW

Diabetes mellitus is a progressive disease that affects nearly 8% of the US population.[1] Diabetes affects patients of all ages and is associated with chronic complications of microvascular, macrovascular, and neuropathic disorders. There are two major types of diabetes: type 1 (T1DM) and type 2 (T2DM). Other subclasses have been identified such as gestational diabetes (GDM) and secondary diabetes associated with hormonal syndromes, medications, diseases of the pancreas, and rare conditions involving insulin receptors.[2] Diabetes is characterized by hyperglycemia due to defects in insulin action, insulin secretion or both. The key differences between T1DM and T2DM are the pathophysiology, etiology of hyperglycemia, and clinical presentation.

T1DM accounts for 5% to 10% of the patient population with diabetes. This cellular-mediated autoimmune process causes destruction of pancreatic β-cells resulting in an absolute deficiency of insulin. Due to the lack of insulin, glucose is not able to be used as energy. The onset of symptoms leading to the diagnosis of T1DM is abrupt in nature occurring within days to weeks. Most often, patients will present with the classic symptoms of polydipsia, polyuria, polyphagia, and weight loss or ketoacidosis due to lipolysis.[2-5]

T2DM is more prevalent in adult populations. Nevertheless, new cases diagnosed at a younger age are occurring at epidemic proportions due to lack of physical activity and obesity in the western culture. Unlike patients with T1DM, patients with T2DM do not necessarily need initial insulin treatment in order to survive. Patients with T2DM have impaired insulin secretion as well as insulin resistance at sites such as the liver, muscles, and adipocytes. Patients with T2DM are able to produce insulin, but the amount may not be sufficient to keep up with the body's glucose metabolism, or the insulin that is produced by a patient with T2DM may not work appropriately at its receptor sites.

It is recommended that pregnant and all overweight adults and children who are at risk for diabetes be screened for diabetes (Table 58-1).[2] Screening efforts are used to identify patients who are likely to develop or have diabetes. The American Diabetes Association (ADA) does not recommend obtaining fasting plasma glucose levels as a measure of screening every patient. It is recommended to have patients fill out the ADA Diabetes Risk Screening Tests first and, if a patient scores a 10 or greater on this test, a finger stick blood sample would be appropriate. The online version of this screening tool is available at www.diabetes.org/risk-test.jsp. The diagnosis of diabetes or classification of prediabetes can be obtained by a laboratory measurement of a hemoglobin A1c, fasting plasma glucose level, or with the administration of an oral glucose tolerance test (OGTT) followed by a plasma glucose level (Table 58-2).[2] Once diagnosed with diabetes, clinicians can use the A1c to explain to patients their long-standing glucose control over the last 2 to 3 months by expressing the A1c into the estimated average glucose (eAG) level. The eAG is the recommended way to express A1c values, as the eAG is expressed in simple measures of blood glucose levels which patients measure at home. The calculation to determine the eAG is expressed as the following equation:

$$\text{eAG (mg/dL)} = 28.7 \times \text{A1c} - 46.7$$

PREVENTION

Considerable efforts are placed on early detection for diabetes, especially T2DM. Studies have indicated that treatment may delay the onset of diabetes and/or modify the risk of complications.[6-21] Lifestyle interventions have demonstrated a reduction in insulin resistance for obese patients with impaired glucose tolerance.[9,22] In the Diabetes Prevention Program (DPP), study patients were randomized to receive intensive lifestyle modifications or metformin compared to placebo. It was found that people who followed the intensified lifestyle interventions (which consisted of a physical activity for 150 minutes per week and a healthy diet) were able to reduce their risk of developing diabetes by 58%, while those who used metformin had a 31% reduction in risk.[9] Other studies since then, have confirmed the findings of a reduction in the risk for developing diabetes with intensive lifestyle modification.[23-26] Oral agents such as metformin, acarbose, rosiglitazone, and orlistat have been proven to be effective for diabetes prevention.[9,15,19,21,25] Based on the results of the aforementioned prevention trials, the ADA Consensus Development Panel states recommendations for lifestyle interventions similar to the DPP study should be provided to all patients at risk for diabetes. Furthermore, due to the side-effect

TABLE 58-1 Screening Recommendations for Diabetes in Adults, Children, and Pregnancy (GDM)

Adults[a]	Children[b]	Pregnancy[c,d,e]
All adults who have a BMI ≥25 kg/m² and other risk factors below: ▪ Physical inactivity ▪ First-degree relative with diabetes ▪ Ethnic population—African-American, Asian-American, Latino, Native American, Pacific islander ▪ IFG or IGT ▪ HTN (>140/90 mm Hg or on antihypertensive agents) ▪ HDL-C <35 mg/dL and or TG ≥250 mg/dL ▪ Women with PCOS ▪ Pregnancy resulting in baby >9 lb at birth ▪ GDM ▪ History of CVD ▪ Acanthosis nigricans	All children who have a BMI >85th percentile for age and sex, weight for height >85th percentile or weight >120% of ideal height *plus* at least two risk factors below: ▪ Ethnic population—African-American, Asian-American, Latino, Native American, Pacific islander ▪ Family history of T2DM in first- or second-degree relative ▪ Maternal history of diabetes or GDM during the child's gestation ▪ Signs of insulin resistance or condition associated with insulin resistance (PCOS, HTN, dyslipidemia, small-for-gestational-age birth weight, acanthosis nigricans)	All women during wk 24-28 of pregnancy with any of the following below: ▪ >25 y of age ▪ Weight higher than normal before pregnancy ▪ Member of an ethnic population of high prevalence for diabetes ▪ Diabetes in first-degree relative ▪ History of abnormal glucose tolerance ▪ History of poor obstetrical outcome

[a]Screening for prediabetes and diabetes should begin at the age of 45, if the patient lacks the above criteria.

[b]Screening should occur at age 10 or at the onset of puberty, if puberty occurs at a younger age.

[c]Low-risk status indicates the patient must have *all* of the following: age <25 years, normal weight before pregnancy, member of an ethnic group with low prevalence of diabetes, no known diabetes in first-degree relative, no history of abnormal glucose tolerance, no history of poor obstetrical outcome. According to the ADA, these patients do not have to be screened for GDM.

[d]High-risk status includes severe obesity, prior history of GDM or delivery of large-for-gestational-age infant, presence of glucosuria, diagnosis of PCOS, or strong family history of type 2 diabetes. These patients should be screened as soon as possible after pregnancy confirmation and if negative with initial screening should be rescreened at weeks 24 to 28 of pregnancy.

[e]Women with the diagnosis of GDM should be screened 6 to 12 weeks postpartum for prediabetes or diabetes.

Abbreviations: BMI, body mass index; CVD, cardiovascular disease; GDM, gestational diabetes mellitus; HDL-C, high-density lipoprotein cholesterol; HTN, hypertension; IFG, impaired fasting glucose; IGT, impaired glucose tolerance; PCOS, polycystic ovarian syndrome; TG, triglycerides.

profiles and the risk versus benefit profiles of the studied therapies, only metformin is recommended for the prevention of diabetes and only if the patient has both impaired fasting glucose (IFG) and impaired glucose tolerance (IGT), is obese and is under the age of 60 years with one other risk factor for diabetes.[27] In order to prevent further cardiovascular complications or other negative health outcomes, the ADA recommends goal attainment for hypertension and hyperlipidemia, use of antiplatelet therapy, smoking cessation, screening and treatment for nephropathy, retinopathy and neuropathy, proper foot and dental care, and appropriate vaccinations (Table 58-3).[28]

TABLE 58-2 Diagnosis of Diabetes or Classification of Prediabetes

	Plasma Glucose Levels	Methods for Diagnosis
Normoglycemia	FPG: 60 mg/dL–99 mg/dL	
Prediabetes	IFG: 100 mg/dL–125 mg/dL *or* IGT: 140 mg/dL–199 mg/dL *or* Hemoglobin A1c 5.7-6.5%	IFG: Sample obtained to measure a fasting plasma glucose level; fasting defined as no caloric intake for at least 8 h prior to blood sample IGT: Sample obtained 2 h after a 75-g anhydrous glucose OGTT
Diabetes	FPG: ≥126 mg/dL[a] *or* 2-h plasma glucose ≥200 mg/dL[a] *or* Random plasma glucose ≥200 mg/dL plus symptoms of hyperglycemia *or* Hemoglobin A1c ≥ 6.5%	Fasting defined as no caloric intake for at least 8 h prior to blood sample 2-h plasma glucose level should be obtained after a 75-g anhydrous glucose OGTT Random plasma glucose defined as a glucose sample obtained at any time of the day without regard to meals Symptoms of hyperglycemia include polyuria, polydipsia, and unexplained weight loss

[a]In the absence of unequivocal hyperglycemia, these criteria should be confirmed by repeating a test on a different day.

Abbreviations: FPG, fasting plasma glucose; IFG, impaired fasting glucose; IGT, impaired glucose tolerance; OGTT, oral glucose tolerance test.

TABLE 58-3 **Prevention and Management of Complications**

	Goals	Screening/Diagnosis	Treatment
Macrovascular Complications			
Hypertension[a]	SBP <130 mm Hg DBP <80 mm Hg	Screening: Measure BP at every visit Diagnosis: >130 mm Hg/>80 mm Hg on confirmed separate days	LSM ACEi or ARB in addition to LSM *Thiazide diuretic* may be added if BP is not controlled with LSM and ACEi or ARB if CrCl >30 mL/min or *loop diuretic* if CrCl <30mL/min Multiple antihypertensive therapies are usually required to attain goal BP Review special populations to make sure no contraindications or unwanted side effects occur
Hyperlipidemia[b]	TC <200 mg/dL TG <150 mg/dL HDL-C >50 mg/dL in women HDL-C >40 mg/dL in men LDL-C <100 mg/dL in patients without overt CVD LDL-C <70 mg/dL in patients with overt CVD or patients with DM and other uncontrolled risk factors (optional)	Screening: Yearly fasting lipid panel for most patients. In patients with low-risk lipid profiles (LDL-C <100 mg/dL, HDL-C >50 mg/dL, and TG <150 mg/dL) at least every 2 y	LSM focusing on reduced saturated fats, trans fats, and cholesterol intake in addition to physical activity *Statin* therapy regardless of baseline LDL-C levels for patients with diabetes who have overt CVD or are without CVD, but are over the age of 40 and have one or more other CVD risk factors[c] Review special populations to make sure no contraindications or unwanted side effects occur
Antiplatelet therapy	To be on therapy if no contraindications or specific population concerns are present	Screening: Advised to assess each visit for antiplatelet therapy	Patients with a Framingham score calculation > 10%, males > 50 y old, and females >60 ys old with at least one additional risk factor of HTN, smoking, dyslipidemia, family history of CVD, or albuminuria should start aspirin therapy of 75-162 mg daily for primary cardiovascular prevention in T1DM and T2DM Aspirin therapy is recommended at the dosage of 75-162 mg daily for secondary prevention in those with a history of CVD In the presence of a documented aspirin allergy, clopidogrel therapy may be used Review special populations to make sure no contraindications or unwanted side effects occur
Smoking cessation	Complete cessation	Screening: Advised to assess smoking status at each visit	Include smoking cessation counseling and forms of treatment for cessation
Microvascular Complications			
Nephropathy	Reduce the risk or slow the progression leading to chronic kidney disease or dialysis Achieve BP and glucose goals	Screening: Obtain annual test to assess excretion of urine albumin in patients with T1DM with duration of diabetes ≥5 y and in all T2DM at diagnosis	ACEi or ARBs should be used in nonpregnant patients with diabetes who have micro- or macroalbuminuria
Retinopathy	Reduce the risk or slow progression leading to blindness or other complications Achieve BP and glucose goals	Screening: 1. All adults and children of ages 10 y or older with T1DM within 5 y after diagnosis 2. All patients with T2DM shortly after diagnosis of diabetes Further follow-up examinations should be performed yearly[d] 3. Women with preexisting diabetes who are planning pregnancy or become pregnant should have an examination within the first trimester	Laser photocoagulation may be an option

(Continued)

TABLE 58-3 **Prevention and Management of Complications (*Continued*)**

	Goals	Screening/Diagnosis	Treatment
Neuropathy	Reduce the risk or slow progression leading to distal symmetric polyneuropathy (DPN) Obtain glucose goals	Screening: 1. Assess annually using simple clinical tests (pinprick sensation, vibration perception [128-Hz tuning fork], and 10-g monofilament pressure sensation at the distal plantar region of both great toes and metatarsal joints for DPN 2. At diagnosis for T2DM and 5 y after diagnosis for T1DM, patients should be screened for cardiovascular autonomic neuropathy	Medical relief of symptoms related to DPN and autonomic neuropathies are recommended: TCA (amitriptyline, nortriptyline, imipramine), anticonvulsants (gabapentin, carbamazepine, pregabalin,[e] duloxetine[e]) or capsaicin cream Surgical options Smoking cessation
Foot care	Reduce the risk of infection or amputation Achieve glucose goals	Screening: All patients with diabetes should have an annual comprehensive foot examination/ inspection which includes screening recommendations for neuropathies Initial screening for PAD is recommended	Provide education to patients Smoking cessation
Dental care	Reduce the risk of infection or gingival disorders Achieve glucose goals	Screening: Yearly to twice yearly	Preventative measures Good oral hygiene
Infectious Disease			
Influenza vaccination	Reduce the risk of infection or death	Screening: Identify those who have not received the vaccine It is important to start talking with patients about this in the summer and throughout influenza season	Provide influenza vaccine yearly during influenza season
Pneumococcal vaccination	Reduce the risk of infection or death	Screening: Identify those who have not received the vaccine	Provide vaccine twice throughout the lifetime. Revaccinate patients who are >65 y of age and received initial dose ≥5 y ago and were <65 y of age at that time

[a]Diagnostic blood pressure is lower in patients with diabetes than in those without diabetes.

[b]If drug-treated patients are not able to obtain LDL-C goal, it is recommended to target a reduction in LDL-C by about 30% to 40% from baseline.

[c]Statin therapy may be considered in addition to LSM for low-risk patients if LDL-C is above 100 mg/dL or in those with multiple CVD risk factors.

[d]Less frequent examination may be appropriate following one or more normal eye examination.

[e]FDA-approved treatment for painful diabetic neuropathy.

Abbreviations: ACEi, angiotensin converting enzyme inhibitor; ARB, angiotensin receptor blocker; BP, blood pressure; CrCl, creatinine clearance; CVD, cardiovascular disease; DBP, diastolic blood pressure; HDL-C, high-density lipoprotein cholesterol; HTN, hypertension; LDL-C, low-density lipoprotein cholesterol; LSM, lifestyle modifications; PAD, peripheral arterial disease; SBP, systolic blood pressure; TC, total cholesterol; TG, triglycerides.

TREATMENT

The ADA clinical practice recommendations suggest that patients should be treated with a therapeutic goal of obtaining normal glucose levels in order to prevent microvascular complications.[28] Therapeutic interventions should be made with careful consideration in order that glucose control may be achieved without increasing the patient's risk for complications of hypoglycemia. In recent years, studies have been conducted to address the question regarding tight glucose control and its ability to reduce the risk of cardiovascular complications.[29,30-33] Due to the results of these trials, continuance of treatment goals to obtain an A1c near or below 7% in the years soon after the diagnosis of diabetes is recommended.[33] Patients are encouraged to self monitor blood glucose, achieve glucose goals, and follow up with their health care provider to address issues of hyperglycemia or hypoglycemia (Table 58-4).

The current Food and Drug Administration (FDA) approved pharmacologic agents for glycemic control in T1DM are insulin and amylin analogs. Glycemic control for T2DM can

TABLE 58-4 **Glucose Goals[a,b]**

A1c	<7%
Fasting SMBGs	70–130 mg/dL
Postprandial SMBGs	<180 mg/dL, 1-2 h after the start of the meal

[a]For nonpregnant adults

[b]Select populations may not choose to target these goals due to increased risk for complications or hypoglycemia.

Abbreviations: SMBGs, self-monitoring blood glucose.

be obtained with oral antihyperglycemic agents, GLP-1 receptor agonists, or pramlintide with or without insulin therapy. It is recommended to consider antihyperglycemic agents due to their effectiveness in lowering glucose, extraglycemic effects that may reduce diabetes-related complications, safety profiles, tolerability, ease of use and expense.[4] At this time, there is insufficient data to support a recommendation of one class of glucose-lowering agents or one combination of medications over the others with regard to effects on complications; however, data are supportive of their differential effects on glycemia.[34]

Injectable Therapy

Insulin[4-5,34-43]

Insulin preparations can be classified by three parameters: onset and duration of action, purity, and concentration. Beef and pork insulins are no longer used in the United States as all animal products have been discontinued from the US market. Two types of human insulins are available: biosynthetic human insulin produced with recombinant DNA technology by genetically altering microorganisms and biosynthetic human insulin produced with recombinant DNA technology in baker's yeast cells. Human insulins are less antigentic, therefore the risk of allergies to the product is reduced as compared with animal insulins. Impurities are not a concerning issue since animal-sourced insulin is no longer available. US available insulins come in concentrations of U-100 and U-500. This represents the number of insulin units per milliliter. U-500 cannot be stocked in pharmacies unless the pharmacy has a patient currently receiving that concentration. U-500 insulin and insulin analogues (lispro, aspart, glulisine, glargine, and detemir) are only available by prescription. The mechanism of action for insulin is multifactorial (Table 58-5). The pharmacokinetic profile of each insulin preparation determines its use in dosage regimens. It is recommended to choose regimens that mimic normal physiological release of insulin. Therefore, the use of basal and bolus insulin is recommended for patients with T1DM and in some patients with T2DM requiring insulin therapy. There are currently four pharmacokinetic profiles available: rapid-, short-, intermediate-, and long-acting insulins (Table 58-6). The most common adverse effect of insulin is hypoglycemia; however, weight gain due to the anabolic effects of insulin and peripheral edema due to sodium retention may occur in some patients. Local allergies may occur presenting with erythema, swelling, and urticaria at the injection site. Systemic allergies are not common, but allergic reactions may occur with all forms of insulin. Some patients may develop lipodystrophy at the injection site including lipohypertrophy (thickening of adipose tissue) and lipoatrophy (thinning of adipose tissue). Lipodystrophy may be reduced by educating the patient to rotate injection sites.

TABLE 58-5 **Mechanism of Action for Insulin[4-5]**

- Stimulates glucose uptake into muscles and adipose tissue
- Stimulates hepatic glucose uptake
- Stimulates amino acid uptake and protein synthesis
- Inhibits hepatic glucose production
- Inhibits breakdown of triglycerides in adipose tissue
- Inhibits protein degradation

Amylin Analog[4-5,34,44,46]

Amylin is a neurohormone that is cosecreted with insulin in the secretory granules of pancreatic β-cells. Pramlintide is a synthetic analog of amylin used to reduce postprandial blood glucose levels by suppressing postprandial glucagon release to limit gluconeogenesis, slowing gastric emptying and inducing postprandial satiety. Pramlintide is indicated for use in both T1DM and T2DM. Gastrointestinal adverse effects are common in patients taking pramlintide. Nausea occurs in 20% of patients with T2DM and even higher (40%-50%) in patients with T1DM. Anorexia and vomiting may occur in roughly 10% of patients with T1DM or T2DM. These adverse effects may be limited by commencing therapy at a lower dose and titrate upward once the adverse effects from the previous dose have subsided. In monotherapy, hypoglycemia does not seem to be of concern due to the glucose-dependent mechanism of action. If used in combination with preprandial rapid- or short-acting insulin, it is recommended to reduce the insulin dose by 50%. Disease states or concomitant medications affected by or causing changes in gastric motility may interact with pramlintide. If rapid absorption of the medication is necessary, it is recommended to take the medication 1 hour before or 3 hours after administration of pramlintide (Table 58-7).

Glucagon-Like Peptide (GLP-1) Receptor Agonist[4-5,34,45-47]

GLP-1 is released from the bowel to stimulate glucose-dependent insulin release. Circulating endogenous GLP-1 is rapidly degraded within minutes by the dipeptidyl peptidase IV enzyme (DPP-IV). The mechanism for lowering fasting and postprandial blood glucose level is glucose-dependent. Exenatide is able to suppress glucagon release, thereby reducing hepatic glucose production, improving first-phase insulin release, slowing gastric emptying, and decreasing appetite. Due to the alteration of gastric emptying, many adverse effects are similar to pramlintide. Gastrointestinal effects subside over time. However, 5% of exenatide patients may have continued intolerance to these effects. Patients should be instructed to

TABLE 58-6 Pharmacokinetic Profile of Insulins[4-5,34-43]

Insulin	Trade Name (Manufacturer)	Onset (h)	Peak (h)	Duration (h)	Comments
Rapid-Acting					
Insulin aspart	NovoLog (Novo Nordisk)	≤0.25	0.5-1.5	3-4	▪ Bolus-type insulin ▪ Route of administration: SC, IV, CSII ▪ Available in insulin-delivery devices (pens) ▪ Concentration: U-100 ▪ Formulations: 1. NovoLog 2. NovoLog 70/30 (insulin aspart protamine/aspart) ▪ Mix only with NPH (inject immediately after mixing) ▪ Unopened refrigerated vial/device: good until expiration date ▪ Opened vial/device: good for 28 d regardless of refrigeration (once device is open, should *not* be refrigerated) ▪ Pregnancy category B ▪ Lactation: unknown if excreted in human milk
Insulin lispro	Humalog (Eli Lilly)	≤0.25	0.5-1.5	3-4	▪ Bolus-type insulin ▪ Route of administration: SC, IV, CSII ▪ Available in insulin-delivery devices (pens) ▪ Concentration: U-100 ▪ Formulations: 1. Humalog 2. Humalog 50/50 (insulin lispro protamine/lispro) 3. Humalog 75/25 (insulin lispro protamine/lispro) ▪ Mix only with NPH (inject immediately after mixing) ▪ Unopened refrigerated vial/device: good until expiration date ▪ Opened vial/device: good for 28 d regardless of refrigeration (once device is open, should *not* be refrigerated) ▪ Pregnancy category B ▪ Lactation: unknown if excreted in human milk
Insulin glulisine	Apidra (Sanofi-aventis)	≤0.25	0.5-1.75	1-3	▪ Bolus-type insulin ▪ Administered: SC, IV, CSII ▪ Available in insulin-delivery device (pens) ▪ Concentration: U-100 ▪ Mix only with NPH (inject immediately after mixing) ▪ Unopened refrigerated vial/device: good until expiration date ▪ Opened vial/device: good for 28 d regardless refrigeration (once opened pens should *not* be refrigerated) ▪ Pregnancy category C ▪ Lactation: unknown if excreted in human milk
Short-Acting					
Regular	Humulin R (Eli Lilly) Novolin R (Novo Nordisk)	0.5-1	2-3	3-6	▪ Bolus-type insulin ▪ Administered: SC, IV, CSII ▪ Available in insulin-delivery device (pens): ▪ Concentration: U-100 and U-500 (only Humulin R) ▪ Formulations: 1. Humulin R 2. Humulin 70/30 (insulin isophane suspension/regular) 3. Novolin R 4. Novolin 70/30 (insulin isophane suspension/regular) ▪ Mix only with NPH (may store mixture for <7 d) ▪ Unopened refrigerated vial/device: good until expiration date ▪ Opened vial/device: see individual package inserts (once opened pens should *not* be refrigerated) ▪ Pregnancy category: B ▪ Lactation: unknown if excreted in human milk

(Continued)

TABLE 58-6 **Pharmacokinetic Profile of Insulins[4-5,34-43] (*Continued*)**

Insulin	Trade Name (Manufacturer)	Onset (h)	Peak (h)	Duration (h)	Comments
			Intermediate-Acting		
NPH	Humulin N (Eli Lilly) Novolin N (Novo Nordisk)	1-4	4-10	10-16	▪ Basal-type insulin ▪ Administered: SC ▪ Available in insulin-delivery device (pens) ▪ Formulation: 1. Humulin N 2. Humulin 70/30 (insulin isophane suspension/regular) 3. Novolin N 4. Novolin 70/30 (insulin isophane suspension/regular) ▪ Concentration: U-100 and U-500 (only Humulin R) ▪ Mix only with short-rapid acting insulin. ▪ Unopened refrigerated vial/device: good until expiration date ▪ Opened vial/device: see individual package inserts (once opened pens should *not* be refrigerated) ▪ Pregnancy category B ▪ Lactation: unknown if excreted in human milk
			Long-Acting		
Insulin glargine	Lantus (Sanofi-aventis)	1.5	None	20-24	▪ Basal-type insulin ▪ Administered: SC ▪ Available in insulin-delivery device (pens) ▪ Concentration: U-100 ▪ Do *not* mix with any other insulins/solutions ▪ Unopened refrigerated vial/device: good until expiration date ▪ Opened vial/device: good for 28 d regardless of refrigeration (once opened pens should *not* be refrigerated) ▪ Pregnancy category C ▪ Lactation: unknown if excreted in human milk
Insulin detemir	Levemir (Novo Nordisk)	1.5	Relatively none	12-24	▪ Basal-type insulin ▪ Administered: SC ▪ Available in insulin-delivery device (pens) ▪ Concentration: U-100 ▪ Do *not* mix with any other insulins/solutions ▪ Unopened refrigerated vial/device: good until expiration date ▪ Opened vial/device: good for up to 42 d regardless of refrigeration (once opened pens should *not* be refrigerated) ▪ Pregnancy category C ▪ Lactation: unknown if excreted in human milk

Abbreviations: CSII, continuous subcutaneous insulin infusion; IV, intravenously; SC, subcutaneously.

eat slowly and limit portion sizes as satiety will occur sooner. Hypoglycemic reactions may be increased when used in combination with oral insulin secretagogues or insulin. Disease states or concomitant medications affected by or causing changes in gastric motility may interact with exenatide. If rapid absorption of the medication is necessary, it is recommended to take the medication 1 hour before or 3 hours after administration of exenatide (see Table 58-7).

Oral Therapies

Insulin Secretagogues[4-5,34,46]

Sulfonylureas Sulfonylureas were the first oral antihyperglycemic agents available and are classified as first- or second-generation agents. This classification indicates the differences in potential side effects, protein binding, and relative potency. Second-generation sulfonylureas (glyburide, glipizide, and glimepiride) are 100 to 200 times more potent than first-generation sulfonylureas (acetohexamide, chlorpropamide, tolazamide, and tolbutamide). However, when prescribed in equipotent doses, all sulfonylureas are equally effective at glucose lowering. Sulfonylureas bind to the sulfonylurea receptor 1 (SUR1) on pancreatic β-cells and block the ATP-sensitive K^+ channel causing a decrease in potassium efflux and depolarization of the membrane. Calcium channels open allowing an influx of Ca^{2+}. This increase of intracellular Ca^{2+} relocates the secretory granules of insulin to the cell surface and results in exocytosis of insulin. Sulfonylureas also reduce

TABLE 58-7 **Noninsulin Agents for Use in the Management of T1DM and T2DM**

Generic Name	Trade Name	Class	FDA Indication	Dose	Pharmacokinetics	Pregnancy Category	Monitoring	Clinical Concerns
Pramlintide	Symlin	Amylin analog	T1DM T2DM	**T1DM:** starting dose of 15 μg tid with meals titrated to maximum dose of 60 μg tid with meals **T2DM:** starting dose of 60 μg tid with meals titrated to maximum dose of 120 μg tid with meals	**A:** 30%-40% BA **D:** not extensively PPB **M:** Renal **E:** Renal	C	Renal function A1c	1. Reduce preprandial insulin by 50% if started on pramlintide 2. Use caution in patients with GI motility disorders 3. Use caution in patients receiving oral medication requiring rapid GI absorption 4. Should not be considered in patients with A1c >9%
Exenatide	Byetta	Incretin mimetic	T2DM	Starting dose of 5 μg bid for 4 wk titrated to maximum dose of 10 μg bid Dosing should be spaced 6 h apart, normally given before the morning and evening meals up to 60 min before meals	**A:** 65%-76% BA **D:** ND **M:** ND **E:** Renal	C	Renal function A1c Signs and symptoms of acute pancreatitis	1. No dosage adjustments indicated in mild-moderate renal or hepatic insufficiency 2. Not recommended for use in CrCl <30 m/min 3. Use caution in patients with GI motility disorders 4. Use caution in patients receiving oral medication requiring rapid GI absorption 5. Positive outcomes with weight loss (reduction 0.3-2.6 kg) 6. Postmarketing cases of acute pancreatitis 7. Should not be considered in patients with A1c >9%
Acetohexamide	Dymelor	Sulfonylurea (first generation)	T2DM	Starting dose of 250 mg qd-bid titrated to maximum dose of 1500 mg daily	**A:** ND **D:** 60%-90% PPB **M:** Liver, (inactive/ active metabolites) **E:** Renal 80%	C	Renal and hepatic function A1c Electrolytes	1. Should not be used in renal dysfunction due to renal clearance of parent drug and active metabolites 2. Dosage adjustment may be needed for hepatic impairment 3. Should not be used due to side-effect profile and risk of hypoglycemia compared to second-generation sulfonylureas
Chlorpropamide	Diabinese	Sulfonylurea (first generation)	T2DM	Starting dose of 250 mg qd titrated to maximum dose of 750 mg daily Plateau effect: 500 mg daily for most patients	**A:** ND **D:** 60%-90% PPB **M:** Liver, moderate **E:** Renal 80%-90% (unchanged in urine)	C	Renal and hepatic function A1c Electrolytes	1. Use caution with renal and hepatic dysfunction; dosage recommendations are not provided 2. Should not be used due to side-effect profile and risk of hypoglycemia compared to second-generation sulfonylureas

Tolazamide	Tolinase	Sulfonylurea (first generation)	T2DM	Starting dose of 100 mg daily and titrated to maximum dose of 1000 mg daily	**A:** ND **D:** ND **M:** Liver, extensive (active metabolites) **E:** Renal 85% Feces 7%	C	Renal and hepatic function A1c Electrolytes	1. Caution use in renal and hepatic dysfunction; dosage recommendations are not provided 2. Should not used due to side-effect profile and risk of hypoglycemia compared to second-generation sulfonylureas
Tolbutamide	Orinase	Sulfonylurea (first generation)	T2DM	Starting dose of 1-2 g qd or in divided doses titrated to maximum dose of 3 g daily	**A:** ND **D:** 80%-99% PPB **M:** Liver, extensive (inactive metabolites) **E:** Renal, extensive	C	Renal and hepatic function A1c Electrolytes	1. Caution use in renal and hepatic dysfunction; dosage recommendations are not provided 2. Should not be used due to side-effect profile and risk of hypoglycemia compared to second-generation sulfonylureas
Glipizide	Glucotrol	Sulfonylurea (second generation)	T2DM	Starting dose of 2.5-5 mg qd-bid titrated to maximum dose of 40 mg daily (qd or divided doses)	**A:** 100% BA **D:** 97%-99% PPB **M:** Liver, extensive (inactive metabolites) **E:** Renal 63%-89% Feces 11%	C	Renal and hepatic function A1c	1. Possibly less hypoglycemic reactions with glipizide than with glyburide and similar hypoglycemic reactions with glimepiride 2. First choice of sulfonylurea therapy in renal dysfunction 3. Good agent to use early in disease progression due to MOA
Glipizide	Glucotrol XL	Sulfonylurea (second generation)	T2DM	Starting dose of 5-10 mg daily titrated to maximum dose of 20 mg daily	**A:** 100% BA **D:** 97%-99% PPB **M:** Liver, extensive (inactive metabolites) **E:** Renal 63%-89% Feces 11%	C	Renal and hepatic function A1c	1. Possibly less hypoglycemic reactions with glipizide than with glyburide and similar hypoglycemic reactions with glimepiride 2. First choice of sulfonylurea therapy in renal dysfunction. 3. Good agent to use early in disease progression due to MOA
Glyburide	Dia Beta Micronase	Sulfonylurea (second generation)	T2DM	Starting dose of 1.25-5 mg qd-bid titrated to maximum of 20 mg daily (qd or in divided doses)	**A:** ND **D:** 99% PPB **M:** Liver, extensively (active metabolites) **E:** Renal 50%	B	Renal and hepatic function A1c	1. Not recommended with CrCl <50mL/min because as much as 50% of a dose may be eliminated unchanged in the urine

(Continued)

TABLE 58-7 **Noninsulin Agents for Use in the Management of T1DM and T2DM (*Continued*)**

Generic Name	Trade Name	Class	FDA Indication	Dose	Pharmacokinetics	Pregnancy Category	Monitoring	Clinical Concerns
Micronized glyburide	Glynase	Sulfonylurea (second generation)	T2DM	Starting dose of 1.5-3 mg qd-bid titrated to maximum of 12 mg daily (qd or in divided doses)	**A:** ND **D:** 99% PPB **M:** Liver, extensively (active metabolites) **E:** Renal 50%	B	Renal and hepatic function A1c	1. Not recommended with CrCl <50 mL/min because as much as 50% of a dose may be eliminated unchanged in the urine
Glimepiride	Amaryl	Sulfonylurea (second generation)	T2DM	Starting dose of 1-2 mg daily titrated to maximum dose of 8 mg daily	**A:** 100% BA **D:** > 99% PPB **M:** Liver (CYP 2C9) **E:** Renal 60%	C	Renal and hepatic function A1c	1. Caution use with renal and hepatic dysfunction; dosage recommendations are not provided
Nateglinide	Starlix	Meglitinides	T2DM	Starting and maximum dose of 120 mg tid Do not take if not administering a meal	**A:** 72%-75% BA **D:** 97%-99% PPB **M:** Liver, extensively (CYP 3A4/2C9) **E:** Renal (13%-14% unchanged in urine)	C	Renal and hepatic function A1c	1. Not recommended to be used with sulfonylureas due to similar MOA 2. Caution with moderate-to-severe hepatic impairment 3. Displacement of protein-bound drugs may cause interactions and complications
Repaglinide	Prandin	Meglitinides	T2DM	A1c <8%: starting dose of 0.5 mg with each meal titrated to maximum dose of 16 mg dailyA1c >8%: starting dose of 1-2 mg with each meal titrated to maximum dose of 16 mg daily Do not take if not administering a meal	**A:** 56% BA **D:** > 98% PPB **M:** Liver, extensively (CYP 3A4 and 2C8) **E:** Fecal 90%; renal 8% (0.1% unchanged in urine)	C	Renal and hepatic function A1c	1. Not recommended to be used with sulfonylureas due to similar MOA 2. Caution with moderate-to-severe hepatic impairment 3. Displacement of protein-bound drugs may cause interactions and complications
Acarbose	Precose	α-Glucosidase inhibitors	T2DM	Starting dose of 25 mg qd-tid with meals titrated up to maximum dosage of 50 mg tid[a] Do not take if not administering a meal	**A:**<2% BA **D:** ND **M:** Exclusively GI: intestinal bacteria **E:** Fecal 51% Renal 34%	B	Renal and hepatic function A1c	1. Treatment of hypoglycemia must be with simple glucose 2. Use in patients with SCr >2 mg/dL has not been studied, therefore not recommended 3. May not be drug of choice for reduction in postprandial blood glucose in patients with GI issues due to side-effect profile

Miglitol	Glyset	α-Glucosidase inhibitors	T2DM	Starting dose of 25 mg qd-tid with meals titrated to maximum dose of 100 mg tid Do not take if not administering a meal	**A:**50%-100% BA; depending on dose **D:**<4% PPB **M:** Not metabolized **E:** Renal >95% (unchanged in urine)	B	Renal function A1c	1. Treatment of hypoglycemia must be with simple glucose 2. Plasma miglitol levels had a two-fold increase in patients with CrCl <25 mL/min 3. May not be drug of choice for reduction in postprandial blood glucose in patients with GI issues due to side-effect profile
Metformin	Glucophage	Biguanide	T2DM	Starting dose of 500 mg twice daily or 850 mg daily titrated to maximum dose of 2550 mg daily	**A:** 50%-60% BA **D:**90% PPB **M:** Not metabolized **E:** Renal 90%	B	Renal and hepatic function A1c Signs and symptoms of lactic acidosis	1. Due to the risk of lactic acidosis, metformin is contraindicated in females with SCr >1.4 mg/dL and males with SCr >1.5 mg/dL 2. Other conditions or medications causing hypoprofusion and concomitant use of metformin may increase the risk of lactic acidosis and caution should be exercised
Extended-release metformin	Glucophage XR	Biguanide	T2DM	Starting dose of 500 mg daily titrated to maximum dose of 2000 mg daily				
Pioglitazone	Actos	TZD	T2DM	Starting dose of 15-30 mg daily titrated to maximum dose of 45 mg daily	**A:** ND BA **D:**>90% PPB **M:** Hepatic (CYP 2C8/3A4; active metabolites) **E:** Fecal metabolite/ unchanged Renal 15%-30%: Metabolites/ conjugates	C	Liver function Edema Signs/ symptoms of HF	1. May cause or exacerbate HF 2. Not recommended in patients with symptomatic HF 3. Contraindicated in NYHA III/IV 4. Pioglitazone provides a more positive lipid-profile effect than rosiglitazone
Rosiglitazone	Avandia	TZD	T2DM	Starting dose of 4 mg qd or in divided doses titrated to maximum dose of 8 mg daily	**A:** 99% BA **D:** 99.8% PPB **M:** Liver, extensive (CYP 2C8/9) **E:** Renal 64%, (no unchanged drug in urine) Feces: 23%	C	Liver function Edema Signs/ symptoms of HF	1. May cause or exacerbate HF 2. Not recommended in patients with symptomatic HF 3. Contraindicated in NYHA III/IV 4. Increased risk of MI associated with rosiglitazone therapy

(Continued)

TABLE 58-7 **Noninsulin Agents for Use in the Management of T1DM and T2DM (*Continued*)**

Generic Name	Trade Name	Class	FDA Indication	Dose	Pharmacokinetics	Pregnancy Category	Monitoring	Clinical Concerns
Sitagliptin	Januvia	DPP-IV inhibitor	T2DM	Starting and maximum dose of 100 mg daily Renal adjustments: 1. 50 mg daily. CrCl ≥30 mL/min-<50 mL/min or SCr in men >1.7 mg/dL-≤3.0 mg/dL or in women >1.5 mg/dL-≤2.5 mg/dL 2. 25 mg daily: Severe and ESRD CrCl <30 mL/min or SCr in men >3.0 mg/dL or in women >2.5 mg/dL or on dialysis	**A:** 87% BA **D:** 38% PPB **M:** Liver, minimal (CYP3A4/2C8) **E:** ~ Renal 87% (79% unchanged in urine)	B	Renal function A1c	1. Lower dosage of sulfonylurea if used in combination 2. SJS, Angioedema, anaphylaxis has been documented 3. Renal adjustments necessary
Saxagliptin	Onglyza	DPP-IV inhibitor	T2DM	Starting dose of 2.5 mg or 5 mg daily titrated to maximum dose of 5 mg daily Renal djustments: 1. 2.5 mg daily: CrCl <50 mL/min	**A:** ND **D:** Negligible PPB **M:** Liver (CYP 3A4/5, active metabolite) **E:** Renal/hepatic	B	Renal function A1c	1. Lower dosage of sulfonylurea if used in combination 2. Renal adjustments necessary
Bromocriptine	Cycloset	Dopamine receptor agonist	T2DM	Starting dose of 0.8 mg daily titrated weekly to maximum dose of 1.6-4.8 mg daily	**A:** 65%-95% BA **D:** 90%-96% PPB **M:** Extensively by GI and liver (CYP 3A4) **E:** Bile	B	Renal/hepatic function A1c BP	1. Hypotension 2. Somnolence 3. Psychiatric disorders treated with a bromocriptine may exacerbate the disorder or diminish the effectiveness of drugs used to treat the disorder 4. Interaction with dopamine receptor antagonists 5. Caution with renal/hepatic impairment—no dosage adjustment recommendations 6. Neutral effects on lipids

[a]If the patient is >60 kg, then maximum dose is 100 mg tid.

Abbreviations: BA, bioavailability; bid, twice daily; CrCl, creatinine clearance; CYP, cytochrome P450; ESRD, end-stage renal disease; GI, gastrointestinal; HF, heart failure; MI, myocardial infarction; MOA, mechanism of action; ND, not documented; NYHA, New York Heart Associations; PPB, plasma protein binding; qd, once daily; SCr, serum creatinine; SJS, Stevens-Johnson syndrome; tid, three times daily; T1DM, type 1 diabetes mellitus; T2DM, type 2 diabetes mellitus.

the secretion of glucagon due to their ability to stimulate the release of somatostatin. All sulfonylureas are metabolized by the liver to some extent with active and inactive metabolites. Sulfonylureas with parent drugs or active metabolites that are renally excreted require dosage adjustments in the presence of renal dysfunction to reduce the risk of hypoglycemia. Hypoglycemia is more common in sulfonylureas with longer half-lives (chlorpropamide and glyburide). Other adverse effects may include skin rash, erythema, urticaria, pruritus, dyspepsia, nausea and vomiting, and weight gain. A disulfiram-like reaction may be noted with the usage of the first-generation sulfonylureas, chlorpropamide and tolbutamide. Chlorpropamide may induce hyponatremia by enhancing the effects of antidiuretic hormone on the collecting ducts in the kidney causing a syndrome of inappropriate antidiuretic hormone (SIADH) reaction. Possible mechanisms for drug interactions involving the sulfonylureas include alterations in protein binding and coadministration of drugs that induce or inhibit cytochrome P-450 (CYP) 2C9. In clinical practice today, due to the increased likelihood of side effects with first-generation agents and concerns related to the use of these agents in patients with hepatic and renal disorders, it is recommended to use second-generation sulfonylureas (see Table 58-7).

Short-Acting Secretagogues[4-5,34,46]

Meglitinides Nateglinide, a phenylalanine amino acid derivative, and repaglinide, a benzoic acid derivative, have a mechanism of action similar to sulfonylureas except that the stimulation of insulin release from the β-cells is glucose dependent, thereby lowering postprandial glucose excursions. This glucose-dependent mechanism allows glucose levels to reduce to normal while also decreasing the release of insulin. This mechanism and short duration of action are responsible for the low incidence of hypoglycemia associated with this class as compared to sulfonylureas. Weight gain may also be noted in patients on these agents. Due to the short duration of action, agents in this class should be taken 30 minutes preprandial. Drug interactions may be seen more frequently with repaglinide use due to its metabolism by CYP 3A4. Concomitant use of gemfibrozil with repaglinide may cause excessive hypoglycemia. However, this does not mean that gemfibrozil is contraindicated in a patient on repaglinide, but rather that more frequent monitoring of blood glucose levels may be needed. Nateglinide is metabolized by the cytochrome P-450 pathway with approximately 70% being metabolized by CYP 2C9 and 30% by CYP 3A4. Short-acting secretagogues should not be used in combination with sulfonylurea therapy. Nateglinide and repaglinide are beneficial for patients who are close to the A1c goal of less than 7% and who have elevated postprandial blood glucose values (see Table 58-7).

Enzyme Inhibitors[4-5,34,46]

α-Glucosidase Inhibitors Acarbose and miglitol delay the breakdown of sucrose and complex carbohydrates in the intestinal brush border by competitively inhibiting enzymes such as maltase, isomaltase, sucrose, and glucoamylase. Their primary place in therapy is for reducing postprandial blood glucose. Hypoglycemia is not a side effect of concern for monotherapy since this class does not stimulate insulin release. If hypoglycemia occurs during monotherapy or in combination with other antihyperglycemic agents, it is recommended to treat the hypoglycemic reaction with oral glucose or milk with lactose sugar. The most common side effects are gastrointestinal in nature such as abdominal bloating, diarrhea, and flatulence. Often times, starting with a low dose and titrating slowly may decrease or eliminate these symptoms. These agents are poorly absorbed. Therefore, drug interactions are minimal and tend to not have clinical significance (see Table 58-7).

Insulin Sensitizers[4-5,34,46]

Biguanide Metformin is a insulin sensitizer that increases insulin action at the site of muscle and adipose tissue. Metformin also decreases hepatic glucose production. Metformin is renally eliminated by tubular secretion and glomerular filtration. Metformin is contraindicated in patients with renal insufficiency, defined by a serum creatinine of 1.4 mg/dL or greater in women and 1.5 mg/dL or greater in men due to the increased risk for lactic acidosis. Although the occurrence of lactic acidosis is rare, conditions that affect the production or accumulation of lactic acid, such as shock, heart failure, recent myocardial infarction, chronic obstructive lung disease (COPD), may predispose patients to this deadly condition. Approximately 30% of patients using metformin complain of gastrointestinal side effects including diarrhea and abdominal discomfort. In order to reduce this side effect, it is recommended for patients to take metformin after a meal, commence therapy with lower doses, titrate the dose over several weeks or consider the extended-release formulation. Patients may experience a metallic taste from metformin. Metformin is the only agent that has been recommended by the ADA for the treatment of prediabetes with the addition of intensive lifestyle modifications. For most patients, metformin is recommended as first line in the treatment of T2DM (see Table 58-7).

Thiazolidinediones (TZDs or Glitazones)[48-50] TZDs are insulin sensitizers due to their indirect effect at muscle, liver, and adipose tissue. Second-generation TZDs, pioglitazone and rosiglitazone bind to the peroxisome proliferator-activated receptor-γ (PPAR-γ) located on adipose and vascular cells. These receptors regulate carbohydrate and lipid metabolism. Pioglitazone has shown beneficial effects on triglycerides and high density lipoprotein cholesterol (HDL-C) levels possibly due to increased activity of PPAR-α with the use of the agent. Cardiovascular effects have been of concern for this class of antidiabetic agents. A meta-analysis indicated an associated risk of myocardial infarction, angina, and sudden death with rosiglitazone. Conversely, a meta-analysis of pioglitazone trials indicated beneficial effects in lowering the risk of death, myocardial infarction, and stroke. Both of these agents have been linked with fluid retention and edema causing or exacerbating heart failure symptoms in patients. The use of TZDs is contraindicated in patients with New York Heart Association (NYHA) class III and IV heart failure. The warning labels for both of these products recommend exercising caution in patients with NYHA class I and II heart failure or other underlying cardiac diseases. Weight gain of 2 to 4 kg is common; however, it has been noted that weight gain positively predicts a larger reduction in A1c. In postmenopausal women, TZDs have been associated with an increased fracture rate in the upper and lower limbs. Hepatotoxicity is rare, but it is recommended to obtain baseline aminotransferase measurements and then to periodically monitor liver function during treatment. Neither pioglitazone nor rosiglitazone have significant drug interactions. The ADA recommends pioglitazone as the agent of choice for this class due to the cardiac effects associated with rosiglitazone (see Table 58-7).

Dipeptidyl Peptidase-IV (DPP-IV) Inhibitors[3-5,34,46]

Sitagliptin and saxagliptin are DPP-IV inhibitors. These agents block the DPP-IV enzymes activity for at least 12 hours. In a glucose-dependent manner, prolongation of the half-life for endogenous glucagonlike peptide 1 (GLP-1) causes enhanced insulin secretion along with a reduction of inappropriately elevated postprandial glucagon. While the mechanism of action is similar to amylin analogs and incretin mimetics, it does not alter gastric emptying. Mild hypoglycemia may occur and is increased when used in combination with a sulfonylurea or metformin. Adverse effects consist of upper respiratory tract infections, nasopharyngitis, headache, and urinary tract infections. Cases of urticaria and angioedema have been documented. Due to the hepatic metabolism, it is recommended to reduce the dose of saxagliptin when used in combination with strong inhibitors of CYP 3A4/3A5. For patients on concomitant digoxin and sitagliptin, it is recommended to monitor for signs and symptoms of digoxin toxicity. However, no empiric dosage adjustments are necessary for either agent when digoxin and sitagliptin are used together. Both sitaglipitin and saxagliptin have been studied in renal impairment including end-stage renal disease. These agents can be used in extensive renal disease, however, starting doses are recommended to be reduced (see Table 58-7).

Dopamine Receptor Agonist[4-5,34,46]

Bromocriptine This ergot derivative is a sympatholytic dopamine D_2 subtype receptor agonist that has been recently approved for use in diabetes. The mechanism of action is unknown. It has been postulated that this agent may provide inhibitory effects on serotonin turnover in the central nervous system (CNS) resulting in alterations in hypothalamic circadian activity, thereby improving insulin sensitivity. Side effects include headache, dizziness, and gastrointestinal intolerance (nausea). Hypoglycemia may occur with monotherapy though the risk of this adverse effect is increased when used in combination with sulfonylureas. Orthostatic hypotension may be observed upon the initiation of therapy and with escalating dosage. Bromocriptine is not advised in patients with psychotic disorders due to its mechanism of action. Patients on potent inhibitors or inducers of CYP 3A4 may have increased circulating levels of bromocriptine. Any advantage of bromocriptine over other agents used to treat T2DM is unknown (see Table 58-7).

CASE Application

Use the following patient profile to answer questions 1 to 5

JR is a 38-year-old obese African American man with a new diagnosis of T2DM. He was classified as having prediabetes 5 years before the diagnosis and has a strong family history of diabetes. JR's blood pressure was 140/92 mm Hg. His laboratory results revealed an A1c of 8.2%, normal cholesterol panel and normal renal/hepatic function.

1. What risk factor(s) does JR display for the development of diabetes?
   a. Obesity
   b. African American
   c. Family history of diabetes
   d. Prediabetes
   e. All of the above

2. What is JR's goal blood pressure?
   a. <150/90 mm Hg
   b. <140/90 mm Hg
   c. <130/80 mm Hg
   d. <110/70 mm Hg

3. JR's blood pressure was elevated at the next visit and he was diagnosed with hypertension. Which agent would be the best to start in order to achieve blood pressure control and to prevent microvascular complications?
   a. Clonidine 0.1 mg twice daily
   b. Terazosin 10 mg at bedtime
   c. Lisinopril 5 mg daily
   d. Isosorbide mononitrate 60 mg daily

4. Which of the following antihyperglycemic agents would be recommended for JR to use as first-line therapy to obtain glycemic control?
   a. Pramlintide 15 μg twice daily
   b. Gemfibrozil 600 mg twice daily
   c. Metformin 500 mg daily with meals and titrate up over a few weeks
   d. Acarbose 100 mg three times daily with each meals

5. What preventative measures should JR be educated on to reduce the risk of complications associated with diabetes?
   a. Perform daily foot examination
   b. See a dentist/dental hygienist routinely throughout the year
   c. Receive the yearly influenza vaccine
   d. All of the above

Use the following patient profile for questions 6 to 8.

PT is a 68-year-old white woman with a body mass index (BMI) of 32 kg/m^2. She was recently referred to a dietitian for weight reduction and lost 40 lb over the past 8 months. She is very dedicated to getting her blood glucose under control. At this time she is not willing to go on insulin therapy. She is testing her blood sugars at home: fasting blood glucose readings are all <130 mg/dL and her 2-hour postprandials are in the range of 190 to 200 mg/dL.

Her past medical history (PMH) is hypertension, hyperlipidemia, T2DM, sleep apnea, and depression; family history (FHx) is unknown (patient was adopted); and social history (SHx) is (+) tobacco use—1.5 packs per day for 52 years, (+) alcohol use—2 sifters (60 oz) of gin and tonic daily. Her medications are metformin 1000 mg twice daily, enalapril 10 mg twice daily, hydrochlorothiazide 25 mg daily, citalopram 40 mg daily, rosuvastatin 5 mg daily, and gemfibrozil 600 mg twice daily. Her laboratory results revealed normal electrolyte and cholesterol panels, normal renal and hepatic function. A1c 7.9%

6. What therapy is the best option to help lower her A1c and improve glycemic control considering her specific patient profile concerns?
   a. Nateglinide 120 mg three times daily with meals
   b. Chlorpropamide 250 mg daily
   c. Increase metformin to 2000 mg twice daily
   d. Start insulin NPH 10 units at bedtime

7. Which of the following is/are common side effect(s) of Glucophage?
   a. Weight gain
   b. Diarrhea
   c. Lactic acidosis
   d. Pancreatitis

8. Which of the following treatment would be the most appropriate method to treat a severe hypoglycemic reaction that PT might have?
   a. 2 to 3 glucose tablets
   b. 1can (8 oz) of soda
   c. One-half of a banana
   d. Glucagon intramuscular (IM) injection

9. Commercially available Symlin should be administered by which route?
   a. Intravenously
   b. Intramuscularly
   c. Subcutaneously
   d. Via insulin pump

10. Insulin detemir can be mixed with which of the following insulins?
    a. Insulin aspart
    b. Insulin regular
    c. Insulin glargine
    d. Insulin detemir cannot be mixed with any insulins

11. How should a patient on acarbose therapy treat a hypoglycemic episode?
    a. Inject 3 units of insulin NPH at the time of episode
    b. 3 to 4 glucose tablets
    c. 1 candy bar
    d. All of the above are suitable choices

12. Which drug would not be recommended for a patient with an ejection fraction of 32% and in symptomatic heart failure documented by a NYHA class III?
    a. Rosiglitazone
    b. Byetta
    c. Saxagliptin
    d. Starlix

13. How many minutes before a meal should a patient administer glulisine insulin?
    a. 15 minutes before the start of a meal
    b. 30 minutes before the start of a meal
    c. 60 minutes before the start of a meal
    d. Glulisine is a basal insulin and administration should be regardless of the mealtime.

14. Which of the following is true regarding the action of insulin?
    a. Enhances ketone production
    b. Stimulates glucose uptake in the periphery
    c. It activates peroxisome-proliferator-activated receptor-γ (PPAR-γ)
    d. Increases amylin production

15. What baseline laboratory results need to be obtained prior to the prescribing of Januvia?
    a. Basic metabolic panel
    b. Prothrombin time (PT)/International normalized ratio (INR)
    c. Cholesterol panel
    d. A1c
    e. a and d

16. Adjustments in antihyperglycemic drug therapy should be based on which of the following concerns?
    i. Liver function tests if the patient is on a TZD
    ii. Blood glucose levels
    iii. Gynecologic examinations
    iv. Dietary habits/physical activity

    a. i only
    b. ii only
    c. i and ii only
    d. i, ii, and iv

17. All of the following are true of repaglinide *except*:
    a. Dosage of repaglinide should be administered regardless of meal
    b. Normal treatment of hypoglycemia is recommended for patients on repaglinide
    c. Caution for hypoglycemic in concomitant therapy with gemfibrozil
    d. Maximum dose of repaglinide is 16 mg daily (divided with meals)

18. Glipizide has which of the following mechanisms of action?
    a. Inhibits and delays carbohydrate metabolism by inhibition of intestinal/pancreatic enzymes.
    b. Improves insulin sensitivity at adipose tissue.
    c. Causes gene transcription at adipose tissue.
    d. Stimulates pancreatic β-cells to release insulin.

19. Exenatide is not recommended in patients with which of the following diagnoses?
    a. Vitamin B12 deficiency
    b. Gastroparesis
    c. A1c >9%
    d. a and b
    e. b and c

20. Which drug therapy may mask the signs of hypoglycemia?
    a. Atenolol
    b. Valsartan
    c. Hydrochlorothiazide
    d. Pioglitazone

TAKEAWAY POINTS ››

- Type 1diabetes mellitus (T1DM) is an autoimmune disorder that results in absolute insulin deficiency.
- Type 2 diabetes mellitus (T2DM) has many genetic and environmental factors that lead to its pathophysiology.
- Diabetes management does not only consist of glycemic control, but rather a multifactorial approach to reduce the risk of microvascular, macrovascular, and neuropathic complications.
- An A1c test is recommended on a quarterly basis to reflect the status of long-term glucose control (until glucose control is achieved at which time biannual measurement of A1c is recommended). The eAG is recommended to be used when educating patient about the result of the A1c.
- Intensive lifestyle modification and metformin therapy have been recommended by the ADA for the treatment of prediabetes in a specific patient population.
- There are different pharmacokinetic profiles of available insulin products which aid in mimicking normal physiologic release of insulin.
- Only short- or rapid-acting insulin can be mixed with NPH.
- Long-acting insulins cannot be mixed with any other insulin.
- Insulin therapy is essential for survival in patients with T1DM
- Metformin, TZDs, and α-glucosidase inhibitors do not induce hypoglycemic reactions when used as monotherapy.
- First-generation sulfonylureas are rarely used due to side effect profile and their increased risk of hypoglycemia.
- Patients on metformin need to be educated about diarrhea and the signs and symptoms of lactic acidosis. These patients need to have continual monitoring for renal dysfunction or signs and symptoms of organ hypoprofusion.
- Patients on TZDs should have liver function tests periodically and should be educated about possible signs and symptoms for heart failure.
- New agents such as DPP-IV inhibitors, pramlintide and exenatide, and bromocriptine do not have distinct roles in diabetes management, however, subpopulations may benefit from these therapies.

REFERENCES

1. Centers for Disease Control and Prevention. *National Diabetes Fact Sheet: General Information and National Estimates on Diabetes in the United States, 2007.* Atlanta, GA: U.S. Department of Health and Human Services, Centers for Disease Control and Prevention, 2008.
2. American Diabetes Association. Diagnosis and classification of diabetes mellitus. *Diabetes Care.* 2009;32(suppl 1):S62-S67.
3. Assemi M, Morello CM. Diabetes mellitus. In: Berardi RR, McDermott JH, Newton GD, et al., eds. *Handbook of Nonprescription Drugs: An Interactive Approach to Self Care.* 16th ed. Washington, DC: American Pharmacists Association; 2009:837-867.
4. Triplitt CL, Reasner CA, Isley WL. Endocrine disorders: diabetes mellitus. In: Dipiro JT, Talbert RL, Yee GC, et al., eds.

Pharmacotherapy: A Pathophysiologic Approach. 7th ed. New York, NY: McGraw-Hill; 2008: 1205-1241.

5. Davis SN. Insulin, oral hypoglycemic agents, and the pharmacology of the endocrine pancreas. In: Brunton LL, Lazo JS, Parker KL, eds. *Goodman & Gilman's: The Pharmacological Basis of Therapeutics*. 11th ed. New York, NY: McGraw-Hill; 2006: 1613-1645.
6. UK Prospective Diabetes Study (UKPDS) Group. Intensive blood-glucose control with sulphonylureas or insulin compared with conventional treatment and risk of complications in patients with type 2 diabetes (UKPDS 33). *Lancet*. 1998;352:837-853.
7. UK Prospective Diabetes Study (UKPDS) Group. Effect of intensive blood-glucose control with metformin on complications in overweight patients with type 2 diabetes (UKPDS 34). *Lancet*. 1998;352:854-865.
8. The Diabetes Control and Complications Trial Research Group. The effect of intensive treatment of diabetes on the development and progression of long-term complications in insulin-dependent diabetes mellitus. *N Engl J Med*. 1993;329:977-986.
9. Knowler WC, Barrett-Conner E, Fowler SE, et al. Reduction in the incidence of type 2 diabetes with lifestyle intervention or metformin. *N Engl J Med*. 2002;346:393-403.
10. Diabetes Prevention Program Research Group. Effects of withdrawal from metformin on the development of diabetes in the diabetes prevention program. *Diabetes Care*. 2003;26:977-980.
11. Maggs DG, Buchanan TA, Burant CF, et al. Metabolic effects of troglitazone monotherapy in type 2 diabetes mellitus. A randomized, double-blind, placebo-controlled trial. *Ann Intern Med*. 1998;128:176-185.
12. Nolan JJ, Ludvik B, Beerdsen P, et al. Improvement in glucose tolerance and insulin resistance in obese subjects treated with troglitazone. *N Engl J Med*. 1994;331:1188-1193.
13. Azen SP, Peters RK, Berkowitz K, et al.. TRIPOD (Troglitazone in the Prevention Of Diabetes): a randomized, placebo-controlled trial of troglitazone in women with prior gestational diabetes mellitus. *Controlled Clin Trials*. 1998;19:217-231.
14. Chiasson JL, Josse RG, Gomis R, et al. Acarbose treatment and the risk of cardiovascular disease and hypertension in patients with impaired glucose tolerance: the STOP-NIDDM Trial. *JAMA*. 2003;290:486-494.
15. Chiasson JL, Josse RG, Gomis R, et al. Acarbose for prevention of type 2 diabetes mellitus: the STOP-NIDDM randomized trial. *Lancet*. 2002;359:2072-2077.
16. Chiasson JL, Josse RG, Leiter LA, et al. The effect of acarbose on insulin sensitivity in subjects with impaired glucose tolerance. *Diabetes Care*. 1996;19:1190-1193.
17. Keating GM, Jarvis B. Orlistat: in the prevention and treatment of type 2 diabetes mellitus. *Drugs*. 2001;61:2107-2119.
18. Heymsfield SB, Segal KR, Hauptman J, et al. Effects of weight loss with orlistat on glucose tolerance and progression to type 2 diabetes in obese adults. *Arch Intern Med*. 2000;160:1321-1326.
19. Torgerson JS, Hauptman J, Boldrin MN, et al. XENical in the prevention of diabetes in obese subjects (XENDOS) study: a randomized study of orlistat as an adjunct to lifestyle changes for the prevention of type 2 diabetes in obese patients. *Diabetes Care*. 2004;27:155-161.
20. Saloranta C, Guitard C, Pecher E,et al. Nateglinide improves early insulin secretion and controls postprandial glucose excursions in a prediabetic population. *Diabetes Care*. 2002; 25:2141-2146.
21. DREAM (Diabetes Reduction Assessment with ramipril and rosiglitazone Medication) Trial Investigators. Effect of rosiglitazone on the frequency of diabetes in patients with impaired glucose tolerance or impaired fasting glucose: a randomised controlled trial. *Lancet*. 2006;368:1096-1105.
22. Uusitupa M, Lindi V, Louheranta A, et al. Long-term improvement in insulin sensitivity by changing lifestyles of people with impaired glucose tolerance: 4-year results from the Finnish Diabetes Prevention Study. *Diabetes*. 2003;52:2532-2538.
23. Tuomilehto J, Lindstrom J, Eriksson JG, et al. Prevention of type 2 diabetes mellitus by changes in lifestyle among subjects with impaired glucose tolerance. *N Engl J Med*. 2001; 344:1343-1350.
24. Pan XR, Li GW, Hu YH, et al. Effects of diet and exercise in preventing NIDDM in people with impaired glucose tolerance The Da Qing IGT and Diabetes Study. *Diabetes Care*. 1997;20:537-544.
25. Ramachandran A, Snehalatha C, Mary S, et al. The Indian Diabetes Prevention Programme shows that lifestyle modifications and metformin prevent type 2 diabetes in Asian Indian subjects with impaired glucose tolerance (IDPP-1). *Diabetologia*. 2006;49:289-297.
26. Kosaka K, Noda M, Kuzuya T. Prevention of type 2 diabetes by lifestyle intervention: a Japanese trial in IGT males. *Diabetes Res Clin Pract*. 2005;67:152-162.
27. Nathan DM, Davidson MB, DeFronzo RA, et al. Impaired fasting glucose and impaired glucose tolerance: implications for care. *Diabetes Care*. 2007;30:753-759.
28. American Diabetes Association. Standards of Medical Care in Diabetes—2010. *Diabetes Care*. 2010;33(supp 1):S11-S60.
29. Gerstein HC, Miller ME, Byington RP, et al. Effects of intensive glucose lowering in type 2 diabetes. *N Engl J Med*. 2008;358:2545-2559.
30. Patel A, MacMahon S, Chalmers J et al. Intensive blood glucose control and vascular outcomes in patients with type 2 diabetes. *N Engl J Med*. 2008;258:2560-2572.
31. Meyers CD, McCarren M, Wong ND, et. al. Baseline achievement of lipid goals and usage of lipid medications in patients with diabetes mellitus (from the Veterans Affairs Diabetes Trial). *Am J Cardiol*. 2006;98:63-65.
32. Abraira C, Duckworth W, McCarren M, et al. Design of the cooperative study on glycemic control and complications in diabetes mellitus type 2: Veterans Affairs Diabetes Trial. *J Diabetes Complications*. 2003;6:314-322.
33. Skyler JS, Bergenstal R, Bonow RO, et al. Intensive glycemic control and the prevention of cardiovascular events: implications of the ACCORD, ADVANCE, and VA diabetes trials: a position statement of the American Diabetes Association and a scientific statement of the American College of Cardiology Foundation and the American Heart Association. *Diabetes Care*. 2009;32:187-192.
34. Nathan DM, Buse JB, Davidson MB, et al. Medical management of hyperglycemia in type 2 diabetes: a consensus algorithm for the initiation and adjustment of therapy: a consensus statement of the American Diabetes Association and the European Association for the Study of Diabetes. *Diabetes Care*. 2009;32:193-203.
35. Apidra [package insert]. Bridgewater, NJ: Sanofi-aventis; February, 2009.
36. NovoLog [package insert]. Princeton, NJ: Novo Nordisk Inc; July, 2009.

37. Humalog [package insert]. Indianapolis, IN: Eli Lilly and Co; March, 2009.
38. Novolin R [package insert]. Princeton, NJ: Novo Nordisk, Inc; June, 2009.
39. Humulin R [package insert]. Indianapolis, IN: Eli Lilly and Co; August, 2007.
40. Novolin N [package insert]. Princeton, NJ: Novo Nordisk, Inc; June, 2009.
41. Humulin N [package insert]. Indianapolis, IN: Eli Lilly and Co; August, 2007.
42. Lantus [package insert]. Bridgewater, NJ: Sanofi-aventis; March, 2007.
43. Levemir [package insert]. Princeton, NJ: Novo Nordisk, Inc; July, 2009.
44. Symlin [package insert]. San Diego, CA: Amylin Pharmaceuticals, Inc; July, 2008.
45. Byetta [package insert]. San Diego, CA: Amylin Pharmaceuticals, Inc; June, 2008.
46. DRUGDEX® System: Klasco RK, ed: DRUGDEX® System (electronic version). Thomson Micromedex, Greenwood Village, Colorado, USA. http://www.thomsonhc.com Accessed 08/12/2009.
47. Victoza [package insert]. Princeton, NJ: Novo Nordisk, Inc; January, 2010.
48. Nissen SE, Wolski K. Effects of rosiglitazone on the risk of myocardial infarction and death from cardiovascular cause. *N Engl J Med*. 2007;356:2457-2471.
49. Mannucci E, Monami M, Lamanna C, et al. Pioglitazone and cardiovascular risk. A comprehensive meta analysis of randomized clinical trials. *Diabetes Obes Metab*. 2008;10: 1221-1238.
50. Lincoff AM, Welski K, Nicholls SJ, et al. Pioglitazone and risk cardiovascular events in patients with type 2 diabetes mellitus: a meta analysis of randomized trials. *JAMA*. 2007;298: 1180-1188.

CHAPTER

59 Thyroid Disorders

Elizabeth W. Blake

FOUNDATION OVERVIEW

The thyroid gland, located in the front of the neck, has two main functions—to secrete thyroid hormones and to secrete calcitonin.[1] The thyroid gland operates via a negative feedback mechanism to synthesize thyroid hormones.[2] The hypothalamus produces thyrotropin-releasing hormone (TRH) which then stimulates the pituitary to release thyroid-stimulating hormone (TSH). TSH, also known as thyrotropin, then stimulates the synthesis and release of thyroid hormones from the thyroid gland. Formation of thyroid hormones requires iodination of tyrosine residues by thyroid peroxidase to produce monoiodinated and diiodinated residues that couple to form triiodothyronine (T_3) and levothyroxine (T_4).[3] Circulating levels of these hormones regulate the amount of TSH secreted. While the thyroid gland is responsible for the production of all T_4, only 20% of T_3 is secreted by the thyroid. Peripheral conversion of T_4 to T_3 forms the majority of T_3. T_3 is more potent, less bound to plasma proteins, and has a greater affinity for the thyroid receptor.[2,3] Thyroid hormones affect multiple organ systems throughout the body (Table 59-1).[1-4] Alterations in these hormone concentrations along with changes in TSH will lead to hyper- or hypothyroidism.[2] (Table 59-2)

HYPERTHYROIDISM

Pathophysiology/Epidemiology

Hyperthyroidism occurs when excessive thyroid hormones are produced.[5] The majority of cases of hyperthyroidism (50%-80%) occur due to Graves disease, an autoimmune condition in which antibodies form against the thyrotropin receptor and stimulate the production of thyroid hormones.[5,6] The remaining cases of hyperthyroidism occur due to a wide variety of reasons.[2,5,6,7] (Table 59-3)

Clinical Presentation/Signs and Symptoms

Patients with hyperthyroidism typically present with nervousness or anxiety, palpitations and tachycardia, weight loss, sleep disturbances, frequent bowel movements, and heat intolerance.[5,7] Women can experience irregular menses or decreased fertility, while men may have decreased libido or gynecomastia. Graves disease may induce ophthalmopathies including exophthalmos.[6,7] Few patients present with thyroid storm, a rare and life-threatening form of hyperthyroidism.

Diagnosis

In order to diagnose hyperthyroidism, patients should undergo a thorough evaluation including a comprehensive history and physical examination and laboratory evaluation of thyroid hormones.[5,6] TSH concentrations as determined by a sensitive TSH assay will typically be decreased to less than 0.1 mIU/L, while unbound T_3 and T_4 concentrations will be elevated. Subclinical hyperthyroidism results when thyroid hormone concentrations remain within the normal reference range but serum TSH is decreased.[8] Though rarely needed for diagnosis, the presence of thyrotropin-receptor antibodies or thyroid-stimulating immunoglobulins (TSI) may indicate Graves disease.[6,7]

Treatment

General Overview

Due to the potential for the development of atrial fibrillation and an increase in all-cause mortality associated with subclinical hyperthyroidism, current recommendations suggest that even subclinical hyperthyroidism should be treated.[9] Since Graves disease remains the most common cause of hyperthyroidism, treatment recommendations focus on this disease state.[5-7,9] Available treatment options include surgery, radioiodine therapy, and antithyroid drugs. Surgical intervention with thyroidectomy remains a last-line option, reserved for treatment-refractory patients or the presence of a large goiter or malignant thyroid nodule.

Specific Agents

Radioactive Iodine Radioactive iodine remains the optimal treatment for Graves disease as it reduces the chance of recurrence of Graves disease.[5-7,9] This treatment, however, induces permanent hypothyroidism within 4 to 12 months in most cases. Thyroid replacement therapy should begin while patients are euthyroid prior to the development of hypothyroidism and its associated symptoms.[7] Less than 20% of patients may need a second dose of radioactive iodine.[6] Prior to starting radioiodine therapy, a 24-hour radioiodine-uptake study may be performed to calculate the dose needed, but a fixed-dose of radioiodine may be given. Patients must take

TABLE 59-1 Effects of Thyroid Hormones

Organ or Organ System	Effects
Skeletal system	Stimulate bone turnover—increase bone resorption and bone formation
Cardiovascular system	Inotropic and chronotropic Decrease systemic vascular resistance Increase resting heart rate Increase left ventricular contractility Increase blood volume
Nervous system	Promote normal brain development
Adipose tissue	Stimulate lipolysis
Muscle	Increase protein breakdown
Liver	Regulate cholesterol and triglyceride metabolism
Gastrointestinal	Increase rate of carbohydrate absorption
All tissues	Increase oxygen consumption and heat production Increase metabolic rate

TABLE 59-3 Causes of Hyperthyroidism and Hypothyroidism

Hyperthyroidism	Hypothyroidism
Graves disease	Chronic autoimmune thyroiditis (Hashimoto disease)
Toxic adenoma	Surgical removal of the thyroid gland
Toxic multinodular goiter	Thyroid gland ablation with radioactive iodine
Painful subacute thyroiditis	External irradiation
Silent thyroiditis	Biosynthetic defect in iodine organification
Iodine-induced hyperthyroidism	Replacement of the thyroid gland by tumor
Ectopic thyroid tissue	Drugs—amiodarone, lithium, excess antithyroid hormones, interferon-α
Excessive pituitary TSH or trophoblastic disease	
Drugs—excess levothyroxine, amiodarone	

several necessary precautions after treatment with radioactive iodine to prevent transference of radioactive iodine to others.[7] Pregnant women should avoid treatment with radioiodine as it crosses the placenta and can be taken up by the fetal thyroid hormone with serious consequences. Additionally, women of childbearing age should avoid getting pregnant for 6 to 12 months after treatment. For patients with underlying cardiovascular disease and some elderly patients, pretreatment with antithyroid drugs may reduce the risk of cardiovascular events associated with posttreatment exacerbation of hyperthyroidism. However, recent studies have shown that use of antithyroid drugs may lead to a higher rate of treatment failure after radioiodine therapy.[9] These medications must be discontinued 3 to 7 days prior to radioiodine therapy to minimize the risk of treatment failure.[6]

Antithyroid Drugs The thionamides, methimazole, and propylthiouracil are given as monotherapy for hyperthyroidism or in preparation for radioactive iodine therapy.[5,6,9,10]

TABLE 59-2 Overview of Thyroid Disorders

Disorder	TSH	T_4 and T_3
Hyperthyroidism	↓↓	↑
Subclinical hyperthyroidism	↓	Normal
Hypothyroidism	↑↑	↓
Subclinical hypothyroidism	↑	Normal

These agents block the formation of thyroid hormones by preventing the incorporation of iodine into tyrosine residues by thyroid peroxidase.[6,10] Additionally, propylthiouracil blocks the peripheral conversion of T_4 to T_3. Over the course of therapy, thionamides may provide immunosuppressive effects, including the reduction in the concentrations of thyrotropin-receptor antibodies.

Both methimazole and propylthiouracil are given orally, with rapid gastrointestinal absorption.[5,6,10] Due to a longer duration of action, methimazole can be administered once daily, while propylthiouracil requires dosing two to three times daily. Other benefits of methimazole include more rapid clinical effects, with faster reductions in serum concentrations of T_4 and T_3.

Initial treatment of hyperthyroidism requires higher doses of antithyroid medications (Table 59-4).[5,6,10] Inadequate dosing of antithyroid medications may lead to continuation of hyperthyroidism or, conversely, development of hypothyroidism. Symptom and laboratory improvement can be seen about 3 to 4 weeks after initiation of medication. While T_4 and T_3 normalize quickly, serum concentrations of TSH might take months to normalize. Thyroid function tests should be checked every 4 to 6 weeks during the first 4 to 6 months. As symptoms improve and thyroid function returns to normal, doses of antithyroid medications may be reduced. Monotherapy should be continued for 12 to 18 months to induce remission. However, some patients may require longer durations of therapy.

TABLE 59-4 **Antithyroid Medications**

	Methimazole	Propylthiouracil
Mechanism of action	Blocks formation of T_4 and T_3	Blocks formation of T_4 and T_3 Blocks peripheral conversion of T_4 to T_3
Starting dose	10-30 mg daily	200-400 mg divided in 2-3 daily doses
Maintenance dose	5-10 mg daily	100-200 mg divided in 2-3 daily doses
Half-life	2-28 h	0.9-4.3 h
Protein binding	None	80%
Major side effects	Agranulocytosis, cholestasis, arthralgias	Agranulocytosis, vasculitis, hepatotoxicity (black box warning), arthralgias

The goal of monotherapy with antithyroid drugs is to achieve remission, defined as the ability to maintain normal thyroid function for 1 year without antithyroid medication.[6,10] Remission can be achieved in 30% to 50% of patients, but relapse occurs in more than half of patients treated with antithyroid medications. Most relapses occur within the first 6 months after stopping therapy. Factors such as male sex, older age (>40 years old), a large goiter, higher baseline T_4 and T_3 concentrations, and higher levels of thyrotropin-receptor antibodies reduce the likelihood of remission. Strategies to improve remission rates, such as longer duration of therapy (>1 year), higher doses of antithyroid medications, and addition of thyroxine, have not proven to be successful. Radioactive iodine therapy remains an alternative for patients who fail antithyroid medications.

Side effects of antithyroid medications occur in about 5% of patients and include cutaneous reactions, gastrointestinal upset, and arthralgias.[5,6,10] The occurrence of arthralgias must be taken seriously and antithyroid medication must be stopped as it may signal the development of a severe polyarthritis. Other side effects occur infrequently but produce severe reactions. Agranulocytosis occurs in approximately 0.3% of patients treated with antithyroid medications. Most cases occur within the first 3 months of therapy but may develop after more than a year. Routine monitoring of white blood cells is not recommended as agranulocytosis rarely occurs and usually develops rapidly. Patients should be advised to discontinue antithyroid medications and seek medical attention if they develop fever, sore throat, or mouth ulcers as hospitalization and treatment with broad-spectrum antibiotics are required. Cross-reactivity between methimazole and propylthiouracil for agranulocytosis can occur. As a result, patients must pursue an alternative therapy for the treatment of hyperthyroidism.

Vasculitis can occur as drug-induced lupus or with the development of antineutrophil cytoplasmic antibodies (ANCA). Though rare, it occurs more frequently in Asian patients treated with propylthiouracil. Patient presentation includes acute renal dysfunction, arthritis, skin ulceration, and upper and lower respiratory symptoms. Antithyroid medication must be discontinued. Severe cases require additional treatment with glucocorticoids or cyclophosphamide.

Hepatotoxicity may occur with methimazole and propylthiouracil but in differing forms.[5,10] Methimazole can induce a cholestasis that is slowly reversed with discontinuation of the drug. Propylthiouracil can induce liver failure that is fatal in a small portion of patients, typically developing in the first 3 months of therapy if it occurs. The FDA added a black box warning for propylthiouracil in April 2010, warning of the risk of severe liver injury and acute liver failure. As a result, methimazole should be recommended as the first-line antithyroid medication. Routine monitoring of liver function tests is not recommended but the development of hepatotoxicity symptoms including fatigue, jaundice, dark urine, and easy bruising should prompt patients to seek medical attention. Discontinuation of propylthiouracil is required. The development of any life-threatening side effects including agranulocytosis, vasculitis, or hepatotoxicity precludes future use of antithyroid medications.

Beta-adrenergic blocking drugs Beta-adrenergic blocking agents are used as adjunctive therapy to ameliorate the symptoms of hyperthyroidism, including anxiety, palpitations, and tremor, until thyroid hormone levels normalize.[5,6] Propranolol and nadolol minimally inhibit the conversion of T_4 to T_3. Choice of beta-adrenergic blocking agent can depend on concomitant disease states and frequency of dosing.

Special Considerations

Pregnancy and Lactation

Hyperthyroidism can develop during pregnancy.[5,6,10] Due to the risk of miscarriage, preeclampsia, and preterm delivery, treatment must be started. The use of radioactive iodine is contraindicated, and surgery should be avoided; therefore, antithyroid drugs should be used.[5] Both methimazole and propylthiouracil can be used, although both are categorized as class D agents by the FDA due to the risk of fetal hypothyroidism.[10] Propylthiouracil is preferred over methimazole, as methimazole has been associated with congenital abnormalities like aplasia cutis and gastrointestinal defects.[5,6] Thyroid levels should be maintained at the upper limit of normal with the lowest dose possible to reduce the risk of neonatal hypothyroidism. In some patients, symptoms improve during the third trimester such that antithyroid medications can be discontinued, but hyperthyroidism may worsen during the postpartum period. Both antithyroid drugs are secreted in breast milk in low concentrations, but may be safe in nursing mothers.

Thyroid Storm

Thyroid storm is a life-threatening event that results from the exaggerated effects of elevated thyroid hormones.[11,12] The condition occurs rarely but has a 20% to 30% mortality rate. Contributing factors include infection, trauma, diabetic ketoacidosis, certain medications, and inappropriate administration of antithyroid hormones or levothyroxine. Patients present with exaggerated symptoms of hyperthyroidism, and usually have fever, tachycardia, confusion or coma, and gastrointestinal disturbances. Laboratory evaluation reveals undetectable TSH concentrations with elevations in free T_4 and T_3 that appear similar to uncomplicated hyperthyroidism. Hyperglycemia and elevated liver enzymes may also be present. Treatment recommendations include high-dose beta-adrenergic blocking agents administered concomitantly with propylthiouracil, glucocorticoids, stable iodide, and supportive care. Propylthiouracil is recommended preferentially over methimazole due to its ability to block the peripheral conversion of T_4 to T_3. The precipitating event should also be managed appropriately.

HYPOTHYROIDISM

Pathophysiology/Epidemiology

Hypothyroidism occurs when the thyroid gland does not secrete sufficient amounts of thyroid hormones.[7,13] Myxedema can occur with overt hypothyroidism that is severe or complicated. Autoimmune thyroiditis (Hashimoto disease) remains the most common cause of hypothyroidism in the United States.[7,13,14] Congenital hypothyroidism occurs frequently in other parts of the world due to iodine deficiency. Hypothyroidism results from many more conditions (Table 59-3).

Clinical Presentation/Signs and Symptoms

Hypothyroidism usually develops slowly, so most patients may not notice an acute onset of symptoms.[7,13,14] In one study, only 30% of patients newly diagnosed with hypothyroidism complained of symptoms.[13] Symptoms associated with hypothyroidism include fatigue, cold intolerance, constipation, dry skin, weight gain, goiter, or hoarseness.[7,13,14] Depression and slow mental cognition may also occur. Cardiovascular effects include bradycardia, dyslipidemia, and edema. Women may experience irregular or heavy menses and infertility. Other rare developments include coma, seizure, and hypothermia.

Diagnosis

Primary hypothyroidism can be identified by elevated TSH concentrations with a decrease in serum free T_4 concentrations.[7,13,14] Patients with overt symptomatic hypothyroidism will have TSH levels greater than 10 mIU/L. Patients with autoimmune thyroiditis will usually test positive for thyroid antibodies, including antithyroid peroxidase antibodies and antithyroglobulin antibodies. Subclinical hypothyroidism can be diagnosed by slightly elevated TSH concentrations between 5 and 10 mIU/L while T_4 concentrations remain within the normal reference range. Additionally, a 30% diurnal variation in TSH concentrations may occur with the lowest levels occurring mid-afternoon further confounding the diagnosis of hypothyroidism.[14] Controversy remains whether subclinical hypothyroidism should be treated.

Nonthyroidal illnesses and drugs may also affect TSH concentrations.[7,14,15] Even in the presence of hypothyroidism, certain drugs including glucocorticoids, dopamine, and dobutamine will suppress TSH concentrations.[7,13] Phenytoin and carbamazepine may suppress both serum T_4 and TSH, resembling central hypothyroidism. Euthyroid sick syndrome may occur when the body is under acute stress.[7] In this situation, thyroid hormone concentrations decrease while TSH concentrations remain normal or also decrease.

Treatment

General Overview

Production of desiccated animal thyroid hormone to treat hypothyroidism began in the mid-1890s.[15] Treatment with desiccated thyroid continued until the 1960s when synthetic levothyroxine (T_4) and liothyronine (T_3) became available. Since synthetic T_4 still undergoes peripheral conversion to T_3 in the body, use of synthetic T_3 has declined. Additionally, recent studies have shown that the combination of T_4 and T_3 produces no significant benefit compared to T_4 alone. The treatment of choice for hypothyroidism remains levothyroxine.[7,13-15] Treatment goals revolve around improvement in patient's symptoms and maintaining TSH concentrations in the lower half of the reference range, around 0.4 to 2.5 mIU/L. Free T_4 levels may be assessed as well.

Specific Agents

Levothyroxine Traditionally, initial doses of oral levothyroxine start low, around 25 to 50 μg daily, with gradual titration of dose, especially in patients greater than 60 years of age and those with ischemic heart disease.[13,14] Recent information indicates that initial therapy may begin with full treatment doses of levothyroxine 1.6 μg /kg in most healthy patients, titrated to optimal TSH levels.[7,13,14,16] Due to the long half-life of levothyroxine (7 days), assessment of TSH concentrations must wait for 4 to 6 weeks to allow medication to reach steady state. Once optimal TSH concentrations have been achieved, follow-up assessments can be deferred to every 6 to 12 months. Patients should be reminded that it may take months for symptoms of hypothyroidism to resolve and that treatment continues indefinitely.

Thyroid hormone replacement can be complicated by many factors. Age and malabsorption states like celiac disease affect absorption. Taking levothyroxine alone on an empty stomach maximizes absorption. Certain drugs, including calcium salts, ferrous sulfate, aluminum hydroxide, and cholestyramine, prevent the absorption of levothyroxine. Other medications, particularly anticonvulsants and rifampin, increase the clearance of levothyroxine.

Most patients require oral replacement with levothyroxine, but parenteral administration, intravenously or intramuscularly, may be needed if the patient cannot take oral medication for an extended time or for the treatment of myxedema coma.[17] The parenteral replacement dose should be 80% of the usual oral dose due to bioavailability differences. Reconstituted parenteral doses must be given immediately due to poor stability.

Due to a narrow therapeutic index, inadequately dosed levothyroxine increases the risk of adverse effects.[7,13-17] Excessive levothyroxine may precipitate atrial fibrillation and worsen osteoporosis. Consequently, patients with cardiac disease should start levothyroxine at low doses with a slow titration to normal TSH concentrations. Unresolved symptoms of hypothyroidism will continue with subtherapeutic doses of levothyroxine. Use of levothyroxine for nontoxic diffuse goiter or nodular thyroid disease may precipitate thyrotoxicosis. Additionally, levothyroxine should be avoided in patients with acute myocardial infarction, thyrotoxicosis, and adrenal insufficiency. Inappropriate use of levothyroxine for the treatment of obesity or for weight reduction should also be avoided.

Special Considerations

Pregnancy

Serious consequences can occur in the mother and fetus if overt hypothyroidism remains untreated.[7] As levothyroxine has been determined safe and effective during pregnancy, hypothyroidism should be treated with thyroid replacement hormone. Pregnancy changes thyroid function, so TSH concentrations should be assessed every 6 weeks.

Bioequivalency of Oral Levothyroxine Preparations

Levothyroxine first became available in 1962, without a new drug application through the Food and Drug Administration (FDA).[18] In 1997, the FDA mandated that all marketed levothyroxine products submit a new drug application. At that time, the FDA did not recognize these products to be safe and effective due to lack of data showing consistent potency and stability. Levothyroxine products were not considered therapeutically interchangeable, as well. In July 2001, the FDA determined standards for bioequivalency of levothyroxine products, based on the absorption of T_4 rather than the effect on TSH concentrations. Currently, nine levothyroxine products are approved for use by the FDA (Table 59-5).[19] Regardless of the product used, patients should be maintained on one particular brand of levothyroxine.[7,14] TSH concentrations should be monitored frequently if a patient changes brands of levothyroxine.

TABLE 59-5 **FDA-Approved Levothyroxine Products**

Proprietary Name	Applicant
Levo-T	Alara Pharm
Levothroid	Lloyd (distributed by Forest)
Levoxyl	Jones Pharma/King
Synthroid	Abbott
Tirosint	Institute Biochimique
Unithroid	Jerome Stevens
Generic Formulations	**Applicant**
Levothyroxine sodium	Genpharm
Levothyroxine sodium	Mylan

AMIODARONE AND THE THYROID

A potent antiarrhythmic, amiodarone can induce thyroid dysfunction in 14% to 18% of treated patients.[7,20,21] Amiodarone contains a significant amount of iodine (75 mg iodine per a 200-mg dose) that may inhibit thyroid function. Amiodarone also blocks the conversion of T_4 to T_3 throughout the body. As a result, it may induce either hypothyroidism or hyperthyroidism. Baseline TSH levels should be obtained prior to starting amiodarone and should be reassessed every 6 months during treatment. Even after discontinuation, amiodarone may continue to exert its effect on the thyroid due to its long half-life.

In iodine-sufficient areas of the world, amiodarone-induced hypothyroidism is more common and occurs after 6 to 12 months of treatment with amiodarone.[20,21] Similar to other forms of hypothyroidism, treatment with levothyroxine remains the therapy of choice. Once amiodarone has been discontinued, thyroid levels may return to normal in 2 to 4 months. The development of antithyroid antibodies may allow hypothyroidism to persist despite the discontinuation of amiodarone.

Amiodarone-induced hyperthyroidism can occur in two forms—type 1 and type 2—and is more common in iodine-deficient areas of the world.[20,21] Type 1 occurs in patients treated with amiodarone who have underlying thyroid disease. Radioactive iodine cannot be used due to low radioiodine uptake associated with this form. Antithyroid medications may offer some benefit, but resumption of a euthyroid state may take discontinuation of amiodarone. Type 2 amiodarone-induced hyperthyroidism is caused by an inflammatory process that results in a destructive thyroiditis that may last for 1 to 3 months. Patients may be treated with corticosteroids, and amiodarone may be continued. Rarely, surgery to remove the thyroid gland may be necessary.

CASE Application

1. Which of the following statements regarding thyroid hormones is true?
   a. The majority of T_4 is formed in the periphery.
   b. T_3 has greater potency than T_4.
   c. Iodine is not involved in the formation of thyroid hormones.
   d. The concentrations of circulating hormones do not affect the secretion of TSH.
2. Hyperthyroidism typically presents with which laboratory result?
   a. Increased TSH, increased thyroid hormones
   b. Decreased TSH, increased thyroid hormones

c. Increased TSH, decreased thyroid hormones
d. Decreased TSH, decreased thyroid hormones

3. What is the most common cause of hyperthyroidism?
   a. Graves disease
   b. Hashimoto disease
   c. Silent thyroiditis
   d. Excessive ingestion of levothyroxine

4. MM is a 27-year-old woman who is 28 weeks pregnant who has just been diagnosed with hyperthyroidism. Which symptoms might MM be experiencing due to her diagnosis?
   a. Bradycardia and cold intolerance
   b. Tachycardia and heat intolerance
   c. Depression and cognition difficulties
   d. Weight gain and constipation

5. What is the optimal treatment for MM?
   a. Surgery
   b. Radioactive iodine
   c. Methimazole
   d. Propylthiouracil

6. Dr. M wants to know which antithyroid medication would be preferred in a nonpregnant patient with hyperthyroidism and why. What is your response?
   a. Propylthiouracil is preferred due to fewer side effects and less frequent dosing.
   b. Methimazole is preferred due to fewer side effects and less frequent dosing.
   c. Methimazole is preferred since it blocks the peripheral conversion of T_4 to T_3.
   d. Propylthiouracil is preferred since it blocks the peripheral conversion of T_4 to T_3.

7. TS is a 35-year-old woman started on methimazole for treatment of hyperthyroidism. Which of the following side effects might she experience that would require discontinuation of her medication?
   a. Agranulocytosis
   b. Insomnia
   c. Gastrointestinal upset
   d. Cutaneous reaction

8. LR is a 32-year-old woman who is still experiencing symptoms of hyperthyroidism despite treatment with propylthiouracil. Which medication can be added to provide additional symptomatic relief?
   a. Nifedipine
   b. Prednisone
   c. Propranolol
   d. Ibuprofen

9. YD presents to the emergency room in a coma with fever and tachycardia. Based on results of his thyroid function tests, YD is diagnosed with thyroid storm. Which therapy would be preferred for treatment of YD?
   a. Radioactive iodine
   b. Propylthiouracil
   c. Methimazole
   d. Surgical thyroidectomy

10. What is the most common cause of hypothyroidism in the United States?
    a. Graves disease
    b. Congenital hypothyroidism
    c. Surgical thyroidectomy
    d. Autoimmune thyroiditis

11. GB is a 55-year-old woman recently diagnosed with hypothyroidism. Which symptoms might she be experiencing?
    a. Bradycardia and cold intolerance
    b. Anxiety and nervousness
    c. Weight loss and insomnia
    d. Frequent bowel movements and edema

12. What would thyroid function tests reveal in GB?
    a. Increased TSH, increased thyroid hormones
    b. Decreased TSH, increased thyroid hormones
    c. Increased TSH, decreased thyroid hormones
    d. Decreased TSH, decreased thyroid hormones

13. What would be the optimal treatment for GB?
    a. Desiccated thyroid hormone
    b. Liothyronine
    c. Levothyroxine
    d. The combination of liothyronine and levothyroxine

14. Which of the following patient counseling tips is accurate regarding levothyroxine?
    a. Levothyroxine should be taken with food to maximize absorption.
    b. Levothyroxine should be taken on an empty stomach to maximize absorption.
    c. Levothyroxine produces immediate symptomatic relief of hypothyroidism.
    d. Levothyroxine will only be needed until symptoms of hypothyroidism resolve.

15. As GB picks up her first prescription of levothyroxine, she asks you when she should have her thyroid function tests rechecked. What is your response?
    a. 1 week
    b. 1 month
    c. 3 months
    d. 6 months

16. Dr. Z in your clinic asks you what are the most recent dosing recommendations for initiating levothyroxine

for the treatment of hypothyroidism. What is your response?

a. Full treatment doses of levothyroxine may be started in all patients.
b. Levothyroxine must be started at low doses and titrated up slowly in all patients.
c. Patients with ischemic heart disease may begin levothyroxine at full treatment doses.
d. Full treatment doses of levothyroxine should be started only in younger healthy patients.

17. PR is a 35-year-old woman admitted for uncontrollable nausea and vomiting during the first trimester of her pregnancy. Her past medical history is significant for hypothyroidism and gastroesophageal reflux disease (GERD). How should her hypothyroidism be managed during her hospitalization?

a. Levothyroxine should be held until PR can restart her oral medication.
b. Levothyroxine should be given intravenously until PR can restart her oral medication.
c. Levothyroxine should be given orally at a lower dose to reduce nausea and vomiting.
d. Levothyroxine should be changed to liothyronine to reduce nausea and vomiting.

18. FN is diagnosed with Hashimoto disease during the second trimester of her pregnancy. Which medication would be preferred for FN?

a. Desiccated thyroid hormone
b. Liothyronine alone
c. Levothyroxine alone
d. Levothyroxine in combination with liothyronine

19. What is the treatment of choice for amiodarone-induced hypothyroidism?

a. Desiccated thyroid hormone
b. Liothyronine alone
c. Levothyroxine alone
d. Levothyroxine in combination with liothyronine

20. Which of the following is true?

a. Radioactive iodine will adequately treat type 1 amiodarone-induced hyperthyroidism.
b. Amiodarone must be discontinued to adequately treat type 1 amiodarone-induced hypothyroidism.
c. Amiodarone must be discontinued to adequately treat type 2 amiodarone-induced hypothyroidism.
d. Antithyroid medications may offer some benefit in type 2 amiodarone-induced hypothyroidism.

TAKEAWAY POINTS ››

- A negative feedback system based on circulating thyroid hormone concentrations determines that amount of thyroid-stimulating hormone produced.
- All of levothyroxine (T_4) is produced in the thyroid gland while the majority of triiodothyronine (T_3) is produced by peripheral conversion of T_4 to T_3.
- The most common cause of hyperthyroidism is Graves disease.
- Symptoms of hyperthyroidism include tachycardia, weight loss, nervousness, heat intolerance, and exophthalmos.
- In hyperthyroidism, TSH concentrations may be undetectable while free thyroid concentrations are elevated above the normal reference range.
- Treatment options for hyperthyroidism include surgery, radioactive iodine, and antithyroid medications.
- Radioactive iodine is the treatment of choice for Graves disease in most patients, but special precautions should be taken after treatment.
- Antithyroid medications, methimazole and propylthiouracil, are preferred in pregnant patients and those patients unable to undergo radioactive iodine treatment. Propylthiouracil is preferred over methimazole in treating hyperthyroidism in pregnancy.
- Both methimazole and propylthiouracil block the formation of thyroid hormones, but propylthiouracil also blocks the peripheral conversion of T_4 to T_3.
- Serious side effects associated with antithyroid medications include agranulocytosis, hepatotoxicity, and vasculitis.
- Beta-adrenergic blocking drugs may be given as adjunctive therapy to provide symptomatic relief.
- Treatment recommendations for thyroid storm include propylthiouracil, beta-adrenergic blocking agents, glucocorticoids, stable iodide, and supportive care.
- The most common cause of hypothyroidism is autoimmune thyroiditis (Hashimoto disease).
- Symptoms of hypothyroidism include cold intolerance, weight gain, depression, and fatigue.
- Serum TSH concentrations are elevated in hypothyroidism while free T_4 concentrations are decreased.
- The treatment of choice for hypothyroidism is levothyroxine though it may take 4 to 6 weeks to reach steady state with levothyroxine due to the long half-life of 7 days.
- Full treatment doses of levothyroxine should be started as initial therapy in most healthy patients. Levothyroxine should be initiated at lower doses to prevent adverse effects in patients over the age of 60 and those with ischemic heart disease.
- Levothyroxine is safe and effective for the treatment of hypothyroidism in pregnancy.

- Amiodarone may induce hypo- or hyperthyroidism due to a significant iodine content that inhibits thyroid function and by blocking conversion of T_4 to T_3.
- Amiodarone-induced hypothyroidism may be treated with levothyroxine along with discontinuation of amiodarone.
- Amiodarone may induce two types of hyperthyroidism. Type 1 may be treated with antithyroid medication, but may require discontinuation of amiodarone. Type 2 may be treated with glucocorticoids, and therapy with amiodarone may continue.

REFERENCES

1. Barrett KE, Barman SM, Boitano S, Brooks H. The thyroid gland. In: Barrett KE, Barman SM, Boitano S, et al eds. *Ganong's Review of Medical Physiology*. 23rd ed. New York, NY: McGraw-Hill; 2010. Available at: http://www.accessmedicine.com/content.aspx?aID=5244652. Accessed August 31, 2009.
2. Jameson J. L, Weetman Anthony P.. Disorders of the thyroid gland. In: Fauci AS, Braunwald E, Kasper DL, et al. eds. *Harrison's Principles of Internal Medicine.* 17th ed. New York, NY: McGraw-Hill; 2008. Available at: http://www.accessmedicine.com/content.aspx?aID=2877285. Accessed September 1, 2009.
3. Yen PM. Physiological and molecular basis of thyroid hormone action. *Physiol Rev.* 2001;81(3):1097-1142.
4. Molina PE. Thyroid gland. In: Molina PE, ed. *Endocrine Physiology*, 2nd ed. New York, NY: McGraw-Hill; 2006. Available at: http://www.accessmedicine.com/content.aspx?aID=2364507. Accessed August 31, 2009.
5. Cooper DS. Hyperthyroidism. *Lancet.* 2003;362(9382):459-68.
6. Brent GA. Graves' disease. *N Engl J Med.* 2008;358(24):2594-605.
7. AACE Thyroid Task Force. American Association of Clinical Endocrinologists: medical guidelines for clinical practice for the evaluation and treatment of hyperthyroidism and hypothyroidism. *Endocr Pract.* 2002;8:(6)457-469.
8. Surks MI, Ortiz E, Daniels GH, et al. Subclinical thyroid disease: scientific review and guidelines for diagnosis and management. *JAMA*. 3004;291(2):228-238.
9. Kharlip J, Cooper DS. Recent developments in hyperthyroidism. *Lancet.* 2009;373(9679):1930-1932.
10. Cooper DS. Antithyroid drugs. *N Engl J Med.* 2005;352(9):905-917.
11. Sarlis NJ, Gourgiotis L. Thyroid emergencies. *Rev Endocrinol Metab Disorders.* 2003;4(2):129-136.
12. Pimentel L, Hansen KN. Thyroid disease in the emergency department: a clinical and laboratory review. *J Emerg Med.* 2005;28(2):201-209.
13. Roberts CGP, Ladenson PW. Hypothyroidism. *Lancet.* 2004; 363(9411):793-803.
14. Vaidya B, Pearce SHS. Management of hypothyroidism in adults. *BMJ.* 2008;337(7664):284-289.
15. Surks MI. Primary hypothyroidism: new issues and controversies. *The Endocrinologist.* 2006;16(4):203-207.
16. Roos A, Linn-Rasker SP, van Domburg RT, et al. The starting dose of levothyroxine in primary hypothyroidism treatment. *Arch Intern Med.* 2005;165(15):1714-1720.
17. DRUGDEX® System [internet database]. Greenwood Village, CO: Thomson Reuters (Healthcare) Inc. Updated periodically.
18. Hennessy JV. Levothyroxine a new drug? Since when? How could that be? *Thyroid.* 2003;13(3):279-282.
19. U.S. Food and Drug Administration (2009). Table of approved levothyroxine sodium oral formulations (tablet or capsule). Available at: http://www.fda.gov/Drugs/DrugSafety/PostmarketDrugSafetyInformationforPatientsandProviders/ucm161275.htm. Accessed August 28, 2009.
20. Klein I, Danzi S. Thyroid disease and the heart. *Circulation.* 2007;116(15):1725-1735.
21. Basaria S, Cooper DS. Amiodarone and the thyroid. *Am J Med.* 2005;118(7):706-714.

PART

11

Health and Wellness and Other Topics

CHAPTER

60 Contraception

Shareen Y. El-Ibiary

FOUNDATION OVERVIEW

Unintended pregnancies account for about 49% of pregnancies in the United States.[1] About half of these unintended pregnancies result in abortions.[1] Currently, it has been reported that over 11.2 million women in the United States use oral contraceptives and reported that about 20% of women use condoms.[2,3] Whether contraceptive methods are over the counter or prescription only, pharmacists play an important role in providing contraception counseling for proper use and adherence to attain desired outcomes.

There are a variety of contraceptives available. Over-the-counter (OTC) contraceptives commonly include condoms and spermicides. Prescription contraceptives are usually hormone based. There are a variety of factors that go into method selection. Factors to consider include effectiveness, cost, accessibility, side effects, return to fertility rate, frequency of sexual activity, sexually transmitted infection prevention, past medical history, and concomitant medications.

PRODUCT OVERVIEW

Nonhormonal Contraception

Most nonhormonal contraceptives are OTC with the exception of the copper-T (ParaGard) intrauterine device (IUD) and diaphragm. One of the more common nonhormonal contraceptives is the condom. Male latex condoms are the most common and protect the best against sexually transmitted infections (STIs).[4] However, use of oil-based lubricants can breakdown latex condoms and should not be used together. For those with allergies to latex, polyurethane and lamb cecum condoms are available. Both of these condoms are thought to increase heat conduction and provide more sensitivity.[5] They can both be used with water-based or oil-based lubricants.[6] Polyurethane condoms may break easier than latex condoms.[7,8] Lamb cecum condoms are porous, cost more than the others, and do not protect against some STIs such as human immunodeficiency virus (HIV).[9] Overall, male condoms have typical use failure rate of about 15% in preventing pregnancy.[5,6] This percentage may decrease if spermicides are used in conjunction.

The female condom (Reality) is also an option for contraception and prevention of STIs. The female condom is made of polyurethane and is inserted vaginally. Female condoms have a 21% typical use failure rate in preventing pregnancy.[6] In addition, the condom may be worn up 8 hours prior to intercourse. Only one condom should be used for each act of intercourse and then discarded carefully by closing the bottom of the condom and removing it from the vagina while closed. Disadvantages of the product include its "squeaks" during intercourse, appearance, irritation, decreased sensitivity, and difficulty inserting the condom.[5,6] Male and female condoms should not be used together as they stick together causing friction and may break.

Spermicides are also available OTC in a variety of formulations. These include jellies, gels, foams, suppositories, and films. The active ingredient in spermicides available in the United States is nonoxynol-9. Nonoxynol-9 is a noniconic detergent that inhibits sperm motility and function.[6] Nonoxynol-9 is not a microbicide and does not kill viruses such as HIV.[10] In some reports, it has been shown to increase the risk of HIV transmission by causing irritation to the mucosal lining of vagina or rectum, which may allow passage of the virus into the bloodstream.[11] The highest concentration is generally found in the film (28%), foams (8%-12%), suppository (2.3%-5.6%), and jelly/gels (2%-5%).[6] The typical use failure rate of spermicides use alone is 5%-29%.[6] Key counseling points for spermicides include not douching within 6 hours of use, apply within 1 hour of intercourse, and each application only works for one act of intercourse. In addition, the vaginal film and suppository must dissolve completely for at least 15 minutes before intercourse. The film is activated by the female secretions, therefore it is not best for women who have trouble with lubrication. Nonoxynol-9 may be irritating to the skin. If irritation occurs, another product with lower concentration of nonoxynol-9 is recommended.

Another form of OTC contraception is the sponge. Taken off the market in 1995, the sponge was re-released in 2003. The sponge contains a polyurethane foam and 1 gram of nonoxynol-9. After moistening the sponge with two teaspoons of water, it is inserted vaginally, placed against the cervix, and may be worn up to 24 hours. After intercourse, the sponge should remain in place for 6 hours. It acts as a spermicide, mechanical barrier, and absorbs semen. The typical failure rate reported is 18% for nulliparous women and 36% for parous women.[6] Side effects may include irritation or ulceration of the cervix and vaginal mucosa. In addition, toxic shock syndrome may be a concern if the sponge is not removed within 24 hours or if particles remain after removal.

Other nonhormonal contraceptives include the copper-T IUD and diaphragm. Both require prescription and are usually

TABLE 60-1 Side Effects of Hormones

Too Much Estrogen	Not Enough Estrogen	Too Much Progestin [a]Associated with Androgenic Properties		Not Enough Progestin
Bloating Breast tenderness Mood changes Headache Nausea Heavy menses Fibroid growth Melasma Vision changes Cyclic weight gain	Breakthrough bleeding early in cycle Light menses Vaginal dryness Spotting No withdrawal bleeding	Decrease in sex drive Less energy Depression Increased appetite Noncyclical weight gain Yeast infections	Acne[a] Hirsutism[a] Cholestatic jaundice[a] Hair loss[a] Swelling in arms/legs[a] Increase in sex drive[a]	Breakthrough bleeding late in cycle No withdrawal bleeding Heavy menses

Reproduced with permission from: *A Pharmacotherapeutic Approach to Women's Health Across the Lifespan*, American Society of Health Systems Pharmacists. Washington, DC; 2010.[34]

provided by the prescriber. The copper-T IUD is a device that is placed in the uterus and prevents implantation. The copper in the IUD has an acrosomal enzyme that stops the sperm from moving. The copper-T may be used for up to 10 years. It is very effective with a typical use failure rate of 0.8%.[6] Some side effects include breakthrough bleeding, cramping, pain, and expulsion. The diaphragm is inserted vaginally and acts as a barrier device to sperm. It has a typical use failure rate of 16%.[6]

Hormonal Contraception

Combined Hormonal Contraception

There are two main types of hormonal contraceptives, progestin-only (progestin) and combined (estrogen and progestin) with ethinyl estradiol (EE) as the main estrogen used in products. Combined hormonal contraceptives (CHCs) work primarily by inhibiting ovulation. All CHCs have an FDA-indicated use for the prevention of pregnancy, have a typical failure rate of approximately 8%, and a reasonable return to fertility averaging around 3 months.[6] Some CHCs are indicated for uses other than preventing pregnancy. YAZ (EE/drospirenone), Yasmin (EE/drospirenone), Ortho Tri-Cyclen (EE, norgestimate), and Estrostep (EE/norethindrone) are products that contain the FDA indication for acne treatment. YAZ also has the FDA-approved indication for the treatment of premenstrual dysphoric disorder (PMDD). Off-label uses for most CHCs include, regulation of menstrual cycle, iron deficiency anemia, polycystic ovary syndrome, hirsutism, dysmenorrhea, and decreased risk of ovarian cancer.[12]

Unfortunately, CHCs are not without side effects. Some side effects may be attributed to the estrogen or the progestin component (Table 60-1). Most commonly seen side effects include: nausea, breakthrough bleeding, mood changes, and weight gain.[13] Generally, it is recommended that a woman try a product for at least 3 months before changing to a new one.[6] It takes a few months for the body to adjust to the CHC. If after 3 months, side effects continue to be bothersome, a product switch is recommended.

As with many medicines, CHCs are not without drug interactions. Estrogens and progestins are metabolized by the CYP-450 enzymes and concomitant medications that affect these enzymes may also alter the effectiveness of hormonal contraceptives (Table 60-2). The most well known interactions that may decrease the effectiveness of combined hormonal contraceptives include antiepileptics, antibiotics, antiretrovirals, protease inhibitors, and herbal products such as St. John's wort.[14,15] Depending on the interaction, higher doses of

TABLE 60-2 Selected Drug Interactions with CHCs[a]

Drugs That Increase Effect of CHCs	Drugs/Herbals That Decrease the Effect of CHCs	Drugs That *May* Decrease the Effect of CHCs (Controversial)	Metabolism or Clearance Altered by CHCs
Atorvastatin Atazanavir Indinavir	Amprenavir Barbiturates Carbamazepine Felbamate Griseofulvin Lopinavir Modafinil Nelfinavir Nevirapine Oxcarbazepine Phenobarbital Phenytoin Primidone Rifamycins Ritonavir Saquinavir St. John's wort Tipranavir	Ampicillin Amoxicillin Ciprofloxacin Clarithromycin Doxycycline Erythromycin Fluconazole Metronidazole Minocycline Ofloxacin Tetracycline Topiramate	Acetaminophen Antidepressants, tricyclic Aspirin Benzodiazepines Beta blockers Caffeine Corticosteroids Cyclosporine Lamotrigine Theophyllines

[a]Drug list is not all inclusive. Some drug interactions may exist that are not cited in this table.

Reproduced with permission from: *A Pharmacotherapeutic Approach to Women's Health Across the Lifespan*, American Society of Health Systems Pharmacists. Washington, DC; 2010.[34]

hormonal contraceptives may be needed or alternate forms of contraception may be recommended. In particular, controversies surround the use of antibiotics and hormonal contraceptives. Most conservative approaches suggest using a back-up method while using antibiotics and for a week following the discontinuation of antibiotics.[16]

Combined Oral Contraceptives

Combined hormonal contraceptives come in a few different dosage forms that include oral tablets, transdermal patch, and vaginal ring. Oral tablets are available in three different types of formulations: monophasic, biphasic, and triphasic (Table 60-3). Monophasic regimens contain the same strength of the hormones in the active tablets throughout the pill pack. Biphasic regimens usually contain 10 days of hormones and 11 days of an increased amount of hormones. Triphasic regimens vary each week of the cycle with different amount of hormones. For most formulations, the estrogen dose stays the same while progestin dose increases each week. The benefit of these formulations was thought to decrease the exposure to progestins. Some products such as Cyclessa (EE/desogestrel) and Estrostep (EE/norethindrone) have varying estrogen doses each week while the progestin remains the same. The benefits of these products decrease the exposure to estrogens and their side effects. All prevent pregnancy with equal effectiveness.

There are various doses of CHCs based on the estrogen content. They are classified as very low dose (20-25 μg EE), low dose (30-35 μg EE), and high dose (50 μg EE). The low dose and very low dose are prescribed more frequently due to fewer side effects associated with estrogen. The high-dose CHCs are generally only prescribed when there are drug interactions or breakthrough bleeding issues that require higher levels of estrogen.

There are varying regimens of active pills as well. Most combined oral contraceptives (COCs) are formulated for 21 days of active tablets with 7 days of placebo. Newer COCs such as YAZ (EE/drospirenone) and Loestrin 24 (EE/norethindrone) have 24 days of active tablets and 4 days placebo to help decrease breakthrough bleeding and minimize bleeding at menses. Others such as Seasonique (EE/levonorgestrel) and Seasonale (EE/levonorgestrel) contain 84 active tablets allowing for four menses per year. Another formulation, Lybrel (EE/levonorgestrel), allows for one mense a year. Monophasic formulations, the vaginal ring and transdermal patch may also be used by continuing on active hormones without a hormone-free interval.[17,18] Benefits of extended regimens include decreased menstrual migraines during the hormone-free interval, less bleeding, and decreased premenstrual syndrome (PMS) symptoms.

Counseling is very important to ensure maximum effectiveness. There are three ways of initiating COCs (Table 60-4). Ideally, COCs should be taken at the same time everyday. If nausea occurs, it is recommended to take the COCs at bedtime. If more than 24 hours have passed since the last dose of a COC, it is considered a missed dose (Table 60-5). If a woman forgets to take her tablet one day, she may double up the next day and take two with no necessary backup method. If she forgets two tablets in a row during the first or second week of the active tablets, she needs to take two tablets for 2 days and use a backup method for 7 days (note the difference for products less than 30 μg of EE). If she misses two tablets on week 3 or misses three tablets at anytime, she needs to restart a new pack and use a backup method for 7 days. For products that contain less than 30 μg of EE, missing two tablets anytime in the cycle should be treated as if three tablets are missed. If unprotected intercourse occurred within the last 5 days, emergency contraception (EC) is also an option.[6]

Transdermal Patch The contraceptive patch (Ortho Evra) is an adhesive square (1.75 in, 20 cm^2 surface area) applied to skin once weekly that delivers norelgestromin 0.15 mg/d (progestin) and EE 20 μg/d (estrogen). The hormones pass into the skin and are metabolized by liver. Norelgestromin is converted to norgestimate in the liver.[19] It has a perfect use failure rate of 0.3%.[19] Use in obese women has not been recommended since some studies concluded that the contraceptive patch is less effective (3% pregnancy rate vs 0.6%) in women who weigh more than 198 lb (90 kg).[19]

The patch should be placed on a clean, dry, hairless skin area either on the shoulder, upper arm, abdomen, or buttock, but not on the breasts, and rotated each week to prevent irritation.[19] Initiating the contraceptive patch is similar to initiation of COCs (see Table 60-4). One new patch is applied each week for 3 weeks. The patch is worn for 7 days and then changed on day 8, which is known as the "patch change day."[19] A backup birth control method should be used for the first 7 days after applying the patch. The patch is removed during the fourth week and menses generally occur at that time. The patch may be worn while taking showers, swimming, exercising, or sitting in a sauna.

If the patch falls off for more than 24 hours, then a new patch should be applied. This will be considered a new cycle and a new "patch change day." Since this is considered a new cycle, a backup birth control method for 7 days is recommended.[19] EC is also a consideration if unprotected intercourse occurred in the last 5 days. If the patch falls off for less than 24 hours, it should be reapplied as soon as possible and no backup birth control method is necessary.[19]

Side effects of the contraceptive patch include those of other CHCs. Side effects commonly reported with the patch (9%-20%) include: breast symptoms, headache, application site reaction, nausea, upper respiratory infection, menstrual cramps, and abdominal pain.[19] More recently, it has been suggested that risks for venous thromboembolism (VTE) with the transdermal patch is higher than other CHCs; although, this is controversial.[20,21] The pharmacokinetic profile of the contraceptive patch differs from that of COCs in that it has a higher steady state concentration and lower peak concentrations. The product labeling states that amount of EE from the patch is about 60% higher than that of a COC containing 35 μg increasing the risk of VTE.[19] In 2008, the labeling was changed stating that women concerned about blood clots should talk to their providers about alternate methods.[19] Drug-drug interactions are also considered to be similar to COCs.

TABLE 60-3 Selected Oral Contraceptives With Hormone Activities[27, 35–39]

Phase Type	Brand Names	Hormone Content	Estrogen Activity	Progestin Activity	Androgen Activity	Comments
Monophasic						
Products with levonorgestrel	Levlen, Levora, Nordette, Portia	0.15 mg levonorgestrel/ 30 μg EE	+	++	++	
	Seasonale (91-d pack), Seasonique (91-d pack with 10 μg instead of placebo)					Four menstrual periods/y
	Alesse, Aviane, Lessina, Levlite	0.1 mg levonorgestrel/ 20 μg EE	+	+	+	Very low estrogen
	LoSeasonique (91-d pack with 10 μg instead of placebo)					Four menstrual periods/y
	Lybrel (1-y formulation)	90 μg levonorgestrel/ 20 μg EE	No data	No data	No data	One menstrual period/y
Products with norgestimate	Ortho-Cyclen, Sprintec	0.25 mg norgestimate/ 35 μg EE	++	+	+	
Products with norethindrone	Brevicon, Modicon, Necon 0.5/35, Nortrel 0.5/35	0.5 mg norethindrone/ 35 μg EE	+++	+	+	
	Ovcon-35, Femcon Fe	0.4 mg norethindrone/ 35 μg EE	+++	+	+	Fe = iron tablets instead of placebo, Femcon-chewable tablet
	Necon 1/35, Norinyl 1+35, Nortrel 1/35 Ortho-Novum 1/35	1 mg norethindrone/ 35 μg EE	+++	++	++	
	Ovcon-50	1 mg norethindrone/ 50 μg EE	+++	++	++	High estrogen
	Necon 1/50, Norinyl 1+50, Ortho-Novum 1/50	1 mg norethindrone/ 50 μg mestranol	++	++	++	High estrogen
Products with norethindrone acetate	Loestrin 21 1/20, Loestrin Fe 1/20,Microgestin Fe 1/20	1 mg norethindrone acetate/20 μg EE	+	+++	++	Fe = iron tablets instead of placebo
	Loestrin 21 1.5/30, Loestrin Fe 1.5/30, Microgestin Fe 1.5/30	1.5 mg norethindrone acetate/30 μg EE	+	+++	+++	Fe = iron tablets instead of placebo
Products with norgestrel	Cryselle, Lo-Ovral, Low-Ogestrel Ovral, Ogestrel	0.3 mg norgestrel/ 30 μg EE 0.5 mg norgestrel/ 50 μg EE	+ +++	++ +++	++ +++	

(Continued)

TABLE 60-3 **Selected Oral Contraceptives With Hormone Activities[27,35-39] (*Continued*)**

Phase Type	Brand Names	Hormone Content	Estrogen Activity	Progestin Activity	Androgen Activity	Comments
Products with drospirenone	Yasmin	3 mg drospirenone/ 30 µg EE	++	No data	No data	Best for acne, hirsutism, bloating (YAZ approved for acne, PMDD)
	YAZ	3 mg drospirenone/ 20 µg EE	No data	No data	No data	
Products with desogestrel	Kariva, Mircette	Desogestrel/EE 0.15 mg-20 µg and EE 10 µg	+	+++	+	Very low estrogen
	Apri, Desogen, Ortho-Cept	0.15 mg desogestrel/ 30 µg EE	+++	++	+	
Products with ethynodiol	Demulen 1/35, Zovia 1/35E	1 mg ethynodiol diacetate/35 µg EE	+	+++	+	
	Demulen 1/50, Zovia 1/50E	1 mg ethynodiol diacetate/50 µg EE	++	+++	+	High estrogen
Biphasic						
	Necon 10/11, Ortho-Novum 10/11	Norethindrone/EE 0.5-35/1-35 mg-µg	+++	++	+	
Triphasic						
Products with desogestrel	Cyclessa	Desogestrel/EE 0.1-25/0.125-25/ 0.15-25 mg-µg	+	+++	+	
Products with levonorgestrel	Enpresse, Tri-Levlen, Triphasil, Trivora	Levonorgestrel/EE 0.05-30/0.075-40/ 0.125-30 mg-µg	++	+	+	
Products with norethindrone	Tri-Norinyl	Norethindrone/EE 0.5-35/1-35/0.5-35 mg-µg	+++	+	+	
	Necon 7/7/7, Ortho-Novum 7/7/7	Norethindrone/EE 0.5-35/0.75-35/1-35 mg-µg	+++	++	+	
	Estrostep[a] 21, Estrostep Fe	Norethindrone/EE 1-20/1-30/1-35 mg-µg	+	+++	++	Best for women who suffer from estrogen side effects, indicated for acne, Fe = iron tablets instead of placebo
Products with norgestimate	Ortho Tri-Cyclen Lo	Norgestimate/EE 0.18-25/0.215-25/0.25-25 mg-µg	+	+	+	
	Ortho Tri-Cyclen	Norgestimate/EE 0.18-35/0.215-35/0.25-35 mg-µg	++	+	+	Approved for acne

[a]Indicates estrophasic.

Abbreviation: EE, ethinyl estradiol.

Reproduced with permission from: *A Pharmacotherapeutic Approach to Women's Health Across the Lifespan*, American Society of Health Systems Pharmacists. Washington, DC; 2010.[34]

TABLE 60-4 Initiation of CHC Products

Initiation Method	Description
First day	Woman starts method the first day of her menses and uses a backup method for 7 d (some sources say no backup method is necessary, however, this is most conservative approach)
Sunday start	Woman starts method the Sunday after her menses begin (for ring best if within 5 d of menses), uses a backup method for 7 d
Quick start	Woman starts method in the clinic regardless of date of the menses, uses a backup method for 7 d

Vaginal Ring The contraceptive ring (NuvaRing) is inserted vaginally and left in place for 3 weeks at a time releasing etonogestrel 0.120 mg/d (progestin) and EE 0.015 mg/d. It has a perfect use rate of 0.3%.[22] The exact location of the ring is not important as long as it rests inside the vagina.[22] During the fourth week, the ring is removed and menses will usually begin 2 to 3 days later. Douching or use of a diaphragm is not recommended with the ring. The ring may be left in place during sexual intercourse, while using a tampon for breakthrough bleeding, and with use of antifungal creams or spermicides. The ring is removed by grasping the ring with an index and middle finger and pulling it out.[22]

Initiation of the ring should be within the first 5 days of the menstrual cycle, preferably the first day of menses for women who are not currently using a hormonal contraceptive, and a backup birth control method should be used for at least 7 days after insertion of the ring. Side effects include those of CHCs but may also include vaginitis, headache, and sensations of the ring (5%-14%).[22]

If removed or expelled, the ring should be rinsed with cool to lukewarm water and reinserted as soon as possible within 3 hours (see Table 60-5). If the ring is left out of the vagina for longer than 3 hours, a backup birth control method should be used until the ring has been in place for at least 7 days.[22] EC could be considered at this time if a woman had unprotected intercourse in the last 5 days.

Progestin-Only Hormonal Contraceptives

For patients who cannot use hormonal contraception containing estrogen, there are alternatives such as progestin-only hormonal contraceptives. Progestin-only contraceptives work by thickening cervical mucus, altering the environment in the uterus making it less suitable for implantation, and at times preventing ovulation. There are different formulations available which include a pill, injection, intrauterine device, and implant.

The progestin pill is an oral tablet taken once daily, also known as the minipill. There are no placebo pills with the progestin-only tablets. They should be taken at the same time everyday. A missed dose is considered 3 hours after the scheduled dose (see Table 60-5).[23] The missed tablet should be taken as soon as possible and a backup method is recommended for 48 hours.[23] Side effects include progestin-associated adverse effects such as acne, weight gain, depression, and male pattern balding. The return to fertility with progestin pill is fairly rapid with ovulation occurring within 1 to 3 months after discontinuation of the pill.[6]

The progestin-only injection (Depo-Provera) is also known as depot medroxyprogesterone acetate (DMPA) available as

TABLE 60-5 Missed Doses

Product	Missed Dose	Remedy
Birth control pills (combined)[6]	Missed one dose (over 24 h)	Take two tablets the next day, no backup necessary, but best if used
	Missed two doses in wk 1 or 2	Take two tablets for the next 2 d, backup method for 7 d, alternatively use EC if had unprotected sex during those days If taking a very low dose COC (<30 μg EE), treat two missed doses as missing three doses.
	Missed two doses in week 3 or three doses anytime	Discard pack, start new pack, and use backup method for 7 d, may use EC if had unprotected sex during those days
	Missed three doses in extended cycle	Skip missed pills and start taking pills for current day. Continue taking pills until pack is finished and use a backup method for 7 d. May use EC if had unprotected sex during those days.
Progestin-only pills[6]	Missed dose is considered 3 h overdue	Continue to take tablets as scheduled, use a backup method for 2 days
Transdermal patch[41]	Fell off <24h	Reapply patch, no backup is necessary
	Off >24 h	Reapply new patch, start new patch day and use backup method for 7 d
Vaginal ring[42]	Left out <3 h	Wash with warm water and reinsert, no backup is needed
	Left out >3 h	Reinsert new ring, use backup method for 7 d
DMPA injection[26]	Missed dose is considered >13 wk since last injection	Use backup method until injection is given and continue to use a backup method for 7 d after injection

TABLE 60-6 **Contraindications to Estrogen**[40]

■ Older than 35 y and smokes 15 cigarettes per day
■ History of DVT
■ Migraine with aura
■ Cardiovascular disease
■ Less than 6 wk postpartum
■ Liver disease
■ Blood pressure >160/100 mm Hg
■ Pregnancy
■ Breast cancer
■ Surgery within 4 wk
■ Gallbladder disease
■ Diabetes with retinopathy, neuropathy, or vascular disease
■ Lactation
■ Coagulopathies (eg, antiphospholipid syndrome, factor V Leiden)

150 mg intramuscular injection or 104 mg subcutaneous injection. The injection is given every 12 weeks ± 1 week. Side effects are similar to other progestins, however, it is thought that there is more weight gain associated with DMPA.[24] In addition, there is a FDA black box warning on DMPA indicating that women who use DMPA may be at risk for low bone density and that DMPA should only be used for long periods of time (>2 years) if an alternate method is not available.[25] A calcium supplement of 1000 to 1200 mg should be recommended while using DMPA. Other side effects include amenorrhea, depression, pain at injection site, and long return to fertility (up to 10 months).[6]

Another progestin-only contraceptive available is the levonorgestrel (Mirena) intrauterine device/system (IUS). The IUS also provides 20 μg/d of levonorgestrel. The IUS is a T-shaped device inserted into the uterus by a health care provider and may be left inside for up to 5 years. The IUS works by blocking implantation and thinning the endometrial lining of the uterus. Side effects are similar to those seen with other progestin agents but in particular may cause more breakthrough bleeding.[26] There is a rapid return to fertility of 1 to 3 months after removal of the IUS which may be desirable for some patients.[6] Due to a small risk of pelvic inflammatory disease, the IUS is recommended for patients in monogamous relationships who have a low risk of contracting STIs.[26]

Lastly, the progestin implant (Implanon) is a rod that is 4 cm in length, 2 mm in diameter, and contains 68 mg of etonogestrel, the active metabolite of desogestrel. It is inserted by a health care provider underneath the skin of the upper arm. It may be left in for up to 3 years and helps prevent pregnancy by suppressing ovulation, thickening cervical mucus, and altering the endometrium. After removal of the rod, return to fertility is relatively short with 24% of women conceiving within 4 months.[6] Side effects of the implant include fibrosis around the device, difficulty removing the device, pain at site, and other side effects associated with progestins (see Table 60-1).[27]

Special Populations

Hormonal contraceptives, in particular CHCs are contraindicated in special populations (see Table 60-6). Because estradiol can increase blood pressure and clotting factors, women with a history of VTE, uncontrolled hypertension, history of migraine with aura, stroke, or cardiovascular disease should avoid the use of CHCs.[28] In addition, women who are older than 35 years and smoke more than 15 cigarettes per day should not use CHCs due to an increased risk of stroke, heart attack, and blood clots.[6]

Women who are 6 weeks postpartum or less should also avoid the use of CHCs, since the risk of blood clots is higher for women recently postpartum. Estradiol may decrease milk production and therefore, progestin-only contraceptives may be recommended if breastfeeding. Currently, the American College of Obstetrics and Gynecology (ACOG) states that a CHC may be used while breast feeding if there is adequate milk production.[28] However, in women who have low milk production or are struggling to produce milk on CHCs, a progestin-only or nonhormonal contraceptive may be more appropriate. Active liver disease is also a contraindication for CHCs since metabolism through the liver is required. Women with a history of breast cancer or other cancer that may be hormone-mediated should also avoid the use of CHCs and possibly progestin-only products. A common pneumonic used to help remember the serious side effects of CHCs is ACHES, where A = abdominal pain (liver), C = chest pain (pulmonary embolism), H = headache (stroke or clot), E = eye pain (stroke), S = swelling in legs (deep vein thrombosis [DVT]).[6]

EMERGENCY CONTRACEPTION

Emergency contraception (EC) is defined by ACOG as a therapy for women who have had unprotected intercourse, including sexual assault. Indications include contraceptive failure, exposure to a teratogen, sexual assault, and unprotected intercourse within 72 to 120 hours.[29] There are different types of emergency contraception. They include the use of the copper IUD, RU-486, or high dose hormones within 5 days of unprotected sex.[30] The copper IUD and RU-486 must be provided by a licensed prescriber and are not used that frequently. Although, RU-486 may be used for emergency contraception, it is considered an abortifacient. High dose hormones are most commonly known and referred to as the "morning after pill" and "EC" to the lay public. The use of high dose hormones is not considered as an abortifacient and works primarily by preventing ovulation, increasing cervical mucus, and preventing implantation. It does not disrupt an implanted fertilized egg.[6,29,30]

Two hormone methods exist, the Yuzpe method which contains two doses of high dose estrogen (100 μg) and high dose progestin (0.5 mg levonorgestrel) and progestin-only (0.75 mg levonorgestrel × 2 doses). Both methods are highly effective in preventing pregnancy (Yuzpe 75% effective and progestin-only 89% effective).[6] EC is not perfect and pregnancy can still occur. EC is most effective the sooner it is taken. EC should be taken within 72 hours of unprotected intercourse, however, studies show that EC is effective up to 120 hours postcoitus.[29]

Currently, Plan B and Next Choice (progestin only) are marketed and available OTC at the pharmacy for those older than 17 years. A prescription is required for those younger than 17 years.[31] In some states such as Alaska, California, Hawaii, Maine, Massachusetts, New Hampshire, New Mexico, Vermont, and Washington, pharmacists may initiate prescriptions under collaborative agreements to women younger than 17 years.[32]

Plan B and Next Choice consist of two tablets, levonorgestrel 0.75 mg each. The tablets may be taken at the same time or 12 hours apart. Another product recently approved is a one tablet formulation called Plan B One-Step (levonorgestrel 1.5 mg) which is taken as one dose and is also available to women who are 17 years of age and older.[33] Common side effects include headache, breast tenderness, nausea, fatigue, and breakthrough bleeding. The incidence of nausea and vomiting is higher with the Yuzpe method.[6] To mediate this side effect, antiemetics such as meclizine, dimenhydrinate, and diphenhydramine may be given 1 hour prior to the EC dose. For women who vomit within 1 to 2 hours of taking an EC dose, another dose should be administered. If a woman does not have her menses within 3 weeks, she should see her provider as pregnancy may have occurred.[6]

Another product recently approved for EC is Ella (ulipristal). Ella is a progesterone-receptor modulator and may be taken by mouth within 120 hours of unprotected intercourse. It will be available by prescription only.[41]

CASE Application

1. TK is a 23-year-old woman who comes to your pharmacy stating that she is taking the mini-pill and missed her dose yesterday. Based on this information, what is the best remedy in this situation?
   a. She should take two tablets today as soon as possible, no backup method is needed.
   b. She should start taking her tablets as scheduled and use a backup method for the next 48 hours.
   c. She should take two tablets today as soon as possible and use a backup method until she gets her period.
   d. She should start taking her tablets as scheduled and use a backup method until she gets her period.

2. AC is a 26 year-old woman who presents to the pharmacy asking to buy emergency contraceptives and says she had unprotected intercourse 3 days ago. Based on the information, select the best statement as it relates to EC.
   a. EC will not be effective for AC because it has been longer than 24 hours since she has had unprotected sex.
   b. EC will not be effective for AC because it has been longer than 48 hours since she has had unprotected sex.
   c. EC cannot be provided to AC without a prescription from her doctor.
   d. EC may still work for AC because it is still within 72 hours since she has had unprotected sex.
   e. EC may still work for AC because it is still within 120 hours since she has had unprotected sex, but she will require a prescription.

3. Which of the following products provides the least amount of estradiol?
   a. Contraceptive ring
   b. Contraceptive patch
   c. Combined oral contraceptive (30 μg EE)
   d. All of the above provide the same amount of estradiol

4. Which of the following has an FDA indication for the treatment of acne?
   a. Depo-Provera
   b. NuvaRing
   c. Ortho-Cept
   d. Estrostep

5. Which of the following is best to avoid in overweight/obese patients due to the side effects of weight gain?
   a. Depo-Provera
   b. NuvaRing
   c. Ortho Evra
   d. Yasmin

6. How often is NuvaRing inserted vaginally?
   a. 1 week
   b. 3 weeks
   c. 2 weeks
   d. 4 weeks

7. BW is a 28-year-old woman who delivered a baby 1 week ago. She does not plan to breast-feed and would like to start combined oral contraceptives as soon as possible. When is the earliest she can start taking combined oral contraceptives without an increased risk of blood clots?
   a. Immediately
   b. 2 weeks postpartum
   c. 6 weeks postpartum
   d. 6 months postpartum

8. AJ is a 22-year-old woman who weighs 220 lb and would like to start hormonal contraception. Which of the following products would not be as effective in preventing pregnancy for AJ?
   a. Depo-Provera
   b. NuvaRing
   c. Ortho Evra
   d. Yasmin

9. Which of the following products contains drospirenone and may increase potassium levels?
   a. Alesse
   b. YAZ
   c. Cyclessa
   d. Nor-QD

10. RS just started a new oral combined oral contraceptive 2 weeks ago and has had some mild nausea when she takes the pill. What is the best recommendation for RS with respect to changing products?

    a. Change the oral combined contraceptive to another agent this week
    b. Wait for 3 months to see if side effects improve, if not change the products
    c. Wait for 2 months to see if side effects improve, if not change the products
    d. Wait for 6 months to see if side effects improve, if not change the products

11. Select the generic name for Plan B.

    a. Levonorgestrel
    b. Desogestrel
    c. Norgestimate
    d. Ethinyl estradiol
    e. Norethindrone

12. Select the contraceptive agent that is formulated as an injection.

    a. Desogen
    b. Mirena
    c. Estrostep
    d. Ortho Evra
    e. Depo-Provera

13. JS is a 21-year-old man who comes to your pharmacy and states, "What can my girlfriend and I use to make sure she doesn't get pregnant and protect ourselves from, you know...diseases?" Select the best regimen to recommend from the following choices below.

    a. Water-based lubricant + male latex condom
    b. Oil-based lubricant + male latex condom
    c. Female condom + male latex condom
    d. Female condom + male lamb cecum condom
    e. Oil-based lubricant + male lamb cecum condom

14. Which of the following condoms conducts heat very well and also protects against STIs?

    a. Polyurethane
    b. Latex
    c. Lamb cecum
    d. All of the above

15. What is the number of active tablets contained in the product Seasonale?

    a. 24
    b. 21
    c. 44
    d. 84
    e. 91

16. CS is a 36-year-old woman who admits to smoking 1 pack of cigarettes per day. She is getting married and would like to start hormonal contraception. Which of the following products is most appropriate for CS?

    a. NuvaRing
    b. Ortho Evra
    c. Mircette
    d. Tri-Levlen
    e. Nor-QD

17. Which of the following drugs may decrease the effectiveness of Ortho-Tri Cyclen?

    a. Atorvastatin
    b. Carbamazepine
    c. Lamotrigine
    d. Acetaminophen
    e. Levothyroxine

18. DL is a 19-year-old woman who calls you and states that she forgot to take her Desogen (EE 30 μg/0.15 mg desogestrel) tablets for the last 2 days. She says she is in her second week of the cycle. Select the following statement that is most appropriate for missed tablets.

    a. DL should take two tablets the next day and use a backup method for 7 days
    b. DL should continue taking her tablets as scheduled, one per day, no backup method is necessary
    c. DL should discard her pill pack and start a new one, use a backup method for 7 days
    d. DL should take two tablets for 2 days and use a backup method for 7 days
    e. DL should take two tablets for 2 days, no backup method is necessary

19. Combined hormonal contraception is contraindicated in which of the conditions?

    a. History of deep vein thrombosis
    b. Migraine with aura
    c. Active liver disease
    d. Uncontrolled hypertension
    e. All of the above

20. Which of the following has an FDA indication for the treatment of premenstrual dysphoric disorder (PMDD)?

    a. YAZ
    b. Ortho Tri-Cyclen
    c. Estrostep
    d. Mircette
    e. Yasmin

TAKEAWAY POINTS »

- Latex condoms are the best choice of condoms for the prevention of STIs and pregnancy, but should not be used with oil-based lubricants.
- The female condom and male condom should not be used together at the same, otherwise breakage may occur.
- Lambskin condoms are not best for preventing the transmission of STIs.
- Factors such as effectiveness, cost, accessibility, return to fertility, side effects, adherence, and comfort need to be considered when selecting a contraceptive agent for a patient.
- The contraceptive patch is less effective in women who weigh more than 198 lb.
- The contraceptive patch provides 60% more estrogen than a 35 μg oral tablet of ethinyl estradiol which may increase the risk of VTE.
- The vaginal ring is inserted vaginally for 3 weeks at a time and provides the least amount of estrogen compared to all other forms of combined hormonal contraception.
- DMPA is an injectable contraceptive agent administered subcutaneously or intramuscularly every 12 weeks.
- Calcium supplements of 1000 to 1200 mg daily should be taken when using DMPA.
- Combined hormonal contraceptives should not be used in patients who have a history of DVT, migraine with aura, stroke, who are 35 years old and smoke more than 15 cigarettes per day, cardiovascular disease, uncontrolled hypertension, or liver disease.
- A missed dose for progestin-only pills is 3 hours.
- Hormonal emergency contraception is also known as the morning after pill, but works up to 5 days after unprotected intercourse.

REFERENCES

1. Brown SS Eisenberg L. *The best intentions: unintended pregnancy and the well-being of children and families.* Washington, DC: National Academy Press; 1995.
2. Mosher WD, Martinez GM, Chandra A, Abma JC, Willson SJ. Use of contraception and use of family planning services in the United States: 1982-2002. *Adv Data.* 2004;350(17-52):1-36.
3. Facts in Brief. Guttmacher Institute Report. January 2008. Available at: http://www.guttmacher.org/pubs/fb_contr_use.html. Accessed July 17, 2009.
4. CDC. Condoms and STDs. *Fact Sheet for Public Health Personnel,* 2009. Available at: http://www.cdc.gov/condomeffectiveness/brief.html. Accessed July 17, 2009.
5. Berardi RM, Kroon, LA. et al. *Handbook of Nonprescription Drugs.* 15th ed. Washington DC: American Pharmacists Association; 2006.
6. Hatcher RA, Trussell J, Stewart F, et al. *Contraceptive Technology.* 18th ed. New York, NY: Ardent Media Inc.; 2004.
7. Potter WD, de Villemeur M. Clinical breakage, slippage and acceptability of a new commercial polyurethane condom: a randomized, controlled study. *Contraception.* 2003;68:39-45.
8. Gallo MF, Grimes DA, Schulz KF. Nonlatex vs. latex male condoms for contraception: a systematic review of randomized controlled trials. *Contraception.* 2003;68:319-326.
9. Carey RF, Lytle CD, Cyr WH. Implications of laboratory tests of condom integrity. *Sex Transm Dis.* 1999;26:216-220.
10. McCormack S, Hayes R, Lacey CJ, Johnson AM. Microbicides in HIV prevention. *BMJ.* 2001;322:410-413.
11. Roddy RE, Cordero M, Cordero C, Fortney JA. A dosing study of nonoxynol-9 and genital irritation. *Int J STD AIDS.* 1993;4:165-170.
12. Jensen JT, Speroff L. Health benefits of oral contraceptives. *Obstet Gynecol Clin North Am.* 2000;27:705-721.
13. Rosenberg MJ, Waugh MS. Oral contraceptive discontinuation: a prospective evaluation of frequency and reasons. *Am J Obstet Gynecol.* 1998;179:577-582.
14. Shenfield GM, Griffin JM. Clinical pharmacokinetics of contraceptive steroids. An update. *Clin Pharmacokinet.* 1991;20:15-37.
15. Murphy PA, Kern SE, Stanczyk FZ, Westhoff CL. Interaction of St. John's Wort with oral contraceptives: effects on the pharmacokinetics of norethindrone and ethinyl estradiol, ovarian activity and breakthrough bleeding. *Contraception.* 2005;71: 402-408.
16. Archer JS, Archer DF. Oral contraceptive efficacy and antibiotic interaction: a myth debunked. *J Am Acad Dermatol.* 2002;46:917-923.
17. Miller L, Verhoeven CH, Hout J. Extended regimens of the contraceptive vaginal ring: a randomized trial. *Obstet Gynecol.* 2005;106:473-482.
18. Stewart FH, Kaunitz AM, Laguardia KD, Karvois DL, Fisher AC, Friedman AJ. Extended use of transdermal norelgestromin/ethinyl estradiol: a randomized trial. *Obstet Gynecol.* 2005;105:1389-1396.
19. Ortho Evra [package insert]. Raritan, NJ: Ortho-McNeil; 2008.
20. Jick SS, Kaye JA, Russmann S, Jick H. Risk of nonfatal venous thromboembolism in women using a contraceptive transdermal patch and oral contraceptives containing norgestimate and 35 microg of ethinyl estradiol. *Contraception.* 2006;73:223-228.
21. Jick SS, Jick H. The contraceptive patch in relation to ischemic stroke and acute myocardial infarction. *Pharmacotherapy.* 2007;27:218-220.
22. NuvaRing [package insert]. Roseland, NJ: Organon; 2004.
23. Ortho-Micronor [package insert]. Raritan, NJ: Ortho-McNeil; 2005.
24. Mangan SA, Larsen PG, Hudson S. Overweight teens at increased risk for weight gain while using depot medroxyprogesterone acetate. *J Pediatr Adolesc Gynecol.* 2002;15:79-82.

25. Depo-Provera [package insert]. New York, NY: Pfizer 2006.
26. Mirena [package insert]. Bayer Pharmaceuticals: Wayne, NJ; 2008.
27. Implanon [package insert]. Roseland, NJ: Organon; 2006.
28. ACOG Practice Bulletin. No. 73. Use of hormonal contraception in women with coexisting medical conditions. *Obstet Gynecol.* 2006;107:1453-1472.
29. Rodrigues I, Grou F, Joly J. Effectiveness of emergency contraceptive pills between 72 and 120 hours after unprotected sexual intercourse. *Am J Obstet Gynecol.* 2001;184:531-537.
30. LaValleur J. Emergency contraception. *Obstet Gynecol Clin North Am.* 2000;4:817-839, vii.
31. FDA Statement, April 22, 2009. Available at: http://www.fda.gov/NewsEvents/Newsroom/PressAnnouncements/ucm149568.htm. Accessed July 17, 2009.
32. www.pharmacyaccess.org. Accessed July 17, 2009.
33. http://planbonestep.com/pdfs/PlanBOneRelease_FINAL.pdf. Accessed July 17, 2009.
34. *A Pharmacotherapeutic Approach to Women's Health Across the Lifespan.* American Society of Health Systems Pharmacists: Washington DC; 2010.
35. Seasonale [package insert]. Pomona, NY:Duramed Pharmaceuticals, Inc.; 2003.
36. Dickey RP. *Managing Contraceptive Pill Patients.* 9th ed. Durant, OK: Essential Medical Information Systems, Inc., 1998.
37. Helms RA, Quan DJ, Herfindal ET, Gourley GK. *Textbook of Therapeutics Drug and Disease Management.* 8th ed. Philidelphia, PA: Lippincott Williams & Wilkins; 2006:420.
38. YAZ [package insert].Wayne, NJ: Bayer HealthCare Pharmaceuticals, Inc.; 2007.
39. Ortho Tri-Cyclen [package insert]. Raritan, NJ: Ortho-McNeil Pharmacetical; 2005.
40. World Health Organization. *Medical Eligibility Criteria for Contraceptive Use.* Geneva: WHO, 2004.
41. FDA News Release, August 13, 2010. Available at: http://www.fda.gov/NewsEvents/Newsroom/PressAnnouncements/ucm222428.htm. Accessed October 8, 2010.

CHAPTER

61 Smoking Cessation

Daniel S. Longyhore

FOUNDATION OVERVIEW: TOBACCO ABUSE AND CESSATION

According to data from the National Center for Health Statistics, smoking is the greatest preventable risk factor for morbidity and mortality in the United States, accounting for approximately 467,000 deaths in 2005.[1] The Center for Disease Control (CDC) estimates that 20% of the US population over the age of 18 currently smokes. The CDC also estimates that 22% of high school students have used cigarettes within the last 30 days.[2] While cigarette smoking remains the most prevalent type of tobacco use, options for nicotine delivery include smokeless tobacco products (chew and snuff) as well as other smoke tobacco products (pipes, cigars, bidis, and hookah pipes).

Nicotine dependence, like any other chemical dependency, is a twofold issue. First is the physiologic dependence a person develops with continued use. Nicotine stimulates the neurotransmitter dopamine and, in turn, activates the dopamine reward pathway in the brain.[3] The purpose of this pathway is to reward the body for pleasurable activity, thereby reinforcing an activity with hopes of continued use. Initially, the person using smoke tobacco is rewarded for using the smoke tobacco with pleasure or a perceived relief from stress. However, with continued use of the smoke tobacco, the person is no longer smoking for pleasurable effects, but smoking to avoid the unpleasant effects of nicotine withdrawal. These symptoms, as well as time of presentation and duration, are located in Table 61-1. Most often, these withdrawal symptoms persist for 1 to 2 weeks after quitting the tobacco product.[4]

The second aspect of nicotine addiction is the psychological addiction. In the absence of the physical reward for smoking, persons who use tobacco smoke begin to experience cravings with certain activities, certain stimuli, or at certain times throughout the day. Unlike the physical component to addiction, which is diminished or alleviated after the first 1 to 2 weeks, the psychological component persists indefinitely. While a person may be able to overcome the psychological drive to regain the reward of smoking, there is always the chance of relapsing due to an event or lapse in judgment.[5]

TREATMENT

Since the only available strategy for preventing tobacco use is public health education and abstinence, there is little to discuss. However, the availability of prescription and over-the-counter nicotine replacement products and prescription oral medications offers a wide array of options to help those who are attempting to quit tobacco use. For most persons who smoke, it will take multiple attempts to quit before they are successful. Also, the addition of cognitive behavioral therapy and increased provider contact increases a person's chance of quitting tobacco products.[6] Health care providers should also utilize the five A's (Table 61-2) each time they come in contact with a person who smokes.

In conjunction with behavior modification, nicotine replacement therapy (NRT) has proven successful for helping persons with tobacco cessation. NRT is available in multiple dosage forms and delivery devices, allowing for various cessation strategies. A compilation of NRT products, doses, and special considerations are provided in Table 61-3. In most cases, combination therapy with a pharmacologic agent or long-acting nicotine replacement product in conjunction with a short-acting nicotine replacement product is superior to either option alone.[7-9] Regardless of NRT choice, persons should not smoke when using any of the NRT products due to an increased risk of nicotine toxicity. Common symptoms of nicotine toxicity include nausea, vomiting, abdominal pain, hypertension, and tachycardia.

Nicotine Transdermal Patch

Nicotine transdermal patches provide a controlled release of nicotine over a 16- to 24-hour period, depending on the product. Its purpose is to control the long-term cravings and diminish the severity of breakthrough cravings in a person quitting smoking. The 24-hour patch may be left on overnight, but may cause insomnia and/or abnormal dreaming. If these effects occur, changing to the 16-hour patch or removing the patch 60 minutes before bedtime will usually correct these adverse reactions.[10] Plasma nicotine levels begin to decline 60 to 120 minutes after removing the patch.[11] Dosing is based on the number of cigarettes per day.

Patients using the nicotine patch should receive adequate counseling on how to use the nicotine patch properly. Users should identify multiple clean, relatively hairless portions of their upper body to apply the patch and rotate application sites each day. When removing old patches, patients should fold the patch over itself to avoid others from coming into contact with the active ingredient and potentially experiencing the adverse events associated with nicotine toxicity. The standard duration of therapy for the nicotine patch is approximately 10 to

TABLE 61-1 Nicotine Withdrawal Symptoms

Symptom	Cause	Duration	Relief Strategy
Chest tightness	Secondary to tension caused by the need for nicotine May also be due to excessive coughing	Few days	Relaxation techniques Deep breathing
Constipation, stomach pain, gas	Slowed intestinal movement	1 to 2 wk	Hydration/fluids Fruits, vegetables, and whole grains
Cough, dry throat, nasal drip	Removing mucus that has blocked airways and affected breathing	Few days	Hydration/fluids Avoiding additional physical stress
Craving for a cigarette	Physiologic urge to stimulate the central reward pathway in the brain	Frequent at first, then less, but long term	Wait out the urge (min) Distract yourself Exercise (walking)
Depressed mood	Common occurrence, most likely secondary to loss of pleasure sensations or stress relief tool	1 to 2 wk	Increase pleasurable activity Extra support from friends and family
Difficulty concentrating	Adjustment to not having nicotine	Few weeks	Plan workloads accordingly Avoid additional stress
Dizziness	Additional oxygen delivery	1 to 2 d	Use extra caution with activity Change positions slowly
Fatigue	Nicotine acted as a stimulant	2 to 4 wk	Schedule rests Do not over exert yourself
Hunger	May be confused with nicotine craving	Several weeks	Drink water Low-calorie options
Insomnia	Brain waves return to normal Coughing and dreaming of smoking	1 wk	Limit caffeine intake Relaxation techniques
Irritability	Body craving for nicotine	2 to 4 wk	Take walks Relaxation techniques

Note: When a person first quits using tobacco, the physiologic and psychological withdrawal manifest as a variety of symptoms. Typically, these symptoms will last for 2 to 4 weeks, with the worst being in the first week of nicotine abstinence. While nicotine replacement therapy may diminish or alleviate these symptoms, they still may present to some degree. It is important to educate patients about these symptoms and how long they are expected to remain.

12 weeks, but patients may alter this timeframe depending on the severity of withdrawal symptoms and overall comfort.

Nicotine Gum

Nicotine polacrilex gum provides an immediate release of nicotine to help control cravings. The dose is absorbed transbuccally after the user has vigorously chewed the gum to release the nicotine. When the user notices a distinguishable taste change, the gum should be parked between the gums and the cheek until a tingling sensation subsides. Persons may use up to 24 pieces of gum daily, but should attempt to use at least nine pieces per day initially. They should also avoid coffee, juices, or other products that would acidify the oral pH for at least 15 minutes before using the product as it will decrease the absorption of the nicotine. Dosing is based on the number of cigarettes per day.[12]

TABLE 61-2 The Five A's of Smoking Cessation

Ask—Ask the patient if they currently use tobacco products.
Advise—Let the patient know about the harms of smoking.
Assess—Evaluate if the person is ready to quit smoking. If he or she is not ready to quit, stop here, continue to use the 5 A's with each additional contact.
Assist—Work with the person to develop a treatment regimen *or* help them over barriers to success if they have just started a smoking cessation program.
Arrange—Stay in contact with the person throughout their quit attempt.

Nicotine Lozenges

Nicotine polacrilex lozenges are an acceptable option for persons with limitations to using gum (orthodontics, temporomandibular joint disorder, social or professional situations, or personal preference). The nicotine from the lozenges is also absorbed transbuccally after the lozenge is parked between the gums and cheek, but patients should not chew the lozenge. Persons should rotate the lozenge to a new site in the mouth periodically to avoid mucosal irritation. Persons may use up to 20 lozenges daily, but should attempt to use at least nine per day initially. As with the nicotine gum, persons should avoid coffee, juices, or other acidic products for at least 15 minutes before using the lozenge. The absorption of the nicotine from the lozenge is highly dependent on oral pH and any alterations to that pH can greatly affect the absorption of active drug. Dosing is based on how soon after waking a patient uses nicotine products.[13]

Nicotine Oral Inhaler

A nicotine inhaler is also available that mimics the nicotine delivery system of a cigarette, without the other caustic inert ingredients. Persons load a cartridge into the inhalation device and puff on the inhaler for the duration of the cartridge

TABLE 61-3 Nicotine Replacement Products

Dosage Form	Doses	Instructions	Special Notes
Patch[b,c]	21 mg, 14 mg, 7 mg (per 24 h)	21 mg daily × 6 wk[a] 14 mg daily × 2 wk 7 mg daily × 2 wk	24-h formulation
	15 mg, 10 mg, 5 mg (per 16 h)	15 mg daily × 6 wk[a] 10 mg daily × 2 wk 5 mg daily × 2 wk	16-h formulation
Gum[b]	2 mg, 4 mg	Wk 1-6: 1 piece every 1-2 h Wk 7-9: 1 piece every 2-4 h Wk 10-12: 1 piece every 4-8 h	Starting dose based on number of cigarettes daily >25 cigarettes: 4 mg <25 cigarettes: 2 mg
Lozenge[b]	2 mg, 4 mg	Wk 1-6: 1 piece every 1-2 h Wk 7-9: 1 piece every 2-4 h Wk 10-12: 1 piece every 4-8 h	Starting dose based on time to first cigarette after waking <30 min: 4 mg >30 min: 2 mg
Nasal spray[c]	0.5 mg (per spray)	Start 1-2 doses per h Max five sprays per h *or* 40 doses per day	Medication should be tapered for discontinuation over 4-6 wk
Inhaler[c]	10 mg cartridge (4 mg available to absorb)	Start 6 cartridges per day May increase to 16 cartridges per day as needed	Cartridge is empty after 20 min of active puffing

[a]If the patient smokes <10 cigarettes daily, then this is only a two-step process. Use step 2 daily for 6 wk and then step down to step 3 daily for 2 wk.

[b]Available as over the counter

[c]Available as prescription

(approximately 20 minutes) or until the craving subsides. Persons using the nicotine inhaler should start using 6 cartridges daily and increase as needed up to 16 cartridges daily for up to 12 weeks. Then, many persons will need up to an additional 12 weeks to taper down inhaler use and stop.[14]

Nicotine Nasal Spray

Nicotine nasal spray is the final option for NRT. Unfortunately, this option is likely to be the least desirable option because of localized, intranasal side effects associated with use. Persons may experience a peppery sensation in their nose or throat, sneezing, coughing, watery eyes, or runny nose. The initial dose is two sprays (0.5 mg nicotine per spray), once to twice per hour. The maximum number of doses is 5 per hour and 40 doses per day. Persons should use at least eight doses per day initially and may require a tapering down of the dose over 4 to 6 weeks before stopping use. Since the dose is absorbed across the nasal mucosa, persons should not inhale and avoid blowing their nose for at least 3 minutes after each dose.[15]

Bupropion and Varenicline

Currently, bupropion and varenicline are the only nonnicotine agents marketed to assist with smoke tobacco cessation. Agents such as nortriptyline and clonidine have been studied and proven effective for tobacco cessation, but have not sought the indication.[16-18]

Bupropion

Bupropion is a weak inhibitor of dopamine, serotonin, and norepinephrine neuronal uptake. Since the pleasurable (and withdrawal) effects of nicotine are mediated by dopaminergic activity, bupropion helps attenuate the rapid fluctuations between pleasure and dysphoria. Through this attenuation, patients are more tolerant of the physical adverse events of nicotine withdrawal. The medication requires 7 to 14 days to reach a steady state. Therefore, bupropion should be started 2 weeks before a person quits smoking. The most commonly used dose is 150 mg twice daily, starting with only once-daily dosing for the first 3 days. Given bupropion's activity on neurotransmitters and neurohormones, its side effect profile includes hypertension, tachycardia, insomnia, weight loss, and headache, which tend to be more pronounced in the first days of therapy if the patient does not titrate to the treatment dose. Bupropion is contraindicated in patients with a history of an eating disorder or seizures as well as those with current or recent use of monoamine oxidase inhibitors (MAOI).[19] Therapy for tobacco cessation usually lasts for 24 to 48 weeks.[20]

Varenicline

Varenicline is a mixed agonist and antagonist of central nervous system nicotinic receptors. In short, the agent mildly stimulates the nicotinic receptors responsible for pleasure (or avoiding withdrawal), but also blocks the same receptors from receiving excessive stimulus, should a person use a nicotine containing product. Varenicline should be titrated up to full dose, starting 7 days before the person's quit date. Patients will start with 0.5 mg daily for days 1 through 3 and then increase to 0.5 mg twice daily for days 4 through 7. Starting in the second week of therapy, patients will use the target dose of 1 mg twice daily. Of note, the treatment dose is adjusted for patients with renal insufficiency and creatinine clearances less than 30 mm/min (target 0.5 mg twice daily) and patient on hemodialysis (target 0.5 mg daily). Therapy should be continued for 12 weeks, but has been studied out to 24 weeks.[21] The most frequent adverse event associated with varenicline is nausea, which is significantly worse in patients who continue to smoke while on the agent. Other common adverse events include insomnia, abnormal dreaming, and headache.[22] Since its approval, the Food and Drug Administration (FDA) has also cautioned practitioners about new suicidal ideations in patients using varenicline.[23]

SPECIAL CONSIDERATIONS

Options for tobacco cessation are very limited in patients for whom NRT, bupropion, and varenicline are contraindicated or strongly cautioned. Such circumstances would include persons with uncontrolled hypertension, unstable angina, cardiac arrhythmias, or are pregnant. Nicotine replacement therapy carries a pregnancy category D rating with the FDA. Agents such as varenicline and bupropion are category C[24]; varenicline lacks study data in pregnant women and bupropion has given mixed results when looking at fetal outcomes with use during pregnancy[25-27].

CASE Application

1. JT is a 42-year-old black man who is interested in quitting smoking. He has smoked 1 pack per day for the last 20 years. He had one successful quit attempt ("cold turkey") in the past that lasted for approximately 16 months, but went back to smoking after starting a new job 3 years ago. Based on the various components of nicotine dependence, which reason most likely caused JT to return to smoking?
   a. Psychological dependence
   b. Physiologic dependence
   c. He did not use a pharmacologic aid to quit smoking
   d. Most persons will relapse within 24 months of a quit attempt

2. HN has decided that she would like to quit smoking, but is not comfortable doing it without some kind of support from a nicotine replacement agent. She decides that the gum will be her best choice because it is easily concealable among friends, family, and coworkers. She has smoked 1 to 1.5 packs per day for the last 16 years. What is the appropriate starting dose for the nicotine polacrilex gum for HN?
   a. 4-mg piece of gum; not to exceed 24 doses in 24 hours
   b. 4-mg piece of gum; not to exceed 20 doses in 24 hours
   c. 2-mg piece of gum; not to exceed 24 pieces in 24 hours
   d. 2-mg piece of gum; not to exceed 20 pieces in 24 hours

3. How long should HN continue to use the first dose/frequency of the gum before titrating down to the next dose/frequency?
   a. 8 weeks
   b. 6 weeks
   c. 4 weeks
   d. 2 weeks

4. AP is 29 years old and starting a new job in a dental clinic. She wishes to quit smoking before she starts her new job because the clinic does not allow employees to smoke during their shift. However, she would also like to quit to preserve her lung health. She smokes approximately 15 cigarettes daily and has her first one in the car on the way to work (about 95 minutes after waking). She wishes to use the lozenges for her quit attempt. What product would you suggest that AP use?
   a. Nicotrol 4 mg
   b. Nicotrol 2 mg
   c. Commit 4 mg
   d. Commit 2 mg

5. AP has chosen the lozenges because she is unable to chew gum at work. She also suffers from which condition that can be made worse using nicotine polacrilex gum?
   a. Temporomandibular joint disorder
   b. Gingival hyperplasia
   c. Oropharyngeal candidiasis
   d. Episodic epistaxis

6. JE is a 68-year-old man with 1 pack per day for the last 40 years smoking history. He has never attempted to quit smoking, but feels he must try after being hospitalized for pneumonia for 3 days. While he was in the hospital he was given a nicotine patch to wear and change daily until discharge. Upon discharge, he was not given the nicotine patch, but wants to continue using it to abstain from smoking. What dose of the patch should JE start?
   a. 21 mg/d patch
   b. 14 mg/d patch
   c. 7 mg/d patch
   d. He does not smoke enough to warrant NRT with a patch

7. JE has been without a cigarette for 3 days with the help of the nicotine patch. On the fourth day, JE is under a great deal of stress and needs to go outside for a cigarette. Since he is still wearing the nicotine replacement patch, what adverse event will he most likely experience?
   a. Excess fatigue
   b. Lower extremity cramping
   c. Nausea, vomiting, and headache
   d. Tinnitus

8. What would be a better choice for JE to use for breakthrough cravings while he is being treated with the nicotine patch?
   a. Nicorette gum
   b. Chantix 1 mg twice daily
   c. Zyban 150 mg twice daily
   d. He should not combine therapies for smoke tobacco cessation

9. OH is a 39-year-old woman with multiple psychiatric medical conditions. She started smoking approximately 5 years ago and has slowly increased her daily cigarette consumption to 2 packs per day. She started using Nicoderm CQ 21 mg patches, but has experienced various abnormal dreams, causing her to lose sleep over the last 3 nights. She will not continue using the patches if the dreams continue. What would be the best alternative for her?

   a. Nicotrol 15 mg/d patch
   b. Habitrol 21 mg/d patch
   c. Habitrol 14 mg/d patch
   d. Nicotine transdermal patch system 21 mg/d patch

10. OH decides not to use the nicotine patches and switches to the Commit nicotine lozenge. Which of the following scenarios for use is the worst with regard to altered pharmacokinetics?

    a. In the morning, immediately after waking
    b. In the afternoon, during her scheduled work break
    c. In the evening, after her dinner and coffee
    d. Before bedtime, watching the evening news

11. OH's provider also decides to use a prescription, nonnicotine, smoking cessation aid because she feels that using lozenges as needed will not be sufficient. Which of the following medications would be discouraged in the patient?

    a. Varenicline
    b. Bupropion
    c. Nortriptyline
    d. Clonidine

12. JM is a 44-year-old woman with a history of dysmenorrhea and tobacco abuse. She has disregarded the advice to quit smoking while she was taking oral contraceptives for the past 10 or more years. Last month, she developed a deep vein thrombosis (DVT) during a long car trip and decided that she needed to quit smoking so as not to be at risk for another one. She is given a prescription for Chantix starter pack and told to start the dose titration _______ week(s) before her quit date.

    a. One
    b. Two
    c. Three
    d. Four

13. The most common adverse event that JM should be warned about is:.

    a. Insomnia
    b. Headache
    c. Abnormal dreaming
    d. Nausea

14. Which disease should JM be screened for before starting varenicline?

    a. Hypertension
    b. Diabetes
    c. Chronic obstructive lung disease
    d. Renal insufficiency

15. TY is a 37-year-old obese man with a medical history significant for hypertension and dyslipidemia. He also smokes cigarettes and has smoked 1.5 packs per day for the last 17 years. His most recent blood pressure was 158/94 mm Hg, which is consistent with his previous three readings. His physician is convinced that if TY were to lose weight and quit smoking, many of his medical issues would be easier to care for. TY requests some assistance to quit smoking. Which of the following medications would be the best choice for TY?

    a. Bupropion
    b. Nicotine polacrilex gum
    c. Nicotine patch
    d. Varenicline

16. Despite the best choice for TY, he starts bupropion 150 mg twice daily. How should TY begin taking this medication?

    a. One tablet daily for 3 days and then one tablet twice daily, 1 week before his quit date
    b. One tablet daily for 3 days and then one tablet twice daily, 2 weeks before his quit date
    c. One tablet daily for 7 days and then one tablet twice daily, 1 week before his quit date
    d. One tablet daily for 7 days and then one tablet twice daily, 2 weeks before his quit date

17. Since insomnia and anxiety are common adverse events with bupropion, which of the following recommendations will help TY the most?

    a. Do not take the second dose after 5 o'clock in the evening.
    b. If the patient develops insomnia, omit the second dose of the day.
    c. Insomnia is a temporary adverse event and will resolve approximately 7 days after increasing the dose to twice daily.
    d. The insomnia and anxiety are most likely due to nicotine withdrawal and will resolve approximately 7 to 10 days after quitting smoking.

18. While combination therapy is ideal for patients attempting to quit smoking, which of the following combinations is *not* appropriate?

    a. Bupropion and nicotine polacrilex gum
    b. Nicotine patches and nicotine polacrilex gum
    c. Varenicline and nicotine polacrilex gum
    d. Nortriptyline and nicotine polacrilex gum

19. LK is a 66-year-old woman with osteoporosis, chronic allergic rhinitis, and a 50- pack-year history of smoking cigarettes. At a recent trip to the dentist, she was told

that due to poor oral hygiene and tooth decay, she would need to have her teeth removed and fitted for dentures. He also recommends that she quit smoking during this time period as it most likely contributed to her current predicament. Which agent listed below would be the best agent for LK to choose?

a. Nicotine polacrilex gum
b. Nicotine lozenge
c. Nicotine nasal inhaler
d. Nicotine transdermal patch

20. AI is a 27-year-old woman with a past medical history significant for polycystic ovarian syndrome (PCOS), hypertriglyceridemia, epilepsy, hyperthyroidism, and tobacco abuse for the last 11 years. Which of her medical conditions is considered a precaution for using bupropion therapy?

a. Polycystic ovarian syndrome
b. Hypertriglyceridemia
c. Epilepsy
d. Hyperthyroidism

TAKEAWAY POINTS ››

- Nicotine dependence is a twofold disease that has both psychological and physiologic obstacles to address.
- Tobacco use and cessation should be continually addressed with patients to maximize their chances of attempting to quit and succeeding.
- While the physical withdrawal symptoms are temporary and can be overcome with pharmacologic assistance, the psychological desire to smoke remains indefinitely. A good treatment plan will include medication(s) in conjunction with behavior modification strategies.
- The nicotine patch is the only long-acting nicotine replacement formulation. It is a good initial choice (with or without bupropion) for tobacco cessation and can be combined with any of the other immediate release preparations.
- Nicotine gum is an appropriate agent to help patients get through cravings, but should be avoided in patients with dental hardware and temporomandibular joint disorder (TMJ). It should be chewed and then parked in the mouth and *not* continuously chewed.
- Nicotine lozenges offer the craving control of the nicotine gum, without the issues of dental hardware or TMJ. Like the nicotine gum, this product is less effective when used within less than 15 minutes after eating or drinking an acidic product such as coffee or juices.
- The nicotine oral inhaler is an ideal option for persons who need to fulfill the hand-to-mouth motion associated with smoking a cigarette.
- The nicotine nasal spray has its limitations for use as its ADRs are usually more cumbersome than the cravings it is intended to treat. With other less abrasive products available, there is limited application for the nasal spray.
- Bupropion is a nonnicotine option for assisting with smoking cessation. It can be combined with the nicotine replacement products for (what might be) superior outcomes. It should be avoided in patients with a history of seizure and/or eating disorders.
- Varenicline is a mixed nicotine agonist and antagonist. Initial results show it to be superior to bupropion for quit rates, but as time continues past 48 weeks, the quit rates between the two agents becomes more similar. It should *not* be combined with nicotine replacement products due to the increased risk of nausea.
- Nortriptyline and clonidine are not approved for tobacco cessation, but may be used if all other products are considered more harmful than beneficial. They may also be used in patients with concurrent comorbidities for which they treat.

REFERENCES

1. Danaei G, Ding EL, Mozaffarian D et al. The preventable causes of death in the United States: comparative risk assessment of dietary, lifestyle, and metabolic risk factors. *P LoS Med.* April 28, 2009;6(4):e1000058.
2. US Department of Health and Human Services. *Health, United States, 2008* (with a special feature on the health of young adults). Atlanta, GA: National Center for Health Statistics. March 1, 2009. Available at: http://www.cdc.gov/nchs/data/hus/hus08.pdf#063. Accessed October 28, 2009.
3. Leshner AI. Addiction is a brain disease, and it matters. *Science.* October 3, 1997;278(5335):45-47.
4. Hatsukami DK, Stead LF, Gupta PC. Tobacco addiction. *Lancet.* June 14, 2008;371(9629):2027-2038.
5. Rigotti NA. Clinical practice. Treatment of tobacco use and dependence. *N Engl J Med.* February 14, 2002;346(7):506-512.
6. US Department of Health and Human Services, Public Health Service. Treating tobacco use and dependence, 2008 update. U S Department of Health and Human Services. May 1, 2008. Available at: http://www.surgeongeneral.gov/tobacco/treating_tobacco_use08.pdf. Accessed October 28, 2009.
7. Shah SD, Wilken LA, Winkler SR, Lin SJ. Systematic review and meta-analysis of combination therapy for smoking cessation. *J Am Pharm Assoc.* September, 2003, 2008;48(5):659-665.
8. Steinberg MB, Greenhaus S, Schmelzer AC et al. Triple-combination pharmacotherapy for medically ill smokers: a randomized trial. *Ann Intern Med.* April 7, 2009;150(7):447-454.
9. Jorenby DE, Leischow SJ, Nides MA et al. A controlled trial of sustained-release bupropion, a nicotine patch, or both for smoking cessation. *N Engl J Med.* March 4, 1999;340(9):685-691.
10. Nicoderm CQ [package insert]. Parsippany, NJ: GlaxoSmith-Kline Consumer Healthcare; 2-13-2009. Ref Type: Pamphlet

11. Henningfield JE. Nicotine medications for smoking cessation. *N Engl J Med.* November 2, 1995;333(18):1196-1203.
12. Nicorette [package insert]. Parsippany, NJ: GlaxoSmithKline Consumer Healthcare; 2-13-2008. Ref Type: Pamphlet
13. Commit Lozenge [package insert]. Parsippany, NJ: GlaxoSmith-Kline Consumer Healthcare; 5-24-2008. Ref Type: Pamphlet
14. Nicotrol Inhaler [package insert]. New York, NY: Pharmacia & Upjohn Company, Pfizer Inc; 2006.Ref Type: Pamphlet
15. Nicotrol Nasal Spray [package insert]. New York, NY: Pharmacia & Upjohn Company, Pfizer Inc; 2006. Ref Type: Pamphlet
16. Prochazka AV, Kick S, Steinbrunn C, Miyoshi T, Fryer GE. A randomized trial of nortriptyline combined with transdermal nicotine for smoking cessation. *Arch Intern Med.* November 8, 2004;164(20):2229-2233.
17. Aveyard P, Johnson C, Fillingham S, Parsons A, Murphy M. Nortriptyline plus nicotine replacement versus placebo plus nicotine replacement for smoking cessation: pragmatic randomised controlled trial. *BMJ.* May 31, 2008;336(7655):1223-1227.
18. Schroeder SA. What to do with a patient who smokes. *JAMA.* July 27, 2005;294(4):482-487.
19. Zyban [package insert]. Greenville, NC: GlaxoSmithKline Consumer Healthcare; 12-1-2008. Ref Type: Pamphlet
20. Eisenberg MJ, Filion KB, Yavin D et al. Pharmacotherapies for smoking cessation: a meta-analysis of randomized controlled trials. *CMAJ.* July 15, 2008;179(2):135-144.
21. Tonstad S, Tonnesen P, Hajek P, Williams KE, Billing CB, Reeves KR. Effect of maintenance therapy with varenicline on smoking cessation: a randomized controlled trial. *JAMA.* July 5, 2006;296(1):64-71.
22. Chantix [package insert]. New York, NY: Pfizer Inc; 5-1-2008. Ref Type: Pamphlet
23. US Food and Drug Administration. FDA issues Public Health Advisory on Chantix. Agency requests that manufacturer add new safety warnings for smoking cessation drug. *US Food and Drug Administration.* February 1, 2008. Available at: http://www.fda.gov/NewsEvents/NewsroomPressAnnouncements/2008/ucm116849.htm. Accessed October 28, 2009.
24. Micormedex. Nicotine. Available at: http://emmerson.csc.wilkes.edu:2060/home/dispatch. Accessed 2009
25. Chan B, Einarson A, Koren G. Effectiveness of bupropion for smoking cessation during pregnancy. *J Addict Dis.* 2005;24(2):19-23.
26. Chun-Fai-Chan B, Koren G, Fayez I et al. Pregnancy outcome of women exposed to bupropion during pregnancy: a prospective comparative study. *Am J Obstet Gynecol.* March, 2005;192(3):932-936.
27. Cole JA, Modell JG, Haight BR, Cosmatos IS, Stoler JM, Walker AM. Bupropion in pregnancy and the prevalence of congenital malformations. *Pharmacoepidemiol Drug Saf.* May, 2007;16(5):474-484.

CHAPTER

62 Glaucoma

Karen H. McGee

INTRODUCTION

Glaucoma is a progressive eye disease. It affects three million Americans and is the second leading cause of blindness in the United States. There are two major types of glaucoma: primary open angle glaucoma (POAG) and angle closure glaucoma. The most common type, POAG, will be the focus of this discussion. Angle closure glaucoma, though less common, is considered a medical emergency. Angle closure glaucoma may result in sudden loss or blurring of vision, significantly elevated eye pressures, nausea and vomiting. Both types of glaucoma may result in optic nerve damage and permanent blindness if not treated. Glaucoma does not cause symptoms in the majority of patients. It is important for pharmacists to counsel patients about routine eye examinations and glaucoma screenings for early detection. There are several risk factors associated with the development of glaucoma. These include age >40 years, African American or Asian race, diabetes, hypertension, elevated intraocular pressure, myopia, and family history in a first-degree relative. Treatment is aimed at reduction in intraocular pressure. Eye drops and surgery are the most common treatments. The most potent eye drops are the prostaglandin analogs. The pharmacist's role in the care of patients with glaucoma includes disease and medication counseling, review of eye drop administration technique, eye drop adherence evaluations, and recommendations for routine eye examinations.[1,2]

PATHOPHYSIOLOGY

Diagnosis and Clinical Presentation

Patients with glaucoma usually do not report symptoms until substantial visual field destruction occurs. Visual field loss occurs in 8% to 20% of patients despite reaching therapy goals. Eighty percent of patients without treatment will develop bilateral blindness. Patients with glaucoma may be involved in a motor vehicle accident because they have blind spots related to peripheral vision field defects. Elderly patients with long-standing glaucoma often experience declining vision, headaches, and eye pain.[3] Some elderly patients continue to use eye drops even after blindness develops to decrease the incidence of eye pain. Glaucoma can be distinguished from other eye diseases, affecting the optic nerve, by performing a dilated eye examination. Ophthalmologists may note during examination that the rim of the optic nerve is thinning. This thinning is caused by loss of retinal nerve cells. The pink color of the eye fields will remain. Other neuropathies of the optic nerve are characterized by loss of the pink color. Optic nerve thinning results in an enlarged cup-to-disc ratio, which is a hallmark visual finding during examination of the eye. The optic disc is the anatomical location where the optic nerve and blood vessels enter the retina. The optic disc can be flat or it can have a certain amount of normal cupping. In glaucoma, increased pressures cause pathological cupping of the optic disc. The pink disc contains nerve fibers. The white cup is a pit with no nerve fibers. As glaucoma advances, the cup enlarges to cover most of the disc. A normal value for the cup-to-disc ratio is 0.3. A greater value indicates glaucoma. Intraocular pressure (IOP) is often elevated. A normal IOP value is between 10 and 21 mm Hg. Elevated IOP in the absence of optic nerve changes may be diagnosed as ocular hypertension. Some patients with glaucoma have normal intraocular pressures.[2,3]

Gonioscopy, perimetry, and tonometry testing provide the ophthalmologist with additional information for the diagnosis of glaucoma. Gonioscopy measures the anterior chamber angle between the iris and cornea and is used to diagnose the type of glaucoma. Automated perimetry testing is used to identify loss of visual fields. Tonometry is also an important assessment tool. Tonometry is the measure of IOP. Applanation tonometry is measured using a small probe to determine the force required to flatten the cornea. This test requires the use of anesthetic eye drops because the small probe is inserted directly onto the eye. Applanation tonometry is very accurate and is used after a simple screening test, such as pneumotonometry or air-puff tonometry, and has indicated an increased IOP. Pneumotonometry does not touch the eye but uses a puff of air to flatten the cornea. This is a more convenient test. It is not as accurate but is used routinely as a screening method.[3]

Eye Physiology

The angle formed by the iris and cornea is measured to define the type of glaucoma present. The most common glaucoma type, POAG, is diagnosed when the angle is not obstructed. Aqueous humor is the fluid that bathes the eye and supplies nutrients.

Aqueous humor, produced by the ciliary body, circulates throughout the anterior chamber of the eye and drains into the eye filter, also known as the trabecular meshwork. Filtration through the meshwork depends on pressure gradients and so blood pressure and IOP changes affect aqueous humor production. The trabecular meshwork may become scarred

TABLE 62-1 Drug-Induced Glaucoma

Medications Associated with Worsening Glaucoma
Corticosteroids
Anticholinergic medications
Antihistamines
Vasodilators
Cimetidine
Benzodiazepines
Topical sympathomimetics
Heterocyclic antidepressants
Phenothiazines
Theophylline
Selective serotonin reuptake inhibitors
Venlafaxine
Topiramate

or clogged with a resultant increase in intraocular pressure. Intraocular pressure elevations may also occur because of reduced aqueous outflow from the trabecular meshwork. The increased pressure results in damage to the ganglion-cell axons that make up the optic nerve. This is a progressive disorder that can lead to blindness. The goal of treatment is to decrease the intraocular pressures to slow the damage caused to the optic nerve.[1-4]

DRUG-INDUCED GLAUCOMA

Glaucoma can also be caused or worsened by certain classes of medications. Pharmacist should review medication regimens and recommend alternatives to improve outcomes for patients with glaucoma. Table 62-1 summarizes medications known to worsen glaucoma.[5]

GOALS OF TREATMENT AND TREATMENT OVERVIEW

The major goals of glaucoma treatment are to preserve vision and decrease intraocular pressure. Medications, the most common treatment, are often used first line to decrease the intraocular pressure. Medication therapy is administered topically using eye drops. Eye drops are absorbed quickly into the eye. This increases efficacy and decreases the incidence of systemic side effects. Oral medications are a second-line option. Surgery is also a treatment option. Medications utilize several different mechanisms to accomplish this goal. For instance, prostaglandin analogs increase uveoscleral outflow. Beta-blockers decrease aqueous humor production and improve aqueous humor outflow. Carbonic anhydrase inhibitors decrease aqueous humor production by inhibiting the enzyme carbonic anhydrase. The two most effective classes of medications are the prostaglandin analogs and the beta-blockers. Each class of medications has their own unique side effects to consider. The most common side effects of these medications are listed in Table 62-2. The incidence of systemic side effects can be significantly decreased by teaching appropriate eye drop administration techniques.[3,4]

Adherence and Persistence

There are several studies addressing the issues of adherence and persistence in the treatment of glaucoma.[6-8] Adherence has been shown to sharply rise 1 week prior to the doctor's appointment. Persistence evaluates the rate of treatment adherence over time. Rates of persistence are generally below 50% at 1 year.[6] The pharmacists should recommend the most effective and least side-effect prone medications. Patients need to be educated about side effects. In most instances, minor eye irritations caused by eye drops improve over time. Patients are more likely to continue treatment despite minor side effects if they understand that the side effects will decrease over time. Patients should be educated about the different classes of eye drops. This would help them understand that other options are available if side effects occur. Prostaglandin analogs are the most commonly prescribed drops for glaucoma. They are the most effective class of eye drops and have few serious side effects. Table 62-2 summarizes the differences in dosing, efficacy, and side effects among the various classes of eye drops. Pharmacists can also monitor refill dates to help monitor and promote adherence.

Eye Drop Administration Technique

Patients should be instructed to wash their hands prior to eye drop administration. They should also avoid touching the tip of the medication bottle to the eye or any other surface to avoid contamination and eye infections. Some eye drops are suspensions, such as brinzolamide (Azopt), betaxolol (Betoptic-S), timolol and dorzolamide combination product (Cozopt), and timolol gel-forming solution (Timoptic XE). These suspensions should be shaken before use. Table 62-3 summarizes the steps for appropriate eye drop technique.[3]

MEDICATIONS

Beta-Blockers

Beta-blockers are very effective options for the treatment of POAG and are considered an appropriate first line of therapy. There are once daily formulations to promote adherence. However, they are not the most commonly prescribed first-line option because side effects may limit their tolerability. Stinging, dry eyes, blurred vision, and blepharitis are common local side effects. Systemic side effects are also very common and include decreased blood pressure, decreased heart rate, and bronchospasm. Systemic side effects are problematic for patients with diabetes, congestive heart failure, heart block, or severe chronic obstructive pulmonary disease. Nasolacrimal occlusion (NLO) helps decrease the frequency of systemic side effects.[2-3]

TABLE 62-2 **Medications for Glaucoma**

Category Generic and Brand Name	Usual Dose	Decrease IOP for the Class (%)	Mechanism for Category	Side Effects for Category (Local and Systemic)
		Beta-Blockers		
Timolol, Timoptic 0.25%, 0.5% Timoptic XE 0.25%, 0.5%	1 drop twice daily 1 drop once daily	18%-34%	↓ Aqueous humor production	Burning, dry eyes, systemic beta-blockade
Betaxolol , Betoptic 0.5, 1% Betoptic S 0.25%	1 drop twice daily			
Carteolol, Cartrol 1% Ocupress	1 drop twice daily			
Levobunolol, Betagan 0.25%, 0.5%	1 drop twice daily			
Metipranolol, Optipranolol 0.3%	1 drop twice daily			
		Prostaglandin Analogs		
Lantanoprost, Xalatan 0.005%	1 drop every night	25%-36%	↑ Uveoscleral outflow	Iris pigmented, hyperpigment, hypertrichosis, itching, hyperemia
Travaprost, Travatan 0.004%	1 drop every night			
Bimatoprost, Lumigan 0.03%	1 drop every night			
Unoprostone, Rescula 0.12%	1 drop every night	14%-23%		
		Alpha-2 Agonist		
Brimonidine, Alphagan 0.15%, 0.1%	1 drop 2-3 times daily	15%-16%	↓ Aqueous humor production	Allergic, lid edema, itching
Apraclonidine, Iopidine 0.5%, 1%	1 drop 2-3 times daily			
		Sympathomimetics		
Dipivefrin, Propine 0.1%	1 drop twice daily	Not available	↑ Outflow of aqueous humor	Tearing, burning, brow ache, headache, tachycardia
		Parasympathomimetics		
Pilocarpine, Pilocar 0.25%-10% Carbachol, Carboptic 1.5%, 3%	1 drop 2-4 times a day Pilocar HS gel 1 drop hs 1 drop 2-4 times a day	20%-30%	↑ Outflow of aqueous humor	Brow ache, headache, myosis, blurred vision, edema
		Carbonic Anhydrase Inhibitor		
Brinzolamide, Azopt 1%	1 drop 2-3 times day	10%-26%	↓ Aqueous humor production	Stinging, bitter taste, acidosis, contains sulfa
Dorzolamide, Trusopt 2%	1 drop 2-3 times day			
Acetazolamide, Diamox 125 mg, 250 mg (sequels), 500 mg	1 tablet 2-4 times day			Systemic acidosis
Methazolamide, Neptazane 25 mg, 50 mg	1 tablet 2-3 times day			Systemic
		Combination Agents		
Timolol/dorzolamide, Cosopt 0.5% and 2%	1 drop twice day	29%	See individual agents	See individual agents
Timolol/brimonidine Combigan 0.5% and 0.2%	1 drop twice day		See individual agents	See individual agents

Prostaglandin Analogs

Prostaglandin analogs have become the most commonly prescribed first-line therapy for POAG. They are extremely effective in lowering IOP and they have a very favorable side effect profile. They can decrease IOP as much as 36%. These medications are also among the first class to demonstrate a diurnal IOP-lowering effect. This means that they are very effective at lowering IOP even at night during sleep when IOP readings are the highest. The most common side effects include hyperpigmentation of the iris and hypertrichosis of the eyelashes. It is believed that these effects are only harmful from a cosmetic point of view. Someone with mixed hazel-brown eyes will probably have more

TABLE 62-3 **Eye Drop Administration Technique with Nasolacrimal Occlusion**

1. Wash hands thoroughly.
2. Pull down lower eyelid to form a pocket with your forefinger.
3. Hold medicine bottle with forefinger and thumb of opposite hand.
4. Brace fingers against the side of the nose, place bottle close to eye.
5. Tilt the head back and administer the correct number of drops.
6. Immediately press finger gently against the inside corner of the eye (nasolacrimal occlusion).
7. Hold pressure to inside corner of eye for one to three minutes.
8. May also close the eye to increase medication absorption.

brown color apparent between 3 to 12 months of use. These eye drops are usually dosed once daily at bedtime.[9-15]

Alpha-2 Agonist

Alpha-2 agonists decrease intraocular pressure by decreasing the production of aqueous humor. They lower IOP 15% and are often combined with other agents. The unique use of alpha-2 agonists is after cataract or laser surgery. They have a rapid onset of effect. They are usually dosed two to three times daily. Side effects include lid edema, foreign body sensation, itching, and hyperemia. Systemic side effects include dizziness, fatigue, and dry mouth. NLO helps decrease the incidence of systemic side effects.[2,3]

Sympathomimetics and Parasympathomimetics

Sympathomimetics and parasympathomimetics are older agents that are used last line due to local and systemic side effects. They decrease IOP 25%. They are usually dosed two to four times daily. Side effects include tearing, blurred vision, brow-ache, and hyperemia. Systemic side effects include headache, increased blood pressure, tachycardia, tremor, and anxiety.[2,3]

Carbonic Anhydrase Inhibitors

Carbonic anhydrase inhibitors inhibit secretion of sodium and bicarbonate by enzyme inhibition. They lower intraocular pressure 10% to 26%.They are usually dosed two to three times daily. Local side effects include stinging, blurred vision, and conjunctivitis. Systemic side effects include acidosis, nausea, weight loss, diaphoresis, and myopia. Oral therapy is a last-line option when eye drops are not effective or when eye drop technique is difficult, such as in patients with mental disabilities. However, close monitoring is required due to the risk of serious systemic side effects.[2,3]

Combination Therapy

Combination therapies such as Cosopt and Combigan help improve compliance and decrease eye drop burden. The combinations are more effective than the individual agents alone. Side effects are a culmination of the two individual agents.[3]

CASE Application

KM is a 44-year-old African American woman with decreased peripheral vision. She was found to have a blind spot on the left side (visual field defect). She was involved in a motor vehicle accident because she did not see the car in the left lane. She complains of brow ache and headaches that have become worse over the past 2 weeks. Intraocular pressure measures 28 in the right eye and 26 in the left eye. She is on a fixed income and buying medications is often difficult. She works odd jobs with varying shifts. Her blood pressure was 140/95 mm Hg.

Diagnosis: Primary open angle glaucoma, hypertension, and insomnia.

Medications: Amlodipine 5 mg daily, pilocarpine 2% in both eyes qid, Tylenol PM 2 at bedtime.

Allergies: Sulfa. Hazel eyes turned brown on Xalatan and she refused treatment.

1. Which of the following are true about KM?
   a. She has at least three risk factors for glaucoma.
   b. Pilocar is first-line therapy for POAG.
   c. She could have drug-induced glaucoma.
   d. Both a and b.
   e. Both a and c.
2. Which of the following could affect KM's glaucoma therapy?
   a. Titration of the blood pressure medication can affect intraocular pressures.
   b. Adherence may be an issue.
   c. Nasolacrimal occlusion should be reviewed.
   d. Both b and c.
   d. a, b, and c.
3. Which glaucoma medication is contraindicated for KM?
   a. Timolol
   b. Iopidine
   c. Brimonidine
   d. Dorzolamide
   e. Both a and b
4. Which medication may be causing KM to have brow aches?
   a. Amlodipine
   b. Acetaminophen
   c. Benadryl
   d. Pilocarpine
   e. Latanoprost
5. Which of the following are good recommendations to improve KM's therapy?
   a. Discontinue Benadryl
   b. Switch to timolol extended release drops
   c. Titrate up to pilocarpine 4% qid
   d. Both a and b
   e. a, b, and c

6. Diagnosis of primary open angle glaucoma includes:
   a. Review of medications
   b. Evaluation of visual fields
   c. Tonometry
   d. Both b and c
   e. a, b, and c

7. The most common type of glaucoma is
   a. Primary open angle
   b. Acute closed angle
   c. Drug-induced glaucoma
   d. Both a and c
   e. Both b and c

8. Goals of treatment for glaucoma include:
   a. Decreasing intraocular pressure
   b. Increasing visual field defects
   c. Decreasing eye pain
   d. both a and b
   e. both a and c

9. Medications reduce intraocular pressure by
   a. Increased aqueous humor outflow
   b. Increased carbonic anhydrase activity
   c. Increased aqueous humor reabsorption
   d. Both a and b
   e. Both a and c

10. Aqueous humor is produced in the
   a. Ciliary body
   b. Trabecular meshwork
   c. Iris
   d. Canal of Schlemm
   e. Pituitary

11. Which glaucoma medication class should be avoided in patients with a sulfa allergy?
   a. Prostaglandin analogs
   b. Beta-blockers
   c. Calcium channel blockers
   d. Carbonic anhydrase inhibitors
   e. Alpha-blockers

12. Which medication class is considered first-line treatment of open angle glaucoma?
   a. Beta-blockers
   b. Calcium channel blockers
   c. Carbonic anhydrase inhibitors
   d. Alpha-blockers
   e. Prostaglandin analog

13. Which class of medications is associated with darker, thicker, and longer eye lashes?
   a. Prostaglandin analogs
   b. Carbonic anhydrase inhibitors
   c. Alpha-blockers
   d. Sympathomimetics
   e. Beta-blockers

14. Which of the following medications can cause drug-induced glaucoma?
   a. Corticosteroids
   b. Antihistamines
   c. Cimetidine
   d. Both a and b
   e. a, b, and c

15. Teaching patients about nasolacrimal occlusion helps:
   a. Improve medication effectiveness
   b. Decrease side effects
   c. Decrease systemic absorption of eye drops
   d. Both a and b
   e. a, b, and c

16. Pharmacist can improve outcomes in glaucoma by:
   a. Reviewing refill histories
   b. Providing medication education
   c. Teaching nasolacrimal occlusion
   d. a, b, and c
   e. Both b and c

17. Which eye disease is characterized by elevated intraocular pressure but normal visual fields?
   a. Open angle glaucoma
   b. Closed angle glaucoma
   c. Hypotensive glaucoma
   d. Ocular hypertension
   e. Both a and c

18. Which glaucoma medication is associated with bronchospasm?
   a. Carbonic anhydrase inhibitors
   b. Epinephrine
   c. Prostaglandin analogs
   d. Mannitol
   e. Alpha-blockers

19. Carbonic anhydrase inhibitors reduce intraocular pressure by:
   a. Miosis
   b. Decreased aqueous humor production
   c. Decreased osmolarity
   d. Increased aqueous humor outflow
   e. Opening of the Canal of Schlemm

20. The most important point of nasolacrimal occlusion includes
   a. Hand washing
   b. Separation of two doses of eye drops by 30 minutes
   c. 3 minutes time for closing the nasolacrimal duct
   d. Both b and c
   e. a, b, and c

TAKEAWAY POINTS ››

- Glaucoma is a progressive eye disease. It affects three million people and is a leading cause of blindness in the United States.
- Early detection and treatment of glaucoma are important for preservation of vision.
- The two major types of glaucoma are primary open angle glaucoma (POAG) and angle closure glaucoma. POAG is the most common type.
- Topical medications are the first choice for treatment of primary open angle glaucoma.
- Prostaglandin analogs and beta-blockers are first-line medication choices. Current prescribing trends favor the prostaglandin analogs.
- Therapy must be individualized. Drug of choice is based on concomitant disease states and medication side effects.
- Carbonic anhydrase inhibitors contain a sulfa moiety. Patients allergic to sulfa should not receive a carbonic anhydrase inhibitor.
- Older agents, such as alpha-2 agonist, sympathomimetics, and pilocarpine cause significant side effects. These agents are last line in the treatment of glaucoma.
- Teaching eye drop administration technique and utilizing nasolacrimal occlusion improves medication efficacy and decreases the risk of systemic absorption and side effects.
- Education about glaucoma and the medications used to treat it, review of eye drop administration technique. and evaluation of medication adherence are all important goals for pharmacists to help patients prevent blindness associated with glaucoma.

REFERENCES

1. Kwon YH, Fingert JH, Kuehn MH, Alward WL. Primary open-angle glaucoma. *N Engl J Med.* 2009 Mar 12;360(11):1113-1124.
2. Sharts-Hopko NC, Glynn-Milley C. Primary open-angle glaucoma. *Am J Nurs.* 2009 Feb;109(2):40-47.
3. Dipiro JT, Talbert RL, Yee GC, Matzke GR, Wells BG, Posey LM. Glaucoma. *Pharmacotherapy: A Pathophysiological Approach.* 7th ed. McGraw-Hill, New York: 1551-1564.
4. Mediero A, Alarma-Estrany P, Pintor J. New treatments for ocular hypertension. *Auton Neurosci.* 2009 May 11;147(1-2): 14-19.
5. Tripathi RC, Tripathi BJ, Haggerty C. Drug-induced glaucomas: mechanism and management. *Drug Safety.* 2003;26(11):749-767.
6. Schwartz GB, Quigley HA. Adherence and persistence with glaucoma therapy. *Surv Ophthalmol.* 2008 Nov;53:suppl. 1:S57-S68
7. Gray TA, Orton LC, Henson, D, Harper R, Waterman H. Interventions for improving adherence to ocular hypotensive therapy. *Cochrane Database Syst Rev.* 2009 April 15(2): CD006132. DOI: 10.1002/14651858.CD006132.pub2.
8. Gurwitz, JH, Glynn RJ, Monane M, et al. Treatment of glaucoma: adherence by the elderly. *Am J Public Health.* 1993:83(5):711-716.
9. Alm A, Nilsson SF. Uveoscleral outflow—a review. *Exp Eye Res.* 2009:Apr;88(4):760-768.
10. Sit AJ, Asrani S. Effects of medications and surgery on intraocular pressure fluctuations. *Surv Ophthalmol.* 2008 Nov;53 suppl 1:S45-S55.
11. Bean GW, Camras CB. Commercially available prostaglandin analogs for the reduction of intraocular pressure: similarities and differences. *Surv Ophthalmol.* 2008 Nov;53 suppl 1:S69-S84.
12. Alm A, Grierson I, Shields MB. Side effects associated with prostaglandin analog therapy. *Surv Ophthalmol.* 2008 Nov;53 suppl 1:S93-S105.
13. Parrish RK, Palmberg P, Wang-Pui S for the XLT Study Group. A comparison of lantanoprost, bimatoprost, and travoprost in patients with elevated intraocular pressure: a 12 week, randomized, masked-evaluator multicenter study. *Am J Ophthalmol.* 2003;135:688-703.
14. Brandt JD, VanDenburgh AM, Whitcup SM. Comparison of once- or twice-daily bimatoprost with twice-daily timolol in patients with elevated IOP. *Ophthalmology.* 2001;108:1023-1032.
15. Toris CB, Gabelt BT, Kaufman PL. Update on the mechanism of action of topical prostaglandins for intraocular pressure reduction. *Surv Ophthalmol.* 2008;53 (suppl 1):S107-S120.

CHAPTER

63 Urology

Matthew A. Cantrell, Michael Kelly, and Scott M. Vouri

FOUNDATION OVERVIEW: BENIGN PROSTATIC HYPERPLASIA

The prostate is a small male organ weighing approximately 15 to 20 g located inferior to the bladder and surrounds the urethra. It produces fluid which contributes to ejaculate volume, but may also prevent infectious processes as this fluid has concentrated quantities of zinc.[1] As men age, the prostate—under the influence of androgenic hormones—may begin to grow which increases risk for benign prostatic hyperplasia (BPH). BPH is the most common urological condition in aging men with histological evidence of its presence approaching 90% in octogenarians.[2,3] Patients with BPH often have increased smooth muscle tissue in the prostate containing α_1-adrenergic receptors resulting in vasoconstriction and subsequent narrowing of the urethral lumen. Patients may also have symptoms of physical obstruction, resulting from an enlarged prostate.

Lower urinary tract symptoms (LUTS) suggestive of BPH are characterized as those associated with impaired bladder emptying or storage.[4] Voiding symptoms are often found early in the disease course and include urinary hesitancy, weak urinary stream, and the sensation of incomplete bladder emptying. Storage symptoms include urinary frequency, nocturia, urinary urgency, and urge incontinence. These symptoms occur after several years of untreated BPH as the bladder smooth muscle hypertrophies and weakens.[5] BPH can increase the risk of urinary tract infections, bladder stones secondary to urinary stasis, and renal impairment, thus adversely affecting quality of life.[6] The most serious complication of BPH is acute urinary retention, which often requires immediate catheterization.

Patients with LUTS should be referred to their physician as a detailed history and physical examination are necessary to exclude other possible etiologies, including other genitourinary tract disorders such as prostate cancer or urinary tract infections, neurological or endocrine disorders. A digital rectal examination (DRE) is necessary to determine prostate size and whether any nodules suggestive of malignancy are present.[7] A urinalysis may also be done to exclude urinary tract infections or bladder stones. Pharmacists should be aware of several medication classes for potentially worsening LUTS, including medications with anticholinergic properties such as antihistamines, tricyclic antidepressants, and opiates. Furthermore, as prostate tissue contains α_1-adrenergic receptors, α-agonists such as pseudoephedrine or other decongestants may exacerbate symptoms or attenuate therapy with α_1-adrenergic antagonists.

TREATMENT

Appropriate treatment depends on multiple factors: LUTS severity, concurrent medical illness that affects hemodynamic stability, prostate size, and presence of BPH-related complications. The American Urological Association (AUA) has developed a scoring system to rate symptoms of BPH.[7] Patients with mild BPH (AUA score of 0-7) may be candidates for watchful waiting if symptoms are not bothersome. This is a reasonable strategy as symptoms of BPH often wax and wane and therefore active treatment may not always be needed.[8] If this strategy is used, patients should be monitored for any potential worsening of symptoms indicating the need for pharmacologic treatment.

For patients with moderate to severe BPH (AUA score 8-35), α_1-adrenergic antagonists are effective in reducing LUTS.[7] This class of medications improves voiding symptoms by relaxing prostatic smooth muscle tissue, thereby allowing passage of urine through the urethra. The primary distinction between these agents is their respective selectivity for the α_{1A}-adrenergic receptor, which ultimately affects tolerability. Agents such as tamsulosin (Flomax) and silodosin (Rapaflo) are uroselective based on their affinity for α_{1A}-receptors and alfuzosin (Uroxatral) is considered "functionally" uroselective largely based on its extended-release formulation preventing peaks in serum concentrations.

While prazosin (Minipress) was once commonly used for BPH, it is no longer recommended due to its short half-life, requiring multiple daily dosing and its quick onset which, along with its lipophilic structure, increases the risk for side effects such as orthostatic hypotension and syncope. Terazosin (Hytrin) and doxazosin (Cardura) are second generation α_1-adrenergic receptor antagonists. Efficacy of these agents is comparable to third-generation or "uroselective" agents. Most clinical trials using α_1-adrenergic receptor antagonists demonstrate a statistically and clinically significant decrease in AUA symptom score (4-6 points) and also improved urinary flow rates up to 25%.[9] Although doxazosin is also available as an extended-release formulation which may improve tolerability, the disadvantages of immediate-release formulations of terazosin and doxazosin include the need to titrate the dose over several days to weeks to prevent cardiovascular side effects, most notably orthostatic hypotension and dizziness. This titration often delays the time to reach an effective dose. Furthermore, unlike the 5-α-reductase inhibitors (5ARI),

TABLE 63-1 **Medications Used to Treat Benign Prostatic Hyperplasia**

α-Adrenergic Antagonists				
Medication	**Starting Dose/ Max Dose (mg)**	**Selectivity for α_{1A}-Receptor**	**Metabolism**	**Common Class-Related Side Effects**
Alfuzosin (Uroxatral)	10/10	No	Hepatic CYP 3A4	Dizziness (6%), fatigue (3%), headache (3%)
Doxazosin (Cardura, Cardura XL)	1/8	No	Hepatic	Dizziness (16%), fatigue (12%), orthostatic hypotension (up to 10%), syncope (2%) Cardura XL: postural hypotension 2% and syncope <1%
Silodosin (Rapaflo)	8	Yes	Hepatic CYP 3A4, CYP 2D6	Abnormal ejaculation 28%, orthostatic hypotension 2.8%[14]
Tamsulosin (Flomax)	0.4/0.8	Yes	Hepatic CYP 3A4, CYP 2D6	Abnormal ejaculation (up to 18%), headache (20%), syncope (0.4%)
Terazosin (Hytrin)	1/10	No	Hepatic	>10%: dizziness, headache, muscle weakness <5%: peripheral edema, orthostatic hypotension

5-α-Reductase-Inhibitors (5ARI)			
Medication	**Dose (mg)**	**Metabolism**	**Side effects**
Dutasteride (Avodart)	0.5	Hepatic CYP 3A4, CYP 3A5	Impotence (3.9%), decreased libido (3.3%), breast tenderness and enlargement (0.9%)
Finasteride (Proscar)	5	Hepatic CYP 3A4	Impotence (19%), decreased libido (10%), gynecomastia (2%)

Data from Lacy CF, Armstrong LL, Goldman MP, Lance LL. *Lexi-Comp Drug Information Handbook.* 14th ed. 2006.

which are discussed below, this class does not reduce the size of the prostate, and does not prevent progression of BPH.[10] Side effects of terazosin and doxazosin include orthostatic hypotension, muscle weakness, and fatigue. Patients should be cautioned about precipitous decreases in blood pressure if they also use phosphodiesterase inhibitors (PDE-5) for erectile dysfunction.

As stated above, novel agents that specifically target α_{1A}-receptors in the prostate have been developed. The first to be marketed was tamsulosin (Flomax) and, more recently, silodosin (Rapaflo). As these agents target α_{1A}-receptors localized to the prostate, they are less likely to cause hypotension or syncope. Since these agents do not require titration, they often improve urinary symptoms within 1 week.[11,12] Ejaculatory disturbances can occur although, in clinical trials, few patients discontinued therapy as a result of this side effect.[13,14] While alfuzosin (Uroxatral) does not specifically target the α_{1A}-receptor, it is considered functionally uroselective. An emerging concern with this class of medications is the propensity to complicate cataract surgery from a condition termed the intraoperative floppy iris syndrome (IFIS).[15] Recent data suggests this class of medications may increase the risk of complications, not only in the operative setting, but also several months after cataract surgery.[16] Pharmacists should counsel patients to inform their ophthalmologist prior to cataract surgery if they take this class of medications.[17] In summary, α_1-adrenergic receptor antagonists are effective first-line agents for symptoms of BPH in patients *without* evidence of an enlarged prostate.

The conversion of testosterone to dihydrotestosterone (DHT) mediated by the enzyme 5-α-reductase is an important stimulus to prostate growth. Inhibiting 5-α-reductase decreases symptoms of BPH by reducing prostate size. Two 5-α-reductase inhibitors are currently available, finasteride (Proscar) and dutasteride (Avodart). The principal difference between agents is that finasteride inhibits type II 5-α-reductase while dutasteride inhibits both type I and II resulting in a faster, more complete decrease in intraprostatic DHT. Despite a greater reduction in DHT due to dutasteride's additional pharmacologic effects, there is no known clinical advantage compared to finasteride. 5ARI therapy will not result in immediate symptom relief; therefore, an appropriate trial of these medications should last a minimum of 6 to 12 months. These agents decrease prostate size by 25% and reduce prostate-specific antigen (PSA) up to 50%. To retain clinical utility of using PSA as a screening tool for prostate cancer, patients should have a baseline PSA measured prior to initiating therapy with subsequent PSA values interpreted two-fold higher to account for the reduction that occurs with 5ARI use.[7] Side effects of 5ARI include reduced libido, other sexual side effects, and rarely gynecomastia.[18] Finasteride and dutasteride are pregnancy category X, so women who are pregnant or of child-bearing age should not handle these medications. Monotherapy with a 5ARI should be considered in patients with BPH due to an enlarged prostate. Combination therapy with a 5ARI and an α-1-adrenergic antagonist improves urinary flow rates and prevents progression of BPH in patients with moderate to severe BPH with evidence of an enlarged prostate (>40 g).[10,19] Additional information regarding prescription medications used to treat BPH is shown in Table 63-1.

Saw palmetto (*Serenoa repens*)—an herbal agent widely used outside the United States—has produced mixed results in clinical trials. Several small studies show a modest effect at reducing BPH symptoms; however, the largest trial to date found no difference compared to placebo after 12 months of therapy.[20-22] It has been suggested that saw palmetto may modestly inhibit 5ARI or have growth factor–inhibiting properties. Based on a lack of clinical studies demonstrating improvement in symptoms, the AUA does not recommend this product. If patients do decide to take saw palmetto, the recommended dose is 160 mg twice daily of the standardized extract. Patients taking saw palmetto along with antiplatelet agents or anticoagulants should be counseled on possible bleeding side effects.

FOUNDATION OVERVIEW: ERECTILE DYSFUNCTION

Defined as the inability to achieve and sustain an erection of sufficient rigidity for intercourse, erectile dysfunction (ED) affects 10 to 20 million men in the United States.[22] It is a disorder associated with increasing patient age with 5% of 40 year olds and 15% to 25% of men ≥65 afflicted with complete or severe dysfunction.[23] The risk of erectile dysfunction is increased in men with diabetes, heart disease, hypertension, and those who smoke.[24,25]

Penile erection is a vascular event mediated by neuronal action under the influence of psychological and hormonal factors. In the flaccid state, arterial vascular smooth muscle is contracted and venules are open and drain freely. Erection occurs when parasympathetic nonadrenergic, noncholinergic neurons and endothelial cells release nitric oxide, triggering a series of reactions which results in relaxation of smooth muscle of the helicine arteries of the penis.[26] Venules, which usually drain blood in the penis, become compressed against the tunica albuginea and entrap blood resulting in an erection.

ED may be a result of organic, psychological factors, or both. Organic causes account for 80% of cases and often present with vascular compromise and decreased penile blood flow.[1] These can include vascular (eg, heart disease, hypertension, dyslipidemia), neurologic (eg, spinal cord injury, Parkinson disease), endocrine disorders (eg, diabetes, hypogonadism), miscellaneous causes (eg, Peyronie disease, prostatic hyperplasia), and psychogenic causes (eg, depression, anxiety, and stress).[27] Use of prescription medications (eg, antihypertensives, antipsychotics, hormones) as well as alcohol and drugs of abuse (eg, cocaine, amphetamine) can also lead to ED.

Evaluation of patients with ED includes a medical history, physical examination, and laboratory tests to exclude serious conditions associated with ED and to identify risk factors. A sexual history should be obtained from the patient and his partner focusing on the nature of the problem (frequency, duration, quality, and duration of erections) and psychosocial factors that may suggest potential causes and the most appropriate approach to treatment.[28] Standardized questionnaires such as the Sexual Health Inventory for Men[29] are also helpful.[26]

TREATMENT

An important treatment goal is to identify and treat any medical or psychological condition that contribute to ED. This would include management of risk factors such as diabetes, hypertension, and dyslipidemia, as well as treatment of hypogonadism with testosterone if necessary. If these causes have been excluded or managed, the main goal is to satisfy the patient's expectations which would include cure, pleasure, partner satisfaction, reproduction, and naturalness.[30] Two measurable dimensions help define this goal: treatment response (consisting of efficacy and tolerability), and treatment satisfaction (ie, how well the treatment meets or exceeds the expectations of the patient and his partner).[31]

Phosphodiesterase Type 5 (PDE-5) Inhibitors

Sildenafil (Viagra), vardenafil (Levitra), and tadalafil (Cialis) enhance the effect of nitrous oxide by selectively inhibiting the phosphodiesterase type 5 enzyme. Randomized clinical trials demonstrate statistically significant response to these agents regardless of cause (organic, psychogenic, or mixed), duration, age, race, or severity. When PDE-5 inhibitors are not effective, secondary causes of ED should be considered. These include incorrect dose, hypogonadism, a possible psychological component, and comorbidities.[32] There is no convincing evidence that one agent is superior to any other.[5] However, in patients unresponsive to on-demand or "as needed" dosing schedules, daily use of tadalafil at doses of 2.5 to 5 mg may improve ED and may be a more acceptable option prior to using second-line treatments such as vasoactive agents.[33] The serum half-life of tadalafil (17.5 hours) is considerably longer than sildenafil (3.7 hours) and vardenafil (3.9 hours) providing extended clinical activity. As such, tadalafil is effective for up to 36 hours following administration, while both sildenafil and vardenafil should be taken 30 to 60 minutes before anticipated intercourse.

Common adverse events include headache, flushing, dyspepsia, and rhinitis; however, drop-out rates due to adverse events did not differ from placebo in clinical trials. Patients receiving concomitant α-adrenergic blockers may experience postural hypotension and dizziness. Since blood pressure is significantly lowered in patients taking concomitant nitrates and PDE-5 inhibitors, the combination is contraindicated. Serious cardiovascular events have been associated temporally with the PDE-5 inhibitors, thus, they should not be used in patients in whom sexual intercourse is inadvisable because of poor cardiac status. These drugs have been associated with temporary difficulty in distinguishing blue and green colors. Sudden vision and hearing loss has been observed in a few patients. Prolonged erections and priapism have been reported infrequently. Patients should seek medical attention for erections lasting more than 4 hours. The PDE-5 inhibitors are metabolized by cytochrome P450 (CYP) 3A4 enzymes. The PDE-5 inhibitor dose should be reduced if coadministered with medications affecting this enzyme system (eg, erythromycin, ketoconazole, ritonavir).

Vasoactive Agents

These agents mimic vascular response in erection and are used when PDE-5 inhibitors fail or are not tolerated. Alprostadil is synthetic prostaglandin E_1 and exerts its activity by relaxing vascular smooth muscle. It is administered by injection into the corpus cavernosa of the penis (Caverject, Edex) or via a medicated transurethral suppository (Muse). Two other vasoactive agents used in ED are phentolamine, an α_1-adrenergic antagonist, and papaverine, a nonspecific phosphodiesterase inhibitor. They are administered by intracavernosal injection usually in combination with alprostadil in patients not responding to alprostadil alone. Use of these agents can be very effective with response rates >70% for alprostadil alone[34] and approaching 90% for the combination.[35]

Pain may be a particular problem with the use of alprostadil and may lead to treatment failure. The combination allows for lower doses of all three agents and better tolerability. Penile fibrosis can occur with intracavernosal injection. Priapism is an adverse effect of particular concern. Patients should seek medical attention for any erection lasting longer than 6 hours. These agents are contraindicated in individuals prone to priapism (patients with sickle cell anemia, multiple myeloma, or leukemia).

Other Treatments

When PDE-5 inhibitors and vasoactive agents fail separately, they have been tried in combination with some success.[32] Vacuum erection devices, which draw blood into the penis with negative pressure to create an erection that is maintained by a constriction ring, may also be effective.[36] Implantation of penile prosthetic devices is another treatment option.[37]

FOUNDATION OVERVIEW: URINARY INCONTINENCE

Urinary incontinence (UI) is an involuntary loss of urine, occurring in the absence of stones or infection. Patients often experience urinary urgency with or without incontinence, urinary frequency, and nocturia.[38-41] In the United States, over 33 million people suffer from UI, with a yearly health-care cost of $26 billion.[42-44] Both men and women 60 years or older have up to a 50% prevalence of this condition.[39,40,44]

Disorders of the lower urinary tract and associated structures can lead to overactivity of the detrusor muscle. These dysfunctional changes in the surrounding nerve structures result in an increased release of acetylcholine (ACh), predominantly in the periphery. ACh acts predominantly on the M_3 muscarinic receptors—which are thought to be responsible for abnormal bladder contractions—and initiates a cascading phenomenon, leading to excessive bladder contractions and sequential symptoms.[43-45] Antimuscarinic medications work by directly inhibiting ACh at the M_3 muscarinic and, to an extent, the M_2 muscarinic receptors of the detrusor muscle—which are thought to be responsible for normal, physiologic bladder contractions—in the afferent pathways of the bladder.[43] These medications allow the bladder to properly fill, thus improving urinary frequency and nocturia.[45]

The four types of UI include stress urinary incontinence (SUI), urge urinary incontinence (UUI), overflow incontinence (OI), and mixed incontinence. SUI occurs during episodes of increased intra-abdominal pressure on the bladder in a patient with a weakened urethral sphincter, typically after an effort or exertion from normal physical activity, sneezing, or coughing.[38,39,46,47] UUI results from increased stimulation and contraction of the bladder detrusor muscle due to an influx of ACh on the M_3 receptors. Patients with UUI typically suffer from bouts of urinary urgency, frequency, and nocturia.[38,39,41] OI is caused by urinary obstruction, most commonly BPH, or bladder underactivity typically from neurological dysfunction. This leads to an inability to completely void urine from the bladder. Mixed incontinence is a combination of any of the three previous types of incontinence.[38,39] Patients with functional or cognitive impairment such as decreased mobility, low physical functioning like arthritis, or decreased mental functioning may become incontinent without classification of UI.[39] Overall, patients presenting with any type of incontinence should undergo tests to rule out bladder infections, bladder cancer, and prostate cancer.[45]

TREATMENT

Nonpharmacologic Treatments

Nonpharmacologic treatments are first line for most patients and can be used in combination with pharmacologic treatment. Prior to evaluation by a practitioner, a voiding diary should be kept to assess the severity of UI. The voiding diary documents the frequency of voiding and the number of episodes of incontinence.[5] In many patients, fluid management and avoidance of caffeine and other bladder irritants will correct UI.[43,45] Obesity is a contributing factor to SUI and a weight loss of 8 kg can provide clinically significant improvements in SUI symptoms.[39,46,48] The most common nonpharmacologic approaches to UI are bladder training, which includes scheduled urination and urge-suppression techniques, and pelvic floor exercises, which include voluntary contraction and relaxation of muscles used to help control urination.[38,45-47] Patients with functional or cognitive impairment may benefit from assistance of caregivers, scheduled bathroom visits, and absorbent pads or garments.[38,45]

Antimuscarinic Agents

Antimuscarinic agents are the most widely prescribed class of drugs for UI and are the first line of therapy unless contraindications such as urinary retention, gastric retention, narrow-angle glaucoma, or hypersensitivity exist.[49-59] As seen in Table 63-2, antimuscarinics are divided into two classes. The tertiary amine antimuscarinics include oxybutynin (Ditropan), tolterodine (Detrol), darifenacin (Enablex), solifenacin (Vesicare), and fesoterodine (Toviaz).

TABLE 63-2 Comparison of Antimuscarinic Medications for Incontinence

Medication	Usual Dose (mg)	Metabolism (CYP)	Renal Dose Adjustments (mg)[a]	Affinity for M3 Receptor	Common Side Effects	Cost[b,c]
Tertiary Amines						
Oxybutynin (Ditropan)	5 po bid	3A4; inhibits 3A4, 2D6 (minor)	None	Moderate	Dry mouth (71%), constipation (12%)	$13.45
Oxybutynin ER (Ditropan XL)	5-10 po daily	3A4; inhibits 3A4	None	Moderate	Dry mouth (29%), constipation (7%)	$86.99,[d] $87.60[e]
Oxybutynin transdermal system (Oxytrol)	3.9/d twice weekly	3A4 (minor)	None	Moderate	Application site reaction (17%), dry mouth (10%)	$135.30[f]
Oxybutynin 10% gel (Gelnique)	1 satchet (1 g) daily	3A4 (minor)	None	Moderate	Dry mouth (8%), application site reaction (6%)	$128.98
Tolterodine (Detrol)	2 po bid	2D6	1 po bid	Nonselective	Dry mouth (37%)	$151.50
Tolterodine ER (Detrol LA)	4 po daily	2D6	2 po daily	Nonselective	Dry mouth (23%)	$138.41
Darifenacin (Enablex)	15 po daily	2D6, 3A4	None	Highly	Dry mouth (35%), constipation (21%)	$138.47
Solifenacin (Vesicare)	10 po daily	3A4	5 po daily	Moderate	Dry mouth (27%), constipation (13%)	$136.38
Fesoterodine (Toviaz)	8 po daily	None	4 po daily	Nonselective	Dry mouth (35%)	$129.99
Quaternary Amines						
Trospium chloride (Sanctura)	20 po bid	None	20 po daily	Nonselective	Dry mouth (20%)	$144.66
Trospium chloride ER (Sanctura XR)	60 po daily	None	Not recommended	Nonselective	Dry mouth (10%)	$136.78

[a]Creatinine clearance <30 mL/min.
[b]Based on 30-day supply.
[c]Prices from www.drugstore.com.
[d]5 mg daily.
[e]10 mg daily.
[f]Four-week supply.

These agents are uncharged, lipophilic entities, which cause more central nervous system (CNS) adverse events as compared to the quaternary amine antimuscarinic, trospium chloride (Sanctura). The latter is a charged species and does not readily penetrate the blood–brain barrier. In general, patients taking antimuscarinics have half the number of incontinent episodes compared to patients taking placebo. Few head-to-head trials between individual agents have been conducted; therefore, one agent is not considered more efficacious than others.[41,43] For relief of UI symptoms, antimuscarinics are designed to specifically antagonize the M_3 receptors. However, M_3 muscarinic receptors are also located in the salivary glands, lower bowel, and ciliary smooth muscle. Therefore, they also commonly cause adverse effects including dry mouth, constipation, and blurred vision.[41] Antimuscarinic agents can also antagonize other muscarinic receptors, such as M_1 muscarinic receptors, which can precipitate delirium or other CNS side effects.[60]

Oxybutynin has higher incidences of dry mouth in the immediate release (IR) formulation due to a higher rate of conversion to the active metabolite, *N*-desethyloxybutynin, as compared to the extended release (ER) formulation.[45] The transdermal patch can be applied to abdomen, hip, or buttock while the gel can also be applied to the upper arm, shoulder, or thigh.[51,52] All four systems are equally effective.[45] Tolterodine, based on pharmacodynamics, is one of the most selective agents in this class for muscarinic receptors located in the bladder.[41] In head-to-head trials with oxybutynin, the two drugs were shown to be equally effective.[45] Darifenacin is the most selective agent for the M_3 receptor. Because of the higher selectivity ratio for M_3 receptors over M_1 receptors, there are very few cognitive function side effects with darifenacin.[41,43,45] Solifenacin and tolterodine are the two most selective medications for muscarinic receptors in the bladder. Solifenacin has the longest half-life of any agent in this class (45-68 hours).[41] Fesoterodine is a prodrug which is hydrolyzed via nonspecific esterases, thus avoiding the CYP system, into the its active ingredient, 5-hydroxymethyl tolterodine.[57,60] Trospium chloride is derived from atropine and has a lower risk for side effects and drug–drug interactions due to its quaternary amine properties and lack of CYP hepatic metabolism.[40,41,43]

Vaginal atrophy is a condition with symptoms of dryness, burning, itching, and an increase in SUI. The vaginal application of micronized 17-beta estradiol (Vagifem) daily for 2 weeks then twice weekly decreases vaginal atrophy symptoms, including UI.[61,62] The deficiency of estrogen in postmenopausal women was once thought to contribute to UUI; however, an increase in UUI symptoms has been demonstrated for patients taking oral estrogen and therefore this route is not recommended.[40,47,63,64]

Duloxetine (Cymbalta), although not FDA approved, may be a viable treatment for SUI. It works by decreasing the frequency of UUI episodes and improving quality of life. It is used in patients after nonpharmacologic treatment has failed.[65,66] This medication increases the urethral striated sphincter-muscle tone, leading to relief of SUI symptoms.[45,65] Duloxetine is typically dosed 40 mg orally twice daily.[66] The most commonly noted side effect is mild to moderate nausea; however, it can also increase blood pressure which should be monitored after initiation.[65,66]

Botulinum toxin, a potent neurotoxin, has efficacy in patients refractory or intolerant to antimuscarinic agents. Injections of 100 to 300 U of botulinum toxin, diluted with normal saline, resulted in improvements in UUI for 12 to 24 weeks.[67,68]

There are many medications previously used for UI that are no longer recommended due to lack of efficacy or poor tolerance. These include other antimuscarinic agents (propantheline, methantheline, emepronium, dicyclomine, terodiline), antispasmodic agents (flavoxate), tricyclic antidepressants (imipramine), and prostaglandin synthetase inhibitors (indomethacin).

CASE Application

1. Which of the following is the brand name for dutasteride?
   a. Hytrin
   b. Flomax
   c. Proscar
   d. Avodart
   e. Cardura

2. An 82-year-old patient who is taking 2 mg of terazosin for BPH comes into the pharmacy complaining of dizziness and generalized muscle weakness and persistent LUTS. What would you recommend to his physician?
   a. Add finasteride 5 mg daily to his regimen.
   b. Switch his terazosin to doxazosin 4 mg.
   c. Switch his terazosin to tamsulosin 0.4 mg daily.
   d. Lower the dose of his terazosin to 1 mg.
   e. Add saw palmetto twice daily.

3. What pregnancy category is finasteride?
   a. A
   b. B
   c. C
   d. D
   e. X

4. A patient reports that he has been taking his finasteride daily for the last 6 months for BPH. His last PSA was 2.6 ng/mL. Today it is 1.3 ng/mL. This can be best explained by which of the following?
   a. Finasteride stops the prostate from producing PSA.
   b. Finasteride can cause erroneous results in laboratory testing for PSA.
   c. PSA levels are often significantly decreased in patients taking 5ARI.
   d. Both a and b.
   e. All of the above.

5. A patient planning on having cataract surgery next week presents with a prescription for tamsulosin. His symptoms are not particularly bothersome but he reports some urinary hesitancy and straining. You decide to:
   a. Fill the prescription and counsel the patient on risk of sexual side effects.
   b. Call his physician and ophthalmologist and get his order changed to finasteride.
   c. Call his physician and ophthalmologist to determine if treatment with tamsulosin should be deferred until after his cataract surgery.
   d. Fill the prescription and counsel on risk of dizziness and orthostatic hypotension.
   e. Call his physician and get his order changed to terazosin.

6. Which of the following is *not* an advantage of tamsulosin when compared to doxazosin?
   a. Increased efficacy in reducing LUTS.
   b. Improved tolerability, especially cardiovascular side effects.
   c. Quicker onset of action in lowering symptoms.
   d. Both b and c.
   e. All of the above are advantages of tamsulosin for LUTS.

7. Which of the following is mainly responsible for increased prostate growth?
   a. PSA.
   b. DHT.
   c. 5-α-reductase.
   d. Testosterone.
   e. All of the above are directly responsible for prostate growth.

8. Select the statement that correctly describes erectile dysfunction.
   a. Individuals with diabetes are at higher risk.
   b. It is uncommon in the United States.
   c. It generally afflicts younger men.
   d. Individuals with above normal blood pressure are protected.
   e. Smokers are less likely to develop the condition.

Vasoactive Agents

These agents mimic vascular response in erection and are used when PDE-5 inhibitors fail or are not tolerated. Alprostadil is synthetic prostaglandin E_1 and exerts its activity by relaxing vascular smooth muscle. It is administered by injection into the corpus cavernosa of the penis (Caverject, Edex) or via a medicated transurethral suppository (Muse). Two other vasoactive agents used in ED are phentolamine, an α_1-adrenergic antagonist, and papaverine, a nonspecific phosphodiesterase inhibitor. They are administered by intracavernosal injection usually in combination with alprostadil in patients not responding to alprostadil alone. Use of these agents can be very effective with response rates >70% for alprostadil alone[34] and approaching 90% for the combination.[35]

Pain may be a particular problem with the use of alprostadil and may lead to treatment failure. The combination allows for lower doses of all three agents and better tolerability. Penile fibrosis can occur with intracavernosal injection. Priapism is an adverse effect of particular concern. Patients should seek medical attention for any erection lasting longer than 6 hours. These agents are contraindicated in individuals prone to priapism (patients with sickle cell anemia, multiple myeloma, or leukemia).

Other Treatments

When PDE-5 inhibitors and vasoactive agents fail separately, they have been tried in combination with some success.[32] Vacuum erection devices, which draw blood into the penis with negative pressure to create an erection that is maintained by a constriction ring, may also be effective.[36] Implantation of penile prosthetic devices is another treatment option.[37]

FOUNDATION OVERVIEW: URINARY INCONTINENCE

Urinary incontinence (UI) is an involuntary loss of urine, occurring in the absence of stones or infection. Patients often experience urinary urgency with or without incontinence, urinary frequency, and nocturia.[38-41] In the United States, over 33 million people suffer from UI, with a yearly health-care cost of $26 billion.[42-44] Both men and women 60 years or older have up to a 50% prevalence of this condition.[39,40,44]

Disorders of the lower urinary tract and associated structures can lead to overactivity of the detrusor muscle. These dysfunctional changes in the surrounding nerve structures result in an increased release of acetylcholine (ACh), predominantly in the periphery. ACh acts predominantly on the M_3 muscarinic receptors—which are thought to be responsible for abnormal bladder contractions—and initiates a cascading phenomenon, leading to excessive bladder contractions and sequential symptoms.[43-45] Antimuscarinic medications work by directly inhibiting ACh at the M_3 muscarinic and, to an extent, the M_2 muscarinic receptors of the detrusor muscle—which are thought to be responsible for normal, physiologic bladder contractions—in the afferent pathways of the bladder.[43] These medications allow the bladder to properly fill, thus improving urinary frequency and nocturia.[45]

The four types of UI include stress urinary incontinence (SUI), urge urinary incontinence (UUI), overflow incontinence (OI), and mixed incontinence. SUI occurs during episodes of increased intra-abdominal pressure on the bladder in a patient with a weakened urethral sphincter, typically after an effort or exertion from normal physical activity, sneezing, or coughing.[38,39,46,47] UUI results from increased stimulation and contraction of the bladder detrusor muscle due to an influx of ACh on the M_3 receptors. Patients with UUI typically suffer from bouts of urinary urgency, frequency, and nocturia.[38,39,41] OI is caused by urinary obstruction, most commonly BPH, or bladder underactivity typically from neurological dysfunction. This leads to an inability to completely void urine from the bladder. Mixed incontinence is a combination of any of the three previous types of incontinence.[38,39] Patients with functional or cognitive impairment such as decreased mobility, low physical functioning like arthritis, or decreased mental functioning may become incontinent without classification of UI.[39] Overall, patients presenting with any type of incontinence should undergo tests to rule out bladder infections, bladder cancer, and prostate cancer.[45]

TREATMENT

Nonpharmacologic Treatments

Nonpharmacologic treatments are first line for most patients and can be used in combination with pharmacologic treatment. Prior to evaluation by a practitioner, a voiding diary should be kept to assess the severity of UI. The voiding diary documents the frequency of voiding and the number of episodes of incontinence.[5] In many patients, fluid management and avoidance of caffeine and other bladder irritants will correct UI.[43,45] Obesity is a contributing factor to SUI and a weight loss of 8 kg can provide clinically significant improvements in SUI symptoms.[39,46,48] The most common nonpharmacologic approaches to UI are bladder training, which includes scheduled urination and urge-suppression techniques, and pelvic floor exercises, which include voluntary contraction and relaxation of muscles used to help control urination.[38,45-47] Patients with functional or cognitive impairment may benefit from assistance of caregivers, scheduled bathroom visits, and absorbent pads or garments.[38,45]

Antimuscarinic Agents

Antimuscarinic agents are the most widely prescribed class of drugs for UI and are the first line of therapy unless contraindications such as urinary retention, gastric retention, narrow-angle glaucoma, or hypersensitivity exist.[49-59] As seen in Table 63-2, antimuscarinics are divided into two classes. The tertiary amine antimuscarinics include oxybutynin (Ditropan), tolterodine (Detrol), darifenacin (Enablex), solifenacin (Vesicare), and fesoterodine (Toviaz).

effect at reducing BPH symptoms; however, the largest trial to date found no difference compared to placebo after 12 months of therapy.[20-22] It has been suggested that saw palmetto may modestly inhibit 5ARI or have growth factor–inhibiting properties. Based on a lack of clinical studies demonstrating improvement in symptoms, the AUA does not recommend this product. If patients do decide to take saw palmetto, the recommended dose is 160 mg twice daily of the standardized extract. Patients taking saw palmetto along with antiplatelet agents or anticoagulants should be counseled on possible bleeding side effects.

FOUNDATION OVERVIEW: ERECTILE DYSFUNCTION

Defined as the inability to achieve and sustain an erection of sufficient rigidity for intercourse, erectile dysfunction (ED) affects 10 to 20 million men in the United States.[22] It is a disorder associated with increasing patient age with 5% of 40 year olds and 15% to 25% of men ≥65 afflicted with complete or severe dysfunction.[23] The risk of erectile dysfunction is increased in men with diabetes, heart disease, hypertension, and those who smoke.[24,25]

Penile erection is a vascular event mediated by neuronal action under the influence of psychological and hormonal factors. In the flaccid state, arterial vascular smooth muscle is contracted and venules are open and drain freely. Erection occurs when parasympathetic nonadrenergic, noncholinergic neurons and endothelial cells release nitric oxide, triggering a series of reactions which results in relaxation of smooth muscle of the helicine arteries of the penis.[26] Venules, which usually drain blood in the penis, become compressed against the tunica albuginea and entrap blood resulting in an erection.

ED may be a result of organic, psychological factors, or both. Organic causes account for 80% of cases and often present with vascular compromise and decreased penile blood flow.[1] These can include vascular (eg, heart disease, hypertension, dyslipidemia), neurologic (eg, spinal cord injury, Parkinson disease), endocrine disorders (eg, diabetes, hypogonadism), miscellaneous causes (eg, Peyronie disease, prostatic hyperplasia), and psychogenic causes (eg, depression, anxiety, and stress).[27] Use of prescription medications (eg, antihypertensives, antipsychotics, hormones) as well as alcohol and drugs of abuse (eg, cocaine, amphetamine) can also lead to ED.

Evaluation of patients with ED includes a medical history, physical examination, and laboratory tests to exclude serious conditions associated with ED and to identify risk factors. A sexual history should be obtained from the patient and his partner focusing on the nature of the problem (frequency, duration, quality, and duration of erections) and psychosocial factors that may suggest potential causes and the most appropriate approach to treatment.[28] Standardized questionnaires such as the Sexual Health Inventory for Men[29] are also helpful.[26]

TREATMENT

An important treatment goal is to identify and treat any medical or psychological condition that contribute to ED. This would include management of risk factors such as diabetes, hypertension, and dyslipidemia, as well as treatment of hypogonadism with testosterone if necessary. If these causes have been excluded or managed, the main goal is to satisfy the patient's expectations which would include cure, pleasure, partner satisfaction, reproduction, and naturalness.[30] Two measurable dimensions help define this goal: treatment response (consisting of efficacy and tolerability), and treatment satisfaction (ie, how well the treatment meets or exceeds the expectations of the patient and his partner).[31]

Phosphodiesterase Type 5 (PDE-5) Inhibitors

Sildenafil (Viagra), vardenafil (Levitra), and tadalafil (Cialis) enhance the effect of nitrous oxide by selectively inhibiting the phosphodiesterase type 5 enzyme. Randomized clinical trials demonstrate statistically significant response to these agents regardless of cause (organic, psychogenic, or mixed), duration, age, race, or severity. When PDE-5 inhibitors are not effective, secondary causes of ED should be considered. These include incorrect dose, hypogonadism, a possible psychological component, and comorbidities.[32] There is no convincing evidence that one agent is superior to any other.[5] However, in patients unresponsive to on-demand or "as needed" dosing schedules, daily use of tadalafil at doses of 2.5 to 5 mg may improve ED and may be a more acceptable option prior to using second-line treatments such as vasoactive agents.[33] The serum half-life of tadalafil (17.5 hours) is considerably longer than sildenafil (3.7 hours) and vardenafil (3.9 hours) providing extended clinical activity. As such, tadalafil is effective for up to 36 hours following administration, while both sildenafil and vardenafil should be taken 30 to 60 minutes before anticipated intercourse.

Common adverse events include headache, flushing, dyspepsia, and rhinitis; however, drop-out rates due to adverse events did not differ from placebo in clinical trials. Patients receiving concomitant α-adrenergic blockers may experience postural hypotension and dizziness. Since blood pressure is significantly lowered in patients taking concomitant nitrates and PDE-5 inhibitors, the combination is contraindicated. Serious cardiovascular events have been associated temporally with the PDE-5 inhibitors, thus, they should not be used in patients in whom sexual intercourse is inadvisable because of poor cardiac status. These drugs have been associated with temporary difficulty in distinguishing blue and green colors. Sudden vision and hearing loss has been observed in a few patients. Prolonged erections and priapism have been reported infrequently. Patients should seek medical attention for erections lasting more than 4 hours. The PDE-5 inhibitors are metabolized by cytochrome P450 (CYP) 3A4 enzymes. The PDE-5 inhibitor dose should be reduced if coadministered with medications affecting this enzyme system (eg, erythromycin, ketoconazole, ritonavir).

application of micronized 17-beta estradiol (Vagifem) daily for 2 weeks then twice weekly decreases vaginal atrophy symptoms, including UI.[61,62] The deficiency of estrogen in postmenopausal women was once thought to contribute to UUI; however, an increase in UUI symptoms has been demonstrated for patients taking oral estrogen and therefore this route is not recommended.[40,47,63,64]

Duloxetine (Cymbalta), although not FDA approved, may be a viable treatment for SUI. It works by decreasing the frequency of UUI episodes and improving quality of life. It is used in patients after nonpharmacologic treatment has failed.[65,66] This medication increases the urethral striated sphincter-muscle tone, leading to relief of SUI symptoms.[45,65] Duloxetine is typically dosed 40 mg orally twice daily.[66] The most commonly noted side effect is mild to moderate nausea; however, it can also increase blood pressure which should be monitored after initiation.[65,66]

Botulinum toxin, a potent neurotoxin, has efficacy in patients refractory or intolerant to antimuscarinic agents. Injections of 100 to 300 U of botulinum toxin, diluted with normal saline, resulted in improvements in UUI for 12 to 24 weeks.[67,68]

There are many medications previously used for UI that are no longer recommended due to lack of efficacy or poor tolerance. These include other antimuscarinic agents (propantheline, methantheline, emepronium, dicyclomine, terodiline), antispasmodic agents (flavoxate), tricyclic antidepressants (imipramine), and prostaglandin synthetase inhibitors (indomethacin).

CASE Application

1. Which of the following is the brand name for dutasteride?
   a. Hytrin
   b. Flomax
   c. Proscar
   d. Avodart
   e. Cardura

2. An 82-year-old patient who is taking 2 mg of terazosin for BPH comes into the pharmacy complaining of dizziness and generalized muscle weakness and persistent LUTS. What would you recommend to his physician?
   a. Add finasteride 5 mg daily to his regimen.
   b. Switch his terazosin to doxazosin 4 mg.
   c. Switch his terazosin to tamsulosin 0.4 mg daily.
   d. Lower the dose of his terazosin to 1 mg.
   e. Add saw palmetto twice daily.

3. What pregnancy category is finasteride?
   a. A
   b. B
   c. C
   d. D
   e. X

4. A patient reports that he has been taking his finasteride daily for the last 6 months for BPH. His last PSA was 2.6 ng/mL. Today it is 1.3 ng/mL. This can be best explained by which of the following?
   a. Finasteride stops the prostate from producing PSA.
   b. Finasteride can cause erroneous results in laboratory testing for PSA.
   c. PSA levels are often significantly decreased in patients taking 5ARI.
   d. Both a and b.
   e. All of the above.

5. A patient planning on having cataract surgery next week presents with a prescription for tamsulosin. His symptoms are not particularly bothersome but he reports some urinary hesitancy and straining. You decide to:
   a. Fill the prescription and counsel the patient on risk of sexual side effects.
   b. Call his physician and ophthalmologist and get his order changed to finasteride.
   c. Call his physician and ophthalmologist to determine if treatment with tamsulosin should be deferred until after his cataract surgery.
   d. Fill the prescription and counsel on risk of dizziness and orthostatic hypotension.
   e. Call his physician and get his order changed to terazosin.

6. Which of the following is *not* an advantage of tamsulosin when compared to doxazosin?
   a. Increased efficacy in reducing LUTS.
   b. Improved tolerability, especially cardiovascular side effects.
   c. Quicker onset of action in lowering symptoms.
   d. Both b and c.
   e. All of the above are advantages of tamsulosin for LUTS.

7. Which of the following is mainly responsible for increased prostate growth?
   a. PSA.
   b. DHT.
   c. 5-α-reductase.
   d. Testosterone.
   e. All of the above are directly responsible for prostate growth.

8. Select the statement that correctly describes erectile dysfunction.
   a. Individuals with diabetes are at higher risk.
   b. It is uncommon in the United States.
   c. It generally afflicts younger men.
   d. Individuals with above normal blood pressure are protected.
   e. Smokers are less likely to develop the condition.

TABLE 63-2 **Comparison of Antimuscarinic Medications for Incontinence**

Medication	Usual Dose (mg)	Metabolism (CYP)	Renal Dose Adjustments (mg)[a]	Affinity for M3 Receptor	Common Side Effects	Cost[b,c]
Tertiary Amines						
Oxybutynin (Ditropan)	5 po bid	3A4; inhibits 3A4, 2D6 (minor)	None	Moderate	Dry mouth (71%), constipation (12%)	$13.45
Oxybutynin ER (Ditropan XL)	5-10 po daily	3A4; inhibits 3A4	None	Moderate	Dry mouth (29%), constipation (7%)	$86.99,[d] $87.60[e]
Oxybutynin transdermal system (Oxytrol)	3.9/d twice weekly	3A4 (minor)	None	Moderate	Application site reaction (17%), dry mouth (10%)	$135.30[f]
Oxybutynin 10% gel (Gelnique)	1 satchet (1 g) daily	3A4 (minor)	None	Moderate	Dry mouth (8%), application site reaction (6%)	$128.98
Tolterodine (Detrol)	2 po bid	2D6	1 po bid	Nonselective	Dry mouth (37%)	$151.50
Tolterodine ER (Detrol LA)	4 po daily	2D6	2 po daily	Nonselective	Dry mouth (23%)	$138.41
Darifenacin (Enablex)	15 po daily	2D6, 3A4	None	Highly	Dry mouth (35%), constipation (21%)	$138.47
Solifenacin (Vesicare)	10 po daily	3A4	5 po daily	Moderate	Dry mouth (27%), constipation (13%)	$136.38
Fesoterodine (Toviaz)	8 po daily	None	4 po daily	Nonselective	Dry mouth (35%)	$129.99
Quaternary Amines						
Trospium chloride (Sanctura)	20 po bid	None	20 po daily	Nonselective	Dry mouth (20%)	$144.66
Trospium chloride ER (Sanctura XR)	60 po daily	None	Not recommended	Nonselective	Dry mouth (10%)	$136.78

[a]Creatinine clearance <30 mL/min.
[b]Based on 30-day supply.
[c]Prices from www.drugstore.com.
[d]5 mg daily.
[e]10 mg daily.
[f]Four-week supply.

These agents are uncharged, lipophilic entities, which cause more central nervous system (CNS) adverse events as compared to the quaternary amine antimuscarinic, trospium chloride (Sanctura). The latter is a charged species and does not readily penetrate the blood–brain barrier. In general, patients taking antimuscarinics have half the number of incontinent episodes compared to patients taking placebo. Few head-to-head trials between individual agents have been conducted; therefore, one agent is not considered more efficacious than others.[41,43] For relief of UI symptoms, antimuscarinics are designed to specifically antagonize the M_3 receptors. However, M_3 muscarinic receptors are also located in the salivary glands, lower bowel, and ciliary smooth muscle. Therefore, they also commonly cause adverse effects including dry mouth, constipation, and blurred vision.[41] Antimuscarinic agents can also antagonize other muscarinic receptors, such as M_1 muscarinic receptors, which can precipitate delirium or other CNS side effects.[60]

Oxybutynin has higher incidences of dry mouth in the immediate release (IR) formulation due to a higher rate of conversion to the active metabolite, *N*-desethyloxybutynin, as compared to the extended release (ER) formulation.[45] The transdermal patch can be applied to abdomen, hip, or buttock while the gel can also be applied to the upper arm, shoulder, or thigh.[51,52] All four systems are equally effective.[45] Tolterodine, based on pharmacodynamics, is one of the most selective agents in this class for muscarinic receptors located in the bladder.[41] In head-to-head trials with oxybutynin, the two drugs were shown to be equally effective.[45] Darifenacin is the most selective agent for the M_3 receptor. Because of the higher selectivity ratio for M_3 receptors over M_1 receptors, there are very few cognitive function side effects with darifenacin.[41,43,45] Solifenacin and tolterodine are the two most selective medications for muscarinic receptors in the bladder. Solifenacin has the longest half-life of any agent in this class (45-68 hours).[41] Fesoterodine is a prodrug which is hydrolyzed via nonspecific esterases, thus avoiding the CYP system, into the its active ingredient, 5-hydroxymethyl tolterodine.[57,60] Trospium chloride is derived from atropine and has a lower risk for side effects and drug–drug interactions due to its quaternary amine properties and lack of CYP hepatic metabolism.[40,41,43]

Vaginal atrophy is a condition with symptoms of dryness, burning, itching, and an increase in SUI. The vaginal

9. Select a vascular cause of erectile dysfunction.
   a. Depression
   b. Parkinson disease
   c. Hypogonadism
   d. Anxiety
   e. Dyslipidemia

10. Select the item that should be part of an evaluation of erectile dysfunction.
    a. A sexual history from the patient and partner
    b. A medical history
    c. A physical examination
    d. A psychosocial assessment
    e. All of the above

11. KR is a 62-year-old Hispanic man with a history of hypertension. He complains of ED for which he seeks treatment. There is no identifiable organic cause for his ED. Select the statement that correctly describes the approach to treatment in this patient.
    a. PDE-5 inhibitors would not be the treatment of choice in this patient.
    b. PDE-5 inhibitors are less efficacious in Hispanics.
    c. The use of a PDE-5 inhibitor is not likely to be effective in this patient with hypertension.
    d. A PDE-5 inhibitor would exert its activity by enhancing the effect of nitric oxide.
    e. He should not receive a PDE-5 inhibitor because sexual intercourse would not be advisable because of his cardiac status.

12. DL is a 59-year-old Caucasian man with a history of benign prostatic hyperplasia (BPH) which is adequately managed with doxazosin. He comes to the office with concerns about ED. His workup is unremarkable and a decision is made to start treatment with a PDE-5 inhibitor. Select the statement that correctly describes treatment in this patient.
    a. DL should be advised to take the medication immediately prior to sexual intercourse.
    b. Use of a PDE-5 inhibitor could lead to postural hypotension.
    c. PDE-5 inhibitors are contraindicated in patients with BPH.
    d. The medication of choice would be sildenafil.
    e. The use of a PDE-5 inhibitor is contraindicated in a patient receiving doxazosin.

13. JC is a 72-year-old African American man with erectile dysfunction and no contraindication to the use of a PDE-5 inhibitor. Which of the following medications could potentially interact and lead to increased serum concentrations of the PDE-5 inhibitor?
    a. Erythromycin
    b. Aspirin
    c. Ampicillin
    d. Haloperidol
    e. Influenza vaccine

14. Select the brand name for tadalafil.
    a. Relenza
    b. Viagra
    c. Enzyte
    d. Cialis
    e. Levitra

15. Which statement best describes alprostadil?
    a. It should be the first agent tried for the treatment of ED.
    b. It is a nonspecific PDE-5 inhibitor.
    c. It can be administered via a medicated transurethral suppository.
    d. Priapism has not been reported with the use of alprostadil.
    e. It exerts its activity by constricting smooth muscle in the penis.

16. LT, a 75-year-old woman, has severe renal impairment (CrCl <30 mL/min). All of the following are viable options for urge urinary incontinence *except*:
    a. Oxybutynin transdermal patch
    b. Tolterodine ER
    c. Solifenacin
    d. Oxybutynin IR
    e. Trospium chloride ER

17. Which subtype of muscarinic receptor is the primary target of antimuscarinics in patients with urge urinary incontinence?
    a. M_1
    b. M_2
    c. M_3
    d. M_4
    e. M_5

18. TV, a 55-year-old woman, is postmenopausal. Along with urinary incontinence, this patient is also suffering from symptoms of vaginal dryness, burning, and itching. Which of the following would be the best pharmacologic option for her?
    a. Oral estrogen
    b. Duloxetine
    c. Botulinum toxin
    d. Topical estrogen
    e. None of the above

19. All of the following are nonpharmacologic options for a patient with urinary incontinence *except*:
    a. Weight reduction
    b. Decrease fluid intake
    c. Increase intake of caffeine
    d. Pelvic floor exercises
    e. All of the above

20. What type of incontinence can be described as having urinary urgency, frequency, and nocturia along with leakage during exercise?
    a. Stress urinary incontinence
    b. Urge urinary incontinence
    c. Overflow incontinence
    d. Mixed incontinence
    e. None of the above

21. What is the brand name for darifenacin?
    a. Detrol LA
    b. Ditropan
    c. Enablex
    d. Vesicare
    e. Sanctura XR

TAKEAWAY POINTS ››

- BPH is the most common urological condition in older men although not all patients will exhibit bothersome LUTS.
- Symptoms of BHP may include urinary hesitancy, weak urinary stream, urinary frequency, nocturia, and incontinence.
- Serious complications of long-standing BPH include urinary retention, urinary tract infections, bladder stones, and renal failure.
- α-Adrenergic antagonists including terazosin, doxazosin, tamsulosin, alfuzosin, and silodosin are effective at reducing LUTS suggestive of BPH.
- In patients with evidence of enlarged prostate (>40 g), 5-α-reductase therapy with either finasteride or dutasteride can be used to shrink the prostate, slow disease progression, and reduce the need for urgency.
- A therapeutic trial of a 5-α-reductase should last at least 6 to12 months.
- Phytotherapy with saw palmetto is not recommended by the AUA based on a lack of quality clinical data.
- Erectile dysfunction is the inability to achieve and sustain an erection of sufficient rigidity for intercourse.
- Prevalence of ED increases with increasing age and is associated with conditions that affect the vascular, hormonal, or neurological system.
- Evaluation of an individual with ED is directed at identifying potentially treatable organic and psychological causes.
- PDE-5 inhibitors are first-line agents for ED and work by enhancing the effect of nitric oxide on smooth muscle in the penis, resulting in arterial vasodilation and erection.
- Sildenafil and vardenafil should be taken 30 to 60 minutes before anticipated intercourse.
- PDE-5 inhibitors may cause dizziness and postural hypotension in patients receiving α-blockers, therefore, patients should be monitored carefully. PDE-5 inhibitors are contraindicated in patients receiving nitrates because of potential for significant blood pressure reduction.
- PDE-5 inhibitors are metabolized by the CYP 3A4 hepatic enzyme system and may interact with inhibitors of this enzyme.
- The vasoactive agents, alprostadil, phentolamine, and papaverine, work by relaxing vascular smooth muscle and are injected directly into the penis.
- Pain and priapism may occur with the use of the vasoactive agents and they are contraindicated in patients prone to priapism.
- The four types of UI include stress urinary incontinence (SUI), urge urinary incontinence (UUI), overflow incontinence (OI), and mixed incontinence.
- Nonpharmacologic treatments are first line for most patients and can be used in combination with pharmacologic treatment.
- Antimuscarinics are designed to specifically antagonize the M_3 muscarinic receptor in the bladder and block the effects of acetylcholine.
- Antimuscarinic agents are the most widely prescribed class of drugs for urge urinary incontinence and are the first line of therapy unless contraindicated.
- The most common adverse effects of antimuscarinics are dry mouth, constipation, and blurred vision.
- There are several other pharmacologic agents for the other types of urinary incontinence including micronized 17-beta estradiol, duloxetine, and botulinum-A toxin.

REFERENCES

1. Fair WR, Parrish RF. Antibacterial substances in prostatic fluid. *Prog Clin Biol Res*. 1981;75A:247-264.
2. Berry SJ, Coffey DS, Walsh PC, Ewing LL. The development of human benign prostatic hyperplasia with age. *J Urol*. 1984;32:474-479.
3. Napalkov P, Maisonneuve P, Boyle P. Worldwide patterns of prevalence and mortality from benign prostatic hyperplasia. *Urology*. 1995;46 (suppl 3A):41-46.
4. Thorpe A, Neal D. Benign prostatic hyperplasia. *Lancet*. 2003;361:359-367.
5. McConnell JD. The pathophysiology of benign prostatic hyperplasia. *J Androl*. 1991;12:356-363.
6. Barry MJ. Evaluation of symptoms and quality of life in men with benign prostatic hyperplasia. *Urology*. 2001;58(6 suppl 1):25-32.
7. American Urological Association Practice Guidelines Committee. AUA guidelines on management of benign prostatic hyperplasia (2003). Chapter 1: diagnosis and treatment recommendations. *J Urol*. 2003;170:530-547.
8. Wiygul J, Babayan RK. Watchful waiting in benign prostatic hyperplasia. *Curr Opin Urol*. 2009;19:3-6.

9. Djavan B, Marberger M. A meta-analysis on the efficacy and tolerability of alpha1-adrenoceptor antagonists in patients with lower urinary tract symptoms suggestive of benign prostatic obstruction. *Eur Urol.* 1999;36:1-13.
10. McConnell JD, Roehrborn CG, Bautista OM, et al, Medical Therapy of Prostatic Symptoms (MTOPS) Research Group. The long-term effect of doxazosin, finasteride, and combination therapy on the clinical progression of benign prostatic hyperplasia. *N Engl J Med.* 2003;349(25):2387-2398.
11. Tomita M, Egawa S, Ikemoto I, et al. One-week effects of tamsulosin on benign prostatic hyperplasia assessed with a daily symptom score. *Hinyokika Kiyo.* 2009;55:193-197.
12. Takao T, Tsujimura A, Kiuchi H, et al. Early efficacy of silodosin in patients with lower urinary tract symptoms suggestive of benign prostatic hyperplasia. *Int J Urol.* 2008;15:992-996.
13. Marks LS, Gittelman MC, Hill LA, Volinn W, Hoel G. Rapid efficacy of the highly selective alpha1A-adrenoceptor antagonist silodosin in men with signs and symptoms of benign prostatic hyperplasia: pooled results of 2 phase 3 studies. *J Urol.* 2009;181:2634-2640.
14. Schulman CC, Cortvriend J, Jonas U, Lock TM, Vaage S, Speakman MJ. Tamsulosin: 3-year long-term efficacy and safety in patients with lower urinary tract symptoms suggestive of benign prostatic obstruction: analysis of a European, multinational, multicenter, open-label study. European Tamsulosin Study Group. *Eur Urol.*1999;36:609-620.
15. Chang DF, Campbell JR. Intraoperative floppy-iris syndrome associated with tamsulosin. *J Cataract Refract Surg.* 2005;31:664-673.
16. Bell CM, Hatch WV, Fischer HD, et al. Association between tamsulosin and serious ophthalmic adverse events in older men following cataract surgery. *JAMA.* 2009;301:1991-1996
17. Chang DF, Braga-Mele R, Mamalis N, et al, ASCRS Cataract Clinical Committee. ASCRS White Paper: clinical review of intraoperative floppy-iris syndrome. *J Cataract Refract Surg.* 2008;34:2153-2162.
18. Marberger MJ. Long-term effects of finasteride in patients with benign prostatic hyperplasia: a double-blind, placebo-controlled, multicenter study. PROWESS Study Group.*Urology.* 1998;51:677-686.
19. Roehrborn CG, Siami P, Barkin J, et al; CombAT Study Group. The effects of dutasteride, tamsulosin and combination therapy on lower urinary tract symptoms in men with benign prostatic hyperplasia and prostatic enlargement: 2-year results from the CombAT study.*J Urol.* 2008;179:616-621.
20. Champault G, Patel JC, Bonnard AM. A double-blind trial of an extract of the plant *Serenoa repens* in benign prostatic hyperplasia. *Br J Clin Pharmacol.* 1984;18:461-462.
21. Gerber GS, Kuznetsov D, Johnson BC, Burstein JD. Randomized, double-blind, placebo-controlled trial of saw palmetto in men with lower urinary tract symptoms. *Urology.* 2001;58:960-964.
22. Bent S, Kane C, Shinohara K, et al. Saw palmetto for benign prostatic hyperplasia. *NEJM.* 2006;354:557-566.
22. NIH Consensus Development Panel on Impotence. NIH Consensus Conference: impotence. *JAMA.* 1993;270:83-90.
23. Feldman HA, Goldstein I, Hatzichristou DG, Krane RJ, McKinlay JB. Impotence and its medical and psychosocial correlates: results of the Massachusetts Male Aging Study. *J Urol.* 1994;151:54-61.
24. Johannes CB, Araujo AB, Feldman HA, Derby CA, Kleinman KP, McKinlay JB. Incidence of erectile dysfunction in men 40 to 69 years old: longitudinal results from the Massachusetts Male Aging Study. *J Urol.* 2000;163:460-463.
25. McVary KT, Carrier S, Wessells H. Smoking and erectile dysfunction: evidence based analysis. *J Urol.* 2001;166: 1624-1632.
26. McVary KT. Erectile dysfunction. *N Engl J Med.* 2007;357: 2472-2481.
27. University of Ottawa Evidence-based Practice Center, Ottawa, Canada. Diagnosis and treatment of erectile dysfunction. AHRQ, U.S. Department of Health & Human Services, 2009. Available at: http://www.ahrq.gov/downloads/pub/evidence/pdf/erectiledys/erecdys.pdf. Accessed January 15, 2010.
28. Beckman TJ, Abu-Lebdeh HS, Mynderse LA. Evaluation and medical management of erectile dysfunction. *Mayo Clin Proc.* 2006;81:385-390.
29. Cappelleri JC, Rosen RC. The Sexual Health Inventory for Men (SHIM): a 5-year review of research and clinical experience. *Int J Impot Res.* 2005;17:307-319.
30. Hanson-Divers C, Jackson SE, Lue TF, et al. Health outcomes variables important to patients in the treatment of erectile dysfunction. *J Urol.* 1998;159:1541-1547.
31. Carson C, Giuliano F, Goldstein I, et al. The 'effectiveness' scale—therapeutic outcome of pharmacologic therapies for ED: an international consensus panel report. *Int J Impot Res.* 2004;16:207-213.
32. McMahon DN, Smith CJ, Shabsigh R. Treating erectile dysfunction when PDE5 inhibitors fail. *BMJ.* 2006;332:589-592.
33. McMahon C. Efficacy and safety of daily tadalafil in men with erectile dysfunction previously unresponsive to on-demand tadalafil. *J Sex Medicine.* 2004;1:292-300.
34. Urciuoli R, Cantisani TA, Carlini IM, Giuglietti M, Botti FM. Prostaglandin E1 for treatment of erectile dysfunction. *Cochrane Database Syst Rev.* 2004;2:CD001784.
35. McMahon CG. A comparison of the response to the intracavernosal injection of a combination of papaverine and phentolamine, prostaglandin PGE1 and a combination of all three agents in the management of impotence. *Int J Impot Res.* 1991;3:113-121.
36. Chen Y, Dai Y, Wang R. Treatment strategies for diabetic patients suffering from erectile dysfunction. *Expert Opin Pharmacother.* 2008;9:257-266.
37. Montague DK, Angermeier KW. Contemporary aspects of penile prosthesis implantation. *Urol Int.* 2003;70:141-146.
38. Abrams P, Cardozo L, Fall M, et al. The standardization of terminology of lower urinary tract function: report from the standardization sub-committee of the International Continence Society. *Neurourol Urodyn.* 2002;21:167-178.
39. Hunskaar S, Arnold EP, Burgio K, et al. Epidemiology and natural history of urinary incontinence. *Int Urogynecol J.* 2000;11:301-319.
40. Wagg AS, Cardozo L, Chapple CR, et al. Overactive bladder syndrome in older people. *BJU Int.* 2007;99:502-509.
41. Abrams P, Andersson KE. Muscarinic receptor antagonists for overactive bladder. *BJU Int.* 2007;100:987-1006.
42. Brown JS, Nyberg LM, Kusek JW, et al. Proceedings of the National Institute of Diabetes and Digestive and Kidney Disease Symposium on epidemiologic issues in urinary incontinence in women. *Am J Obstet Gynecol.* 2003;188: S77-S88.
43. Staskin DR. Overactive bladder in the elderly: a guide to pharmacological management. *Drug Aging.* 2005;22:1013-1028.

44. Jackson RA, Vittinghoff E, Kanaya AM, et al. Urinary incontinence in elderly women: findings from the health, aging, and body composition. *Obstet Gynecol.* 2004;104:301-307.
45. Ouslander JG. Management of overactive bladder. *N Engl J Med.* 2004;350:786-799.
46. Rogers RG. Urinary stress incontinence. *N Engl J Med.* 2008;358:1029-1036.
47. Holroyd-Leduc JM, Straus SE. Management of urinary incontinence in women: scientific review. *JAMA.* 2004;291(8);986-995.
48. Subak LL, Wing R, West DS, et al. Weight loss to treat urinary incontinence in overweight and obese women. *N Engl J Med.* 2009;360:481-490.
49. Ditropan [package insert]. Raritan, NJ; Ortho-McNeil Pharmaceutical, Inc.; 2003.
50. Ditropan XL [package insert]. Raritan, NJ; Ortho-McNeil Pharmaceutical, Inc.; 2008.
51. Oxytrol [package insert]. Corona, CA. Watson Pharmaceuticals, Inc.; 2006.
52. Gelnique [package insert]. Corona, CA; Watson Pharmaceuticals, Inc.; 2008.
53. Detrol [package insert]. New York, NY; Pfizer, Inc.; 2008.
54. Detrol LA [package insert]. New York, NY; Pfizer, Inc.; 2008.
55. Enablex [package insert]. East Hanover, NJ; Novartis Pharmaceuticals Corporation; 2006.
56. Vesicare [package insert]. Research Triangle Park, NC; GlaxoSmithKline; 2008.
57. Toviaz [package insert]. New York, NY; Pfizer, Inc.; 2008.
58. Sanctura [package insert]. Irvine, CA; Allergan, Inc.; 2006.
59. Sanctura XR [package insert]. Irvine, CA; Allergan, Inc.; 2008.
60. Hegde SS, Mammen M, Jasper JR. Antimuscarinics for the treatment of overactive bladder: current options and emerging therapies. *Curr Opin Investig Drugs.* 2004;5:40-49.
61. Eriksen PS, Rasmussen H. Low-dose 17β-estradiol vaginal tablets in the treatment of atrophic vaginitis: a double-blind placebo controlled study. *Eur J Obstet Gynecol Reprod Biol.* 1992;44:137-144.
62. Simunic V, Banovic I, Ciglar S. Local estrogen in patient with urogenital symptoms. *Int J Gynaecol Obstet.* 2003;82:187-197.
63. Andersson KE, Wein AJ. Pharmacology of the lower urinary tract: basis for current and future treatments of urinary incontinence. *Pharmacol Rev.* 2004;56:581-631.
64. Hendrix SL, Cochrane BB, Nygaard IE, et al. Effects of estrogen with and without progestin on urinary incontinence. *JAMA.* 2005;293:935-948.
65. Millard RJ, Moore K, Rencken R, et al. Duloxetine vs placebo in the treatment of stress urinary incontinence: a four-continent randomized clinical trial. *BJU Int.* 2004:93;311-318.
66. Van Kerrebroeck P, Abrams P, Lange R, et al. Duloxetine versus placebo in the treatment of European and Canadian women with stress urinary incontinence. *Br J Obstet Gynaecol.* 2004;111:249-257.
67. Werner M, Schmid DM, Schüssler B. Efficacy of botulinum-A toxin in the treatment of detrusor overactivity incontinence: a prospective nonrandomized study. *Am J Obstet Gynecol.* 2005;192:1735-1740.
68. Schulte-Baukloh H, Weib C, Stolze T, et al. Botulinum-A toxin detrusor and sphincter injection in treatment of overactive bladder syndrome: objective outcome and patient satisfaction. *Eur Urol.* 2005;48:984-990.

CHAPTER

64 Allergic Rhinitis

Nancy Borja-Hart and Karen Whalen

FOUNDATION OVERVIEW

Allergic rhinitis is a chronic inflammatory disease of the upper airways.[1-4] It is characterized by one or more of the following symptoms: nasal congestion, rhinorrhea, sneezing, and itching. This disease affects 10% to 30% of all adults and up to 40% of children.[2] In the United States, allergic rhinitis affects nearly 50 million people. Allergic rhinitis can significantly impact quality of life. Subjects who suffer from this disorder complain of missed work and schooldays and sleep disturbance.

Allergic reactions in the nose are mediated by immunoglobulin E (IgE).[5] In patients with allergic rhinitis, airborne allergens react with antigen-specific IgE bound to mast cells, thereby triggering release of inflammatory mediators such as histamine and leukotrienes. Both early (immediate) and late-phase allergic reactions occur following allergen exposure. The early-phase reaction happens within seconds to minutes and is mainly due to the release of histamine, leukotrienes, tryptase, and cytokines. Sneezing, itching, rhinorrhea, and congestion are typical symptoms. The release of cytokines results in the infiltration of inflammatory cells such as basophils and eosinophils. This produces a late-phase reaction that usually occurs 4 to 8 hours after allergen exposure. With continued exposure to the allergen, the late-phase inflammatory response results in chronic symptoms of allergic rhinitis.

Patients with allergic rhinitis may present with the following symptoms: clear rhinorrhea, nasal congestion, allergic conjunctivitis, sneezing, postnasal drip, and itchiness in the nose, ears, and/or eyes.[1] Allergic shiners (swelling and darkening of circles under the eyes due to nasal obstruction and venous congestion) and allergic salute (upward rubbing of the nose) are less reported signs.

Allergic rhinitis can be differentiated from other types of rhinitis by a thorough history and physical examination. Chief concerns, symptoms, patterns, and triggers of nasal and related symptoms should be obtained from the patient. Percutaneous skin testing or allergen-specific IgE antibody testing (eg, radioallergosorbent test [RAST]) are the most common tests used to confirm the diagnosis of allergic rhinitis.

Two classification schemes exist to grade the severity of allergic rhinitis. The Allergic Rhinitis and its Impact on Asthma (ARIA) organization has designated four categories of allergic rhinitis: mild intermittent, mild persistent, moderate-severe intermittent, and moderate-severe persistent.[6] Patients who experience symptoms <4 d/wk or for less than 4 consecutive weeks meet the criteria for *intermittent* allergic rhinitis. The *persistent* classification applies to patients whose allergic rhinitis symptoms occur more than 4 d/wk and for more than 4 consecutive weeks. If symptoms do not impact daily activities, sleep patterns, work, or school, then the disease is considered *mild*. If these areas are impacted by allergic rhinitis, then the patient has a *moderate-severe* form. In a second classification scheme, the Joint Task Force on Practice Parameters categorizes allergic rhinitis as *seasonal*, *perennial*, or *episodic*.[2] *Seasonal* allergic rhinitis refers to those patients with symptoms primarily during the spring and fall (high pollen seasons). Patients with *perennial* allergic rhinitis have symptoms throughout the year. Patients with *episodic* allergic rhinitis experience symptoms by sporadic exposures to inhalant aeroallergens.

PREVENTION

Patients should be advised to try and avoid offending allergens (pollen, fungi, dust mites, and animals) if possible.[2,6] During high pollen seasons, patients should limit outside exposure. To further assist with allergen avoidance, subjects may take the following additional precautions to minimize exposure to indoor allergens: use a high-efficiency particulate air (HEPA) filter, vacuum with a HEPA filter, wash laundry in hot water, use barrier protection on pillow and mattresses, and use a pest control system to avoid insect emanations.[2]

TREATMENT

The management of allergic rhinitis includes the following three components: allergen avoidance (as above), pharmacotherapy, and immunotherapy.[2] The goals of therapy for patients with allergic rhinitis are to improve symptoms, improve the patient's quality of life, and provide the patient with a medication (if needed) with minimal adverse effects.[2,6] Six different classes of medication are available for the management of allergic rhinitis. These include antihistamines, decongestants, intranasal corticosteroids, intranasal mast cell stabilizers, intranasal anticholinergic agents and leukotriene modifiers (Table 64-1). When considering monotherapy or combination therapy, presenting symptoms, severity of symptoms, patient age, and comorbidities should be taken into consideration.

TABLE 64-1 **Available Medications for Allergic Rhinitis**

Medication (Brand Name)	Normal Adult Dosage
Antihistamines	
Oral first-generation	
Brompheniramine[a]	4 mg po every 4 to 6 h prn
(BroveX chewable tablets)[b]	12-24 mg po every 12 h
(LoHist-12extended release tabs)[b]	6-12 mg po every 12 h
Chlorpheniramine[a] (Aller-Chlor)	4 mg po every 4 to 6 h
Clemastine[a] (Tavist Allergy)	1.34 mg po every 12 h po every 12 h
Diphenhydramine[a] (Benadryl, Diphenhist)	25-50 mg po every 4 to 6 h prn
Triprolidine (Zymine)[b]	2.5 mg po every 4 to 6 h
Oral second-generation[a]	
Cetirizine[a] (Zyrtec)	10 mg po once daily
Desloratadine[a] (Clarinex)[b]	5 mg po once daily
Fexofenadine[a]	
(Allegra)[b]	60 mg po twice daily
(Allegra 180 mg tablet)[b]	180 mg po once daily
Levocetirizine (Xyzal)[b]	5 mg po once daily in the evening
Loratadine[a] (Claritin)	10 mg po once daily
Intranasal	
Azelastine 137 μg/spray (Astelin)[b]	1-2 sprays per nostril twice daily
Azelastine 0.1% (Astepro 0.1%)[b]	1-2 sprays per nostril twice daily
Azelastine 0.15% (Astepro 0.15%)[b]	1-2 sprays per nostril twice daily *or* 2 sprays per nostril once daily
Olopatadine 665 μg/spray (Patanase)[b]	2 sprays per nostril twice daily
Ocular	
Azelastine 0.05% (Optivar)[b]	1 drop in affected eye twice daily
Ketotifen fumarate 0.025% (Zaditor, Zyrtec Itchy Eye)	1 drop in affected eye every 8-12 h
Olopatadine 0.1% (Patanol)[b]	1-2 drops in affected eye twice daily
Olopatadine 0.2% (Pataday)[b]	1 drop in affected eye once daily
Decongestants	
Oral	
Phenylephrine (Sudafed PE)	10 mg po every 4 to 6 h
Pseudoephedrine (Sudafed)	60 mg po every 4 to 6 h
(Sudafed 12 h extended-release tablet)	120 mg po every 12 h
(Sudafed 24 h extended-release tablet)	240 mg po every 24 h
Intranasal	
Phenylephrine 0.1% (4-way fast acting)	2-3 sprays per nostril every 3-4 h
Oxymetazoline 0.05% (Afrin)	2 sprays per nostril twice daily
Intranasal Corticosteroids	
Beclomethasone 42 μg/spray (Beconase AQ)[b]	1-2 sprays per nostril twice daily
Budesonide 32 μg /spray (Rhinocort Aqua)[b]	1-2 sprays per nostril daily in the AM
Flunisolide 25 μg/spray (generic only)[b]	2 sprays per nostril twice daily
Fluticasone furoate 27.5 μg/spray (Veramyst)[b]	2 sprays per nostril once daily; may reduce to 1 spray per nostril once daily
Fluticasone propionate 50 μg/spray (Flonase)[b]	2 sprays per nostril once daily *or* 1 spray per nostril twice daily; may reduce to 1 spray per nostril once daily
Mometasone furoate 50 μg/spray (Nasonex)[b]	2 sprays per nostril once daily

TABLE 64-1 **Available Medications for Allergic Rhinitis (*Continued*)**

Medication (Brand Name)	Normal Adult Dosage
Mast Cell Stabilizer	
Intranasal	
Cromolyn sodium 5.2 mg/spray (Nasalcrom)	1 spray per nostril 3-4 times per day
Ocular	
Cromolyn sodium 4% (Crolom)[b]	1-2 drops in each eye 4-6 times per day
Intranasal Anticholinergic	
Ipratropium bromide 0.03% (Atrovent)[b]	2 sprays per nostril 2-3 times per day
Leukotriene Receptor Antagonist	
Montelukast (Singulair)[b]	10 mg po once daily

[a]Antihistamines also available as a combination product with a decongestant.
[b]Product available by prescription only (Rx).
Abbreviations: po, by mouth (per os); prn, as needed (pro re nata).

Antihistamines

Antihistamines are histamine (H_1)-receptor antagonists. Oral, intranasal, and ocular dosage forms are available for the treatment of allergic rhinitis. Oral antihistamines are efficacious for management of rhinorrhea, sneezing, itching, and allergic conjunctivitis. These agents are more effective at preventing symptoms of allergic rhinitis than alleviating symptoms once they have occurred. As such, they are best taken prior to anticipated allergen exposure.

Among the oral antihistamines, the second-generation agents (eg, desloratadine, fexofenadine) are preferred. In general, the first-generation antihistamines are nonselective and considerably more sedating than the second-generation antihistamines.[2] In children, the first-generation oral antihistamines can cause paradoxical agitation rather than sedation. Additionally, the first-generation antihistamines have more anticholinergic adverse effects (dry mouth, constipation) compared to the second-generation agents. Some of the second-generation antihistamines can be sedating at usual doses (eg, cetirizine and intranasal azelastine) or when usual doses are exceeded (eg, loratadine and desloratadine). Intranasal antihistamines (azelastine and olopatadine) are effective in patients with seasonal allergic rhinitis. Azelastine has a rapid onset of action, which allows patients to administer the dose shortly before contact with a known allergen. Ketotifen fumarate is an over-the-counter (OTC) ophthalmic antihistamine that provides ocular itch relief.[7] It is indicated for children as young as 3 years of age.

Decongestants

Decongestants produce vasoconstriction due to sympathomimetic effects. In allergic rhinitis, decongestants are most effective for patients who present with nasal congestion.[6] For years, pseudoephedrine was the most common oral decongestant; however, abuse of pseudoephedrine has resulted in substitution of phenylephrine as the decongestant in many over-the-counter products. Concerns with abuse of pseudoephedrine stem from the fact that pseudoephedrine can be used to make methamphetamine. Therefore, it is only available behind the counter.[8] At higher than recommended doses, pseudoephedrine can increase blood pressure. Additional adverse effects include insomnia and irritability.[9] The adverse effect profile of phenylephrine is similar to that of pseudoephedrine.[10] Oral decongestants should be avoided in patients with uncontrolled hypertension, coronary artery disease, closed-angle glaucoma, and urinary retention. These agents may be used cautiously in patients with diabetes, controlled hypertension, and renal impairment.

Topical decongestants are available as nasal sprays or nasal drops. Topical products can cause burning, stinging, sneezing, or dryness of the nasal mucosa. When using topical decongestants, patients should be advised to use them infrequently and to avoid prolonged usage. Use for greater than 3 to 5 days may lead to the development of *rhinitis medicamentosa* or rebound nasal congestion.

Intranasal Corticosteroids

Intranasal corticosteroids inhibit allergic inflammation in the nose. This class of agents target the four hallmark symptoms of allergic rhinitis including sneezing, itching, rhinorrhea, and nasal congestion. Intranasal corticosteroids are the most effective medications for treating allergic rhinitis and improve nasal congestion more than oral antihistamines.[6,11] The likelihood of significant systemic absorption of intranasal corticosteroids causing hypothalamic-pituitary-adrenal (HPA) axis suppression is minimal.[12] Growth retardation has been associated with the use of intranasal beclomethasone in children; however, growth suppression has not been observed with agents that have a lower systemic bioavailability such as fluticasone propionate and mometasone furoate.[13,14] Local irritation of the nasal mucosa (burning, drying, and irritation) is common with intranasal corticosteroids. Following application, patients should be instructed not to blow the nose for at least 10 minutes.

Mast Cell Stabilizer

Cromolyn sodium is an intranasal mast cell stabilizer that is modestly effective in the prevention and treatment of allergic rhinitis. Cromolyn works by inhibiting mast cell degranulation and release of inflammatory leukotrienes.[15] It should be administered intranasally four times a day to be most effective. Cromolyn must cover the entire nasal lining. Therefore, patients should be instructed to blow the nose prior to administration. Patients may experience the peak effect of cromolyn in 1 to 2 weeks. Cromolyn sodium is also available as an ophthalmic solution for allergic conjunctivitis; however, it needs to be administered four to six times daily for maximum effect.

Intranasal Anticholinergic Agent

Intranasal anticholinergic agents such as ipratropium are effective in managing rhinorrhea and may be even more effective for this symptom when given in combination with an intranasal corticosteroid.[2]

Leukotriene Receptor Antagonists

Montelukast is a good choice in patients with coexisting asthma and is the only antileukotriene agent approved for managing the symptoms of allergic rhinitis. Montelukast can be used in children as young as 6 months of age.[16] It is available in a tablet or granule formulation. The granules can be given directly into the mouth, dissolved in baby formula or breast milk, or mixed with a spoonful of applesauce, carrots, rice, or ice cream for children 6 months to 5 years of age.

Nasal Saline

Nasal saline is effective for rhinorrhea associated with mild intermittent allergic rhinitis. It may also be useful for clearing blocked nasal passages prior to the administration of other intranasal medications.[6]

Allergen Immunotherapy

Allergen immunotherapy should be considered for patients whose symptoms are not improved with pharmacologic management and for those who are experiencing undesirable adverse effects.[17] Immunotherapy is the gradual administration of antigens to induce tolerance with the intended outcome of reduced symptoms with allergen exposure. The optimal patients to receive immunotherapy are patients with specific IgE antibodies to clinically relevant allergens.

Special Populations

Infants and children >6 months of age can use montelukast,[16] cetirizine, levocetirizine, desloratadine, or fexofenadine for mild allergic rhinitis symptoms. Loratadine is also approved for use in children 2 years of age and up. If symptoms become more severe, this population may benefit from intranasal corticosteroids, some of which are approved for children 2 years of age or older.[6]

The FDA has established five categories to determine the potential harm of medications in pregnancy (Table 64-2). Antihistamines, particularly loratadine, cetirizine, and levocetirizine can be used in pregnant patients (all three antihistamines are pregnancy category B).[18] Budesonide is the only intranasal corticosteroid that is pregnancy category B.[2] Pseudoephedrine can be used following the first trimester, but it is classified as a pregnancy category C drug.[19] Women should not initiate immunotherapy during pregnancy; however, it may be continued during pregnancy.[20]

TABLE 64-2 **FDA Pregnancy Categories**

A	Adequate, well-controlled studies in pregnant women have failed to demonstrate risk to the fetus.
B	Either animal findings show risk (but human findings do not) or, if no adequate human studies have been done, animal findings are negative.
C	Human studies are lacking and animal studies are either positive for fetal risk or lacking as well. However, potential benefits may justify the potential risk.
D	Investigational or postmarketing data show risk to fetus. Nevertheless, potential benefits may outweigh the risk.
X	Studies in animals or humans, or investigational or postmarketing reports have shown fetal risk which clearly outweighs any possible benefit to the patient.

CASE Application

1. All of the following are classic symptoms of allergic rhinitis *except*
   a. Rhinorrhea
   b. Congestion
   c. Sneezing
   d. Thick nasal discharge

2. Which of the following is a potential adverse effect when using oral antihistamines for the management of allergic rhinitis in a 3-year-old child?
   a. HPA axis suppression
   b. Paradoxical agitation
   c. Rebound congestion
   d. Medication tolerance

3. JB is a 45-year-old man with a history of chronic nasal stuffiness nearly daily and all year round. His only other medical condition is high blood pressure. In addition to stuffiness, he has been sneezing a lot at work (which he finds very embarrassing). Also, his allergies have caused him to cancel park outings with his family. Using the ARIA guidelines, which of the following best classifies JB's symptoms?
   a. Mild intermittent
   b. Moderate to severe intermittent
   c. Mild persistent
   d. Moderate to severe persistent

4. Which therapeutic option would be best for JB?
   a. Oral decongestant
   b. Nonselective antihistamine
   c. Intranasal corticosteroid
   d. Intranasal decongestant

5. If the patient in Question 3 were a 30-year-old pregnant (first trimester) woman, how would the management change?
   a. The management would be the same.
   b. Initiate nonselective antihistamine.
   c. Initiate oral decongestant.
   d. Initiate mast cell stabilizer.

6. Select the brand name for montelukast.
   a. Clarinex
   b. Zaditor
   c. Xyzal
   d. Singulair

7. The use of pseudoephedrine is concerning in a patient with which of the following disease states?
   a. Diabetes mellitus
   b. Chronic kidney disease
   c. Hypertension
   d. All of the above

8. Which of the following antihistamines is available by prescription only?
   a. Diphenhydramine
   b. Ketotifen fumarate
   c. Levocetirizine
   d. Loratadine

9. Which of the following classes of medication can be used for management of allergic rhinitis in pregnancy?
   a. Oral antihistamines
   b. Intranasal corticosteroids
   c. Oral decongestants
   d. All of the above

10. JS is a 23-year-old man with a history of seasonal allergic rhinitis. He complains of bothersome nasal stuffiness each year during the fall when ragweed pollen is prevalent. Which of the following medications is most appropriate to provide immediate relief of his nasal congestion?
    a. Cetirizine
    b. Chlorpheniramine
    c. Fluticasone
    d. Oxymetazoline

11. Which of the following allergen avoidance techniques would be most appropriate to help reduce allergic symptoms caused by ragweed pollen?
    a. Encase pillow and mattress in allergen-proof cover.
    b. Keep windows closed and minimize outdoor activities.
    c. Reduce indoor humidity to <50%.
    d. Wash bedding in hot water.

12. Which of the following medications is beneficial in reducing symptoms of seasonal allergic rhinitis when started prior to allergen exposure?
    a. Intranasal corticosteroid
    b. Leukotriene antagonist
    c. Oral antihistamine
    d. All of the above

13. CW is an 8-year-old boy with seasonal allergic rhinitis and mild persistent asthma. Which of the following medications would be most appropriate to manage symptoms of both his asthma and allergic rhinitis?
    a. Intranasal beclomethasone
    b. Intranasal cromolyn
    c. Cetirizine
    d. Montelukast

14. Sedation would most likely occur with which of the following antihistamines when used at recommended dosages for adult patients?
    a. Desloratadine
    b. Diphenhydramine
    c. Fexofenadine
    d. Olopatadine

15. Which of the following antihistamines is available in an intranasal formulation?
    a. Azelastine
    b. Ketotifen fumarate
    c. Levocetirizine
    d. Loratadine

16. Which of the following categories of allergic rhinitis medications is most likely to be associated with rhinitis medicamentosa (rebound nasal congestion) with prolonged use?
    a. Intranasal corticosteroid
    b. Intranasal decongestant
    c. Oral antihistamine
    d. Oral decongestant

17. Which of the following medications must be kept behind the pharmacy counter since it may be used in the production of methamphetamine?
    a. Brompheniramine
    b. Chlorpheniramine
    c. Phenylephrine
    d. Pseudoephedrine

18. NB is a 28-year-old woman who is taking a combination of cetirizine, intranasal fluticasone, pseudoephedrine, and montelukast to manage symptoms of persistent allergic rhinitis. She complains of feeling jittery and having palpitations after taking all of her medications in the morning. Which of the following medications is most likely causing her complaints?
    a. Cetirizine
    b. Fluticasone
    c. Montelukast
    d. Pseudoephedrine

19. TR is a 6-year-old boy with persistent allergic rhinitis. He is experiencing symptoms despite the use of an oral antihistamine, and the physician would like to add an intranasal corticosteroid. Which of the following is correct regarding the use of an intranasal corticosteroid for TR?
    a. Intranasal corticosteroids should not be combined with oral antihistamines in pediatric patients.
    b. Newer intranasal corticosteroids with low systemic bioavailability are unlikely to cause growth suppression in TR.
    c. The use of intranasal corticosteroids is contraindicated in children <12 years of age.
    d. TR should obtain relief of his symptoms within minutes of using the intranasal corticosteroid.

20. KW is a 39-year-old woman who experiences daily rhinorrhea despite the use of cetirizine and intranasal flunisolide. Which of the following medications would be the most appropriate to add to target the symptoms of rhinorrhea?
    a. Azelastine
    b. Ipratropium
    c. Oxymetazoline
    d. Phenylephrine

TAKEAWAY POINTS ››

- Allergic rhinitis is a common inflammatory disorder of the nasal mucosa characterized by one or more of the following nasal symptoms: rhinorrhea, itching, sneezing, and nasal congestion. Symptoms of allergic conjunctivitis often accompany allergic rhinitis.
- Avoidance of allergens (eg, encasing mattresses and pillows, getting rid of carpets, using HEPA filters) may help reduce or prevent symptoms of allergic rhinitis.
- Selection of allergic rhinitis pharmacotherapy should be based on the presenting symptoms and consideration of the patient's age and coexisting medical conditions.
- Overall, intranasal corticosteroids are the most effective medication for allergic rhinitis. They target multiple symptoms of allergic rhinitis including rhinorrhea, itching, sneezing, and nasal congestion. Intranasal corticosteroids may also be beneficial in reducing ocular symptoms.
- Growth suppression in children has been a concern with intranasal beclomethasone; however, this has not been associated with newer intranasal corticosteroids with low systemic bioavailability.
- Oral antihistamines target multiple symptoms of allergic rhinitis, although, they are less effective than intranasal corticosteroids for managing nasal congestion. For optimal efficacy, antihistamines should be taken prior to exposure to the allergen.
- In general, first-generation antihistamines have more anticholinergic and sedative properties than the second-generation antihistamines.
- Intranasal topical antihistamines have a rapid onset of action and are an alternative to oral antihistamines. They do not target ocular symptoms. Thus, the addition of topical ocular antihistamines may be needed for management of allergic conjunctivitis.
- Oral and topical decongestants are only effective for management of the nasal congestion aspect of allergic rhinitis. Patients should be advised not to use topical decongestants for greater than 3 to 5 days due to the possibility of developing rhinitis medicamentosa.
- The leukotriene antagonist montelukast is indicated for seasonal allergic rhinitis and is a reasonable choice for patients with allergic rhinitis and asthma.
- Intranasal ipraptropium may be considered for patients with persistent rhinorrhea despite other therapies, or those intolerant of other treatments.
- Effective agents for seasonal allergic rhinitis include oral and topical antihistamines, intranasal corticosteroids, leukotriene antagonists (montelukast), and intranasal cromolyn. For maximal efficacy, these agents should be started prior to the expected onset of allergic symptoms.

REFERENCES

1. Skoner DP. Allergic rhinitis: definition, epidemiology, pathophysiology, detection, and diagnosis. *J Allergy Clin Immunol.* 2001;108(suppl):S2-S8.
2. Wallace DV, Dykewicz MS, Bernstein DI, et al; Joint Task Force on Practice; American Academy of Allergy; Asthma & Immunology; American College of Allergy; Asthma and Immunology; Joint Council of Allergy, Asthma and Immunology. The diagnosis and management of rhinitis: an updated practice parameter. *J Allergy Clin Immunol.* 2008;122(2 suppl):S1-S84.
3. Meltzer EO, Szwareberg J, Pill MW. Allergic rhinitis, asthma, and rhinosinusitis: diseases of the integrated airway. *J Manag Care Pharm.* 2004;10:310-317.
4. Nathan RA. The burden of allergic rhinitis. *Allergy Asthma Proc.* 2007;28:3-9.
5. Bousquet J, Vignola AM, Campbell AM, et al. Pathophysiology of allergic rhinitis. *Int Arch Allergy Immunol.* 1996;110(3): 207-218.
6. Bousquet J, Khaltaev N, Cruz AA, et al; World Health Organization; GA(2)LEN; AllerGen. Allergic Rhinitis and its Impact on Asthma (ARIA) 2008 update (in collaboration with the World Health Organization, GA(2)LEN and AllerGen). *Allergy.* 2008;63(suppl 86):8-160.
7. Zaditor (ketotifen fumurate). www.zaditor.com. Accessed August 18, 2009.

8. FDA—US Food and Drug Administration. Legal requirements for the sale and purchase of drug products containing pseudoephedrine, ephedrine, and phenylpropanolamine. Available at: www.fda.gov/ Drugs/DrugSafety/InformationbyDrugClass/ ucm072423.htm. Accessed August 3, 2009.
9. Greiner AN, Meltzer EO. Pharmacologic rationale for treating allergic and nonallergic rhinitis. *J Allergy Clin Immunol.* 2006;118:985-998.
10. Eccles R. Substitution of phenylephrine for pseudoephedrine as a nasal decongestant. An illogical way to control methamphetamine abuse. *Br J Clin Pharmacol.* 2006;63:10-14.
11. Weiner JM, Abramson MJ, Puy RM. Intranasal corticosteroids versus oral H1 receptor antagonists in allergic rhinitis: systematic review of randomised controlled trials. *BMJ.* 1998;317(7173):1624-1629.
12. Benninger MS, Ahmad N, Marple BF. The safety of intranasal steroids. *Otolaryngol Head Neck Surg.* 2003;129:739-750.
13. Allen DB, Meltzer EO, Lemanske RF, Jr, et al. No growth suppression in children treated with the maximum recommended dose of fluticasone propionate aqueous nasal spray for one year. *Allergy Asthma Proc.* 2002;23:407-413.
14. Schenkel EJ, Skoner DP, Bronsky EA, et al. Absence of growth retardation in children with perennial allergic rhinitis after one year of treatment with mometasone furoate aqueous nasal spray. *Pediatrics.* 2000;105:E22.
15. Nasalcrom (cromolyn sodium). www.nasalcrom.com. Accessed August 18, 2009.
16. Singulair [package insert]. Whitehouse Station, NJ. Merck & Co., Inc., July 2008.
17. Joint Task Force on Practice Parameters. Allergen immunotherapy: a practice parameter, second update. *J Allergy Clin Immunol.* 2007;120 (suppl):S25-S85.
18. Gilbert C, Mazzotta P, Loebstein R, Koren G. Fetal safety of drugs used in the treatment of allergic rhinitis: a critical review. *Drug Saf.* 2005;28:707-719.
19. National Asthma Education Program. *Management of asthma during pregnancy: report of the Working Group on Asthma and Pregnancy.* Bethesda, MD: National Institutes of Health; 1993. NIH Publication No. 93-3279.
20. Piette V, Daures JP, Demoly P. Treating allergic rhinitis in pregnancy. *Curr Allergy Asthma Rep.* 2006;6:232-238.

CHAPTER

65 Geriatrics

Rachel S. Cathey

FOUNDATION OVERVIEW: GERIATRICS

Geriatrics is defined as 65 years of age and older. With the baby boomer adult population entering their "golden years," the population of older adults is steadily increasing in the United States.[1] According to the Center for Disease Control's (CDC) review of public health and aging, the median age of the world's population is increasing.[1] The percentage of the population of 65 years and older in the United States is projected to increase from 12.4% in the year 2000 to 19.6% in the year 2030, which will increase demands in medical care.[1] This chapter will focus on appropriate prescribing principles in the elderly, as well as provide an overview of the management of Alzheimer dementia and Parkinson disease.

Polypharmacy

Polypharmacy is defined as taking nine or more medications.[2-3] Chronic illness among geriatric patients comes with a risk for increased numbers of medications, which potentially lead to polypharmacy and adverse events such as falls, constipation, confusion, and delirium.[2-3] Medication-related side effects can often be mistaken as the onset of a new chronic illness or simply the normal aging process. As medications are prescribed for these perceived new conditions, it may precipitate a "prescribing cascade" in which the provider prescribes one drug to treat the side effects of another medication the patient is taking.[4] It has been estimated in the geriatric population, for every dollar spent on medications, as much as $1.30 is spent on treating medication-related side effects.[5] Key facts about medication use are:

- Approximately 30% of hospital admissions in geriatric adults are directly related to medications.[6]
- Studies have also shown that a 4% chance of experiencing an adverse drug reaction exists with administration of five medications.[7]
- The risk of a medication-related adverse event increases to as high as 28% when taking 11 to 15 medications.[7]

These data significantly support the need for pharmacist intervention in prescribing to the older adult population. Appropriate prescribing of medications is vital to prevent medication-related adverse events due to duplications in therapy, drug-drug and drug-food interactions, inappropriate dosing, as well as polypharmacy.

Appropriate Prescribing in the Older Adult

Special consideration must be taken when prescribing medications in the geriatric population.[8] The original Beers criteria outlined medications to *avoid* in the elderly[9-11] (Table 65-1). The Beers list includes medications such as propoxyphene and cyclobenzaprine.[9] Propoxyphene, which is considered ineffective for pain management, causes very similar side effects in the elderly as other narcotic analgesics.[9] Cyclobenzaprine is also on the Beers list due to an unfavorable side effect profile and metabolism to a tricyclic antidepressant.[9] The 2009 publication by Beers and colleagues identifies *preferred* medications when prescribing central nervous system targeted medications[9-11] (Table 65-2). Examples of these agents include extended-release galantamine, memantine as add-on therapy for advanced dementia, as well as citalopram for treatment of depression in the elderly.[11]

Pathophysiologic Changes

Pathophysiologic changes associated with aging significantly impacts the need for tailored prescribing for geriatric patients. Differences in geriatric pharmacology include the effects of aging on pharmacokinetics. Pharmacokinetics includes the processes of absorption, distribution, metabolism, and elimination of medications.[12] Geriatric patients are more sensitive to benzodiazepines causing increased sedation and psychomotor dysfunction due to decreased clearance and higher plasma levels.[12]

Absorption Absorption of medications may be affected in the elderly by the chosen route of administration, comorbidities, and concomitantly administered medications.[12-15] For example, when administered with enteral feedings, the absorption of phenytoin may be decreased.[12,15] Reduction in gastric acid secretion by the use of H2-antagonists and proton pump inhibitors may affect absorption of medications that require an acidic environment such as itraconazole.[13] Gastric motility, including slowed gastric emptying and decreased peristalsis, is also affected by the aging process due to reduction of neuronal function to the GI tract as well as decreased intestinal blood flow.[15] These changes in gastric motility in the elderly can affect the absorption of potentially toxic medications such as digoxin.[14]

Distribution Volume of distribution is also affected by aging. As one ages, body fat increases by 20% to 40% and body water decreases by 10% to 15%.[12,15] Thus, hydrophilic medications will

TABLE 65-1 **Beers Criteria for Inappropriate Medication Use in the Older Adult**[1]

Drug Class	Medication Examples	
Antiemetics	Trimethobenzamide: least effective antiemetic and may cause extrapyramidal side effects Promethazine: anticholinergic and antihistamine properties	
Antihistamines	Diphenhydramine: may cause sedation and confusion; do not use for insomnia in the elderly Chlorpheniramine Hydroxyzine Cyproheptadine Class effects: all antihistamines may have potent anticholinergic properties; nonanticholinergic antihistamines preferred (such as loratadine)	
Antispasmodics and muscle relaxants	Cyclobenzaprine: metabolized to a tricyclic antidepressant Carisoprodol Methocarbamol Oxybutynin Class effects: poorly tolerated due to anticholinergic side effects, sedation, and weakness	
Benzodiazepines	*Long-acting:* Chlordiazepoxide Diazepam Chlorazepate *Short-acting:* Alprazolam Lorazepam Oxazepam	Use all benzodiazepines with caution due to risk of falls, sedation, and confusion Avoid long-acting benzodiazepines due to very long half-life in elderly patients Avoid use of alprazolam due to highly lipophilic and euphoric properties If use of a benzodiazepine is required, use very low doses of a short or intermediate-acting agent
Narcotic	Propoxyphene: poor analgesic properties; adverse effects similar to other narcotics	
NSAIDs	Indomethacin: most central nervous system (CNS) effects of nonsteroidal anti-inflammatory drugs (NSAIDs) Other examples include: ketorolac, naproxen, oxaprozin, piroxicam Class effects: significant risk of gastrointestinal side effects; risk of bleeding, renal failure, hypertension, and heart failure	
Tricyclic antidepressant	Amitriptyline: strong anticholinergic and sedative properties	

have a lower volume of distribution (V_d) and lipophilic drugs will have a higher V_d and longer elimination half-life.[12,15] For example, the V_d of benzodiazepines is much higher in older adults due to their highly lipophilic properties.[9,12,15]

Metabolism The plasma protein albumin is also reduced by approximately 10% in the aging adult. This reduction in albumin results in increased amounts of unbound (free) drug available in the circulation for medications that are highly protein bound such as phenytoin.[12,15] Despite the liver being the primary avenue of drug metabolism, it is not exempt from the aging process. Due to an estimated 40% decrease in blood flow to the liver resulting in reduced liver mass, drug metabolism can be significantly reduced in the geriatric patient.[12,15] This is particularly true with medications that undergo phase I metabolism in which the drug is converted to an active metabolite, such as glyburide.[12,17] Phase I metabolism medications are more likely to accumulate and cause adverse events, such as hypoglycemia in the case of glyburide.[17] Thus, drugs that undergo phase II metabolism, such as glipizide, are preferred in the elderly because they are converted to inactive metabolites.[12, 16-17]

TABLE 65-2 **2009 Beers Criteria for Preferred Central Nervous System Medications in the Elderly**[11]

Disease State	Preferred Medications
Dementia	Donepezil hydrochloride Galantamine hydrochloride extended-release Memantine hydrochloride, as adjunct therapy
Depression	Citalopram hydrochloride Escitalopram oxalate Duloxetine hydrochloride Bupropion hydrochloride extended release Mirtazapine
Parkinson disease	Entacapone, as adjunct therapy Ropinirole hydrochloride Carbidopa and levodopa
Psychosis	Risperidone Haloperidol, only for acute psychosis

Elimination Elimination of medications is proportionately dependent upon renal function as the majority of medications exit the body through the kidneys. As with the liver, blood flow and mass of the kidneys is also reduced with the aging process. Common comorbid illnesses, such as hypertension and diabetes, can also impair renal function in the elderly.[12,15] A reduction in functioning nephrons and renal tubular secretion combined with a decrease in overall muscle mass and creatinine production in the elderly, leads to an inaccurate reflection of measured serum creatinine. Thus, in clinical practice when using the Cockcroft-Gault equation to estimate creatinine clearance, the recommendation is to estimate the measured serum creatinine to 1.0 mg/dL if the actual serum creatinine value is less than 1.0 mg/dL.[16] Another consideration when using the Cockcroft- Gault equation is

TABLE 65-3 Principles for Prescribing in Geriatrics[4,5,7,13]
Helpful Hints for Prescribing in the Elderly
■ Start with low doses and titrate slowly.
■ Avoid starting two medications at the same time.
Before Prescribing a New Medication
■ Assess if the medication is absolutely necessary.
■ Ask if the new medication is being prescribed to treat side effects of another drug.
■ Reassess if the benefits of the drug outweigh the risks of its side effects.
■ Set realistic goals and outcomes for your patient.
■ Consider drug-drug and drug-disease interactions.
■ Evaluate if one drug could be used to treat two conditions.
■ Educate the patient about dosing, indications, and potential side effects.
■ Encourage compliance with medications.

the patient's body weight. If the patient's actual body weight is less than ideal body weight, the actual body weight should be used to calculate the estimated creatinine clearance.[12,15]

The most commonly used adage to describe appropriate prescribing in geriatrics is "start low, go slow."[12] This method takes into account the pharmacokinetic changes previously discussed, and will allow for correct dosing and titration of medications. Another concept for prescribing in geriatrics is to avoid starting two medications at the same time. This practice may circumvent potential medication-related side effects as well as avoid confusion if the patient does experience an adverse event. Successful pharmacotherapy in the older adult has been described as prescribing the correct drug, at the correct dose, for the correct patient, for the correct condition.[12] Obtaining a thorough and accurate medication history, as well as assessment of compliance plays a vital role in successful pharmacotherapy in the older adult patient (Table 65-3).

FOUNDATION OVERVIEW: ALZHEIMER DISEASE

Alzheimer disease (AD) is defined as a progressive and ultimately fatal disease in which nerve cells in vulnerable areas of the brain degenerate and die causing irreversible memory loss, behavioral and personality changes as well as decline in thinking abilities. The cause of AD is unknown, but is a leading cause of mortality in the United States. The pathology of AD is characterized by hallmark neurofibrillary tangles and senile plaques as well as cerebrocortical atrophy and degeneration of cholinergic neurons.[18-20] AD is the most common form of dementia and affects approximately 5.2 million Americans; it is estimated that by the year 2030, 7.7 million elderly Americans will have AD.[18-20] Described as a disease of the elderly, statistics indicate that more than 14% of individuals over the age of 65 have AD.[18-20] The prevalence of AD is estimated to increase to 40% in patients over the age of 80.[18-20]

TABLE 65-4 Ten Warning Signs of Alzheimer Disease from the Alzheimer's Association
■ Memory changes that interfere with daily life
■ Problems with planning or solving problems
■ Difficulty with accomplishing familiar tasks at work, home, or leisure
■ Confusion with orientation to time or place
■ Problems comprehending visual images and spatial relationships
■ Problems with language (verbal or written) and word-finding
■ Misplacing items and inability to retrace one's steps
■ Decrease in judgment and decision making abilities
■ Withdrawal from work and social activities
■ Changes in behavior, mood, and personality

Information from the Alzheimer's Association. www.alz.org.[15]

Clinical Presentation

Initial symptoms of AD may mimic the aging process as patients in the early stages may be able to function appropriately. Patients notice problems with memory function but family members and close friends are often first to recognize the symptoms their loved one is experiencing. The Alzheimer's Association has identified 10 warning signs of AD (Table 65-4). Initial symptoms of AD include difficulty performing familiar tasks, forgetting recently learned information, disorientation to time and place, poor judgment, difficulty with abstract thinking (ie, balancing a checkbook), changes in mood, behavior or personality, as well as loss of interest in usual activities.[18-21]

Alzheimer disease is a diagnosis of exclusion. The two most commonly used criteria for the diagnosis of AD are those found in the *Diagnostic and Statistical Manual of Mental Disorders, Fourth Edition* (DSM-IV).[21-23] The DSM-IV criteria describe the diagnosis of AD as an insidious onset with continuous decline in cognitive function that results in inhibition of social and occupational activities. DSM-IV criteria for diagnosis of AD also include memory impairment and at least one other cognitive deficit that cannot be due to other psychiatric, neurological, or systemic causes.[21-23] Treatable conditions that should be examined and ruled out prior to the diagnosis of AD include depression, side effects of medications, thyroid disease, vitamin deficiencies, neurosyphilis or other infections, as well as brain lesions, subdural hematomas, and hydrocephalus.[19-25] The routine workup for AD should include cranial imaging with either CT scan or preferably MRI of the brain, a complete blood count, chemistry panel, thyroid function tests, and serum vitamin B_{12} level.[19-25] Once other causes have been ruled out, testing using tools such as the Mini-Mental State Examination (MMSE), Blessed Dementia Scale, and Alzheimer's Disease Assessment Scale (ADS-Cog) can provide staging and evaluation guidance.[19-25] Mild AD is often associated with an MMSE score of greater than or equal to 20 out of the 30 possible points. Moderate dementia correlates with an MMSE score of 10-19 points, and patients with severe AD often score less than 10 points.[25]

TREATMENT

Goals of therapy include preservation of cognitive and functional abilities, minimizing behavioral disturbances, and slowing disease progression coupled with maintenance of patient and caregiver's quality of life. Response to therapy would not be defined as an improvement from baseline but rather long-term stabilization and slowed progression of the disease process.[25] There are two medication classes available for treatment of AD and include cholinesterase inhibitors and the *N*-methyl-D-aspartate (NMDA) glutamate receptor antagonist, memantine.[23-26] As the pathophysiology of AD primarily involves degeneration of cholinergic neurons, cholinesterase inhibitors were designed to inhibit the centrally acting enzyme cholinesterase which is responsible for the hydrolysis of acetylcholine.[23-26] Inhibition of this enzyme increases synaptic availability of acetylcholine (Figure 65-1). Cholinesterase inhibitors have been the gold standard of therapy for over a decade with the marketing of tacrine in 1993.[23-26] Due to its intolerable side effects, difficult dosing (four times per day), and significant hepatotoxicity, tacrine is rarely used in clinical practice.[23-26] Donepezil, rivastigmine, and galantamine are widely used and all approved for use in mild to moderate AD, with exception of donepezil which is approved for use in mild, moderate, and severe AD.[23-26] Although tolerability has significantly improved with these newer agents, due to increased availability of acetylcholine, their primary side effect involves gastrointestinal symptoms such as nausea, vomiting, and diarrhea.[23-26] Newer dosage forms such as extended-release tablets and patches have shown improved tolerability for these agents. Also note the latest Beers criteria for preferred CNS agents include the extended release dosage form of galantamine[23-26] (Table 65-5).

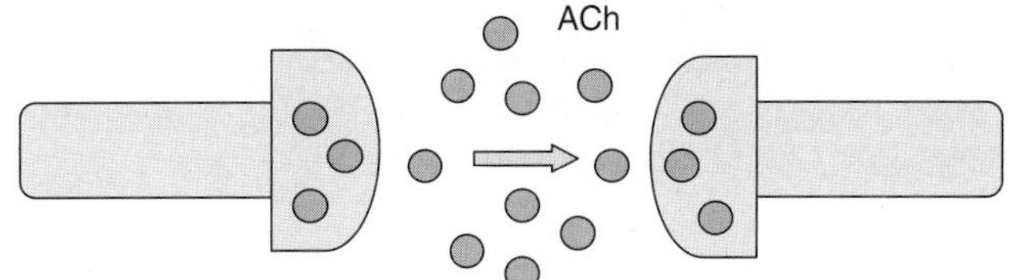

FIGURE 65-1 Cholinesterase Inhibitors block the cholinesterase enzyme and inhibit breakdown of acetylcholine (ACh), thus increasing synaptic availability of acetylcholine.
Illustration created by Rachel S. Cathey, Pharm D, CGP.

TABLE 65-5 Medications for Alzheimer Disease[15-19,22]

Medication	Drug Class	Mechanism of Action	Dose Titration	Side Effects	Considerations
Donepezil (Aricept)	Cholinesterase inhibitor	Inhibits action of cholinesterase enzyme, increasing synaptic availability of acetylcholine	Starting dose: 5 mg daily at bedtime After a minimum of 4-6 wk titrate to maximum dose of 10 mg at bedtime	Diarrhea Nausea Vomiting Insomnia Headache Dizziness	Dose-related GI side effects usually resolve in 1-3 wk Tablets and orally disintegrating tablets (ODT) available Take with food
Galantamine (Razadyne)	Cholinesterase inhibitor	Inhibits action of cholinesterase enzyme, increasing synaptic availability of acetylcholine	Starting dose: 4 mg twice daily (immediate release [IR]) or 8 mg daily (extended-release [ER]) After a minimum of 4 wk, titrate to 8mg twice daily (IR) or 16 mg daily (ER) After an additional 4 wk and if tolerated by patient may titrate to 12 mg twice daily (IR) or 24 mg daily (ER)**	Nausea Vomiting Diarrhea Dizziness Headache Insomnia	Extended-release dosage form noted in Beers Criteria as preferred CNS agent Take with meals IR = Tablets ER = Capsules Also available in liquid form **Do *not* titrate to 24 mg/d if patient has moderate renal or hepatic impairment
Rivastigmine (Exelon)	Cholinesterase inhibitor	Inhibits action of cholinesterase enzyme, increasing synaptic availability of acetylcholine	*Oral:* Starting dose: 1.5 mg twice daily May titrate by 3 mg/d (1.5 mg/dose) every 2-4 wk as tolerated by patient, up to maximum dose of 6 mg twice daily *Transdermal:* Starting dose: 4.6 mg/24 h After a minimum of 4 wk and if well tolerated may titrate to maximum dose of 9.5 mg/24 h	Nausea Vomiting Dizziness Diarrhea Headache	Also FDA approved for use in dementia related to Parkinson disease Take with meals Available as capsules, oral solution, and transdermal patches
Memantine (Namenda)	NMDA receptor antagonist	Blocks NMDA glutamate receptors preventing excessive stimulation and potential cell death	Week 1: 5 mg daily Week 2: 5 mg twice daily Week 3: 10 mg each AM, 5 mg each PM Week 4: 10 mg twice daily	Dizziness Headache Constipation Hypertension	Maximum dose for patients with severe renal impairment (CrCl = 5-29 mL/min) is 5 mg twice daily

TABLE 65-6 Comparison of Alzheimer Dementia and Parkinson Disease[15-20,22,24-26]

	Alzheimer Disease	Parkinson Disease
Usual age of onset	≥ 65 years old	≥ 60 years old
Neurotransmitter	Acetylcholine	Dopamine
Primary symptom	Irreversible memory loss	Tremor, slowed movement and cogwheel rigidity
Goals of therapy	Slow disease progression Promote quality of life	Alleviate symptoms that interfere with ADLs Promote quality of life
Medication classes	Cholinesterase inhibitors NMDA glutamate receptor antagonist	Drugs that increase dopamine Dopamine agonists Monoamine oxidase B inhibitors Catechol-*O*-methyltransferase (COMT) inhibitors Anticholinergic agents Antiviral: Amantadine

Glutamate is the primary excitatory neurotransmitter in the central nervous system and is thought to contribute to the pathogenesis of AD by overstimulating glutamate receptors leading to toxicity and cell death. Memantine is an uncompetitive antagonist of the NMDA-type glutamate receptors located throughout the brain.[25] Excessive receptor activation is theorized to occur during the process of AD. Memantine functions to block the NMDA receptors but only during periods of excessive stimulation; thus memantine does not affect normal neurotransmission.[25] In clinical practice, memantine is thought to be well tolerated by patients and is generally considered an adjunctive therapy. Most clinical trials with memantine showed benefit when adding it on to a cholinesterase inhibitor. Memantine has been approved and marketed for patients with moderate to severe AD. Memantine is well tolerated by most patients with the most commonly reported side effects including dizziness, headache, and confusion.[27]

FOUNDATION OVERVIEW: PARKINSON DISEASE

Despite also being considered a disease of the elderly, Parkinson disease (PD) is not as prevalent as Alzheimer disease. Parkinson disease is thought to affect approximately 0.3% of the US population, with an average age of onset of 60 years old.[28] The incidence of disease is estimated to increase to 4% to 5% of Americans over the age of 85 years.[28] In 2004, it was estimated that approximately 500,000 patients were diagnosed with PD, and that another 50,000 new cases were being reported each year.[28-30] Table 65-6 shows a comparison between AD and PD.

Although the exact pathophysiology underlying PD is unknown, most theories converge on the reduction in transmission of dopamine within the basal ganglia in the substantia nigra of the midbrain which leads to cellular death. Several causative factors have been hypothesized including genetics, environmental causes (eg, pesticides), and oxidative stress.[28,30] Parkinson disease is a debilitating disorder affecting not only the patient, but their family and friends.[28]

Clinical Presentation

The cardinal signs of PD include bradykinesia (slowed movements), akinesia (unable to initiate movement), tremor at rest, and cogwheel rigidity (ratchet-like resistance with range of motion) that present in a unilateral fashion.[28-30] Later in the disease, other manifestations of PD include postural instability, shuffling gait, increased falling, impaired balance and coordination, reduced olfaction, as well as micrographia (small, irregular writing).[28-30] Patients may present with difficulty with performing activities of daily living (ADLs) such as brushing their teeth or buttoning their shirt.[28-30] Patients may also complain of muscle weakness or stiffness. Poor postural reflexes have also been described in PD patients; patients may fall when moved even slightly in a forward or backward direction.[30]

Diagnosis

Parkinson disease, similar to AD, is a diagnosis of exclusion. There are no disease-specific laboratory tests or imaging used to diagnose PD. The differential diagnosis should rule out other causes among which include drug-induced parkinsonism, essential tremor, normal pressure hydrocephalus, lacunar infarcts, and Huntington disease[28-33] (Table 65-7). For the clinical diagnosis of PD, patients must exhibit the hallmark signs of distal tremor at rest, bradykinesia, and rigidity

TABLE 65-7 Drugs That May Induce Parkinsonian-Type Symptoms[24-26]

Haloperidol	Risperidone
Metoclopramide	Olanzapine
Reserpine	Lithium
Valproic acid	Ondansetron

TABLE 65-8 **Medications for Parkinson Disease**[23,26,30,31]

Drug Class	Medication	Mechanism of Action	Side Effects	Considerations
Drugs that increase dopamine	Levodopa/carbidopa (Sinemet) Available as immediate release, extended-release, sustained-release, and orally disintegrating tablets	Carbidopa blocks peripheral dopa decarboxylase allowing levodopa to reach the blood-brain barrier	Orthostasis Nausea Hallucinations Confusion Dizziness	Most effective therapy for symptom control Almost all patients respond Does not stop disease progression
	Amantadine (Symmetrel)	Antiviral agent that acts synergistically with levodopa Thought to block reuptake of presynaptic dopamine and stimulate postsynaptic receptors	Orthostasis Nausea Hallucinations Confusion Dizziness	Benefits are limited Patients may develop tolerance Cognitive side effects
Dopamine agonists	Bromocriptine (Parlodel) Pergolide (Permax) Pramipexole (Mirapex) Ropinirole (Requip)	Drug structure similar to dopamine, thus stimulates dopamine receptors	Orthostasis Nausea Vomiting Hallucinations Abnormal dreams Dyskinesia	Very useful adjuncts for patients already taking levodopa Effective for motor complications Also can be used as monotherapy Do not treat freezing
	Apomorphine (Apokyn)	Stimulates postsynaptic dopamine receptors in the brain	Orthostasis Chest pain Somnolence Dizziness Nausea Vomiting Hallucinations	Subcutaneous injection only For advanced PD patients only Test dose must be given with physician supervision For sudden, resistant "off" periods
Inhibitors of dopamine metabolism	Selegiline (Eldepryl)	Inhibits breakdown of dopamine in the CNS by inhibiting monoamine oxidase B	Headache Sweating Insomnia Nausea Hypotension Hallucinations	Used as adjunctive therapy to levodopa Methamphetamine metabolite may cause psychomotor stimulation
	Entacapone (Comtan)	Inhibits breakdown of dopamine in the periphery by blocking peripheral COMT	Nausea Vomiting Hypotension Hallucinations Dyskinesia	Extends therapeutic effect of levodopa No dose titration, easily administered Increased "on" time Decreased motor complications
	Tolcapone (Tasmar)	Inhibits breakdown of dopamine in the periphery by blocking COMT centrally and peripherally	Nausea Vomiting Hypotension Hallucinations Dyskinesia Explosive diarrhea Hepatotoxicity	Extends therapeutic effect of levodopa Rarely used due to hepatotoxic side effects
Anticholinergics	Trihexyphenidyl (Artane) Benztropine (Cogentin) Diphenhydramine (Benadryl)	Mechanism unclear, possibly related to location of dopamine receptors on cholinergic neurons in the striatum	Memory impairment Confusion Hallucinations Sedation Dry mouth Constipation Nausea Urinary retention	Only for patients without cognitive impairment Use in younger patients only (< 60 years old) with dominant feature of resting tremor

with asymmetrical onset that responds to an adequate trial of levodopa or a dopamine agonist.[28-33] Depression, anxiety, sleep disturbances as well as psychosis often accompany PD and should be considered during management of these patients. It has been estimated that up to 40% to 45% of patients with PD have concomitant depression, and 20% to 40% of patients experience psychosis during the course of their disease process due to potential for concomitant psychiatric disorders as well as the medication therapy for their PD.[28] The Unified Parkinson's Disease Rating Scale (UPDRS) is an assessment tool that is often used to monitor disease progression and treatment response.[28] The components of this rating scale include effects on mental capacity, limitations in ADLs, impairment of motor skills, as well as complications from medications or the disease process itself.[28]

TREATMENT

The primary goal of drug therapy in patients with PD involves alleviating symptoms of the disease that interfere with the patient's ADLs.[28-29] Several classes of medications exist for management of PD symptoms including those that increase dopamine levels, dopamine agonists, monoamine oxidase B inhibitors, catechol-*O*-methyltransferase (COMT) inhibitors, anticholinergics and the antivirals amantadine[28-29] (Table 65-8). Dopamine does not readily cross the blood-brain barrier, thus it is administered as its precursor levodopa. However, levodopa is readily broken down in the periphery by the enzyme dopa decarboxylase.[28-29] Thus, carbidopa is always administered with levodopa to block decarboxylation in the periphery and increase availability of levodopa at the blood-brain barrier.[28-29]

Combinations of levodopa and carbidopa remain the gold standard of therapy for PD, specifically for symptomatic patients.[28-29] Because carbidopa saturates the dopa decarboxylase enzyme at doses of 70 to 100 mg, it is essential that patients receive this dose to prevent levodopa-related side effects such as nausea and vomiting.[29] Although MAO-B inhibitors, amantadine and anticholinergics may improve less severe symptoms initially, levodopa or a dopamine agonist will be required for symptom management in the majority of PD patients.[27-29] Levodopa has been shown to best improve motor disability (bradykinesia and rigidity), whereas dopamine agonists cause fewer motor complications and may reduce the risk of motor fluctuations during the first 4 to 5 years of therapy.[28-29] Essentially, dopamine agonists are best prescribed in younger patients with mild disease, whereas levodopa therapy is required for older patients with more severe symptoms.[27-29]

Pharmacotherapy for treatment of PD is described by referring to the medication classes that are most effective for the point at which the patient is in their disease process, that is, early or late stage.[29] Early-stage PD includes patients who have been diagnosed for less than 5 years or those who have not yet experienced motor fluctuations from prolonged levodopa use.[29] Late-stage PD includes patients who have been on carbidopa/levodopa therapy and who have experienced motor complications.[29] It is estimated that after 5 years of therapy with levodopa, approximately 40% of patients experience dyskinesia and motor fluctuations. Some patients undergo a "wearing-off" effect in which they experience a lessened duration of therapy and increased disease-related symptoms prior to their next dose of levodopa.[29-33] PD patients can also experience what is described as an "on-off" phenomenon in which they experience spontaneous fluctuations in motor symptoms where the medication is effective ("on") for a period of time, and conversely where their PD signs are prevalent ("off") and symptoms worsen. This phenomenon can be treated by adding a dopamine agonist, COMT inhibitor or an MAO-B inhibitor to the current levodopa dosage regimen.[30-35] A fine balance must be kept between dose titrations and precipitation of medication-related side effects. With adjunctive therapies as well as dose titration of monotherapy, caution must be taken as dose-related side effects may occur such as nausea, vomiting, hypotension, and hallucinations, at which point the dose must be reduced until tolerated.[27-29]

CASE Application

1. Factors affecting medication absorption in the older adult include
   a. Elevated gastric pH
   b. Shortened gastric emptying time
   c. Increased plasma albumin
   d. Decreased elimination

2. Pharmacotherapy management in geriatric patients is challenging. Which of the following best describes the statement and why?
   a. Physiologic changes with aging affect how medications are metabolized.
   b. Reduced renal and hepatic function affect elimination of medications.
   c. Side effects can often be mistaken for a new medical condition.
   d. All of the above.

3. What types of medications are preferred to use in the older adult?
   a. Tricyclic antidepressants.
   b. Drugs that undergo phase I metabolism.
   c. Medications that undergo phase II metabolism.
   d. Those that do not go through the CYP-450 system.

4. What is the term defined by the following: When an adverse drug event is misinterpreted as a new medical condition in which the provider prescribes an additional medication to treat the side effect of the original medication?
   a. Prescribing downfall
   b. Prescribing cascade

c. Domino effect
d. Provider cascade

5. Which of the following medications is found on the Beers list of medications to avoid in the elderly?

a. Acetaminophen
b. Ramipril
c. Propoxyphene
d. Fosinopril

6. Which of the following medications are among those recommended by the Beers list of the preferred medications to use in the elderly?

a. Propoxyphene
b. Amitriptyline
c. Galantamine extended release
d. Indomethacin

7. Which of the following are pathologic signs of Alzheimer disease?

a. Cogwheel rigidity
b. Neurofibrillary tangles
c. Senile plaques
d. Essential tremor
e. Both b and c

8. Which of the following is one of the 10 warning signs (ie, initial symptoms) of Alzheimer disease identified by the Alzheimer's Association?

a. Changes in vision
b. Difficulty hearing
c. Difficulty with abstract thinking (ie, balancing a checkbook)
d. Constipation

9. Which of the following scales is commonly used to assess the level of dementia in Alzheimer patients?

a. MMSA
b. MMSE
c. Geriatric Depression Scale
d. Delirium Index

10. Which of the following classes of medications are used in Alzheimer disease?

a. Dopamine agonists
b. Cholinesterase inhibitors
c. NMDA-antagonist
d. Anticholinergics
e. b and c

11. Which neurotransmitter is primarily involved in the disease process of Alzheimer disease?

a. Serotonin
b. Acetylcholine
c. Norepinephrine
d. Dopamine

12. What side effect(s) do patients complain of most often with cholinesterase inhibitors?

a. Nausea, vomiting, diarrhea
b. Dizziness
c. Hypotension
d. Headache

13. Select the potential cause of decreased serum creatinine in elderly patients.

a. Increased stores of body fat
b. Decreased renal production of creatinine
c. Loss of muscle mass
d. Increased body mass

14. Which of the following best describes the place in therapy for memantine?

a. As an adjunct therapy to Sinemet for Parkinson patients without cognitive impairment
b. As monotherapy for Parkinson disease
c. As an augmentation to an Alzheimer patient's cholinesterase inhibitor
d. In Alzheimer patients with heart disease

15. Which neurotransmitter is involved in the neuronal degradation of Parkinson disease?

a. Acetylcholine
b. GABA
c. COMT
d. Dopamine

16. Which of the following is the primary goal of drug therapy in patients with Parkinson disease?

a. Provide comfort measures only
b. To alleviate symptoms of disease that interfere with ADLs
c. To prevent further memory loss
d. To reverse neuronal degradation

17. Which medication is considered the gold standard for treating Parkinson disease?

a. Ropinirole
b. Pramipexole
c. Levodopa/carbidopa
d. Bromocriptine

18. Which of the following medications would be the most likely to cause a Parkinson patient's nausea and vomiting?

a. Simvastatin
b. Diphenhydramine
c. Levodopa/carbidopa
d. Furosemide

19. Mrs. J is a 78-year-old Parkinson patient with cognitive changes who has been experiencing worsening symptoms over the past months despite her dose of Sinemet

being maximized. Which would be a reasonable recommendation to her physician?

a. Start apomorphine orally as adjunctive therapy.
b. Start tolcapone at the highest possible dose.
c. Consider adding ropinirole to augment the treatment she is currently receiving.
d. None of the above.

20. What side effect is most likely to occur with ropinirole?

a. Possible explosive diarrhea
b. Liver toxicity
c. Nausea, hallucinations, and abnormal dreams
d. Worsening memory loss

TAKEAWAY POINTS ››

- Geriatrics is defined as 65 years of age and older. This demographic in the United States is steadily increasing due to aging of the baby boomer generation.
- Polypharmacy is defined as taking nine or more medications and can lead to a "prescribing cascade" in which the provider prescribes a new medication to treat the side effect of another medication.
- Beers criteria describes inappropriate medications in the elderly, and more recently published preferred CNS medications to use in the older adult.
- Pharmacokinetic and pharmacodynamic changes occur as the aging process ensues including loss of muscle mass as well as decreased function of the kidneys and liver.
- Alzheimer dementia is thought to be caused by degeneration of cholinergic neurons in the brain. It is characterized by irreversible memory loss, poor judgment, difficulty performing familiar tasks as well as changes in mood and personality.
- The MMSE is a commonly used tool for assessment of cognitive function in all elderly patients and is helpful in staging patients who have been diagnosed with Alzheimer disease.
- Cholinesterase inhibitors and the NMDA-antagonist memantine are the only medication therapies available for Alzheimer disease.
- Parkinson disease is thought to be due to a deficiency in dopamine and is characterized by the cardinal signs of tremor, bradykinesia, and cogwheel rigidity. Other symptoms may include shuffling gait, impaired balance, postural instability, decreased olfaction as well as micrographia.
- Sinemet remains the gold standard of therapy for most patients with Parkinson disease, although dopamine agonists can be used as monotherapy in younger patients with mild symptoms.

REFERENCES

1. Public Health and Aging: Trends in Aging—United States and World Wide. *MMWR Weekly.* 2003;52(06): 101-106.
2. Brummel-Smith K. Polypharmacy and the elderly patient. *Instructional Course Lectures.* 1997;46:409-416.
3. Linjakumpu T, Hartikainen S, Klaukka T, Veijola J, Kivela SL, Isoaho R. Use of medications and polypharmacy are increasing among the elderly. *J Clin Epidemiol.*2002;55:809-817.
4. Williams, Cynthia M. Using medications appropriately in older adults. *Am Fam Physician.* 2002;66(10):1917-1924.
5. Zarowitz BJ, Stebelsky LA, Muma BK, Romain TM, Peterson EL. Reduction of high-risk polypharmacy drug combinations in patients in a managed care setting. *Pharmacotherapy.* 2005;25(11):1636-1645.
6. Fick DM, Cooper JW. Updating the Beers criteria for potentially inappropriate medication use in older adults. *Arch Intern Med.*2003;163(22):2716-2724.
7. Nash DB, Koenig JB, Chatterton ML. Why the elderly need individualized pharmaceutical care. *Office of Health Policy and Clinical Outcomes, Thomas Jefferson University.* 2000.
8. Budnitz DS, Shehab N, Kegler SR, Richards CL. Medication use leading to emergency department visits for adverse drug events in older adults. *Ann Intern Med.* 2007;147(11):755-765.
9. Beers MH. Explicit criteria for determining potentially inappropriate medication use by the elderly. *Arch Intern Med.*1997;157:1531-1536.
10. Fick DM, Cooper JW, Wade WE, Waller JL, Maclean JR, Beers MH. Updating the Beers criteria for potentially inappropriate medication use in older adults. *Arch Intern Med.* 2003;163:2716-2724.
11. Stefanacci RG, Cavallaro E, Beers MH, Fick DM. Developing explicit positive Beers criteria for preferred central nervous system medications in older adults. *Consult Pharm.* 2009;24(8):601-610.
12. Raitt BB, Blackstone K, Cobbs EL, et al. Pharmacotherapy. *GRS.* 5th ed. American Geriatrics Society; 2002.
13. Chin TW, Loeb M, Fong IW. Effects of an acidic beverage on absorption of ketoconazole. *Antimicrob Agents Chemother.* 1995;39(8):1671-1675.
14. Ujhelyi MR, Robert S. Pharmacokinetic aspects of digoxin-specific Fab therapy in the management of digitalis toxicity. *Clin Pharmacokinet.* 1995;28(6):483-493.
15. McLean AJ, LeCouteur GL. Aging biology and geriatric clinical pharmacology. *Pharmacol Rev.* 2004;56(2):163-184.
16. Smythe M, Hoffman J, Kizy K, et al. Estimating creatinine clearance in elderly patients with low serum creatinine concentrations. *Am J Hosp Pharm.* 1994;51:189-204.
17. Brodows RG. Benefits and risks with glyburide and glipizide in elderly NIDDM patients. *Diabetes Care.* 1992;15(1):75-80.
18. The Alzheimer's Association. Website information for professional care providers. Available at: www.alz.org. Accessed February 12, 2010.

19. Cherry D, Segal-Gidan F, Fox P, et al. California Workgroup on Guidelines for Alzheimer's Disease Management. *Guideline for Alzheimer's disease management.* Chicago, IL: Alzheimer's Association; April 2008.
20. American Psychiatric Association (APA). *Practice guideline for the treatment of patients with Alzheimer's disease and other dementias.* Arlington, VA: American Psychiatric Association (APA); October 2007.
21. Anderson HS. Alzheimer's disease. *Behavioral neurology and dementia: Alzheimer disease.* Available at: www.emedicine.medscape.com. August 27, 2009.
22. Cummings JL, Frank JC, Cherry D, et al. Guidelines for managing Alzheimer's disease: Part I assessment. *Am Fam Physician.* 2002;65(11):2263-2272.
23. McKhann G, Drachman D, Folstein M, Katzman R, Price D, Stadlan EM. Clinical diagnosis of Alzheimer's disease: report of the NINCDS-ADRDA work group under the auspices of Department of Health and Human Services Task Force on Alzheimer's disease. *Neurology.* 1984;34:939-944.
24. Knopman DS, DeKosky ST, Cummings JL, et al. Practice parameter: management of dementia (an evidence-based review). Report of the Quality Standards Subcommittee of the American Academy of Neurology. *Neurology.* 2001;56:1143-1153.
25. Geldmacher DS. Treatment Guidelines for Alzheimer's disease: redefining perceptions in primary care. *J Clin Psychiatry.* 2007;9(2):113-121.
26. Lexi-Comp Online Drug Information Resource. Available at: www.crlonline.com. 2009. Accessed February 10, 2010.
27. Orgogozo JM, Rigaud AS, Stoffler A, et al. Efficacy and safety of memantine in patients with mild to moderate vascular dementia: a randomized, placebo-controlled trial (MMM 300). *Stroke.* 2002;33:1834-1839.
28. Scott DM, Brown DA. Parkinson's disease: a review. *Drug Topics.* 2009;153(8):40-47.
29. Rao SS, Hofmann LA, Shakil A. Parkinson's disease: diagnosis and treatment. *Am Fam Physician.* 2006;74(12):2046-2054.
30. Young R. Update on Parkinson's disease. *Am Fam Physician.* April 1999; 15:1-16.
31. Suchowersky O, Reich S, Perlmutter J, et al. Practice parameter: diagnosis and prognosis of new onset Parkinson disease (an evidence-based review): report of the Quality Standards Subcommittee of the American Academy of Neurology. *Neurology.* April 2006;66:967-975.
32. Suchowersky O, Gronseth G, Perlmutter J, et al. Practice parameter: neuroprotective strategies and alternative therapies for Parkinson disease (an evidence-based review): report of the Quality Standards Subcommittee of the American Academy of Neurology. *Neurology.* April 2006;66:976-982.
33. Pahwa R, Factor A, Lyons KE, et al. Practice parameter: treatment of Parkinson disease with motor fluctuations and dyskinesia (an evidence-based review): report of the Quality Standards Subcommittee of the American Academy of Neurology. *Neurology.* April 2006;66:983-995.
34. Swope DM. Rapid treatment of "wearing off" in Parkinson's disease. *Neurology.* 2004;62(S4):S27-S31.
35. Olanow CW, Watts RL, Koller WC. An algorithm (decision tree) for the management of Parkinson's disease (2001): treatment guidelines. *Neurology.* 2001;56(11S5):S1-S88.

CHAPTER

66 Clinical Toxicology

Keith R. McCain and Howell R. Foster

FOUNDATION OVERVIEW

Clinical toxicology involves the assessment and management of disease caused by exposure to an agent(s) in which adverse effects may develop. All natural and synthetic xenobiotics are capable of causing toxicity in humans. It is paramount to recognize that all substances can be poisonous in a specific situation. Paracelsus, the father of modern toxicology, identified this principle in stating that "solely the dose determines that a thing is not a poison."[1] As such, some agents are capable of severe consequence at microgram dose (botulinum toxin) while others are typically viewed as harmless, but at extremes can be lethal (water intoxication).[2]

Poisoning affects all ages, is associated with varying cause (ie. unintentional, environmental, therapeutic error, suicide attempt, malicious), can occur by numerous routes (ie, ingestion, dermal, inhalation, parenteral), and can be due to acute, acute-on-chronic, or chronic exposure. Unintentional and intentional poisoning is a significant source of morbidity and mortality in the United States. In 2007 over 2.4 million exposure calls were made to US poison centers (PCs). More than half of calls involved children less than age 6. The reason for exposure was unintentional in 83.2% and the route of exposure was ingestion in 78.4% of these cases.[3] In the most recent report detailing injury mortality, poisoning was the second leading cause of injury death in the United States. Fatalities due to poisoning were found to be more likely unintentional (72%), drug related (91%), and involving patients age 20 to 54 (80%).[4] It is estimated there were over 1.7 million patient visits to emergency departments due to drug-related issues in 2006.[5]

Key Definitions

ABCs: Airway, breathing, and circulation
ABG: Arterial blood gases
ACLS: Advanced cardiac life support
APAP: Acetaminophen
AST: Aspartate aminotransferase
BZD: Benzodiazepine
CNS: Central nervous system
EKG: Electrocardiogram
GABA: Gamma amino butyric acid
NAPQI: N-acetyl-p-benzoquinone imine
NAC: N-acetylcysteine
PC: Poison center(s)
PPPA: Poison Prevention and Packaging Act

PREVENTION

Multiple avenues have been developed to reduce the incidents of unintentional poisoning. National Poison Prevention Week is designated by law (1961) as the third week in March and is used to increase public awareness of the incidents and dangers of poisoning. The Poison Prevention and Packaging Act (1970) (PPPA) requires some hazardous household products as well as oral prescription medications and some over-the-counter medications to utilize child-resistant containers. Additionally, the PPPA limits the quantity for packaging of some products. The Poison Control Center Enhancement and Awareness Act (2000) established a toll-free number (1-800-222-1222) to allow nationwide 24 hour access to PC consultation in the United States. Table 66-1 provides select tips that should be emphasized to the public to prevent poisoning emergencies.

GENERAL MANAGEMENT

General Approach to the Poisoned Patient

While at times diagnosis may appear obvious, a broad differential should always be employed early on in the course of care. In the setting of actual or suspected overdose, patients commonly present with inadequate and unreliable histories. As such, the potential for rapid patient deterioration should be anticipated and aggressive supportive care should be instituted early with first consideration given to the "ABCs" (airway, breathing, circulation). In patients with concerning histories or abnormalities, interventions should also include administration of oxygen, establishment of intravenous access, obtaining a 12-lead electrocardiogram (EKG) and continuous cardiac monitoring, and determination of arterial blood gases (ABGs), blood glucose, and electrolyte values. Additionally, empiric administration of an intravenous "Coma Cocktail" consisting of 100 mg of thiamine, 25 to 50 g of dextrose, and 0.05 to 2 mg of naloxone should be considered early in the management of patients with altered mental status.

Seizure and dysrhythmia potential should be realized and potential need for treatment with a benzodiazepine (intravenous lorazepam or diazepam) and standard advanced cardiac life support (ACLS) measures, respectively, anticipated. Upon stabilization, attention can be turned toward a more detailed physical examination, laboratory results, history of exposure, and potential decontamination measures.[2]

TABLE 66-1 Poison Prevention Tips[2,40]

1. Identify all potentially hazardous items in the home and workplace.
2. Keep all chemicals and medicines locked up and out of sight.
3. Do not transfer products from original containers.
4. Utilize and ensure proper use of child-resistant closures.
5. Do not store chemicals and medications with food items.
6. Read product labels prior to use.
7. Avoid taking medicine in front of children; never refer to medicine as candy.
8. Return products and medicine to proper storage immediately after use.
9. Do not take/administer medicine in the dark, check the dose with every use.
10. Keep the Poison Center number (1-800-222-1222) readily available.

Physical Examination

A thorough history and physical examination are essential in treating toxicologic emergencies. Close and ongoing evaluation of patient's vital signs and physical findings can provide invaluable information in determining appropriate supportive care as well as aid in diagnosis. After the primary survey of the toxic patient and assuring that the ABCs have been addressed, a more detailed secondary survey should be performed. Recognition of a pattern or syndrome of symptoms may narrow the diagnosis to a particular class or group of offending agents. Several "toxidromes" have been developed and are described in Table 66-2. It is important to note that not all patients will be "classic" representations of the toxidrome, further some share overlapping characteristics, as such they should be utilized carefully in patient assessment with their limitations recognized.[6]

Laboratory Results

In conjunction with history and physical examination, laboratory results can provide important clues in treatment of the poisoned patient. While "toxicology" screens are commonly ordered in the setting of the poisoned patient, there is significant debate about their utility. These tests are limited to a handful of agents, associated with false-positive and negative results, do not prove impairment, and are rarely associated with significant impact on overall patient management. Proving of more benefit are the results from a basic metabolic panel, ABGs, EKG, and occasionally specific x-rays.[7] Additionally, in all patients with suspected self-poisoning, an acetaminophen level and possibly a salicylate level should be determined.[8] Serum levels of specific agents may prove useful and should be obtained depending on history or suspicion (ie, toxic alcohols, lithium, digoxin, heavy metals, etc). Other potentially useful determinations from laboratory data include evidence of an anion gap acidosis, osmolal gap, or oxygen saturation gap.[9]

TABLE 66-2 Select Syndromes of Toxicity[2]

Toxidrome	Symptoms
Opiate	CNS depression, respiratory depression, miosis, decreased bowel motility
Cholinergic	Salivation, lacrimation, urination, defecation, GI distress, emesis, bronchorrhea, bradycardia
Anticholinergic	Delirium/hallucinations, urinary retention, decreased bowel motility, mydriasis, tachycardia, hyperthermia, flushed skin, dry mucous membranes
Sympathomimetic	Agitation, mydriasis, tachycardia, hyperthermia, diaphoresis, tremor, hypertension

Decontamination

Dermal and ocular exposures should initially be managed with prompt and thorough irrigation of contaminated surfaces. Patients with inhalation exposure should be moved to fresh air. As 80% of exposures are associated with ingestion, the need and method of gastric decontamination following poisoning is a common decision associated with poisoning. There is extreme variance and controversy associated with the practice of gastric decontamination.[10] Position papers have been developed by leading toxicology groups after evaluation of the available literature evidence with regard to gastric decontamination. These papers indicate there is limited evidence to support routine use of ipecac, gastric lavage, single dose– or multiple dose–activated charcoal, cathartics, or whole bowel irrigation.[11-16] The decision for gastric decontamination should be made on an individual case basis with full understanding of the benefits and risk as well as attention to the indications and contraindications for individual technique utilization. Table 66-3 outlines the variables and conditions that should be utilized in assessing if gastric emptying would be indicated. The indications and contraindications for orogastric lavage, syrup of ipecac, single dose–activated charcoal, multiple dose–activated charcoal, and whole bowel irrigation are detailed in Tables 66-4, 66-5, 66-6, 66-7, and 66-8 respectively.

Antidotes

Among the 2007 reports to PCs there were approximately 70,000 instances of specific antidote administration among more than 2.4 million cases.[3] This would indicate antidotal therapy at a maximum was utilized in <3% of patients represented in the database. While this underscores the importance that supportive care is the mainstay of treatment in the poisoned patient, there are instances in which antidotal therapy can be significant in reducing morbidity and mortality. Ideally antidotes would be highly effective in reversing or attenuating toxicity, readily available, associated with a low adverse effect profile, and inexpensive. Unfortunately, these characteristics are difficult to obtain as insufficient stocking of multiple antidotes has historically been an issue, several therapies have high acquisition cost, and antidotes often have adverse effect profiles that must be weighed against potential benefit.[17,18] The most recent consensus guidelines recommend 24 antidotes that should be stocked by hospitals.[18] Common antidote and associated toxins are detailed in Table 66-9.

TABLE 66-3 **Risk Assessment: When to Consider Gastric Emptying**

Gastric Emptying Is Usually Not Indicated If[a]	Gastric Emptying May Be Indicated If[b]
The xenobiotic has limited toxicity at any dose	There is reason to believe that, given the time of ingestion, a significant amount of the ingested xenobiotic is still present in the stomach
Although the xenobiotic ingested is potentially toxic, the dose ingested is less than that expected to produce significant illness	The ingested xenobiotic is known to produce serious toxicity *or* the patient has obvious signs or symptoms of life-threatening toxicity
The ingested xenobiotic is well adsorbed by activated charcoal, and the amount ingested is not expected to exceed the adsorptive capacity of activated charcoal	The ingested xenobiotic is not adsorbed by activated charcoal
Significant spontaneous emesis has occurred	Although the ingested xenobiotic is adsorbed by activated charcoal, the amount ingested exceeds the activated charcoal-to-xenobiotic ratio of 10:1 even with a double-standard dose of activated charcoal
The patient presents many hours postingestion and has minimal signs or symptoms of poisoning	The patient has not had spontaneous emesis
The ingested xenobiotic has a highly efficient antidote (such as acetaminophen)	No highly effective specific antidote exists or alternative therapies (such as hemodialysis) pose a significant risk to the patient

[a]Patients who fulfill these criteria can be decontaminated safely with activated charcoal alone or may require no decontamination at all.

[b]Patients who fulfill these criteria should be considered candidates for gastric emptying *if* there are no contraindications. For individuals who meet some of these criteria but who are judged not to be candidates for gastric emptying, single or multiple-dose activated charcoal, and/or whole-bowel irrigation should be considered.

TABLE 66-4 **Indications and Contraindications to Orogastric Lavage**

Indications	Contraindications
The patient meets criteria for gastric emptying (Table 66-3)	The patient does not meet criteria for gastric emptying (Table 66-3)
The benefits of gastric emptying outweigh the risks	The patient has lost or will likely lose his/her airway protective reflexes and has not been intubated. (Once intubated, orogastric lavage can be performed if otherwise indicated.) Ingestion of an alkaline caustic Ingestion of a foreign body (such as a drug packet) Ingestion of a xenobiotic with a high aspiration potential (such as a hydrocarbon) in the absence of endotracheal intubation The patient is at risk of hemorrhage or gastrointestinal perforation because of underlying pathology, recent surgery, or other medical condition that could be further compromised by the use of orogastric lavage Ingestion of a xenobiotic in a form known to be too large to fit into the lumen of the lavage tube (such as many modified-release preparations)

TABLE 66-5 **Indications and Contraindications for Syrup of Ipecac**

Indications	Contraindications
The patient meets criteria for gastric emptying (Table 66-3)	The patient does not meet criteria for gastric emptying (Table 66-3)
Orogastric lavage cannot be performed or is contraindicated because of the size of the xenobiotic formulation	Either activated charcoal or another oral agent is expected to be necessary in the next few hours
The history and/or physical examination suggest that there is likely to be a clinically significant amount of xenobiotic remaining in the stomach	Airway protective reflexes might be lost within the next 30-60 min Ingestion of a caustic Ingestion of a foreign body such as a drug packet or sharp item
The benefits of gastric emptying outweigh the risks from the contraindications	Ingestion of a xenobiotic with a high aspiration potential such as a hydrocarbon The patient is younger than 6 mo of age, elderly, or debilitated The patient has a premorbid condition that would be compromised by vomiting

TABLE 66-6 **Indications and Contraindications for Single-Dose Activated Charcoal Therapy Without Gastric Emptying**

Indications	Contraindications
The patient does not meet criteria for gastric emptying (Table 66-3) or gastric emptying is likely to be harmful	Activated charcoal is known not to adsorb a clinically meaningful amount of the ingested xenobiotic
Ingestion of a toxic amount of a xenobiotic that is known to be adsorbed by activated charcoal	Airway protective reflexes are absent or expected to be lost and the patient is not intubated
The ingestion has occurred within a time frame amenable to adsorption by activated charcoal or clinical factors are present that suggest that not all of the xenobiotic has already been systemically absorbed	Gastrointestinal perforation is likely as in cases of caustic ingestions Therapy may increase the risk and severity of aspiration, such as in the presence of hydrocarbons with a high aspiration potential Endoscopy will be an essential diagnostic modality (acid or alkaline caustics)

TREATMENT OF SELECT TOXINS

Acetaminophen

Acetaminophen (APAP) is perhaps the most common cause of poisoning worldwide.[19] Excessive acute or chronic doses can result in hepatic injury. Toxicity is due to production of the metabolite *N*-acetyl-p-benzoquinone imine (NAPQI), a potent electrophile by CYP2E1. Under therapeutic conditions, the small amount of NAPQI generated is detoxified by endogenous stores of glutathione. In excessive dose glutathione stores are depleted allowing NAPQI to bind with hepatocytes leading to liver injury, which can range from mild transaminitis to fulminant failure.[20] As toxicity is related to metabolite production, symptoms are delayed from time of ingestion and nausea and vomiting may be the only apparent symptoms in the first 24 hours following overdose. Acute ingestions of >10 g or 200 mg/kg (whichever is lower) warrant medical attention. Chronic ingestions of doses >10 g or 200 mg/kg (whichever is less) over a 24-hour period, 6 g or 150 mg/kg (whichever is less) per 24-hour period for the prior 48 hours, or for children <6 years a dose of 100 mg/kg/24-hour period for the preceding 72 hour or longer period prompt need for medical evaluation. Patients potentially at increased risk of hepatic injury (alcoholism, concurrent therapy with CYP2E1 inducers, malnourished) should have medical evaluation at chronic doses >4 g or 100 mg/kg (whichever is less) per day.[21] Medical evaluation should include determination of a serum APAP level and baseline liver function test. In acute overdose, the APAP level and known time postingestion can be plotted on the Rumack-Matthew nomogram to determine potential risk of hepatic injury and need for antidotal therapy with *N*-acetylcysteine (NAC, Acetadote, Mucomyst). NAC likely serves to maintain/restore glutathione stores or as an alternate substrate for NAPQI. For optimal liver protective effect, acetylcysteine should be administered within the first 8 hours of ingestion as efficacy progressively diminishes further into the course of toxicity.[22] NAC can be administered intravenously or orally; however the dose and duration of treatment are different, with IV administration consisting of three different dose bags given over a 21-hour treatment period compared to the oral protocol of a 140 mg/kg loading dose followed by an every 4 hour maintenance dose of 70 mg/kg for 72 hours to complete a full oral course of NAC. Outside of patients with irretractable vomiting or pregnant women, in which intravenous administration is recommended, debate exist about which route of administration should be preferred. The intravenous course is of shorter duration, requires fewer doses, and eliminates issues associated with nausea and vomiting, a common symptom of early toxicity. However it has a higher acquisition cost, increased incidence of adverse effect, and there is some concern about the shorter duration of therapy in some scenerios.[20,23] The nomogram is not applicable to chronic poisoning and should not be utilized. There is less definitive standard for treatment following repeated supratherapeutic doses but one author recommends treatment with NAC in patients with twice normal AST values; elevated AST associated with symptoms or APAP level >10 μg/mL; or APAP level higher than expected. All other

TABLE 66-7 **Indications and Contraindications for Multiple-Dose Activated Charcoal Therapy**

Indications	Contraindications
Ingestion of a life-threatening amount of carbamazepine, dapsone, phenobarbital, quinine, or theophylline	Any contraindication to single dose–activated charcoal
Ingestion of a life-threatening amount of another causes of xenobiotic that undergoes enterohepatic or enteroenteric recirculation that is adsorbed to activated charcoal	The presence of an ileus or other diminished peristalsis
Ingestion of a significant amount of any slowly released xenobiotic, or of a xenobiotic known to form concretions or bezoars	

TABLE 66-8 **Indications and Contraindications for Whole-Bowel Irrigation**

Indications	Contraindications
Potentially toxic ingestions of sustained-release drugs	Airway-protective reflexes are absent or expected to become so in a patient who has not been intubated
Ingestion of a toxic amount of a xenobiotic that is not adsorbed to activated charcoal when other methods of gastrointestinal decontamination are not possible or not efficacious	Gastrointestinal tract is not intact
Removal of packets of illicit drugs (eg, from body packers)	Signs of ileus obstruction, significant gastrointestinal hemorrhage, or hemodynamic instability that might compromise gastrointestinal motility Persistent vomiting Signs of leakage from illicit cocaine packets (indication for surgical removal)

patients should be instructed to return to medical attention if symptoms develop.[2]

Toxic Alcohols

Ethylene glycol and methanol are dangerous nonethanol alcohols. Small ingestions of either are capable of producing significant toxicity. Ethylene glycol is a common ingredient in antifreeze. Methanol can be found in windshield-washer fluid, canned fuel, paint removers, and deicer products. The toxicity of both is related to their metabolites. The initial metabolism of both occurs primarily via alcohol dehydrogenase, with ethylene glycol yielding glycolic and oxalic acids, and methanol yielding formic acid. These organic acid metabolites can result in profound metabolic acidosis with an elevated anion gap ($[Na^+]) - ([Cl^-]+[HCO_3^-]$) and/or presence of an osmolal gap (measured serum osmolality – calculated osmolarity). Additionally, oxalic acid can complex with systemic calcium leading to calcium oxalate precipitates, causing renal and other organ dysfunction and hypocalcemia. Formic acid attacks the retinal and optic nerves and can result in visual impairment including blindness.[24] Prompt treatment to minimize formation of toxic metabolites is imperative. Ethanol and fomepizole (Antizol) are both inhibitors of alcohol dehydrogenase and effectively prevent formation of ethylene glycol and methanol metabolites. Fomepizole is preferred over alcohol as it does not cause inebriation or other additive toxicity, does not require blood monitoring, and has standardized dosing.[25] Fomepizole is given as a 15 g/kg loading dose then a 10 mg/kg maintenance dose every 12 hours for four doses, then maintenance dose are increased to 15 mg/kg every 12 hours as it induces its own metabolism. Hemodialysis may be a required concurrent therapy depending on patient disposition and serum glycol or methanol levels.[26]

Benzodiazepines

Benzodiazepines (BZD) facilitate enhanced binding of gamma amino butyric acid (GABA) binding to the $GABA_A$ receptor, resulting in hyperpolarization of postsynaptic neuron causing central nervous system (CNS) inhibition.[27] BZD are frequent agents involved in overdose. Symptoms of BZD toxicity include: CNS depression ranging from ataxia, confusion, and drowsiness to coma, hypotension, and respiratory depression. As a sole ingestant BZD poisoning has low mortality, but in multidrug overdose with other CNS depressants their additive toxicity increases the risk of respiratory depression and mortality.[10,17] Flumazenil (Romazicon) is an intravenous competitive antagonist of BZDs on the CNS, and is classified as an antidote for BZD overdose. However, the utility of flumazenil in the overdose and nonspecific coma setting is associated with caveats and debate. Prior to utilization, thought should be given to the potential that it may precipitate a withdrawal syndrome, including seizures, or unmask coingestant toxicity.[27,28] Flumazenil is given at an initial dose of 0.2 mg over 1 minute with cautious titration to limit risk of precipitating withdrawal or unmasking coingestant toxicity. Titration doses should be in 0.5 mg/min increases until desired effect or total of 3 to 5 mg have been administered. Doses greater than this are not expected to be of benefit. Due to short half-life, patients administered flumazenil should be closely observed for resedation.[29]

Beta-Adrenergic Antagonist

Beta-blockers competitively antagonize adrenergic beta-receptors. Blockade of these receptors results in decreased intracellular phosphokinase A activation and ultimately a reduction in inotropy and chronotropy.[17] The individual agents have significant inherent difference with regard to overall pharmacologic profiles. Potential differences within the class include cardioselectivity, intrinsic sympathomimetic activity, alpha-antagonism, membrane-stabilizing activity, and lipophilicity. Beta-blocker receptor selectivity is lost in overdose and effects not seen with standard therapeutic use can develop.[30] Hypotension and bradycardia are the most common clinical findings associated with beta-blocker toxicity. Other potential complications include seizures, CNS depression, ventricular dysrhythmia due to sodium channel blockade, heart block, pulmonary edema, hypoperfusion, and bronchospasm. CNS depression, seizures, and dysrhythmia are particularly problematic with the more lipophilic agents (ie, propranolol).[24] Classically glucagon has been considered antidotal therapy for beta-blocker overdose. Stimulation of the glucagon receptor located on the beta-receptor complex effectively bypasses the blockade of beta-blocker antagonism, thus activating a

TABLE 66-9 **Select Antidotes**

Antidote	Drug/Toxin	Comment
Acetylcysteine/NAC (IV = Acetadote, PO = Mucomyst or generic)	Acetaminophen	If IV route necessary and Acetadote unavailable, oral NAC can be given through appropriate filter IV Oral dose should be diluted to max 5% concentration
Crotalidae polyvalent immune Fab, ovine (CroFab)	North American crotaline snake (rattlesnakes, cottonmouth, copperheads)	Dosing is not weight based Reconstitution may take up to 1 h Potential for allergic reaction in patients with papaya or papain hypersensitivity
Antivenin (*Latrodectus mactans*)	Black widow spider	Horse serum–derived antitoxin, caution for immunogenic reactions and serum sickness
Antivenin (*Micrurus fulvius*)	Eastern/Texas coral snake	Product discontinued by manufacturer, some supply remains Horse serum–derived antitoxin
Atropine sulfate	Organophosphate and carbamate pesticides, nerve agents, drug/toxin-induced bradycardia	Cholinesterase inhibitor (CI) toxicity may require large doses Endpoint of therapy in CI toxicity is dry bronchial tree not mydriasis or tachycardia
Calcium chloride 10% Calcium gluconate 10%	Calcium channel blockers, hydrofluoric acid/fluoride	CaCl should be given through central IV if possible due to vascular irritating properties For hydrofluoric acid burns topical 2.5% CaGlu can be compounded from parenteral GaGlu and a water-based jelly
Calcium disodium EDTA (Versenate)	Lead	Potential for medication error due to confusion with disodium EDTA
Calcium trisodium pentetate	Internal contamination with plutonium, americium, curium	Potential components of a radiological dispersal device ("dirty bomb")
Cyanide antidote kit or Cyanokit	Cyanide	Cyanide kit contains: amyl nitrite inhalant, parenteral sodium nitrite sodium thiosulfate Cyanokit contains: parenteral hydroxocobalamin and does not utilize induction of methemoglobinemia as any portion of its mechanism of action
Deferoxamine (Desferal)	Iron (acute)	Change in urine color is not always detected Use >24 h has been associated with acute respiratory distress syndrome (ARDS)
Digoxin immune Fab fragments (DigiFab, Digibind)	Digoxin/cardiac glycosides	Multiple methods of calculating dose, dependent on variables of specific case, consult prescribing information Fab product will interfere with digoxin level measurements after administration Potential for allergic reaction in patients with papaya or papain hypersensitivity, previous digoxin immune Fab therapy, and ovine protein or latex allergy
Dimercaprol (BAL in Oil)	Arsenic, gold, mercury, lead	Must combine with calcium disodium EDTA for lead Formulated with peanut oil
Ethanol	Methanol or ethylene glycol	Difficult to obtain, dose, and monitor levels Associated with multiple negative side effects if utilized
Fomepizole (Antizol)	Methanol or ethylene glycol	Requires dose increase on fifth dose Manufacturer will replace expired stock
Flumazenil (Romazicon)	Benzodiazepines	Should utilize with caution if at all in the setting of acute overdose due to potential to precipitate withdrawal seizures or unmask coingestant toxicity Primary indication should be in the setting of iatrogenic oversedation Short duration of action
Glucagon	Beta-blockers, calcium channel blockers	Nausea and vomiting common, caution in patients with decreased level of consciousness and unprotected airway
Methylene blue	Methemoglobinemia	Contraindicated in patients with G6PD deficiency as hemolysis may result
Naloxone (Narcan)	Opioids, opiates	Start with low dose to reduce potential to precipitate withdrawal Short duration of action
Octreotide (Sandostatin)	Oral sulfonylurea-induced hypoglycemia	Suppress sulfonylurea-induced insulin secretion Subcutaneous or IV administration, may require multiple doses over 24-48 h period

(Continued)

TABLE 66-9 Select Antidotes (*Continued*)

Antidote	Drug/Toxin	Comment
Physostigmine (Antilirium)	Anticholinergic syndrome, especially antimuscarinic delirium	Inhibits acetylcholinesterase, resulting in increased cholinergic tone Significant debate about appropriate use, especially in the setting of multidrug overdose or agents that may prolong QRS/QT intervals (tricyclics, neuroleptics) Side-effect potentials include seizures and SLUDGE syndrome
Potassium iodide	Thyroid radioiodine prophylaxis	Risk of associated cancer is most concerning in the very young <18 y/o with the exception of pregnant persons Persons >40 y/o have extremely small associated risk Treatment is indicated in lactating mothers regardless of age
Pralidoxime/2-PAM (Protopam)	Organophosphate pesticides, nerve agents	Reactivates cholinesterase which have been inactivated by organophosphate pesticides and related compounds
Pyridoxine/Vitamin B_6	Isoniazid, hydrazines	Empiric 5 g dose requires #50 100 mg/mL 1 mL vials
Sodium bicarbonate	Agents producing wide QRS, urine, or serum alkalization	Multiple roles/mechanisms of action Attention to systemic pH, sodium, and potassium levels

shared G protein and increasing intracellular phosphokinase A activity. Glucagon should be given as a 3 to 5 mg IV bolus, additional boluses or a continuous infusion may be required due to short duration of effect. Nausea and vomiting should be anticipated from glucagon administration. Additionally, aggressive supportive care consisting of a combination of measures including fluid resuscitation, atropine, external pacing, vasopressor support, and high-dose insulin and dextrose therapy maybe required.[17,24,30]

Calcium Channel Antagonist

Calcium channel blockers reduce calcium flow through voltage-gated calcium channels. These channels are found in myocardial, smooth muscle, and pancreatic cells. Blockade of these channels results in reduction in intracellular calcium, leading to reduced actin-myosin interaction producing reduced vascular and myocardial contractility. Additionally a reduction in intracellular calcium causes a reduction in sinoatrial and atrioventricular nodal tone.[30,31] At therapeutic doses the dihydropyridines have peripheral action with vasodilatory effect, where the nondihydropyridines (verapamil, diltiazem) express more direct cardiac effect.[17] In overdose these differences are lost. Common symptoms include hypotension, bradycardia, and conduction disturbances. Elevated blood glucose may be noted because of blockade of pancreatic islet cell, calcium channels, and a resultant decrease in insulin secretion. This metabolic impairment reduces carbohydrate supply to cardiac muscle and compounds myocardial dysfunction. Other potential symptoms include nausea and vomiting, CNS depression, hypoperfusion, and pulmonary edema.[30] Initial therapies in the setting of calcium channel blocker toxicity should include intravenous fluids, atropine, and administration of calcium salts (10-20 mL 10% calcium gluconate via peripheral line or 5-10 mL 10% calcium chloride via central venous access). These methods commonly do not improve patient hemodynamics in moderate to severe poisoning and vasopressor support is required. If response remains inadequate glucagon and/or amrinone are additional treatment options.[30] There is increasing support for early intervention using high-dose insulin and dextrose therapy (hyperinsulinemia-euglycemia therapy) in the setting of calcium channel blocker overdose. Insulin has positive inotropic activity and improves the carbohydrate delivery to cardiac myocytes. Current suggested dosing recommends a 1 U/kg bolus dose of regular insulin, followed by a 0.5 to 1 U/kg/h infusion adjusted to response. A dextrose infusion should be initiated at time of insulin bolus to maintain euglycemia, and close monitoring of glucose and potassium should be carried out throughout the therapy. Prior to initiating therapy, blood glucose and potassium levels should be checked and if <200 mg/dL or <2.5 mEq/L respectively, supplementation should be provided.[30,31]

Digoxin

Digoxin is a cardiac glycoside that inhibits the sodium/potassium ATPase pump. This effect increases inotropy and contractility as a result of increased intracellular calcium. Additionally, digoxin decreases heart rate via activity on both vagal and sympathetic tone. Digoxin has a narrow therapeutic window, and a multitude of drug interactions (verapamil, carvedilol, spironolactone, alprazolam, macrolide antibiotics, etc) and comorbid conditions (renal dysfunction, reduced lean body mass) can precipitate toxicity.[32] Symptoms of toxicity may be nonspecific and a high degree of suspicion should be utilized. Early clinical symptoms of excess commonly include nausea, vomiting, and fatigue. Other effects may include hyperkalemia, visual disturbances, confusion, and a broad array of cardiovascular toxicity.[17,32]

Digoxin toxicity can produce virtually every known dysrhythmia.[2] With exception of the administration of calcium salts to treat hyperkalemia and use of Class IA antidysrhythmics, both of which may increase mortality in the setting of suspected digoxin toxicity, standard supportive care measures should be utilized. More significant cardiac glycoside toxicity can be treated with digoxin immune Fab. This antibody fragment antidote binds digoxin with higher affinity than the target pump, effectively blocking and reversing associated toxicities. Each vial of Fab fragment will bind approximately 0.5 mg of digoxin.[33]

Antidotal treatment is indicated with potassium levels >5 mEq/L, life-threatening dysrhythmia, significant/refractory hemodynamic instability, acute ingestions of >10 mg in adults or >4 mg in children, a serum digoxin level of ≥15 ng/mL at any time postingestion, or a serum digoxin level ≥10 ng/mL 6 hours after ingestion.[2,10,17,32] However, there is support for antidotal treatment as a first-line therapy.[34] Determining appropriate antidote dose can be accomplished by the following methods:

1. Empirically, with recommended doses of 10 vials for acute overdose and 3 vials for chronic toxicity for all patient ages.
2. Based on a known dose ingested, as one vial of digoxin Fab fragments will complex 0.5 mg of digoxin.
3. Based on a steady-state serum level (must be drawn 4-6 hours postingestion to allow complete distribution) and calculations listed in the product package insert.[33]

Digoxin levels can rise dramatically following administration of digoxin immune Fab fragment as the levels indicate both bound and unbound drug. As such, total digoxin levels are not useful in guiding patient management after administration of Fab fragment antidote.

Tricyclic Antidepressants

Tricyclic antidepressants (TCAD) produce toxicity by multiple mechanisms: sodium channel antagonism, alpha-receptor antagonism, anticholinergic effects, and inhibition of norepinephrine and serotonin uptake. Moderate to severe toxicity can develop with doses of 10 to 20 mg/kg, with doses >20 mg/kg potentially fatal. Clinical manifestations of toxicity can have abrupt onset and include CNS depression, respiratory depression, seizures, anticholinergic effects, conduction disturbances (particularly prolongation of the QRS interval), dysrhythmias, and profound hypotension.[35,36] QRS duration >100 ms in the setting of TCAD poisoning is associated with a higher risk of seizure and durations >160 ms with malignant dysrhythmias. Hypotension is largely due to alpha-blockade and direct-acting alpha agonists (norepinephrine or phenylephrine) are the vasopressors of choice. In addition to aggressive supportive care, serum alkalinization using sodium bicarbonate is utilized in TCAD poisoning with evidence of QRS prolongation or seizure activity with a goal of establishing a systemic pH of 7.45 to 7.55.[17] In addition to providing higher levels of sodium in the setting of competitive sodium channel blockade, increased systemic pH is theorized to increase TCAD volume of distribution and enhance recovery time of blocked sodium channels.[35] Alkalinization will potentially be of aid in correcting disturbances related to sodium channel blockade as well as treating metabolic acidosis associated with TCAD-induced seizure or hypotension, but it will not address other mechanisms of TCAD toxicity, as such it is only a component of intervention.

Opioids

Opioids were associated with the second largest number of fatalities reported to US PCs in 2007.[3] The hallmarks of toxicity include CNS and respiratory depression. Other potential complications include vomiting, hypoxia, decreased bowel motility, pulmonary edema, hypotension, bradycardia, seizures (meperidine, propoxyphene, and tramadol), dysrhythmia (propoxyphene, methadone), and acidosis.[24,37] The degree of interpatient tolerance can significantly effect the severity of symptoms observed related to dose. In addition to good ABCs, naloxone, an antagonist of opioid receptors, can reverse the CNS and respiratory depression related to opioid overdose. The lowest effective dose should be utilized initially (0.4-2 mg IV) with incremental titration (0.1 mg) to desired response in attempt to avoid opiate withdrawal syndrome.[6,10] If no significant improvement in CNS/respiratory state has been achieved after administration of 10 mg of naloxone, other causes should be investigated. Duration of antagonism by naloxone may be shorter than opioid effect; as such patients should be monitored closely for resedation and may require continuous naloxone infusion.[17] Toxicities of agents commonly formulated in combination with opioids should also be investigated.

Salicylates

Salicylates are ingredients of a number of prescription and over-the-counter products in the United States. Toxicity is typically related to ingestion, but can occur due to improper dermal use.[38] Toxicity can result following acute overdose as well as chronic use either in supratherapeutic dose or in the setting of patients with decreased metabolism or renal function.[2] In order to determine potential toxicity, individual agents must be converted to appropriate aspirin equivalents by multiplying the ingested dose by a corresponding individual salicylate aspirin equivalent factor (ie, aspirin = 1, methyl salicylate = 1.4, bismuth subsalicylate = 0.5, magnesium salicylate = 1.21, etc). Current guidelines recommend emergency department evaluation for all symptomatic patients and ingestions >150 mg/kg or 6.5 g of aspirin equivalents in asymptomatic patients.[38] Acute and chronic salicylate poisoning can result in gastrointestinal, CNS, and metabolic dysfunction. Potential symptoms include nausea and vomiting, tinnitus, tachypnea, diaphoresis, hypoglycemia, hyperthermia, altered mental status, seizures, CNS depression, a respiratory alkalosis (early), mixed respiratory alkalosis and metabolic acidosis (late), pulmonary edema, and cerebral edema.[24,36,38] Chronic toxicity is often not recognized early in diagnosis as the symptoms and salicylate blood levels may not be as pronounced or syndromic as acute toxicity. Delay in recognition of salicylism can prove lethal, and as such salicylate toxicity should be investigated in all patients with unexplained altered mental status and metabolic disturbance.[38,39] Serum salicylate concentrations interpretation is complex. Salicylates have the potential for delayed or continual absorption due to formulation, pylorospasm or concretion formation. For this reason serial levels are typically indicated in acute overdose. Decreasing levels do not always indicate resolving toxicity. While intuitively falling levels would seem to correspond with improving condition, this cannot be determined solely based on salicylate serum levels. This is because in the setting of salicylate-induced acidemia, the volume of distribution will increase and tissue penetration into vital organs, especially the CNS, increases resulting in more significant clinical toxicity. For these reasons salicylate levels should never be the sole factor in assessing toxicity.[39] Additionally, the Done nomogram is not considered appropriate for determination of salicylate toxicity and should not be utilized.[2,24] There is no true antidote for salicylate poisoning. Treatment is aimed at decreasing absorption and enhancing elimination. Urinary alkalinization by administration of sodium bicarbonate with goal of maintaining a urinary pH of 7.5 to 8 is an effective means of increasing renal elimination of salicylates as it increases the portion of ionized salicylate in the urine.[36] Hemodialysis effectively removes salicylate and is indicated in the salicylate-toxic patients with CNS dysfunction, renal failure, pulmonary edema, severe acid-base or electrolyte disturbance, or salicylate levels >100 mg/dL regardless of symptoms.[39]

SPECIAL POPULATIONS

Children, elderly, and the pregnant patient are groups in which special considerations may be required in the management of toxicity. Poisoning in toddlers are not attempts at self-harm, typically involve small dose, and a single ingredient compared to exposures in older children and adults. However, due to their small size relative to dose, several medications or chemicals can be lethal in single tablet or mouthful ingestions. In elderly patients, drug toxicity may not be readily apparent or investigated as cause of clinical symptoms. However, changes in hepatic or renal function may alter kinetics and elimination leading to increased serum levels. Additionally, older patients tend to take multiple pharmacologically active agents and have comorbid conditions that increase the risk of drug-drug interactions and additive clinical effects. In the pregnant patient as a general rule, treatment that is deemed necessary for the mother should not be held out of concern for the fetus. Of note in this population is the fact that intravenous acetylcysteine is recommended over oral acetylcysteine and that carbon monoxide is significantly more toxic to the fetal hemoglobin and hyperbaric oxygen therapy is recommend at lower carboxyhemoglobin levels compared to nonpregnant patients.[2]

CASE Application

1. Which of the following is an appropriate poisoning first aid measure?
   a. Cutaneous acid exposures should be neutralized with an alkaline product.
   b. Emesis should be routinely induced.
   c. Patients should be observed for abnormal symptoms for 30 minutes.
   d. Poison control should be called if the patient is having difficulty in breathing.
   e. If the poison was swallowed, any residual should be removed from the mouth.

2. RC is a 35-year-old, 170 lb man. He reports a toothache for which he has been taking four 500-mg acetaminophen tablets every 3 to 4 hours for the last 3 days without relief. Additionally, he complains of nausea and new onset of right upper quadrant pain. He denies use of any other medications or other significant past medical history, but does report consuming a 12 pack of beer daily. His last dose of acetaminophen was 2 hours prior to physical examination. Which of the following would be an appropriate measure in the evaluation/treatment of RC?
   a. Acetaminophen level should be plotted on the Rumack-Matthew nomogram to determine if antidote therapy is indicated.
   b. Antidote therapy should be initiated immediately.
   c. Acetaminophen level should be ordered to determine need for antidote therapy.
   d. Activated charcoal should be administered and acetaminophen level should be ordered to determine need for antidote therapy.

3. How much aspirin equivalent is contained in 5 mL of the topical analgesic, oil of wintergreen (100% methyl salicylate)?
   a. 140 mg
   b. 500 mg
   c. 1400 mg
   d. 5 g
   e. 7 g

4. Select the agent that would be associated with the toxidrome mnemonic: mad as a hatter, blind as a bat, red as a beet, hot as a hare, dry as a bone.
   a. Methylphenidate
   b. Amitriptyline
   c. Donepezil
   d. Hydromorphone

5. Early in the course of salicylate toxicity, arterial blood gases would most likely indicate which of the following acid-base derangements
   a. Metabolic acidosis
   b. Respiratory alkalosis
   c. Partially compensated metabolic acidosis
   d. Partially compensated respiratory acidosis

6. Which toxin antidote combination pairing is not correct?
   a. Butorphanol and naloxone
   b. Cyanide and hydroxocobalamin
   c. Fomepizole and isopropyl alcohol
   d. Pyridoxine and isoniazid
   e. Deferoxamine and iron

7. PM is a 23-year-old woman that presents to the emergency department with a history of ingesting #60 digoxin 0.25-mg tablets 6 hours ago. The tablets came from a brand new #60 count prescription for her grandfather. On presentation she is lethargic and reported to have vomited multiple times in the last 1 to 2 hours by her family. Her electrocardiogram revealed high-degree heart block with a ventricular rate of 40 to 50 beats/min and her potassium was found to be 5.8 mEq/L and a digoxin concentration of 12 ng/mL. Her urine pregnancy test was negative and her past medical history is significant for depression. The treating physician initiated antidote therapy with digoxin immune Fab fragments in an appropriate dose for the given ingestion. Within 60 minutes the patients' clinical status improved significantly but repeat digoxin concentration 6 hours after Fab administration returned at 19 ng/mL. What is the best answer to explain the increase in digoxin concentration?

   a. Continued absorption of digoxin.
   b. The time frame of ingestion was incorrect and ingestion was closer to time of presentation.
   c. Administration of digoxin immune Fab fragment has increased serum levels of total digoxin.
   d. Endogenous digoxin-like immunoreactive substance.

8. Which of the following should caution for anaphylactoid reaction be used with digoxin immune Fab fragments' administration.

   a. Papaya or papain allergy
   b. Patients treated previously with digoxin immune Fab fragments
   c. Sheep protein allergy
   d. Latex allergy
   e. All of the above

9. The administration of which of the following agents would be indicated in the setting of tricyclic antidepressant overdose associated with seizures or QRS interval >115 ms?

   a. Sodium bicarbonate
   b. Flumazenil
   c. Physostigmine
   d. Procainamide
   e. Both a and c

10. Which vasopressor would be the best choice for hypotension due to tricyclic antidepressant toxicity that is refractory to fluid and sodium bicarbonate support?

    a. Norepinephrine
    b. Epinephrine
    c. Dopamine
    d. Isoproterenol
    e. Dobutamine

11. Which of the following is a form of acetylcysteine that can be giving intravenously as antidote therapy in acetaminophen poisoning?

    a. Mucomyst
    b. Acetadote
    c. 10% acetylcysteine
    d. 20% acetylcysteine
    e. All of the above

12. Which of the following are differences between calcium gluconate and calcium chloride parenteral preparations?

    a. The mechanism of action of calcium chloride is superior in calcium channel blocker poisoning.
    b. The mechanism of action of calcium gluconate is superior in calcium channel blocker poisoning.
    c. Calcium chloride provides three times more cation compared to calcium gluconate on an equal volume basis.
    d. Calcium gluconate is more irritating when given intravenously than calcium chloride.
    e. Both c and d

13. HF presents to the emergency department and states that he took an overdose of his "heart medication." He does not remember the name of the medication but states he took a handful of tablets approximately 3 hours ago and now feels lethargic and sick in his stomach. His vitals reveal a heart rate of 45 beats/min, blood pressure of 85/40 mm Hg, respiratory rate of 12 breaths/min, and temperature of 98.6 F°. The ED staff contacts the patient's pharmacy and is told the patient has prescriptions for atenolol, amlodipine, and digoxin. Laboratory test is ordered and is pending. Which of the following agents should not be administered prior to return of digoxin serum concentration determination?

    a. Atropine
    b. Fluid bolus
    c. Calcium salt
    d. Glucagon
    e. All of the above

14. RC is a 36-year-old man brought to the emergency department by his wife. She states that RC has been vomiting for the last 2 hours and acting abnormal following an argument approximately 4 hours ago. RC has a history of peptic ulcer disease for which he takes omeprazole and uses minoxidil topically. In the ED he complains of nausea, vomiting, abdominal pain, and is diaphoretic. On physical examination the patient is awake and oriented but lethargic. His blood pressure is 135/80 mm Hg, heart rate is 111 beats/min, respiratory rate is 33 breaths/min, and temperature is 100.1°F. HEENT was unremarkable, chest was clear to auscultation, no murmurs, rubs, or gallops detected, bowels sounds were present, but abdomen was tender, stool guaiac test was negative. ECG was normal. Initial laboratory data results include: sodium of 144 mEq/L, potassium 3.8 mEq/L, bicarbonate 8 mEq/L, chloride 98 mEq/L, BUN 23 mg/dL, creatinine 0.7 mg/dL, glucose 93 mg/dL, calcium 9.6 mg/dL, and albumin 4 g/dL.

Arterial blood gas values on room air were determined to be: pH 7.34, Pco_2 11 mm Hg, Po_2 93 mm Hg. What is the calculated anion gap for this patient?

a. 23
b. −49.8
c. 147
d. 38
e. 14

15. Which opioid is associated with both proconvulsant and prodysrhythmic activity in overdose?

a. Meperidine
b. Methadone
c. Hydrocodone
d. Heroin
e. Propoxyphene

16. Which of the following gastric decontamination method and toxin pairs would be appropriate?

a. Syrup of ipecac and amitriptyline; 30 minutes postexposure
b. Activated charcoal and lithium; <30 minutes postexposure
c. Multiple dose–activated charcoal and carbamazepine
d. Whole bowel irrigation and acetaminophen; 30 minutes postexposure
e. Sorbitol and atenolol; 30 minutes postexposure

17. Which of the following is a first-line agent in the management of beta-blocker toxicity and associated with a high incidence of nausea and vomiting?

a. Atropine
b. Normal saline intravenous fluid
c. Calcium gluconate
d. Glucagon
e. Milrinone

18. Following acute ingestion of 10 g of acetaminophen, what is the earliest time postingestion that an acetaminophen level can be drawn and plotted on the Rumack-Matthew nomogram to appropriately determine potential hepatotoxic risk and need for antidote administration?

a. 30 minutes postingestion
b. 1 hour post ingestion
c. 2 hours postingestion
d. 4 hours postingestion
e. 8 hours postingestion

19. ZM is a 44-year-old, 170 lb man who was found unresponsive in the middle of a city street and brought to the emergency department by ambulance. He is noted to have a blood pressure of 115/60 mm Hg, a heart rate of 61 beats/min, and a respiratory rate of 6 breaths/min; his ECG reveals a normal sinus rhythm, he is afebrile, has no apparent trauma, and is noted to have an odor of alcohol on his breath. Prescription bottles for methadone and clonazepam were found in his shirt pocket. The attending physician requests recommendations on the administration of flumazenil, naloxone, thiamine, and dextrose. Which of these agents would not be appropriate with ZM's history?

a. Flumazenil
b. Naloxone
c. Thiamine
d. Dextrose

20. Which of the following are correct statements with regard to the Poison Prevention Packaging Act of 1970?

a. Child-resistant effectiveness of not <85% without demonstration and not <80% after demonstration.
b. Senior adults must have ease in opening of not <90%.
c. Single package forms of acetaminophen of <1 g do not require child-resistant closures.
d. It is estimated that over 900 children's lives have been saved due to implementation of child-resistant packaging of aspirin and oral prescription medications.
e. All of the above.

TAKEAWAY POINTS ››

- All substances can produce untoward and toxic effect in sufficient dose. Sufficient dose can be highly variable from patient to patient.
- All patients regardless of symptoms or expected toxicity should have medical evaluations following exposures that are attempts at self-harm.
- Urine drug screens are associated with a number of pitfalls, have limited utility, and rarely change treatment. Traditional laboratory tests generally provide better aid in diagnosis and treatment than "tox screens."
- There are significant limitations and little evidence to support routine utilization of gastric decontamination. Decisions to employ these techniques should thoroughly assess the risk-to-benefit ratio on an individual patient basis.
- There are limited circumstances and toxins in which antidotal therapy is available. As such, symptomatic and supportive care is the cornerstone in management of the poisoned patient.
- Acetaminophen overdose can produce hepatotoxicity to the point of fulminant failure. Acute doses >10 g or 200 mg/kg necessitate medical evaluation.
- Ethylene glycol and methanol can produce significant morbidity and mortality in very small dose. Toxicity can

be prevented by inhibition of alcohol dehydrogenase by fomepizole or ethanol if given early in the course of poisoning prior to significant metabolite generation and resultant acidosis.

- Due to the potential for precipitating benzodiazepine withdrawal or unmasking of coingestant toxicity, flumazenil should not be routinely utilized in the treatment of benzodiazepine poisoning.
- Glucagon utilizes a mechanism of action that bypasses antagonized beta-receptors in the setting of beta-blocker toxicity.
- Calcium channel blockers can produce severe cardiovascular toxicity. High-dose insulin and dextrose therapy has increasingly been employed early in the course of toxicity.
- Digoxin inhibits the sodium-potassium ATPase pump resulting in increased intracellular calcium stores and increased extracellular potassium levels. Digoxin immune Fab fragments are extremely effective in reversing digoxin toxicity.
- Tricyclic antidepressants can cause severe CNS depression and block sodium channels leading to prolonged QRS interval and significant dysrhythmia risk in 10 to 20 mg/kg dose.
- Opioid-toxic patients that respond to naloxone with improved level of consciousness or increased respiratory effort require close observation for resedation as the duration of action for naloxone may be as short as 45 minutes. Overdose of long-acting opiates may require a continuous naloxone infusion.
- Ion trapping with urinary alkalinization is an effective measure to increase salicylate elimination, but is not as effective as hemodialysis which should be utilized for more significant toxicity.
- Proper management of the poisoned patient necessitates sound understanding of the pathophysiology and pharmacology of poisoning and the risks and benefits associated with potential interventions. Consultation with a regional poison center (1-800-222-2222) provides free, 24-hour immediate expert advice.

REFERENCES

1. Borzelleca JF. Paracelsus: herald of modern toxicology. *Toxicol Sci.* 2000;53:2-4.
2. Flomenbaum NE, Goldfrank LR, Hoffman RS, et al. *Goldfrank's Toxicologic Emergencies.* 8th ed. New York, NY: McGraw-Hill Companies; 2006.
3. Bronstein AC, Spyker DA, Cantilena JR, et al. 2007 Annual Report of the American Association of Poison Control Centers' National Poison Data System (NPDS): 25th Annual Report. *Clin Toxicol.* 2008;46:927-1057.
4. Fingerhut LA, Anderson RA. *The Three Leading Causes of Injury Mortality in the United States, 1999-2005.* Hyattsville, MD: National Center for Health Statistics; March 2008. http://www.cdc.gov/nchs/products/pubs/pubd/hestats/injury99-05/injury99-05.pdf. Accessed August 1, 2009.
5. Substance Abuse and Mental Health Services Administration, Office of Applied Studies. *Drug Abuse Warning Network, 2006: National Estimates of Drug-Related Emergency Department Visits.* DAWN Series D-30, DHHS Publication No. (SMA) 08-4339, Rockville, MD; 2008.
6. Boyle JS, Bechtel LK, Holstege CP. Management of the critically poisoned patient. *Scand J Trauma Resusc Emerg Med.* 2009;17:29. doi: 10.1186/1757-7241-17-29.
7. Tenebein M. Do you really need that emergency drug screen? *Clin Toxicol.* 2009;47:286-291.
8. Sporer KA, Khayam-Bashi H. Acetaminophen and salicylate serum levels in patients with suicidal ingestion or altered mental status. *Am J Emerg Med.* 1996:14:443-446.
9. Mokhlesi B, Leiken JB, Murray P, et al. Adult toxicology in critical care: part 1: general approach to the intoxicated patient. *Chest.* 2003;123;577-592.
10. Holstege CP, Dobmeier SG, Bechtel LK. Critical care toxicology. *Emerg Med Clin North Am.* 2008;26:715-739.
11. American Academy of Clinical Toxicology, European Association of Poison Centers and Clinical Toxicologists. Position paper: ipecac syrup. *J Toxicol Clin Toxicol.* 2004;42:133-143.
12. American Academy of Clinical Toxicology, European Association of Poison Centers and Clinical Toxicologists. Position paper: single-dose activated charcoal. *Clin Toxicol.* 2005; 43:61-87.
13. American Academy of Clinical Toxicology, European Association of Poison Centers and Clinical Toxicologists. Position statement and practice guidelines on the use of multi-dose activated charcoal in the treatment of acute poisoning. *J Toxicol Clin Toxicol.* 1999;37:731-751.
14. American Academy of Clinical Toxicology, European Association of Poison Centers and Clinical Toxicologists. Position paper: cathartics. *J Toxicol Clin Toxicol.* 2004;42:243-253.
15. American Academy of Clinical Toxicology, European Association of Poison Centers and Clinical Toxicologists. Position paper: whole bowel irrigation. *J Toxicol Clin Toxicol.* 2004;42:843-854.
16. American Academy of Clinical Toxicology, European Association of Poison Centers and Clinical Toxicologists. Position paper: gastric lavage. *J Toxicol Clin Toxicol.* 2004;42:933-943.
17. Betten DP, Vohra RB, Cook MD, et al. Antidote use in the critically ill poisoned patient. *J Intensive Care Med.* 2006;21:255-277.
18. Dart RC, Borron SW, Caravati EM, et al. Expert consensus guidelines for stocking of antidotes in hospitals that provide emergency care [published online ahead of print May 5 2009]. *Ann Emerg Med.* doi:10.1016/j.annemergmed.2009.01.023.
19. Gunnell D, Murray V, Hawton K. Use of paracetamol (acetaminophen) for suicide and nonfatal poisoning: worldwide patterns of use and misuse. *Suicide Life Threat Behav.* 2000;30:313-326.
20. Heard KJ. Acetylcysteine for acetaminophen poisoning. *N Engl J Med.* 2008;359:285-292.
21. Dart RC, Erdman AR, Olson KR, et al. Acetaminophen poisoning: an evidence-based consensus guideline for out-of-hospital management. *Clin Toxicol.* 2006;44:1-18.

22. Acetadote (acetylcysteine injection) [package insert]. Nashville, TN: Cumberland Pharmaceuticals Inc.; 2008.
23. Yarema MC, Johnson DW, Berlin RJ, et al. Comparison of the 20-hour intravenous and 72-hour oral acetylcysteine protocols for the treatment of acute acetaminophen poisoning. [published online ahead of print June 25 2009]. *Ann Emerg Med. doi:*10.1016/j.annemergmed.2009.05.010.
24. Mokhlesi B, Leikin JB, Murray P, et al. Adult toxicology in critical care: part II: specific poisonings. *Chest.* 2003;123; 897-922.
25. Brent J. Fomepizole for ethylene glycol and methanol poisoning. *N Engl J Med.* 2009;360:2216-2223.
26. Antizol (fomepizole injection) [package insert]. Palo Alto, CA: Jazz Pharmaceuticals, Inc.; 2006.
27. Seger DL. Flumazenil-treatment or toxin. *J Toxicol Clin Toxicol.* 2004;42:209-216.
28. Ngo AS, Anthony CR, Samuel M, et al. Should a benzodiazepine antagonist be used in unconscious patients presenting to the emergency department? *Resuscitation.* 2007;74:27-37.
29. Romazicon (flumazenil injection) [package insert]. Nutley, NJ: Roche Laboratories Inc.; 2007.
30. Shepherd G. Treatment of poisoning caused by beta-adrenergic and calcium-channel blockers. *Am J Health-Syst Pharm.* 2006;63:1828-1835.
31. Harris NS. Case records of the Massachusetts General Hospital. Case 24-2006: a 40-year-old woman with hypotension after an overdose of amlodipine. *N Engl J Med.* 2006;355:602-611.
32. Vivo RP, Krim SR, Perez J, et al. Digoxin: current use and approach to toxicity. *Am J Med Sci.* 2008;336:423-428.
33. Digifab (digoxin immune fab (ovine)) [package insert]. Melville, NY: Savage Laboratories; 2005.
34. Lapostolle F, Borron SW, Verdier C, et al. Digoxin-specific Fab fragments as single first-line therapy in digitalis poisoning. *Crit Care Med.* 2008;36:3014-3018.
35. Kerr GW, McGuffie AC, Wilkie S. Tricyclic antidepressant overdose: a review. *Emerg Med J.* 2001;18:236-241.
36. Greene SL, Dargan PI, Jones AL. Acute poisoning: understanding 90% of cases in a nutshell. *Postgrad Med J.* 2005;81:204-216.
37. Forti RJ, Adam HM. Opiate overdose. *Pediatr Rev.* 2007;28:35-36.
38. Chyka PA, Erdman AR, Christianson G, et al. Salicylate poisoning: an evidence-based consensus guideline for out-of-hospital management. *Clin Toxicol.* 2007;45:95-131.
39. Fertel BS, Nelson LS, Goldfarb DS. The underutilization of hemodialysis in patients with salicylate poisoning. *Kidney Int.* 2009;75:1349-1353. doi:10.1038/ki.2008.443; published online August 20, 2008.
40. Poison Prevention Week Council Web site http://www.poisonprevention.org. Accessed August 1, 2009.

CHAPTER

67 All Hazards Preparedness

Howell R. Foster and Keith R. McCain

FOUNDATION OVERVIEW

Paraphrasing the great scientist Louis Pasteur, "Luck favors the prepared!" When an event occurs there will be a response. That response will begin locally and radiate. While most events are small and local, some are incidences of national significance. The collapse of the I-35 bridge in Minneapolis in 2007 is a great example of local tragedy with a well-executed local response. According to Director of Pharmacy, University of Minnesota Medical Center, Scott Knoer, "All of the disaster training really pays off." "While this was a horrible tragedy for our city," reflected Knoer, "it was rewarding to see such a well-orchestrated response as our community pulled together."[1]

It is the authors' opinion that as health care professionals it is pharmacists' ethical duty to assist during a disaster. Hospital pharmacists most likely have the easiest role to define because their participation in the hospital disaster plan should be clear and during a disaster their service should be to their home institution. Pharmacists not associated with a health care facility will have to make their desire to volunteer known at the local or state level. Contacting your states department of health, pharmacy association, or department of emergency management would be good places to start.

Organization at the local or state level will vary, but virtually all plans will be based on the National Incident Management System (NIMS). NIMS provides a systematic, proactive approach to guide departments and agencies at all levels of government, nongovernmental organizations, and the private sector. The guide allows agencies to work seamlessly to prevent, protect against, respond to, recover from, and mitigate the effects of incidents, regardless of cause, size, location, or complexity, in order to reduce the loss of life and property and harm to the environment.[2] Preparedness is achieved and maintained through a continuous cycle of planning, organizing, training, equipping, exercising, evaluating, and taking corrective action.[3]

The Strategic National Stockpile (SNS) Program provides pharmaceuticals and medical supplies to the public free of charge in the event of a disaster. The governor of the afflicted state must ask for the SNS. If the request is granted, the material will be on site within 12 hours, hence they are often referred to as 12-Hour Push Packs.[4] It is the requesting states' responsibility to manage the housing, dissemination, and administration of the material once it is received. However, this response time is inadequate for a nerve agent event, as treatment must be accomplished in <12 hours. The CHEMPACK container system is responsible for allowing storage of nerve agent antidote by various local and state agencies.[5]

The pharmaceuticals initially found in the SNS were based on Category A threat agents. Presently, the pharmaceuticals are targeted for biologicals (smallpox, anthrax, botulism, viral hemorrhagic fevers, plague, and tularemia), chemical agents (nerve agents), radiologicals, and recently pandemic influenza.[4] Pediatric dosing cards have been developed for the majority of these threats and would be extremely useful in the field.[6]

BIOLOGICAL CATEGORY A AGENTS

The biologicals are typically referred to as the Category A threat agents. In regards to anthrax, plague, and tularemia, active cases will require IV antibiotics. These IV regimens will vary depending on the available agents prior to SNS delivery. The focus in this section will be on oral postexposure antibiotic prophylaxis for these infections. The use of ciprofloxacin and doxycycline in the pediatric population is not a common occurrence. However, the risk of mortality is so great with an exposure to a Category A Agent that pediatric use of the antibiotics is warranted.

Anthrax Inhalation Exposure

Bacillus anthracis is an encapsulated, aerobic, gram-positive, spore-forming, rod-shaped bacterium. The bacterium is known to cause cutaneous, gastrointestinal, respiratory, and oropharyngeal infections. Ciprofloxacin or doxycycline is indicated as initial therapy for postexposure prophylaxis to prevent inhalational anthrax from inhaled spores. There is presently no evidence to support either agent over the other for prophylaxis. Therefore a patient's individual history will be the determining factor.[7,8]

Postexposure Prophylaxis (Adults)[7,8]

Ciprofloxacin (Cipro) 500 mg every 12 hours for 60 days. Dose adjustment will be required for patients with a CrCL <50 mL/min.

or

Doxycycline (Doryx, Doxy, Monodox, Vibramycin, and Vibra-Tabs) 100 mg every 12 hours for 60 days.

Postexposure Prophylaxis (Children)[7,8]

Ciprofloxacin (Cipro) 10 to 15 mg/kg every 12 hours for 60 days.[a]

[a]If ciprofloxacin and doxycycline are contraindicated, then amoxicillin (Amoxil; Polymox; Trimox) 80 mg/kg/d in divided doses every 8 hours.

or

Doxycycline[a] (Doryx, Doxy, Monodox, Vibramycin, and Vibra-Tabs)

>8 year old and ≥45 kg: 100 mg every 12 hours for 60 days.

>8 year old and <45 kg: 2.2 mg/kg every 12 hours for 60 days.

≤8 year old: 2.2 mg/kg every 12 hours for 60 days.

Plague

Yersinia pestis is a gram-negative, rod-shaped facultative anaerobe that is known to cause bubonic and pneumonic plague. These diseases, although caused by the same organism, are different, but both carry a high mortality. The pneumonic form is the greatest concern as a biologic weapon. The bacteria are aerosolized and once inhaled the incubation period is 2 to 3 days. Pneumonia develops and patients often display stridor, cyanosis, and dyspnea. Pneumonic patients are highly contagious. Although it occurs naturally, bubonic plague could cause a mass casualty outbreak as it is considered the cause of the "Black Death" during the Middle Ages. Patients develop fever, malaise, and painful adenopathy (buboes). Patients can progress to the pneumonic form. Due to *Yersinia's* ability to replicate at a high rate and its pathogenesis, mortality is nearly 50% even with treatment and nearly 100% if untreated.[9] Therefore, antibiotic therapy should be started immediately and it should not be delayed while awaiting laboratory results.[10,11]

Tularemia

Francisella tularensis is a gram-negative rod facultative intracellular pathogen. Tularemia is a naturally occurring disease most commonly associated with tick bites; however, it could be weaponized as an aerosol.[12] Naturally occurring tularemia usually presents with a local skin ulcer, fever, chills, headache and regional lymphadenopathy; progression to the pneumonic form is rare. Aerosolized tularemia is a potent entity, inoculums as low as 25 colony-forming units/mL are capable of causing debilitating or fatal disease.[8] The pneumonic form carries the highest mortality.[13] An outbreak of the pneumonic form of tularemia should be considered an intentional event until proven otherwise.

Plague and Tularemia Postexposure Prophylaxis[8,12,14]

Postexposure Prophylaxis (Adults)

Ciprofloxacin (Cipro) 500 mg every 12 hours for 7 days. Dose adjustment will be required for patients with a CrCL <50 mL/min.

or

Doxycycline (Doryx, Doxy, Monodox, Vibramycin, and Vibra-Tabs) 100 mg every 12 hours for 7 days.

Postexposure Prophylaxis (Children)

Ciprofloxacin (Cipro) 10 to 15 mg/kg every 12 hours for 7 days.

or

Doxycycline (Doryx, Doxy, Monodox, Vibramycin, and Vibra-Tabs) ≤45 kg: 2.2 mg/kg every 12 hours for 7 days.

Botulism

Clostridium botulinum is an anaerobic, gram-positive, spore-forming rod that produces a potent neurotoxin. The spores are heat-resistant and can survive in foods that are incorrectly or minimally processed. Seven types (A, B, C, D, E, F, and G) of botulism are recognized, based on the antigenic specificity of the toxin produced by each strain. Types A, B, E, and F cause human botulism naturally, human cases of other types would be suggestive of an act of terrorism.[15] Types C and D cause most cases of botulism in animals. Animals most commonly affected are wild fowl and poultry, cattle, horses, and some species of fish.[16] Botulinum-infected patients with extensive muscle weakness, ptosis, dysphagia, great frequency of gastrointestinal effects, and urinary retention are at a greater risk of developing respiratory failure.[17] Mechanical ventilation may be required. Botulism is not communicable.[15] There is a bivalent antitoxin preparation containing types A and B, and a monovalent antitoxin preparation type E (suggestive of contaminated seafood) for treatment of botulism caused by the aforementioned toxins. (The trivalent antitoxin [types A, B, and E] is no longer available). The monovalent type E is given only when it is suspected. To obtain the antitoxin preparations call the CDC at 770-488-7100. There is also an investigational heptavalent antitoxin maintained by the US military.[15]

VIRAL HEMORRHAGIC FEVERS

Viral hemorrhagic fevers (VHFs) are caused by viruses of four distinct families: arenaviruses (Lassa fever), filoviruses (Ebola and Marburg), bunyaviruses (Rift Valley fever), and flaviviruses (Yellow fever and dengue).[18] They require a host and are RNA viruses. Naturally, VHFs are restricted geographically by their host. Human cases or outbreaks of VHFs caused by these viruses occur sporadically since humans are not their natural hosts. However once infected, human to human transmission is possible with some of the viruses. There are no cures, however ribavirin may be useful against arenaviruses and bunyaviruses.[18,19] Treatment is otherwise symptomatic and supportive.

Smallpox

The orthopoxvirus variola (smallpox) causes an acute febrile illness with a corresponding rash that develops into small, pus-filled blisters. Mortality rates are as high as 30%. Survivors are often severely scarred and ocular involvement may lead to blindness in some. Prolonged face-to-face contact is generally required for transmission. A person is considered infectious to others from the onset of fever until the last pox scab sloughs off.[20]

On the first day of a documented outbreak, the SNS will distribute smallpox vaccine to anyone who has been exposed.

Then over the next 5 to 6 days the CDC will oversee the vaccination of the rest of the country as needed.[20]

NERVE AGENTS

Organophosphate Compounds

These compounds are divided into the militarized agents GA (tabun), GB (sarin), GD (soman), and VX and the nonmilitarized or agricultural agents parathion, malathion, diazinon, and many other derivatives. The latter are considered less potent, but with a large dose they can be formidable substances.[21,22]

Organophosphates are toxic by all routes of exposure. Regardless of the route of exposure, signs and symptoms are cholinergic in nature and will be muscarinic or nicotinic. Salivation, lacrimation, urination, defecation, gastrointestinal symptoms, and emesis form the acronym SLUDGE to assist in remembering the basic signs and symptoms. Pinpoint pupils, chest tightness, shortness of breath, excessive sweating, muscle twitching, confusion, seizures, paralysis, coma, respiratory paralysis, and death may also occur. With the more potent military agents, the incapacitating effects can occur within 1 minute and fatal effects can occur within 1 to 10 minutes. Fatigue, irritability, nervousness, and memory defects may persist for as long as 6 weeks after recovery from an exposure episode.[21,23]

As a result of the rapid onset of severe signs and symptoms, nerve agents are stored and shipped differently than other treatments found in the SNS. As previously stated, they are stored under CHEMPACK. CHEMPACK is a voluntary program of the SNS operated by the CDC for the benefit of the US civilian population. Its mission is to provide state and local governments a sustainable nerve agent antidote cache. The CHEMPACK only contains materials for a nerve agent exposure and does not contain any other materials.

In the event of an organophosphate (OP) poisoning, three agents need to be readily available (atropine, pralidoxime, and diazepam). Atropine will be used to counter the muscarinic effects commonly seen. However, it has little affinity for nicotinic receptors and will not reverse respiratory paralysis, fasciculation, or general muscle weakness.[23] Pralidoxime will be used to reverse the binding of the OP to the acetylcholinesterase as long as aging has not occurred. Aging is the process by which the OP covalently binds the acetylcholinesterase rending it useless. Aging can occur in <12 hours with some of the militarized OPs, this is the principal reason for the CHEMPACK. Diazepam will be used to prevent or treat seizures.[21,22,23]

Atropine[a]

Adult: 2 to 6 mg (0.02-0.04 mg/kg) repeated every 2 to 30 minutes.

Pediatric: 0.05 to 0.1 mg/kg bolus every 2 to 30 minutes.

Pralidoxime (Protopam)

Adult: 1 to 2 g in 100 mL of 0.9% NS, IV, over 15 to 30 minutes followed by a continuous infusion of 500 mg/h. The infusion should be continued until symptoms have resolved for at least 24 hours.

Pediatric: 20 to 40 mg/kg in 100 mL of 0.9% NS over 30 minutes up to a maximum of 1 g followed by a continuous infusion of 10 to 20 mg/kg/h. The infusion should be continued until symptoms have resolved for at least 24 hours.

CNS damage from OP poisoning is currently thought to be due to seizure activity rather than a direct toxic effect. Prevention and treatment of seizures with diazepam is an important aspect of patient management. Seizures are more common in pediatric poisoning with cholinesterase inhibitors.[21,22,23,]

Diazepam (Dizac; Valium)

Adult: 5 to 10 mg, IV, every 5 to 10 minutes (one, 10-mg autoinjector, every 10 minutes × 3 maximum)

Pediatric: 0.2 mg/kg, IV, every 5 to 10 minutes.

RADIOLOGICS

Radioactive materials cannot be seen, tasted, felt, or smelled. It takes special equipment to detect them. Because of the unknown, they make an ideal weapon of terror. While a dirty bomb has been the focus of media reports in recent years, the biggest threat to life is most likely from the incendiary device used in the explosion and not the radiation itself. An atomic bomb is very different from a dirty bomb and the detonation of an atomic weapon would have very grave consequences. The following are recommendations for individuals near the blast area of a dirty bomb.[24]

Dirty Bomb

If You Are Outside and Close to the Incident[24]

- Cover your nose and mouth with a cloth to reduce the risk of breathing in radioactive dust or smoke.
- Don't touch objects thrown off by an explosion—they might be radioactive.
- Quickly go into a building where the walls and windows have not been broken. This area will shield you from radiation that might be outside.
- Once you are inside, take off your outer layer of clothing and seal it in a plastic bag if available. Put the cloth you used to cover your mouth in the bag, too. Removing outer clothes may get rid of up to 90% of radioactive dust.
- Put the plastic bag where others will not touch it and keep it until authorities tell you what to do with it.

[a]Dosing until someone has tachycardia, mydriasis, and dry membranes should be avoided. Clinically significant control is best described as a decrease in bronchorrhea and bronchoconstriction with a corresponding increase in oxygenation and ventilation.[21,22,23]

- Shower or wash with soap and water. Be sure to wash your hair. Washing will remove any remaining dust.
- Tune to the local radio or television news for more instructions.

If You Are Inside and Close to the Incident[24]

- If the walls and windows of the building are not broken, stay in the building and do not leave.
- To keep radioactive dust or powder from getting inside, shut all windows, outside doors, and fireplace dampers. Turn off fans and heating and air-conditioning systems that bring in air from the outside. It is not necessary to put duct tape or plastic around doors or windows.
- If the walls and windows of the building are broken, go to an interior room and do not leave. If the building has been heavily damaged, quickly go into a building where the walls and windows have not been broken. If you must go outside, be sure to cover your nose and mouth with a cloth. Once you are inside, take off your outer layer of clothing and seal it in a plastic bag if available. Store the bag where others will not touch it.
- Shower or wash with soap and water, removing any remaining dust. Be sure to wash your hair.
- Tune to local radio or television news for more instructions.

Treatment for many patients postexposure to radioactive materials will be symptomatic and supportive. However if an individual has been exposed to I131, or Cs137, there may be an antidote.[25,26]

Potassium Iodide KI is used for I131 acute exposures. Children are significantly more susceptible to the thyroid effects of I131. KI has to be given rapidly to be of benefit. Up to 90% of I131 uptake can be blocked in the first 2 hours postexposure. By 4 hours postexposure only 50% of I131 is blocked. Maintenance doses may be given daily for 7 to 14 days to prevent recycling of I131 into the thyroid. Adults 40 years of age or older have low risk of thyroid damage and KI therapy is not warranted. If you live within 50 miles of a nuclear facility that produces or is capable of releasing I131, you should work with your medical association, local or state public health department, emergency response organizations, and elected representatives to ensure that a stockpile of KI is available and a distribution plan is in place.[25]

Prussian Blue Prussian blue traps radioactive cesium in the intestines preventing reabsorption. The bound Cs is then excreted. Prussian blue reduces the T½ of Cs137 from about 110 days to about 30 days. Because Prussian blue reduces the time that radioactive Cs137 stays in the body, it helps limit the amount of time the body is exposed to radiation.[26]

Nuclear Attack Under the National Response Plan and the Nuclear/Radiological Annex, HHS has the major role in protecting people's health by monitoring, assessing, and following up on people's health. Ensuring the safety of workers by assessing the amount of time they can safely work in an area contaminated with radioactive materials and providing them protective equipment such as respiratory devices and monitoring devices. Maintaining and ensuring the safety of the area's food and water supply will be paramount. Medical and public health advice will be disseminated and the deployment of the SNS will occur if necessary.[27]

PANDEMIC FLU

An influenza pandemic is a global disease outbreak that occurs when a new influenza A virus emerges for which there is little or no immunity in the human population. Since immunity is low, the virus can spread quickly. In late March and early April 2009 novel swine influenza A (properly called 2009 H1N1) was detected in the United States for the first time. At the end of June, novel or 2009 H1N1 had infected over 1 million people in the United States alone.[28] Pharmacist should be aware of two websites dedicated to the flu: (1) www.cdc.gov/flu/weekly provides weekly surveillance updates by region and is designed for the health care professional. (2) www.pandemicflu.gov is a one-stop site for all things flu. It is well designed and has useful information for the public and professionals.[28,29,30,31]

During the fall 2009 flu season it was recommended that individuals receive both the seasonal influenza vaccine as well as the 2009 or novel H1N1 vaccine.

The Advisory Committee on Immunization Practices recommended that novel H1N1 flu vaccine be made available first to the following five groups:

- Pregnant women
- Health care workers and emergency medical responders
- People caring for infants under 6 months of age
- Children and young adults from 6 months to 24 years
- People aged 25 to 64 years with underlying medical conditions (eg, asthma, diabetes)

Combined, these groups would equal approximately 159 million individuals.[28]

Antiviral drugs are being stockpiled by HHS as part of the SNS. Production capacity for both oseltamivir and zanamivir has been increased and now is sufficient to support expanded recommendations. However, these recommendations do not obligate the Federal Government or public sector to purchase or stockpile antiviral drugs for all recommended uses and implementation will depend on the actions of other sectors of society. Pandemic preparedness is a shared responsibility of all levels of government, businesses, families, and individuals. The majority of 2009 influenza A (H1N1) viruses are susceptible to the neuraminidase inhibitor antiviral medication oseltamivir; however rare sporadic cases of oseltamivir resistant 2009 influenza A (H1N1) viruses have been detected worldwide, including two viruses in the United States. All tested

TABLE 67-1 **Interim Recommendations for the Selection of Antiviral Treatment Using Laboratory Test Results and Viral Surveillance Data, United States, 2008-2009 Season**[a] [32]

Rapid Antigen or Other Laboratory Test	Predominant Virus(es) in Community	Preferred Medication(s)	Alternative (Combination Antiviral Treatment)
Not done or negative, but clinical suspicion for influenza	H1N1 or unknown	Zanamivir	Oseltamivir + Rimantadine[b]
Not done or negative, but clinical suspicion for influenza	H3N2 or B	Oseltamivir or zanamivir	None
Positive A	H1N1 or unknown	Zanamivir	Oseltamivir + rimantadine[b]
Positive A	H3N2 or B	Oseltamivir or zanamivir	None
Positive B	Any	Oseltamivir or zanamivir	None
Positive A+B[c]	H1N1 or unknown	Zanamivir	Oseltamivir + rimantadine[b]
Positive A+B[c]	H3N2 or B	Oseltamivir or zanamivir	None

[a]Influenza antiviral medications used for treatment are most beneficial when initiated within the first 2 days of illness. Clinicians should consult the package insert of each antiviral medication for specific dosing information, approved indications and ages, contraindications/warnings/precautions, and adverse effects.

[b]Amantadine can be substituted for rimantadine but has increased risk of adverse events. Human data are lacking to support the benefits of combination antiviral treatment of influenza; however, these interim recommendations are intended to assist clinicians treating patients who might be infected with oseltamivir-resistant influenza A (H1N1) virus.

[c]Positive A+B indicates a rapid antigen test that cannot distinguish between influenza and influenza B viruses

viruses retain their sensitivity to the other neuraminidase inhibitor zanamivir.[28,29,30,31] See Table 67-1 for antiviral therapy recommendations.

CASE Application

1. Preparedness is achieved and maintained by which of the following?
   a. Planning
   b. Organizing
   c. Training
   d. Exercising
   e. All of the above

2. Virtually all disaster plans are based on what national system?
   a. National Planning System (NPS)
   b. National Incidence Management System (NIMS)
   c. Federal Incidence Bureau System (FIBS)
   d. Strategic National Planning System (SNPS)

3. The Strategic National Stockpile provides what during an incidence of national significance?
   a. Highly trained medical personal from around the country to disseminate supplies.
   b. Pharmaceuticals only to the state.
   c. Active military medical personnel to support the public.
   d. Pharmaceuticals and medical supplies to the state in need.

4. What government official must request the SNS?
   a. President of the United States
   b. Director of Health and Human Services
   c. Governor
   d. Speaker of the House

5. The CHEMPACK Program stores nerve agent antidotes with participating local or state entities. What are the antidotes provided by this program?
   a. Atropine and pralidoxime
   b. Atropine, pyridoxine, and diazepam
   c. Atropine, pralidoxime, and diazepam
   d. Atropine and pyridoxine

6. Which of the following is not considered a Category A threat agent?
   a. Smallpox
   b. H1N1
   c. Anthrax
   d. Arenavirus

7. Which agent is found in the SNS and is indicated for postexposure prophylaxis to inhaled *B. anthracis*?
   a. Dapsone
   b. Difloxacin
   c. Doxycycline
   d. Dicloxacillin

8. Antibiotic therapy for postexposure prophylaxis to inhaled *B. anthracis* should last for how many days?
   a. 30
   b. 40
   c. 60
   d. 90

9. An 18-year-old patient has been diagnosed with a pneumonic form of *Y. pestis*. What is the best course of action for the individuals exposed to the patient?

   a. Start ciprofloxacin 500 mg every 12 hours once symptoms appear.
   b. Start doxycycline 100 mg every 12 hours for 7 days in all individuals exposed during the patient's clinical course.
   c. Await the patient's culture and sensitivity results and start the most appropriate antibiotic as prophylaxis in the exposed individuals.
   d. Prophylaxis is not beneficial

10. A pharmacist working in local retail pharmacy that is adjacent to a hospital complex receives a call during a bioterrorism drill from an emergency department physician at that health care facility. He states they have a confirmed case of pneumonic tularemia. The patient states a former coworker threatened everyone in the workplace. Upon questioning from the police it was determined the coworker had released *F. tularensis* into the air ducts of his former workplace approximately 3 days prior. There are six individuals in that area and he has written them each a prescription for ciprofloxacin 500 mg every 12 hours for 7 days as prophylaxis. However the air duct system is shared with a daycare and eight children have been potentially exposed. All of the children are <30 kg. The physician asks for an antibiotic recommendation. Which of the following is the best treatment recommendation for all of the children?

    a. Doxycycline 50 mg every 12 hours for 7 days
    b. Doxycycline 2.2 mg/kg every 12 hours for 7 days
    c. Ciprofloxacin 500 mg once daily for 7 days
    d. Ciprofloxacin 25 mg/kg every 12 hours for 7 days

11. Which of the following botulism types can potentially be treated with an antitoxin obtained from the CDC?

    a. Types A and B only
    b. Types A, B, C, D, E, and F
    c. Types A, B, and E
    d. Type B only

12. Twelve patients with type G botulism have been found in the United States in the past 24 hours. All had recently flown through Toronto Pearson International Airport in the last 72 hours from various destinations. All are experiencing a rapid descending paralysis. What is the most likely reason for the outbreak?

    a. Contaminated seafood at an airport vendor
    b. Deliberate release of toxin within the airport
    c. Person to person contamination
    d. Serendipity

13. What is presently the best course of treatment for Ebola?

    a. Fluid replacement, ventilation, and additional supportive care as needed
    b. High-dose ribavirin
    c. Cryotherapy to drop the core temperature to < 95 F
    d. A cocktail of acyclovir, protease inhibitor, and interferon

14. A person with smallpox is no longer considered infectious when what event occurs?

    a. Defervescence
    b. The last pustule scabs over
    c. Sloughing of the last pustule scab
    d. When the rash turns to pustules

15. Which of the following signs and symptoms are considered clinically significant control with atropine in a postexposure organophosphate patient?

    a. Miosis, salivation, and muscle twitching
    b. Mydriasis, dry mucous membranes, flushing, and tachycardia
    c. Tachycardia, bronchorrhea, and salivation
    d. Decreased bronchial secretions and increased ease of ventilation

16. An adult patient with sarin poisoning has been decontaminated and is now in the triage area. He has small pupils, sweating, and copious salivation and nasal secretions. He begins having a seizure almost immediately after being brought to the triage area. Which is the best course of treatment?

    a. Administer diazepam 10 mg, followed by a 2 mg bolus of atropine, and then pralidoxime 2 g in 100 cc of NS infused over 30 minutes.
    b. A 2 mg bolus of atropine and repeat as needed, then pralidoxime 2 g in 100 cc of NS infused over 30 minutes. If the seizure activity has not abated post pralidoxime then give 5 mg of diazepam.
    c. Administer 10 mg of diazepam for the seizure, then no additional therapy as the other signs and symptoms are not concerning.
    d. Administer 5 g of pralidoxime via IVP since it will replenish GABA, then give atropine 2 g prn until bronchorrhea decreases.

17. A 3-year-old child and her 65-year-old grandmother were riding in car that was involved in a three-vehicle accident at 3 am. They have only minor injuries, but one of the other vehicles was carrying I131 for use as an imaging agent. The I131 container was not properly stored or sealed and it entered the side window of the vehicle with the child and grandmother. Many of the compounded I131 capsules were ruptured and dispersed throughout the car. They are 20 minutes post accident and no one is answering the phone at the nuclear pharmacy, there is no paperwork with the product, and the delivery driver is unconscious. Which is the best advice for the grandmother and child?

    a. Treat both with potassium iodide.
    b. Treat the grandmother with potassium iodide and leave the child untreated.

c. Treat the child with potassium iodide and leave the grandmother untreated.
d. Treat both with Prussian blue.
e. Treat neither.

18. Which of these is not considered a representative of the first five groups recommended to receive the novel H1N1 vaccine?

a. Healthy but pregnant 28-year-old
b. Emergency room physician
c. 55-year-old healthy male accountant
d. 23-year-old woman with type I diabetes
e. 32-year-old healthy daycare worker

19. As of 2009 according to the CDC guidelines which is considered the preferred agent for influenza in the United States regardless of *viral type*?

a. Rimantadine
b. Amantidine
c. Oseltamivir
d. Zanamivir

20. The first case of novel H1N1 was reported in the United States in late March-early April 2009. By the end of June, reported cases topped 1 million US residents. The logical reason for rapid dissemination of the disease is mostly likely which of the following?

a. The seasonal flu vaccine weakened the immune system.
b. The wet spring months are better for viral survival.
c. The population lacks immunity.
d. Antivirals are infective.

TAKEAWAY POINTS »

- Organization at the local or state level will vary, but virtually all plans will be based on the National Incident Management System (NIMS). NIMS provides a systematic, proactive approach to guide departments and agencies at all levels of government, nongovernmental organizations, and the private sector.
- The Strategic National Stockpile (SNS) Program provides pharmaceuticals and medical supplies to the public free of charge in the event of a disaster.
- *Bacillus anthracis* is an encapsulated, aerobic, gram-positive, spore-forming, rod-shaped bacterium. The bacterium is known to cause cutaneous, gastrointestinal, respiratory, and oropharyngeal infections. Ciprofloxacin or doxycycline is indicated as initial therapy for postexposure prophylaxis to prevent inhalational anthrax from inhaled spores.
- *Yersinia pestis* is a gram-negative, rod-shaped facultative anaerobe that is known to cause bubonic and pneumonic plague. Treatment or prophylaxis on Yersinia consists of ciprofloxacin or doxycycline.
- *Francisella tularensis* is a gram-negative rod facultative intracellular pathogen. Tularemia is a naturally occurring disease most commonly associated with tick bites; however it could be weaponized as an aerosol. Treatment or prophylaxis on Tularemia consists of ciprofloxacin or doxycycline.
- *Clostridium botulinum* is an anaerobic, gram-positive, spore-forming rod that produces a potent neurotoxin.
- VHFs are caused by viruses of four distinct families: arenaviruses (Lassa fever), filoviruses (Ebola and Marburg), bunyaviruses (Rift Valley fever), and flaviviruses (Yellow fever and dengue). There are no cures; however ribavirin may be useful against arenaviruses and bunyaviruses. Treatment is otherwise symptomatic and supportive.
- The orthopoxvirus variola (smallpox) causes an acute febrile illness with a corresponding rash that develops into small, pus-filled blister. On the first day of a documented outbreak, the SNS will distribute smallpox vaccine to anyone who has been exposed. Then over the next 5 to 6 days the CDC will oversee the vaccination of the rest of the country as needed.
- In the event of an organophosphate (OP) poisoning, three agents need to be readily available (atropine, pralidoxime, and diazepam).

REFERENCES

1. Sheffer JU. Minnesota hospital pharmacist lend a hand in bridge crisis. *Pharm Today*. 2007;13(9):1. Available at: http://www.pharmacytoday.org/index.htm#. Accessed August 28, 2009.
2. http://www.fema.gov/emergency/nims/. Accessed August 28, 2009.
3. http://www.fema.gov/emergency/nims/Preparedness.shtm. Accessed August 28, 2009.
4. http://www.bt.cdc.gov/stockpile/. Accessed August 28, 2009.
5. http://emergency.cdc.gov/planning/continuationguidance/pdf/chempack-attachj.pdf. Accessed August 28, 2009.
6. Montello MJ, Tarosky M, Pincock L, et al. Dosing cards for treatment of children exposed to weapons of mass destruction. *Am J Health-Syst Pharm*. 2006;63:944-949.
7. Update: Investigation of Anthrax Associated with Intentional Exposure and Interim Public Health Guidelines. *MMWR*. October 2001;50(41):889-893. Available at: http://www.cdc.gov/mmwr/preview/mmwrhtml/mm5041a1.htm. Accessed August 29, 2009.
8. Update: Investigation of Bioterrorism-Related Anthrax and Interim Guidelines for Exposure Management and Antimicrobial Therapy. *MMWR*. October 26, 2001;50(42):909-919.

9. Gage K, Dennis D, Tsai T. Prevention of plague: recommendations of the advisory committee on immunization practices (ACIP). *MMWR*. December 13, 1996;45(RR-14):1-15.
10. http://emergency.cdc.gov/agent/plague/faq.asp. Accessed August 29, 2009.
11. Chang M, Glynn M, Groseclose S. Endemic, notifiable bioterrorism-related diseases, United States, 1992-1999. *Emerg Infect Diseases*. 2003;9(5):556-564.
12. Dennis DT, Inglesby TV, Henderson DA, et al. Tularemia as a biological weapon. *JAMA*. 2001;285(21):2763-2773.
13. Oyston PC, Sjostedt A, Titball RW. Tularaemia: bioterrorism defence renews interest in *Francisella tularensis*. *Nat Rev Microbiol*. 2004 Dec;2(12):967-978.
14. Riedel S. Plague: from natural disease to bio-terrorism. *Proc Bayl Univ Med Cent*. 2005;18(2):116-124.
15. Abrutyn E. Chapter 134: botulism. In: Fauci AS, Braunwald E, Kasper DL, et al, eds. *Harrison's Principles of Internal Medicine*. 17th ed. New York, NY: McGraw-Hill Inc; 2008.
16. http://emergency.cdc.gov/agent/botulism/factsheet.asp. Accessed August 30, 2009.
17. Schmidt-Nowara WW, Samet JM, Rosario PA. Early and late pulmonary complications of botulism. *Arch Intern Med*. 1983;143:451-456.
18. Barlam TF, Kasper DL. Chapter 115: approach to the acutely ill infected febrile patient. In: Fauci AS, Braunwald E, Kasper DL, et al, eds. *Harrison's Principles of Internal Medicine*. 17th ed. New York, NY: McGraw-Hill Inc; 2008.
19. http://www.cdc.gov/ncidod/dvrd/spb/mnpages/dispages/vhf.htm. Accessed August 30, 2009.
20. http://emergency.cdc.gov/agent/smallpox. Accessed August 30, 2009.
21. Leikin JB, Thomas RG, Walter FG, et al. A review of nerve agent exposure for the critical care physician. *Crit Care Med*. 2002;30(10):2346.
22. http://www.atsdr.cdc.gov/csem/cholinesterase. Accessed August 30, 2009.
23. Wiener S, Hoffman R. Nerve agents: a comprehensive review. *J Int Care Med*. 2004;19(1):22-37.
24. http://emergency.cdc.gov/radiation/dirtybombs.asp. Accessed August 30, 2009.
25. http://emergency.cdc.gov/radiation/isotopes/iodine/. Accessed August 30, 2009.
26. http://emergency.cdc.gov/radiation/isotopes/cesium.asp. Accessed August 30, 2009.
27. http://emergency.cdc.gov/radiation/cdcrole.asp. Accessed August 30, 2009.
28. http://www.pandemicflu.gov/faq/pandemicinfluenza/2008.html. Accessed August 31, 2009.
29. http://www.cdc.gov/h1n1flu/surveillanceqa.htm#2. Accessed August 31, 2009.
30. http://www.cdc.gov/h1n1flu/updates/us/. Accessed August 31, 2009.
31. http://www.cdc.gov/flu/weekly/. Accessed August 31, 2009.
32. http://www2a.cdc.gov/HAN/ArchiveSys/ViewMsgV.asp?AlertNum=00279. Accessed August 31, 2009.

CHAPTER

68 Ergogenic Aids and Sports Pharmacy

Vince Colucci

FOUNDATION OVERVIEW

Introduction

Performance-enhancing substances will remain utilized and their ethical existence will spur debate as long as desire and pressure to win and the financial reward for winning remain key incentives. As competition in athletics grows and becomes more lucrative, so does the temptation to use chemical performance enhancers. The use of drugs and supplements to enhance performance is almost ubiquitous across athletic competition. The use of ergogenic aids stretches from the professional athlete to adolescent competitors without regard to gender.[1-4] This large prevalence suggests education and monitoring is required at all levels.

Definitions

Ergogenic aid (EA)—chemical, pharmaceutical, or neutraceutical product introduced into the body for the specific purpose of enhancing athletic performance

Exogenous substance—substance not ordinarily capable of being produced by the body naturally (xenobiotic); or a naturally occurring substance administered externally in addition to that produced internally

Endogenous substance—substance capable of being produced by the body naturally

Masking agent—substance used to hide or mask the substance in question from detection

Doping control—regulating, restricting, and testing for substances determined to be illicit for an athlete or competition

Analytical/testing methods—methods used to detect EA in blood, urine, or other body fluids that include, but are not limited to, gas chromatography, mass spectrometry, liquid chromatography, and isoelectric focusing

World Anti-Doping Agency (WADA)—multinational organization created to develop standards, definitions, testing, and regulations with regards to doping control on a world wide basis for athletic competition[5,6]

The WADA stance on the presence of a prohibited substance or its metabolite(s) or marker(s) in an athlete's bodily specimen(s) or sample is clear: *it is each athlete's personal duty to ensure that no prohibited substance enters his or her body.*[6]

WADA also informs athletes about drug testing programs and provides a prohibited drug list, information about drug use, drug actions, adverse drug actions, side effects, and ethics.[5,6] Different compounds may represent banned substances in different competitive sports and, thus, prohibitive lists are sport specific. For example, archers and competitive marksmen are banned from using antiadrenergic agents such as beta-adrenergic-blocking agents,[5] whereas other athletic endeavors may suffer from the negative inotrope or chronotrope properties of beta-adrenergic-blocking agents. (See Table 68-1 for a partial list of agents.)

Athletic organizations may have specific regulation standards and banned substance policies, lists, and testing policies (National Football League [NFL], Major League Baseball [MLB], National Collegiate Athletic Association [NCAA], United States Olympic Committee [USOC], etc) and it is the athlete's responsibility to understand and know the organizational rules and restrictions.

Agents may also be classified as training augmentation agents (eg, anabolic steroids; oxygen enhancers such as erythropoietin) versus agents that produce a relatively immediate effect (eg, amphetamines, bronchodilating drugs). (See Table 68-2 for summary reference.)

Doping control and regulation remains difficult and at times elusive because of the need for improved techniques to stay ahead of designer drugs, masking agents, or chemicals designed to thwart detection or camouflage the active EA.[7]

PREVENTION/DETECTION/ ANALYTICAL TESTING METHODS

1. Testing and analytical methods. Detection of foreign substances requires diligence, organization, and the analytical ability to ascertain the presence of the prohibitive substance or its metabolite(s) in body fluid samples. Some substances are allowed to be present but are prohibited to reach a certain (serum or urine) threshold. Below threshold, it is believed the substance lacks ergogenic potential (eg, caffeine) or is naturally occurring (eg, testosterone). Some testing methodology involves the use of surrogate markers or measuring the pharmacodynamic effect (eg, measuring hematocrit and hemoglobin as a test for oxygen-enhancing effects of erythropoietin).

TABLE 68-1 Partial List of Prohibited Substances and Methods

Substance Class	Substance Examples
Anabolic agents—endogenous	1-Androstenedione, bolasterone, boldenone, clostebol, danazol, fluoxymesterone, gestrinone, mestanolone, methyltestosterone, nandrolone oxandrolone quinbolone, stanozolol, tetrahydro-gestrinone, trenbolone
Anabolic agents—endogenous but administered exogenous	Androstenedione, dihydrotestosterone, testosterone, prasterone
Hormones and related substances	Erythropoietin, darbepoetin, growth hormone, insulin-like growth factors, chorionic gonadotropin, luteinizing hormone, insulins[a]
Beta-2 agonists	All beta-2 agonists including D-, L- isomers [a,b]
Hormone antagonists and modulators	Aromatase inhibitors (eg, anastrozole) selective estrogen receptor modulators (eg, tamoxifen)
Diuretics/masking agents	Loop diuretics (eg, furosemide), thiazides (eg, chlorthalidone, HTCZ), probenecid, plasma expanders (eg, albumin)
O_2 transfer enhancement	Blood doping, autologous transfusion, RBC products
Chemical and physical manipulation	Sample tampering; IV infusions
Gene doping	Peroxisome proliferator-activated receptor δ agonists
Stimulants	Amphetamine and derivatives; epinephrine and derivatives[c]
Narcotics	Morphine and opioid derivatives
Cannabinoids	Hashish, marijuana
Glucocorticoids#	Prednisone, methylprednisolone, and others
Alcohol	In-competition only; threshold = 0.1 g/L
Beta-blockers	In-competition only, specific sports

[a]Requires therapeutic use exemption when used as necessary medicine.
[b]Urine salmeterol concentration >1 μg/mL is an *adverse analytical finding* unless athlete proves otherwise.
[c]Adrenaline with local anesthetics or by local administration (nasal, ophthalmologic) is not prohibited.

2. Collection and chain-of-custody.[6,8] Chain-of-custody protocols are documents constructed to ensure appropriate collection, transportation, and laboratory analysis of the human specimen. The specimen must remain unadulterated or uncontaminated and is handled, manipulated, or analyzed as directed per protocol. Notably, drug testing is distinctly different than biomedical testing and should be acknowledged and differentiated by clinicians. It is important that body fluid collection must be witnessed (by one of the same sex if it is a urine test) and two samples (sample A and sample B) are provided. The sample collection is based on three principles

   i. Random athlete selection
   ii. Direct observation by same sex validator
   iii. Specimen integrity checks (eg, urine specific gravity and pH)

After the sample is collected, it is transported to an accredited laboratory for WADA—sponsored for international competition (WADA has only certified 35 laboratories

TABLE 68-2 Common Ergogenics Reference

Drug	Anticipated Effect	Immediate Response	Training Response	Testing Method
AAS	↑ Muscle mass		X	Drug identification (GC-MS, LC-MS) urine, T:E ratio
Stimulants	↓ Fatigue; ↑ metabolism	X		Urine GC-MS
Erythropoietin	↑ O_2 carrying capacity and endurance		X	IEF
HGH	↑ Muscle mass		X	IEF(?)
Creatine	↑ Muscle mass, ↑ATP		X	None
Androstenedione	↑ Muscle mass		X	Threshold; T:E ratio
Diuretics	Lose weight, masking	X		GC-MS

Abbreviations: AAS, androgenic-anabolic steroids; GC-MS, gas chromatography-mass spectrometry; LC-MS, liquid chromatography-mass spectrometry; T:E, testosterone to epitestosterone ratio; IEF, isoelectric focusing; HGH, human growth hormone.

throughout the world; three in North America: Los Angeles, Salt Lake City, Montreal) or a laboratory accredited by the sponsoring sports organization (eg, NCAA, NFL, MLB). The accredited laboratory personnel examine the sample(s) to ensure that no break in the custody chain has occurred. If sample A is found to be positive, then a repeat analytical procedure is performed for sample B.

3. Therapeutic use exemption (TUE).[9] TUE for a drug can be granted but cases are reviewed and assessed individually. It must be determined that (1) the medication in question is necessary for the athlete's condition and diagnosis was appropriate and accurate, (2) no benefit (performance enhancing) from the drug treatment is gained other than a return to a baseline state of health, (3) no reasonable therapeutic alternative is available, (4) the TUE cannot be for an effect from a prior nontherapeutic use of a prohibited substance (eg, therapy for a previous exogenous testosterone-induced gonadal atrophy), and (5) a TUE cannot be granted for "low levels" of endogenous hormone. Diseases do not lend themselves to quantitative measure.
4. Principal assays and analytical tests. The following are the assays and tests used to detect prohibited substances:
   a. Gas chromatography/mass spectrometry (GC/MS)—involves separating components of drug mixtures to specific ions based on chromatogenic characteristics. With GC/MS, submitted sample(s) must be compared with known reference standard(s).
   b. Liquid chromatography/mass spectrometry (LC/MS)—separation phase occurs in the liquid phase rather than in the gas phase with GC/MS.
   c. Qualification (eg, GC/MS), then ratio analysis (eg, testosterone: epitestosterone ratio).
   d. Use of endogenous compounds (erythropoietin, human chorionic gonadotropin, testosterone) is difficult to detect because exogenous and endogenous compounds have identical MS patterns; therefore, advanced techniques have been developed:
      i. Carbon isotope ratio testing (isotope ratio MS [IRMS])— designed to differentiate the exogenous compound from that which is naturally occurring, using isotopic differences in carbon (exogenous testosterone vs naturally produced testosterone).
      ii. Isoelectric focusing (IEF)—technique using a chemical moiety (eg, glycosylation) to separate exogenous substance from endogenous in a pH gradient electric field (this has been developed for recombinant erythropoietin detection).
5. Detection of a banned substance in one sample (A) warrants confirmation testing in a second sample (B). Analytical detection can be used for both exogenous and endogenous substance identification (testosterone, erythropoietin, human growth hormone). Analytical detection can also identify dietary and nutritional supplements if they have previously been identified and are on the prohibited list (eg, androstenedione). In some instances, analytical testing may not be able to distinguish exogenous from endogenous substances in the case of "naturally occurring chemicals" (eg, testosterone). Therefore, WADA or other organizations can establish thresholds or "cutoff" levels due to these naturally occurring substances or their metabolites (eg, 19-norandrosterone [testosterone metabolite] urine threshold is 2 ng/mL).

SPECIFIC ERGOGENIC AGENTS

Testosterone and Anabolic/Androgenic Steroids (AAS)

Overview

- Most widely abused substances; adolescent use estimates range from 4% to 12%.[2-4]
- Includes "designer" steroids such as tetrahydrogestrinone (THG).[10]

Pharmacology

Testosterone is responsible for secondary male sex characteristics and skeletal muscle anabolism and accretion. AAS were designed by modifying the chemical structure of testosterone and were produced to increase anabolic effects but reduce the androgenic effects of testosterone.

The pharmacologic actions of AAS mimic testosterone: skeletal muscle cell binding which allows cell entry and eventual nucleus binding. This then stimulates RNA messenger synthesis and produces an increase in structural and contractile proteins.

Both testosterone and AAS combat the catabolic effects of cortisol through competitive inhibition of the glucocorticoid receptor.

Ergogenic Evidence/Performance Evaluation

Well-designed clinical trials evaluating performance enhancement of AAS are lacking. Those that exist contain numerous methodological and design flaws. Results of small doses of AAS have shown equivocal results compared to placebo.[1] Studies have not taken into account the effects of multiple AAS given simultaneously or the extraordinarily large doses many athletes consume.

One study demonstrated an increase in lean body mass (LBM) and strength when administered in supraphysiologic doses to normal men.[11] This was not designed to demonstrate an enhancement in athletic performance.

Most experts agree that supraphysiologic doses of AAS or testosterone, when combined with strength training, lead to an increase in LBM, muscle size, and strength in normal men. Whether this will lead to improved athletic performance has not been demonstrated in research studies; however, this continues to be a contentious area of debate as most athletes that use and abuse anabolic steroids argue that their performance was significantly enhanced. AAS have been shown to reduce recovery time from strenuous exercise, thus, indirectly improving performance.[10] Clearly, ethical reasoning for future studies limits research.

Side Effects (SE) and Adverse Reactions

AAS are banned substances and unethical in athletic competition, therefore, quantifying SE is difficult. Once again, existing studies contain poor methodology and analysis of the SE profile proves difficult to quantify accurately.

There is an association between atherogenic lipid profiles (↓HDL, ↑LDL) and endothelial dysfunction/risk for atherosclerosis. Androgens are known to worsen atherogenic profiles. Whether this has contributed to cardiovascular events is unknown but case reports exist. AAS have also been shown to increase blood pressure, especially diastolic blood pressure (~25%) and will increase the risk for liver transaminasemia. AAS side effects appear to be reversible with drug cessation; however, anecdotal deaths (cardiovascular, sudden cardiac death, hypertensive crisis) have been reported throughout the literature.

AAS have the potential to induce or unmask significant psychoses.[12] Evidence exists suggesting AAS use may be associated with an increased risk of violent death from impulsive, aggressive, or depressive behaviors.[12] Whether this is a direct causal relationship or the effect of unveiling underlying disorders has not been ascertained.

Regulation and Testing

AAS and testosterone products are classified by the DEA as Schedule III substances because of their abuse potential. They are banned and tested substances in organizations that include but are not limited to: WADA, NCAA, USOC, NBA, MLB, and the NFL. GC/MS is often used to identify the substances in urine samples.

The use of exogenous testosterone presents a specific problem because the exogenous product and the endogenous compound have identical spectrometric patterns.

A testosterone: epitestosterone ratio is commonly used as an analytical test:

- Normally, this ratio is 1:1; the *allowable* threshold is usually 4:1.
- One can subvert this analysis by taking exogenous epitestosterone to increase its concentration, allowing an increase in testosterone, either endogenous or exogenous, thus, a urine concentration threshold exists for epitestosterone (200 ng/mL).
- Random testing will occur (WADA).

A ketoconazole test has also been used. Healthy, adult males will demonstrate a decrease in testosterone concentrations and T:E ratio when administered ketoconazole. If one is taking exogenous testosterone, no decrease in testosterone concentrations occurs and the T:E ratio increases.

Carbon isotope ratio testing: Isotope ratio MS (IRMS) is a new technique that may be a new analytical testing approach. IRMS is able to differentiate exogenous testosterone and/or epitestosterone from that which is endogenous by utilizing isotopic differences in structure carbons, which could have significant utility.

Human Growth Hormone (HGH)

Overview

- HGH is an endogenous peptide with metabolic functions generally considered anabolic and growth promoting.
- Athletes will attempt to stimulate muscular growth by supplementing with exogenous hormone, now available by recombinant techniques.
- There is a large underground market that traffics HGH.

Pharmacology

HGH is a 22,000-Dalton peptide that is released from the anterior pituitary gland. Endogenous release and regulation is by growth hormone–releasing hormone, sleep, exercise, L-dopamine and arginine.[1,13] HGH stimulates hepatic gluconeogenesis and lipolysis and facilitates the transport of amino acids across cell membranes, increasing RNA amounts leading to increased protein synthesis.[13] GH, thus, predominantly causes cellular hyperplasia whereas AAS tends to cause skeletal muscle cell hypertrophy. Growth hormone works synergistically with other growth factors (eg, insulin-like growth factor).

Ergogenic Evidence/Performance Evaluation

Animal studies have shown recombinant HGH leads to skeletal hyperplasia and hypertrophy but this increase in muscle mass is not associated with proportionate increases in strength. This is further evidenced by acromegalics that have increased GH levels and larger muscle mass but functionally and proportionally weaker muscles.[13] There are little research data with regard to human performance evaluation or muscle accretion with HGH. A recent systematic review of the scientific literature does not support ergogenic claims.[14] Limited evidence suggests that HGH can increase lean body mass, but may not improve strength. Much of the hypertrophy is thought to be an increase in fluid/water volume in the skeletal muscle cell. Other evidence suggests it may *worsen* exercise capacity and increase adverse effects.[14]

Side Effects and Adverse Reactions

Based on studies of agromegalics, high levels of HGH over long periods of time can lead to myopathies, fluid retention, diabetes, and heart failure, all of which are irreversible.[13] Fatigue, arthralgias, and carpal tunnel syndrome occur more often in individuals treated with HGH than those not treated.[14]

Regulation and Testing

The use of HGH to enhance athletic performance is prohibited by WADA[5] and other organizations. Exogenous injection of recombinant HGH is undetectable after 24 hours. Because HGH exerts most of its effects through receptors at target cells, marker or mediators are sometimes tracked (eg, insulin-like growth factor or somatomedin-C). Recent new technology has been able to ascertain exogenous use of HGH from nonusers; however, this test has not been forensically challenged.[8]

Amphetamines/Stimulants

Overview

- Historically, these are drugs of abuse with track and field, MLB and NFL athletes.
- These compounds are congeners of amphetamine and epinephrine and exist throughout the prescription drug, OTC, herbal, and dietary supplement markets.

Pharmacology

Amphetamines are chemically related to catecholamines and stimulate the release of epinephrine and norepinephrine from sympathetic nerve endings resulting in increases in HR, BP, vasoconstriction, and bronchodilation. Amphetamines promote a relative "immediate" effect and are short lived. They do not produce long-lasting "training" effects. They can elevate mood and promote short-term fatigue resistance, likely via dopaminergic pathway modification.

Ergogenic Evidence/Performance Evaluation

There is a paucity of data with regard to exercise performance assessment and much is anecdotal. Studies exist demonstrating a moderate resistance to fatigue but no increase in VO_{2max} or strength. Some have suggested a mild, short-term increase in strength; the combination of ephedrine and caffeine has been shown to increase endurance secondary to glycogen sparing (increased lipolysis).[15-17]

Side Effects

Cardiovascular side effects (HTN, stroke, TIA, ventricular dysrhythmias) occur at a rate two- to threefold greater than placebo.[15] CNS effects such as anxiety, paranoia, and hallucinations are also increased with stimulant use. Dependence and addiction can occur with relative frequency.

Regulation and Testing

Amphetamine and its congeners are listed in the WADA Prohibitive List[5] and most other amateur and professional organizations ban their use (eg, NFL, USOC). Traditional analytical methods such as GC/MS are most often used to detect substances. Many amphetamine and stimulant derivatives and congeners are OTC and are in herbal and dietary supplement preparations and it is the athlete's responsibility to know what they are ingesting.

Erythropoietin, Darbepoetin, and Blood Doping

Overview

- Used and abused by endurance athletes seeking to increase oxygen-carrying capacity of the red blood cells (RBC)
- Exogenous administration of erythropoietin (rhEPO) or darbepoetin (rDPO) produces similar response to that of living/training at high altitudes or autologous transfusion of previously phlebotomized blood after a period of hematocrit recovery

Pharmacology

Erythropoietin is a natural, growth-type hormone produced in the kidneys that stimulates the bone marrow to produce RBC. It has been suggested that an increase in hemoglobin concentration by 1g/dL with an athletic cardiac output of 25 L/min and a normal VO_{2max} of 4 L/min can increase oxygen transport by up to 335 mL or approximately 8%.[1] Animal studies suggest an increase in glycogen stores as well. This would suggest that energy substrate use during exercise is affected by enhanced O_2 availability (ie, supplementation with rhEPO or rDPO results in lower contribution of anaerobic metabolism to energy production).[1,18]

Ergogenic Evidence/Performance Evaluation

Autologous transfusions or blood doping has been associated with approximately a 7% increase in hemoglobin concentration, a 5% increase in VO_{2max} and a 34% increase in time to exhaustion at 95% VO_{2max} and 44-second decrease in 5-mile treadmill run time.[1] Other studies have confirmed these increases and also demonstrate that aerobically fit individuals experience approximately twice the maximal uptake than that of normal individuals.[1,19-21]

Side Effects and Adverse Reactions

Increasing hematocrit/hemoglobin by exogenous use of rEPO and rDPO or by blood doping can produce abnormally high concentrations of RBC and can increase the risk of cerebrovascular events such as stroke or TIA, myocardial infarction, systemic and pulmonary HTN, pulmonary emboli, and both arterial and venous thromboembolic disease. Blood doping also carries an infectious risk as well, despite reinfusion of one's own blood.

Regulation and Testing

Oxygen enhancement drugs and invasive methods are prohibited by WADA.[5,8] Other competitive organizations may vary but it is incumbent upon the athlete to be aware of specific organizational rules. There is no specific test currently for detecting exogenous erythropoietin. Most commonly, it is assessed by monitoring indirect or pharmacodynamic markers (hematocrit, hemoglobin concentration). Recently, an IEF urine test has been developed to detect exogenous administration. Darbepoetin is chemically different than endogenous erythropoietin and can be detected with both GC/MS and IEF.

Creatine

Overview

- Creatine has become a very popular ergogenic aid in the nutraceutical market. There is no federal assessment of quality or quantity within this market.
- Creatine is popular in anaerobic, short-energy burst athletic performance.

Pharmacology

Creatine is a naturally occurring nitrogenous amino acid peptide synthesized in the liver, pancreas, and kidney and stored in skeletal muscle. The creatine–energy associated equation is as follows:

$$\text{Phosphocreatine} + \text{ADP} + \text{H}^+ \leftrightarrow \text{ATP} + \text{Creatine}$$

- ADP = adenosine diphosphate
- ATP = adenosine triphosphate
- Catalyzed by creatine phosphokinase

In short, phosphorylated creatine contributes to rapid resynthesis of ATP during short-term episodes of strenuous physical exertion. Phosphocreatine supplementation has been shown to increase muscles stores up to 50%. Studies have demonstrated decreased anaerobic glycolysis during brief but maximal exercise.[1,22]

Ergogenic Evidence/Performance Evaluation

Weight-resistance exercises, mainly single-repetition maximal amounts, have shown increases of approximately 25% in small cohort studies.[22] Whether this extrapolates to improved athletic performance has not been demonstrated. With sprint cyclists, most studies have suggested that creatine supplementation is effective in maintaining muscle force and power output.[22] However, sprint swimming has demonstrated equivocal results with some results showing a decrease in sprint times and others demonstrating no benefit.[1,22]

Track and field athletes have found minimal benefit overall. Similarly, older athletes have found little improvement in athletic performances. Studies have found that creatine, as a training aid supplement, appears to increase LBM about 1-2 kg over a short-term supplementing cycle (eg, 6-8 weeks).[1,22]

Creatine can be an effective mass-accreting, potentially ergogenic, supplement when used for simple, short duration, maximal effort, anaerobic events.[1] The major exception seems to be with sprint swimming.

Side Effects and Adverse Reactions

There have been isolated case reports of renal SE including acute renal failure, although no cause-effect has been established. None of the short term randomized controlled trials with creatine have demonstrated adverse SE profiles in healthy athletes; however, this should not be extrapolated beyond this cohort.

Long-term administration concerns include down-regulation of the internal feedback control of creatine transporter proteins and resistance to the compound. Long-term safety with regard to other organ toxicity has not been fully assessed.

Regulation and Testing

Phosphocreatine is widely available in OTC and dietary supplements. Currently, it is not banned by WADA or other competitive organizations. The NCAA stipulates that none of its member teams are to provide creatine to their players[1]. Currently, there is no active test for detection of exogenous creatine.

Androstenedione

Overview

- Androstenedione is a precursor of and directly converted to testosterone. It is marketed as a dietary supplement that can increase testosterone levels, thus, acting as an alternative to testosterone administration.

Pharmacology

Chemically, androstenedione is the immediate precursor to testosterone and is thought to work by being degraded to testosterone. Effectiveness of androstenedione is based on the functionality of testosterone, assuming it can increase testosterone concentrations.

Little evidence supports that the "nutraceutically" marketed dose of androstenedione increases testosterone concentrations significantly. Increasing the androstenedione dose can increase testosterone concentrations but also increases estrogen concentrations, producing antiandrogenic effects.[23]

Ergogenic Evidence/Performance Evaluation

Studies evaluating the performance-enhancing effects and the anabolic effects of androstenedione supplementation have revealed no significant ergogenic or mass accretion effect of any kind.[1,23,24,]

Side Effects and Adverse Reactions

Because of its androgenic pharmacology, it is not surprising that lipid profiles have been shown to be adversely affected (decreased HDL) and may increase cardiovascular risk.[1] One study demonstrated increased estrogenic effects and down-regulation of endogenous testosterone synthesis.[23]

Regulation and Testing

Androstenedione is nonprescription and is available in many OTC, dietary, and herbal supplements. It is banned by the WADA[5] but may vary in other organizations. It is currently banned by the NFL, USOC, NCAA, and most recently, MLB.

Monitoring and testing for androstenedione occurs mainly through sensitive GC/MS and threshold determination, including T:E ratio determinations.

EDUCATION AND PROGRAM CONTROL[25]

The primary focus of an educational program to abate, minimize, and prevent illicit EA use begins with the development of a mission and purpose for the program and making sure all parties within the system understand and buy into the program. Second, securing adequate resources for collection and testing aspects of the program is very important.

The athlete-testing protocol should include at minimum, the following components:

- Establishment of a correct chain-of-custody
- Use of third party administrators to collect samples to prevent inherent conflict of interest

- Use of a high-quality laboratory or an accredited one, if available
- Involvement of important stakeholders in the testing development process: coaches, athletes, administrators, certified athletic trainers, legal counsel, etc

Drug education and counseling resources should be available to all coaches, athletes, and athletic trainers with regard to the pharmacology and pharmacodynamics of the tested agents. This should be offered early and routinely. Evidence-based medicine and pharmacy, ethics, and adverse effects should be integral components of the education program.[7]

CASE Application

1. A female swimmer preparing for the US National Championships has been notified that she is required to submit a random urine sample for analysis. She calls you and asks if she can provide the sample herself or if she must consent to the collector's protocol. Your best response to this question is:

   a. Yes, you can prepare a sample and send it in to the appropriate laboratory.
   b. Yes, but your coach must witness the sample.
   c. No, according to the USOC policy, all chain-of-custody protocols must be followed.
   d. No, you must report to the nearest hospital laboratory to submit the sample.

2. JM is a competing cyclist and will likely compete on the European circuit this summer. He has an underlying asthma disorder that you help to manage. He was previously managing his asthma with formoterol/budesonide 4.5 μg/80 μg actuation inhalation aerosol: two inhalations twice daily and an occasional albuterol inhalation as needed for rescue. He has recently experienced some mild worsening. His asthma medications have changed to formoterol/budesonide 4.5 μg/160 μg actuations by aerosol (Symbicort) two inhalations twice daily with albuterol as a rescue inhaler. Last year he obtained a "therapeutic use exemption" (TUE). He asks you if he will require another TUE. Your best response to this question is:

   a. Yes, he will require a new TUE.
   b. No, since he has already obtained one, he need not obtain another.
   c. No, asthma medicines have been removed from the "prohibited list" for international competition.
   d. Yes, but only for the albuterol since it is short acting.

3. A competitor in a cross-country ski race is consuming caffeine and pseudoephedrine prior to his competition. He is likely using this combination for what purpose?

   a. To increase his heart rate
   b. To increase his blood pressure
   c. To increase his alertness
   d. To spare his glycogen stores

4. Androstenedione (Andro) is a dietary supplement touted to act as an anabolic agent. The purported basic science behind this theory is best described by which of the following?

   a. Androstenedione blocks the breakdown of endogenous testosterone.
   b. Androstenedione is a natural anabolic steroidal compound that acts at the androgenic receptors with a higher affinity than testosterone.
   c. Androstenedione is a precursor in the cascade of steps that produces testosterone.
   d. Androstenedione has no anabolic potential.

5. The most common analytical test used to assess whether exogenous testosterone or one of its derivatives has been used is which of the following?

   a. Androstenedione: testosterone ratio
   b. Testosterone: epitestosterone ratio
   c. Urine sample of 19-Nandrolone
   d. Blood specimen of 19-NA

6. JS is college football player who is training during the off-season. He asks you about supplementing his dietary regimen with creatine monophosphate. He specifically asks if the creatine supplementation will positively affect his exercise performance. Of the following, which factor is the *least* likely to affect creatine's effect on exercise performance?

   a. Dose
   b. Trained versus untrained individuals
   c. Laboratory studies versus actual studies
   d. Concomitant medications

7. BB is a 24-year-old body builder that presents to you complaining of female-like breast development that is somewhat painful. Upon questioning him, you discover that he takes 2 mg daily of stanozolol, 20 mg of methandrostenolone (Dianabol), and an injection of testosterone cypionate IM once weekly. He also takes a multitude of multivitamins and supplements and eats about 6000 kcal daily. He is 5'10" and weighs 225 lb; his HR is 80 beats/min and BP is 162/94 mm Hg. He states that he feels he is dependent on the steroids for his muscle mass and appearance. His laboratory values include Scr 1.3 mg/dL, BUN 32 mg/dL, Na 138 mEq/L, K 4.4 mEq/L, Cl 99 mEq/L, CO_2 22 mEq/L, ALT 120 U/L, AST 80 U/L, HDL 34 mg/dL, LDL 180 mg/dL, and TC 220 mg/dL. Assuming you cannot convince BB to abate his steroid abuse, what do you think his greatest risk from long-term use would be?

   a. Cardiovascular risk
   b. Hepatotoxicity
   c. Breast cancer
   d. Psychoses

8. LL is a 34-year-old single woman who likes to compete in local cycling events. She has a history of a leg DVT 3 years ago, thought secondary to her use of oral contraceptives. She currently takes no prescription medications but does take a calcium supplement and a multivitamin. She is otherwise healthy. She is employed as an LPN at an oncology clinic where she was asked to label for destruction and shipping some outdated darbepoetin. She confides in you that she took a couple of vials because she had read somewhere that substances like this can improve cycling performance. Of the following, what do you think the best response would be?
   a. Turn her to the DEA immediately.
   b. Inform her that the increase in hematocrit will likely induce a pulmonary embolus in her given her history.
   c. Educate and encourage clean competition and to disclose what she did to her superiors.
   d. The drug was outdated, it will have no effect.

9. To gain an alleged ergogenic benefit from anabolic steroids, they must be used
   a. Immediately (30 minutes) before competition.
   b. 2 weeks before competition.
   c. Cyclically in one's training regimen months before competition.
   d. They offer no ergogenic benefit.

10. Fostering an antidrug mentality in sports and athletics means focusing on
   a. The ill effects and adverse reactions of the agents involved
   b. Denying any purported benefit from the drugs
   c. An appeal to communities through "town hall" meetings
   d. Behavior, drug education, and athletes' social sphere of influence

11. LA is a competitive cyclist. Recently his random urine sample revealed a testosterone: epitestosterone (T:E) ratio of 12:1. His sample from 10 days ago revealed a T:E ratio of 4:1. A reasonable explanation for the difference between these two ratios would be which of the following?
   a. T:E ratios can vary widely between stages of rest and intense exercise. One of the values was likely during a rest cycle.
   b. This may be indicative of a pathology where he cannot metabolize his testosterone.
   c. This sample likely indicates exogenous testosterone supplementation.
   d. There is likely an error in the testing process.

12. KM comes into your pharmacy with a prescription for propranolol 20 mg. The signatura (SIG) on the prescription reads "take as directed." As you question KM about this, you determine the propranolol is only taken during her archery competitions. She states that the competition increases her blood pressure. The most likely conclusion you should glean from this would be which of the following?
   a. Competition does, indeed, increase the BP of many competitors and, thus, for medical and safety reasons, you should dispense the prescription.
   b. KM is using the beta-adrenergic blocking drug, propranolol, to block adrenergic response peripherally (decrease tremors) and thus using the drug unethically.
   c. KM is using the beta-adrenergic blocking drug, propranolol, to block beta-2 receptors in her lung bed to control her breathing while she competes, thus using the drug unethically.
   d. KM is using the drug as an ergogenic aid to boost her performance, but it is permissible under international competition rules.

13. You have been asked to serve as a consultant on a panel analyzing competitor samples. A "sample A" specimen turns up positive for the drug probenecid. The panel asks your assessment of this drug. Of the following, which would be the best response?
   a. Probenecid blocks the tubular secretion of many drugs including some AAS and their metabolites and was used to mask the sample. Sample B should be tested and the appropriate administrative authorities should be notified.
   b. Probenecid can act as an anabolic agent. Sample B should be tested and the appropriate administrative authorities should be notified.
   c. Probenecid can act as an oxygen enhancer. Sample B should be tested and the appropriate administrative authorities should be notified.
   d. Probenecid prevents catabolic breakdown of skeletal proteins in athletes, helping them to recover from training. It is not on the 2009 Prohibited List and the sample should be disregarded.

14. Which of the following would be considered *least* likely to be an ergogenic substance that produces an "immediate" effect?
   a. Marijuana
   b. Albuterol
   c. Modafinil
   d. Erythropoietin

15. A group of parents approach you because they are concerned some student-athletes may be using human growth hormone (HGH) in an attempt to increase muscle mass. They inquire how to test for this agent. Of the following, what would be your best response?
   a. Currently, there is no definitive test for exogenously administered recombinant HGH and surrogate markers must be utilized.

b. While there may be some lean mass accretion, there are no data to confirm an actual ergogenic benefit, so the parents should not be concerned.
c. Currently, there is no definitive test for exogenously administered recombinant HGH; monitoring for a SE profile is the best way to detect its use.
d. Set up a program and threshold levels and begin measuring serum levels of HGH.

16. Which of the following is not considered legitimate criteria for granting a therapeutic use exemption (TUE)?
    a. The athlete would experience significant health problems without taking the prohibited substance or method.
    b. The substance is needed to treat the side effects of previously administered ergogenic aids (eg, testosterone for gonadal atrophy from previous abuse of AAS).
    c. There is no reasonable therapeutic alternative to the use of the otherwise prohibited substance or method.
    d. The therapeutic use of the substance would produce no additional enhancement of a performance other than that which might be anticipated by a return to a state of normal health.

17. A 22-year-old female cross-country skier is planning on national and international competition and asks you if she can consume caffeine on daily basis without concern. Which of the following provides the best response?
    a. No, caffeine exists on the WADA prohibited use.
    b. Yes, caffeine is monitored on an in-competition basis only and even then, can be consumed to a certain urine threshold.
    c. Yes, caffeine is monitored on an in-competition basis but must be discontinued 24 hours prior to any competition.
    d. Yes, but evidence exists suggesting caffeine is deleterious to endurance performance.

18. JS is a football player alleged to have taken AAS. Which of the following would not be considered a confirmatory test to monitor for exogenous AAS?
    a. Gas chromatography
    b. T:E ratio
    c. Ketoconazole administration
    d. Polygraph test

19. RJ, an aspiring baseball player, states that he has been taking nutraceuticals and dietary supplements so as to avoid prescription drugs that are prohibited in organized baseball. He asks you what your opinion is about this. Of the following, your best response would be:
    a. This is a good plan for maintaining nutrition but avoiding prohibited substances.
    b. This is a good plan for avoiding prohibited substances but will not improve his performance.
    c. This is not a good plan. Many prohibited substances are components of dietary supplements and nutraceuticals.
    d. This is not a good plan. Many nutraceuticals and dietary supplements can be identified in the urine.

20. JR is a long-distance cyclist that recently suffered a transient ischemic attack (TIA). He reported to the emergency department (ED) where he related no prescription drug use. His vitals in the ED were: BP 164/90 mm Hg, RR 20 breaths/min, HR 52 beats/min and regular, temperature 99°F. His BUN was 18 mg/dL and his Scr was 1.1 mg/dL. Of note, his hemoglobin was 19 g/dL and his hematocrit was 57.2%. He was assessed as being well hydrated but not fluid overloaded. He was no longer suffering from any neurologic deficit. He did not lose consciousness. A urine test using isoelectric focusing would likely be positive for which exogenously administered substance?
    a. Testosterone
    b. Recombinant human growth hormone
    c. Recombinant erythropoietin
    d. Recombinant human chorionic gonadotropin

TAKEAWAY POINTS ››

- Promotion of education and program control needs to involve stakeholders: administrators, coaches, athletes, trainers, physicians, pharmacists, legal counsel. Other components of a good educational program include banned substances lists, who is tested, how often the testing can and will occur, consequences of positive tests, and chain-of-custody methods.
- The spirit of ethics and competition should prevail over cheating and it is incumbent upon athletes, coaches, and health-care professionals to become educated on the use and abuse of pharmaceuticals and nutraceuticals and on sport/organizational-specific restrictions.
- The emphasis on athletic performance and more importantly, winning, will drive athletes, coaches, trainers, and, in some cases, administrators and owners, to use, encourage the use of, and allow the use of ergogenic substances.
- Physicians, pharmacists, sports psychologists, and exercise physiologist researchers are frequently asked to serve as medical directors or education/review officers for drug testing, athlete education, results interpretation, or therapeutic use exemption.
- Different compounds may represent banned substances in different competitive sports and, thus, prohibitive lists are sport specific.

- Agents may be classified as training augmentation agents or those that produce a relative immediate effect (eg, amphetamines, bronchodilating drugs)
- It is imperative that athletes competing within a certain sport understand the governing organization's rules about performance enhancers. Generally, athletes are responsible for any prohibited substance or its metabolites or markers found to be present in their samples.
- Randomized, controlled trials to ascertain performance enhancement properties are unlikely to be constructed and evidence-based conclusions and recommendations will unlikely be forthcoming because of the ethical component of fair competition in sports.

REFERENCES

1. Tokish JM, Kocher MS, Hawkins RJ. Ergogenic aids: a review of basic science, performance, side effects, and status in sports. *Am J Sports Med*. 2004;32:1543-1553
2. Bahrke MS, Yesalis CE, Brower KJ. Anabolic-androgenic steroid abuse and performance-enhancing drugs among adolescents. *Child Adolesc Psychiatr Clin N Am*. 1998;7: 821-838.
3. Faigenbaum AD, Zaichkowsky LD, Gardner DE, Micheli LJ. Anaboic steroid use by male and female middle school students. *Pediatrics*. 1998;101(5). Available at: http://www.pediatrics.org/cgi/content/full/101/5/e6. Accessed July 20,2009.
4. Yesalis CE, Barsukiewicz CK, Kopstein AN, Bahrke MS. Trends in anabolic-androgenic steroid use among adolescents. *Arch Ped Adol Med*. 1997;151:1197-1206.
5. World Anti-Doping Agency. The 2009 Prohibited List International Standard. Available at: http://www.wada ama.org/rtecontent/document/2009_Prohibited_list_Eng_Final_20_Sept_08_pdf. Accessed July 18, 2009.
6. World Anti-Doping Agency. World Anti-Doping Code. Available at: http://www.wada-ama.org/rtecontent. Accessed July 18, 2009.
7. Goldberg L, Elliot DL, Clarke GN, et al. Effects of a multidimensional anabolic steroid prevention intervention: the Adolescents Training and Learning to Avoid Steroids (ATLAS) Program. *JAMA*. 1996;276:1555-1562
8. Green GA. Doping control for the team physician. A review of drug testing procedures in sport. *Am J Sports Med*. 2006;34:1690-1698.
9. World Anti-Doping Agency. Therapeutic Use Exemption International Standard. Available at: http://www.wada-ama.org/rtecontent/document. Accessed July 18, 2009.
10. FDA Statement on THG. Available at: http://www.fda.gov/bbs/topics/NEWS/2003/NEW00967.html. Accessed November 15, 2003.
11. Bhasis S, Storer TW, Berman N, et al. The effects of supraphysiologic doses of testosterone on muscle size and strength in normal men. *N Engl J Med*. 1996;335:1-7.
12. Reents S. Androgenic—anabolic steroids. In: Bahrke MS, McEntire C, Wentworth J, eds. *Sport and Exercise Pharmacology*. Champaign, IL: Human Kinetics; 2000: 161.
13. Reents S. Human growth hormone. In: Bahrke MS, McEntire C, Wentworth J, eds. *Sport and Exercise Pharmacology*. Champaign, IL: Human Kinetics; 2000: 149.
14. Liu H, Bravata DM, Olkin I, et al. Systematic review of growth hormone on athletic performance. *Ann Intern Med*. 2008;148:747-758.
15. Shekelle PG, Hardy ML, Morton SC, et al. Efficacy and safety of ephedra and ephedrine for weight loss and athletic performance. *JAMA*. 2003;289:1537-1545.
16. Bell DG, McLellan TM, Sabiston CM. Effect of ingesting caffeine and ephedrine of 10-km run performance. *Med Sci Sport Exerc*. 2002;34:344-349.
17. Jacobs I, Pasternak H, Bell DG. Effects of ephedrine, caffeine, and their combination on muscular endurance. *Med Sci Sport Exerc*. 2003;35:987-994.
18. Reents S. Iron and erythropoietin (Epoetin Alfa). In: Bahreke MS, McEntire C, Wentworth J, eds. *Sport and Exercise Pharmacology*. Champaign, IL: Human Kinetics; 2000:203.
19. Sawka MN, Young AJ, Muza SR, Gonzalez RR, Pandolf KB. Erythrocyte Reinfusion and Maximal Aerobic *Power JAMA*. 1987;257:1496-99
20. Ekblom B. Blood doping and erythropoietin. *Am J Sports Med*. 1996;24(suppl):S40-S42.
21. Audran M, Gareau R, Matecki S, et al. Effects of erythropoietin administration in training athletes and possible indirect detection in doping control. *Med Sci Sports Exerc*. 1999;31:639-645.
22. Reents S. Creatine. In: Bahreke MS, McEntire C, Wentworth J, eds. *Sport and Exercise Pharmacology*. Champaign, IL, Human Kinetics; 2000;p185
23. Leder BZ, Longcope C, Catlin DH, Ahrens B, Achoenfeld DA, Finkelstein JS. Oral androstenedione administration and serum testosterone concentrations in young men. *JAMA*. 2000;283:779-782.
24. Broeder CE, Quindry J, Brittingham K, et al. The andro project. *Arch Int Med*. 2000;160:3093-3104.
25. Goldberg L, Elliot DL, Clarke GN, et al. Effects of a multidimensional anabolic steroid prevention intervention: the Adolescents Training and Learning to Avoid Steroids (ATLAS) Program. *JAMA*. 1996;276:1555-1562.

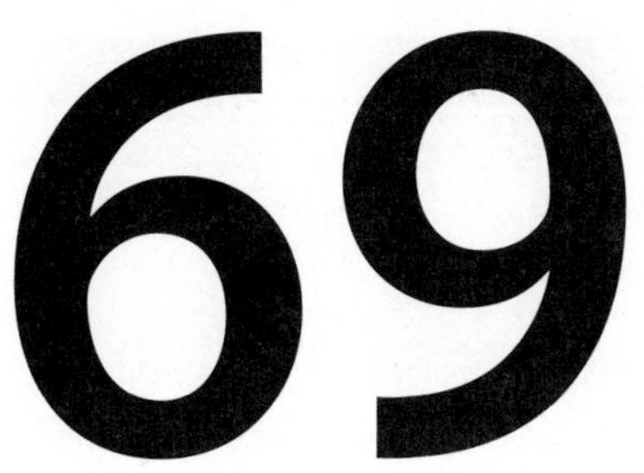

Vaccines and Immunizations

Patricia H. Powell and Catherine H. Kuhn

VACCINE PREVENTABLE DISEASES

Rates of vaccine preventable diseases in the United States are at an all time low due to the routine vaccination of infants, children, and adults.[1] Unfortunately, gaps in coverage still exist. Providers are not only responsible for the appropriate administration of vaccines; they are also responsible for ensuring patients receive appropriate vaccinations as recommended by the ACIP. Only routine childhood, adolescent, and adult vaccines are covered in this chapter. Readers are encouraged to visit the CDC vaccines website (http://www.cdc.gov/vaccines/) for information regarding travel and bioterrorism vaccines.

Indications

Indications and target populations for the vaccines available for use in the United States are listed in Table 69-1.

Key Definitions

ACIP = Advisory Committee on Immunization Practices
CDC = Centers for Disease Control and Prevention
DTaP = pediatric diphtheria toxoid, tetanus toxoid, and acellular pertussis vaccine
DT = pediatric diphtheria-tetanus toxoid vaccine
GBS = Guillain-Barré syndrome
GSK = GlaxoSmithKline
Hep A = hepatitis A
Hep B = hepatitis B
Hib = *Haemophilus influenzae* type b
HIV = human immunodeficiency virus
HPV = human papillomavirus
IM = intramuscularly
IPV = inactivated poliovirus
MCV = meningococcal conjugate vaccine
MPSV = meningococcal polysaccharide vaccine
MMR = measles, mumps, rubella
MMWR = *Morbidity and Mortality Weekly Report*
PCV = pneumococcal conjugate vaccine
PPSV = pneumococcal polysaccharide vaccine
RV = rotavirus
SC = subcutaneously
SP = Sanofi Pasteur
Td = adult tetanus-diphtheria toxoid vaccine
Tdap = tetanus, diphtheria toxoids, and acellular pertussis vaccine
Varicella = varicella zoster virus
Zoster = herpes zoster virus

Diphtheria, Tetanus, and Pertussis (DTaP, DT, Td, and Tdap)

Diphtheria is a disease caused by a toxin produced by *Corynebacterium diphtheriae.* The bacterium is transmitted person-to-person through respiratory droplets and most commonly infects the pharynx and tonsils. Symptoms include fever, sore throat, and a bluish-white membrane on the soft palate.[2] The membrane can grow leading to respiratory obstruction. Systemic absorption of the toxin can occur and causes tachycardia, stupor, coma, and death. More serious complications, such as myocarditis, neuritis, thrombocytopenia, and proteinuria, are caused by the toxin produced by certain strains of diphtheria. A diphtheria toxoid is available in different combinations with tetanus toxoid and pertussis vaccine. Diphtheria toxoid, tetanus toxoid, and acellular pertussis (DTaP) and diphtheria-tetanus toxoid (DT) vaccines contain a larger amount of diphtheria toxoid and are indicated in children <7 years of age. Children who have had an anaphylactic reaction to the pertussis vaccine should receive DT as their primary diphtheria-tetanus vaccine. Adults receive Td or Tdap because these products contain a smaller dose of the diphtheria toxoid.[2]

Tetanus is a disease caused by an exotoxin produced by *Clostridium tetani.* The spores are found in soil and generally enter the body through a wound. Tetanus commonly presents with trismus (lockjaw) and difficulty swallowing which progresses as descending paralysis, muscle rigidity, and convulsions.[3] Major complications include laryngospasm and spine or hip fractures due to the convulsions. A tetanus toxoid was developed in the 1920s and is currently available in combination with diphtheria toxoid and pertussis vaccine.[3]

Pertussis, or "whooping cough," is a highly contagious respiratory infection caused by *Bordetella pertussis.* Patients commonly present with a deep cough that makes it difficult to breathe and the cough can last for more than 3 weeks. Since antibiotics do little to decrease the duration of symptoms, routine vaccination is the primary method used to decrease incidence.[4] In recent years, the number of cases of pertussis in adolescents and adults has increased because immunity to pertussis decreases 5 to 10 years after vaccination. For this reason, ACIP recommends adolescents and adults ages 11 to 64 years obtain one booster dose of the Tdap vaccine to replace a single dose of Td.[5,6]

TABLE 69-1 Vaccine Indications

Vaccine	Indication	Target Population
DTaP	Prevention of diphtheria, tetanus, and pertussis	Children <7 y of age
Td	Booster immunization against tetanus and diphtheria as well as tetanus prophylaxis in wound management	Adolescents and adults >7 y of age
Tdap	Booster immunization against tetanus, diphtheria, and pertussis	Adolescents and adults 10-64 y (Boostrix) or 11-64 y (Adacel)
DT	Prevention of diphtheria and tetanus	Children <7 y of age who are allergic to the pertussis vaccine
Hep A	Prevention of hepatitis A infection	Children >12 mo of age Adults at high risk for Hep A infection
Hep B	Prevention of hepatitis B infection	All infants beginning at birth Unvaccinated children and adolescents Adults at high risk for Hep B infection
Hib	Prevention of invasive bacterial disease caused by *Haemophilus influenzae* type b	Children <5 y of age Adults with sickle cell disease, asplenia, leukemia, or HIV infection
HPV-4	Prevention of cervical cancer, precancerous or dysplastic lesions, and genital warts caused by the human papillomavirus types 6, 11, 16, 18	Females aged 9-26 y Males 9-26 y[a]
HPV-2	Prevention of cervical cancer, cervical intraepithelial neoplasia, and adenocarcinoma in situ caused by HPV types 16 and 18	Females aged 10-25 y
IPV	Prevention of poliomyelitis cause by poliovirus types 1,2,3	All children
MCV, MPSV	Prevention of invasive meningococcal disease caused by *N. meningitidis* serogroups A, C, Y, W135	Adolescents 11-12 y of age Adults at high risk for meningococcal disease
MMR	Prevention of measles, mumps, rubella, and congenital rubella syndrome	Children >12 mo of age
PCV	Prevention of invasive pneumococcal disease caused by *S. pneumoniae*	Children <2 y of age
PPSV	Prevention of invasive pneumococcal disease caused by *S. pneumoniae*	Adults ≥65 y of age Aged 2-64 y with chronic conditions (diabetes, asthma, cardiovascular disease), asplenia, HIV infection, or those who smoke
RV	Prevention of gastroenteritis caused by rotavirus	Infants aged 6 wk to 8 mo
Varicella	Prevention of varicella caused by varicella-zoster	Children >12 mo
Zoster	Prevention of shingles and reducing the pain associated with shingles caused by herpes zoster	Adults over the age of 60 y

[a]HPV-4 vaccine may be used in males to prevent genital warts; however routine vaccine is not recommended.

Haemophilus Influenzae Type b (Hib)

Haemophilus influenza is a bacterium that enters the body through the nasopharynx. There are six different serotypes (a-f), the majority of which remain locally and cause flu-like symptoms.[7] In some cases, the organism enters the bloodstream and causes invasive disease, such as meningitis. Type b was the leading cause of meningitis in children <5 years of age before routine vaccination was recommended.[7,8] Refer to Table 69-2 for the dosing differences between the three Hib vaccines available for use in the United States.[9]

Hepatitis A (Hep A)

Infection with the hepatitis A virus presents as fever, malaise, anorexia, nausea, dark urine, and jaundice. Symptoms are generally worse in adults than in children. The hepatitis A virus replicates in the liver, is excreted in the bile, and shed in the stool.[10] Primary mode of transmission is through the fecal-oral route. Those at greatest risk for Hep A infection are travelers to developing countries, injection drug users, and patients with clotting factor disorders. It is recommended that all children receive the Hep A vaccine series at 1 year of age; children and adolescents over the age of 2 years living in states with specific vaccination programs or those at high risk for infection should be offered the Hep A series. Adults not previously vaccinated, who remain at high risk for infection, should also be offered the series. Currently, it is not recommended that food-service workers receive the Hep A vaccine.[10]

Hepatitis B (Hep B)

Hepatitis B is a bloodborne and sexually transmitted virus that replicates in the liver. Symptoms of Hep B infection, if present, are jaundice, anorexia, nausea, vomiting, and malaise. Patients who engage in risky sexual behavior, use injection drugs, live with someone who has chronic Hep B infection, are at risk for occupational exposure, are on dialysis, and who travel to Hep B–endemic regions are at the greatest risk of contracting Hep B.[11] Previous recommendations to vaccinate only those at increased risk were not successful in reducing Hep B infection rates. Therefore, in addition to vaccination of at-risk populations, routine vaccination of all infants beginning at birth is now recommended.[12]

Human Papillomavirus (HPV)

Human papillomavirus is the most common sexually transmitted infection in the United States. Most infections do

TABLE 69-2 **Vaccine Dose and Administration**

Vaccine	Brand Name (Manufacturer)	Dose	Route	Series
DTaP	Daptacel (SP) Infanrix (GSK) Tripedia (SP)	0.5 mL	IM	Five-dose series given at 2, 4, 6, 12-18 mo, and 4-6 y of age
Td	Decavac (SP)	0.5 mL	IM	Booster dose every 10 y
Tdap	Boostrix (GSK) Adacel (SP)	0.5 mL	IM	Single dose as a substitute for *one* Td booster
DT	*Available generic*	0.5 mL	IM	Five-dose series given at 2, 4, 6, 12-18 mo, and 4-6 y of age
Hep A	Havrix (GSK) Vaqta (Merck)	≤18 y: 0.5 mL ≥ 19 y: 1.0 mL	IM	Two-dose series given 6 mo apart
Hep B	Engerix-B (GSK) Recombivax HB (Merck)	≤19 y: 0.5 mL ≥20 y: 1.0 mL	IM	Three-dose series given 0, 1, and 6 mo apart
Hib	ActHIB (SP)	0.5 mL	IM	Three -dose series given at 2, 4, and 6 mo of age *plus* one booster dose at 12-15 mo of age
Hib	PedvaxHIB (Merck)	0.5 mL	IM	Two-dose series given at 2 and 4 mo of age *plus* one booster dose at 12-15 mo of age
Hib	Hiberix (GSK)	0.5 mL	IM	Substitute for booster dose at 12-15 mo of age and children aged 15 mo to 4 y who have not received a booster dose
HPV-4	Gardasil (Merck)	0.5 mL	IM	Three-dose series given 0, 2, and 6 mo apart
HPV-2	Cervarix (GSK)	0.5 mL	IM	Three-dose series given at 0, 1, and 3 mo apart
IPV	Ipol (SP)	0.5 mL	IM or SC	Four-dose series given at 2, 4, 6-18 mo, and 4-6 y
MCV	Menactra (SP) Menveo (Novartis)	0.5 mL 0.5 mL	IM IM	Single dose Single dose
MPSV	Menomune (SP)	0.5 mL	SC	Single dose
MMR	M-M-R II (Merck)	0.5 mL	SC	Two-dose series given at 12-15 mo and 4-6 y
PCV	Prevnar (Wyeth)	0.5 mL	IM	Four-dose series given at 2, 4, 6, and 12-15 mo of age
PPSV	Pneumovax 23 (Merck)	0.5 mL	IM or SC	Single dose[a]
RV	RotaTeq (Merck)	2 mL	Oral	Three-dose series given at 2, 4, and 6 mo[b]
RV	Rotarix (GSK)	1 mL	Oral	Two-dose series given at 2 and 4 mo[b]
Varicella	Varivax (Merck)	0.5 mL	SC	Two-dose series given at 12-15 mo and 4-6 y
Zoster	Zostavax (Merck)	0.65 mL	SC	Single dose

[a]A second dose is recommended 5 years after the first for patients ≥2 years who are immunocompromised, have sickle cell disease, asplenia, or received their first dose prior to age 65.

[b]First dose of RV vaccine cannot be administered after 14 weeks and 6 days of age; maximum age to receive any RV vaccine dose is 8 months.

not cause symptoms; however, persistent infection can lead to genital warts in both men and women as well as cervical, vaginal, and vulvar cancers. Over half of cervical cancer cases are caused by HPV types 16 and 18. In 2006, an HPV vaccine against types 6, 11, 16, and 18 was licensed for use in the United States. Current recommendations are to vaccinate females between 11 and 26 years.[13] In 2009, the FDA approved an HPV-2 vaccine. See Tables 69-1 and 69-2 for differences between the two commercially available HPV vaccines. In October 2009, the FDA approved the use of HPV-4 vaccines in males aged 9 to 26 years. Postmarketing safety analysis has shown an increase incidence in syncope following administration of the HPV vaccine.[14] It is recommended that patients remain seated or lie down for at least 15 minutes right after receiving the vaccine.

Measles, Mumps, and Rubella (MMR)

The measles rash generally appears 14 days after exposure. Measles can cause diarrhea, otitis media, encephalitis, mental retardation, and death.[15] Mumps cause bilateral or unilateral parotitis (swollen parotid gland). Mumps can lead to permanent sequelae, including paralysis, seizures, and deafness.[16] Rubella can cause an erythematous, pruritic rash, arthralgia, and low-grade fever. Most severe complications of rubella occur when pregnant women become infected in the first trimester. Congenital rubella syndrome (CRS) can lead to deafness, cataracts, and mental retardation.[17] Routine vaccination is recommended for all children at least 1 year of age. A second dose at age 4 to 6 years is recommended for all children because a small percentage of patients fail to respond to the first vaccination. If necessary, the second dose of the MMR vaccine may be administered 28 days after the first dose.[18]

Meningo[coccal Infection (MCV, MPSV)

Neisseria meningitides is transmitted through respiratory droplets and is the leading cause of bacterial meningitis in the United States. The fatality rate is 10% to 14% despite the availability of effective antibiotics.[19] Persons at risk for meningococcal disease are college freshmen living in dormitories, military recruits, travelers to countries in which infection is widespread, and patients with functional or anatomical asplenia. Three vaccines are available—a tetravalent polysaccharide vaccine (MPSV), a tetravalent conjugate vaccine (MCV), and an oligosaccharide diphtheria CRM 197 conjugate vaccine (MCV). Current recommendations are to routinely vaccinate all children at the age of 11 or 12 years of age as well as previously unvaccinated adults who are at high risk for infection. The conjugate vaccine is the preferred vaccine. If it is necessary to vaccinate with MPSV, revaccination with MCV 5 years later is recommended for patients who remain at risk.[20]

Pneumococcal Infection (PCV, PPSV)

Streptococcus pneumoniae, a bacterial pathogen, can cause upper respiratory tract infections (otitis media, sinusitis), lower respiratory tract infections (pneumonia), and invasive disease (bacteremia, meningitis). Persons at greatest risk for invasive disease are children <5 years of age, adults >65 years, patients with chronic lung disease, chronic cardiovascular disease, diabetes mellitus, chronic liver disease, functional or anatomic asplenia, and smokers.[21] Two vaccines are licensed for use in the United States—a pneumococcal conjugate vaccine (PCV) and a pneumococcal polysaccharide vaccine (PPSV). The conjugate vaccine can be used in children <5 years of age.[22] The polysaccharide vaccine is indicated for patients >2 years who are at high risk for developing severe complications from *S. pneumoniae* infection.[23]

Poliomyelitis (IPV)

Poliomyelitis is a highly contagious disease caused by the poliovirus that is mainly transmitted by the fecal-oral route.[24] Symptoms of polio range from a fever to meningitis and paralysis. Poliovirus replicates in the motor neurons and may cause asymmetric paralysis. However, the majority of polio infections are asymptomatic. The ratio of asymptomatic to paralytic illness ranges from 100:1 to 1000:1 (usually 200:1).[24] Several decades after infection, patients can develop post-polio syndrome which is characterized by muscle pain and weakness and even paralysis. Due to routine vaccination, the United States is free from indigenous polio. Therefore, the oral polio vaccine is no longer included in the recommendations. All children should receive four doses of the inactivated polio vaccine (IPV) starting at age 2 months.[24]

Rotovirus (RV)

Rotovirus is the most common cause of severe gastroenteritis in infants and young children and is responsible for over 50,000 hospitalizations every year. It infects the small intestine causing diarrhea, vomiting, and fever leading to dehydration. Two RV vaccines are available in the United States—a monovalent human vaccine (Rotarix) and a pentavalent human-bovine reassortant vaccine (RotaTeq). A previous RV vaccine (Rotashield) was removed from the market due to an increased incidence of intussusception. Currently licensed RV vaccines have not been shown to increase the risk of intussusception. It is recommended that the first dose of the RV vaccine be administered to all infants before the age of 14 weeks and 6 days. The last dose in the RV vaccine series should be administered before the age of 8 months.[25]

Varicella Zoster Virus (Varicella, Zoster)

The varicella zoster virus causes two conditions—varicella (chickenpox) and herpes zoster (shingles). The varicella zoster virus enters the respiratory tract and replicates in the nasopharynx.[26] Varicella, the primary infection, is a contagious rash that is common among children. It can present with fever and general malaise before the characteristic rash appears. Varicella is generally mild and self-limiting, but complications can occur. They include bacterial skin infections, pneumonia, meningitis and encephalopathy.[27]

The varicella zoster virus can lie dormant in the sensory dorsal root ganglia of the spine. It can reactivate years later to cause herpes zoster, a localized painful rash. The rash occurs unilaterally and does not cross the center of the body. The pain is described as aching and shock-like. The rash will typically disappear within 4 weeks, but postherpetic neuralgia (PHN), a complication of herpes zoster, can last for weeks to months or even years. Postherpetic neuralgia is a debilitating pain that persists after the rash dissipates.[28]

Three live attenuated viral vaccines for the varicella zoster virus are available for use in the United States—a varicella vaccine, a combination vaccine with MMR and varicella, and a vaccine to prevent herpes zoster infection. See Table 69-1.

VACCINE ADMINISTRATION

Injection Route and Site

Most vaccines are administered intramuscularly (IM) or subcutaneously (SC). A 1-in needle should be used for IM injections in most adults. Intramuscular injections are administered at a 90° angle in the deltoid muscle of the arm for adults and children or the anterolateral thigh for infants. A 5/8-in needle should be used for subcutaneous injections.[29] Subcutaneous injections are administered at a 45° angle in the outer aspect of the triceps. Table 69-2 lists the dosages and routes of administration for most of the vaccines available in the United States.

Simultaneous Administration

Simultaneously administering all vaccines a patient is eligible for in one office visit has been shown to increase vaccination rates without decreasing vaccine efficacy.[29] Therefore, it is recommended that all age-appropriate vaccinations be administered on the same day unless contraindications/precautions are present. Whether the vaccine is live or inactivated does not affect simultaneous administration. Inactivated vaccines can be administered without regard to spacing. A live and inactivated vaccine may be administered without regard to spacing, as well. There is evidence suggesting that the varicella vaccine is not effective when administered <28 days after the MMR vaccine, but is effective if administered on the same day as the MMR vaccine.[30] Therefore, it is recommended to administer

TABLE 69-3 Inactivated and Live Vaccines

Inactivated	Live Attenuated
DTaP, DT, Td, Tdap	MMR
Hep B	Varicella
Hib	Zoster
Hep A	RV
HPV	LAIV[a]
PCV	Yellow fever[a]
PPSV	Oral typhoid[a]
IPV	
MCV	
MPSV	
Influenza[a]	

[a]Vaccines not covered in this chapter.
Abbreviation: LAIV, live attenuated influenza vaccine.

two live vaccines on the same day or separated by at least 28 days.[30] The exception to this recommendation is with oral live vaccines—they may be administered at any interval from previous vaccination with either live or inactivated vaccines. Vaccines that require a series of doses have specific recommendations regarding spacing intervals. Administering a dose in a series earlier than recommended may decrease vaccine efficacy and should be avoided. Table 69-3 lists the inactivated and live vaccines available for use in the United States.

Contraindications and Precautions

Prior to administering a vaccine it is important to screen the patient for potential contraindications and precautions. A contraindication is a patient condition that greatly increases the likelihood that a serious adverse reaction will occur if the vaccine is administered. Vaccines are contraindicated in a patient who has experienced an anaphylactic reaction to a prior dose or any component of that vaccine. A precaution is a condition that might increase the risk of a serious adverse reaction or decrease the effectiveness of the vaccine.[31] Generally, the vaccination should be withheld until the precaution has resolved. In some instances the benefit of administering the vaccine outweighs the risk and can be administered. Administration of any vaccine should be cautioned in patients with moderate to severe acute illness with or without a fever. Contraindications and precautions for most of the vaccines available in the United States are listed in Table 69-4. Health care professionals are encouraged to visit the CDC vaccine website for the latest safety information on vaccines.

TABLE 69-4 Vaccine Contraindications and Precautions

Vaccine	Contraindication	Precautions
DTaP, Tdap	Encephalopathy within 7 d of a previous dose Progressive neurologic disorder—infantile spasms, uncontrolled epilepsy, encephalopathy	Seizure within 3 d of receiving a previous dose Any of the following within 48 h of a previous dose: Fever >40.5°C Collapse or shock-like state Persistent, inconsolable crying for >3 h
Hep A		Pregnancy
Hep B	Allergy to baker's yeast	Infant weighing <2000 g
Hib	Age <6 wk	
HPV	Pregnancy Allergy to yeast	
IPV	Allergy to neomycin, streptomycin, or polymyxin B	Pregnancy
MMR	Allergy to gelatin or neomycin Pregnancy Severe immunodeficiency	Receipt of antibody-containing blood product within 11 mo History of thrombocytopenia or thrombocytopenic purpura
RV	Severe latex allergy (Rotarix only)	Immunodeficiency Acute gastroenteritis Preexisting chronic gastrointestinal disease History of intussusception Spinal bifida or bladder exstrophy
Varicella	Pregnancy Immunodeficiency Untreated active tuberculosis Allergy to gelatin or neomycin	Receipt of antibody-containing blood product within 11 mo
Zoster	Pregnancy Immunodeficiency Allergy to gelatin or neomycin	

TABLE 69-5 **Vaccine Adverse Events**

Vaccine	Adverse Events
DTaP	Injection site reactions (pain, swelling, erythema), fever, fatigue, vomiting, anorexia, febrile seizures (rare)
Td, Tdap	Injection site reactions, headache, myalgias, fatigue, neuropathy (rare), and paralysis (rare)
Hep A	Injection site reactions, headache, malaise, fever, Guillain-Barré syndrome(GBS)
Hep B	Injection site reactions, fever, GBS
Hib	Injection site reactions, fever
HPV	Injection site reactions, syncope, fever, nausea, headache, GBS, thromboembolism
IPV	Injection site reactions, fever
MCV, MPSV	Injection site reactions, fever, diarrhea, anorexia, drowsiness, GBS[a]
MMR	Injection site reactions, thrombocytopenia, febrile seizures, GBS
PCV	Injection site reactions, fever, febrile seizures
PPSV	Injection site reactions, fever, myalgias
RV	Mild diarrhea and vomiting, irritability
Varicella	Injection site reactions, varicella-like rash
Zoster	Injection site reactions, fever, arthralgias, varicella-like reactions

[a]MCV has a higher incidence of GBS than MPSV.

Adverse Events

Adverse events for most vaccines available in the US are listed in Table 69-5. Health care professionals administering vaccinations are required to report any adverse event that occurs after vaccine administration. The CDC requires that the provider complete the Vaccine Adverse Event Reporting System (VAERS) form. The form is available from: http://vaers.hhs.gov. Personnel administering vaccinations should be prepared to handle emergency situations that may arise from vaccine administration. Epinephrine, diphenhydramine, and CPR may need to be administered if a patient has an anaphylactic reaction.[29] Practitioners will need to be CPR and first aid certified.

Combination Vaccines

Combination vaccines approved for use in the United States are listed in Table 69-6. The main advantage of using combination vaccines is the decrease in the number of injections. The ACIP recommends the use of combination vaccines whenever possible based upon provider assessment, patient preference, safety, availability, and cost.[32]

Vaccine Storage

Proper storage is important to maintain vaccine potency.[29] Package inserts contain recommended storage temperatures as well as instructions for reconstitution (if necessary). Most vaccines require refrigeration; however some need to be kept frozen (eg, zoster). Recommended storage temperature for refrigerated vaccines is 35°F to 46°F (2°C-8°C). Frozen vaccines should be stored at ≤5°F (≤15°C).[29]

TABLE 69-6 **Combination Vaccines**

Brand Name (Manufacturer)	Vaccines	Dose	Route
Pediarix (GSK)	DTaP/IPV/Hep B	0.5 mL	IM
Pentacel (SP)	DTaP/IPV/Hib	0.5 mL	IM
TriHIBit (SP)	DTaP/Hib	0.5 mL	IM
Kinrix (GSK)	DTaP/IPV	0.5 mL	IM
Twinrix (GSK)	Hep A/Heb B	1 mL	IM
Comvax (Merck)	Hep B/Hib	0.5 mL	IM
ProQuad (Merck)	MMR/Varicella	0.5 mL	SC

VACCINE SCHEDULES

The 2009 recommended vaccination schedule for children, adolescents, and adults are provided in Appendices 69-1 and 69-2. Changes to vaccine schedules are made annually. Readers are encouraged to visit the CDC vaccines website for the most current vaccination schedule (http://www.cdc.gov/vaccines/recs/schedules/default.htm).

CASE Application

1. Which of the following can safely be given to a 6-month-old child who had an allergic reaction to the pertussis vaccine?
   a. DTaP
   b. Tdap
   c. Td
   d. DT
2. KS, a 5-year-old girl, has an appointment today with her pediatrician to receive vaccines. Her vaccination record shows the following: Hep B at birth, 2 months, and 6 months; RV at 2, 4, and 6 months; DTaP at 2, 4, 6, and 15 months; Hib (ActHIB) at 2, 4, 6, and 15 months; PCV at 2, 4, 6, and 15 months; IPV at 2, 4, and 6 months; MMR at 15 months; Varicella at 15 months; and Hep A at 15 months. She does not have any medical conditions and is not allergic to any medications or vaccines. What vaccines should KS receive today?
   a. DT, PPSV, IPV, MMR, MCV, and Hep A
   b. DTaP, IPV, MMR, Varicella, and Hep A
   c. Tdap, IPV, MMR, Varicella, and Hep A
   d. DTaP, PPSV, IPV, MMR, Varicella, and Hep A
3. Which of the following vaccines is given as a single dose?
   a. PCV
   b. Zoster
   c. RV
   d. Td

4. Which of the following pediatric vaccines are administered orally?

   a. IPV
   b. PCV
   c. RV
   d. Varicella

5. A 69-year-old man comes into your pharmacy after receiving a letter advertising your immunization program. He has diabetes and hypertension and smokes a pack of cigarettes a day. He does not have any medication or vaccine allergies. His vaccination record shows that he completed all of his childhood vaccinations (DTaP, Hib, PCV, IPV, and MMR) as well as the Hep B series. He had chickenpox when he was 5 years old and received his last Td booster 11 years ago. Which vaccines should this patient receive?

   a. Td, Zoster, PPSV, and Hep A
   b. Tdap, Varicella, and PPSV
   c. Tdap, Zoster, and Hep A
   d. Td, Zoster, and PPSV

6. Which of the following diphtheria and tetanus vaccines should be used in adults as a one-time booster dose?

   a. Td
   b. DT
   c. Tdap
   d. DTaP

7. Which of the following adults under the age of 65 would require a pneumococcal polysaccharide vaccine (PPSV)?

   a. Pregnant women
   b. Smokers
   c. Health care workers
   d. Splenic patients

8. How should the hepatitis B vaccine (Hep B) be administered?

   a. In the deltoid muscle at a 90° angle.
   b. In the deltoid muscle at a 45° angle.
   c. In the outer aspect of the triceps at a 45° angle.
   d. In the anteriolateral thigh at a 45° angle.

9. EP is pregnant and in her second trimester. Which of the following vaccines can EP receive?

   a. HPV
   b. Hep B
   c. MMR
   d. DTaP

10. An 11-year-old girl fainted after receiving her 11- to 12-year-old routine vaccinations. Which of the following vaccines most likely caused her to faint?

    a. Tdap
    b. HPV
    c. MCV
    d. Hep B

11. Herpes zoster vaccine should be stored at what temperature?

    a. ≤5°F
    b. 6°F to 35°F
    c. 36°F to 46°F
    d. 47°F to 77°F

12. JM, a 6-month-old infant, is seeing his pediatrician today in order to receive his 6 month vaccinations. His vaccination records are as follows: Hep B at birth and 2 months; DTaP at 2 and 4 months; Hib (PedvaxHIB) at 2 and 4 months; PCV at 2 and 4 months; IPV at 2 and 4 months. JM does not have any medical conditions or allergies to medications or vaccines. Which vaccines should JM receive today?

    a. Hep B, RV, DTaP, Hib, PCV, and IPV
    b. Hep B, RV, DTaP, PCV, and IPV
    c. Hep B, DTaP, Hib, PCV, and IPV
    d. Hep B, DTaP, PCV, and IPV

13. Which of the following vaccines require a booster dose?

    a. HPV
    b. MMR
    c. MCV
    d. Hib

14. The Haemophilus influenza type b (Hib) vaccine can be administered to all of the following, *except*:

    a. A 4-month-old infant
    b. A 20-year-old smoker
    c. A 58-year-old man with leukemia
    d. A 26-year-old with asplenia

15. How should the herpes zoster vaccine (Zoster) be administered?

    a. In the deltoid muscle at a 90° angle.
    b. In the deltoid muscle at a 45° angle.
    c. In the outer aspect of the triceps at a 45° angle.
    d. In the anteriolateral thigh at a 45° angle.

16. LM is an 18-year-old woman who is leaving for her first semester of college next month. She would like to know what vaccinations she needs before going to college. Her vaccination record shows the following: DTaP at 2, 4, 6, and 15 months, and 5 years; Hib (ActHIB) at 2, 4, and 6 months; PCV at 2, 4, 6, and 15 months; IPV at 2, 4, and 6 months, and 5 years; MMR at 15 months and 5 years; Varicella at 15 months and 5 years; Hep A at 12 and 18 months; Hep B at 11 years, 11 years 2 months, and 11 years 6 months; Tdap at 15 years. LM does not have any medical conditions and is not allergic to any medications or vaccines. What vaccines should LM receive today?

a. MCV and HPV
b. Tdap, MCV, and HPV
c. Tdap and MCV
d. MPSV and HPV

17. TR, a 4-year-old girl, is in the doctor's office for her 4- to 6-year-old vaccinations. She has completed her Hep B, Hib, PCV, and Hep A series. She has no medical conditions and is not allergic to any medications or vaccines. Five days ago she received the live-attenuated influenza vaccine. Which vaccines should TR receive today?

a. DTaP, IPV, MMR, and Varicella
b. DTaP, PPSV, IPV, and MMR
c. IPV only
d. DTaP and IPV

18. When should the second dose of the Hepatitis A (Hep A) vaccine be administered?

a. 28 days after the first dose
b. 2 months after the first dose
c. 6 months after the first dose
d. 30 days after the first dose

19. All of the following are patients at risk for hepatitis B (Hep B) infection, *except*:

a. A man who has sex with men
b. A woman with diabetes
c. An injection-drug user
d. A wound-care nurse

20. Which of the following patients should receive the herpes zoster vaccine?

a. A 58-year-old diabetic
b. A 37-year-old without a spleen
c. A 68-year-old with hypertension
d. A 72-year-old allergic to neomycin

TAKEAWAY POINTS ››

- DTaP is indicated for the prevention of diphtheria, tetanus, and pertussis in children <7 years of age. DT is indicated for the prevention of diphtheria and tetanus in children <7 years of age who have a history of anaphylactic reaction to the pertussis vaccine.
- Adults should receive one Td booster every 10 years. Patients aged 11 to 64 years should replace one Td dose with Tdap once in their lifetime.
- The three Hib vaccines available in the United States have different dosing guidelines and are not interchangeable.
- All children over the age of 12 months, travelers to developing countries, injection drug users, and patients with clotting factor disorders should receive two doses of the Hep A vaccine separated by 6 months.
- Hep B is given in a three-dose series at 0, 1, and 6 months. It is the only vaccine that can be given at birth.
- Administration of the HPV vaccine can cause syncope. Therefore, patients should remain seated for at least 15 minutes after receiving the vaccine.
- The MMR vaccine requires two doses—one at 12 to 15 months of age and another at 4 to 6 years of age because a small percentage of patients do not respond to the first dose.
- Adolescents 11 to 12 years of age, college freshman living in dormitories, military recruits, travelers to countries with wide-spread meningococcal disease, and asplenic patients should receive one dose of MCV. If MPSV is administered, re-vaccination with MCV is recommended in patients who remain at high risk 5 years later.
- PCV is recommended in all children <5 years of age. PPSV is recommended in patients >2 years who are at high risk for invasive disease, adults >65 years, patients with chronic lung, cardiovascular or, liver diseases, smokers, and asplenic patients.
- The first dose of the RV vaccine should be given before 14 weeks and 6 days. The last dose should be administered before 8 months.
- IM vaccines are administered in adults at a 90° angle in the deltoid muscle using a 1-in needle. SC vaccines are given at a 45° angle in the outer aspect of the triceps using a 5/8-in needle.
- Most vaccines may be administered without regard to spacing. However, two live vaccines should be given on the same day *or* 28 days apart.
- Administration of any vaccine should be cautioned in patients with moderate to severe acute illness.
- The CDC requires that immunizing practitioners report any adverse event that occurs after vaccine administrations using the VAERS form.
- Refrigerated vaccines should be stored at 35°F to 46°F (2°C to 8°C). Frozen vaccines should be stored at ≤5°F (−15°C).

REFERENCES

1. Centers for Disease Control and Prevention. Immunization strategies for healthcare practices and providers. In: Atkinson W, Wolfe S, Hamborsky J, McIntyre L, eds. *Epidemiology and Prevention of Vaccine-Preventable Diseases.* 11th ed. Washington DC: Public Health Foundation; 2009: 31-44
2. Centers for Disease Control and Prevention. Diphtheria. In: Atkinson W, Wolfe S, Hamborsky J, McIntyre L, eds. *Epidemiology and Prevention of Vaccine-Preventable Diseases.* 11th ed. Washington DC: Public Health Foundation; 2009: 59-70.
3. Centers for Disease Control and Prevention. Tetanus. In: Atkinson W, Wolfe S, Hamborsky J, McIntyre L, eds. *Epidemiology and Prevention of Vaccine-Preventable Diseases.* 11th ed. Washington DC: Public Health Foundation; 2009: 273-282.

4. Centers for Disease Control and Prevention. Pertussis. In: Atkinson W, Wolfe S, Hamborsky J, McIntyre L, eds. *Epidemiology and Prevention of Vaccine-Preventable Diseases.* 11th ed. Washington DC: Public Health Foundation; 2009: 199-216.
5. Centers for Disease Control and Prevention. Preventing tetanus, diphtheria, and pertussis among adolescents: use of tetanus toxoid, reduced diphtheria toxoid and acellular pertussis vaccines: recommendations of the Advisory Committee on Immunization Practices (ACIP). *MMWR.* 2006;55(No. RR-3):1-43.
6. Centers for Disease Control and Prevention. Preventing tetanus, diphtheria, and pertussis among adults: use of tetanus toxoid, reduced diphtheria toxoid and acellular pertussis vaccine: recommendations of the Advisory Committee on Immunization Practices (ACIP). *MMWR.* 2006;55(No. RR-17):1-36.
7. Centers for Disease Control and Prevention. *Haemophilus influenzae.* In: Atkinson W, Wolfe S, Hamborsky J, McIntyre L, eds. *Epidemiology and Prevention of Vaccine-Preventable Diseases.* 11th ed. Washington DC: Public Health Foundation; 2009: 71-84.
8. Centers for Disease Control and Prevention. Haemophilus b conjugate vaccines for prevention of *Haemophilus influenzae* Type b disease among infants and children two months of age and older: recommendations of the Advisory Committee on Immunization Practices (ACIP). *MMWR.* 1991;40(No. RR-01):1-7.
9. Centers for Disease Control and Prevention. Updated recommendations for use of *Haemophilus influenzae* Type b (Hib) vaccine: reinstatement of the booster dose at ages 12-15 months. *MMWR.* 2009;58(No. RR-24):673-674.
10. Centers for Disease Control and Prevention. Prevention of Hepatitis A through active or passive immunization: recommendations of the Advisory Committee on Immunization Practices (ACIP). *MMWR.* 2006;55(No. RR-7):1-18.
11. Centers for Disease Control and Prevention. A comprehensive immunization strategy to eliminate transmission of hepatitis B virus infection in the United States: recommendations of the Advisory Committee on Immunization Practices (ACIP); Part 1: immunization of adults. *MMWR.* 2006;55(No. RR-16):2-26.
12. Centers for Disease Control and Prevention. A comprehensive immunization strategy to eliminate transmission of hepatitis B virus infection in the United States: recommendations of the Advisory Committee on Immunization Practices (ACIP); Part 1: immunization of infants, children, and adolescents. *MMWR.* 2005;54(No. RR-16):1-32.
13. Centers for Disease Control and Prevention. Quadrivalent human papillomavirus vaccine: recommendations of the Advisory Committee on Immunization Practices (ACIP). *MMWR.* 2007;56(No. RR-2):1-19.
14. Slade BA, Leidel L, Vellozzi C, et al. Postlicensure safety surveillance for quadrivalent human papillomavirus recombinant vaccine. *JAMA.* 2009;302(7):750-757.
15. Centers for Disease Control and Prevention. Measles. In: Atkinson W, Wolfe S, Hamborsky J, McIntyre L, eds. *Epidemiology and Prevention of Vaccine-Preventable Diseases.* 11th ed. Washington DC: Public Health Foundation; 2009: 157-176.
16. Centers for Disease Control and Prevention. Mumps. In: Atkinson W, Wolfe S, Hamborsky J, McIntyre L, eds. *Epidemiology and Prevention of Vaccine-Preventable Diseases.* 11th ed. Washington DC: Public Health Foundation; 2009: 189-198.
17. Centers for Disease Control and Prevention. Rubella. In: Atkinson W, Wolfe S, Hamborsky J, McIntyre L, eds. *Epidemiology and Prevention of Vaccine-Preventable Diseases.* 11th ed. Washington DC: Public Health Foundation; 2009: 257-272.
18. Centers for Disease Control and Prevention. Measles, mumps, and rubella—vaccine use and strategies for elimination of measles, rubella, and congenital rubella syndrome and control of mumps: recommendations of the Advisory Committee on Immunization Practices (ACIP). *MMWR.* 1998;47(No. RR-8):1-48.
19. Centers for Disease Control and Prevention. Prevention and control of meningococcal disease: recommendations of the Advisory Committee on Immunization Practices (ACIP). *MMWR.* 2005;54(No. RR-7):1-17.
20. Centers for Disease Control and Prevention. Meningococcal disease. In: Atkinson W, Wolfe S, Hamborsky J, McIntyre L, eds. *Epidemiology and Prevention of Vaccine-Preventable Diseases.* 11th ed. Washington DC: Public Health Foundation; 2009: 177-188.
21. Centers for Disease Control and Prevention. Pneumococcal disease. In: Atkinson W, Wolfe S, Hamborsky J, McIntyre L, eds. *Epidemiology and Prevention of Vaccine-Preventable Diseases.* 11th ed. Washington DC: Public Health Foundation; 2009: 217-230.
22. Centers for Disease Control and Prevention. Preventing pneumococcal disease among infants and young children: recommendations of the Advisory Committee on Immunization Practices (ACIP). *MMWR.* 2000;49(No. RR-9):1-29.
23. Centers for Disease Control and Prevention. Prevention of pneumococcal disease: recommendations of the Advisory Committee on Immunization Practices (ACIP). *MMWR.* 1997;46(No. RR-8):1-19.
24. Centers for Disease Control and Prevention. Poliomyelitis prevention in the United States: updated recommendations of the Advisory Committee on Immunization Practices (AICP). *MMWR.* 2000;49(No. RR-5):1-19.
25. Centers for Disease Control and Prevention. Prevention of rotavirus gastroenteritis among infants and children: recommendations of the Advisory Committee on Immunization Practices (ACIP). *MMWR.* 2009;58(No. RR-2):1-21.
26. Centers for Disease Control and Prevention. Varicella. In: Atkinson W, Wolfe S, Hamborsky J, McIntyre L, eds. *Epidemiology and Prevention of Vaccine-Preventable Diseases.* 11th ed. Washington DC: Public Health Foundation; 2009: 283-304.
27. Centers for Disease Control and Prevention. Prevention of varicella: recommendations of the Advisory Committee on Immunization Practices (ACIP). *MMWR.* 2007;56(No. RR-4):1-38.
28. Centers for Disease Control and Prevention. Prevention of herpes zoster: recommendations of the Advisory Committee on Immunization Practices (ACIP). *MMWR.* 2008;57(No. RR-5):1-23.
29. Centers for Disease Control and Prevention. General recommendations on immunization: recommendations of the Advisory Committee on Immunization Practices (ACIP). *MMWR.* 2006;55(No. RR-15):1-46.
30. Centers for Disease Control and Prevention. General recommendations on immunizations. In: Atkinson W, Wolfe S, Hamborsky J, McIntyre L, eds. *Epidemiology and Prevention of Vaccine-Preventable Diseases.* 11th ed. Washington DC: Public Health Foundation; 2009: 9-30.
31. Centers for Disease Control and Prevention. Contraindications to Vaccines Chart. Available at: http://www.cdc.gov/vaccines/recs/vac-admin/contraindications-vacc.htm. Accessed September 11, 2009.
32. ACIP Provisional Recommendations for the Use of Combination Vaccines. Available at: www.cdc.gov/vaccines/recs/provisional/default.htm. Accessed September 11, 2009.

APPENDIX 69-1 2009 Childhood and Adolescent Immunization Schedules

Recommended Immunization Schedule for Persons Aged 0 Through 6 Years—United States • 2009

For those who fall behind or start late, see the catch-up schedule

Vaccine ▼ Age ▶	Birth	1 month	2 months	4 months	6 months	12 months	15 months	18 months	19–23 months	2–3 years	4–6 years
Hepatitis B[1]	HepB	HepB		*see footnote 1*	HepB						
Rotavirus[2]			RV	RV	*RV*[2]						
Diphtheria, Tetanus, Pertussis[3]			DTaP	DTaP	DTaP	*see footnote 3*	DTaP				DTaP
Haemophilus influenzae type b[4]			Hib	Hib	*Hib*[4]	Hib					
Pneumococcal[5]			PCV	PCV	PCV	PCV				PPSV	
Inactivated Poliovirus			IPV	IPV	IPV						IPV
Influenza[6]					Influenza (Yearly)						
Measles, Mumps, Rubella[7]						MMR		*see footnote 7*			MMR
Varicella[8]						Varicella		*see footnote 8*			Varicella
Hepatitis A[9]						HepA (2 doses)				HepA Series	
Meningococcal[10]										MCV	

Range of recommended ages

Certain high-risk groups

This schedule indicates the recommended ages for routine administration of currently licensed vaccines, as of December 1, 2008, for children aged 0 through 6 years. Any dose not administered at the recommended age should be administered at a subsequent visit, when indicated and feasible. Licensed combination vaccines may be used whenever any component of the combination is indicated and other components are not contraindicated and if approved by the Food and Drug Administration for that dose of the series. Providers should consult the relevant Advisory Committee on Immunization Practices statement for detailed recommendations, including high-risk conditions: http://www.cdc.gov/vaccines/pubs/acip-list.htm. Clinically significant adverse events that follow immunization should be reported to the Vaccine Adverse Event Reporting System (VAERS). Guidance about how to obtain and complete a VAERS form is available at http://www.vaers.hhs.gov or by telephone, 800-822-7967.

1. **Hepatitis B vaccine (HepB).** ***(Minimum age: birth)***
   At birth:
   - Administer monovalent HepB to all newborns before hospital discharge.
   - If mother is hepatitis B surface antigen (HBsAg)-positive, administer HepB and 0.5 mL of hepatitis B immune globulin (HBIG) within 12 hours of birth.
   - If mother's HBsAg status is unknown, administer HepB within 12 hours of birth. Determine mother's HBsAg status as soon as possible and, if HBsAg-positive, administer HBIG (no later than age 1 week).

   After the birth dose:
   - The HepB series should be completed with either monovalent HepB or a combination vaccine containing HepB. The second dose should be administered at age 1 or 2 months. The final dose should be administered no earlier than age 24 weeks.
   - Infants born to HBsAg-positive mothers should be tested for HBsAg and antibody to HBsAg (anti-HBs) after completion of at least 3 doses of the HepB series, at age 9 through 18 months (generally at the next well-child visit).

   4-month dose:
   - Administration of 4 doses of HepB to infants is permissible when combination vaccines containing HepB are administered after the birth dose.
2. **Rotavirus vaccine (RV).** ***(Minimum age: 6 weeks)***
   - Administer the first dose at age 6 through 14 weeks (maximum age: 14 weeks 6 days). Vaccination should not be initiated for infants aged 15 weeks or older (i.e., 15 weeks 0 days or older).
   - Administer the final dose in the series by age 8 months 0 days.
   - If Rotarix® is administered at ages 2 and 4 months, a dose at 6 months is not indicated.
3. **Diphtheria and tetanus toxoids and acellular pertussis vaccine (DTaP).** ***(Minimum age: 6 weeks)***
   - The fourth dose may be administered as early as age 12 months, provided at least 6 months have elapsed since the third dose.
   - Administer the final dose in the series at age 4 through 6 years.
4. ***Haemophilus influenzae*** **type b conjugate vaccine (Hib).** ***(Minimum age: 6 weeks)***
   - If PRP-OMP (PedvaxHIB® or Comvax® [HepB-Hib]) is administered at ages 2 and 4 months, a dose at age 6 months is not indicated.
   - TriHiBit® (DTaP/Hib) should not be used for doses at ages 2, 4, or 6 months but can be used as the final dose in children aged 12 months or older.
5. **Pneumococcal vaccine.** ***(Minimum age: 6 weeks for pneumococcal conjugate vaccine [PCV]; 2 years for pneumococcal polysaccharide vaccine [PPSV])***
   - PCV is recommended for all children aged younger than 5 years. Administer 1 dose of PCV to all healthy children aged 24 through 59 months who are not completely vaccinated for their age.
   - Administer PPSV to children aged 2 years or older with certain underlying medical conditions (see *MMWR* 2000;49[No. RR-9]), including a cochlear implant.
6. **Influenza vaccine.** ***(Minimum age: 6 months for trivalent inactivated influenza vaccine [TIV]; 2 years for live, attenuated influenza vaccine [LAIV])***
   - Administer annually to children aged 6 months through 18 years.
   - For healthy nonpregnant persons (i.e., those who do not have underlying medical conditions that predispose them to influenza complications) aged 2 through 49 years, either LAIV or TIV may be used.
   - Children receiving TIV should receive 0.25 mL if aged 6 through 35 months or 0.5 mL if aged 3 years or older.
   - Administer 2 doses (separated by at least 4 weeks) to children aged younger than 9 years who are receiving influenza vaccine for the first time or who were vaccinated for the first time during the previous influenza season but only received 1 dose.
7. **Measles, mumps, and rubella vaccine (MMR).** ***(Minimum age: 12 months)***
   - Administer the second dose at age 4 through 6 years. However, the second dose may be administered before age 4, provided at least 28 days have elapsed since the first dose.
8. **Varicella vaccine.** ***(Minimum age: 12 months)***
   - Administer the second dose at age 4 through 6 years. However, the second dose may be administered before age 4, provided at least 3 months have elapsed since the first dose.
   - For children aged 12 months through 12 years the minimum interval between doses is 3 months. However, if the second dose was administered at least 28 days after the first dose, it can be accepted as valid.
9. **Hepatitis A vaccine (HepA).** ***(Minimum age: 12 months)***
   - Administer to all children aged 1 year (i.e., aged 12 through 23 months). Administer 2 doses at least 6 months apart.
   - Children not fully vaccinated by age 2 years can be vaccinated at subsequent visits.
   - HepA also is recommended for children older than 1 year who live in areas where vaccination programs target older children or who are at increased risk of infection. See *MMWR* 2006;55(No. RR-7).
10. **Meningococcal vaccine.** ***(Minimum age: 2 years for meningococcal conjugate vaccine [MCV] and for meningococcal polysaccharide vaccine [MPSV])***
    - Administer MCV to children aged 2 through 10 years with terminal complement component deficiency, anatomic or functional asplenia, and certain other high-risk groups. See *MMWR* 2005;54(No. RR-7).
    - Persons who received MPSV 3 or more years previously and who remain at increased risk for meningococcal disease should be revaccinated with MCV.

The Recommended Immunization Schedules for Persons Aged 0 Through 18 Years are approved by the Advisory Committee on Immunization Practices (www.cdc.gov/vaccines/recs/acip), the American Academy of Pediatrics (http://www.aap.org), and the American Academy of Family Physicians (http://www.aafp.org).

DEPARTMENT OF HEALTH AND HUMAN SERVICES • CENTERS FOR DISEASE CONTROL AND PREVENTION

CS103164

Recommended Immunization Schedule for Persons Aged 7 Through 18 Years—United States • 2009

For those who fall behind or start late, see the schedule below and the catch-up schedule

Vaccine ▼ Age ▶	7–10 years	11–12 years	13–18 years
Tetanus, Diphtheria, Pertussis[1]	*see footnote 1*	Tdap	Tdap
Human Papillomavirus[2]	*see footnote 2*	HPV (3 doses)	HPV Series
Meningococcal[3]	MCV	MCV	MCV
Influenza[4]		Influenza (Yearly)	
Pneumococcal[5]		PPSV	
Hepatitis A[6]		HepA Series	
Hepatitis B[7]		HepB Series	
Inactivated Poliovirus[8]		IPV Series	
Measles, Mumps, Rubella[9]		MMR Series	
Varicella[10]		Varicella Series	

Range of recommended ages

Catch-up immunization

Certain high-risk groups

This schedule indicates the recommended ages for routine administration of currently licensed vaccines, as of December 1, 2008, for children aged 7 through 18 years. Any dose not administered at the recommended age should be administered at a subsequent visit, when indicated and feasible. Licensed combination vaccines may be used whenever any component of the combination is indicated and other components are not contraindicated and if approved by the Food and Drug Administration for that dose of the series. Providers should consult the relevant Advisory Committee on Immunization Practices statement for detailed recommendations, including high-risk conditions: http://www.cdc.gov/vaccines/pubs/acip-list.htm. Clinically significant adverse events that follow immunization should be reported to the Vaccine Adverse Event Reporting System (VAERS). Guidance about how to obtain and complete a VAERS form is available at http://www.vaers.hhs.gov or by telephone, 800-822-7967.

1. **Tetanus and diphtheria toxoids and acellular pertussis vaccine (Tdap).** ***(Minimum age: 10 years for BOOSTRIX® and 11 years for ADACEL®)***
   - Administer at age 11 or 12 years for those who have completed the recommended childhood DTP/DTaP vaccination series and have not received a tetanus and diphtheria toxoid (Td) booster dose.
   - Persons aged 13 through 18 years who have not received Tdap should receive a dose.
   - A 5-year interval from the last Td dose is encouraged when Tdap is used as a booster dose; however, a shorter interval may be used if pertussis immunity is needed.
2. **Human papillomavirus vaccine (HPV).** ***(Minimum age: 9 years)***
   - Administer the first dose to females at age 11 or 12 years.
   - Administer the second dose 2 months after the first dose and the third dose 6 months after the first dose (at least 24 weeks after the first dose).
   - Administer the series to females at age 13 through 18 years if not previously vaccinated.
3. **Meningococcal conjugate vaccine (MCV).**
   - Administer at age 11 or 12 years, or at age 13 through 18 years if not previously vaccinated.
   - Administer to previously unvaccinated college freshmen living in a dormitory.
   - MCV is recommended for children aged 2 through 10 years with terminal complement component deficiency, anatomic or functional asplenia, and certain other groups at high risk. See *MMWR* 2005;54(No. RR-7).
   - Persons who received MPSV 5 or more years previously and remain at increased risk for meningococcal disease should be revaccinated with MCV.
4. **Influenza vaccine.**
   - Administer annually to children aged 6 months through 18 years.
   - For healthy nonpregnant persons (i.e., those who do not have underlying medical conditions that predispose them to influenza complications) aged 2 through 49 years, either LAIV or TIV may be used.
   - Administer 2 doses (separated by at least 4 weeks) to children aged younger than 9 years who are receiving influenza vaccine for the first time or who were vaccinated for the first time during the previous influenza season but only received 1 dose.
5. **Pneumococcal polysaccharide vaccine (PPSV).**
   - Administer to children with certain underlying medical conditions (see *MMWR* 1997;46[No. RR-8]), including a cochlear implant. A single revaccination should be administered to children with functional or anatomic asplenia or other immunocompromising condition after 5 years.
6. **Hepatitis A vaccine (HepA).**
   - Administer 2 doses at least 6 months apart.
   - HepA is recommended for children older than 1 year who live in areas where vaccination programs target older children or who are at increased risk of infection. See *MMWR* 2006;55(No. RR-7).
7. **Hepatitis B vaccine (HepB).**
   - Administer the 3-dose series to those not previously vaccinated.
   - A 2-dose series (separated by at least 4 months) of adult formulation Recombivax HB® is licensed for children aged 11 through 15 years.
8. **Inactivated poliovirus vaccine (IPV).**
   - For children who received an all-IPV or all-oral poliovirus (OPV) series, a fourth dose is not necessary if the third dose was administered at age 4 years or older.
   - If both OPV and IPV were administered as part of a series, a total of 4 doses should be administered, regardless of the child's current age.
9. **Measles, mumps, and rubella vaccine (MMR).**
   - If not previously vaccinated, administer 2 doses or the second dose for those who have received only 1 dose, with at least 28 days between doses.
10. **Varicella vaccine.**
    - For persons aged 7 through 18 years without evidence of immunity (see *MMWR* 2007;56[No. RR-4]), administer 2 doses if not previously vaccinated or the second dose if they have received only 1 dose.
    - For persons aged 7 through 12 years, the minimum interval between doses is 3 months. However, if the second dose was administered at least 28 days after the first dose, it can be accepted as valid.
    - For persons aged 13 years and older, the minimum interval between doses is 28 days.

The Recommended Immunization Schedules for Persons Aged 0 Through 18 Years are approved by the Advisory Committee on Immunization Practices (www.cdc.gov/vaccines/recs/acip), the American Academy of Pediatrics (http://www.aap.org), and the American Academy of Family Physicians (http://www.aafp.org).

DEPARTMENT OF HEALTH AND HUMAN SERVICES • CENTERS FOR DISEASE CONTROL AND PREVENTION

CS103164

APPENDIX 69-2 2009 Adult Immunization Schedule

FIGURE 1. Recommended adult immunization schedule by vaccine and age group — United Sates, 2009

VACCINE ▼ AGE GROUP ▶	19–26 years	27–49 years	50–59 years	60–64 years	≥65 years
Tetanus, diphtheria, pertussis (Td/Tdap)[1,*]	Substitute 1-time dose of Tdap for Td booster; then boost with Td every 10 yr				Td booster every 10 yrs
Human papillomavirus (HPV)[2,*]	3 doses (females)				
Varicella[3,*]	2 doses				
Zoster[4]				1 dose	
Measles, mumps, rubella (MMR)[5,*]	1 or 2 doses		1 dose		
Influenza[6,*]	1 dose annually				
Pneumococcal (polysaccharide)[7,8]	1 or 2 doses				1 dose
Hepatitis A[9,*]	2 doses				
Hepatitis B[10,*]	3 doses				
Meningococcal[11,*]	1 or more doses				

*Covered by the Vaccine Injury Compensation Program.

For all persons in this category who meet the age requirements and who lack evidence of immunity (e.g., lack documentation of vaccination or have no evidence of prior infection)

Recommended if some other risk factor is present (e.g., on the basis of medical, occupational, lifestyle, or other indications)

No recommendation

NOTE: The above recommendations must be read along with the footnotes on pages Q2–Q4 of this schedule.

1. Tetanus, diphtheria, and acellular pertussis (Td/Tdap) vaccination

Tdap should replace a single dose of Td for adults aged 19 through 64 years who have not received a dose of Tdap previously

Adults with uncertain or incomplete history of primary vaccination series with tetanus and diphtheria toxoid–containing vaccines should begin or complete a primary vaccination series. A primary series for adults is 3 doses of tetanus and diphtheria toxoid–containing vaccines; administer the first 2 doses at least 4 weeks apart and the third dose 6–12 months after the second. However, Tdap can substitute for any one of the doses of Td in the 3-dose primary series. The booster dose of tetanus and diphtheria toxoid–containing vaccine should be administered to adults who have completed a primary series and if the last vaccination was received 10 or more years previously. Tdap or Td vaccine may be used, as indicated.

If a woman is pregnant and received the last Td vaccination 10 or more years previously, administer Td during the second or third trimester. If the woman received the last Td vaccination less than 10 years previously, administer Tdap during the immediate postpartum period. A dose of Tdap is recommended for postpartum women, close contacts of infants aged less than 12 months, and all health-care personnel with direct patient contact if they have not previously received Tdap. An interval as short as 2 years from the last Td is suggested; shorter intervals can be used. Td may be deferred during pregnancy and Tdap substituted in the immediate postpartum period, or Tdap may be administered instead of Td to a pregnant woman after an informed discussion with the woman.

Consult the ACIP statement for recommendations for administering Td as prophylaxis in wound management.

2. Human papillomavirus (HPV) vaccination

HPV vaccination is recommended for all females aged 11 through 26 years (and may begin at age 9 years) who have not completed the vaccine series. History of genital warts, abnormal Papanicolaou test, or positive HPV DNA test is not evidence of prior infection with all vaccine HPV types; HPV vaccination is recommended for persons with such histories.

Ideally, vaccine should be administered before potential exposure to HPV through sexual activity; however, females who are sexually active should still be vaccinated consistent with age-based recommendations. Sexually active females who have not been infected with any of the four HPV vaccine types receive the full benefit of the vaccination. Vaccination is less beneficial for females who have already been infected with one or more of the HPV vaccine types.

A complete series consists of 3 doses. The second dose should be administered 2 months after the first dose; the third dose should be administered 6 months after the first dose.

HPV vaccination is not specifically recommended for females with the medical indications described in Figure 2, "Vaccines that might be indicated for adults based on medical and other indications." Because HPV vaccine is not a live-virus vaccine, it may be administered to persons with the medical indications described in Figure 2. However, the immune response and vaccine efficacy might be less for persons with the medical indications described in Figure 2 than in persons who do not have the medical indications described or who are immunocompetent. Health-care personnel are not at increased risk because of occupational exposure, and should be vaccinated consistent with age-based recommendations.

3. Varicella vaccination

All adults without evidence of immunity to varicella should receive 2 doses of single-antigen varicella vaccine if not previously vaccinated or the second dose if they have received only one dose, unless they have a medical contraindication. Special consideration should be given to those who 1) have close contact with persons at high risk for severe disease (e.g., health-care personnel and family contacts of persons with immunocompromising conditions) or 2) are at high risk for exposure or transmission (e.g., teachers; child care employees; residents and staff members of institutional settings, including correctional institutions; college students; military personnel; adolescents and adults living in households with children; nonpregnant women of childbearing age; and international travelers).

Evidence of immunity to varicella in adults includes any of the following: 1) documentation of 2 doses of varicella vaccine at least 4 weeks apart; 2) U.S.-born before 1980 (although for health-care personnel and pregnant women, birth before 1980 should not be considered evidence of immunity); 3) history of varicella based on diagnosis or verification of varicella by a health-care provider (for a patient reporting a history of or presenting with an atypical case, a mild case, or both, health-care providers should seek either an epidemiologic link to a typical varicella case or to a laboratory-confirmed case or evidence of laboratory confirmation, if it was performed at the time of acute disease); 4) history of herpes zoster based on health-care provider diagnosis or verification of herpes zoster by a health-care provider; or 5) laboratory evidence of immunity or laboratory confirmation of disease.

Pregnant women should be assessed for evidence of varicella immunity. Women who do not have evidence of immunity should receive the first dose

FIGURE 2. Vaccines that might be indicated for adults based on medical and other indications — United States, 2009

VACCINE ▼ / INDICATION ▶	Pregnancy	Immuno-compromising conditions (excluding human immunodeficiency virus [HIV])[13]	HIV infection[3,12,13] CD4+ T lymphocyte count <200 cells/μL	HIV infection[3,12,13] CD4+ T lymphocyte count ≥200 cells/μL	Diabetes, heart disease, chronic lung disease, chronic alcoholism	Asplenia[12] (including elective splenectomy and terminal complement component deficiencies)	Chronic liver disease	Kidney failure, end-stage renal disease, receipt of hemodialysis	Health-care personnel
Tetanus, diphtheria, pertussis (Td/Tdap)[1,*]	Td	Substitute 1-time dose of Tdap for Td booster; then boost with Td every 10 yrs							
Human papillomavirus (HPV)[2,*]		3 doses for females through age 26 yrs							
Varicella[3,*]	Contraindicated			2 doses					
Zoster[4]	Contraindicated				1 dose				
Measles, mumps, rubella (MMR)[5,*]	Contraindicated			1 or 2 doses					
Influenza[6,*]	1 dose TIV annually								1 dose TIV or LAIV annually
Pneumococcal (polysaccharide)[7,8]	1 or 2 doses								
Hepatitis A[9,*]	2 doses								
Hepatitis B[10,*]	3 doses								
Meningococcal[11,*]	1 or more doses								

*Covered by the Vaccine Injury Compensation Program.

For all persons in this category who meet the age requirements and who lack evidence of immunity (e.g., lack documentation of vaccination or have no evidence of prior infection)

Recommended if some other risk factor is present (e.g., on the basis of medical, occupational, lifestyle, or other indications)

No recommendation

NOTE: The above recommendations must be read along with the footnotes on pages Q2–Q4 of this schedule.

of varicella vaccine upon completion or termination of pregnancy and before discharge from the health-care facility. The second dose should be administered 4–8 weeks after the first dose.

4. Herpes zoster vaccination

A single dose of zoster vaccine is recommended for adults aged 60 years and older regardless of whether they report a prior episode of herpes zoster. Persons with chronic medical conditions may be vaccinated unless their condition constitutes a contraindication.

5. Measles, mumps, rubella (MMR) vaccination

Measles component: Adults born before 1957 generally are considered immune to measles. Adults born during or after 1957 should receive 1 or more doses of MMR unless they have a medical contraindication, documentation of 1 or more doses, history of measles based on health-care provider diagnosis, or laboratory evidence of immunity.

A second dose of MMR is recommended for adults who 1) have been recently exposed to measles or are in an outbreak setting; 2) have been vaccinated previously with killed measles vaccine; 3) have been vaccinated with an unknown type of measles vaccine during 1963–1967; 4) are students in postsecondary educational institutions; 5) work in a health-care facility; or 6) plan to travel internationally.

Mumps component: Adults born before 1957 generally are considered immune to mumps. Adults born during or after 1957 should receive 1 dose of MMR unless they have a medical contraindication, history of mumps based on health-care provider diagnosis, or laboratory evidence of immunity.

A second dose of MMR is recommended for adults who 1) live in a community experiencing a mumps outbreak and are in an affected age group; 2) are students in postsecondary educational institutions; 3) work in a health-care facility; or 4) plan to travel internationally. For unvaccinated health-care personnel born before 1957 who do not have other evidence of mumps immunity, administering 1 dose on a routine basis should be considered and administering a second dose during an outbreak should be strongly considered.

Rubella component: 1 dose of MMR vaccine is recommended for women whose rubella vaccination history is unreliable or who lack laboratory evidence of immunity. For women of childbearing age, regardless of birth year, rubella immunity should be determined and women should be counseled regarding congenital rubella syndrome. Women who do not have evidence of immunity should receive MMR vaccine upon completion or termination of pregnancy and before discharge from the health-care facility.

6. Influenza vaccination

Medical indications: Chronic disorders of the cardiovascular or pulmonary systems, including asthma; chronic metabolic diseases, including diabetes mellitus, renal or hepatic dysfunction, hemoglobinopathies, or immunocompromising conditions (including immunocompromising conditions caused by medications or human immunodeficiency virus [HIV]); any condition that compromises respiratory function or the handling of respiratory secretions or that can increase the risk of aspiration (e.g., cognitive dysfunction, spinal cord injury, or seizure disorder or other neuromuscular disorder); and pregnancy during the influenza season. No data exist on the risk for severe or complicated influenza disease among persons with asplenia; however, influenza is a risk factor for secondary bacterial infections that can cause severe disease among persons with asplenia.

Occupational indications: All health-care personnel, including those employed by long-term care and assisted-living facilities, and caregivers of children less than 5 years old.

Other indications: Residents of nursing homes and other long-term care and assisted-living facilities; persons likely to transmit influenza to persons at high risk (e.g., in-home household contacts and caregivers of children aged less than 5 years old, persons 65 years old and older and persons of all ages with high-risk condition[s]); and anyone who would like to decrease their risk of getting influenza. Healthy, nonpregnant adults aged less than 50 years without high-risk medical conditions who are not contacts of severely immunocompromised persons in special care units can receive either intranasally administered live, attenuated influenza vaccine (FluMist®) or inactivated vaccine. Other persons should receive the inactivated vaccine.

7. Pneumococcal polysaccharide (PPSV) vaccination

Medical indications: Chronic lung disease (including asthma); chronic cardiovascular diseases; diabetes mellitus; chronic liver diseases, cirrhosis; chronic alcoholism, chronic renal failure or nephrotic syndrome; functional or anatomic asplenia (e.g., sickle cell disease or splenectomy [if elective splenectomy is planned, vaccinate at least 2 weeks before surgery]); immunocompromising conditions; and cochlear implants and cerebrospinal fluid leaks. Vaccinate as close to HIV diagnosis as possible.

Other indications: Residents of nursing homes or other long-term care facilities and persons who smoke cigarettes. Routine use of PPSV is not recommended for Alaska Native or American Indian persons younger than 65 years unless they have underlying medical conditions that are PPSV indications. However, public health authorities may consider recommending PPSV for Alaska Natives and American Indians aged 50 through 64 years who are living in areas in which the risk of invasive pneumococcal disease is increased.

8. Revaccination with PPSV

One-time revaccination after 5 years is recommended for persons with chronic renal failure or nephrotic syndrome; functional or anatomic asplenia (e.g., sickle cell disease or splenectomy); and for persons with immunocompromising conditions. For persons aged 65 years and older, one-time revaccination if they were vaccinated 5 or more years previously and were aged less than 65 years at the time of primary vaccination.

9. Hepatitis A vaccination

Medical indications: Persons with chronic liver disease and persons who receive clotting factor concentrates.

Behavioral indications: Men who have sex with men and persons who use illegal drugs.

Occupational indications: Persons working with hepatitis A virus (HAV)–infected primates or with HAV in a research laboratory setting.

Other indications: Persons traveling to or working in countries that have high or intermediate endemicity of hepatitis A (a list of countries is available at http://wwwn.cdc.gov/travel/contentdiseases.aspx) and any person seeking protection from HAV infection.

Single-antigen vaccine formulations should be administered in a 2-dose schedule at either 0 and 6–12 months (Havrix®), or 0 and 6–18 months (Vaqta®). If the combined hepatitis A and hepatitis B vaccine (Twinrix®) is used, administer 3 doses at 0, 1, and 6 months; alternatively, a 4-dose schedule, administered on days 0, 7, and 21 to 30 followed by a booster dose at month 12 may be used.

10. Hepatitis B vaccination

Medical indications: Persons with end-stage renal disease, including patients receiving hemodialysis; persons with HIV infection; and persons with chronic liver disease.

Occupational indications: Health-care personnel and public-safety workers who are exposed to blood or other potentially infectious body fluids.

Behavioral indications: Sexually active persons who are not in a long-term, mutually monogamous relationship (e.g., persons with more than 1 sex partner during the previous 6 months); persons seeking evaluation or treatment for a sexually transmitted disease (STD);current or recent injection-drug users; and men who have sex with men.

Other indications: Household contacts and sex partners of persons with chronic hepatitis B virus (HBV) infection; clients and staff members of institutions for persons with developmental disabilities; international travelers to countries with high or intermediate prevalence of chronic HBV infection (a list of countries is available at http://wwwn.cdc.gov/travel/contentdiseases.aspx); and any adult seeking protection from HBV infection.

Hepatitis B vaccination is recommended for all adults in the following settings: STD treatment facilities; HIV testing and treatment facilities; facilities providing drug-abuse treatment and prevention services; health-care settings targeting services to injection-drug users or men who have sex with men; correctional facilities; end-stage renal disease programs and facilities for chronic hemodialysis patients; and institutions and nonresidential daycare facilities for persons with developmental disabilities.

If the combined hepatitis A and hepatitis B vaccine (Twinrix®) is used, administer 3 doses at 0, 1, and 6 months; alternatively, a 4-dose schedule, administered on days 0, 7, and 21 to 30 followed by a booster dose at month 12 may be used.

Special formulation indications: For adult patients receiving hemodialysis or with other immunocompromising conditions, 1 dose of 40 μg/mL (Recombivax HB®) administered on a 3-dose schedule or 2 doses of 20 μg/mL (Engerix-B®) administered simultaneously on a 4-dose schedule at 0,1, 2 and 6 months.

11. Meningococcal vaccination

Medical indications: Adults with anatomic or functional asplenia, or terminal complement component deficiencies.

Other indications: First-year college students living in dormitories; microbiologists routinely exposed to isolates of Neisseria meningitidis; military recruits; and persons who travel to or live in countries in which meningococcal disease is hyperendemic or epidemic (e.g., the "meningitis belt" of sub-Saharan Africa during the dry season [December–June]), particularly if their contact with local populations will be prolonged. Vaccination is required by the government of Saudi Arabia for all travelers to Mecca during the annual Hajj.

Meningococcal conjugate vaccine (MCV) is preferred for adults with any of the preceding indications who are aged 55 years or younger, although meningococcal polysaccharide vaccine (MPSV) is an acceptable alternative. Revaccination with MCV after 5 years might be indicated for adults previously vaccinated with MPSV who remain at increased risk for infection (e.g., persons residing in areas in which disease is epidemic).

12. Selected conditions for which Haemophilus influenzae type b (Hib) vaccine may be used

Hib vaccine generally is not recommended for persons aged 5 years and older. No efficacy data are available on which to base a recommendation concerning use of Hib vaccine for older children and adults. However, studies suggest good immunogenicity in patients who have sickle cell disease, leukemia, or HIV infection or who have had a splenectomy; administering 1 dose of vaccine to these patients is not contraindicated.

13. Immunocompromising conditions

Inactivated vaccines generally are acceptable (e.g., pneumococcal, meningococcal, and influenza [trivalent inactivated influenza vaccine]) and live vaccines generally are avoided in persons with immune deficiencies or immunocompromising conditions. Information on specific conditions is available at http://www.cdc.gov/vaccines/pubs/acip-list.htm.

CHAPTER

70 Pharmacy Math

S. Scott Sutton, Nancy Culberson Taylor, and L. Clifton Fuhrman

FOUNDATION OVERVIEW

Units of Measure

Pharmaceutical calculations involve four different systems of measure: the International System of Units (SI), formerly known as the metric system, apothecaries', avoirdupois', and household. SI is an international decimalized system of measurement that uses the following units: gram, liter, and meter. SI is a decimal system, in the sense that all multiples and submultiples of the base units are factors of powers of ten of the unit. Examples of the SI system include:

- Mega: 10^6
- Kilo = 10^3
- Deci = 10^{-1}
- Centi = 10^{-2}
- Milli = 10^{-3}
- Micro = 10^{-6}
- Nano = 10^{-9}
- Pico = 10^{-12}

The apothecaries' system is a traditional system of measurement using drams (liquids) and grains (solids) and is occasionally found in prescriptions. For example, a prescribed medicine being sold in four ounce (℥ iv) bottles or five grains (V gr.) of aspirin. The system consists of two basic units, grains for solids and minims for liquids. Examples of the apothecaries' system are listed in Table 70-1.

The avoirdupois system is a system of weights or mass commonly used in the United States for measuring body weight and in selling products. The avoirdupois ounce equals 437.5 grains. Sixteen ounces (7000 grains) corresponds to 1 pound (lb) (Table 70-2).

A common household unit of measure includes the teaspoon and tablespoon. A teaspoon is equivalent to 5 mL and a tablespoon is equivalent to 3 teaspoons. Other household liquid measurements are listed in Table 70-3.

Number Systems

Pharmaceutical calculations utilize two systems of numbers, Arabic and Roman. The Arabic system is more commonly used; however, the Roman system is occasionally utilized. The Roman numeral system uses letters to represent quantities and amounts. Common examples of Roman numerals include:

- ss = ½
- I = 1
- V = 5
- X = 10
- L = 50
- C = 100
- D = 500
- M = 1000

Roman numerals may be grouped together to express different quantities. To interpret these numbers, addition and subtraction may be needed. Key issues for Roman numerals include:

- When a numeral is repeated or a smaller numeral follows a larger one, the values are added together.
  - ii = 2 (1 + 1 = 2)
  - CXIII = 113 (100 + 10 + 1+ 1 + 1 = 113)
- When a smaller numeral comes before a larger numeral, subtract the smaller value.
  - IV = 4 (5 − 1 = 4)
  - IX = 9 (10 − 1 = 9)
- Numerals are never repeated more than three times in a sequence.
  - III = 3
  - IV = 4
- When a smaller numeral comes between two larger numerals, subtract the smaller numeral from the numeral following.
  - XIV = 14 (10 − 1+5 = 14)
  - XIX = 19 (10 + 10 − 1) = 19

The Arabic system is a decimal system. The decimal point serves as the anchor. Each place to the left of the decimal signals a 10-fold increase and each place to the right signals a 10-fold decrease.

Percentage and Ratio Strengths

Medications are administered as dosage forms that contain active and inactive ingredients; however, the amount of the active ingredient in a preparation needs to be expressed. A preparation may be a solution, but may also refer to a powder

TABLE 70-1 Apothecaries' System of Measure[a]

Weight

- 20 grains = 1 scruple
- 60 grains = 3 scruples = 1 dram
- 480 grains = 24 scruples = 8 drams = 1 ounce
- 5760 grains = 288 scruples = 96 drams = 12 ounces = 1 pound

Pound (lb)	Ounce (℥)	Dram	Scruple	Grain
1	12	96	288	5760
	1	8	24	480
		1	3	60
			1	20

Volume

- 60 minims = 1 fluidram
- 480 minims = 8 fluidrams = 1 fl oz
- 7680 minims = 128 fluidrams = 16 fl oz = 1 pt
- 15360 minims = 256 fluidrams = 32 fl oz = 2 pt = 1 qt
- 61440 minims = 1024 fluidrams = 128 fl oz = 8 pt = 4 quarts = 1 gallon

Gallon (gal)	Quart (qt)	Pint (pt)	Fluidounce (f℥)	Fluidram	Minim
1	4	8	128	1024	61440
	1	2	32	256	15360
		1	16	128	7680
			1	8	480
				1	60

[a]Note: Apothecary and avoirdupois systems of measure have common terms—grain, pounds, and ounces. Pounds and ounces each have different values in each system. The grain, however, has the same value in both the avoirdupois and apothecary system.

mixture, ointment, etc. There are several ways to do this and they include: (1) amount per individual dosage form (capsule, tablet); (2) concentration per dosing volume; (3) percent; (4) ratio strength; (4) parts per million.

TABLE 70-2 Avoirdupois System of Measure[a]

- 1 ounce = 437.5 grains
- 16 ounces = 1 pound (lb) = 256 drams = 7000 grains

Pound (lb)	Ounce (oz)	Grains (gr)
1	16	7000
	1	437.5

[a]Note: Apothecary and avoirdupois systems of measure have common terms—grain, pounds, and ounces. Pounds and ounces each have different values in each system. The grain, however, has the same value in both the avoirdupois and apothecary system.

Percentage specifies the number of active parts per 100 parts (eg, the number of parts of solute in 100 total parts of solution). In pharmacy, this is expressed in three ways:

- Percent weight-in-weight: % (w/w) = grams of ingredient in 100 grams of product; assumed for mixtures of solids and semisolids
- Percent volume-in-volume: % (v/v) = milliliters of ingredient in 100 milliliters of product; assumed for solutions of liquids in liquids
- Percent weight-in-volume: % (w/v) = grams of ingredient in 100 milliliters of product; assumed for solutions, or suspensions of solids in liquids, or gases in liquids

Note: In performing calculations, percentages may be changed to a decimal fraction by eliminating the % sign and dividing the numerator by 100.

$$0.05\% = 0.05/100 \text{ or } 0.0005$$

In reverse, a concentration expressed as a decimal can be converted to a % by multiplying by 100.

$$0.50 \times 100 = 50\%$$

Ratio and proportions are frequently encountered calculations in pharmacy. Ratio strength expresses concentration in terms of parts of active ingredient related to parts of the whole. When expressing a ratio strength, the numerator is preferably set as 1. It is written with a colon between the numbers. The expression 1:2 means there is 1 part in a total of 2 parts. A ratio of 1:100 means there is 1 part of a drug to 100 parts of a mixture or preparation.

Example: 5 ounces of drug A mixed with water to make 20 ounces of mixture is 5:20 or 1:4. The ratio may be written as 1:4 or as a fraction ¼.

A proportion is the expression of two ratios which are equal. It is usually written in one of two ways: two equal fractions (a/b = c/d) or using a colon (a:b = c:d).

Parts per million is a special case of ratio strength used to express very dilute solution concentrations. Instead of fixing the numerator as 1, you fix the denominator as 1,000,000. Parts per notation is used to denote relative proportions in measured quantities; particularly in low-value (high-ratio) proportions.

ppm (parts per million) represents the number of parts of solute in 10^6 parts of solution

ppb (parts per billion) represents the number of parts of solute in 10^9 parts of solution

ppt (parts per trillion) represents the number of parts of solute in 10^{12} parts of solution

TABLE 70-3 Household System of Measure

1 tablespoon (T) = 15 mL
1 teaspoon (tsp) = 5 mL
2 tablespoons = 1 fluid ounce (fl oz) = 1/8 cup
1 cup = 8 fl oz
1 pint = 16 fl oz = 2 cups
1 quart = 32 fl oz = 4 cups
1 gallon = 128 fl oz = 16 cups

Preparations of Solutions—Dilution, Concentration, and Alligation

Dilution

Medications are often prepared by pharmaceutical manufacturers with adult usage as the primary intent. Pharmacists will encounter clinical situations in which patients are children or small in stature requiring the medication to be diluted.

Example: An aminoglycoside antibiotic injection is available as a 10 mg/mL preparation and the infant is to receive 4 mg. Volumes <1 mL are considered too small to measure accurately. Therefore, you must dilute the preparation. Prepare the dilution to a final concentration of 1 mg/mL. How much medication and how much diluent will you need if the aminoglycoside comes as 10 mg/mL in a 1 mL vial, and the entire contents of the vial are to be used?

- $\frac{1 \text{ mg}}{1 \text{ mL}} = \frac{10 \text{ mg}}{x \text{ mL}}$ x = 10 mL (total volume of the preparation)
- 10 mL − 1 mL (aminoglycoside) = 9 mL diluent Solution will then be 10 mg/10 mL (1 mg/mL).
- $\frac{1 \text{ mg}}{1 \text{ mL}} = \frac{4 \text{ mg}}{x \text{ mL}}$ x = 4 mL of solution will contain 4 mg of aminoglycoside

Concentration

A solution is a mixture of two or more substances. Solutions exist in three states: gas, liquid, or solid. A solution may exist in which the components are: (1) both liquids (a mixed drink); (2) a gas in a liquid (soda water); (3) solid in a liquid (salt water). In a solution, the substance dissolved in the liquid is the solute and the liquid is the solvent. If both substances are liquids, the component with the least amount is the solute. Concentration may be defined as follows:

Concentration = Quantity of solute/Quantity of preparation

Examples:

- A 9% solution means there are 9 parts of the drug in 100 parts of solution.
- When the drug is a liquid, 1:50 means 1 mL of drug in 50 mL of solution.
- When the drug is a solid or in dry form, 1:50 means 1 g of drug in 50 mL of solution.

Powder Volume

A medication in a solid or dry form has a weight that is taken into account when preparing solutions or suspensions; however, when this solid or dry powder is added to the diluent, it also occupies a certain volume of space. When dealing with dry pharmaceuticals, this space is called powder volume. Powder volume is equivalent to the difference between the final volume and the volume of diluent added.

Example: QP is a cystic fibrosis patient prescribed a broad-spectrum antibiotic to treat a *Pseudomonas aeruginosa* infection. You are to reconstitute a dry powder that is 500 mg. The label states that you are to add 9.3 mL and the resultant solution will be 50 mg/mL. What is the powder volume?

$$\frac{500 \text{ mg}}{x \text{ mL}} = \frac{50 \text{ mg}}{1 \text{ mL}} \quad x = 10 \text{ mL}$$

10 mL is the final volume. You added 9.3 mL, therefore the difference (10 mL − 9.3 mL = 0.7 mL) is the powder volume.

The same calculations may be made to determine powder volume for both dry powders intended for oral use and those intended for parenteral solution.

Alligation

The mixing of solutions or solids possessing different percentage strengths presents a calculation problem which may be solved using an arithmetic method called alligation. In setting up an alligation formula, you must express the strength of each component as a percentage. Then you will determine how many parts of each different percent strength product you will need to create the final desired concentration of your product. Finally, you will be able to calculate the exact quantity of each beginning product you will need to create the final product. Alligation involves changing the percentages to parts and by using ratio and proportion, solving for the unknown amount of each initial product.

Example: Prepare 500 mL of dextrose 7.5% using dextrose 5% and dextrose 50%. How many milliliter of each solution will be needed?

Cross subtract smaller number from larger number:

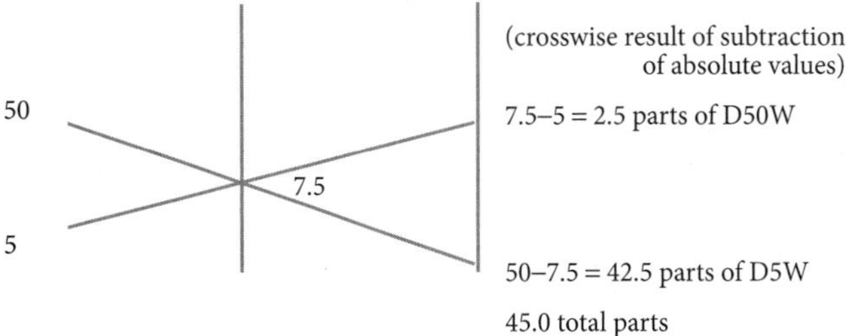

Step 1:

$$\frac{45 \text{ parts}}{500 \text{ mL}} = \frac{2.5 \text{ parts}}{x \text{ mL D50W}} \quad x = 27.78 \text{ mL D50W}$$

Step 2:

$$\frac{45 \text{ parts}}{500 \text{ mL}} = \frac{42.5 \text{ parts}}{x \text{ mL D5W}} = 472.22 \text{ mL D5W}$$

Step 3: Check to see if the two volumes of the two ingredients are equal to the total required volume

472.22 mL + 27.78 mL = 500 mL

Step 4: Another method to check your answer involves comparing the grams of dextrose of the three solutions. The grams of dextrose from the resultant 7.5% solution should equal the sum of the grams from the 50% and 5% solution.

(a) 500 mL total solution × 0.075 (7.5% solution was the desired final concentration) = 37.5 g of dextrose is the amount made in the solution. When we compare the grams of dextrose contributed by the D50W and the D5W, it should equal the 37.5 g.
(b) 27.78 mL × 0.50 (D50W) = 13.89 g of dextrose.
(c) 472.22 mL × 0.05 (D5W) = 23.61 g of dextrose.
(d) 13.89 g + 23.61 g = 37.5 g of dextrose

Other Units of Measure

Density and Specific Gravity

Density describes the relationship between the mass of a substance and the volume it occupies.

$$\text{Density} = \frac{\text{Mass}}{\text{Volume}}$$

Utilization of density allows conversion from a volume measure to a weight measure or vice versa and is usually expressed as grams per cubic centimeter or g/mL.

The specific gravity (sp gr) is a ratio of the weight of a material to the weight of the same volume of standard material. For liquids, the standard material is water, which has a density of 1 g/mL. Specific gravity is unit-less, because it is equal to the density divided by density of standard material; therefore, the units cancel out.

$$\text{Specific gravity} = \frac{\text{Weight of substance}}{\text{Weight of equal volume of water}}$$

Thus,

$$\text{Weight of substance} = \text{Volume of substance} \times \text{Specific gravity}$$

or,

$$\text{g} = \text{mL} \times \text{sp gr}$$

Examples:

- Water is the volume of standard material. It weighs 100 g/100 mL or a specific gravity of 1. Therefore, everything is compared to it.
- If the weight of 100 mL of a 50% solution of dextrose is 117 g, what is the specific gravity of the dextrose solution?
  - 117 g (weight of the dextrose solution)/100 g (weight of a 100 mL of water) = 1.17 specific gravity
- If a liquid has a specific gravity of 0.75. What is the weight of 150 mL?
  - g = mL × sp gr
  - g = 150 × 0.75 = 112.5 g

Milliequivalents

A milliequivalent (mEq) describes the ability of an inorganic molecule to dissociate in a liquid and is a measurement of the chemical activity of an electrolyte based on its valence. The equivalent weight of an ion is the atomic weight of the ion divided by the absolute value of its valence. Thus the equivalent weight of ferric ion, Fe^{3+} (atomic weight 55.9, valence 3) is 18.6. A milliequivalent is one-thousandth of an equivalent weight (eg, there are 1000 milliequivalent weights in 1 equivalent weight). For a molecule, the equivalent weight is obtained from the gram molecular weight (formula weight) divided by the total cation or the total anion charge.

Examples: Most electrolytes are measured by the milliequivalent method (the measure of the ion's combining power). The valence of an ion determines how many other ions it must combine with to form a stable compound. The valence is important, but not the positive or negative charge.

- Water (H_2O): Hydrogen has a valence of 1 and oxygen has a valance of 2. It takes two hydrogen ions to form a stable compound with 1 oxygen ion.
- Molecular weight, formula weight, and atomic weights are just numbers with no units attached.
- The atomic weight (with the unit of grams attached) and the valence determine the equivalent weight.
  - Equivalent weight (in grams) = atomic weight/valence.
  - Sodium has an atomic weight of 22.99 and a valence of 1.
  - 1 equivalent weight of sodium = 22.99/1 = 22.99 g or 23 g.
- The milliequivalent (mEq) weight is one-thousandth the equivalent weight. The milliequivalent formula is similar to the equivalent weight formula; however, mEq weight is expressed in milligrams.
  - Milliequivalent weight (in mg) = atomic weight/valence.
  - Sodium has an atomic weight of 22.99 and a valence of 1.
  - 1 mEq weight of sodium = 22.99/1 valence = 22.99 mg or 23 mg.
- The mEq weight may be used to convert between mg and mEq using the equation:
  - mg = mEq × molecular weight (atomic weight)/ valence or
  - mEq = mg × valence/molecular weight (atomic weight)
- Sodium has an atomic weight of 23 and a valence of 1. How many mEq are present in 115 mg of sodium?
  - Using the equation above: $\text{mEq} = \text{mg} \times \frac{\text{Valence}}{\text{Atomic weight}}$
    - mEq = 115 × 1/23
  - mEq = 5, so 115 mg of Na is equivalent to 5 mEq of Na
  - Or solving by proportion:

$$\frac{\text{115 mg sodium}}{\text{x mEq}} = \frac{\text{23 mg sodium (atomic weight)}}{\text{1 mEq}}$$

$$= \text{5 mEq in 115 mg sodium}$$

Moles and Millimoles

A mole = the molecular weight of a substance in grams.

A millimole (mmol) = the molecular weight or formula weight of a substance in milligrams. A one molar solution contains 1 g of molecular weight (1 GMW = 1 mole = weight in grams of Avogadro's number of particles) per liter of solution. The molarity expresses the number of moles per liter. The millimolarity (millimoles/liter) is 1/1000 times the molarity of a solution.

Examples: Magnesium has an atomic weight of 24. What is the weight of 1 millimole (mmol)?

$$1 \text{ mmol} = 24/1000 = 0.024 \text{ g or } 24 \text{ mg}$$

Milliosmoles

Osmotic concentration is a measure of the total number of particles in solution and is expressed in milliosmoles (mOsmol). Thus the number of milliosmoles is based on the total number of cations and total number of anions. The milliosmolarity of a solution is the number of milliosmoles per liter of solution (mOsm/L):

$$\text{mOsmol/L} = \frac{\text{Weight of substance (g/L)} \times \text{number of species} \times 1000}{\text{Molecular weight (g)}}$$

Number of species = number of ionic species on complete dissociation (dextrose = 1; NaCl = 2, $MgCl_2$ = 3).

The total osmolarity of a solution is the sum of the osmolarities of the solute components of the solution. When calculating osmolarities in the absence of other information, assume that salts (eg, NaCl) dissociate completely. Be aware of the difference between osmolarity (milliosmoles of solute per liter of solution) and osmolarity (milliosmoles of solute per kilogram of solvent).

CASE Application

1. Identify the Roman numeral with a value of 50.
   a. X
   b. M
   c. I
   d. L

2. Identify the Arabic value of DCXXIV.
   a. 624
   b. 626
   c. 1024
   d. 1026

3. If 120 mL of a cough syrup contains 0.4 g of dextromethorphan, how many milligrams are contained in 1 teaspoonful?
   a. 0.016 mg
   b. 16 mg
   c. 160 mg
   d. 1.6 mg

4. Interferon injection contains 5 million U/mL. How many units are in 0.65 mL?
   a. 3,250 U
   b. 32,500 U
   c. 325,000 U
   d. 3,250,000 U

5. An inhalant solution contains 0.025% w/v of a drug in 5 mL. Calculate the number of milligrams in this solution.
   a. 0.125 mg
   b. 1.25 mg
   c. 12.5 mg
   d. 0.0125 mg

6. How many milligrams of a drug would be contained in a 10 mL container of a 0.65% w/v solution of a drug?
   a. 0.65
   b. 6.5
   c. 65
   d. 650

7. How many milliequivalents of potassium are in 240 mL of a 10% solution of KCL? The gram molecular weight is 74.5 g (K^+ 39 atomic weight; Cl 35.5 atomic weight).
   a. 24 mEq
   b. 0.0745 mEq
   c. 2.4 mEq
   d. 322 mEq

8. How many milliosmoles of sodium chloride are there in 1 L of a 0.9% solution of normal saline solution? Molecular weight of NaCl = 58.5.
   a. 58.5 mOsmol
   b. 308 mOsmol
   c. 1 mOsmol
   d. 9000 mOsmol

9. What is the percentage concentration (w/v) of a 250 mL solution containing 100 mEq of ammonium chloride? Molecular weight of NH_4Cl is 53.5.
   a. 53.5%
   b. 5.35%
   c. 2.14%
   d. 21.4%

10. How many millimoles of HCl are contained in 130 mL of a 10% solution? Molecular weight = 36.5.
    a. 361 mmol
    b. 34 mmol
    c. 36.5 mmol
    d. 13 mmol

11. How many 60 mg tablets of codeine sulfate should be used to make this cough syrup?

    Rx: Codeine SO_4 30 mg/teaspoon
    Cherry Syrup qs ad 150 mL
    Sig: 1 teaspoonful every 6 hours as needed for cough

a. 7
b. 15
c. 20
d. 24

12. How many milliliters of a 17% solution of benzalonium chloride are required to prepare 350 mL of a 1:750 w/v solution?

a. 2.75 mL
b. 0.275 mL
c. 27.5 mL
d. 275 mL

13. If 10 mL of a diluent is added to an injectable containing 0.5 g of a drug with a final volume of 7.3 mL, what is the final concentration of the parenteral solution in mg/mL?

a. 6.85 mg/mL
b. 0.069 mg/mL
c. 685 mg/mL
d. 68.5 mg/mL

14. A medication order of a drug calls for a dose of 0.6 mg/kg to be administered to a child weighing 31 lb. The drug is to be supplied from a solution containing 0.25 g in 50 mL bottles. How many milliliters of this solution are required to fill this order?

a. 8.45 mL
b. 0.00845 mL
c. 1.69 mL
d. 0.25 mL

15. A solution contains 2 mEq of KCl/mL. If a TPN order calls for the addition of 180 mg of K^+, how many milliliters of this solution should be used to provide the potassium required. Atomic weight of K = 39 and the atomic weight of Cl = 35.5.

a. 343.85 mL
b. 2.3 mL
c. 39 mL
d. 74.5 mL

16. A TPN solution contains 750 mL of D5W. If each gram of dextrose provides 3.4 kcal, how many kcals would the TPN solution provide?

a. 127.5 kcal
b. 37.5 kcal
c. 34 kcal
d. 75 kcal

17. Select the definition of specific gravity.

a. Ratio of the weight of a material to the weight of the same volume of standard material.
b. The mixing of solutions or solids possessing different percentage strengths.
c. The expression of two ratios which are equal.
d. Grams of ingredient in 100 g of product; assumed for mixtures of solids and semisolids.

18. Select the apothecary measure of volume.

a. Grain
b. Scruple
c. Dram
d. Minim

19. 480 minims equals:

i. 8 fluidrams
ii. 1 fl oz
iii. 1 gallon

a. i and ii
b. i and iii
c. ii and iii
d. All of the above

20. 437.5 grains equal how many ounces?

a. 1 oz
b. 16 oz
c. 30 oz
d. 38 oz

TAKEAWAY POINTS ››

- Pharmaceutical calculations involve four different systems of measure: metric, apothecaries, avoirdupois, and household.
- The International System of Units (SI), formerly called the metric system, is the most common system of measure in pharmacy and uses the following units: gram, liter, and meter. The metric system is decimal, in the sense that all multiples and submultiples of the base units are factors of powers of ten of the unit.
- The apothecaries' system is a traditional system of measurement occasionally found in prescriptions, for example: a prescribed medicine being sold in four ounce (℥iv) bottles or five grains (V gr.) of aspirin. The system consists of two basic units, grains for solids, and minims for liquids.
- The avoirdupois system is a system of weights or mass. The avoirdupois ounce equals 437.5 grains. Sixteen ounces (7000 grains) correspond to 1 pound (lb).
- Common household units of measure include the teaspoon and tablespoon. A teaspoon is equivalent to 5 mL and a tablespoon is equivalent to three teaspoons.

- Pharmaceutical calculations utilize two systems of numbers: Arabic and Roman. The Arabic system is more commonly used; however, the Roman system is occasionally utilized.
- Medications are administered as dosage forms that contain active and inactive ingredients; however, the amount of the active ingredient needs to be expressed. There are several ways to do this and they include: (1) amount per individual dosage form (capsule, tablet); (2) concentration per dosing volume; (3) percentage; (4) ratio strength; (5) parts per million.
- Percent weight-in-weight: %(w/w) = grams of ingredient in 100 g of product; assumed for mixtures of solids and semisolids
- Percent volume-in-volume: %(v/v) = milliliters of ingredient in 100 milliliters of product; assumed for solutions of liquids in liquids.
- Percent weight-in-volume: %(w/v) = grams of ingredient in 100 mL of product; assumed for solutions or suspensions of solids in liquids, or gases in liquids.
- Medications are often prepared by pharmaceutical manufacturers with adult usage as the primary intent. Pharmacists will encounter clinical situations in which patients are children or small in stature requiring the medication to be diluted.
- A medication in a solid or dry form has a weight that is taken into account when preparing solutions; however, when this solid or dry powder is added to the solution, it also occupies a certain volume of space. When dealing with dry pharmaceuticals, this space is called powder volume. Powder volume is equivalent to the difference between the final volume and the volume of diluent added.
- Alligation is an arithmetic method of product preparation that involves using two initial products of differing percentage concentrations. Alligation involves changing the percentages to parts and by using ratio and proportion, solving for the unknown amount of each initial product.
- Density describes the relationship between the mass of a substance and the volume it occupies. Utilization of density allows conversion from a volume measure to a weight measure or vice versa.
- The specific gravity is a ratio of the weight of a material to the weight of the same volume of standard material. For liquids, the standard material is water, which has a density of 1 g/mL.
- A milliequivalent (mEq) is the measurement of the chemical activity of an electrolyte based on its valence and its ability to dissociate in a liquid. The equivalent weight of an ion is the atomic or formula weight of the ion divided by the absolute value of its valence.
- A one molar solution contains 1 g of molecular weight (1 GMW = 1 mole = weight in grams of Avogadro's number of particles) per liter of solution.
- Osmotic concentration is a measure of the total number of particles in solution and is expressed in milliosmoles (mOsmol).

REFERENCES

1. HC Ansel. *Pharmaceutical Calculations.* 13th ed. Philadelphia, PA: Lippincott Williams & Wilkins; 2010.
2. JL Zatz, M Teixeira. *Pharmaceutical Calculations.* 3rd ed. New York: NY: John Wiley and Sons, Inc., 2005.

CASE Application ANSWERS

CHAPTER 1 | Acute Decompensated Heart Failure

Questions 1 through 3 pertain to the following case.

JP is a 73-year-old man with nonischemic cardiomyopathy (EF 30%-35%) presenting to the emergency department (ED) with an acute HF exacerbation. His vital signs include BP 145/80 mm Hg, heart rate (HR) 92 beats per minute (bpm), RR 23 rpm, and O_2 sat 96% on 4 L/min of oxygen by nasal cannula (NC). Physical examination reveals 16 cm jugular venous distension (JVD), regular rate and rhythm (RRR), crackles bilaterally, and 3+ bilateral lower extremity edema. He admits to a 20-lb weight gain in the past 3 weeks since his carvedilol dose was increased and reports strict adherence to both dietary restrictions and medications. In the ED, he has already received a furosemide 40 mg IV ×1 dose with minimal response in urine output. Pertinent laboratory results include potassium 4.1 mmol/L, BNP 950 pg/mL, BUN 41 mg/dL, and creatinine 1.5 mg/dL (baseline). JP's home medications include enalapril 10 mg twice daily, carvedilol 12.5 mg twice daily, digoxin 0.125 mg/d, and furosemide 40 mg orally twice daily.

1. Based on the BNP result, JP is experiencing which one of the following?

   a. Active myocardial ischemia
   b. Shortness of breath due to a noncardiac etiology
   c. Significant volume overload and ventricular wall stretch
   d. Renal insufficiency

Answer c is correct. Common laboratory tests for assessing active myocardial ischemia (Answer a) include creatinine kinase, creatinine kinase-myocardial fraction, and troponin. Brain natriuretic peptide (BNP) is released and elevated in the setting of significant volume overload causing stretch of the ventricular wall (Answer c). It may be used to rule out other etiologies of shortness of breath due to a noncardiac etiology (Answer b), in which cases the BNP level will be normal. While BNP may be altered in the setting of renal insufficiency (Answer d), it is not to the same degree as the level of elevations which occurs in the setting of fluid overload.

---

2. Which one of the following interventions is the best for JP on arrival to the intensive care unit (ICU)?

   a. Dobutamine 2.5 μg/kg/min infusion
   b. Milrinone 0.375 μg/kg/min infusion
   c. Furosemide 80 mg IV twice daily
   d. Metolazone 10 mg po now and then daily

Answer c is correct. JP is clearly experiencing fluid overload secondary to ADHF. Currently, he is not exhibiting any signs or symptoms of low cardiac output which would necessitate administration of an inotropic agent such as dobutamine (Answer a) or milrinone (Answer b). JP has failed an initial dose of intravenous furosemide but the dose, while a reasonable initial attempt, is small. And thus, it is appropriate to try a higher dose of intravenous furosemide such as 80 mg IV twice daily (Answer c). Metolazone (Answer d) is a thiazide diuretic which will act synergistically with a loop diuretic in the setting of refractory fluid overload; however, JP has yet to be proven to be refractory to higher furosemide doses.

---

3. Which of the following is appropriate management of JP's beta-blocker at this time?

   a. Continue carvedilol 12.5 mg twice daily.
   b. Increase carvedilol to 25 mg twice daily.
   c. Decrease carvedilol to 6.25 mg twice daily.
   d. Discontinue carvedilol.

Answer c is correct. JP experienced fluid accumulation in association with recent up-titration of his beta-blocker dose. And thus, continuation of this same dose, carvedilol 12.5 mg twice daily (Answer a), is inappropriate at this time. An increase to carvedilol 25 mg twice daily (Answer b) would only be warranted if JP was tolerating the current dose with no fluid accumulation or worsening HF. A decrease to carvedilol 6.25 mg twice daily (Answer c), the previously tolerated dose, should be indicated in this situation. The decision to discontinue carvedilol (Answer d) should occur only in the setting of cardiogenic shock.

---

4. Which of the following should be closely monitored during IV diuretic administration?

   a. Hypernatremia
   b. Hypertension
   c. Hypokalemia
   d. Hypouricemia

Answer c is correct. Aggressive diuretic administration may result in hyponatremia rather than hypernatremia (Answer a). Hyponatremia frequently preexists and is a predictor of poor outcome in HF patients. Diuretic administration may cause hypotension rather than hypertension (Answer b) especially if over diuresis occurs. Hypokalemia (Answer c) is a common side effect of loop and thiazide diuretics. Hyperuricemia rather than hypouricemia (Answer d) may occur with diuretic use.

Questions 5 and 6 pertain to the following case.

AL is a 68-year-old woman complaining of "always tired these days." Her exercise tolerance is significantly less than it was 3 months ago; she now has to rest during daily activities. This has come on gradually. She has a history of hypertensive cardiomyopathy (LVEF 30% by ECHO 1 year ago). She is compliant with both diet restrictions and medications and her daughter confirms this as she prepares all meals for AL and fills her pillbox weekly. Vital signs include BP 92/57 mm Hg, HR 95 bpm (symptomatic orthostasis), and RR 16 rpm. AL has no complaints of dizziness or palpitations and her electrocardiogram (ECG) is normal. On physical examination, she has no jugular venous distention, clear lungs, and no ascites or lower extremity edema. Laboratory analysis reveals sodium 132 mmol/L, potassium 3.9 mmol/L, BUN 52 mg/dL, and serum creatinine (SCr) 1.8 mg/dL (baseline BUN/SCr 32/0.9). AL has been stable on the following oral regimen for several months: valsartan 80 mg twice daily, metoprolol XL 50 mg/d, furosemide 40 mg twice daily, amiodarone 200 mg/d, and digoxin 0.125 mg/d.

5. Which one of the following clinical categories best describes AL?
   a. Warm and dry
   b. Warm and wet
   c. Cold and dry
   d. Cold and wet

Answer c is correct. AL is not experiencing any signs of pulmonary or peripheral edema (ie, wet) based upon physical examination and thus she is not warm and wet (Answer b) or cold and wet (Answer d). In fact, the presence of orthostasis and a BUN/SCr ratio > 20 suggests volume depletion. AL is complaining of fatigue which is a common symptom of low cardiac output (ie, cold). And thus, she is not warm and dry (Answer a). AL's worsening renal function may be associated with low output. Being cold and dry (Answer c) best describes her current status. Administration of fluid would assist with correcting her volume depletion. In addition, it may or may not correct her low output.

---

6. Which one of the following is the optimal initial intervention for AL?
   a. Change furosemide to 80 mg intravenously twice daily.
   b. Hold furosemide and begin cautious hydration with IV fluids.
   c. Hold metoprolol and begin dobutamine at 2 μg/kg/min.
   d. Increase metoprolol XL to 100 mg/d.

Answer b is correct. Since AL is volume depleted, a decision to change furosemide to the more aggressive IV route (Answer a) would be incorrect. At a minimum, her diuretic dose should be held and administration of IV fluids should be reasonable (Answer b), especially given worsening renal function. Since recent up-titration of beta-blocker has not occurred and symptomatic hypotension or cardiogenic shock is not present, the beta-blocker should be continued at the current dose. In addition to not holding the beta-blocker, inotropic therapy (Answer c) would not be indicated until AL's low volume status and filling pressures are corrected. Beta-blocker up-titration (Answer d) would not be indicated until low output has been corrected.

Question 7 pertains to the following case.

After your intervention, AL feels much better. Her vital signs today include BP 126/86 mm Hg, HR 83 bpm, and RR 21 rpm and orthostasis has resolved. An ECHO (done today) reveals an EF of 15% with increasing ventricular dilation. Her relevant laboratory values are sodium 125 mmol/L, potassium 4.9 mmol/L, BUN 38 mg/dL, and SCr 1.4 mg/dL.

7. Which one of the following most likely explains AL's decompensation?
   a. Acute arrhythmia
   b. Dietary nonadherence
   c. Renal insufficiency
   d. Progression of heart failure

Answer d is correct. AL's ECG was normal and thus acute arrhythmia (Answer a) is not the cause of her decompensation. Also, the patient report strict adherence with her medications (Answer b). While renal insufficiency (Answer c) did occur in the setting of volume overload, the elevated BUN/SCr ratio did improve. Unfortunately, AL's SCr did not return to baseline suggesting that some level of HF progression may exist (Answer d). Also, the presence of hyponatremia also suggests worsening HF.

Questions 8 through 12 pertain to the following case.

CJ is an 81-year-old woman who presents to the hospital with ADHF. Vital signs include BP 92/63 mm Hg, HR 72 bpm, and RR 19 rpm. Physical examination reveals JVP elevated to the jawline, $+S_3$, bilateral rales on auscultation, 1+ abdominal ascites, and 3+ bilateral edema extending to her thighs. Chest radiograph reveals pulmonary edema and pleural effusions. Hemodynamic measurements obtained by pulmonary artery catheter (PAC) include PCWP 31 mm Hg, CI 1.9 L/min/m^2, and SVR 1400. Her laboratory values are all normal, except sodium 128 mmol/L, BUN 34 mg/dL, and SCr 1.5 mg/dL (baseline BUN/SCr 32 and 0.9). Her drugs on admission include lisinopril 20 mg/d, carvedilol 12.5 mg twice daily, bumetanide 2 mg twice daily, hydralazine 25 mg three times daily, isosorbide dinitrate 20 mg three times daily, and aspirin 325 mg/d.

8. Which one of the following is a reasonable choice for diuretic therapy in CJ?
   a. CJ should not receive diuretic therapy because she is volume-depleted.
   b. Intravenous loop diuretic therapy should be given to provide a net fluid loss of 500 to 2000 mL/d.
   c. Metolazone should be considered a first-line option because of CJ's impaired renal function.
   d. Nesiritide therapy should be used as a replacement for diuretic therapy because CJ is volume overloaded.

Answer b is correct. Avoiding diuretic administration (Answer a) in CJ is not an option as she is clearly volume overloaded. Loop diuretics are the mainstay of initial diuretic therapy for fluid overload and 500 to 2000 mL/d net fluid loss (Answer b) is very appropriate. In addition, a loop diuretic is the diuretic of choice in patients with renal insufficiency and thus metolazone (Answer c) should only be considered in addition to loop diuretic in the setting of refractory volume overload. CJ's low BP precludes nesiritide administration since this agent is a potent vasodilator. Also, the price of nesiritide prohibits it from being used first-line for diuresis.

---

9. Which of the following best describes what PCWP represents in CJ?

   a. Fluid status
   b. Inotropy
   c. Afterload
   d. Chronotropy

Answer a is correct. Pulmonary capillary wedge pressure or PCWP reflects fluid status (Answer a). The term preload rather than afterload (Answer c) represents the pressure stretching the ventricle of the heart and also reflects fluid status. Inotropy (Answer b) or the force of myocardial contraction is reflected in cardiac output (CO) and cardiac index (CI). Chronotropy (Answer d) reflects the time or rate of the heart or heart rate (HR).

---

10. What is the desired PCWP for CJ?

    a. Less than 2.2 L/min/m^2
    b. Greater than 2.2 L/min/m^2
    c. Between 6 and 12 mm Hg
    d. Between 15 and 18 mm Hg

Answer d is correct. For patients with normal cardiac function, the desired PCWP is between 6 and 12 mm Hg (Answer c). For patients with left ventricular dysfunction, the optimal PCWP is 15 to 18 mm Hg (Answer d) as maintaining mildly elevated filling pressures is essential to optimizing the Starling curve and assuring optimal cardiac output. A cardiac index of greater than 2.2 L/min/m^2 is necessary to maintain adequate tissue perfusion.

---

11. Once CJ has undergone successful diuresis, her CI and SVR do not change substantially and her vital signs and oral HF medications remain essentially unchanged with the exception of her diuretic dose. Which of the following therapies are now appropriate to manage CJ's ADHF?

    a. Nitroprusside
    b. Nesiritide
    c. Dobutamine
    d. Milrinone

Answer d is correct. Nitroprusside (Answer a) and Nesiritide (Answer b) are potent vasodilators and CJ's current BP preclude their safe use. In the setting of low blood pressure and worsening renal function, current guidelines recommend inotropic therapy. CJ is currently receiving beta-blocker therapy and thus the effectiveness of dobutamine (Answer c) will be minimal unless rather high doses are utilized. While milrinone is an inodilator and does have some vasodilatory properties, it is the best option for CJ at this time. Clinically, the increase in CO that should occur with milrinone will commonly prevent a decrease in BP (recall BP = CO × SVR) and this is more likely to be the case with an inodilator than a pure vasodilator.

---

12. Discharge for CJ is planned with outpatient inotropic therapy based on your recommendations. According to the American College of Cardiology/American Heart Association (ACC/AHA) Inpatient HF performance measures, which one of the following should be completed prior to CJ's discharge?

    a. Beta-blocker therapy in left ventricular systolic dysfunction (LVSD)
    b. Written documentation of her EF
    c. Care of her IV access site
    d. Advance directives

Answer b is correct. Addressing beta-blocker for LVSD (Answer a), intravenous access site care (Answer c), and advance directives (Answer d) are all important to addressed prior to discharging a patient for ADHF. However, written documentation of EF (Answer b) is one of several performances recommended by ACC/AHA to be obtained prior to discharge for ADHF. While beta-blocker therapy for LVSD is not required, use of an ACE inhibitor or ARB in LVSD is a current performance measure.

---

13. Which of the following should be assured prior to administering intravenous inotropes and vasodilators?

    a. Adequate filling pressures with a PCWP 6 to 12 mm Hg
    b. Adequate filling pressures with a PCWP >15 mm Hg
    c. Adequate filling pressure with an SVR > 1200 dyne/s/cm^5
    d. Adequate filling pressure with an SVR >1500 dyne/s/cm^5

Answer b is correct. Adequate filling pressures as reflected by a PCWP 15 to 18 mm Hg (Answer b) should be assured prior to safely administering IV inotropes or vasodilators. While a PCWP 6 to 12 mm Hg (Answer a) would suggest adequate filling pressures in a patient with normal cardiac function, patients with LVSD require a higher filling pressure to optimize cardiac output (starling curve). An SVR measurement (Answers c and d) reflects vascular tone or afterload and not filling pressure.

---

14. Which of the following would be a contraindication to intravenous vasodilators?

    a. Heart rate >90 bpm
    b. Heart rate >110 bpm
    c. Systolic blood pressure <90 mm Hg
    d. Systolic blood pressure <110 mm Hg

Answer c is correct. Vasodilators typically do not affect heart rate unless extreme hypotension occurs. In this setting, a reflex tachycardia would occur. And thus, a heart rate >90 bpm (Answer a) or 110 bpm (Answer b) would not be a contraindication to therapy. A blood pressure <100 mm Hg is a relative contraindication to therapy but certainly not 110 mm Hg (Answer d), a blood pressure <90 mm Hg (Answer c) is a definite contraindication to therapy.

15. Which of the following are well-known adverse effects of dobutamine?

    a. Hyponatremia
    b. Renal dysfunction
    c. Hyperkalemia
    d. Arrhythmia

Answer d is correct. If inotropic therapy improves cardiac output, it could potentially improve hyponatremia (Answer a) and renal dysfunction (Answer b), which are both markers of poor outcome in HF patients. Hypokalemia rather than hyperkalemia (Answer c) has been reported with dobutamine and is likely associated with direct stimulation of beta-receptors. Arrhythmia (Answer d) is a well known adverse effect of inotropes.

16. Which of the following is referred to as an "inodilator," having both inotropic and vasodilatory properties?

    a. Milrinone
    b. Dobutamine
    c. Nesiritide
    d. Nitroprusside

Answer a is correct. Milrinone (Answer a) is often referred to as an "inodilator" since it has both inotropic and vasodilatory properties. Dobutamine (Answer b) is an inotrope. While Dobutamine does stimulate beta-2 receptors in the periphery which can cause some mild vasodilation, it also stimulates alpha receptors, which counteracts such with mild vasoconstriction. And thus, the decrease in SVR that may occur with dobutamine administration is most likely a reflexive response to the increase in cardiac output that occurs with its use. Nesiritide (Answer c) and nitroprusside (Answer d) are potent arterial and venous vasodilators. When these agents vasodilate the arterial vessels the decrease in SVR may cause a reflexive increase in cardiac output.

17. MJ is a 45-year old man (70 kg) admitted for ADHF refractory to aggressive outpatient titration of oral diuretics, including torsemide and metolazone. He is now receiving intravenous furosemide 30 mg/h and chlorothiazide 500 mg twice daily. While MJ's vital signs and renal function appear stable (BP 110/65 mm Hg, HR 85 bpm, SCr 1.3 mg/dL), his urine output is unchanged despite over 24 hours of the above regimen, and review of continuous telemetry demonstrates multiple 10-beat runs of ventricular tachycardia. Which of the following is an appropriate next step in therapy?

    a. Initiate milrinone 0.1 μg/kg/min
    b. Initiate dobutamine 2.5 μg/kg/min
    c. Initiate nesiritide 0.01 μg/kg/min
    d. Increase furosemide to 60 mg/h

Answer c is correct. MJ is demonstrating refractory fluid overload. While the inotropic agents, milrinone (Answer a) and dobutamine (Answer b), can be considered in this setting, ventricular tachycardia precludes use of these proarrhythmic agents. The continuous infusion of furosemide can be up-titrated to the maximal target dose of 0.4 mg/kg/h, and thus, infusion rate of furosemide can be increased from 30 to 60 mg/h (Answer d). However, this is not expected to significantly further enhance diuresis. Alternative options include adding a drug with an alternative mechanism of action such as a thiazide diuretic or nesiritide (Answer c). MJ's systolic blood pressure is >100 mm Hg, making nesiritide a safe option.

18. AS is a 54-year old woman with NICM who is admitted to the critical care unit (CCU) for transplant work-up. A pulmonary artery catheter reveals elevated pulmonary pressures with a PAS 75 mm Hg despite normal fluid status. To best assess AS's appropriateness for transplant, her pulmonary pressures must be proven as reversible. Which of the following medications is commonly used for such purposes, given a short half-life and potent pulmonary vasodilator effects?

    a. Dobutamine
    b. Milrinone
    c. Hydralazine
    d. Nitroprusside

Answer d is correct. Dobutamine (Answer a) is an inotrope with minimal vasodilatory effects. While milrinone does have vasodilatory properties in addition to inotropic effects, it has a half-life of 1 hour in patients with normal renal function and up to 3 hours in patients with renal dysfunction. Thus, rapid titration of this agent is not feasible. Hydralazine is an arterial vasodilator and its half-life also precludes its use for this purpose. Nitroprusside (Answer d) is a potent mixed vasodilator with direct effects on the pulmonary vasculature. It also has an extremely short half-life.

CHAPTER 2 | Chronic Heart Failure

1. JB is a 45-year-old man with cardiomyopathy (LVEF 35%) following an acute MI. Immediately following his MI, he developed signs and symptoms of HF including shortness of breath (SOB) at rest. Which of the following best characterizes JB's current ACC/AHA HF stage and New York Heart Association (NYHA) class?

a. Stage A, NYHA class not applicable
b. Stage B, NYHA class I
c. Stage C, NYHA class II
d. Stage C, NYHA class IV

Answer d is correct. Using the ACC/AHA staging system, patients who are Stage A are at risk for developing left ventricular dysfunction and heart failure (eg, hypertension, coronary artery disease). Patients who are Stage B have developed structural heart disease but have not developed signs and symptoms of heart failure. Patients such as JB who are Stage C have developed signs and/or symptoms of heart failure. JB meets the criteria for Stage C. The NYHA classification system categorizes patients as class I if they are relatively asymptomatic and physical activity is not limited by the heart failure disease process. Patients who are NYHA class II and III are symptomatic with moderate and minimal physical activity, respectively. Finally, patients such as JB who have symptoms at rest are classified as NYHA class IV.

2. Which of the following is the best predictor of fluid status and should be monitored daily by all HF patients?
   a. Fatigue
   b. Shortness of breath
   c. Weight change
   d. Lower extremity edema

Answer c is correct. Patients with fluid overload may present with signs and symptoms of pulmonary congestion such as shortness of breath (Answer b) or peripheral congestion such as lower extremity edema (Answer d). Signs and symptoms of low cardiac output are less readily identified and may be very subjective. Vague symptoms of fatigue (Answer a) are common. Weight gain (Answer c) is the best predictor of fluid status since weight change often precedes overt HF signs and symptoms.

3. Which of the following laboratory values may be helpful in differentiating HF from other disease states that cause similar symptoms?
   a. Sodium
   b. Creatinine
   c. B-type natriuretic peptide (BNP)
   d. Hematocrit

Answer c is correct. Decreased sodium (Answer c) or hyponatremia may occur in HF and is a predictor of worse outcome. Increased creatinine (Answer b) or worsening renal function is a common objective measure of low output. Increased BNP (Answer c) is elevated in the setting of left ventricular stretch secondary to fluid overload. It may be helpful in differentiating HF from other disease states that cause similar symptoms (eg, pneumonia). In response to a decline in cardiac output, numerous compensatory mechanisms are activated to maintain adequate CO, including activation of the SNS with increased norepinephrine (Answer d). Other disease states may also cause elevated norepinephrine levels.

4. AF is a 63-year-old woman with HF (NYHA class I) receiving furosemide 40 mg twice daily, lisinopril 10 mg daily, metoprolol XL 50 mg daily, digoxin 0.125 mg daily, and spironolactone 25 mg daily. During her routine clinic visit today, pertinent findings include: BP 120/80 mm Hg, HR 70 bpm, RR 14 rpm, K^+ 5.1 mmol/L, BUN 35 mg/dL, creatinine 1.2 mg/dL (baseline), and SDC 0.7 ng/mL. Which of the following is the most appropriate change to optimize AF's medical regimen?
   a. Increase ACE inhibitor dose
   b. Increase beta-blocker dose
   c. Increase digoxin dose
   d. Increase spironolactone dose

Answer b is correct. For heart failure management, ACE inhibitor and beta-blocker therapy should be titrated to target doses demonstrated in clinical trials to improve outcomes. This patient has adequate blood pressure to increase either therapy. In addition, heart rate is adequate to further titrate beta-blocker. Unfortunately, ACE inhibitors (Answer a) are associated with dose-related hyperkalemia and this patient already has borderline high serum potassium. The desired serum digoxin concentration is less than 1 ng/mL, and thus, this patient's digoxin dose should not be changed (Answer c). Finally, aldosterone antagonists such as spironolactone (Answer d) are also associated with hyperkalemia. Thus, the spironolactone dose should not be increased and may even need to be reduced to 12.5 mg daily if hyperkalemia persists or worsens. Up-titration of beta-blocker therapy is the safest medication change for this patient (Answer b).

Questions 5 through 8 pertain to the following case.

IH is a 54-year-old African American man with systolic heart failure presenting with a 2-week history of SOB which limits his normal daily activities and increases lower extremity edema. His weight has recently increased by 10 lb. His physical examination is notable for BP 148/72 mm Hg, HR 88 bpm, RR 24 rpm, rales, and 3+ lower extremity edema. Pertinent laboratory values include: sodium 138 mmol/L, potassium 5.4 mmol/L, BUN 35 mg/dL, creatinine 0.9 mg/dL, and digoxin 2.1 ng/mL. Past medical history is significant for hypertension (HTN), gout, COPD. Current medications include lisinopril 20 mg daily, diltiazem CD 120 mg daily, digoxin 0.250 mg daily salmeterol/fluticasone 250/50, two puffs bid. IH recently began taking naproxen 220 mg tid for gout pain.

5. In addition to counseling on salt and fluid restriction, which of the following pharmacologic options is most appropriate for managing IH's fluid overload?
   a. Initiate hydrochlorothiazide 50 mg daily.
   b. Initiate furosemide 40 mg twice daily.
   c. Initiate metolazone 2.5 mg daily.
   d. Initiate spironolactone 25 mg daily.

Answer b is correct. Loop diuretics, such as furosemide (Answer b), are the treatment of choice for managing volume overload in HF patients. Thiazide diuretics such as hydrochlorothiazide (Answer a) and metolazone (Answer c) are not effective options for monotherapy; however, these therapies may be added if patients are not responding adequately to loop diuretic dose escalation. In the setting of refractory fluid overload, combined use of a loop and thiazide diuretic work synergistically through complementary mechanisms of action. Spironolactone (Answer d) has been shown to be effective in reducing mortality when added to standard HF therapy in moderately severe to severe (NYHA class III-IV) patients. The low doses (eg, 12.5-25 mg/d) used to manage HF typically do not result in clinically significant diuresis.

6. Within the following 24 hours, IH experiences a brisk diuresis with considerable improvement in HF signs and symptoms. What additional medication changes should be considered?
    a. Continue current regimen and initiate hydrochlorothiazide 50 mg daily.
    b. Continue current regimen and initiate spironolactone 25 mg daily.
    c. Discontinue lisinopril and initiate combination hydralazine 25 mg and isosorbide dinitrate 20 mg tid.
    d. Discontinue over-the-counter naproxen and initiate colchicine 0.6 mg tid until gout pain resolves.

Answer d is correct. Medications that may exacerbate fluid retention should be avoided in HF patients. The nonsteroidal anti-inflammatory drug (NSAID) that IH is taking for gout pain should be discontinued and colchicine initiated as a safe alternative for managing IH's acute gout flares (Answer d). Addition of hydrochlorothiazide (Answer a) would not be indicated unless IH demonstrated refractoriness to loop diuretic therapy. Spironolactone (Answer b) should not be considered until IH continues to have moderately severe to severe symptoms (NYHA class III-IV) and IH is not yet receiving beta-blocker therapy. In addition, current hyperkalemia would also preclude use of this potassium-sparing diuretic. Combination hydralazine and isosorbide dinitrate should only be used in lieu of ACE inhibitor therapy (Answer c) if IH exhibits intolerable hypotension, renal dysfunction, or hyperkalemia. In addition, combination hydralazine and isosorbide dinitrate may be added to ACE inhibitor in African American patients with NYHA class III to IV symptoms despite standard HF therapy.

7. Once optimal fluid status has been achieved, which of the following represents the best option to manage IH's hypertension?
    a. Discontinue diltiazem and initiate amlodipine 5 mg daily.
    b. Initiate carvedilol 3.125 mg twice daily.
    c. Discontinue diltiazem and initiate carvedilol 3.125 mg twice daily.
    d. Initiate prazosin 2 mg daily.

Answer c is correct. In addition to assisting with managing IH's HTN, carvedilol is one of the three beta-blockers shown to reduce mortality in HF patients. Amlodipine (Answer a) has not been shown to reduce mortality and would not be considered until other HF medications that also reduce blood pressure but have been shown to reduce mortality have been initiated. In addition to initiating beta-blocker therapy, diltiazem should be discontinued (Answer c) due to its negative inotropic effect which would likely cause worsening HF. Prazosin (Answer d) may be useful for controlling HTN, however, it has been shown to not benefit HF patients.

8. What additional medication change should be considered to decrease morbidity (ie, hospitalizations) outcomes for IH?
    a. Increase lisinopril to 40 mg daily.
    b. Reduce digoxin to 0.125 mg daily.
    c. Initiate spironolactone 25 mg daily.
    d. Initiate candesartan 4 mg daily.

Answer b is correct. While digoxin does not reduce mortality in HF, it has been shown to reduce hospitalization and improve symptoms. The goal serum digoxin concentration is < 1 ng/mL and serum digoxin concentrations >1 ng/mL may negatively impact IH's mortality. IH's digoxin dose should be reduced to 0.125 μg daily in an attempt to lower his serum digoxin concentration <1 ng/mL (Answer b). Although up-titration of ACE inhibitors (Answer a) to target doses reduces mortality, IH's current potassium level does not allow for the up-titration because hyperkalemia secondary to ACE inhibitor therapy is dose related. Adding spironolactone (Answer c) is not indicated unless IH has moderately severe to severe (NYHA class III-IV) symptoms despite standard HF therapy. In addition, current hyperkalemia precludes initiation of this potassium-sparing therapy. Candesartan (Answer d) is also likely to worsen IH's current hyperkalemia and should be avoided at this time. The benefit of adding an ARB to standard HF therapy is not as clinically meaningful as adding an aldosterone antagonist. In addition, dual therapy with both an ARB and aldosterone antagonist in addition to background ACE inhibitor therapy is discouraged due to the additive risk of hyperkalemia with all three agents. In fact, such "triple therapy" is given a class III recommendation (harm > benefit) in the ACC/AHA guidelines.

Questions 9 and 10 pertain to the following case.

RJ is a 71-year-old woman with a history of ischemic cardiomyopathy who presents to clinic with symptoms consistent with NYHA class IV HF. Past medical history includes hyperlipidemia, diabetes mellitus, myocardial infarction, and hypothyroidism. RJ complains of progressive weight gain (~6 lb increase since her previous visit 3 months ago), SOB at rest, 2 pillow orthopnea, and occasional paroxysmal nocturnal dyspnea (PND) Her physical examination is positive for 1+ pitting edema in her ankles and minimal JVD. Vital signs include BP 105/70 mm Hg and HR 91 bpm. Laboratory results include: potassium 3.6 mmol/L, BUN 39 mg/dL, and creatinine 1.4 mg/dL. RJ's

current medications are levothyroxine 0.05 mg daily, furosemide 40 mg twice daily, lisinopril 20 mg daily, atorvastatin 40 mg daily, aspirin 81 mg daily, insulin glargine 46 units at bedtime, and insulin aspart 6 units before meals.

9. Which of the following is the best treatment option to manage RJ's hypokalemia and fluid overload?

   a. Continue furosemide 40 mg twice daily.
   b. Increase furosemide to 80 mg twice daily
   c. Initiate spironolactone 25 mg once daily.
   d. Increase furosemide to 80 mg twice daily and initiate spironolactone to 25 mg once daily.

Answer d is correct. RJ is experiencing fluid overload based upon her signs and symptoms and the current loop diuretic dose in inadequate (Answer a). Increasing the furosemide dose alone (Answer b) is inappropriate as it will worsen RJ's relatively low serum potassium. While the addition of a potassium supplement could be considered, the addition of spironolactone along with the diuretic dose increase (Answer d) would provide additional mortality benefit as well as result in potassium retention. When added to standard HF therapy in patients with NYHA class III or IV HF symptoms, spironolactone has been shown to reduce mortality. Spironolactone alone (Answer c) at the low doses used to reduce mortality in HF does not commonly result in clinically meaningful diuresis. It is important to recognize that spironolactone alone may be insufficient to maintain adequate serum potassium levels and close monitoring is indicated.

---

10. RJ is approaching euvolemia and the medical team anticipates another 2 to 3 days of aggressive diuresis prior to achieving euvolemia. Which of the following represents the next best option to manage RJ's heart failure?

   a. Initiate metoprolol succinate 25 mg daily immediately.
   b. Initiate metoprolol succinate 25 mg daily once euvolemia is achieved.
   c. Initiate metoprolol tartrate 12.5 mg bid immediately.
   d. Initiate digoxin 0.25 mg daily.

Answer b is correct. Given the mortality benefit associated with beta-blockers in heart failure, this medication should be a part of the patient's medical regimen. However, beta-blockers should only be initiated once euvolemia is obtained and thus Answers a and c are incorrect. In addition, it is important to only use one of three beta-blockers shown to reduce mortality. Metoprolol succinate (Answer b) but not metoprolol tartrate (Answer c) has been shown to reduce mortality. Digoxin (Answer d) is indicated for patients who remain symptomatic despite standard HF therapy with both an ACE inhibitor and a beta-blocker. In addition, a lower digoxin dose should be initiated in an elderly patient to achieve a serum digoxin concentration less than 1 ng/mL.

---

11. Which of the following are absolute contraindications to the use of beta-blockers?

   a. Asthma with active bronchospasm
   b. Diabetes
   c. Chronic obstructive pulmonary disease
   d. Peripheral vascular disease

Answer a is correct. There are very few absolute contraindications to beta-blocker therapy: asthma with active bronchospasm (Answer a) and symptomatic hypotension. Relative contraindications to beta-blocker therapy include: diabetes with recurrent hypoglycemia, asthma without active bronchospasm, heart rate <55 bpm, second- or third-degree heart block, and systolic blood pressure <80 mm Hg. Given the benefit being greater than the risk, beta-blockers should not be avoided in patients with diabetes mellitus (Answer b), chronic obstructive pulmonary disease (Answer c), asthma, and peripheral vascular disease (Answer d).

Questions 12 and 13 pertain to the following case.

BT is a 54-year-old African American man recently diagnosed with nonischemic cardiomyopathy. His past medical history is notable for moderate asthma since childhood and hypertension. Current medications include salmeterol, one inhalation twice daily; fluticasone 88 μg, inhaled twice daily; furosemide 80 mg twice daily; enalapril 20 mg twice daily; and spironolactone 25 mg daily.

12. Which of the following beta-blockers is the best option to treat BT's heart failure and minimize aggravating his asthma?

   a. Carvedilol
   b. Metoprolol succinate
   c. Propranolol
   d. Atenolol

Answer b is correct. Only three beta-blockers have been demonstrated to reduce mortality in heart failure: carvedilol (Answer a), metoprolol succinate (Answer b), and bisoprolol. Propranolol (Answer c) and atenolol (Answers d) have not been studied in heart failure. Carvedilol (Answer a) is a nonselective beta-blocker, and thus, it would be more likely to aggravate underlying lung disease while metoprolol (Answer b) is beta-1 selective. It is important to recognize that beta-receptor selectivity may be less as dose is up-titrated.

---

13. Which of the following medication changes may provide further mortality benefit for BT?

   a. Digoxin 0.125 mg daily
   b. Combination hydralazine 25 mg and isosorbide dinitrate 10 mg three times daily
   c. Candesartan 8 mg daily
   d. Amlodipine 5 mg daily

Answer b is correct. The combination of hydralazine and isosorbide dinitrate has shown a significant mortality benefit in African Americans receiving optimal HF therapy with beta-blockers and ACE inhibitors (Answer b). Digoxin (Answer a) improves symptoms and reduces hospitalization but is not associated with a mortality benefit. Candesartan (Answer c) reduces cardiovascular mortality, but not all-cause mortality when added to an ACE inhibitor. Amlodipine (Answer d) has neutral effects on mortality in HF patients.

14. Which of the following is an appropriate rationale to switch an ACE inhibitor to an ARB?
    a. Hypotension
    b. Renal dysfunction
    c. Hyperkalemia
    d. None of the above

Answer d is correct. Hypotension (Answer a), renal dysfunction (Answer b), and hyperkalemia (Answer c) are all likely to reoccur with an ARB if patients experience these side effects with an ACE inhibitor. Although ACE inhibitors and ARBs have different mechanisms of action, their overall function is to inhibit the effects of angiotensin II. Blocking this pathway is responsible for the side effects listed above. An ARB may be considered for patients who have a cough or angioedema with an ACE inhibitor. These side effects are mediated by the elevation in bradykinin caused by ACE inhibitors which is not as likely with an ARB. It is important to exert extreme caution if an ARB is initiated following ACE inhibitor-induced angioedema as cross sensitivity has been reported.

15. TH is a 34-year-old man presenting with dizziness and orthostatic hypotension. His laboratory values reveal the following: potassium 5.8 mmol/L, BUN 60 mg/dL (baseline 18), creatinine 2.0 mg/dL (baseline 0.9). TH's medications include furosemide 80 mg twice daily, ramipril 5 mg twice daily, and metoprolol XL 50 mg daily. Which of the following immediate medication adjustments are appropriate?
    a. Temporarily hold furosemide.
    b. Temporarily hold metoprolol XL.
    c. Temporarily hold furosemide and ramipril.
    d. Continue current regimen with no changes.

Answer c is correct. TH's vital signs and laboratory values suggest mild to moderate dehydration with orthostatic hypotension and an elevated BUN/creatinine ratio, and thus, temporarily holding furosemide (Answer a) is indicated until TH becomes euvolemic. However, the patient is also experiencing hyperkalemia secondary to renal dysfunction, and thus, temporarily holding furosemide and ramipril (Answer c) is the most optimal response. Temporarily holding metoprolol XL (Answer b) or down-titration of dose should be considered if recent initiation or up-titration results in fluid retention or worsening HF. To continue current regimen with no changes (Answer d) would be inappropriate.

16. Which of the following beta-blocker regimens would be a goal for most HF patients?
    a. Metoprolol succinate XL 150 mg once daily
    b. Carvedilol 25 mg twice daily
    c. Atenolol 100 mg once daily
    d. Bisoprolol 2.5 mg once daily

Answer b is correct. Three beta-blockers have been shown to reduce mortality in HF patients. In these studies, target doses of these therapies included: metoprolol XL 200 mg once daily, carvedilol 25 mg twice daily (Answer b), and bisoprolol 10 mg once daily. Metoprolol XL 150 mg once daily (Answer a) is the mean dose achieved in the HF study demonstrating it's mortality benefit; however, the target dose in this study was 200 mg once daily. The mortality benefit of beta-blocker is dose-related, and thus, reaching target dose as tolerated is important. Atenolol (Answer c) has not been studied in a randomized controlled trial of HF patients, and thus, should not be considered. Bioprolol 2.5 mg once daily (Answer d) is an appropriate starting dose to consider in HF patients.

17. Which of the following are important to consider when initiating combination hydralazine and isosorbide dinitrate in an African American patient with HF?
    a. Initiate hydralazine 37.5 mg and isosorbide dinitrate 20 mg one tablet three times daily.
    b. Discontinue background ACE inhibitor therapy.
    c. Utilize a nitrate-free interval.
    d. Therapy is commonly well tolerated.

Answer a is correct. In African American patients with HF, hydralazine 37.5 mg and isosorbide dinitrate 20 mg tid (Answer a) is the appropriate starting dose while hydralazine 75 mg and isosorbide dinitrate 40 mg tid is the appropriate target dose. This combination therapy should be initiated in addition to background ACE inhibitor therapy in this patient population, and thus, Answer b is incorrect. A nitrate-free interval (Answer c) is not indicated in patients taking concomitant hydralzine. Dizziness and headache are common dose-limiting side effects of this therapy and thus, Answer d is incorrect.

18. Which of the following is the primary cost driver in HF?
    a. Medication
    b. Physician visits
    c. Home health care
    d. Hospitalizations

Answer d is correct. While medication (Answer a), physician visits (Answer b), and home health care (Answer c) are not inexpensive, hospitalization (Answer d) is the primary cost driver in HF.

19. Which of the following are important to monitor for when initiating beta-blocker therapy?
    a. Tachycardia
    b. Dehydration
    c. Fatigue
    d. Hyperkalemia

Answer c is correct. When initiating beta-blocker therapy, it is important to monitor for worsening HF including fluid retention (rather than dehydration or Answer b) as well as fatigue (Answer c). Worsening HF may occur as a result of the acute negative inotropic effects of therapy. Bradycardia rather than tachycardia (Answer a) is a common side effect of beta-blocker. Hyperkalemia occurs with many HF therapies including ACE inhibitors, ARBs, and ARAs but not with beta-blockers.

20. In which HF patients should aldosterone antagonists be avoided?
    a. Serum potassium <3.5 mmol/L
    b. Creatinine clearance is <30 mL/min
    c. Concomitant ARB therapy
    d. NYHA class III to IV despite standard HF therapy

Answer b is correct. Aldosterone antagonists (ARA) can cause hyperkalemia and renal dysfunction and thus should be avoided in patients with a serum potassium >5 mmol/L and could be safely prescribed in a patient with a serum potassium <3.5 mmol/L (Answer a). Patients with creatinine clearance <30 mL/min (Answer b) are at higher risk of hyperkalemia and thus is a contraindication to ARA therapy. Therapy with an ARA may be initiated with concomitant ARB (Answer c) or ACE inhibitor as long as hyperkalemia is not present. Combination ACE inhibitor plus ARB plus ARA is not recommended due to a perceived increased risk of hyperkalemia. This therapy is recommended in patients who are NYHA class III to IV despite standard HF therapy (Answer d).

CHAPTER 3 | Hypertension

1. What is the BP goal for a hypertensive patient without any comorbid conditions and who is at low risk for heart disease based on the Framingham risk score?
    a. <120/80 mm Hg
    b. <140/90 mm Hg
    c. <130/80 mm Hg
    d. <125/75 mm Hg
    e. <160/100 mm Hg

Answer a is incorrect. This is the cutoff for normal BP. It is important to counsel that cutoffs, including normal BP, should be viewed as the ceiling recommendation. Some studies show damage to vessels beginning at a systolic BP of 115, so 120/80 is really the maximum acceptance for normal.

Answer b is correct. In the absence of other disease states, this is the goal for a hypertensive patient.

Answer c is incorrect. This is the goal for patients with comorbid heart disease, such as diabetes or post-myocardial infarction.

Answer d is incorrect. This is the new goal recommended by the kidney foundation for patients with proteinuria.

Answer e is incorrect. This BP represents a person with stage 1 hypertension because it is less than 160/100. If the systolic is 160 or greater or the diastolic is 100 or greater, it becomes stage 2.

2. Which of the following recommendations for lifestyle modification is correct?
    a. Weight loss of at least 15 lb.
    b. Sodium restriction of 4 g or less per day.
    c. Moderation of alcohol to no more than two drinks a day for a woman, one for a man.
    d. Exercise for at least 30 minutes most days of the week.
    e. Adopt an eating plan low in potassium and carbohydrates.

Answer a is incorrect. Although many patients may require a weight loss of 15 lb or more, the recommendation is to maintain normal body weight, which is a BMI of 18.5-24.9 kg/m^2. Maintaining normal body weight can lower BP by 5 to 20 mm Hg/10 kg weight loss.

Answer b is incorrect. The recommendation is no more than 2.4 g of sodium per day. This is the same recommended daily intake for normotensive patients. Restriction of sodium can decrease BP by 2 to 8 mm Hg.

Answer c is incorrect. Alcohol should be moderated to no more than one drink per day for a woman and two drinks per day for a man. A drink is considered to be a 24 oz beer, a 10 oz glass of wine, or 3 oz of 80-proof whiskey. Moderating the intake of alcohol can lower BP by 2 to 4 mm Hg.

Answer d is correct. Thirty minutes per day is the minimum recommendation for exercise such as brisk walking. Exercise should be attempted most days of the week. Regular physical activity can lower BP by 2 to 9mm Hg.

Answer e is incorrect. The DASH plan is low in sodium and fat (saturated and total) and high in potassium, fruits and vegetables, and low-fat dairy products. Adopting the DASH eating plan can lower BP by 8 to 14 mm Hg.

3. JD is a 55-year-old African American woman with newly diagnosed hypertension. Her average BP is 167/92 mm Hg. Which of the following is the best recommendation for JD?

a. Begin hydrochlorothiazide and return to clinic in 3 months.
b. Begin metoprolol and prescribe monitoring blood pressure at home.
c. Begin two medications since most patients with stage 2 hypertension will not reach goal with one agent alone.
d. Prescribe lifestyle modifications first, and return to clinic in 1 month to determine if pharmacotherapy is warranted.
e. Begin clonidine patch since a once weekly patch increases patient compliance.

Answer a is incorrect. Although JD will most likely require two medications as she has stage 2 hypertension, it is equally logical to begin one and add the other at follow-up to determine efficacy of the first agent. However, follow-up should be monthly until the patient is at goal.

Answer b is incorrect. At home BP monitoring should be prescribed and implemented for any hypertensive patient who is willing and able. However metoprolol is not the best initial choice for this patient. Results are more inconsistent with beta-blockers than other medication classes for the treatment of hypertension, and JD does not have any concomitant conditions that would warrant starting with a beta-blocker (eg, post-MI, heart failure).

Answer c is correct. This is the best option for JD She has stage 2 hypertension, and in order to reach her goal of 140/90 mm Hg she will most likely require two medications.

Answer d is incorrect. Lifestyle modifications are essential to the treatment and management of hypertension. They should always be prescribed. However JD definitely requires medications with a BP of 167/92 mm Hg as she will most likely not reach goal with lifestyle modifications alone.

Answer e is incorrect. Although transdermal systems are good options for patients with compliance problems, clonidine and other centrally acting agents are reserved as last-line options for patients who do not respond to first-line agents. RAS agents, CCBs, and BBs should be tried before centrally acting medications.

---

4. JD was started on a new medication for her blood pressure. About a week later she noticed a persistent cough. Which of the following medications could be the cause?

a. Maxzide
b. Bystolic
c. Vasotec
d. Diovan
e. Catapres

Answer a is incorrect. Maxide is triamterene and hydrochlorothiazde, a combination of two diurectics. Cough is not a common side effect. Both may cause electrolyte abnormalities, glucose and lipid intolerance, and sexual dysfunction.

Answer b is incorrect. Bystolic is nebivolol, a BB. Cough is not a common side effect. BBs cause glucose and lipid disturbances, fatigue, bradycardia, exercise intolerance, and sexual dysfunction.

Answer c is correct. Vasotec is enalapril, an ACEI. ACEIs inhibit the breakdown of bradykinin, a vasodilator that is in high concentrations in the lungs. Increased levels of bradykinin by ACEI are hypothesized to cause the side effect of a nagging, unproductive cough. According the CHEST journal, this occurs in 5% to 35% of patients and usually resolves in 1 to 4 weeks, though in some it has been reported to last up to 3 months.

Answer d is incorrect. Diovan is valsartan, an ARB. ARBs do not inhibit the breakdown of bradykinin like ACEIs and are good alternatives for patients with ACE-induced cough.

Answer e is incorrect. Catapres is clonidine, which does not cause a cough as a side effect. The most common adverse reaction is orthostatic hypotension.

---

5. You have identified the cause of the cough. At the next visit, JD wants to change the medication as she cannot tolerate the cough. Unfortunately, she missed her follow-up and returns to you in 6 months. In between appointments she was admitted to the hospital and diagnosed with type 2 diabetes. Which of the following recommendations is best for JD?

a. Switch to Lopressor.
b. Switch to Atacand.
c. Switch to Altace.
d. Switch to Cardizem.
e. Continue her current medication as this side effect usually resolves in a couple of months, and may take up to a year.

Answer a is incorrect. Although a BB (Lopressor = metoprolol) is an alternative option for the treatment of hypertension, other medications are more appropriate to try next in this patient. In addition, JD's diabetes may be worsened due to glucose intolerance caused by BBs. However, this would not be a reason to avoid BB in the case of compelling indications (eg, HF or post-MI) or if nothing else is a viable option to reach BP goal.

Answer b is correct. JD is a diabetic with hypertension and should be on an RAAS agent, either an ACEI or an ARB (Atacand = candesartan). RAAS agents are proven to slow the progression of target organ damage in diabetics and should be used unless contraindicated. Since cough was the reason for discontinuing the ACEI, switching to an ARB is the best option to control JD's hypertension. ARBs do not cause the breakdown of bradykinin and therefore do not induce a nagging cough.

Answer c is incorrect. Altace is another ACEI (ramipril). Switching to another medication of the same class will not provide relief for JD.

Answer d is incorrect. Although calcium channel blockers are viable hypertensive agents (Cardizem = diltiazem), JD is a diabetic and if not contraindicated requires the addition of a RAAS agent.

Answer e is incorrect. Documentation of an ACEI-induced cough has shown resolution occurs as late as 3 months. Being it is 6 months post initiation of the medication, the chances of JD's cough going away are very slim. Important to note is that the cough is nonproductive and essentially benign. If a patient is not bothered by the cough, the ACEI does not necessarily have to be discontinued.

---

6. FS is a 50-year-old woman diagnosed with osteoporosis and hypertension. Which of the following antihypertensives is most likely to help the patient's osteoporosis in addition to lowering her BP?
   a. Dyazide
   b. Demadex
   c. Microzide
   d. Capoten
   e. Toprol XL

Answer a is incorrect. Dyazide is a combination of triamterene and HCTZ. Currently the doctor wants to start only one blood pressure medication.

Answer b is incorrect. Demadex (torsemide) is a loop diuretic. These agents are generally not used as monotherapy for hypertension. In addition, these agents increase the excretion of calcium, rendering this agent least appropriate for a patient with osteoporosis.

Answer c is correct. Microzide (HCTZ) is a thiazide diuretic, the preferred initial therapy for the treatment of hypertension. Unlike loop diuretics, thiazide diuretics decrease the excretion of calcium, and added benefit in a patient with concomitant osteoporosis.

Answer d is incorrect. Capoten (captopril) is an ACE inhibitor. Although ACE inhibitors are viable first-line options for the treatment of hypertension, there are no compelling indications to use this agent over HCTZ, which will also benefit the patient's osteoporosis.

Answer e is incorrect. Toprol XL (metoprolol) is a beta-blocker. This class of medications is not currently recommended as first-line agents for the treatment of hypertension in the absence of compelling comorbid conditions.

---

7. Which of the following statements is true regarding lifestyle modifications?
   a. They only decrease the risk for cardiovascular disease.
   b. They decrease the risk for renal disease but not stroke.
   c. Morbidity, not mortality, is decreased.
   d. They are critical for the prevention of hypertension but not the treatment.
   e. Risk for cardiovascular and renal disease and stroke are all decreased.

Answer a is incorrect. All forms of cardiovascular disease, renal disease, and stroke are decreased.

Answer b is incorrect.

Answer c is incorrect. Both morbidity and mortality are decreased through lifestyle modifications.

Answer d is incorrect. Hypertension represents a major public health challenge. Lifestyle modifications are essential to the management and prevention of hypertension. They decrease the risk for all forms of heart disease, renal disease, and stroke. These modifications simply represent a healthy lifestyle and should be adopted by all regardless of health status.

Answer e is correct. Lifestyle modifications decrease the risk for all forms of cardiovascular disease, renal disease, and stroke. Such modifications can benefit any patient's overall health even in the absence of disease states.

---

8. A patient presents to the emergency room (ER) with signs and symptoms of hyperkalemia. Electrolyte testing reveals serum potassium of 6.7 mmol/L. All of the following agents could cause or exacerbate the situation *except* for which one?
   a. Bumex
   b. Mavik
   c. Dyrenium
   d. Aldactone
   e. Cozaar

Answer a is correct. Bumex (bumetanide) is a loop diuretic. Loop diuretics profoundly increase the excretion of potassium, lowering the serum concentration.

Answer b is incorrect. Mavik (trandolapril) is an ACE inhibitor. This class causes an increase in serum potassium.

Answer c is incorrect. Dyrenium (triamterene) is a potassium-sparing diuretic which also increases the concentration of serum potassium.

Answer d is incorrect. Aldactone (spironolactone) is an aldosterone antagonist. Blocking aldosterone increases the concentration of serum potassium.

Answer e is incorrect. Cozaar (losartan) is an angiotensin-receptor blocker (ARB). Like ACE inhibitors, these agents also increase the serum concentration of potassium.

---

9. Which of the following is true regarding the use of combination treatment with an ACE inhibitor and an ARB for the treatment of hypertension?
   a. The combination significantly reduces the risk of cardiovascular events in this setting.
   b. The combination increases the risk of hyperkalemia but is otherwise safe in this setting.
   c. The combination improves renal function in this setting.
   d. The combination is very effective for controlling blood pressure in this setting.
   e. This combination is not currently recommended because it does not reduce cardiovascular events in this setting.

Answer a is incorrect. Although additional blood pressure lowering was achieved, it is at the expense of increased syncope, hypotension, renal dysfunction, and hyperkalemia.

Answer b is incorrect. If this combination is to be used, prudent electrolyte monitoring is required. However there is also an increased risk for syncope, renal dysfunction, and hypotension.

Answer c is incorrect. This statement is false—the combination does not significantly lower BP compared with monotherapy

Answer d is incorrect. An ACE-I does not inhibit all forms of angiotensin production. It would theoretically make sense to test the effect of additional blockade by adding an ARB, which blocks angiotensin at the receptor directly.

Answer e is correct. Until more evidence demonstrates an increase in benefit to risk ratio, this combination is not currently recommended.

10. DL is a 35-year-old man recently diagnosed with diabetes, hypertension, hyperlipidemia, and sexual dysfunction induced by diabetic neuropathy. Which of the following two-drug regimens is most appropriate to initiate in DL for antihypertensive therapy?

    a. Amlodipine + lisinopril
    b. Short-acting nifedipine + trandolapril
    c. Doxazosin + HCTZ
    d. Pindolol + losartan
    e. HCTZ + lisinopril

Answer a is correct. A RAAS agent, such as an ACE-I or an ARB, is indicated for renal protection in diabetic patients. Therefore lisinopril is an appropriate first-line option for the treatment of hypertension in this patient. A CCB such as amlodipine is appropriate, given that calcium channel blockers have equal antihypertensive efficacy (compared to an ACE-I or a diuretic) and have neutral effects on glucose homeostasis and on the lipid profile. This regimen is also least likely to worsen sexual function.

Answer b is incorrect. Although an ACE-I (trandolapril) is a good choice, short-acting CCBs should be avoided because of an increase in side effects from the immediate release formulations (flushing, headache, etc).

Answer c is incorrect. The alpha-1 blocker doxazosin would be a viable option in patients with concomitant BPH, however it is less effective in lowering blood pressure and not a first-line agent. HCTZ, normally the agent of choice, would not be appropriate in this patient since diuretics have negative effects on the lipid and glucose profile. In addition, other agents are available (CCBs). Diabetes and hyperlipidemia are not absolute contraindications for diuretics but if they can be avoided they should be. In ALLHAT, approximately 30% of patients developed lipid abnormalities but this did not translate into lower morbidity or mortality.

Answer d is incorrect. Losartan is a viable option since diabetic patients should be on an ACE-I or an ARB. However pindolol is not the best option since BBs are not first-line and they often cause sexual dysfunction. BBs with ISA, such as pindolol, seem to have neutral effects on the lipid profile but can still worsen glucose homeostasis. In addition, BBs can mask signs and symptoms of hypoglycemia (except for sweating).

Answer e is incorrect. This would be a good first-line regimen, except HCTZ can worsen glucose intolerance and the lipid profile, whereas CCBs have neutral effects. Since a CCB like amlodipine is not contraindicated in this patient, it is a better choice than HCTZ.

11. The risk for cardiovascular events increases sharply when blood pressure exceeds:

    a. 100/60 mm Hg
    b. 115/75 mm Hg
    c. 130/80 mm Hg
    d. 140/90 mm Hg
    e. 160/100 mm Hg

Answer b is correct. The study by Lewington et al demonstrated this in one million persons.

12. Which of the following is most correct regarding the pathophysiology of hypertension?

    a. Most patients with hypertension have an identifiable secondary cause such as hyperaldosteronism.
    b. Peripheral vascular resistance is often increased because the activity of the renin-angiotensin system is decreased.
    c. Cardiac output and peripheral vascular resistance are the two key factors that determine blood pressure.
    d. Stroke volume and heart rate are the two key factors that determine blood pressure.
    e. In the elderly, cardiac output rises, increasing the risk of hypertension, especially diastolic hypertension.

Answer a is incorrect since 90% of patients have essential hypertension.

Answer b is incorrect because the RAAS is activated in hypertension and Ang II increases PVR.

Answer c is correct. The stroke volume multiplied by the heart rate is the cardiac output.

Answer d is incorrect. Stroke volume and heart rate are the parameters that determine cardiac output. Blood pressure is determined by cardiac output and peripheral vascular resistance.

Answer e is incorrect. Isolated systolic hypertension accounts for more than two-thirds of hypertensive cases in the elderly population. As individuals age, their risk of developing systolic hypertension increases while diastolic hypertension tends to stabilize or decrease.

13. AC is a 46-year-old white man with a medical history significant for type 2 diabetes (4 years), obesity, and new-onset hypertension. He is treated for his diabetes and his current HA1c is 7.2%.

He was started on lisinopril 10 mg 4 weeks ago and the dose was increased after 2 weeks to 20 mg. His BP is now 146/94 mm Hg and his heart rate is 67 beats per minute (bpm). Which of the following is the most appropriate recommendation for AC?

a. Continue current regimen with no changes.
b. Discontinue lisinopril and start diltiazem.
c. Discontinue lisinopril and start HCTZ.
d. Add atenolol.
e. Add amlodipine.

Answer a is incorrect. The patient's blood pressure is not at goal and requires intervention. BP reductions are required to decrease morbidity and mortality associated with hypertension.

Answers b and c are incorrect. ACE inhibitor therapy is warranted in a hypertensive diabetic and should be continued unless the patient has contraindications to ACE inhibitor therapy (this patient does not have any contraindications).

Answer d is incorrect. Beta blocker therapy is controversial in the management of hypertension, except when the patient has a compelling indication (eg, myocardial infarction).

Answer e is correct. The calcium channel blocker amlodipine is the best option.

---

14. TJ is a 64-year-old man with long-standing hypertension. He has recently been diagnosed with chronic kidney disease and his estimated glomerular filtration rate (GFR) is 24 mL/min. He is currently taking ramipril 10 mg/d and verapamil ER 240 mg/d. His blood pressure is 138/86 mm Hg, heart rate (HR) is 58 bpm, and electrolytes notable for a potassium of 5.1 mEq/L. Which of the following would be the best recommendation?

a. Continue current therapy and monitor BP regularly.
b. Add HCTZ 12.5 mg daily.
c. Add furosemide 20 mg twice daily.
d. Increase verapamil ER to 360 mg daily.
e. Add spironolactone 25 mg qd.

Answer a is incorrect. The patient's blood pressure is not at goal and requires intervention.

Answer b is incorrect. HCTZ is unlikely to be effective because the patient has kidney dysfunction (CrCl < 30 mL/min).

Answer c is correct. Loop diuretics such as furosemide may be used in hypertensive patients with reduced CrCl. Loop diuretics are filtered and secreted, so when a patient loses kidney filtration ability (ie, CrCl < 30 mL/min), the loop diuretics may still be effective (thiazide diuretics would most likely not be effective in this setting because they are only filtered).

Answer d is incorrect. Increasing the verapamil would not be appropriate given the patient's heart rate. Verapamil is a negative chronotrope and requires monitoring of heart rate.

Answer e is incorrect. Spironolactone use in the setting of renal dysfunction would increase the risk of hyperkalemia. The patient's potassium level is already on the high end of the normal range.

---

15. RH is a 47-year-old white woman who has been seen by her family physician twice in the last 2 weeks, and her BP (measured properly) was similar at both visits, averaging 138/98 mm Hg. RH has no significant medical history or risk factors for cardiovascular disease; she is relatively active and likes to exercise. Which of the following would be the most appropriate recommendation for RH?

a. She should be seen again by her physician within 2 months to see if she has hypertension.
b. She should be counseled to undertake an intensive weight reduction program, with follow-up in 2 months.
c. Initiate treatment with ramipril.
d. Initiate treatment with atenolol.
e. Initiate treatment with clonidine.

Answers a and b are incorrect. Drug therapy is warranted in patients with diastolic hypertension. While lifestyle modifications are indicated, the patient should also be started on antihypertensive medications.

Answer c is correct. ACE inhibitors are effective first-line options for the management of hypertension.

Answer d is incorrect. Beta blocker therapy is controversial as initial therapy, except when there is a compelling indication present (eg, previous myocardial infarction). Atenolol might also impair the exercise tolerance in this active patient.

Answer e is incorrect. Clonidine is not recommended as initial therapy for hypertension. Clonidine is reserved for hypertension not responding to traditional agents (eg, ACE inhibitors, diuretics, calcium channel blockers).

---

16. In a patient with risk factors for hyperkalemia and history of hyperkalemia, which of the following agents would be the least likely to increase potassium?

a. Amiloride
b. Amlodipine
c. Enalapril
d. Spironolactone
e. Valsartan

Answer a is incorrect. Amiloride is a potassium sparing diuretic (similar to triamterene).

Answer b is correct. Calcium-channel blockers (such as amlodipine) are not associated with hyperkalemia.

Answer c is incorrect. ACE inhibitors (such as enalapril) are associated with hyperkalemia because of their effects on aldosterone.

Answer d is incorrect. Spironolactone is a potassium-sparing diuretic (aldosterone antagonist).

Answer e is incorrect. Angiotensin receptor blockers (such as valsartan) are associated with hyperkalemia because of their effects on aldosterone.

---

17. Which of the following agents is the least likely to increase blood glucose?
    a. Chlorthalidone
    b. Furosemide
    c. Hydrochlorothiazide
    d. Lisinopril
    e. Propranolol

Answers a, b, c, and e are incorrect. These are all associated with blood glucose effects and would not be the answer to this question because the questions asks to select the medication least likely to effect blood glucose.

Answer d is correct. ACE inhibitors (such as lisinopril) are not associated with hyperglycemia. ACE inhibitors are beneficial in diabetic patients.

18. FS is a 56-year-old man with diabetes mellitus and newly diagnosed hypertension. His mean blood pressure in clinic today after three proper measurements is 158/101 mm Hg. He is not currently on treatment. Which of the following drug regimens would be the most appropriate to treat FS?
    a. Chlorthalidone
    b. Quinapril
    c. Benazepril + amlodipine
    d. Benazepril + losartan
    e. Atenolol + HCTZ

Answer a is incorrect. While chlorthalidone is an effective hypertensive medication, ACE inhibitors are preferred in a hypertensive patient with diabetes. Also, combination therapy is warranted in patients with a BP goal < 130/80 mm Hg that is more than 20 mm Hg from goal.

Answer b is incorrect. ACE inhibitor therapy is warranted in this patient; however, since this patient is more than 20 mm Hg away from BP goal, combination therapy should be used.

Answer c is correct. Because the patient has diabetes, ACE inhibitor therapy should be part of the combination regimen. The addition of a calcium channel blocker has been shown to be beneficial in this setting.

Answer d is incorrect. While this patient should be given an ACE inhibitor, combination therapy with an angiotensin-receptor blocker is not warranted in hypertension.

Answer e is incorrect. Because the patient has a history of diabetes, the combination regimen needs to include an ACE Inhibitor.

19. How would you classify an average blood pressure of 158/104 mm Hg (it is taken properly and averaged over two clinical visits)?
    a. Normal
    b. Prehypertension
    c. Stage 1 hypertension
    d. Stage 2 hypertension
    e. None of the above

Answer a is incorrect. Normal BP would be < 120/80.

Answer b is incorrect. Prehypertension is systolic BP 120-139 and diastolic BP 80-89.

Answer c is incorrect. Stage 1 is systolic BP 140-159 and diastolic BP 90-99.

Answer d is correct. Stage 2 is systolic BP greater than or equal to 160 and diastolic BP is greater than or equal to 100. While the systolic BP appears to be stage 1, the diastolic BP is stage 2. Classification is driven by which one is the highest.

Answer e is incorrect. The patient has stage 2 hypertension.

20. Which of the following does *not* require monitoring in a patient on HCTZ?
    a. Renal function
    b. Hepatic function
    c. Electrolytes
    d. Uric acid
    e. Blood glucose

Answers a, c, d, and e are incorrect. These are all effects of HCTZ and should be monitored or followed.

Answer b is correct. HCTZ is not associated with liver effects and therefore hepatic function does not need to be monitored.

21. Which of the following should be considered in patients with resistant hypertension?
    a. Volume overload is a common cause.
    b. Spironolactone might be effective.
    c. Minoxidil might be effective.
    d. A loop diuretic might be necessary.
    e. All of the above.

Answer a is correct. Patients with volume overload may have resistant hypertension.

Answer b is correct. Spironolactone may be used in the treatment of resistant hypertension.

Answer c is correct. Minoxidil is a direct acting vasodilator that may be used in the treatment of resistant hypertension.

Answer d is correct. Diuretic therapy might be necessary in resistant hypertension.

Answer e is the correct and best answer.

CHAPTER 4 | Dyslipidemia

1. MM is a 74-year-old woman with a past medical history (PMH) of unstable angina, hypertension, and diabetes. She smokes two packs of cigarettes daily. Her LDL-C is 120 mg/dL, HDL-C 48 mg/dL, and TG 220 mg/dL. Which of the following is *not* an acceptable LDL-C goal for MM?

1. <70 mg/dL
2. <100 mg/dL
3. A 20% to 30% decrease
4. A 30% to 40% decrease

Answer a is incorrect. This goal is acceptable. The ADA recommends a lower optional goal of <70 mg/dL for patients with diabetes and overt CVD. She also meets the criteria for "very high risk" with an optional goal of <70 mg/dL per the ATP III update.

Answer b is incorrect. This goal is acceptable. ADA guidelines recommend a goal of <100 mg/dL for patients with diabetes.

Answer c correct. A 20% to 30% reduction is an insufficient goal for this high-risk patient.

Answer d is incorrect. This goal is acceptable. A 30% to 40% reduction is recommended by the ATP III update for higher risk patients.[4] The ADA also allows a 30% to 40% reduction as an alternative therapeutic goal in patients with diabetes who do not reach target LDL-C on maximally tolerated statin.

---

2. KW is a 53-year-old Asian woman with an LDL-C of 210 mg/dL, HDL-C 56mg/dL, and TG 182 mg/dL. Her PMH is notable for hypertension with a recent BP of 118/70 mm Hg on lisinopril monotherapy. She is a nonsmoker. Her father died of a myocardial infarction at age 58. Which of the following are ATP III major risk factors for CHD that modify her LDL-C goal?

   a. Her age
   b. Family history of heart disease
   c. Hypertension
   d. Low HDL-C

Answer a is incorrect. Only age ≥55 years in women and ≥45 years in men is a major risk factor.

Answer b is incorrect. Only a family history of premature CHD (CHD in male first-degree relative <55 years of age or in female first-degree relative <65 years of age) is a major risk factor.

Answer c is correct. Hypertension (BP ≥140/90 mm Hg) or use of antihypertensive medication, even with well-controlled blood pressure, is a major risk factor.

Answer d is incorrect. Only HDL-C <40 mg/dL is a major risk factor. HDL-C >60 mg/dL allows removal of one risk factor from the total count.

---

3. KW's physician elects to use rosuvastatin to treat her hyperlipidemia and requests a dosing recommendation. Select the most appropriate starting dose for this patient, keeping in mind genetic factors.

   a. 5 mg daily
   b. 10 mg daily
   c. 20 mg daily
   d. 40 mg daily
   e. 80 mg daily

Answer a is correct. Asian patients have a twofold increase in median exposure to rosuvastatin compared to Caucasians. The recommended starting dose is 5 mg in these patients.

Answers b, c, and d are incorrect. The starting doses are too high for an Asian patient. The 40-mg dose in Answer d is reserved for patients who have not met therapeutic goals on the 20-mg dose.

Answer e is incorrect. The maximum daily dose is 40 mg daily. Proteinuria was observed in patients receiving rosuvastatin 80 mg daily in clinical trials.

---

4. LE is a 33-year-old woman currently attempting to become pregnant. Her physician decides that benefits of hyperlipidemia treatment outweigh fetal risks. Her LDL-C is 240 mg/dL, HDL-C 64 mg/dL, and TG 132 mg/dL. Her PMH includes recent cholelithiasis. What is the most appropriate medication for LE?

   a. Rosuvastatin
   b. Niacin
   c. Colesevelam
   d. Gemfibrozil
   e. Omega-3-acid ethyl esters

Answer a is incorrect. Statins are pregnancy category X and should only be given to women of childbearing age if they are highly unlikely to conceive.

Answer b is incorrect. Niacin is pregnancy category C and insufficiently studied in pregnancy.

Answer c is correct. Cholesterol and cholesterol derivatives are critical for normal fetal development. Because BAS are not systemically absorbed, they are considered the treatment of choice for women of childbearing age who are lactating or pregnant, or could become pregnant. Colesevelam is pregnancy category B and also not expected to be excreted in breast milk. Clofibrate and cholestyramine are pregnancy category C.

Answer d is incorrect. Gemfibrozil is pregnancy category C and contraindicated in patients with gallstones.

Answer e is incorrect. Omega-3-acid ethyl esters (Lovaza) is pregnancy category C and may actually increase LDL-C further.

---

5. MJ has a history of subtherapeutic anticoagulation on warfarin (due to poor adherence) until the administration time was changed from evening to morning. The patient also frequently skips meals and takes antacids for reflux. Which of the following statins is optimal for this patient?

   a. Pravastatin
   b. Atorvastatin
   c. Lovastatin
   d. Rosuvastatin
   e. Fluvastatin

Answer a is incorrect. Pravastatin has a short half-life and should be dosed in the evening since cholesterol synthesis is maximal at night.

Answer b is correct. Atorvastatin has a longer half-life and can be dosed at any time of day. Atorvastatin is also unlikely to interact with warfarin.

Answer c is incorrect. Lovastatin should be dosed in the evening with food, while other statins may be given with or without food. Both lovastatin and simvastatin can increase the effects of warfarin through CYP3A4 inhibition.

Answer d is incorrect. Rosuvastatin has the longest half-life and can be given at any time of day. However, it may cause a pronounced prothrombin increase in patients on warfarin due to CYP-3A4 and possibly CYP-2C9 inhibition. Rosuvastatin should also be dosed at least 2 hours apart from antacids due to reduced absorption.

Answer e is incorrect. Fluvastatin must also be dosed in the evening and potently inhibits CYP-2C9, which could result in increased warfarin effects.

---

6. CE is a 74-year-old man with a PMH of CHD, stroke, and hypothyroidism. He currently takes aspirin, levothyroxine, and simvastatin and has now been prescribed cholestyramine. What will you discuss with the patient?
   a. Take on an empty stomach once daily.
   b. Mix each dose with at least 12 oz of juice or soda.
   c. Sip slowly to reduce side effects.
   d. Take other medications at least 1 to 2 hours before or 4 to 6 after cholestyramine.

Answer a is incorrect. BAS should be taken with or just after meals in 2 to 3 divided doses daily, with the exception of colesevelam (625 mg, six tablets per day), which may be dosed all at once if tolerated.

Answer b is incorrect. Cholestyramine (and colestipol) powder should be mixed with 2 to 6 oz of water, a noncarbonated beverage such as orange, apple or grape juice, or a high moisture content pulpy fruit (eg, applesauce).

Answer c is incorrect. Powdered resins may cause teeth discoloration, erosion, and decay and must be swallowed quickly.

Answer d is correct. Cholestyramine and colestipol can bind a wide array of medications, including digoxin, warfarin, levothyroxine, phenytoin, niacin, oral contraceptives, ezetimibe, fibrates, statins, and aspirin.[31] Interacting medications should be given 1 to 2 hours before or 4 to 6 hours after these resins. Colesevelam has the lowest likelihood of interactions, but the manufacturer still recommends either closely monitoring or separating medications with a narrow therapeutic index by 4 hours.

---

7. Select the brand name for fenofibrate.
   a. Fenoglide
   b. Tricor
   c. Triglide
   d. Lipofen
   e. All of the above

Answer e is correct and the best answer. All are brand names for fenofibrate so all options from Answer a to d are correct. Generic fenofibrate is also available.

---

8. What medication for hyperlipidemia may be used in a patient with active hepatic disease?
   a. Colesevelam
   b. Simvastatin
   c. Ezetimibe
   d. Niacin
   e. Gemfibrozil

Answer a is correct. BAS are not contraindicated in hepatic disease, although these patients may be sensitive to GI side effects. No dose adjustment is necessary for drugs in this class.

Answer b is incorrect. Statins are contraindicated in patients with active hepatic disease.

Answer c is incorrect. Ezetimibe is not recommended in patients with moderate or severe hepatic impairment.

Answer d is incorrect. Niacin is contraindicated in patients with active hepatic disease.

Answer e is incorrect. Fibrates are contraindicated in patients with hepatic dysfunction.

---

9. JM is a 64-year-old woman with a PMH of pancreatitis (when TGs were 2200 mg/dL), uncontrolled gout, severe psoriasis, recurrent infections requiring hospitalization, and lovastatin-associated myopathy. Her current medications include rosuvastatin, prednisone, and allopurinol. Colchicine was also added a few days ago for a gout exacerbation. She reports an anaphylactic reaction after eating seafood in college. Her LDL-C is 96 mg/dL, HDL-C 42 mg/dL, and TG 540 mg/dL. Which of the following is the safest addition to her therapy?
   a. Niacin
   b. Colesevelam
   c. Fish oil
   d. Gemfibrozil
   e. Fenofibrate

Answer a is incorrect. There is no convincing evidence that the niacin-statin combination results in greater risk of myopathy over statin monotherapy. There is also only weak, largely anecdotal evidence linking niacin monotherapy to myopathy. However, niacin should be avoided in this patient with uncontrolled gout since it may increase uric acid.

Answer b is incorrect. BAS can increase TG and are contraindicated in patients with TG >500 mg/dL or history of pancreatitis caused by elevated TG.

Answer c is incorrect. Fish oil is best avoided considering her severe allergic reaction to seafood. EPA and DHA in doses >3 g/d may also suppress T- and B-cell function and lead to more infections in combination with prednisone.

Answer d is incorrect. Gemfibrozil is a potent inhibitor of several components of statin metabolism, inhibiting glucuronidation, OATP1B1-mediated uptake of statin acids, and biliary excretion. Gemfibrozil increases myopathy risk by increasing the plasma concentrations of most statins. Myopathy risk is also increased when gemfibrozil is combined with colchicine.

Answer e is correct. Fenofibrate does not appear to interfere with statin metabolism and has a rate of reported rhabdomyolysis 15 times lower than that of gemfibrozil when combined with statins.

---

10. Select the brand name for lovastatin.
    a. Lescol
    b. Crestor
    c. Mevacor
    d. Pravachol
    e. Zocor

Answer a is incorrect. Lescol is the brand name for fluvastatin.

Answer b is incorrect. Crestor is the brand name for rosuvastatin.

Answer c is correct. Mevacor is the brand name for lovastatin.

Answer d is incorrect. Pravachol is the brand name for pravastatin.

Answer e is incorrect. Zocor is the brand name for simvastatin.

---

11. Which of the following statins should be temporarily discontinued for a patient starting a short course of clarithromycin?
    a. Simvastatin
    b. Pravastatin
    c. Lovastatin
    d. Atorvastatin
    e. a and c

Answer a is correct. Simvastatin is metabolized by the CYP-3A4 isoenzyme and should not be coadministered with clarithromycin.

Answer b is incorrect. Pravastatin does not require dose adjustment. It is metabolized through non-CYP enzymes.

Answer c is correct. Lovastatin is metabolized by the CYP-3A4 isoenzyme and should not be coadministered with clarithromycin.

Answer d is incorrect. Although atorvastatin is metabolized by CYP-3A4 to a small extent, there are no specific recommendations for therapy adjustment with clarithromycin.

Answer e is correct and the best answer. Simvastatin and lovastatin should never be given with itraconazole, ketoconazole, telithromycin, clarithromycin, erythromycin, protease inhibitors, and nefazodone. Patients especially taking higher doses of simvastatin and lovastatin should also avoid grapefruit juice in quantities over 1 quart per day, which has been associated with rhabdomyolysis.

---

12. Which of the following statin doses may be dispensed to a patient also taking gemfibrozil?
    a. Rosuvastatin 20 mg
    b. Simvastatin 20 mg
    c. Lovastatin 40 mg
    d. Fluvastatin 40 mg

Answer a is incorrect. Although rosuvastatin has few drug interactions since 90% is eliminated unchanged, doses should not exceed 5 mg for patients on cyclosporine and 10 mg for those on gemfibrozil, ritonavir, lopinavir, and oral contraceptives.

Answer b is incorrect. Simvastatin doses should not exceed 10 mg for patients on gemfibrozil, danazol, and cyclosporine and 20 mg for those on amiodarone and verapamil.

Answer c is incorrect. Lovastatin doses should not exceed 20 mg for patients on gemfibrozil, fenofibrate, cyclosporine, and niacin (≥ 1 g/d) and 40 mg for those on amiodarone and verapamil.

Answer d is correct. There is no dose limit for fluvastatin in combination with gemfibrozil. Studies suggest that fluvastatin is the only statin that may be safely combined with gemfibrozil, although caution is still advised.

---

13. LR is a 54-year-old woman with elevated TG who wants to substitute OTC fish oil instead of omega-3-acid ethyl esters (Lovaza) to save money. Her physician approves this change. She mentions past GI problems with dietary fish. What should you advise the patient regarding a product with 180 mg of EPA and 120 mg of DHA per capsule?
    a. Change to the more concentrated cod liver oil.
    b. Six capsules a day will equal the dose of the prescription product.
    c. Take on an empty stomach to improve tolerability.
    d. Eleven capsules a day will equal the dose of the prescription product.
    e. Have your mercury levels tested periodically.

Answer a is incorrect. Cod liver oil can cause toxicity with long-term use or large doses due to vitamin A content.

Answer b is incorrect. Since OTC fish oil capsules generally contain only 30% to 50% of EPA and DHA per 1000- to 1200-mg capsule, an even larger number of capsules would be needed to lower TG.

Answer c is incorrect. Fish oil tolerability may be improved by dosing with meals, spacing doses apart, using enteric-coated products, and freezing capsules (however, the manufacturer recommends against freezing Lovaza).

Answer d is correct. Lovaza contains 840 mg of EPA and DHA per 1000-mg capsule and is dosed four capsules once daily or two capsules tid with meals. Since at least 11 capsules a day of this fish oil would provide an equivalent therapeutic dose, a higher potency product should be considered.

Answer e is incorrect. The majority of OTC products have no detectable levels of mercury and other toxins.

---

14. RR is a 56-year-old Asian man with an LDL-C of 180 mg/dL, HDL-C 28 mg/dL, and TG 140 mg/dL. His fasting glucose is 96 mg/dL, waist circumference 41 in, and BP 128/82 mm Hg. His medications include hydrochlorothiazide and gemfibrozil. Which of the following does *not* potentially indicate metabolic syndrome in R.R.?

 a. HDL-C
 b. TG
 c. Fasting glucose
 d. Waist circumference
 e. BP

Answer a is incorrect. HDL-C <40 mg/dL in men and <50 mg/dL in women is defined as a potential risk factor. ATP III guidelines classify a patient with *three* such risk factors as having metabolic syndrome.

Answer b is incorrect. Although ATP III only defines TG ≥150 mg/dL as a potential risk factor, the diagnostic criteria were recently expanded to include drug treatment of elevated TG.

Answer c is correct. Although ATP III considers fasting glucose ≥110 mg/dL as a potential risk factor, the definition was lowered to ≥100 mg/dL based on the ADA's revised definition of impaired fasting glucose. RR's fasting glucose is currently <100 mg/dL, so glucose is not a risk factor at this time.

Answer d is incorrect. ATP III defines abdominal obesity (waist circumference >40 in. in men, >35 in women) as a risk factor. Newer diagnostic criteria also recommend using a lower waist of >35 in. in men and >31 in, in women for Asian Americans.

Answer e is incorrect. Although ATP III only defines BP ≥130/85 mm Hg as a potential risk factor, diagnostic criteria were expanded to include drug treatment of hypertension.

---

15. Which of the following key ATP III therapeutic lifestyle changes (TLC) should be recommended to patients with hyperlipidemia?

 a. Increase soluble fiber to at least 50 g/d.
 b. Limit cholesterol intake to <400 mg/d.
 c. Reduce trans fat and limit saturated fat to <15% of calories.
 d. Engage in regular physical activity.
 e. Eat one serving per week of fatty fish.

Answer a is incorrect. Patients should be advised to increase soluble fiber to 10 to 25 g/d. Plant stanols/sterols at a dose of 2 g/d may also be helpful.

Answer b is incorrect. Cholesterol intake should be kept <200 mg/d.

Answer c is incorrect. Although trans fat should be reduced or preferably eliminated, the recommended saturated fat intake is <7% of calories.

Answer D is correct. Increased activity should be recommended to all patients without physical restrictions. Regular physical activity and weight loss can raise HDL-C, reduce TG, and lower LDL-C.

Answer e is incorrect. The American Heart Association recommends consuming at least two servings of fish per week for the general population and approximately 1 g of EPA + DHA daily (preferably from oily fish) for those with documented CHD. ATP III guidelines support including fish in the diet but do not recommend a specific amount of dietary omega-3 fatty acids.

---

16. Select a patient risk factor for development of myopathy on statin therapy.

 a. Larger body size
 b. Hyperthyroidism
 c. Male sex
 d. Vitamin D deficiency
 e. Young age

Answer a is incorrect. Small body frame and frailty are risk factors.

Answer b is incorrect. Hypothyroidism is a risk factor, and thyroid-stimulating hormone should be screened at baseline or checked in patients who develop symptoms.

Answer c is incorrect. Women have greater risk.

Answer d is correct. Vitamin D deficiency has been found to predispose patients to statin-induced myopathy, with resolution in the majority of patients after replacement.

Answer e is incorrect. Advanced age is a risk factor. Other risk factors are alcoholism, major surgery, trauma, strenuous physical activity, multisystem disease, history of myopathy with another lipid-lowering therapy, history of CK elevation, unexplained cramps, family history of myopathy or myopathy while receiving lipid-lowering therapy, higher statin dose, and the presence of concomitant interacting drugs.

---

17. CL is a 10-year-old boy with familial hyperlipidemia (FH). His physician wishes to use drug therapy since TLC has failed. His LDL-C is 320 mg/dL. Which of the following medications would you recommend?

 a. Atorvastatin
 b. Colesevelam
 c. Ezetimibe
 d. Niacin
 e. Fenofibrate

Answer a is correct. Atorvastatin is approved for treatment of FH in children 10 years of age and older. Pravastatin and simvastatin are also approved for treatment of FH in children 8 and 10 years of age and older, respectively.

Answer b is incorrect. Colesevelam is not recommended in this population due to the large tablet size. Cholestyramine is approved for treating hypercholesterolemia in children but has poor adherence.[6,34]

Answer c is incorrect. Although ezetimibe appears effective and tolerable in children ages 10 to 17 years, it is not FDA-approved in this population. It also causes only a modest LDL-C reduction compared to atorvastatin.

Answer e is incorrect. Niacin has not been adequately studied in this population and is not generally recommended.[29,34]

Answer d is incorrect. The fibrates have not been adequately studied in this population and are not generally recommended.

---

18. Select the lipid-lowering medication that requires adjustment in a patient with renal impairment.

    a. Atorvastatin
    b. Gemfibrozil
    c. Ezetimibe
    d. Cholestyramine
    e. Niacin

Answer a is incorrect. Atorvastatin and fluvastatin (≤40 mg) are confirmed to be safe in this population. Atorvastatin has even been shown safe in patients with diabetes on dialysis. Although statins at currently approved doses are not considered nephrotoxic, all other drugs in this class should be given at lower doses to reduce myopathy risk.

Answer B is correct. Fibrates require renal adjustment in patients with mild to moderate renal impairment. Fibrates are also contraindicated in patients with severe renal impairment, defined by manufacturers as <30 mL/min for fenofibrate and <10 mL/min for gemfibrozil.

Answer c is incorrect. Ezetimibe does not require adjustment.

Answer d is incorrect. Cholestyramine and other BAS do not require adjustment.

Answer e is incorrect. There are no specific renal adjustments for niacin, although niacin should be used with caution in this population.

---

19. A patient on simvastatin complains of muscle pain, weakness, and cramps since running a marathon this past weekend. His CK is 1760 U/L today (normal range, 50-160) and 280 U/L when checked 3 months ago. His Cr is 1.0 mg/dL. How should you manage this patient?

    a. Continue therapy and closely monitor the CK.
    b. Stop simvastatin until symptoms and CK improve, then try another statin.
    d. Add coenzyme Q10.
    e. Change simvastatin to ezetimibe.

Answer a is incorrect. Experts generally agree that statins should be stopped for intolerable muscle complaints, progressively increasing CK, and/or moderate CK elevations (>10 times ULN). If symptoms are tolerable, the National Lipid Panel Muscle Safety Expert Panel recommends continuing therapy for CK elevations <10 times ULN with closer CK monitoring (however, many clinicians prefer discontinuation even when the CK is more than times the ULN). Milder CK elevations less than five times the ULN with tolerable symptoms may be followed every 3 to 6 months.

Answer b is correct. Many patients tolerate another statin without problems. No studies have directly compared incidence of myopathy but there are likely differences. For example, fluvastatin was associated with lower incidence of muscle-related symptoms in a large observational trial. There have also been no documented cases of fatal rhabdomyolysis associated with fluvastatin. Less lipophilic statins with fewer drug interactions (ie, pravastatin and rosuvastatin) theoretically may have reduced risk. Retrospective studies and case reports also suggest benefit from altered dosing regimens of atorvastatin and rosuvastatin (ie, 1-3 times a week).

Answer c is incorrect. Statins block the synthesis of coenzyme Q10, and a small trial found a significant 40% reduction in pain severity when 100 mg/d was added to therapy. Coenzyme Q10 can be considered for patients with no benefit from other approaches, but is not generally recommended due to variable response and insufficient evidence.

Answer d is incorrect. Although he may tolerate ezetimibe better, this option should be reserved for patients who fail other strategies.

---

20. JT is a 62-year-old woman with low HDL-C who was prescribed niacin. She did not fill her prescription because of the expense and instead took five 100-mg immediate-release niacin tablets at bedtime. She complains of flushing and dizziness after the first dose that almost caused her to fall. What is the best recommendation to improve overall tolerability?

    a. Change to a "no flush" formulation.
    b. Take 81 mg of aspirin 30 to 60 minutes before each dose.
    c. Start with 100 mg tid.
    d. Take with food and a hot liquid.
    e. Change to sustained-release OTC formulation.

Answer a is incorrect. "No flush" niacin products are not effective for cholesterol lowering.

Answer b is incorrect. A higher dose of 325 mg of aspirin is recommended to prevent flushing.

Answer c is correct. Niacin should be slowly titrated to reduce flushing. A common starting dose for immediate-release niacin is 100 mg 3 times a day or 250 mg twice daily.

Answer d is incorrect. Although dosing with food can improve tolerability, concomitant hot liquids, alcohol, and spicy foods can worsen symptoms.

Answer e is incorrect. Although this product may reduce flushing, hepatic toxicity occurs more frequently with sustained-release formulations (with the exception of prescription extended-release niacin).

CHAPTER 5 | Stroke

1. A 47-year-old white man with a PMH significant for hypertension, diabetes, and chronic alcoholism comes to your clinic for routine follow-up. His social history is significant for alcohol and tobacco abuse. He currently drinks one case of beer per night and smokes two packs per day. Pertinent laboratory findings are as follows: TC 182 mg/dL, TG 218 mg/dL, LDL 96 mg/dL, HDL 52 mg/dL, glucose 146 mg/dL. Current blood pressure is 158/94 mm Hg and HR is 92 beats per minute (bpm). He is 69 in tall and weighs 232 lb. Which of the following is a risk factor for ischemic stroke in this patient?

i. Hypertension
ii. Obesity
iii. Diabetes

a. Only i is correct.
b. Only iii is correct.
c. Only i and ii are correct.
d. Only ii and iii are correct.
e. i, ii, and iii are all correct.

Answer e is correct. All of the above are risk factors for ischemic stroke. Dyslipidemia and atrial fibrillation are also commonly cited modifiable risk factors. Men have a greater risk than women and African Americans are at greater risk than Caucasians.

---

2. Which of the following statements most accurately describes the acute presentation of ischemic stroke?

a. Focal neurological deficit lasting <24 hours, one-sided weakness, systolic blood pressure >200 mm Hg
b. Focal neurological deficit lasting >24 hours, one-sided weakness, visual impairment
c. Diffuse neurological deficit lasting <24 hours, one-sided weakness, visual impairment
d. Diffuse neurological deficit lasting >24 hours, one-sided weakness, blood glucose >200 mg/dL

Answer a is incorrect. Focal neurological deficit lasting <24 hours is a transient ischemic attack (TIA). Patients do commonly present with one-sided weakness; however, they may or may not present with elevated blood pressure. Further, there is not an upper limit of systolic blood pressure that is indicative of acute ischemic stroke.

Answer b is correct. Acute ischemic stroke is caused by a local thrombus formation leading to a focal neurological deficit. By definition, a stroke is neurological deficit lasting >24 hours. A transient ischemic attack (TIA) is neurological deficit lasting <24 hours. Visual impairment, weakness on one side of the body, and inability to speak are all other common symptoms of acute stroke.

Answer is c is incorrect. Acute ischemic stroke is caused by a local thrombus formation leading to a focal neurological deficit, not diffuse. Further neurological deficit lasting <24 hours is a transient ischemic attack (TIA). Patients do commonly present with one-sided weakness and visual impairment. They may also present with the inability to speak.

Answer is d is incorrect. Acute ischemic stroke is caused by a local thrombus formation leading to a focal neurological deficit, not diffuse. Patients do commonly present with one-sided weakness, and, while diabetes is a risk factor for having an ischemic stroke, there is not a correlation with elevated blood glucose levels and acute stroke.

---

3. JS is a 78-year-old white woman with a PMH significant for atrial fibrillation, systolic heart failure with an ejection fraction of 35%, and hypertension. She presents to the emergency department with symptoms of right-sided paralysis. She is not able to communicate, but her family member states that the symptoms began approximately 5 hours ago. MRI of the brain confirms the patient has had an ischemic stroke. At home she takes metoprolol 100 mg po bid, lisinopril 40 mg po daily, and furosemide 20 mg po daily. Which of the following medications would be the most appropriate for secondary stroke prevention in JS?

a. Aspirin
b. Clopidogrel
c. Warfarin
d. Extended-release dipyridamole plus aspirin
e. Ticlopidine

Answers a, b and d are incorrect. Aspirin, clopidogrel, and extended-release dipyridamole plus aspirin are all appropriate options of secondary prevention of ischemic stroke if the patient does not have a cardioembolic source.

Answer c is correct. Warfarin is the most effective treatment option for the secondary prevention of stroke in patients with a cardioembolic source (atrial fibrillation). All patients with atrial fibrillation should be on either aspirin or warfarin for primary stroke prevention. The decision to use one over the other is made based on a patients risk for having a stroke. Patients at higher risk are candidates for warfarin therapy.

Answer e is incorrect. Ticlopidine is not currently recommended by the American Heart Association Stroke Council due to its significant side effect profile. It can cause severe gastrointestinal side effects and there have been reports of neutropenia, agranulocytosis, aplastic anemia, and thrombotic thrombocytopenic purpura.

---

4. HB is a 54-year-old African American man who presents to the emergency department with symptoms of left-sided paralysis and visual impairment. He has a PMH significant for hypertension, hyperlipidemia, and benign prostatic hyperplasia. MRI of the brain confirms the patient has had an ischemic stroke. Which of the following medications would be the most appropriate for secondary stroke prevention in HB?

a. Ticlopidine
b. Dipyridamole
c. Aspirin
d. Clopidogrel plus aspirin
e. Warfarin

Answer a is incorrect. Ticlopidine is not currently recommended by the American Heart Association Stroke Council due to its significant side-effect profile. It can cause severe gastrointestinal side effects and there have been reports of neutropenia, agranulocytosis, aplastic anemia, and thrombotic thrombocytopenic purpura.

Answer b is incorrect. Dipyridamole should not be used as monotherapy in the secondary prevention of ischemic stroke. The combination of extended-release dipyridamole plus aspirin is an acceptable antiplatelet option for initial therapy.

Answer c is correct. Aspirin is the most well-studied antiplatelet agent used in the secondary prevention of stroke. Currently, aspirin, clopidogrel, and extended-release dipyridamole plus aspirin are all antiplatelet anti-platelet options for initial therapy. Currently, the American Heart Association Stroke Council recommends the use of extended-release dipyridamole plus aspirin over aspirin monotherapy.

Answer d is incorrect. The American Heart Association Stroke Council currently does not recommend the combination of clopidogrel with aspirin as there is an increased risk of hemorrhage when used together.

Answer e is incorrect. Warfarin should only be used when there is a cardioembolic source such as atrial fibrillation.

---

5. Which of the following is a common side effect of extended-release dipyridamole plus aspirin?

   a. Agranulocytosis
   b. Visual disturbances
   c. Pancreatitis
   d. Headache

Answer a is incorrect. Extended-release dipyridamole plus aspirin has not been shown to cause agranulocytosis. Anemia has been reported in approximately 1% of patients. Agranulocytosis is a side effect of ticlopidine.

Answer b is incorrect. Extended-release dipyridamole plus aspirin has not been shown to cause visual disturbances.

Answer c is incorrect. Extended-release dipyridamole plus aspirin has not been shown to cause pancreatitis. It has been shown to cause abdominal pain, indigestion, and diarrhea with incidences approaching 20%.

Answer d is correct. The incidence of headache in patients taking extended-release dipyridamole plus aspirin approaches 40% and is the most common reason for discontinuation.

---

6. A 63-year-old African American man with a PMH significant for hyperlipidemia presented to the emergency department several days ago with symptoms of an acute stroke. The physician you are working with wants your recommendations on what to send this patient home on for blood pressure control. Current vitals are as follows: BP 138/88 mm Hg, HR 86 bpm. What do you recommend?

   a. Beta-blocker.
   b. Nondihydropyridine calcium channel blocker.
   c. Angiotensin-converting enzyme inhibitor plus a diuretic.
   d. Angiotensin-converting enzyme inhibitor.
   e. No blood pressure medication. The patient's blood pressure is at goal.

Answer a is incorrect. There is no data to support the use of a beta-blocker post ischemic stroke, and this patient does not have any compelling indications that warrant a beta-blocker use. Currently the American Heart Association Stroke Council recommends the use of diuretics or the combination of diuretics plus an angiotensin-converting enzyme inhibitor.

Answer b is incorrect. There is no data to support the use of a calcium channel blocker, both nondihydropyridine and dihydropyridine, post ischemic stroke. Currently the American Heart Association Stroke Council recommends the use of diuretics or the combination of diuretics plus an angiotensin-converting enzyme inhibitor.

Answer c is correct. Currently the American Heart Association Stroke Council recommends the use of diuretics or the combination of diuretics plus an angiotensin-converting enzyme inhibitor.

Answer d is incorrect. The American Heart Association Stroke Council does not recommend the use of ACEI monotherapy post ischemic stroke. Currently it recommends the use of diuretics or the combination of diuretics plus an angiotensin-converting enzyme inhibitor.

Answer e is incorrect. Per the American Heart Association Stroke Council, antihypertensive treatment is recommended for all patients with a history of ischemic stroke regardless of whether or not the patient has a history of hypertension.

---

7. What is the brand name of extended-release dipyridamole 200 mg plus aspirin 25 mg?

   a. Angiomax
   b. Aggrastat
   c. Aggrenox
   d. Abraxane
   e. Anaprox

Answer a is incorrect. The generic name for Angiomax is bivalirudin. Bivalirudin is a direct thrombin inhibitor.

Answer b is incorrect. The generic name for Aggrastat is tirofiban. Tirofiban is a glycoprotein IIb/IIIa inhibitor.

Answer c is correct. The generic name for Aggrenox is extended-release dipyridamole 200 mg plus aspirin 25 mg. The dose used in the secondary prevention of stroke is one capsule po bid.

Answer d is incorrect. The generic name for Abraxane is paclitaxel. Paclitaxel is an antineoplastic agent.

Answer e is incorrect. The generic name for Anaprox is naproxen. Naproxen is a nonsteroidal anti-inflammatory agent.

---

8. A 49-year-old white man with a PMH significant only for osteoarthritis was diagnosed with an ischemic stroke several days ago. The patient drinks one to two beers per day and denies smoking. Family history is unremarkable. His current lipid panel is as follows: TC 168 mg/dL, TG 88 mg/dL, HDL 44 mg/dL, LDL 116 mg/dL. Vitals: BP 136/84 mm Hg, HR 78 bpm. The physician you are working with wants to know if this patient needs to be placed on statin therapy. What do you recommend?

   a. This patient's only major risk factor for coronary heart disease is his age. His goal LDL is <160 mg/dL. He does not need to be placed on statin therapy.
   b. This patient's only major risk factors for coronary heart disease are his age and history of previous ischemic stroke. His goal LDL is <130 mg/dL. He does not need to be placed on statin therapy.
   c. This patient's only major risk factors for coronary heart disease are his age and history of previous ischemic stroke. His goal LDL is <100 mg/dL. He does not need to be placed on statin therapy. Therapeutic lifestyle recommendation should be initiated.

d. Statin therapy is recommended for all patients with an ischemic stroke. His LDL goal is <100 mg/dL with a preference of <70 mg/dL. He should be put on statin therapy.

Answers a, b, and c are incorrect. If this patient had not had a previous stroke, his only major risk factor would be age >45 (he does not have an HDL <40 mg/dL, a history of hypertension, a history of smoking, or a significant family history). For patients with only one risk factor, the goal LDL is <160 mg/dL. However, he does have a previous history of ischemic stroke and all patients with atherosclerotic, ischemic stroke should receive statin therapy to reduce the risk of recurrent events.

Answer d is correct. On the basis of the SPARCL trial, all patients with atherosclerotic, ischemic stroke should receive statin therapy to reduce the risk of recurrent events. Patients should be treated to a goal LDL cholesterol level of 100 mg/dL with an optional goal of <70 mg/dL.

---

9. Which of the following medications inhibit platelet activity?

i. Clopidogrel
ii. Aspirin
iii. Dipyridamole

a. Only i is correct.
b. Only iii is correct.
c. Only i and ii are correct.
d. Only ii and iii are correct.
e. i, ii, and iii are all correct.

Answer e is correct. Aspirin causes irreversible inhibition of platelet cyclooxygenase ultimately leading to a reduction in platelet aggregation. Clopidogrel works through selective, irreversible inhibition of adenosine diphosphate–induced platelet aggregation. Dipyridamole is an inhibitor of phosphodiesterase.

---

10. Which of the following is the most appropriate way for you to tell your patient to take extended-release dipyridamole plus aspirin therapy?

a. Extended-release dipyridamole 200 mg plus aspirin 25 mg po daily
b. Extended-release dipyridamole 25 mg plus aspirin 200 mg po daily
c. Extended-release dipyridamole 200 mg plus aspirin 25 mg po bid
d. Extended-release dipyridamole 25 mg plus aspirin 200 mg po bid
e. Extended-release dipyridamole 200 mg plus aspirin 25 mg two capsules po bid

---

Answer c is correct. Aggrenox is supplied as a capsule containing extended-release dipyridamole 200 mg plus aspirin 25 mg. This capsule is given twice daily.

---

11. CS is a 61-year-old white woman who has a PMH significant for hypertension and diabetes mellitus. She presented to the emergency department yesterday with signs and symptoms of an ischemic stroke. CT of the brain confirmed this diagnosis. Which of the following medications would be the most appropriate for secondary stroke prevention in CS?

a. Extended-release dipyridamole 200 mg plus aspirin 25 mg two capsules po bid
b. Aspirin 81 mg po daily
c. Clopidogrel 75 mg po bid
d. Clopidogrel 150 mg po daily
e. Warfarin 5 mg po daily

Answer a is incorrect. The American Heart Association Stroke Council gives preference to Aggrenox (extended-release dipyridamole plus aspirin) over aspirin monotherapy. However, Aggrenox is supplied as a capsule containing extended-release dipyridamole 200 mg plus aspirin 25 mg. This capsule is given twice daily; not two capsules twice daily.

Answer b is correct. Aspirin is an acceptable antiplatelet option for initial therapy. The dosing range varies from 50 to 325 mg/d.

Answer c is incorrect. Clopidogrel is an acceptable antiplatelet option for initial therapy; however, the dose is 75 mg once daily.

Answer d is incorrect. Clopidogrel is an acceptable antiplatelet option for initial therapy; however, the dose is 75 mg once daily.

Answer e is incorrect. Warfarin should only be used when there is a cardioembolic source such as atrial fibrillation.

---

12. Which of the following best describes the mechanism of action of clopidogrel?

a. Irreversible inhibition of adenosine diphosphate–induced platelet aggregation
b. Irreversible inhibition of platelet cyclooxygenase
c. Reversible inhibition of adenosine diphosphate–induced platelet aggregation
d. Reversible inhibition of platelet cyclooxygenase

Answer a is correct. Clopidogrel works via irreversible inhibition of adenosine diphosphate–induced platelet aggregation.

Answer b is incorrect. Aspirin works via irreversible inhibition of platelet cyclooxygenase.

Answer c and d are incorrect. Clopidogrel works via inhibition of adenosine diphosphate–induced platelet aggregation and aspirin works via inhibition of platelet cyclooxygenase; however, both of the medications cause irreversible inhibition, not reversible.

---

13. Which of the following medications works by binding to fibrin and subsequently converting plasminogen to plasmin?

a. Plavix
b. Aggrenox
c. Ticlid
d. Argatroban
e. Activase

Answer a is incorrect. Plavix is the brand name for clopidogrel. It works by irreversibly inhibiting adenosine diphosphate–induced platelet aggregation.

Answer b is incorrect. Aggrenox is the brand name for the combination of extended-release dipyridamole plus aspirin. Dipyridamole inhibits phosphodiesterase, and aspirin irreversibly inhibits cyclooxygenase.

Answer c is incorrect. Ticlid is the brand name for ticlopidine. Similar to clopidogrel, ticlopidine inhibits adenosine diphosphate–mediated platelet aggregation.

Answer d is incorrect. Argatroban is a direct thrombin inhibitor.

Answer e is correct. Activase is the brand name for rtPA. rtPA is a fibrinolytic agent used to dissolve clots associated with acute ischemic stroke.

---

14. Which of the following is the correct dose of aspirin for use during an acute stroke?

    i. Aspirin 81 mg within 48 hours
    ii. Aspirin 160 mg within 48 hours
    iii. Aspirin 325 mg within 48 hours

    a. Only i is correct.
    b. Only ii is correct.
    c. Only iii is correct.
    d. ii and iii are correct.
    e. i, ii, and iii are all correct.

Answer c is correct. All answers include the correct timeframe of aspirin use; however, the only dose approved for the treatment of acute stroke is aspirin 325 mg.

---

15. A 68-year-old man with a PMH significant for diabetes mellitus, DVT 5 years ago, and GI bleed 2 weeks ago presents with right-sided weakness and right facial droop that began 2 hours ago. CT of the head confirms ischemic stroke. Home medications include: warfarin 5 mg po daily, pantoprazole 40 mg po daily, and metformin 1000 mg po bid. Pertinent laboratory values on admission include INR 1.4, hemoglobin 14, hematocrit 41, platelets 175,000, and glucose 200 mg/dL. Blood pressure on admission is 160/90 mm Hg. Which of the following is an exclusion criterion for this patient to receive rtPA?

    a. Elevated INR
    b. Low platelets
    c. Recent GI bleed
    d. Elevated blood pressure on admission
    e. Time elapsed since onset of symptoms

Answer a is incorrect. Patients taking warfarin who have a current INR of ≤1.7 may be considered for rtPA.

Answer b is incorrect. Patients may be considered for rtPA if platelets are >100,000.

Answer c is correct. Gastrointestinal bleeds within the previous 3 weeks qualify as exclusion criteria for rtPA use.

Answer d is incorrect. In order to receive rtPA, blood pressure must remain <185/110 mm Hg.

Answer e is incorrect. Patient is well within the 3 hour window to receive rtPA.

---

16. A 72-year-old woman (68 in, 111 kg) is admitted for acute ischemic stroke confirmed by CT of the head. She presents within 1.5 hours of symptom onset and meets all criteria to receive rtPA. The physician asks you what the appropriate dose is for this patient and how to administer it. Your response is:

    a. 100 mg IV over 1 hour
    b. 90 mg IV over 1 hour
    c. 10 mg IV bolus over 10 minutes and then 90 mg over an hour
    d. 9 mg IV bolus over 1 minute and then 81 mg over an hour
    e. 10 mg IV bolus over 1 minute and then 90 mg over an hour

---

Answer a is incorrect. The maximum rtPA dose is 90 mg in patients over 100 kg.

Answer b is incorrect. The total dose is correct (maximum dose is 90 mg for patients over 100 kg). However, 10% (9 mg) should be given as a bolus dose over 1 minute with the remaining amount (81 mg) given over an hour.

Answer c is incorrect. The maximum total rtPA dose is 90 mg in patients over 100 kg. Also, the bolus dose should be given over 1 minute, not 10 minutes.

Answer d is correct. Because our patient is over 100 kg, the maximum rtPA dose is 90 mg. Ten percent (9 mg) is given as an IV bolus over 1 minute, and the remainder of the dose (81 mg) is given over an hour.

Answer e is incorrect. The maximum total rtPA dose is 90 mg in patients over 100 kg.

---

17. In May 2009, the American Heart Association Stroke Council updated their guidelines to consider the use of rtPA up to 4.5 hours after symptom onset in certain patients. Patients who are not candidates for this extended window of rtPA use include:

    a. Age >80 years
    b. Patients taking oral anticoagulants regardless of INR
    c. Score of >25 on the National Institutes of Health Stroke Scale
    d. History of both stroke and diabetes together
    e. All of the above

Answer e is correct. If patients fall into any of these four groups, they may not be considered for an extended rtPA window of up to 4.5 hours. These patients may still undergo consideration of rtPA if symptom onset is within 3 hours.

---

18. An 81-year-old man with a PMH significant for diabetes, hypertension, and ischemic stroke 3 years ago presents with slurred speech and left-sided weakness that began 3.5 hours ago. NIH stroke score is calculated to be 15. Home medications include lisinopril 40 mg po daily and glipizide 5 mg po bid. Laboratory values are within normal limits and blood pressure is 150/84 mm Hg. The patient weighs 80 kg. Which of the following may be used as initial treatment for ischemic stroke in this patient?

i. rtPA 72 mg (10% IV bolus over 1 minute and the remainder over 1 hour)
ii. Aspirin 325 mg po
iii. Aspirin 162 mg po
iv. Lovenox 1 mg/kg SQ q12h

a. Only i
b. Only ii
c. i and ii
d. ii and iv
e. iii and iv

Answer a is incorrect. This patient does not qualify for rtPA. He presented within the extended 4.5 hour time frame, but is excluded from consideration due to age >80 *and* PMH significant for both a history of diabetes and stroke.

Answer b is correct. He should receive aspirin at a dose of 325 mg within 24 to 48 hours initially.

Answer c is incorrect. This patient does not qualify for rtPA. He presented within the extended 4.5 hour time frame, but is excluded from consideration due to age >80 and PMH significant for both a history of diabetes and stroke. If this patient did qualify for both rtPA and aspirin, it would be important to wait at least 24 hours after rtPA administration to initiate aspirin therapy.

Answer d is incorrect. While this patient should receive aspirin 325 mg within 24 to 48 hours as initial treatment, Lovenox is not beneficial in the treatment of acute stroke and should not be used.

Answer e is incorrect. Lovenox is not beneficial in the treatment of acute stroke and the initial aspirin dose in acute stroke is 325 mg within 24 to 48 hours.

19. Which of the following may be used to treat elevated blood pressure in acute stroke patients who have concomitant renal dysfunction?

i. Labetalol
ii. Nicardipine
iii. Sodium nitroprusside

a. Only i
b. Only ii
c. Only iii
d. i and ii
e. ii and iii

Answer d is correct. Both labetalol and nicardipine may be initiated in patients with renal dysfunction and they both are the preferred medications to use for blood pressure lowering in acute stroke. Sodium nitroprusside's metabolite accumulates in renal insufficiency and can lead to cyanide toxicity.

20. A 62-year-old woman is admitted 2 hours after onset of acute stroke symptoms including blurred vision, slurred speech, and right facial droop. CT of the head confirms ischemic stroke. Past medical history is nonsignificant, and the patient takes no medications at home. All laboratory values are within normal limits. Blood pressure is 200/110 mm Hg. Patient meets all other inclusion criteria for rtPA use. Which of the following is the best option for blood pressure control in this patient?

a. No treatment should be given since the systolic blood pressure is <220 mm Hg and the diastolic blood pressure is <120 mm Hg.
b. Since the patient meets all other inclusion criteria for rtPA, labetalol should be given to lower blood pressure to <185/110 mm Hg so that the patient can receive rtPA.
c. Since the patient meets all other inclusion criteria for rtPA, nicardipine infusion should be initiated to lower blood pressure to <140/90 mm Hg.
d. Since the patient meets all other inclusion criteria for rtPA, sodium nitroprusside should be initiated to lower the blood pressure by 15% to 25% within the first day.

Answer a is incorrect. Normally antihypertensive treatment is not necessary until blood pressure rises above 220/120 mm Hg. However, if blood pressure lowering would result in patient becoming an rtPA candidate, then it is prudent to lower blood pressure to below 185/110 mm Hg.

Answer b is correct. Assuming this patient meets all inclusion criteria for rtPA use, then it is prudent to lower blood pressure to below 185/110 mm Hg. Labetalol is an appropriate first line option.

Answer c is incorrect. Blood pressure should not be dropped to 140/90 mm Hg. Lower blood pressures in the acute setting can cause neurological deterioration. A reasonable goal is to lower the blood pressure by 15% to 25% within the first 24 hours. The goal is to lower the blood pressure to >185/110 mm Hg when a patient is a candidate for rtPA.

Answer d is incorrect. Sodium nitroprusside is typically reserved for situations when blood pressure remains elevated despite adequate use of both labetalol and nicardipine. The goal is to lower the blood pressure to <185/110 mm Hg when a patient is a candidate for rtPA.

CHAPTER 6 | Anticoagulation/Venous Thromboembolism

1. Which of the following agents would be the most appropriate reversal agent to be used in the case of warfarin overdose?

a. Phenprocoumon
b. Protamine sulfate
c. Vitamin K
d. Activated charcoal
e. Ipecac syrup

Answer a is incorrect. Phenprocoumon is a vitamin K antagonist available in countries outside the United States. The addition of this agent would have an additive effect to warfarin and increase the severity of the adverse effects.

Answer b is incorrect. Protamine sulfate is the agent of choice for the reversal of unfractionated heparin (UFH) overdose. The recommended dose for reversal of UFH effects is 1 mg of protamine per 100 U of heparin.

Answer c is correct. Vitamin K reverses the anticoagulant effects of vitamin K antagonists (VKAs) such as warfarin. VKAs reduce thrombus formation by inhibiting the activation of the vitamin K-dependent clotting factors, II, VII, IX, and X. The anticoagulant effect of VKAs is a fine balance between the amount of vitamin K available to activate the clotting factors and ultimately produce thrombin. Ingestion of additional Vitamin K upsets this equilibrium and reverses the anticoagulant effects.

Answer d is incorrect. Activated charcoal is a commonly used antidote for several overdose situations based on its ability to absorb toxins. However, it is ineffective for the treatment of warfarin toxicity.

Answer e is incorrect. Ipecac syrup was once commonly used in many overdose or accidental ingestion situations for its ability to induce emesis. It is less commonly recommended due to the potential harm to occur when used chronically or to induce emesis with certain substances.

---

2. Which of the following is not an adverse reaction associated with vitamin K antagonist use?
   a. Hematochezia
   b. Cardiac arrhythmias (QT prolongation)
   c. Bleeding
   d. Purple toe syndrome
   e. Anemia

Answer a is incorrect. Melena is the medical term used for the passing of black, tarry stools. It is potential sign of a gastrointestinal bleed and/or supratherapeutic level of vitamin K antagonist.

Answer b is correct. Vitamin K antagonists may be used to prevent clot formation in atrial fibrillation. However, they do not impact the rate or rhythm of the heart.

Answer c is incorrect. Bleeding is the most common adverse reaction associated with any of the anticoagulant agents.

Answer d is incorrect. Purple toe syndrome is rare but potentially serious adverse reaction usually associated with warfarin use.

Answer e is incorrect. Anemia may be a sign of potential bleeding which is a common adverse reaction with warfarin use.

---

3. Which of the following agents would result in a major drug interaction in conjunction with warfarin use?
   a. Lisinopril
   b. Metoprolol
   c. Darvon
   d. Lanoxin
   e. Fluconazole

Answer a is incorrect. There is no significant drug interaction noted between lisinopril and warfarin.

Answer b is incorrect. There is no significant drug interaction noted between metoprolol and warfarin.

Answer c is incorrect. Darvon is a brand name for propoxyphene. There is no significant interaction between propoxyphene and warfarin.

Answer d is incorrect. Lanoxin is a brand name for digoxin, which may be used to treat heart failure. While an exacerbation of heart failure can result in elevated INR values, the use of digoxin alone is not expected to interact with warfarin.

Answer e is correct. Fluconazole is a cytochrome P (CYP)-450-2C9 inhibitor and to a lesser extent CYP-3A4 inhibitor. R-warfarin is metabolized by CYP-1A2 and CYP-3A4, while the more potent enantiomer, S-warfarin, is primarily metabolized via the CYP-450-2C9 pathway. Agents that are inhibitors or inducers of the CYP-2C9 pathway can significantly impact the therapeutic effects of warfarin and increase the risk of adverse effects.

---

4. Which of the following would be the best agent for treatment of DVT in a patient with heparin-induced thrombocytopenia?
   a. Enoxaparin
   b. Argatroban
   c. Aspirin
   d. Unfractionated heparin
   e. Fragmin

Answer a is incorrect. LMWH have a documented cross-sensitivity with UFH and may result in reoccurrence of heparin-induced thrombocytopenia (HIT) if administered.

Answer b is correct. Direct thrombin inhibitors, such as Argatroban, are the agents of choice for patients with HIT.

Answer c is incorrect. Aspirin effects mostly platelet aggregation and would not be appropriate alternative to anticoagulation.

Answer d is incorrect. UFH is the most common agent known to cause HIT. Therefore, this agent would be contraindicated for use in any patient with a history of HIT.

Answer e is incorrect. Fragmin is the brand name for dalteparin, an LMWH. See explanation in choice A above.

---

5. JC is a 36-year-old pregnant woman with an active DVT. She takes no other medications and has no significant past medical history. Which of the following agents would be the best choice for the initial treatment of her DVT?
   a. Enoxaparin
   b. Clopidogrel
   c. Aspirin
   d. Warfarin
   e. Apidra

Answer a is correct. UFH or LMWH are the agents of choice for anticoagulation during pregnancy. LMWHs are the agents of choice for outpatient use due to less monitoring and subcutaneous route of administration. UFH requires close monitoring and is generally given intravenously.

Answer b is incorrect. Clopidogrel is used as an antiplatelet medication. Antiplatelet and anticoagulant therapies may often be confused since they both may be used for the prevention of stroke and thrombus formation in certain situations. However, they differ in their mechanisms of action and are not interchangeable.

Answer c is incorrect. Aspirin is also considered an antiplatelet medication. See explanation under choice B above.

Answer d is incorrect. Jantoven is a brand name for warfarin. Warfarin has a pregnancy category of X and is considered teratogenic.

Answer e is incorrect. Apidra is the brand name for insulin glulisine, a rapid-acting insulin, which may be mistaken for Arixtra which is the brand name for fondaparinux, a selective Xa inhibitor. Both medications are administered subcutaneously but may be harmful if given inappropriately.

---

6. Which of the following would be the most appropriate test for monitoring the efficacy of dalteparin in a pregnant female?

   a. International normalized ratio
   b. Liver enzymes
   c. Prothrombin time
   d. Anti-Xa activity
   e. Complete blood count

Answer a is incorrect. The international normalized ratio (INR) is used to monitor the therapeutic effects of warfarin.

Answer b is incorrect. LMWHs are cleared renally and have minimal impact on hepatic function.

Answer c is incorrect. Prothrombin time (PT) is another laboratory test used to primarily assess and monitor the therapeutic effects of warfarin.

Answer d is correct. LMWHs work by inactivating factors Xa and IIa in the clotting cascade. Anti-Xa activity is the laboratory test used to monitor efficacy in select patient populations, such as pregnant women.

Answer e is incorrect. Although a CBC is an appropriate test to monitor for bleeding, it will not measure the efficacy of LMWH therapy.

---

7. Which of the following choices below represents an appropriate initial regimen for a patient weighing 60 kg recently diagnosed with a pulmonary embolism?

   i. Coumadin5 mg po daily
   ii. Lovenox 60 mg SQ bid
   iii. Plavix 75 mg po daily

   a. i only
   b. iii only
   c. i and ii only
   d. ii and iii only
   e. i, ii, and iii

Answer a is incorrect. Although warfarin therapy is appropriate initial therapy for treatment of PE, it has a delayed onset of anticoagulant effect and is not appropriate as monotherapy.

Answer b is incorrect. Plavix, or clopidogrel, is an antiplatelet agent and not appropriate therapy for the treatment of PE.

Answer c is correct. Both options i and ii are appropriate initial therapies in this case. For treatment purposes, both of these agents would be started initially and the LMWH would be discontinued shortly after therapeutic levels of warfarin are achieved. An alternative method of using LMWH monotherapy is an option; however, this option may not be cost-effective. The starting dose for treatment with enoxaparin is 1 mg/kg given subcutaneously every 12 hours or an alternative dose of 1.5 mg/kg given subcutaneously once daily.

Answer d is incorrect. Although enoxaparin is an appropriate initial treatment for PE, clopidogrel is not.

Answer e is incorrect. Only enoxaparin and warfarin are appropriate initial treatment options in this case.

---

8. Which of the following drugs can be used safely in a HIT patient with a creatinine clearance of 25 mL/min?

   a. Lepirudin
   b. Enoxaparin
   c. Dalteparin
   d. Fondaparinux
   e. Argatroban

Answer a is incorrect. Lepirudin, a direct thrombin inhibitor, is renally eliminated and should not be used in patients with creatinine clearance <30 mL/min.

Answers b and c are incorrect. LMWHs should not be used in patients who have developed heparin-induced thrombocytopenia. Although LMWH have a lower incidence of HIT, they still interact with platelets and could worsen HIT. Heparin should also be used over LMWH for treatment of VTE in patients with renal insufficiency and creatinine clearance <30 mL/min.

Answer d is incorrect. Fondaparinux is contraindicated in patients with creatinine clearance <30 mL/min.

Answer e is correct. Argatroban, a direct thrombin inhibitor, should be used to prevent and treat thrombosis associated with HIT. It is metabolized in the liver and therefore, safe to use in patients with renal insufficiency.

---

9. Which of the following agents has a delayed onset of anticoagulant effect?

   a. Unfractionated heparin
   b. Lovenox
   c. Arixtra
   d. Warfarin
   e. Innohep

Answers a, b, c and e are incorrect. These anticoagulants have a rapid onset of anticoagulant effect.

Answer d is correct. The anticoagulant effect of warfarin is dependent on the depletion of vitamin K–dependent clotting factors, II, VII, IX, and X. Factor II, thrombin, is largely responsible for warfarin's anticoagulant effect, and it also has the longest half-life.

10. A 57-year-old woman (65 kg, BMI 28) was just admitted to the hospital for treatment of a pulmonary embolism. An order was written for heparin IV bolus 80 U/kg followed by a continuous infusion of 18 U/kg/h. What are respective heparin bolus dose and continuous infusion rate for this patient?

    a. 5000 U IV bolus; 1200 U/h infusion
    b. 4000 U IV bolus; 800 U/h infusion
    c. 6000 U IV bolus; 1150 U/h infusion
    d. 6000 U IV bolus; 1200 U/h infusion
    e. 4000 U IV bolus; 1150 U/h infusion

Answer a is correct. Heparin is dosed based on actual body weight. For the initial bolus dose, 65 kg × 80 U/kg = 5200 U. The dose is rounded to 5000 U for ease of administration. Heparin is prepared as a 5000 U syringe. Alternatively, it would be difficult to draw up a dose to the nearest 100 U dose. For the continuous infusion, 65 kg × 18 U/kg/h = 1150 U/kg/h. In this case, the dose is rounded to the nearest 100 U because most IV pumps could not be programmed to the nearest 50 U dose.

Answer b is incorrect. Actual body weight and not ideal body weight is used in calculating the dose.

Answer c and d are incorrect. The bolus dose is rounded too high. The IV pump would be unable to program the continuous IV infusion dose for C, and the continuous infusion dose is rounded too high in D.

Answer e is incorrect. The bolus dose is based on actual body weight. The continuous infusion rate should be rounded to the nearest 100 U for purposes of programming the IV pump and accuracy of dosing.

11. Which of the following over-the-counter products can be initiated safely in a patient on chronic warfarin therapy?

    a. Aspirin
    b. Naproxen
    c. Centrum Silver multivitamin
    d. Loratadine
    e. Micatin topical

Answers a and b are incorrect. NSAIDs can increase the risk of bleeding when used in combination with warfarin. In certain situations, aspirin is used in combination with warfarin but only under the supervision of a physician or an anticoagulation-monitoring service.

Answer c is incorrect. Many multivitamins such as this one contain vitamin K. When initiated in a patient receiving chronic warfarin therapy, the INR decreases due to the interaction between warfarin and vitamin K–containing foods and supplements.

Answer d is correct. Loratadine is not known to interact with warfarin.

Answer e is incorrect. Micatin contains miconazole, an azole antifungal. These CYP-2C9 inhibitors can have a significant interaction with warfarin, even when used topically.

12. From which of the following routes of administration may unfractionated heparin be administered?

    i. Intravenously
    ii. Subcutaneously
    iii. Intramuscularly

    a. i and iii
    b. iii only
    c. i and ii only
    d. ii and iii only
    e. i, ii, and iii

Answers a, b, d, and e are incorrect. Heparin may be administered IV and SQ only. Intramuscular administration of heparin may cause hematoma and should be avoided.

Answer c is correct. Both options i and ii are appropriate routes of administration with UFH.

13. Which of the following statements is appropriate for educating patients taking chronic warfarin therapy?

    a. Report any missed warfarin doses to your physician or clinic.
    b. Avoid foods high in vitamin K content.
    c. All herbal therapies are safe in combination with warfarin therapy.
    d. Over-the-counter analgesics are safe in combination with warfarin therapy.
    e. Alcohol consumption does not affect warfarin therapy.

Answer a is correct. Lack of adherence to therapy is a major cause of subtherapeutic INRs in patients receiving warfarin therapy. A decrease in the INR may be seen even after only one missed warfarin dose. For this reason, it is important that patients report any missed doses to their physician or anticoagulation-monitoring service.

Answer b is incorrect. Patients should be educated to maintain a consistent intake of vitamin K–containing foods. Many of these foods are recommended part of our diets and should not be avoided indefinitely. Additionally, small changes in vitamin K intake have a greater impact on warfarin therapy and INR values in patients who consistently receive minimal vitamin K in their diets.

Answer c is incorrect. Many herbal therapies can interact with warfarin and patients should check with their physician or anticoagulation–monitoring service before starting any new herbal therapies.

Answer d is incorrect. Many OTC analgesics, such as NSAIDs, can increase the risk of bleeding when used concomitantly with warfarin. When used in high doses, acetaminophen may also interact with warfarin by increasing the INR value.

Answer e is incorrect. Alcohol use can interfere with warfarin therapy. Chronic excessive alcohol use can result in a decrease in the INR. An acute alcohol binge can cause an increase in the INR due to an inhibition of hepatic microsomal enzymes.

---

14. JT is a 62-year-old man with a history of atrial fibrillation, coronary heart disease, hypertension, and benign prostatic hyperplasia. His current medications include warfarin 5 mg daily, amlodipine 5 mg daily, clopidogrel 75 mg daily, lisinopril 10 mg daily, finasteride 5 mg daily, and acetaminophen 500 mg prn. Which of the medications he is currently taking increases the risk of bleeding with warfarin?

    a. Clopidogrel
    b. Amlodipine
    c. Finasteride
    d. Acetaminophen
    e. Lisinopril

Answer a is correct. Clopidogrel, an antiplatelet agent, can increase bleeding risk when used alone and this risk is increased when it is used concomitantly with warfarin.

Answers b, c, and e are incorrect. Amlodipine, finasteride, and lisinopril do not interact with warfarin.

Answer d is incorrect. Although acetaminophen can increase the INR when used at high doses, occasional use would not be expected to interact with warfarin.

---

15. Which antibiotic would be expected to have the least effect on warfarin therapy in a 32–year-old woman with a urinary tract infection?

    a. Sulfamethoxazole-trimethoprim
    b. Nitrofurantoin
    c. Ciprofloxacin
    d. Dicloxacillin
    e. Metronidazole

Answers a, c, d, and e are incorrect. The antibiotics listed in these choices have been known to interact with warfarin. Sulfamethoxazole-trimethoprim, ciprofloxacin, and metronidazole can increase the INR, while dicloxacillin can decrease it.

Answer b is correct. Nitrofurantoin can be used safely in patients receiving warfarin therapy without interaction.

---

16. A middle-aged woman presents a new prescription for her husband to your pharmacy for enoxaparin (Lovenox) 240 mg subcutaneously twice daily for 7 days for deep venous thrombosis. The patient's weight is 150 kg. Of the following choices, what is the most appropriate action for dispensing the medication?

    a. Dispense 21 80-mg syringes with instructions to inject three 80-mg syringes daily.
    b. Repackage the 240-mg dose in one syringe and dispense seven 220-mg syringes.
    c. Call the prescriber and recommend changing the dose to 150 mg twice daily.
    d. Call the prescriber and recommend changing the dose to 200 mg daily.
    e. Call the prescriber and recommend changing enoxaparin to warfarin 5 mg daily instead.

Answer a is incorrect. It would be difficult and painful for the patient to inject three syringes to make one dose.

Answer b is incorrect. Sterile products cannot be repackaged and dispensed to patients.

Answer c is correct. Enoxaparin has not been adequately studied in doses more than 150 mg. Because this patient is at the upper end of the studied weight, he will be unable to use the 1.5 mg/kg once daily dose and must use the 1 mg/kg bid dosing instead.

Answer d is incorrect. The dose of 200 mg exceeds the maximum number of milligrams that may be given in one dose.

Answer e is incorrect. There is not enough information available to determine if this is an acceptable recommendation.

---

17. In which of the following patient types are lower initial doses of warfarin recommended?

    a. Pediatric
    b. Elderly
    c. Stroke
    d. Atrial fibrillation
    e. Hypothyroidism

Answers a, c, and d are incorrect. These patient characteristics have not been consistently associated with the need for a lower warfarin maintenance dose.

Answer b is correct. Elderly often need maintenance warfarin doses below 5 mg daily that is the recommended starting dose for most patients. Lower warfarin-starting doses are also recommended in patients that are severely malnourished, have moderate to severe heart failure, had recent major surgery, or those receiving drugs that can increase warfarin sensitivity.

Answer e is incorrect because a patient who is profoundly hypothyroid may require higher warfarin doses to achieve a therapeutic anticoagulant effect.

---

18. A patient comes to your pharmacy requesting help in choosing a Boost dietary supplement. In your discussion, she tells you that she is also taking warfarin for recurrent DVT. Which of the following is a likely consequence of starting this dietary supplement in someone who is receiving chronic warfarin therapy?
    a. Increased risk of bleeding
    b. Increase in the INR
    c. Decrease in the INR
    d. Decrease in warfarin dose
    e. Warfarin-induced skin necrosis

Answers a, b, and d are incorrect because these are all consequences for a patient who is taking an interacting medication with warfarin that increases the INR.

Answer c is correct. Boost dietary supplement contains vitamin K which can interact with warfarin and make it more difficult for the patient to be appropriately anticoagulated.

Answer e is incorrect because warfarin-induced skin necrosis is a rare adverse effect of warfarin therapy that is not necessarily related to low INR values or drug–drug interactions.

---

19. Which of the following medications should be avoided in pregnant women (pregnancy category X)?
    a. Unfractionated heparin
    b. Enoxaparin
    c. Fondaparinux
    d. Argatroban
    e. Warfarin

Answer a is incorrect. UFH is pregnancy category C.

Answer b, c, and d are incorrect. Enoxaparin, fondaparinux, and argatroban all are classified in pregnancy category B.

Answer e is correct. Warfarin is classified as pregnancy category X and, therefore, is an absolute contraindication. The primary concern is fetal bleeding risk. Additional risks for CNS abnormalities to the fetus may also occur with use during pregnancy. Unfractionated heparin or low molecular weight heparins are the recommended anticoagulants for use in pregnancy.

---

20. Which of the following is *not* an appropriate counseling point when counseling a patient on Lovenox?
    a. Rotate injection site to minimize bruising and pain.
    b. Inject at least 2 inches from your belly button and out toward your sides.
    c. Prior to injection, gently press the plunger to remove the air bubble from the syringe.
    d. Dispose of used syringe in thick plastic container or biohazard container.
    e. Avoid rubbing site of injection after administration to minimize risk of bruising.

Answers a, b, d, and e are incorrect These statements are accurate.

Answer c is correct. This is a false statement. Attempting to remove the air bubble from the syringe may result in loss of medication.

---

21. Which of the following agents would be the best pain management option in a patient with chronic warfarin therapy?
    a. Celebrex
    b. Ibuprofen
    c. Excedrin
    d. Aspirin
    e. Acetaminophen

Answer a is incorrect. Celebrex is the brand name for celecoxib, a COX-2 inhibitor. COX-2 inhibitors increase bleeding risk in warfarin patients due to their potential to cause gastrointestinal ulceration.

Answer b is incorrect. Ibuprofen, as well as all other NSAIDs, may cause gastrointestinal ulcerations and bleeds. Combination of NSAIDs with warfarin therapy increases the risk for bleeding.

Answer c is incorrect. Excedrin contains aspirin. Aspirin reduces platelet aggregation and increases risk for bleeding.

Answer d is incorrect. Aspirin reduces platelet aggregation and increases risk for bleeding.

Answer e is correct. Although use of high doses of acetaminophen over several days can cause an interaction with warfarin therapy, as needed, doses <1500 mg daily is a safe option. Acetaminophen is the recommended over-the-counter agent for the management of mild–moderate pain with chronic warfarin therapy.

---

22. In which of the following procedures should Lovenox use be avoided?
    a. Computed tomography (CT) scan
    b. Magnetic resonance imaging (MRI) scan
    c. Epidural anesthesia
    d. 24 hour urine collection
    e. Liver biopsy

Answers a, b, and d are incorrect. These procedures are noninvasive and pose no added bleeding risk in patients receiving LMWHs.

Answer c is correct. LMWHs should be avoided in patients undergoing epidural anesthesia due to the potential of developing a spinal hematoma, which can result in long-term or permanent paralysis.

Answer e is incorrect because there is no contraindication to the use of LMWHs in patients undergoing liver biopsy.

CHAPTER 7 | Acute Coronary Syndromes

Questions 1 to 5 refer to the following patient case

TS is a 75-year-old woman who presents to emergency department (ED) via emergency medical system (EMS) to a large academic medical center (with a coronary catheterization laboratory) complaining of sudden onset of diaphoresis and nausea. She states, "About 5 hours ago my chest started hurting and I just don't feel well." TS's weight is 65 kg.

Past medical history: Coronary artery disease and arthritis

Family history: Father died of Acute myocardial infarction at 76 years of age and mother passed away at age 70 from pneumonia

Social history: Does not drink; smokes 1 pack of cigarettes per week.

Medications: Aspirin 81 mg orally once daily, atorvastatin 40 mg orally at bedtime, conjugated estrogens 0.625 mg, and celecoxib 200 mg orally daily

Laboratory data: SCr = 1.9 mg/dL, total cholesterol 250 mg/dL, triglycerides 150 mg/dL, HDL 40 mg/dL, LDL 130 mg/dL, troponin I = 5.7 ng/mL

Electrocardiogram: ST-segment elevation

1. Which one of the following is the preferred approach to reperfuse this patient?

   a. Chew aspirin 81mg, clopidogrel 75 mg, unfractionated heparin (UFH) for 48 hours
   b. Reteplase 10 units IV for two doses 30 minutes apart and UFH for 48 hours
   c. Chew aspirin 324 mg, administer clopidogrel 600 mg orally once, abciximab 16.25 μg IV bolus and percutaneous intervention with coronary stent placement
   d. Streptokinase 1,500,000 units IV over 30 minutes, aspirin 81 mg, clopidogrel 300 mg

---

Answer a is incorrect. TS is experiencing a STEMI and the goal for these patients is always primarily reperfusion. Aspirin, clopidogrel, and UFH will prevent further platelet aggregation and thrombus formation but they do not dissolve current clots.

Answer b is incorrect. A regimen including reteplase is a possibility for TS's treatment since reperfusion can occur either with fibrinolytic or percutaneous coronary intervention (PCI). However, if the facility has PCI capabilities, the patient should receive PCI as it is more effective than thrombolysis.

Answer c is correct. TS is experiencing a STEMI that requires emergent reperfusion and has presented to a hospital with cardiac catheterization capabilities. The patient should be loaded (higher doses) with antiplatelets, and started on abciximab since he will be going to catheterization emergently.

Answer d is incorrect. This is a possibility for treatment since this patient is a STEMI and will need reperfusion either with fibrinolytic or percutaneous transluminal coronary angioplasty (PTCA). However, streptokinase is not a common or highly recommended fibrinolytic due to its lack of specificity and capability of allergic reactions. Newer second generation fibrinolytics are preferred.

---

2. The physicians are debating on whether TS should receive early oral beta- blockers after receiving aspirin, clopidogrel, oxygen, nitrates, and morphine. Which of the following vital signs for TS would be conducive for early beta-blocker use?

   a. Heart rate 110 bpm; systolic blood pressure 85 mm Hg
   b. Heart rate 50 bpm; systolic blood pressure 120 mm Hg
   c. Heart rate 120 bpm; systolic blood pressure 120 mm Hg
   d. Heart rate 120 bpm; systolic blood pressure 120 mm Hg with rales and rhonchi on physical examination

---

Answer a is incorrect. Oral beta-blocker therapy should be initiated in the first 24 hours for patients who do not have any signs of heart failure, evidence of a low-output state (hypotension or cardiogenic shock) or contraindications to beta-blockade (bradycardia or active asthma). These vitals show hypotension a sign of low-output state.

Answer b is incorrect. These vitals show a heart rate of 50 bpm. A normal heart rate is around 70 bpm and so this represents bradycardia. Beta-blocker therapies are not recommended for patients with bradycardia.

Answer c is correct. These vitals show tachycardia and normal systolic so, with the information provided, this patient would be a candidate for beta-blockade.

Answer d is incorrect. This patient is hemodynamically stable but has signs of reactive airway disease or heart failure with the rales and rhonchi.

---

3. Which one of the following statements would you *not* suggest to the attending physician prior to patient discharge regarding her home medication regimen?

   a. Discontinue conjugated estrogens
   b. Discontinue aspirin
   c. Discontinue celecoxib
   d. Start a beta-blocker
   e. All of the above should be suggested prior to discharge.

Answer a is incorrect. Conjugated estrogens should be discontinued prior to discharge. Estrogen therapy was once thought to decrease cardiovascular events, however, the Women's Health Initiative study revealed increased incidence of breast cancer, heart attacks, and strokes in women receiving hormone replacement therapies (HRT). Based on these findings it is now recommended that women take prescribed HRT treatment at the lowest feasible dose, for the shortest possible time. ACS guidelines also recommend discontinuation of therapy post-MI.

Answer b is correct. This patient has extensive coronary artery disease and should remain on an aspirin, at least 75 mg daily.

Answer c is incorrect. Patients routinely taking NSAIDs (except for aspirin), both nonselective as well as COX-2 selective agents, have increase risk of cardiovascular mortality compared to those not receiving these therapies. Upon presentation with STEMI these agents should be discontinued to prevent adverse effects including reinfarction, hypertension, heart failure, and myocardial rupture associated with their use.

Answer d is incorrect. Beta-blocker initiation should be recommended before discharge if the patient is stable.

Answer e is incorrect because aspirin should not be discontinued.

---

4. A patient experiencing chest pain for a few hours decides to take a SL tablet of nitroglycerin (NTG). The first tablet provides no pain relief, so EMS is contacted. The patient continued to take the NTG every 5 minutes. The third tablet she took provided relief. How do nitrates decrease chest pain?
   a. Vasoconstriction of venous vasculature
   b. Vasodilation of arterial vasculature
   c. Vasodilation of venous vasculature
   d. Decreased cardiac output

Answer a is incorrect. Nitrates cause vasodilation of venous vasculature, not constriction

Answer b is incorrect. Nitrates cause vasodilation of the venous vasculature, not arterial.

Answer c is correct. Nitrates cause venous vasodilation as well as peripheral vasodilation at higher doses. This decreases the pressure going into the heart (preload) and decreases the pressure the heart has to push against in the arteries (afterload). This decreases the workload on heart. Nitrates also facilitate collateral flow in coronary arteries.

Answer d is incorrect. Nitrates increase cardiac output by decreasing the work load on the heart and improving coronary perfusion.

---

5. What is the mechanism of clopidogrel's benefit in a STEMI patient that has already received aspirin, oxygen, nitrates, and morphine?
   a. Clopidogrel improves myocardial oxygen supply.
   b. Clopidogrel opens up the infarct-related artery.
   c. Clopidogrel reduces myocardial oxygen demand.
   d. Clopidogrel prevents myocardial reinfarction.

Answer a is incorrect. Clopidogrel cannot dissolve platelets that are already in platelet clot covered by thrombin, therefore, will not improve myocardial oxygen supply by the removal of the clot. It also does not cause vasodilation or improve blood supply to heart.

Answer b is incorrect. Antiplatelets cannot disable platelets that are already in platelet clot covered by thrombin. A fibrinolytic is needed to break up a fibrin-bound clot.

Answer c is incorrect. Clopidogrel will not decrease heart rate or afterload that would decrease myocardial oxygen demand.

Answer d is correct. Clopidogrel along with aspirin will prevent the infarct from expanding further as well as prevent future myocardial infarctions and reinfarction (thrombosis) after reperfusion with thrombolytics or PCI.

Questions 6 to 8 refer to the following patient case.

MS is a 68-year-old man who presents to his local physician's office after eating lunch at McDonald's. He complains of chest pain with radiation to his jaw. His physician has him chew aspirin 325 mg and calls 911. He is transported to the local hospital where electrocardiogram shows ST-segment elevation.

Past medical history: Hypertension, coronary artery disease, chronic obstructive pulmonary disease (COPD), stage IV chronic kidney disease, cerebrovascular accident 2 months ago

Family history: Mother died of a stroke at 85 years and father passed away at 75 years in a car accident.

Social history: Smokes 1.5 pack of cigarette per day for 50 years; no alcohol history

Medications: Hydrochlorothiazide 25 mg orally daily, metoprolol 25 mg orally bid, tiotropium 18 μg inhaled once daily, albuterol inhaler 1 puff every 6 hours PRN, fluticasone/salmeterol 250/50 μg inhaled bid

Vital signs: Blood pressure 150/90 mm Hg, heart rate 98 bpm, respiratory rate 22 rpm, O_2 sat 88%, weight 100 kg

Laboratory data: Unavailable

Allergies: Heparin

6. MS presents at a hospital that does not have a cardiac catheterization laboratory, therefore they have 30 minutes to verify his candidacy for fibrinolytic therapy. Which of the following is a contraindication to MS receiving a fibrinolytic?
   a. MS already received aspirin and clopidogrel.
   b. MS's blood pressure is 150/90 mm Hg.
   c. Ms had a recent cerebrovascular accident.
   d. MS has an allergy to heparin.

Answer a is incorrect. Patients that receive fibrinolytic therapy should also receive antiplatelet therapy with aspirin and a thienopyridine.

Answer b is incorrect. Severe uncontrolled hypertension on presentation is classified as systolic blood pressure (SBP) >180 mm Hg, and is a relative contraindication. Remember that even if MS's BP was >180 mm Hg it should be treated prior to fibrinolysis, but does not preclude treatment.

Answer c is correct. Ischemic stroke in the last 3 months is a contraindication to fibrinolysis. The possibility of having an intracranial hemorrhage in MS outweighs the benefits of administering fibrinolytic therapy.

Answer d is incorrect. Anticoagulation is required with thrombolysis but heparinoids are not the only anticoagulant option.

---

7. Given MS's contraindication to fibrinolytic therapy, he was life-flighted to a hospital with 24 hour cardiac catheterization

capabilities. The plan is for emergent PCI on arrival. Which of the following statements about abciximab (glycoprotein IIb/IIIa inhibitor) is true?

a. Abciximab needs to be renally adjusted.
b. Abciximab can be reversed with platelet transfusion.
c. Abciximab is administered as two subcutaneous boluses.
d. Abciximab is the only glycoprotein IIb/IIIa inhibitor that is indicated as an adjunct to PCI.
e. Abciximab is safe to give in this patient.

Answer a is incorrect. It does not need to be renally adjusted. Eptifibatide and tirofiban however are renally eliminated and do require dosage adjustments.

Answer b is correct. Abciximab is the only glycoprotein inhibitor (GPI) that can be reversed by a platelet infusion.

Answer c is incorrect. Abciximab is dosed as an IV bolus followed by a continuous infusion.

Answer d is incorrect. All GPIs are indicated as an adjunct to PCI.

Answer e is incorrect. Abciximab is contraindicated for 2 years following ischemic stroke or transient ischemic attack (TIA). Eptifibatide is safe after 3 months, while tirofiban can be given 1 month following stroke or TIA.

---

8. Which of the following beta-blockers would be most appropriate in MS?

a. Propranolol ER
b. Atenolol
c. Carvedilol
d. Acebutolol
e. Esmolol

Answer a is incorrect. This patient has COPD and β_1-selective beta-blockers are preferred in this patient population.

Answer b is correct. Atenolol is a β_1-selective beta-blocker with little activity at β_2 receptors.

Answer c is incorrect. Carvedilol is not cardioselective. It has β_1, β_2, and α effects making it less than desirable in MS.

Answer d is incorrect. Acebutolol is β_1-selective but it also has mild intrinsic sympathomimetic activity (ISA) which is not desirable in patients post-MI.

Answer e is incorrect. Esmolol is a short-acting β_1-selective blocker, but it is only available intravenously.

---

9. Which anticoagulant is treatment of choice in a STEMI patient that is also dialysis dependent?

a. Enoxaparin
b. Dalteparin
c. Fondaparinux
d. Heparin

Answer a is incorrect. Enoxaparin is renally eliminated and does not have data for treatment in hemodialysis patients.

Answer b is incorrect. Dalteparin does not have dosing data for hemodialysis patients and is renally eliminated.

Answer c is incorrect. Fondaparinux is contraindicated if creatinine clearance is less than 30 mL/min.

Answer d is correct. Heparin is not renally eliminated.

---

10. What laboratory value is traditionally used to monitor the level of anticoagulation achieved with unfractionated heparin?

a. International normalized ratio (INR)
b. PT (Prothrombin time)
c. Anti-Xa level
d. Activated partial thromboplastin time (aPTT)

Answer a is incorrect. INR is used to monitor vitamin K antagonism therapy (warfarin).

Answer b is incorrect. PT is the unstandardized laboratory value associated with INR. Therefore it is also used to monitor warfarin therapy.

Answer c is incorrect. Anti-Xa levels can be monitored when patients are on low molecular weight heparin. There are also an increasing number of institutions using anti-Xa levels to monitor unfractionated heparin. However, this has not been used historically.

Answer d is correct. aPTTs are used to monitor unfractionated heparin anticoagulation. When treating ACS the goal aPTT is 1.5 to 2 times a patient's baseline (approximately 50 to 70 seconds).

---

11. Which of the following antiplatelet/anticoagulant regimens would be recommended for treatment of a NSTEMI patient with a heparin allergy? The patient is going to receive PCI later in the day.

a. Bivalirudin
b. Eptifibatide and low molecular weight heparin
c. Abciximab and unfractionated heparin
d. Fondaparinux

Answer a is correct. In patients with UA and NSTEMI bivalirudin may be started prior to PCI (if PCI is planned). It is a direct thrombin inhibitor and does not require concomitant use with heparin or glycoprotein IIb/IIIa inhibitors.

Answer b is incorrect. Eptifibatide therapy is appropriate, but administration with LMWH is not appropriate in this patient due to heparin allergy.

Answer c is incorrect. Abciximab may be used in this patient since it is indicated when PCI is planned. However it is not necessary to start it early. Also, this patient has a heparin allergy and should not receive heparin.

Answer d is incorrect. Fondaparinux would be safe to use in patients with heparin allergies, however it is not recommended when PCI is planned.

---

12. Which of the following agents is *not* indicated in the setting of NSTEMI?
    a. Eptifibatide
    b. Unfractionated heparin (UFH)
    c. Aspirin
    d. Reteplase
    e. Clopidogrel

Answer a is incorrect. Eptifibatide can be used as an adjunct for PCI in NSTEMI and for the medical management of ACS.

Answer b is incorrect. Unfractionated heparin is indicated in PCI as well as the medical management of NSTEMI.

Answer c is incorrect. Aspirin should be given to all patients experiencing ACS unless significant contraindication.

Answer d is correct. Fibrinolytics are not indicated in the treatment of NSTEMI or unstable angina. They break fibrin clots, also known as "red clots," that occur with complete occlusion of coronary arteries, which occur with STEMI only.

Answer e is incorrect. Clopidogrel plus aspirin has been found to have added benefit over aspirin alone in treatment of NSEMI.

---

13. Once the acute phase of myocardial infarction has passed, which of the following therapies is most likely to slow the development of heart failure (HF)?
    a. Clopidogrel
    b. Atenolol
    c. Ramipril
    d. Amiodarone
    e. Isosorbide mononitrate

Answer a is incorrect. Clopidogrel prevents recurrent ischemic events and provides an important reduction in morbidity post-MI, however does not alter progression of left ventricular dysfunction.

Answer b is incorrect. Atenolol prevents recurrent ischemic events and provides mortality post-MI, however does not alter progression of left ventricular dysfunction.

Answer c is correct. Angiotensin-converting enzyme inhibitor (ACEI), like ramipril, have been shown to prevent ventricular remodeling. This is the main pathophysiologic change that results in heart failure following myocardial infarction.

Answer d is incorrect. Amiodarone treats atrial and ventricular arrhythmias, which occur with increased frequency following ACS. However, it does not affect heart failure progression.

Answer e is incorrect. Isosorbide mononitrate and other nitrate products should be considered for patients to treat on-going symptoms of ischemic heart disease not relieved with beta-blockers. However, they do not alter cardiovascular mortality or prevent heart failure.

---

14. TL is an 82-year- old woman who is status post drug-eluting stent placement following presentations with a STEMI. She has a past medical history significant for hypertension, dyslipidemia, and hypothyroidism. She has no known drug allergies. Which of the following is the best choice of long-term antiplatelet therapy?
    a. Aspirin 325 mg orally daily
    b. Aspirin 81 mg plus prasugrel 10 mg daily
    c. Prasugrel 5 mg orally daily
    d. Aspirin 81 mg plus clopidogrel 75 mg orally daily
    e. Clopidogrel 75 mg orally daily

Answer a is incorrect. Following treatment with coronary artery stents dual antiplatelet therapy is indicated (aspirin plus thienopyridine).

Answer b is incorrect. Although use of low-dose aspirin is appropriate, use of prasugrel is contraindicated in this patient. Prasugrel has a black box warning regarding increased bleeding and recommends against use in patients > 75 years old, less than 60 kg, and with history of ischemic stroke or TIA. Therefore prasugrel should not be used in this patient.

Answer c is incorrect. Following treatment with coronary artery stents dual antiplatelet therapy is indicated (aspirin plus thienopyridine). Prasugrel use is contraindicated in this patient.

Answer d is correct. This regimen of low-dose aspirin and a thienopyridine represents the best option in this patient. Aspirin plus clopidogrel should be continued for at least a year following drug-eluting stent placement.

Answer e is incorrect. Following treatment with coronary artery stents dual antiplatelet therapy is indicated (aspirin plus thienopyridine). This would be an option for patients with aspirin allergies.

---

15. Which of the following is the most appropriate lipid lowering regimen to give a patient with recent NSTEMI with an LDL of 150 mg/dL, TC of 192 mg/dL, TG of 140 mg/dL, and HDL of 47 mg/dL? The patient has no allergies or intolerances.
    a. Pravastatin 40 mg qhs
    b. Simvastatin 20 mg daily
    c. Atorvastatin 80 mg daily
    d. Niacin 500 mg qhs
    e. Rosuvastatin 10 mg qhs

Answer a is incorrect. Pravastatin would lower this patient's LDL by approximately 25%, bringing it to approximately 110 mg/dL, which do not reach his therapeutic goal.

Answer b is incorrect. Like pravastatin, this dose of simvastatin will not allow this patient to achieve a low enough LDL.

Answer c is correct. Numerous trials have evaluated the use of atorvastatin post-MI. This is the medication of choice to prevent future ischemic events. It would also reduce this patients LDL by approximately 75 mg/dL.

Answer d is incorrect. Niacin alone will not reduce this patient's LDL enough. Niacin can be used in addition to statins in patients with low HDL as a secondary target.

Answer e is incorrect. Rosuvastatin is the most potent statin. This dose correlates with LDL reduction similar to lipitor 20 mg, simvastatin 80 mg, and it too would not decrease enough LDL to reach this patient's therapeutic goal. Rosuvastatin 40 mg would be an option to achieve target LDL, however there have been no prospective trials evaluating the use post-MI.

---

16. Which of the following therapies requires monitoring of serum creatinine and potassium?
    a. Carvedilol
    b. Spironolactone
    c. Atenolol
    d. Pravastatin
    e. Clopidogrel

Answer a is incorrect. Carvedilol is not renally eliminated nor does it has much effect on serum potassium levels.

Answer b is correct. Initiation of spironolactone should only occur in patients with SCr < 2.5 and K < 5.0. Dose reductions are used in patients with SCr 1.5 to 2.5 as well. This medication requires frequent monitoring of both laboratory values during initiation and occasionally thereafter.

Answer c is incorrect. Atenolol is renally eliminated. Therefore it would be appropriate to monitor SCr occasionally. However, effect on potassium is minimal and does not require routine monitoring.

Answer d is incorrect. Pravastatin requires monitoring of hepatic function tests and lipid levels only.

Answer e is incorrect. Clopidogrel is not renally eliminated nor does it affect potassium levels.

---

17. Which of the following is an appropriate fibrinolytic dosing regimen for a 78-kg person with STEMI?
    a. Streptase 1 million units intravenously over 20 minutes.
    b. Reteplase or rPA 10 units IV bolus twice 30 minutes apart.
    c. Tenecteplase or TNK 50 mg IV bolus once.
    d. Alteplase 100 mg IV over 2 hours.

Answer a is incorrect. Streptokinase, SK, or streptase is rarely used, and the dose is 1.5 million units over 60 minutes.

Answer b is correct. Reteplase or rPA is given as to 10 units boluses 30 minutes apart.

Answer c is incorrect. TNK or tenecteplase is given as a single bolus, but is weight-based and this patient's weight would require a bolus of 40 mg.

Answer d is incorrect. This dose of alteplase (tPA) is for treatment of pulmonary embolism. When given for STEMI, it is administered in three phases 15 mg IV bolus followed by 0.75 mg/kg IV over 30 minutes (max 50 mg) followed by 0.5 mg/kg (max 35mg) over 60 minutes.

---

18. PK presents with chest pain, nausea, vomiting, and diaphoresis. He is diagnosed with a NSTEMI. Current blood pressure is 92/56 mm Hg and HR is 105 bpm. Which of the following should be given immediately?
    a. ASA EC 325 mg orally once
    b. ASA 81 mg two tablets chewed once
    c. NTG IV drip at 20 μg/min
    d. IV metoprolol 5 mg IV once
    e. Morphine 2 to 4 mg IV every 2 hours

Answer a is incorrect. Enteric-coated aspirin products by design have delayed absorption. In the setting of ACS it is important to have rapid absorption of aspirin.

Answer b is correct. Aspirin 162 to 325 mg should be chewed upon presentation with ACS.

Answer c is incorrect. This patient is currently hypotensive, the risks of giving nitroglycerin outweigh the benefits.

Answer d is incorrect. This patient does have an elevated heart rate, however IV beta-blockers should be avoided in patients demonstrating signs of reduced cardiac output, like hypotension.

Answer e is incorrect. IV morphine can decrease blood pressure and should be avoided in patients with low blood pressure.

---

19. When completing a home medication evaluation for a patient admitted with unstable angina you notice he is on sildenafil. Which of the following statements is true regarding this medication?
    a. He probably has not taken it in a while so I can disregard the information.
    b. Nitroglycerin IV does not interfere with sildenafil like sublingual tablets.
    c. The patient does not need the medication restarted while he is in the hospital.
    d. a and c
    e. None of the above

Answer a is incorrect. If the patient took this last dose of sildenafil greater than 24 hours ago it should not affect other therapies, like nitrates.

Answer b is incorrect. IV nitroglycerin given with sildenafil can also decrease blood pressure and therefore this combination should be avoided.

Answer c is incorrect. It is important to identify what his indication for therapy is. Sildenafil therapy is also used for treatment of pulmonary hypertension and it would be important to continue treatment and therefore avoid nitrates.

Answer d is incorrect. See above.

Answer e is correct. a, b, and c are incorrect.

---

20. DL is a 62-year-old woman who presents to the ED with NSTEMI. She has no significant past medical history. Pertinent data includes, blood pressure 125/79 mm Hg, heart rate 75 bpm, SCr 1.2 mg/dL, platelet count 142 k/uL, weight 94 kg. She has allergies to penicillin, sulfa, and aspirin. Which of the following regimens are okay to give DL while she waits for her PCI?
    a. Aspirin 324 mg once, then 81 mg daily
    b. Clopidogrel 300 mg once, then 75 mg daily
    c. Aspirin 162 mg once, then 81 mg daily plus clopidogrel 600 mg once, then 75 mg daily
    d. Prasugrel 60 mg once then 5 mg daily
    e. None of the above.

Answer a is incorrect. DL has an aspirin allergy. Although desensitization protocols exist, this is not the time to attempt this ;so aspirin products should be avoided.

Answer b is correct. Clopidogrel alone may be used in patients with aspirin allergies.

Answer c is incorrect. As with answer a, aspirin should be avoided in this patient secondary to aspirin allergy.

Answer d is incorrect. Prasugrel would be an option in this patient, however, the correct dose is 60 mg once followed by 10 mg orally daily.

Answer e is incorrect.

---

21. Which of the following beta-blockers are available in both oral and IV formulations?
    a. Atenolol
    b. Esmolol
    c. Metoprolol
    d. Carvedilol
    e. a and c

Answer a is incorrect. Atenolol is available in both IV solution and oral tablets.

Answer b is incorrect. Esmolol is only available intravenously.

Answer c is incorrect. Metoprolol is available in both IV solution and oral tablets (sustained and immediate release).

Answer d is incorrect. Carvedilol is only available in oral immediate release formulation and in an oral sustained release formulation.

Answer e is correct. Both atenolol and metoprolol are available in IV and oral formulations.

---

22. Secondary prevention of acute coronary syndrome should include which of the following therapies?
    a. HMG-CoA reductase inhibitors
    b. Aspirin
    c. Calcium channel blockers
    d. Fenofibrates
    e. a and b

Answer a is incorrect. Statins are indicated for all patients post-ACS unless contraindicated. They reduced major adverse cardiovascular endpoints. If patients have been intolerant to one statin, another should be tried before moving to another class of cholesterol lowering medication.

Answer b is incorrect. Aspirin should also be used in all patients without contraindications.

Answer c is incorrect. Calcium channel blockers, specifically dihydropyridine calcium channel blockers may be used as third line treatment for hypertension in patients with a history of ACS. Both beta-blockers and ACEI should utilized first.

Answer d is incorrect. Fenofibrates may be added to statins for treatment of hypertriglyceridemia, however, they are not required for secondary prevention.

Answer e is correct.

CHAPTER 8 | Arrhythmias

1. A patient with a HR of 53 bpm is complaining of shortness of breath (SOB), light-headedness, and has a BP of 80/58 mm Hg. Transcutaneous pacing is being prepared. What is the first drug and dose that should be administered?
    a. Epinephrine 1 mg IV
    b. Atropine 0.5 mg IV
    c. Atropine 1 mg IV
    d. Dopamine 1-5 μg/kg/min IV

This patient is in sinus bradycardia with a HR of 53 bpm. The patient is considered unstable due to SOB, light-headedness, and hypotension (BP 80/58 mm Hg). Therefore, intervention is warranted.

Answer a is incorrect. Epinephrine is an appropriate drug to administer for bradycardia, but in the form of an infusion after atropine has failed.

Answer b is correct. Atropine 0.5 mg IV is the first drug and dose that should be administered while transcutaneous pacing is being prepared.

Answer c is incorrect. The dose is too high. Atropine 0.5 mg is the correct dose for symptomatic bradycardia and may be repeated up to 3 mg total.

Answer d is incorrect. Dopamine is an appropriate drug to administer for bradycardia. However it should be tried after atropine has failed and the correct dose range is dopamine 2 to 10 μg/kg/min.

---

2. You respond with the code team to a patient that is in cardiac arrest. High quality chest compressions are being given. The patient is intubated and an IV has been started. ECG reveals that the patient is in asystole. The first IV drug and dose to administer is:

   a. Amiodarone 300 mg IV
   b. Epinephrine 1 mg IV
   c. Dopamine 1 to 5 μg/kg/min
   d. Lidocaine 1 to 1.5 mg/kg IV

Answer a is incorrect. Class III antiarrhythmics have no role in asystole.

Answer b is correct. Epinephrine 1 mg IV is the initial drug and dose to be administered for asystole.

Answer c is incorrect. Dopamine has no role in asystole.

Answer d is incorrect. Class Ib antiarrhythmics have no role in asystole.

---

3. Which of the following antiarrhythmic drugs is *least likely* to cause torsade de pointes?

   a. Quinidine
   b. Sotalol
   c. Lidocaine
   d. Dofetilide

Answer a is incorrect. Class Ia antiarrhythmics prolong the QT interval and can cause torsades.

Answer b is incorrect. Sotalol, a Class III antiarrhythmic can prolong the QT interval and cause torsades.

Answer c is correct. Lidocaine, a Class Ib antiarrhythmic has a low potential of causing torsades.

Answer d is incorrect. Dofetilide, a Class III antiarrhythmic can prolong the QT interval and cause torsade.

---

4. A 78 year-old-woman with recurrent persistent atrial fibrillation is referred to your ambulatory care clinic for consideration for possible anticoagulation therapy. Her current medications include amiodarone 200 mg daily, simvastatin 10 mg HS for hyperlipidemia, lisinopril 10 mg daily for hypertension, and sitagliptin 50 mg daily for diabetes. Based on her risk of stroke, which of the following recommendations would be appropriate?

   a. Aspirin 325 mg daily
   b. Warfarin with a target INR 2.5
   c. Warfarin with a target INR 3.5
   d. None of the above

Answer a is incorrect. Because this patient is in persistent atrial fibrillation, she should be considered for anticoagulation therapy. Her risk factors for ischemic stroke are age >75 years, hypertension, and diabetes. Because she has greater than two risk factors, warfarin is indicated.

Answer b is correct. The goal INR for a patient with atrial fibrillation is 2 to 3 and this patient requires therapy with warfarin for reasons stated above.

Answer c is incorrect. This INR target is too high.

Answer d is incorrect. Warfarin is indicated with a target INR of 2.5.

---

5. A nonresponsive patient in ventricular fibrillation has received multiple appropriate defibrillations, and epinephrine 1 mg IV twice. Which antiarrhythmic drug can be used next?

   a. Cordarone
   b. Isoptin
   c. Brevibloc
   d. Quinidex

Answer a is correct. Once the primary ABCD algorithm for VF/pulseless VT has been followed, drugs should be administered followed by shocks in between. Since the patient has already received the first drug of choice, epinephrine, antiarrhythmic therapy should be initiated. Amiodarone 300 mg IV is a good choice.

Answer b is incorrect. Non-DHP calcium channel blockers have no role in the treatment of VF.

Answer c is incorrect. β-Blockers have no role in the treatment of VF.

Answer d is incorrect. Quinidex (Quinidine), a Class 1a antiarrhythmic, has no role in the treatment of VF.

---

6. A 79-year-old man presents to your hospital emergency room with newly discovered atrial fibrillation with rapid ventricular response and is very symptomatic with little rate control achieved after initiation of a diltiazem drip. It is decided by the attending physician to proceed with electrical cardioversion. The patient's wife reports that he underwent a cardiac workup the day before for routine knee replacement surgery. The ECG from that workup is retrieved and shows normal sinus rhythm. What is the next appropriate step in this patient's care?

   a. Proceed with synchronized direct cardioversion
   b. Anticoagulate with warfarin for 3 weeks, target INR 2.0 to 3.0, then cardioversion
   c. Obtain transesophageal ECHO to rule out thrombus then cardioversion
   d. None of the above

The first goal of managing a patient presenting with atrial fibrillation is rate control. This has been attempted with the diltiazem drip. However, the patient is still very symptomatic. Because of the symptoms, immediate cardioversion should be considered.

Answer a is correct. Because it is very clear that the patient has been in atrial fibrillation for less than 48 hours, it is appropriate to proceed with immediate cardioversion. Anticoagulation with heparin or low molecular weight heparin (LMWH) would be beneficial, but not necessarily required per guidelines.

Answer b is incorrect. Because the patient is still symptomatic despite rate control, an attempt should be made to cardiovert now.

Answer c is incorrect. Because we know that the patient's atrial fibrillation has been occurring for less than 48 hours, it is appropriate to proceed with cardioversion without the TEE.

---

7. Which of the following drug(s) are considered safe and effective when utilized for pharmacologic cardioversion of atrial fibrillation in patients with structural heart disease?

   i. Flecainide
   ii. Sotalol
   iii. Dofetilide

   a. i only
   b. iii only
   c. i and ii
   d. ii and iii
   e. i, ii and iii

Answer b is correct. Dofetilide, a Class III antiarrhythmic is a safe drug to use in patients with structural heart disease and left ventricular dysfunction. Amiodarone is the other antiarrhythmic that is safe in this patient population.

Answers a, c, d, and e are all incorrect. Flecainide and sotalol are not safe for use in patients with structural heart disease.

---

8. Amiodarone requires substantial safety monitoring during long-term therapy due to its numerous side effects. Which of the following does not have to be routinely performed in a patient on long-term amiodarone therapy?

   a. Hepatic function panel
   b. Thyroid function tests
   c. Ophthalmologic examination
   d. B-type natriuretic peptide levels

Answer a is incorrect. Amiodarone can cause elevations in liver function test (LFT) and may require dose adjustment in patients with liver impairment. Hepatic function panels should be monitored routinely.

Answer b is incorrect. Amiodarone can cause both hyperthyroidism and hypothyroidism. Thyroid function tests should be obtained routinely.

Answer c is incorrect. Amiodarone can cause corneal deposits in most patients that take the drug. Amiodarone can also cause macular degeneration. Patients should have annual eye examinations while taking amiodarone.

Answer d is correct. Amiodarone does not affect B-type natriuretic peptide (BNP) levels, which is considered a measurement of heart failure status and response to ventricular stretch.

---

9. Dofetilide is contraindicated in all of the following situations *except:*

   a. A patient initiated in an outpatient setting
   b. A patient with CrCl <20 mL/min
   c. A baseline QTc 510 millisecond
   d. A patient with left ventricular hypertrophy

Answer a is incorrect. Dofetilide must be initiated in an inpatient setting under telemetry.

Answer b is incorrect. Dofetilide is contraindicated in patients with a CrCl<20 mL/min.

Answer c is incorrect. Dofetilide is contraindicated in patients with a QTc > 440 millisecond (or 500 millisecond with a ventricular conduction abnormality).

Answer d is correct. Dofetilide is relatively safe in patients with structural heart disease and ventricular hypertrophy.

---

10. Which antiarrhythmic drug is safe to use for maintenance of sinus rhythm in a patient with atrial fibrillation, heart failure, and an ejection fraction of 15%.

    a. Sotalol
    b. Flecainide
    c. Amiodarone
    d. Procainamide

Answer a is incorrect. Sotalol, a Class III antiarrhythmic, while used often for atrial fibrillation and ventricular arrhythmias, is not safe for use in patients with left ventricular dysfunction and heart failure.

Answer b is incorrect. Flecainide, a Class Ic antiarrhythmic, while used often for atrial fibrillation, is not safe for patients with impaired left ventricular function.

Answer c is correct. Amiodarone is safe for use in patients with heart failure and impaired ventricular output.

Answer d is incorrect. Procainamide, a Class Ia antiarrhythmic is not safe for this patient. Class Ia agents are not typically recommended for atrial arrhythmias any longer.

---

11. RT is a 65-year-old woman who presents with paroxysmal supraventricular tachycardia (PSVT) with a regular rhythm. RT is experiencing mild symptoms and was given unilateral carotid sinus massage with no success. If the patient has a narrow QRS interval, what medication(s) is(are) first-line agent(s) to treat this patient?

   i. Adenosine
   ii. Verapamil
   iii. Procainamide

   a. i only
   b. iii only
   c. i and ii
   d. ii and iii
   e. i, ii, and iii

Answer a is incorrect. Adenosine is indicated for the treatment of patients with PSVT with a narrow QRS interval and a regular rhythm, but verapamil can also be used in these patients.

Answer b is incorrect. Procainamide is used for the treatment of patients with PSVT and an irregular rhythm.

Answer c is correct. The initial treatment for a patient with mild symptoms associated with PSVT is to perform vasovagal maneuvers. If unsuccessful, the next step in treatment is determined by the patient's ECG findings. Patients with a narrow QRS interval and a regular rhythm can be treated with adenosine, verapamil, or diltiazem.

Answer d is incorrect. Adenosine is indicated for the treatment of patients with PSVT with a narrow QRS interval and a regular rhythm, but verapamil can also be used in these patients. Procainamide is used for the treatment of patients with PSVT and an irregular rhythm.

Answer e is incorrect. Adenosine and verapamil are indicated for the treatment of patients with PSVT with a narrow QRS interval and a regular rhythm, but procainamide is used for the treatment of patients with PSVT and an irregular rhythm.

---

12. What antiarrhythmic drug has the potential for causing taste disturbances?

   a. Norpace
   b. Mexitil
   c. Betapace
   d. Rythmol

Answer a is incorrect. Norpace (disopyramide) has not been shown to produce taste disturbances.

Answer b is incorrect. Mexitil (mexiletine) has not been shown to produce taste disturbances.

Answer c is incorrect. Betapace (sotalol) has not been shown to produce taste disturbances.

Answer d is correct. Rythmol (propafenone) can illicit taste disturbances.

---

13. KG is a 55-year-old man who presents with recurrent complaints of shortness of breath and describes feeling like his heart is racing. An ECG is performed and it is determined that he is in atrial fibrillation with a ventricular rate of 160 bpm. An evaluation of his left ventricular function concluded that his ejection fraction is 35%. While the patient was still in the examination room, he reports that his symptoms have subsided and a repeat ECG was completed and it was found that the patient was in normal sinus rhythm. What medication should be prescribed to KG to control his rate?

   a. Digoxin
   b. Amiodarone
   c. Diltiazem
   d. Verapamil

Answer a is incorrect. Due to the fact that the recurrent AF terminated spontaneously, KG is determined to have paroxysmal AF and thus digoxin should not be used.

Answer b is correct. If a patient presenting with AF is stable, the initial focus of therapy is rate control. In patients with decreased LV function (EF ≤ 40%), digoxin or amiodarone are the recommended treatments for rate control. Due to the fact that the recurrent AF terminated spontaneously, KG is determined to have paroxysmal AF and thus digoxin should not be used.

Answer c is incorrect. Diltiazem or other calcium channel blockers are used in AF rate control if the patient has no comorbid conditions.

Answer d is incorrect. Verapamil or other calcium channel blockers are used in AF rate control if the patient has no comorbid conditions. In addition, verapamil is contraindicated in patients with LV dysfunction.

---

14. Potential side effect(s) of dronedarone is (are):

   i. Gingival hyperplasia
   ii. Increased serum creatinine
   iii. QT prolongation

   a. i only
   b. iii only
   c. i and ii
   d. ii and iii
   e. i, ii, and iii

Answer a is incorrect. Gingival hyperplasia is a side effect of verapamil.

Answer b is incorrect. QT prolongation is a potential side effect of dronedarone, but an increased serum creatinine can also occur with dronedarone.

Answer c is incorrect. Gingival hyperplasia is a side effect of verapamil. Increased serum creatinine is a potential side effect of dronedarone, but QT prolongation can also occur with dronedarone.

Answer d is correct. Increased serum creatinine and QT prolongation are potential side effects of dronedarone.

Answer e is incorrect. Increased serum creatinine and QT prolongation are potential side effects of dronedarone. Gingival hyperplasia is a side effect of verapamil and has not been shown to occur with dronedarone.

---

15. CB is a 56-year-old woman who presents with palpitations, dyspnea, and presyncope. An ECG is performed and premature ventricular complexes are found. CB has a past medical history of hypertension, hyperlipidemia, and post-myocardial infarction 2 years ago. What is the treatment of choice for CB?

    a. Flecainide
    b. Propafenone
    c. Metoprolol succinate
    d. Amiodarone

Answer a is incorrect. Class Ic antiarrhythmic agents, such as flecainide, should be avoided in patients with premature ventricular contraction (PVC) due to the increased risk of mortality post-myocardial infarction.

Answer b is incorrect. Class Ic antiarrhythmic agents, such as propafenone, should be avoided in patients with PVCs due to the increased risk of mortality post-myocardial infarction.

Answer c is correct. β-Blockers, such as metoprolol, are indicated for treatment of symptomatic patients with PVCs.

Answer d is incorrect. Amiodarone is not indicated for the treatment of PVCs.

---

16. What is the initial step in therapy for a stable patient presenting with monomorphic VT?

    a. Epinephrine
    b. Amiodarone
    c. Lidocaine
    d. Immediate DCC

Answer a is incorrect. Epinephrine is utilized in the treatment of VF or pulseless VT. Following CPR and DCC, epinephrine 1 mg IV is given every 3 to 5 minutes with no maximum dose.

Answer b is correct. The initial treatment for a stable patient with monomorphic VT is a loading dose of amiodarone (150 mg) over 10 minutes followed by an amiodarone drip.

Answer c is incorrect. Lidocaine is given during the treatment of VF or pulseless VT. Following CPR, DCC, and epinephrine therapy, lidocaine 1 to1.5 mg/kg IV can be given and repeated at a dose of 0.5 mg to 0.75 mg/kg IV every 5 to 10 minutes (maximum dose of 3 mg/kg).

Answer d is incorrect. Immediate DCC is utilized if the patient is unstable.

---

17. Which of the following medications given during the treatment of VF or pulseless VT has no dose maximum?

    i. Vasopressin
    ii. Epinephrine
    iii. Lidocaine

    a. i only
    b. ii only
    c. i and ii
    d. ii and iii
    e. i, ii, and iii

Answer a is incorrect. During the treatment of VF or pulseless VT, vasopressin is given as a 40 IU single dose.

Answer b is correct. During the treatment of VF or pulseless VT, epinephrine is given 1 mg IV every 3 to 5 minutes with no maximum dose.

Answer c is incorrect. During the treatment of VF or pulseless VT, epinephrine is given 1 mg IV every 3 to 5 minutes with no maximum dose, but vasopressin is given as a 40 IU single dose.

Answer d is incorrect. During the treatment of VF or pulseless VT, epinephrine is given 1 mg IV every 3 to 5 minutes with no maximum dose, but lidocaine has a maximum dose of 3 mg/kg.

Answer e is incorrect. During the treatment of VF or pulseless VT, lidocaine 1 to1.5 mg/kg IV is used and can be repeated at a dose of 0.5 to 0.75 mg/kg IV every 5 to 10 minutes with a maximum dose of 3 mg/kg.

---

18. JL is a 58-year-old woman whose past medical history includes atrial fibrillation and seasonal allergies. What is the indicated treatment to prevent thromboembolic complications in JL?

    a. Aspirin 325 mg daily
    b. Warfarin with a target INR 2.5
    c. Warfarin with a target INR 3.5
    d. None of the above

Answer a is correct. Patients, who are less than 75 years of age and have no risk factors for ischemic stroke, it is recommended that they receive long-term aspirin therapy with a dose of 75-325 mg/d for the prevention of thromboembolic complications.

Answer b is incorrect. Warfarin therapy is reserved for use in patients who possess risk factors for ischemic stroke such as: age > 75 years, history of hypertension, diabetes mellitus, moderately or severely impaired left ventricular systolic function, and/or heart failure.

Answer c is incorrect. Warfarin therapy is reserved for use in patients that possess risk factors for ischemic stroke such as: age > 75 years, history of hypertension, diabetes mellitus, moderately or severely impaired left ventricular systolic function, and/or heart failure.

Answer d is incorrect. Patients who are less than 75 years of age and have no risk factors for ischemic stroke, it is recommended that they receive long-term aspirin therapy with a dose of 75 to 325 mg/d for the prevention of thromboembolic complications.

---

19. Which of the following medications slows depolarization through sodium channel blockade?
    a. Brevibloc
    b. Tambocor
    c. Tiazac
    d. Covert

Answer a is incorrect. Brevibloc (esmolol) slows AV nodal conduction through β-blockade.

Answer b is correct. Tambocor (flecainide) slows depolarization through sodium channel blockade.

Answer c is incorrect. Tiazac (diltiazem) slows AV nodal conduction through calcium channel blockade.

Answer d is incorrect. Covert (ibutilide) slows repolarization through potassium channel blockade.

---

20. TG is an 85-year old female who is currently hospitalized for pneumonia. Her current medications include levofloxacin, albuterol via nebulization, zolpidem, and acetaminophen. On the second day of her hospitalization, her ECG reveals that she is experiencing polymorphic VT. If TG remains stable, what would be the first step of treatment?
    a. Immediate DCC
    b. Epinephrine 1 mg IV
    c. Discontinue levofloxacin
    d. Amiodarone 150 mg over 10 minutes

Answer a is incorrect. Immediate DCC is indicated for unstable patients with polymorphic VT.

Answer b is incorrect. Epinephrine 1 mg IV is utilized in the treatment of VF or pulseless VT.

Answer c is correct. If a patient is experiencing polymorphic VT (torsade de pointes) and is stable, the first step is to discontinue any agents that may be causing the arrhythmia. In this case, levofloxacin has the potential for causing polymorphic VT and should be discontinued.

Answer d is incorrect. Amiodarone 150 mg is utilized in the treatment of someone with monomorphic VT.

CHAPTER 9 | Peripheral Arterial Disease

1. Risk factors for the development and progression of PAD include which of the following?
    a. Tobacco abuse
    b. Hypertension
    c. Diabetes mellitus
    d. All of the above

Answer a is correct. Tobacco abuse is a risk factor for PAD.

Answer b is correct. Hypertension is a risk factor for PAD.

Answer c is correct. Diabetes mellitus is a risk factor for PAD.

Answer d is correct. Risk factors for PAD include increasing age, tobacco abuse, diabetes mellitus, hypertension, and hyperlipidemia.

---

2. A 40-year-old smoker with hypertension, diabetes, hypercholesterolemia, and PAD complains of pain in his calves when he walks two to three blocks. What therapy might offer him the greatest benefit in symptom reduction and in overall mortality?
    a. Limb revascularization procedure
    b. Cilostazol
    c. Smoking cessation
    d. Pravastatin

Answer a is incorrect. A limb revascularization procedure is indicated with an acute arterial occlusion that threatens limb viability.

Answer b is incorrect. Cilostazol may help with claudication symptoms but will not affect cardiovascular mortality.

Answer c is correct. Tobacco cessation is the most important intervention to improve cardiovascular morbidity and mortality in high- risk patients and to improve claudication symptoms.

Answer d is incorrect. Pravastatin will not help with claudication symptoms.

---

3. The gold standard diagnostic test for PAD is arteriography. Another test which is useful in the diagnosis is which of the following?
    a. Systolic blood pressure
    b. Diastolic blood pressure
    c. Cardiac angiography
    d. Resting ankle-brachial systolic pressure index (ABI)

Answer a is incorrect. An elevated systolic blood pressure gives no useful information about PAD.

Answer b is incorrect. An elevated diastolic blood pressure gives no useful information about PAD.

Answer c is incorrect. Cardiac angiography is the gold standard diagnostic test for coronary artery disease.

Answer d is correct. An ABI of ≤ 0.90 has a high degree of sensitivity and specificity for the diagnosis of PAD.

---

4. Aspirin carries non-FDA labeled indications (Class IIb, Category B) for PAD, thrombosis, and prophylaxis. Which of the following are contraindications to the use of aspirin in this patient population?
   a. Asthma
   b. Hypersensitivity to NSAIDS
   c. Nasal polyps
   d. All of the above

Answer a is correct. Asthma is a contraindication to the use of aspirin.

Answer b is correct. Hypersensitivity to NSAIDS is a contraindication to the use of aspirin.

Answer c is correct. Nasal polyps a contraindication to the use of aspirin.

Answer d is correct.

---

5. Which of the following is recommended as an effective alternative antiplatelet therapy for patients who do not tolerate aspirin?
   a. Dipyridamole
   b. Clopidogrel, 150 mg a day
   c. Clopidogrel, 75 mg a day
   d. Pentoxifylline

Answer a is incorrect. Patients who do not tolerate aspirin generally do not tolerate dipyridamole. Dipyridamole is only used in combination with aspirin (Aggrenox).

Answer b is incorrect. The recommended dosage of clopidogrel in the treatment of PAD is 75 mg a day, orally.

Answer c is correct. The recommended dosage of clopidogrel in the treatment of PAD is 75 mg a day, orally.

Answer d is incorrect. The use of pentoxifylline in the treatment of PAD is for symptoms of claudication, not to reduce cardiovascular risk. It is not a replacement for aspirin in patients who do not tolerate aspirin, clopidogrel is.

---

6. Which of the following pharmacologic interventions is least appropriate for achieving a reduction in serious vascular events for a patient with established peripheral artery disease?
   a. Aspirin
   b. Clopidogrel
   c. Aspirin plus extended release dipyridamole
   d. Pentoxifylline

Answer a achieves reduction in vascular events. Aspirin carries non-FDA labeled indications (Evidence Class IIb, Category B) for peripheral arterial disease and the medical literature strongly supports the use of low and medium-dose aspirin (75 mg to 325 mg daily).

Answer b achieves reduction in vascular events. Clopidogrel (Plavix) is recommended as an alternative antiplatelet therapy for patients who do not tolerate aspirin. Clopidogrel carries a FDA-labeled indication (Evidence Class IIb, Category A) for the treatment of PAD.

Answer c achieves reduction in vascular events. The efficacy of extended-release dipyridamole plus aspirin (Aggrenox) in the treatment of peripheral arterial occlusive disease has been compared to aspirin, but meta-analysis findings have not revealed a statistically significant advantage for combination therapy.

Answer d does not achieve reduction in vascular events. Pentoxifylline (Trental) is an antiplatelet used in the treatment of PAD. Recent studies have demonstrated no benefit over placebo with walking distance improvements in several trials.

---

7. A 58-year-old man with peripheral artery disease, hypertension, hyperlipidemia, and New York Heart Association class III heart failure is noted to have significant functional impairment due to intermittent claudication. Which of the following pharmacologic interventions should be avoided due to safety issues which led to a black box warning from the FDA?
   a. Aspirin
   b. Clopidogrel
   c. Simvastatin
   d. Cilostazol

Answer a is incorrect. Aspirin may be used in patients with the listed comorbidities.

Answer b is incorrect. Clopidogrel may be used in patients with the listed comorbidities.

Answer c is incorrect. Simvastatin may be used in patients with the listed comorbidities.

Answer d is correct. Cilostazol may not be used in patients with any stage/degree of heart failure.

---

8. Which of the following antiplatelet agents should be monitored with periodic complete blood count testing related to potential hematologic complications that include agranulocytosis and aplastic anemia?
   a. Aspirin
   b. Simvastatin
   c. Ticlopidine
   d. Dipyridamole plus aspirin

Answer a is incorrect. Aspirin does not require periodic monitoring of the complete blood count.

Answer b is incorrect. Simvastatin does not require periodic monitoring of the complete blood count.

Answer c is correct. Ticlopidine has a black box warning—may cause life-threatening hematologic reactions, including neutropenia, agranulocytosis, thrombotic thrombocytopenic purpura (TTP), and aplastic anemia. Routine monitoring is required for ticlopidine. Monitor for signs and symptoms of neutropenia and thrombocytopenia. Discontinue therapy if the absolute neutrophil count falls less than $1200/mm^3$ or if the platelet count falls less than $80,000/mm^3$.

Answer d is incorrect. Dipyridamole plus aspirin does not require monitoring of the complete blood count.

---

9. Which of the following patients should not be given cilostazol as treatment for peripheral artery disease?

   a. A 49-year-old woman with hypertension
   b. A 60-year-old man with a history of benign prostatic hypertrophy
   c. A 48-year-old man with congestive heart failure
   d. A 52-year-old woman with hypothyroidism

Answer a is incorrect. Although cilostazol can cause edema, having hypertension is not an absolute contraindication to cilostazol.

Answer b is incorrect. Benign prostatic hyperplasia (BPH) is not a contraindication to the use of cilostazol.

Answer c is correct. Cilostazol is contraindicated in all degrees of heart failure.

Answer d is incorrect. Hypothyroidism is not a contraindication to cilostazol.

---

10. Which medication(s) should be avoided in a 53-year-old patient with peripheral artery disease, asthma, and allergic rhinitis (with nasal polyps) who is currently taking albuterol as needed and flunisolide for his asthma and loratadine for allergic rhinitis?

    a. Aspirin
    b. Trental
    c. Plavix
    d. a and c

Answer a is correct. Aspirin should be avoided in patients with syndrome of asthma as it can cause bronchospasm.

Answer b is incorrect. Trental does not induce or interfere with syndrome of asthma.

Answer c is incorrect. Plavix does not induce or interfere with syndrome of asthma.

Answer d is incorrect. a is correct because aspirin is to be avoided in patients with asthma, rhinitis, and nasal polyps as it can induce bronchospasm, but b, Trental, does not induce or interfere with syndrome of asthma.

---

11. Which of the following mechanisms of action is associated with pentoxifylline?

    a. Reduces blood viscosity
    b. Improves erythrocyte flexibility
    c. Inhibits platelet aggregation
    d. All of the above

Answers a, b, and c are correct.

Answer d is the best answer. These are all mechanisms of action of pentoxifylline.

---

12. A patient is prescribed cilostazol for diagnosis of peripheral artery disease because he could not tolerate aspirin. What would be appropriate monitoring or evaluation points for patients receiving a prescription for cilostazol?

    a. Evaluation of medications that inhibit the CYP 450 3A4
    b. Evaluation of medications that inhibit the CYP 450 2C19
    c. Evaluation of comorbidities (eg, heart failure)
    d. All of the above

Answer a is correct. The dosing of cilostazol for intermittent claudication is 100 mg orally bid. Cilostazol dosing adjustments are required for concomitant use with diltiazem, ketoconazole, erythromycin, omeprazole, and other cytochrome P450 3A4 or 2C19 inhibitors (decrease dose to 50 mg orally bid).

Answer b is correct. The dosing of cilostazol for intermittent claudication is 100 mg orally bid. Cilostazol dosing adjustments are required for concomitant use with diltiazem, ketoconazole, erythromycin, omeprazole, and other cytochrome P450 3A4 or 2C19 inhibitors (decrease dose to 50 mg orally bid).

Answer c is correct. Contraindications to the use of cilostazol include heart failure of any severity (black box warning).

Answer d is correct and the best answer.

---

13. Select the treatment goal(s) for PAD in patients with intermittent claudication.

    a. Increase maximal walking distance
    b. Increase duration of walking
    c. Increase amount of pain-free walking
    d. All of the above

Answer a is correct. Increasing maximal walking distance is a treatment goal for patients with PAD.

Answer b is correct. Increasing duration of walking is a treatment goal for patients with PAD.

Answer c is correct. Increasing amount of pain-free walking is a treatment goal for patients with PAD.

Answer d is correct and the best answer.

---

14. A 48-year-old cancer patient presents to the clinic and states to feel terrible (weakness, fatigue) after his last chemotherapy session. His medication list includes the antiplatelet ticlopidine (Ticlid) for peripheral arterial disease. Select the condition that may be caused by ticlopidine that may contribute to the patient's symptoms.

    a. Anemia
    b. Reye syndrome
    c. Headache
    d. Rash

Answer a is correct. Anemia is a potential side effect of ticlopidine. Anemia will cause symptoms such as weakness and fatigue. *Note:* The patient is also receiving chemotherapeutic agents which may also cause anemia.

Ticlopidine has a black box warning—may cause life-threatening hematologic reactions, including neutropenia, agranulocytosis, thrombotic thrombocytopenia purpura (TTP), and aplastic anemia. Routine monitoring is required for ticlopidine. Monitor for signs and symptoms of neutropenia and thrombocytopenia. Discontinue therapy if the absolute neutrophil count falls less than 1200/mm^3 or if the platelet count falls less than 80,000/mm^3.

Answer b is incorrect. Reye syndrome is not associated with ticlopidine. It is associated with the use of aspirin in patients less than 16 years of age with flu-like symptoms or chickenpox. Reye syndrome is a potentially fatal disease that causes numerous detrimental effects to many organs, especially the brain and liver. The exact cause is unknown, and while it has been associated with aspirin consumption by children with viral illness, it also occurs in the absence of aspirin use.

Answer c is incorrect. Headache is a potential side effect of ticlopidine and a lot of other medications (most medications have a potential side effect of headache); however, headache associated with ticlopidine has *not* been described as severe. Dipyridamole is an example of an antiplatelet associated with a severe headache. Aggrenox has dosing recommendations for patients that receive the vasodilator dipyridamole and develop a headache. Dosing and administration is one capsule (aspirin 25 mg/extended-release dipyridamole 200 mg) orally bid in the morning and evening. Dosing adjustments for individuals who develop intolerable headaches on this drug regimen should take one capsule (aspirin 25 mg/extended-release dipyridamole 200 mg) orally at bedtime and one low-dose aspirin in the morning will return to usual regimen as soon as possible, usually within a week.

Answer d is incorrect. Ticlopidine is associated with a rash; however, this side effect would not be responsible for the patient's symptoms.

---

15. Select the risk factors (comorbidities) that should be controlled in a patient with PAD.

    a. Hypertension
    b. Hyperlipidemia
    c. Diabetes
    d. All of the above

Answers a, b, and c are correct.

Answer d is correct and the best answer. Risk factor reduction and controlling underlying causes such as diabetes mellitus, hypertension, and hyperlipidemia should be included in the treatment strategy. Improving control of comorbid conditions can result in improvement in overall quality of life and reduction in cardiovascular complications and death.

---

16. Select the primary pharmacologic management for PAD.

    a. Anticoagulant
    b. Antiplatelet
    c. Antihypertensive
    d. Antisympathomimetic

Answer a is incorrect. Anticoagulants (eg, warfarin, heparin) are not utilized in the management of PAD.

Answer b is correct. Primary pharmacologic interventions for PAD involve antiplatelet drug therapies. Antiplatelet therapy is indicated to reduce the risk of myocardial infarction, stroke, or vascular death in individuals with atherosclerotic lower extremity PAD. Aspirin, clopidogrel, cilostazol, and pentoxifylline are commonly prescribed antiplatelet agents for the treatment of PAD.

Answer c is incorrect. Antihypertensives are not utilized in the management of PAD; however, control of blood pressure is a key factor to decreasing complications. Improving control of comorbid conditions (eg, hypertension, hyperlipidemia, and diabetes) can result in improvement in overall quality of life and reduction in cardiovascular complications and death.

Answer d is incorrect. Antisympathomimetics (eg, beta blockers) are not utilized in the management of PAD.

---

17. A 28-year-old mother with no significant medical history states her doctor wants her to start taking low-dose aspirin and thinks it is a good idea to keep a bottle in the house in case anyone in her family gets a headache or has some mild pain. Which of the following would be *inappropriate* counseling points?

    a. Low-dose aspirin is perfectly fine to have around the house. Many people find it works well for mild pains and headache and it is safe for anyone over the age of 12.
    b. Since you will be taking aspirin daily, you should know that some of the common side effects include indigestion and nausea and some of the serious side effects include bleeding, ringing in the ears, and peptic ulcer disease.

c. Should you decide to become pregnant while you are taking aspirin, let your doctor know right away because aspirin may not be safe while pregnant, especially during the third trimester.
d. Do not give aspirin to anyone in your home who has asthma or breathing problems because aspirin can cause bronchospasm.

Answer a is correct. Aspirin should be avoided in anyone under the age of 16 due to the risk of Reye syndrome.

Answer b is incorrect. These are common side effects and serious adverse effects.

Answer c is incorrect. Aspirin is not recommended in pregnancy, especially during the third trimester.

Answer d is incorrect. Aspirin can cause bronchospasm (especially in the triad of asthma, allergic rhinitis with nasal polyps).

---

18. Select the dose(s) of aspirin utilized in the management of PAD.
    a. 81 mg
    b. 162 mg
    c. 325 mg
    d. All of the above

Answer a is correct. Aspirin 81 mg may be used in the management of PAD.

Answer b is correct. Aspirin 162 mg may be used in the management of PAD.

Answer c is correct. Aspirin 325 mg may be used in the management of PAD.

Answer d is correct and the best answer. Aspirin may be dosed 75 to 325 mg for management of PAD. *Note:* Side effects associated with aspirin may be encountered with low dose (81 mg) aspirin.

---

19. Clopidogrel works by which of the following mechanisms?
    a. Selectively and irreversibly inhibits ADP-induced platelet aggregation.
    b. Reversibly inhibits platelet aggregation.
    c. Reduces blood viscosity by inhibiting phosphodiesterase.
    d. Suppresses cyclic adenosine monophosphate (cAMP) degradation, which produces vasodilation.

Answer a is correct. Clopidogrel requires in vivo biotransformation to an active metabolite. The clopidogrel active metabolite inhibits platelet aggregation by selectively and irreversibly inhibiting the binding of adenosine diphosphate (ADP) to its platelet receptor and the subsequent activation of ADP-mediated glycoprotein GPIIb/IIIa complex. Since this action is irreversible, the remainder of the platelet life span is affected.

Answer b is incorrect. Clopidogrel irreversibly inhibits platelets.

Answer c is incorrect. This is the mechanism of action of pentoxifylline.

Answer d is incorrect. This is the mechanism of dipyridamole.

---

20. Which of the following medications is contraindicated in patients with hypersensitivity to xanthenes?
    a. Aspirin
    b. Plavix
    c. Trental
    d. Pletal

Answer a is incorrect. Aspirin is not contraindicated in patients with hypersensitivity to xanthenes.

Answer b is incorrect. Plavix (clopidogrel) is not contraindicated in patients with hypersensitivity to xanthenes.

Answer c is correct. Trental (pentoxifylline) is contraindicated in patients with hypersensitivity to xanthenes.

Answer d is incorrect. Pletal (cilostazol) is not contraindicated in patients with hypersensitivity to xanthenes.

CHAPTER 10 | Anemia

1. Patients with symptomatic anemia may present with:
    a. Fatigue
    b. Shortness of breath
    c. Tachycardia
    d. Neurologic manifestations
    e. All of the above

Answer a is correct. Fatigue may be a symptom of anemia.

Answer b is correct. Shortness of breath may be a symptom of anemia.

Answer c is correct. Tachycardia may be a symptom of anemia.

Answer d is correct. Neurologic manifestations may be a symptom of vitamin B_{12} anemia.

Answer e is correct and the best answer. All of the above symptoms may be present in anemic patients. Fatigue and shortness of breath may present because of the lack of oxygen being delivered due to the low hemoglobin. However, anemic patients may be asymptomatic.

---

2. Select the nutritional factor that may cause a hypo-productive anemia.

a. Iron
b. Cancer
c. Phenytoin
d. Chronic kidney disease
e. Anemia of chronic disease

Answer a is correct. Iron is a nutritional factor that can cause anemia. Other nutritional factors that may cause a hypo-productive anemia include vitamin B_{12} and iron.

Answer b is incorrect. Cancer is a cause of anemia of chronic disease. Other factors related to cancer that may cause anemia of chronic disease include tumors and chemotherapy. Other causes of anemia of chronic disease include chronic kidney disease and inflammatory conditions (rheumatoid arthritis).

Answer c is incorrect. Phenytoin may cause an anemia, however it is not a nutritional cause. Phenytoin may cause a macrocytic anemia.

Answer d is incorrect. Chronic kidney disease is a cause of anemia of chronic disease.

Answer e is incorrect. Anemia of chronic disease is a hypo-productive anemia caused by chronic illnesses.

---

3. Select the hypo-productive anemia that is caused by destruction of proliferating stem cells.
   a. Chronic kidney disease
   b. Iron
   c. Chemotherapy
   d. Folic acid
   e. Anemia of chronic disease

Answer a is incorrect. Chronic kidney disease causes anemia because erythropoietin is produced in the kidneys.

Answer b is incorrect. Iron is a vital nutrient in the development of erythrocytes. Iron deficiency decreases hemoglobin synthesis and ultimately red blood cells.

Answer c is correct. Chemotherapy may cause destruction of proliferating stem cells, thereby decreasing erythrocyte production.

Answer d is incorrect. Deficiencies in folic acid hinder the process of erythrocyte maturation. Folic acid is required for the formation of DNA.

Answer e is incorrect. Anemia of chronic disease causes a blunted production and a diminished response to erythropoietin. Anemia of chronic disease also affects iron homeostasis via iron sequestration, thereby decreasing the amount available to the rest of the body.

---

4. Select the treatment for pernicious anemia.
   a. Oral cyanocobalamin
   b. Parenteral vitamin B_{12}
   c. Iron
   d. Epoetin
   e. Sodium ferric gluconate

Answer a is incorrect. Oral vitamin B_{12} is not the recommended treatment of pernicious anemia. Pernicious anemia is a vitamin B_{12} deficiency anemia caused by impaired absorption of vitamin B_{12}; therefore, the nutrient needs to be administered parenterally. Oral replacement for pernicious anemia is rarely utilized, but if it is utilized, high doses will be required.

Answer b is correct. Parenteral vitamin B_{12} is the treatment of choice for pernicious anemia. The parenteral formulation is desired because pernicious anemia patients have an impaired absorption of vitamin B_{12}.

Answer c is incorrect. Iron supplementation is utilized for iron deficiency anemia. Pernicious anemia is caused by a deficiency in vitamin B_{12}.

Answer d is incorrect. Epoetin-alfa or darbepoetin-alfa is utilized for chemotherapy and chronic kidney disease induced anemia.

Answer e is incorrect. Sodium ferric gluconate (Ferrlecit) is a parenteral formulation of iron. Parenteral formulations of iron are utilized for iron deficient patients unable to tolerate the oral formulation, noncompliance, or nonresponders (Iron dextran [InFED] is the only parenteral formulation with that indication). Sodium ferric gluconate (Ferrlecit) and iron sucrose (Venofer) are indicated to treat anemia associated with CKD in patient receiving erythropoietin products.

---

5. Select the cause(s) of macrocytic, megaloblastic anemia.
   a. Sickle cell anemia
   b. Hemolysis
   c. Anemia of chronic disease
   d. Iron
   e. Vitamin B_{12}

Answer a is incorrect. Sickle cell anemia is genetic anemia with the morphology classification of microcytic. The most common cause of microcytic anemia is iron deficiency anemia.

Answer b is incorrect. The morphology classification of hemolysis is normocytic. Other normocytic anemias include: recent blood loss, bone marrow failure, and anemia of chronic disease.

Answer c is incorrect. Anemia of chronic disease is a normocytic anemia.

Answer d is incorrect. The morphology classification of iron deficiency anemia is microcytic hypochromic.

Answer e is correct. Vitamin B_{12} is a macrocytic, megaloblastic anemia. Folic acid deficiency anemia is also a cause of macrocytic, megaloblastic anemia.

---

6. Select the hemoglobin or hematocrit *normal* range for a 37-year-old male patient.
    a. Hemoglobin 12.3 g/dL
    b. Hematocrit 39%
    c. Hematocrit 44%
    d. Hemoglobin 13.1g/dL
    e. All of the above

Answer a is incorrect. Normal hemoglobin range for males is 14 to 17.5 g/dL.

Answer b is incorrect. Normal hematocrit range for males is 42% to 50%.

Answer c is correct. Normal hematocrit range for males is 42% to 50%.

Answer d is incorrect. Normal hemoglobin range for males is 14 to 17.5 g/dL

Answer e is incorrect.

---

7. Select the laboratory test that measures the size of a red blood cell.
    a. Mean corpuscular volume
    b. Hematocrit
    c. Red cell distribution width
    d. Total iron-binding capacity
    e. Red blood cell

Answer a is correct. Mean corpuscular volume (MCV) is a widely used laboratory value to measure the size of the red blood cell. Higher MCV values indicate macrocytosis and lower values indicate microcytosis.

Answer b is incorrect. Hematocrit is the percent of blood that the erythrocytes encompass.

Answer c is incorrect. Red cell distribution width (RDW), when elevated, means the presence of many different sizes of red blood cells; therefore, the MCV is less reliable.

Answer d is incorrect. Total iron-binding capacity (TIBC) measures the capacity of transferrin to bind to iron. TIBC is elevated in iron deficiency anemia.

Answer e is incorrect. Red blood cell represents the number of erythrocytes in a volume of blood.

---

8. A patient with a low mean corpuscular volume and low serum ferritin would have what type of anemia?
    a. Low mean corpuscular volume and serum ferritin are not associated with anemia
    b. Iron deficiency anemia
    c. Vitamin B_{12} deficiency anemia
    d. Anemia of chronic disease
    e. Aplastic anemia

Answer a is incorrect. Mean corpuscular volume and serum ferritin values are often utilized in differentiating anemia types.

Answer b is correct. Low mean corpuscular volume (MCV) values indicate a microcytic anemia. Types of microcytic anemia are: iron deficiency and genetic (sickle cell, thalassemia, and hemoglobinopathies). The most common type of microcytic anemia is iron deficiency. Ferritin is the protein-iron complex found in macrophages used for iron storage. Low ferritin levels are found in iron deficiency anemia. Therefore, a patient with a low mean corpuscular volume and low serum ferritin would likely have iron deficiency anemia.

Answer c is incorrect. Vitamin B_{12} deficiency anemia would present with an elevated mean corpuscular volume (macrocytic). Remember that MCV values are in single cases of anemia. If a patient has iron deficiency and vitamin B_{12} deficiency anemia, the MCV values are not as helpful. In this situation (two different types of anemia), you would expect to see an elevated red cell distribution width (RDW).

Answer d is not correct. Anemia of chronic disease would present with a normocytic morphology. Other normocytic anemias include: recent blood loss, hemolysis, and bone marrow failure.

Answer e is not correct. Aplastic anemia is characterized by diminished or absent hematopoietic precursors in the bone marrow, most often due to injury to the pluripotent stem cell. Therefore, aplastic anemia is a normocytic anemia (rarely, aplastic anemia may present as macrocytic). The designation "aplastic anemia" is a misnomer because the disorder is defined as pancytopenia (simultaneous presence of neutropenia, thrombocytopenia, and anemia) rather than anemia. Many drugs, such as chloramphenicol, gold, sulfonamides, felbamate, carbamazepine, valproic acid, phenytoin, and nifedipine have been associated with aplastic anemia.

---

9. Select the nonpharmacologic therapy for anemia that exhibits the greatest increase on hemoglobin and hematocrit.
    a. Dietary supplementation with vitamin B_{12}
    b. Dietary supplementation with iron
    c. Dietary supplementation with folic acid
    d. Red blood cell transfusion
    e. All of the above

Answer a is incorrect. Diets lacking key nutrients are rarely the sole cause of anemia in the United States. Therefore, ingesting a diet rich in vitamin B_{12} should not be the only modality of treatment.

Answer b is incorrect. Diets lacking key nutrients are rarely the sole cause of anemia in the United States. Therefore, ingesting a diet rich in iron should not be the only modality of treatment.

Answer c is incorrect. Diets lacking key nutrients are rarely the sole cause of anemia in the United States. Therefore, ingesting a diet rich in folic acid should not be the only modality of treatment.

Answer d is correct. Nonpharmacologic therapy plays a limited role in the management of anemia. However, symptomatic anemia patients with a hemoglobin concentration less than 7 g/dL are candidates for transfusion of red blood cells. Generally, only patients requiring immediate correction receive blood transfusions.

Answer e is incorrect.

---

10. Select the product and dose that would be appropriate for a patient with iron deficiency anemia.

    a. Feosol 325 mg four times per day without food
    b. Niferex capsule 150 mg daily
    c. Niferex 50 mg tablet tid
    d. Feostat 100 mg daily
    e. Fergon 325 mg tid with food

Answer a is correct. Ferrous sulfate (Feosol) 325 mg four times per day would be 260 mg of elemental iron. Treatment of iron deficiency anemia requires 200 mg per day of elemental iron. Each 325 mg tablet of ferrous sulfate has 65 mg of elemental iron.

Answer b is incorrect. Polysaccharide-iron complex (Niferex) 150 mg capsule has 150 mg of elemental iron. Therefore, taking 150 mg daily would not meet the elemental iron requirements for treatment of iron deficiency anemia.

Answer c is incorrect. Polysaccharide-iron complex (Niferex) 50 mg tablets tid would be 150 mg of elemental iron and would not meet the elemental iron requirements for treatment of iron deficiency anemia. Each 50 mg tablet has 50 mg of elemental iron.

Answer d is incorrect. Each 100 mg tablet of ferrous fumarate (Feostat) has 33 mg of elemental iron. Therefore, taking ferrous fumarate 100 mg daily would be 33 mg of elemental iron and would not meet the elemental iron requirements for treatment of iron deficiency anemia.

Answer e is incorrect. Each 325 mg tablet of ferrous gluconate (Fergon) has 39 mg of elemental iron. Therefore, taking ferrous gluconate 325 mg tid would be 117 mg of elemental iron and would not meet the elemental iron requirements for treatment of iron deficiency anemia. Maximal iron absorption is achieved on an empty stomach (1 hour before or 2 hours after a meal); however, patients who cannot tolerate iron on an empty stomach may take it with food.

---

11. Select the iron formulation that may cause the highest rate of anaphylaxis.

    a. Ferrous sulfate
    b. Ferrous gluconate
    c. Iron dextran
    d. Iron sucrose
    e. Sodium ferric gluconate

Answer a is incorrect. Ferrous sulfate (Feosol) is not associated with anaphylaxis. Ferrous sulfate and all other oral iron products are associated with abdominal pain, nausea, constipation, and heartburn.

Answer b is incorrect. The oral iron product ferrous gluconate (Fergon) is not associated with anaphylaxis.

Answer c is correct. Iron dextran (InFED) is a parenteral formulation of iron that is associated with anaphylaxis. A test dose (0.5 mL over 30 seconds) must be administered to patients receiving their first dose of iron dextran because of an anaphylaxis risk. Patients should be monitored for signs of anaphylaxis for at least 1 hour after the test dose before administering the total dose. Other side effects of iron dextran include: arthralgias, arrhythmias, hypotension, flushing, and pruritus.

Answer d is incorrect. Iron sucrose (Venofer) is a parenteral form of iron; however, it is not associated with anaphylaxis. It is appealing to use this agent in the setting of iron deficiency anemia because it is considered safer (compared to iron dextran) owing to a decreased risk of anaphylaxis. However, the high cost of this agent may preclude the routine use in iron-deficiency anemia patients without kidney disorders.

Answer e is incorrect. Sodium ferric gluconate (Ferrlecit) is a parenteral form of iron; however, it is not associated with anaphylaxis. It is appealing to use this agent in the setting of iron deficiency anemia because it is considered safer (compared to iron dextran) owing to a decreased risk of anaphylaxis. However, the high cost of this agent may preclude the routine use in iron-deficiency anemia patients without kidney disorders.

---

12. Select the generic name for polysaccharide-iron complex.

    a. Feostat
    b. Niferex
    c. Feosol
    d. InFED
    e. Fergon

Answer a is incorrect. The generic name of Feostat is ferrous fumarate.

Answer b is correct. The generic name of Niferex is polysaccharide-iron complex.

Answer c is incorrect. The generic name of Feosol is ferrous sulfate.

Answer d is incorrect. The generic name of InFED is iron dextran.

Answer e is incorrect. The generic name of Fergon is ferrous gluconate.

---

13. Calculate the dose of iron dextran in milliliters for a 37-year-old man. Height 6 ft 3 in, weight 80 kg, hemoglobin (observed) 7.0 g/dL, and hemoglobin (desired) 12.0 g/dL.

   a. 367 mL
   b. 410 mL
   c. 514 mL
   d. 574 mL

Note: Iron dextran is available in 50 mg/mL vials and is often ordered in milligrams.

Answer a is correct. Dose (mL) = 0.0442 ($\text{Hemoglobin}_{\text{desired}}$ – $\text{Hemoglobin}_{\text{observed}}$) × (weight in kg) (0.26 × weight in kg). Dose (mL) = 0.0442 (12 – 7) × (80) (0.26 × 80) = 367 mL.

Lean body weight should be used for adults and children weighing more than 15 kg. Actual body weight should be used for children weighing 5 to 15 kg. However, for this patient, actual body weight (80 kg) is lower than ideal body weight (ideal body weight for males = 50 + 2.3 [inches over 60] = 50 + 2.3(15) = 84.5 kg). Therefore, since actual body weight is lower than ideal, actual body weight will be used to calculate the milliliter dose of iron dextran.

Answer b is incorrect. The result of using the ideal body weight is 410 mL. However, since actual body weight is lower than ideal body weight, actual body weight is used for this dose calculation.

Answer c is incorrect.

Answer d is incorrect.

---

14. A patient is to receive 300 mL of iron dextran to treat an iron deficiency anemia not corrected by oral therapy. How many milliliters should the patient receive during the first hour?

   a. 50 mL
   b. 100 mL
   c. 30 mL
   d. 0.5 mL
   e. 300 mL

Note: Iron dextran is available in 50 mg/mL vials and is often ordered in milligrams.

Answer a is incorrect.

Answer b is incorrect.

Answer c is incorrect.

Answer d is correct. A test dose (0.5 mL over 30 seconds) must be administered to patients receiving their first dose of iron dextran because of an anaphylaxis risk. Patients should be monitored for signs of anaphylaxis for at least 1 hour after the test dose before administering the total dose.

Answer e is incorrect.

---

15. Select the disabilities that may occur for vitamin B_{12} deficiency anemia that is not treated appropriately.

   a. Paresthesias
   b. Memory loss
   c. Psychosis
   d. Numbness
   e. All of the above

Answers a, b, c, and d are correct.

Answer e is correct and the best answer. Early treatment is paramount because neurologic damage may be irreversible if the deficiency is not detected and corrected within months.

---

16. Select the pharmacokinetic variable that differentiates subcutaneous administration of vitamin B_{12} as compared to oral administration of vitamin B_{12}.

   a. Absorption
   b. Distribution
   c. Metabolism
   d. Elimination
   e. All of the above

Answer a is correct. Vitamin B_{12} (cyanocobalamin) administered orally or parenterally is effective in treating vitamin B_{12} anemia. Parenteral use is more common because absorption is higher and more predictable. Subcutaneous or intramuscular administration may be given. Oral vitamin B_{12} may be given to treat vitamin B_{12} deficiency.

Answers b, c, d, and e are incorrect.

---

17. Vitamin B_{12} may be administered via which of the following formulations?

   a. Oral
   b. Subcutaneous
   c. Intramuscular
   d. Nasal
   e. All of the above

Answers a, b, c, and d are correct.

Answer e is correct and the best answer.

---

18. Causes of anemia of chronic disease include:

   a. Chemotherapy
   b. Rheumatoid arthritis
   c. Chronic kidney disease
   d. Systemic lupus erythematosus
   e. All of the above

Answers a, b, c, and d are correct.

Answer e is correct and the best answer.

---

19. Select the pharmacokinetic variable(s) that differentiates epoetin-alfa and darbepoetin-alfa.
   a. Absorption
   b. Distribution
   c. Metabolism
   d. Elimination
   e. All of the above

Answers a, b, c, and e are incorrect.

Answer d is correct. Darbepoetin differs from epoetin in that it has a longer elimination half-life.

---

20. Select the target hemoglobin concentration for chronic kidney disease patients receiving epoetin-alfa and darbepoetin-alfa.
   a. 7 g/dL
   b. 8 g/dL
   c. 9 g/dL
   d. 10 g/dL
   e. 11 g/dL

Answer a is incorrect. A hemoglobin concentration of 7 g/dL is the value to consider red blood transfusion, but not the target concentration for epoetin-alfa and darbepoetin-alfa. Symptomatic anemia patients with a hemoglobin concentration less than 7 g/dL are candidates for transfusion of red blood cells.

Answers b, c, and d are incorrect.

Answer e is correct. Patient survival may be decreased if the hemoglobin level is titrated. above 11 to 12 g/dL. Therefore, the target hemoglobin concentration is 11 to 12 g/dL.

---

21. What nutritional factor is required to be normal to maximize effectiveness of epoetin-alfa and darbepoetin-alfa in patients with CKD?
   a. Vitamin B_{12}
   b. Folic acid
   c. Iron
   d. a and b
   e. b and c

Answers a, b, d, and e are incorrect.

Answer c is correct. Iron stores in patients with CKD should be maintained. If iron stores are not maintained, epoetin and darbepoetin will not be effective. Oral iron therapy can be used, but is often ineffective, particularly in dialysis patients. Therefore, IV iron therapy is used extensively in these patients.

CHAPTER 11 | Immune System

1. The immune system is designed to attack and destroy foreign antigens and should be able to differentiate self from nonself. Failure to differentiate self from nonself may lead to:
   a. Addison disease
   b. Rheumatoid arthritis
   c. Systemic lupus erythematosus
   d. All of the above

Failure to differentiate self from nonself may lead to an autoimmune disease. An autoimmune disease is a condition that occurs when the immune system mistakenly attacks and destroys healthy body tissue.

Answer a is correct. Addison disease is an autoimmune disease. Addison disease is a disorder that results when your body produces insufficient amount of certain hormones produced by your adrenal glands. The gradual destruction of the adrenal cortex, the outer layer of the adrenal glands, by the body's immune system causes up to 80% of Addison cases. In autoimmune disorders, the immune system makes antibodies that attack the body's own tissues or organs and slowly destroy them. Adrenal insufficiency occurs when at least 90% of the adrenal cortex has been destroyed. As a result, often both cortisol and aldosterone are lacking.

Answer b is correct. Rheumatoid arthritis (RA) is a chronic disease that leads to inflammation of the joints and surrounding tissues. The cause of RA is unknown, but is considered to be an autoimmune disease. The disease usually begins gradually with fatigue, loss of appetite, morning stiffness, widespread muscle aches, and weakness. Eventually, joint pain appears. When the joint is not used for a while, it can become warm, tender, and stiff. When the lining of the joint becomes inflamed, it gives off more fluid and the joint becomes swollen. Joint pain is often felt on both sides of the body and may affect the fingers, wrists, elbows, shoulders, hips, knees, ankles, toes, and neck. Additional symptoms include: anemia, eye burning, hand and feet deformities, limited range of motion, low-grade fever, lung inflammation (pleurisy), nodules under the skin (sign of severe disease), numbness/tingling, and paleness. Joint destruction may occur within 1 to 2 years after the appearance of the disease.

Answer c is correct. Systemic lupus erythematosus (SLE) is a chronic, inflammatory autoimmune disorder. SLE may affect the skin, joints, kidneys, and other organs. Symptoms vary from person to person, and may come and go. The condition may affect one organ or body system at first. Others may become involved later. Almost all people with SLE have joint pain and most develop arthritis. Frequently affected joints are the fingers, hands, wrists, and knees. Inflammation of various parts of the heart may occur as pericarditis, endocarditis, or myocarditis. Chest pain and arrhythmias may result from these conditions. General symptoms include arthritis, fatigue, fever, general discomfort (malaise), muscle aches, nausea and vomiting, pleural effusions, pleurisy, seizures, sensitivity to sunlight, and skin rash. (A butterfly rash over the cheeks and bridge of the nose, affects about half of those with SLE. The rash gets worse when in sunlight.)

Answer d is the correct and best answer.

---

2. Select the nonspecific functional division of the immune system.

   a. Innate
   b. Adaptive
   c. Granulocytes
   d. Lymphocytes
   e. a and b

Answer a is correct. The innate immune system is the nonspecific functional division of the immune system. There are two functional divisions, innate (nonspecific) and adaptive (specific).

Answer b is incorrect. While the adaptive immune system is a functional division of the immune system, it is the specific division.

Answer c is incorrect. Granulocytes are white blood cells that make up part of the innate (nonspecific) immune system.

Answer d is incorrect. Lymphocytes are white blood cells that make up part of the adaptive (specific) immune system.

Answer e is incorrect.

---

3. The difference between the innate and adaptive immune system is described by:

   a. Specificity
   b. Memory
   c. Strength
   d. a and b
   e. All of the above

Answer a is correct. The adaptive immune exhibits specificity compared to the innate division. The adaptive immune response can evolve with each subsequent infection, whereas the innate immune response stays the same with each infection.

Answer b is correct. The adaptive immune exhibits memory compared to the innate division. The adaptive immune response can evolve with each subsequent infection, whereas the innate immune response stays the same with each infection.

Answer c is incorrect. Both the adaptive and innate immune divisions display a significant amount of strength to fight off pathogens. While we are describing the innate and adaptive systems separately, they work collectively to attack and destroy foreign antigens/pathogens.

Answer d is correct and the best answer.

Answer e is incorrect.

---

4. Physical and chemical defenses compose the innate immune system and consist of:

   a. Skin
   b. Lymphocytes
   c. Granulocytes
   d. a and c
   e. All of the above

Answer a is correct. The skin is an example of physical defenses of the innate immune system. Other examples of physical innate immunity are: pH of the stomach, coughing, cilia lining the epithelium, normal urine flow, normal bacterial flora of the throat and gastrointestinal tract.

Answer b is incorrect. Lymphocytes are part of the adaptive immune system.

Answer c is correct. Granulocytes are part of the chemical defense of the innate immune system. Cells that make up the granulocytes are: neutrophils, basophils, eosinophils, and monocytes.

Answer d is correct and the best answer.

Answer e is incorrect.

---

5. Examples of physical defense innate immunity are:

   a. Skin
   b. Stomach pH
   c. Normal flora of gastrointestinal tract
   d. Coughing
   e. All of the above

Answer a is correct. The skin is an example of physical innate immunity.

Answer b is correct. The pH of the stomach is an example of physical innate immunity.

Answer c is correct. The normal flora of the gastrointestinal tract is an example of physical innate immunity.

Answer d is correct. Coughing is an example of physical innate immunity.

Answer e is correct and the best answer.

---

6. Select the medication that may cause Stevens Johnson syndrome and in turn alter the skin, leading to an easy portal of entry for bacterial pathogens.
   a. Carbamazepine
   b. Lamotrigine
   c. Loratadine
   d. a and b
   e. All of the above

Stevens Johnson syndrome (SJS) is a *rare*, serious disorder in which the skin and mucous membranes react severely to a medication or infection.

Answer a is correct. Carbamazepine has been associated with causing Steven Johnson syndrome.

Answer b is correct. Lamotrigine has been associated with causing Steven Johnson syndrome. Lamotrigine has a black box warning stating: severe and potentially life-threatening skin rashes requiring hospitalization have been reported; risk may be increased by coadministration with valproic acid, higher than recommended starting doses, and rapid dose titration. The majority of the cases occur in the first 8 weeks; however, isolated cases may occur after prolonged treatment. Discontinue at first sign of rash unless rash is clearly not drug related.

Answer c is incorrect. Loratadine has not been associated with Stevens Johnson syndrome.

Answer d is correct and the best answer.

Answer e is incorrect.

---

7. Select the agent(s) that may cause pneumonia by altering the pH of the stomach.
   a. Omeprazole
   b. Ranitidine
   c. Ceftriaxone
   d. a and b
   e. All of the above

Medications with the ability to alter the pH of the stomach may change the gastrointestinal bacterial flora and increase risk of infections. Antisecretory agents such as proton pump inhibitors have been associated with the development of bacterial infections. Given the frequency with which antisecretory agents are utilized, this is a rare adverse reaction (although causal relationship has not been established). Gram-negative nosocomial pneumonia may result from retrograde colonization of the pharynx from the stomach, and this may be more likely when the gastric pH is relatively high.

Answer a is correct. Omeprazole and other proton pump inhibitors may cause infections by altering the normal bacterial flora.

Answer b is correct. Ranitidine and other H_2 antagonists may cause infections by altering the normal bacterial flora.

Answer c is incorrect. Ceftriaxone does not have any effect on the pH of the stomach.

Answer d is correct and the best answer.

Answer e is incorrect.

---

8. Select the medication that may alter the normal flora of the gastrointestinal tract leading to infection.
   a. Lansoprazole
   b. Clindamycin
   c. Pantoprazole
   d. a and c
   e. All of the above

Answer a is correct. Lansoprazole may alter the normal flora of the gastrointestinal tract leading to an infection. Medications with the ability to alter the pH of the stomach may change the gastrointestinal bacterial flora and increase risk of infections. Antisecretory agents such as proton pump inhibitors have been associated with the development of bacterial infections.

Answer b is correct. Clindamycin and other anti-infectives that alter gastrointestinal flora leave the patient at an increased risk of infection (*Clostridium difficile* infection).

Answer c is correct. Pantoprazole may alter the normal flora of the gastrointestinal tract leading to an infection. Medications with the ability to alter the pH of the stomach may change the gastrointestinal bacterial flora and increase risk of infections. Antisecretory agents such as proton pump inhibitors have been associated with the development of bacterial infections.

Answer d is correct.

Answer e is correct and the best answer.

---

9. Select the chemical cell(s) of the innate immune system.
   a. Neutrophils
   b. Eosinophils
   c. Basophils
   d. Granulocytes
   e. All of the above

Answer a is correct. Neutrophils are chemical cells of the innate immune system. Neutrophils may also be known as segs, mature neutrophils, polymorphonuclear cells, and PMNs. Bands or stabs are immature neutrophils.

Answer b is correct. Eosinophils are chemical cells of the innate immune system.

Answer c is correct. Basophils are chemical cells of the innate immune system.

Answer d is correct. Granulocytes are chemical cells of the innate immune system. Granulocytes are composed of neutrophils, basophils, eosinophils, and monocytes. Sometimes the term granulocyte is used incorrectly. Clinicians often use the term granulocytes to refer to neutrophils. This is done because neutrophils make up 80% to 90% of the granulocytes.

Answer e is correct and the best answer.

---

10. Innate cells may be evaluated clinically by ordering which laboratory test?
    a. C-reactive protein
    b. Chemokines
    c. Complete blood cell count
    d. a and c
    e. All of the above

Answer a is correct. C-reactive protein is an innate cell and has become very useful clinically. C-reactive protein is a plasma protein that can increase up to 1000 times its baseline concentration. Clinical evidence found that CRP is also released in response to inflammatory markers present within atherosclerotic plaques and leads to cardiovascular disease. Cholesterol medications (HMG-CoA reductase inhibitors/statins) decrease CRP levels and rosuvastatin was found to decrease cardiovascular disease in patients with elevated CRP levels.

Answer b is incorrect. Chemokines are not part of the innate immune system, but rather play an essential role in linking the innate and adaptive immune response by orchestrating traffic. The chemokine system consists of a group of small polypeptides and their receptors. Chemokines possess four cysteines. Based upon the positions of the cysteines, chemokines fall into one of two categories: (1) CC group or (2) CXC group. Maraviroc selectively and reversibly binds to the chemokine receptor (C-C motif receptor 5 [CCR5]) co-receptors located on CD4 cells. A CCR5 assay must be ordered before a patient can be prescribed maraviroc for HIV. Not all HIV patients will have the CCR5 chemokine on their CD4 cell.

Answer c is correct. The innate cells are one of the most widely monitored clinical laboratory tests. Innate cells may be evaluated by ordering a complete blood count (CBC). When a CBC is ordered, part of the laboratory test reports a tally of the total white blood cells (WBCs) in a given volume of blood plus the relative percentages of each cell type contributes to the total. A CBC also reports lymphocytes, part of the adaptive immune system.

Answer d is correct and the best answer.

Answer e is incorrect.

---

11. Select the innate cell that represents the majority of granulocytes and serves as the primary defense against bacterial infections.
    a. Lymphocytes
    b. Neutrophils
    c. Monocytes
    d. Eosinophils
    e. Basophils

Answer a is incorrect. Lymphocytes are not part of the granulocyte cells; they are key cells for the adaptive immune system and consist of B lymphocytes (humoral) and T lymphocytes (cell-mediated). T lymphocytes are tailored to defend against infections that are intracellular (viral infections), whereas B lymphocytes secrete antibodies that neutralize pathogens prior to their entry into host cells.

Answer b is correct. Neutrophils represent the majority of granulocytes (80%-90%) and leukocytes (40%-70%) and serve as the primary defense against bacterial infections. Neutrophils, also termed as segs or polymorphonuclear cells, migrate from the bloodstream into infected or inflamed tissue. In this migration process known as chemotaxis, neutrophils reach the desired site and recognize, adhere to, and phagocytose pathogens. During phagocytosis, the pathogen is internalized within the phagocyte. The neutrophil releases its granular contents which lead to destruction of the engulfed pathogen.

Answer c is incorrect. Monocytes account for 1% to 10% of circulating granulocytes and leukocytes, remove dead/damaged tissues, destroy cancer cells, and regulate against foreign substances.

Answer d is incorrect. Eosinophils account for less than 7% of circulating granulocytes and leukocytes and are present in the intestinal mucosa and lungs, two locations where foreign proteins enter the body. Eosinophils can phagocytize, kill, and digest bacteria and yeast. Elevations of eosinophil counts are highly suggestive of parasitic infections, or may be associated with allergies and asthma.

Answer e is incorrect. Basophils are the least common granulocyte, accounting for 0.1% to 0.3% of granulocytes. Signs and symptoms of allergic responses are linked to basophil and mast cell products. Basophils may be associated with

immediate hypersensitivity and delayed hypersensitivity reactions, and increase in chronic inflammation and leukemia.

12. Select the innate cell that is immature.
    a. Basophil
    b. Eosinophil
    c. Band
    d. Neutrophil
    e. Macrophage

Answer a is incorrect. Basophils are mature cells.

Answer b is incorrect. Eosinophils are mature cells.

Answer c is correct. The neutrophil (mature and immature) releases its granular content, which leads to destruction of the engulfed pathogen. The less mature form of a neutrophil is a band. During an acute infection, there is an increase in the percentage of neutrophils as they are released from the bone marrow. Less mature band forms may also be released. These immature neutrophils are still considered active. The appearance of band cells is called a shift to the left.

Answer d is incorrect. Neutrophils are mature cells.

Answer e is incorrect. Macrophages are mature cells.

13. Select the cell that is part of cell-mediated immunity.
    a. B lymphocyte
    b. Neutrophil
    c. Macrophage
    d. T lymphocyte
    e. Complement

Answer a is incorrect. B lymphocytes compose the humoral part of the adaptive immune system and secrete antibodies that neutralize pathogens prior to their entry into host cells. B cells, once activated by T cells or antigen presenting cells, become a plasma cell that will produce one of five immunoglobulin types: IgA, IgD, IgE, IgG, or IgM.

Answer b is incorrect. Neutrophils are key cells of the innate chemical immunity that fight off bacterial infections.

Answer c is incorrect. Macrophages are the main scavenger cells of the immune system. In addition to attacking foreign cells, they are involved in the destruction of old erythrocytes, denatured plasma proteins, and plasma lipids.

Answer d is correct. T lymphocytes compose the cell-mediated part of the adaptive functional division and are tailored to defend against infections that are intracellular (viral infections).

Answer e is incorrect. The complement system is a mediator of innate immunity. The complement system consists of multiple proteins that play a key role in immune defense. The complement system serves as an adjunct or "complement" to humoral immunity.

14. B and T lymphocytes may be distinguished from each other by the presence of lineage specific membrane markers termed:
    a. Clusters of differentiation (CD)
    b. Complement
    c. C-reactive protein (CRP)
    d. Chemokines
    e. CCR5 coreceptor

Answer a is correct. Morphologic differentiation of lymphocytes is difficult and visual inspection of a blood smear cannot distinguish between T and B cells. Fortunately, lymphocytes can be distinguished by the presence of lineage-specific membrane markers, termed clusters of differentiation (CD). Mature T cells are CD4 or CD8 and B cells are CD20. Identification of the subtype of lymphocyte is not a routine clinical hematology test; lymphocytes are reported as a total lymphocyte count on the complete blood count (CBC). An exception is the reporting/monitoring of CD4 cells for patients with human immunodeficiency virus (HIV).

Answer b is incorrect. The complement system is a mediator of innate immunity. The complement system consists of multiple proteins that play a key role in immune defense. The complement system serves as an adjunct or "complement" to humoral immunity.

Answer c is incorrect. C-reactive protein is an acute phase reactants produced by the liver during early stages of infection or inflammation. Acute phase reactants or proteins increase in response to inflammatory stimuli such as tissue injury or infection. Recent clinical evidence found that CRP is also released in response to inflammatory markers present within atherosclerotic plaques and leads to cardiovascular disease. Cholesterol medications (HMG-CoA reductase inhibitors/statins) decrease CRP levels and rosuvastatin was found to decrease cardiovascular disease in patients with elevated CRP levels.

Answer d is incorrect. Chemokines play an essential role in linking the innate and adaptive immune response by orchestrating traffic. The chemokine system consists of a group of small polypeptides and their receptors. Chemokines possess four cysteines. Based upon the positions of the cysteines, almost all chemokines fall into one of two categories: (1) CC group or (2) CXC group.

Answer e is incorrect. CCR5 is a chemokine receptor located on CD4 cells. Maraviroc blocks CCR5 and this CCR5 antagonism prevents interaction between the human CCR5 co-receptor and the gp120 subunit of the viral envelope glycoprotein, thereby inhibiting gp120 conformational change required for fusion of CCR5 HIV with the CD4 cell and subsequent entry.

15. A neutrophil count greater than 12,000 cells/mm^3 is termed:
    a. Neutrophilia
    b. Bandemia
    c. Lymphocytosis
    d. a and b
    e. a and b

Answer a is correct. Neutrophilia is an elevated neutrophil count. A normal neutrophil count is 2.3 to 7.7 × 10^3 cells/mm^3. Rarely do you hear clinicians say the term neutrophilia. The term leukocytosis will most likely be used since neutrophils are the predominant white blood cell. The term leukocytosis could be caused by any of the five white blood cells.

Answer b is incorrect. A bandemia is an increase in immature neutrophils and is termed a shift to the left. A normal band count is 0 to 10 × 10^3 cells/mm^3. However, it is possible with a neutrophil count of 12,000 cells/mm^3, that a bandemia may also be present.

Answer c is incorrect. Lymphocytosis is an increase in lymphocytes. A normal lymphocyte count is 1.6 to 2.4 × 10^3 cells/mm^3.

Answer d is incorrect.

Answer e is incorrect.

---

16. Select the cause(s) of neutrophilia.
    a. Acute bacterial infections
    b. G-CSF
    c. Glucocorticoids
    d. a and c
    e. All of the above

Answer a is correct. Acute bacterial infections can increase neutrophils. Neutrophils are the predominate cell that fights bacterial infections.

Answer b is correct. The actions of cytokine medications such as granulocyte colony-stimulating factor (G-CSF) and granulocyte-macrophage colony-stimulating factor (GM-CSF) may intensify neutrophil activity. G-CSF (filgrastim [Neupogen]) is a granulocyte colony-stimulating factor used to stimulate granulocyte production in chemotherapy induced neutropenia and severe chronic neutropenia. GM-CSF (sargramostim [Leukine]) is a granulocyte-macrophage colony-stimulating factor used in acute myelogenous leukemia, bone marrow transplant, and stem cell transplant to shorten time to neutrophil recovery and reduce infections.

Answer c is correct. Glucocorticoids may cause neutrophilia and different glucocorticoids seem to have different effects. Neutrophils are primarily located intravascularly; they do not normally reside extravascularly in the tissues. The total blood granulocyte pool is composed of two equal parts, the circulating pool and the noncirculating pool). Cells in the noncirculating pool are adherent to the vascular endothelium in areas of decreased blood flow. After administration of a glucocorticoid, noncirculating cells are released into the circulating pool, making a neutrophilia. The white blood cell count returns to normal within 24 hours.

Answer d is correct.

Answer e is correct and the best answer.

---

17. Select the drug-induced cause of a neutrophil count less than 1500 cells/mm^3.
    a. Zidovudine
    b. Beta-lactam antibiotics
    c. ACE inhibitors
    d. Ticlopidine
    e. All of the above

Answer a is correct. Zidovudine may cause neutropenia.

Answer b is correct. Beta-lactam antibiotics may cause neutropenia, although this occurs rarely.

Answer c is correct. ACE inhibitors, particularly captopril, may cause neutropenia, although this is a rare occurrence.

Answer d is correct. Ticlopidine may cause neutropenia.

Answer e is correct and the best answer.

---

18. Select the cause(s) of an eosinophil count greater than 350 cells/mm^3.
    a. Asthma
    b. Parasitic infections
    c. Antibiotics (allergic reaction)
    d. All of the above

Answer a is correct. Asthma may cause an eosinophilia.

Answer b is correct. Parasitic infections may cause an eosinophilia.

Answer c is correct. Allergic reactions to antibiotics may cause an eosinophilia.

Answer d is correct and the best answer.

---

19. Human immunodeficiency virus (HIV) is most likely to cause a:
    a. Neutrophilia
    b. Eosinophilia
    c. Monocytosis
    d. Lymphocytosis
    e. Lymphopenia

Answer a is incorrect. HIV may cause neutropenia, but it is not the predominant cell line affected by HIV.

Answer b is incorrect. Eosinophilia may be caused by allergic disorders, asthma, parasitic infections, leukemia, and antibiotics (allergic reaction).

Answer c is incorrect. Monocytosis may be caused by tuberculosis, endocarditis, protozoal infection, and leukemia.

Answer d is incorrect. Lymphocytosis may be caused by mononucleosis, viral infections, pertussis, tuberculosis, syphilis, and lymphoma.

Answer e is correct. Lymphopenia may be caused by HIV since HIV disease attacks and destroys T lymphocytes (CD4 cells). Lymphopenia may also be caused by: radiation exposure, lymphoma, aplastic anemia, and glucocorticoids. Glucocorticoids may cause leukocytosis as well, by demargination (increasing noncirculating white blood cells). However, administration of glucocorticoids may also decrease white blood cell counts.

---

20. A patient that is found to have a granulocyte count less than 500 cells/mm^3 would be classified as:

    a. Lymphopenia
    b. Basophilia
    c. Agranulocytosis
    d. Eosinophilia

Answer a is incorrect. Lymphopenia is a decreased lymphocyte count.

Answer b is incorrect. Basophilia is an increased basophil count. Because basophils represent a small portion of the granulocytes, a basophilia would be unlikely to have an effect on the total granulocyte count.

Answer c is correct. Agranulocytosis is defined as a severe form of neutropenia with a total granulocyte count <500/mm^3.

Answer d is incorrect. Eosinophilia is an increased eosinophil count. Because eosinophils represent a small portion of the granulocytes, an eosinophilia or eosinopenia would be unlikely to have an effect on the total granulocyte count.

---

21. Which of the following functions is performed by neutrophils?

    a. Antigen presentation to T lymphocytes
    b. Engulfing pathogens
    c. Lysing virally infected cells
    d. Secreting antibody

Answer a is incorrect because only APCs (eg, macrophages and dendritic cells) present antigen to T-lymphocytes (specifically helper T lymphocytes).

Answer b is correct. The major role of neutrophils is to engulf and destroy the infectious pathogen.

Answer c is incorrect. Only CD8(+) cytotoxic T lymphocytes have the machinery to lyse cells that are infected with viruses.

Answer d is incorrect. B lymphocytes become activated to plasma cells which secrete antibody or immunoglobulin.

---

22. Which of the following cell types can present peptide fragments from an engulfed pathogen in association with MHC class II to T lymphocytes?

    a. Neutrophils
    b. Basophils
    c. Dendritic cell
    d. Eosinophils

Answer a is incorrect because neutrophils simply engulf and destroy the pathogen. They cannot present antigen to T lymphocytes.

Answer b is incorrect. Basophils play a role in allergic reactions, like other granulocytes, they cannot present antigen.

Answer c is correct. Dendritic cells area a potent APC.

Answer d is incorrect. Eosinophils play an important role in parasitic infections and allergic disorders. Like other granulocytes, they cannot present antigen to T lymphocytes.

---

23. Which of the following cell types plays a critical role in parasitic infections?

    a. Basophil
    b. Macrophage
    c. Plasma cell
    d. Eosinophil

Answer a is incorrect. Basophils play a major role in allergic reactions.

Answer b is incorrect. Macrophages also engulf pathogens and present fragments of the pathogen to T lymphocytes. They do not play a major role in parasitic infections.

Answer c is incorrect. Plasma cells are activated B lymphocytes that secrete antibody.

Answer d is correct. Eosinophils play a major role in parasitic infections.

CHAPTER 12 | Lung Cancer

1. A 62-year-old man who has quit smoking 10 years ago comes to clinic asking, "Should I undergo screening for lung cancer?" His past medical history is significant for hypertension and COPD. His social history is significant for a 30-pack year history of smoking and drinks a beer or two a day. What should you advise?

    a. A chest x-ray annually
    b. A chest x-ray annually plus sputum cytology
    c. A spiral CT annually
    d. Enrollment in a clinical trial of lung cancer screening

---

Answer a is incorrect. Randomized trials did not demonstrate that chest x-rays either every 6 months or annually reduce the mortality associated with lung cancer.

Answer b is incorrect. Randomized trials did not demonstrate chest x-rays plus sputum cytology to reduce the mortality associated with lung cancer.

Answer c is incorrect. Preliminary results of nonrandomized trials of annual spiral CT scans are encouraging; however, we are awaiting the results of a randomized clinical trial comparing an annual spiral CT scan versus annual chest x-ray.

Answer d is correct. Until the randomized trial of an annual spiral CT scan are known, enrollment in clinical trial of lung cancer screening is most appropriate.

2. A 60-year-old woman comes into your pharmacy to pick up her prescription for hydrochlorothiazide for hypertension. She asks you about taking vitamin supplements to decrease her risk of lung cancer. Her social history is significant for smoking a pack of cigarettes a day for 25 years, but she stopped a year ago. Based upon this information, you should recommend which of the following?

   a. No supplement is recommended
   b. β-Carotene
   c. Vitamin E plus β-carotene
   d. β-Carotene plus retinyl palmitate

Answer a is correct. To date, randomized trials of chemopreventive agents (eg, vitamin E, β-carotene, and retinyl palmitate) have not demonstrated any benefit in preventing lung cancer in patients at high risk for developing lung cancer. In two randomized clinical trials, β-carotene has been associated with an increased risk of lung cancer and mortality in patients at high risk for developing lung cancer.

Answer b is incorrect. In two randomized, clinical trials, β-carotene has been associated with an increased risk of lung cancer and mortality in patients at high risk for developing lung cancer.

Answer c is incorrect. In two randomized clinical trials, β-carotene has been associated with an increased risk of lung cancer and mortality in patients at high risk for developing lung cancer. Additionally, vitamin E (tocopherol) offers no benefit in lowering the risk of developing lung cancer.

Answer d is incorrect. In two randomized clinical trials, β-carotene has been associated with an increased risk of lung cancer and mortality in patients at high risk for developing lung cancer. Additionally, retinyl palmitate offers no benefit in lowering the risk of developing lung cancer.

3. A 68-year-old man with recently diagnosed adenocarcinoma of the lung is found to have stage IV disease (liver metastases). At home, he is bedridden due to severe COPD that requires home oxygen. His social history is significant for an 80-pack year history. Which of the following chemotherapy regimens, if any, would be rational?

   a. Cisplatin plus etoposide
   b. Carboplatin plus paclitaxel
   c. Cisplatin plus gemcitabine
   d. Best supportive care

Answer a is incorrect because the patient has a performance status of 4 due to COPD.

Answer b is incorrect because the patient has a performance status of 4 due to COPD.

Answer c is incorrect because the patient has a performance status of 4 due to COPD.

Answer d is correct because the patient has a performance status of 4 due to COPD. A key predictor of survival in lung cancer besides staging is performance status (PS). The Eastern Cooperative Oncology Group (ECOG) PS (see Table 12-2) delineation ranges from fully active to confinement to bed. Generally, patients with a PS of 3 and 4 are not treated, but offered best supportive care.

4. A 59-year-old man with recently diagnosed limited-stage small-cell lung cancer comes to clinic for treatment. Which of the following would be rational therapy for this gentleman?

   a. Surgery followed by four cycles of cisplatin plus etoposide
   b. Six cycles of cisplatin plus pemetrexed
   c. Concurrent radiation therapy, cisplatin, and etoposide
   d. Six cycles of carboplatin plus paclitaxel

Answer a is incorrect because surgery is not a primary treatment option in SCLC.

Answer b is incorrect. Cisplatin plus pemetrexed is a regimen utilized in NSCLC not in SCLC.

Answer c is correct. For limited stage SCLC to maximize survival, one should utilize concurrent radiation therapy and cisplatin plus etoposide.

Answer d is incorrect. Carboplatin plus paclitaxel is a regimen utilized in NSCLC not in SCLC.

5. For a patient receiving etoposide, you should counsel the patient about which of the following side effects?

   a. Severe acute nausea and vomiting within hours of receiving etoposide
   b. Myelosuppression about 1 week after receiving etoposide
   c. Neurotoxicity starting after two or more cycles of etoposide
   d. Nephrotoxicity occurring after three or more cycles of etoposide

Answer a is incorrect. Etoposide is a low-risk agent for causing acute nausea and vomiting.

Answer b is correct. The dose-limiting toxicity of etoposide is myelosuppression, which occurs 7 to 10 days after receiving etoposide.

Answer c is incorrect. Neurotoxicity is not an anticipated toxicity of etoposide. One should closely monitor patients receiving cisplatin and taxanes for neurotoxicity.

Answer d is incorrect. Nephrotoxicity is not an anticipated toxicity of etoposide. One should closely monitor patients receiving cisplatin for nephrotoxicity.

6. A 61-year-old woman presents to clinic with newly diagnosed squamous cell carcinoma of the lung which metastasize to the liver and bone. The EGFR status reveals no mutations. All of her laboratory values are within normal limits, and reports that she is extremely active. Based upon this information, which of the following treatments would be rational?
   a. Best supportive care
   b. Erlotinib
   c. Cisplatin plus pemetrexed
   d. Cisplatin plus gemcitabine

Answer a is incorrect. Because of the patients good performance status either a 0 or 1, she should receive active therapy.

Answer b is incorrect. Because the tumor does not exhibit any EGFR mutations, she is unlikely to benefit from erlotinib.

Answer c is incorrect. Patients with squamous cell carcinoma of the lung have a significantly shorter survival with cisplatin plus pemetrexed as compared to cisplatin plus gemcitabine.

Answer d is correct. Patients with squamous cell carcinoma of the lung have a significantly longer survival when treated with cisplatin plus gemcitabine as compared to cisplatin plus pemetrexed.

7. Which of the following side effects is more common with carboplatin rather than cisplatin?
   a. Tingling in the hands and feet
   b. A lowered platelet count
   c. A rising serum creatinine
   d. Nausea and vomiting

Answer a is incorrect. Neurotoxicity (tingling in the hands and feet) is much more common in patients receiving cisplatin.

Answer b is correct. Thrombocytopenia (a lowered platelet count), as well as neutropenia, is much more common in patients receiving carboplatin.

Answer c is incorrect. Nephrotoxicity (a rising serum creatinine) is much more common in patients receiving cisplatin.

Answer d is incorrect. Nausea and vomiting (both acute and delayed) is much more common in patients receiving cisplatin.

8. What is the best treatment option for a 61-year-old man who is chemotherapy naïve and was recently diagnosed with extensive-stage small-cell lung cancer?
   a. Cisplatin plus vinorelbine
   b. Carboplatin plus paclitaxel
   c. Cisplatin plus etoposide
   d. Carboplatin, paclitaxel, plus bevacizumab

Answer a is incorrect. Cisplatin plus vinorelbine is a regimen utilized in NSCLC not in SCLC.

Answer b is incorrect. Carboplatin plus paclitaxel is a regimen utilized in NSCLC not in SCLC.

Answer c is correct. For extensive-stage SCLC to maximize survival, one should utilize cisplatin plus etoposide regimen.

Answer d is incorrect. Carboplatin, paclitaxel, plus bevacizumab is a regimen utilized in NSCLC not in SCLC.

9. For a patient receiving erlotinib, you should counsel them about which of the following side effects?
   a. Rash
   b. Myelosuppression
   c. Neurotoxicity
   d. Alopecia

Answer a is correct. Developments of a rash and GI upset are the most common side effects in patients receiving erlotinib.

Answer b is incorrect. Myelosuppression is not a common side effect of erlotinib, but it is a common side effect of chemotherapy agents used in the treatment of NSCLC.

Answer c is incorrect. Neurotoxicity is not a common side effect of erlotinib, but it is a common side effect of chemotherapy agents used in the treatment of NSCLC.

Answer d is incorrect. Alopecia is not a common side effect of erlotinib, but it is a common side effect of chemotherapy agents used in the treatment of NSCLC.

10. Which of the following factors predicts a favorable chance to respond to erlotinib?
    a. Adenocarcinoma histology
    b. Squamous histology
    c. EGFR mutations present
    d. *K-ras* mutations present

Answer a is incorrect. The NSCLC histology is not an important predictor of response to erlotinib. Adenocarcinoma NSCLC does respond more often to pemetrexed than gemcitabine.

Answer b is incorrect. The NSCLC histology is not an important predictor of response to erlotinib. Squamous cell NSCLC does respond more often to gemcitabine than to pemetrexed.

Answer c is correct. The best predictor of response to erlotinib is the presence of EGFR mutations.

Answer d is incorrect. In contrast to EGFR mutations, the presence of *K-ras* mutations is associated with poor outcomes in patients treated with erlotinib.

11. Which of the following is the trade name of erlotinib?
    a. Tarceva
    b. Alimta

c. Navelbine
d. Hycamtin

Answer a is correct. Tarceva is the trade name for erlotinib.

Answer b is incorrect. Alimta is the trade name for pemetrexed.

Answer c is incorrect. Navelbine is the trade name for vinorelbine.

Answer d is incorrect. Hycamtin is the trade name for topotecan.

12. A 64-year-old man with a performance status of 1 returns to clinic with relapsed small-cell lung cancer (SCLC), new bone and liver metastases. He completed his previous chemotherapy of carboplatin and etoposide 5 months ago and reports no other medical problems. He and his wife request further treatment if it is reasonable. Based upon this information, which of the following treatments would be rational?

a. Best supportive care
b. Erlotinib
c. Cisplatin, paclitaxel, and bevacizumab
d. Topotecan

Answer a is incorrect. Because his SCLC relapsed > 3 months since completing first-line therapy, his performance status is a one, and he requests therapy, it is rational to give him second-line therapy by offering a clinical trial, topotecan, gemcitabine, or taxanes.

Answer b is incorrect. Erlotinib is utilized for non–small-cell lung cancer (NSCLC) not SCLC.

Answer c is incorrect. Cisplatin, paclitaxel, and bevacizumab is a regimen utilized for NSCLC not SCLC.

Answer d is correct. Topotecan demonstrates activity in patients with relapsed SCLC and has a FDA-approved indication for this patient population.

13. For a patient receiving gemcitabine, you should counsel them about which of the following side effects?

a. Rash after the first and subsequent doses
b. Fever and chills with 1 to 2 days of the infusion
c. Neurotoxicity after four cycles
d. Severe magnesium and potassium wasting after multiple cycles

Answer a is incorrect. A development of a rash is a common side effect in patients receiving erlotinib not gemcitabine.

Answer b is correct. Patients receiving gemcitabine should be counseled on flu-like symptoms (fever and chills) during the infusion but more likely within 1 to 2 days of the infusion.

Answer c is incorrect. Neurotoxicity is not a common side effect of gemcitabine, but it is a common side effect of cisplatin and paclitaxel.

Answer d is incorrect. Severe magnesium and potassium wasting is a common side effect of cisplatin not gemcitabine.

14. For a patient receiving bevacizumab, you should closely monitor the patient for which of the following side effects?

a. Nausea and vomiting, myelosuppression (especially thrombocytopenia), and alopecia
b. Fluid retention, severe myelosuppression, and alopecia
c. Hypertension, thromboembolic events, and proteinuria
d. Arthralgias/myalgias, tingling in the hands and feet, and alopecia

Answer a is incorrect. Nausea/vomiting, myelosuppression (especially thrombocytopenia), and alopecia are common side effects of carboplatin.

Answer b is incorrect. Fluid retention, severe myelosuppression, and alopecia are common side effects of docetaxel.

Answer c is correct. For a patient receiving bevacizumab, one should closely monitor the patient for hypertension, thromboembolic events, and proteinuria.

Answer d is incorrect. Arthralgias/myalgias, tingling in the hands and feet, and alopecia are common side effects of paclitaxel.

15. In which of the following histologies of lung cancer should one avoid bevacizumab due to its association with causing pulmonary hemorrhage in this histology?

a. Adenocarcinoma
b. Large cell
c. Bronchoalveolar
d. Squamous

Answer a is incorrect. Bevacizumab can be safely used in patients with adenocarcinoma of the lung but not squamous cell.

Answer b is incorrect. Bevacizumab can be safely used in patients with large-cell carcinoma of the lung but not squamous cell.

Answer c is incorrect. Bevacizumab can be safely used in patients with bronchoalveolar sub-type of adenocarcinoma of the lung but not squamous cell.

Answer d is correct. Bevacizumab should not be used in squamous cell carcinoma of the lung because of its association with causing pulmonary hemorrhage in this subtype of lung cancer.

16. Which of the following is the trade name of bevacizumab?

a. Gemzar
b. Avastin
c. Taxotere
d. VePesid

Answer a is incorrect. Gemzar is the trade name for gemcitabine.

Answer b is correct. Avastin is the trade name for bevacizumab.

Answer c is incorrect. Taxotere is the trade name for docetaxel.

Answer d is incorrect. VePesid is one of the trade names for etoposide.

17. In addition to a short course of dexamethasone, one should ensure that a patient receiving pemetrexed receives which of the following medications?

    a. Folate and vitamin B_{12} supplementation
    b. Aggressive hydration with normal saline
    c. Oral potassium and magnesium supplementation
    d. β-Carotene and α-tocopherol supplementation

Answer a is correct. Folate and vitamin B_{12} supplementation is required to minimize the myelosuppression associated with pemetrexed. The recommended doses are folate 1 mg po daily and vitamin B_{12} 1 mg SC/IM every 3 months.

Answer b is incorrect. Aggressive hydration with normal saline is needed to prevent the nephrotoxicity of cisplatin.

Answer c is incorrect. Oral potassium and magnesium supplementation maybe needed for patients receiving cisplatin not pemetrexed.

Answer d is incorrect. β-Carotene and α-tocopherol have been used unsuccessfully to prevent lung cancer, and they do not mitigate any of the toxicities of pemetrexed.

18. Which of the following is the trade name of pemetrexed?

    a. Paraplatin
    b. Taxol
    c. Alimta
    d. Taxotere

Answer a is incorrect. Paraplatin is the trade name for carboplatin.

Answer b is incorrect. Taxol is the trade name for paclitaxel.

Answer c is correct. Alimta is the trade name for pemetrexed.

Answer d is incorrect. Taxotere is the trade name for docetaxel.

19. Which of the following patients with small-cell lung cancer should receive prophylactic cranial irradiation?

    a. All patients with limited-stage SCLC.
    b. All patients with extensive-stage SCLC.
    c. Patients with limited-stage SCLC who achieve a complete response to their chemotherapy regimen.
    d. Patients with extensive-stage SCLC who do not respond to their chemotherapy regimen.

Answer a is incorrect. Prophylactic cranial irradiation is only recommended in SCLC, whether limited or extensive stage, if the patient achieves a complete response to their chemotherapy regimen.

Answer b is incorrect. Prophylactic cranial irradiation is only recommended in SCLC, whether limited or extensive stage, if the patient achieves a complete response to their chemotherapy regimen.

Answer c is correct. Whether limited or extensive stage, patients with SCLC who achieve a complete response to their chemotherapy regimen should receive prophylactic cranial irradiation (PCI). In this situation, PCI decreases the incidence of brain metastases and improves overall survival.

Answer d is incorrect. Prophylactic cranial irradiation is only recommended in SCLC, whether limited or extensive stage, if the patient achieves a complete response to their chemotherapy regimen.

20. For a patient receiving docetaxel, you should closely monitor the patient for which of the following side effects?

    a. Acneiform rash, dry skin, and diarrhea
    b. Fluid retention, severe myelosuppression, mucositis, and alopecia
    c. Impaired wound healing, hypertension, proteinuria, and thromboembolic events
    d. Severe nausea/vomiting, nephrotoxicity, neurotoxicity, and ototoxicity

Answer a is incorrect. Acneiform rash, dry skin, and diarrhea are common side effects of erlotinib.

Answer b is correct. Fluid retention, severe myelosuppression, mucositis, and alopecia are common side effects of docetaxel.

Answer c is incorrect. For a patient receiving bevacizumab, one should closely monitor the patient for impaired wound healing, hypertension, proteinuria, and thromboembolic events.

Answer d is incorrect. Severe nausea/vomiting, nephrotoxicity, neurotoxicity, and ototoxicity are common side effects of cisplatin.

CHAPTER 13 | Prostate Cancer

1. Which of the following is the most accurate statement pertaining to prostate cancer?

    a. Prostate cancer is the leading cause of cancer death in both men and women.
    b. Age, race-ethnicity, and family history are known risk factors for prostate cancer.

c. Prostate cancer is related to decreased exposure to testosterone.
d. Squamous cell carcinoma is the major pathologic cell type of prostate cancer.

Answer a is incorrect. Prostate cancer is the second leading cause of cancer deaths in men. Lung cancer is the leading cause of cancer deaths in men and women. Women do not develop prostate cancer because they do not have a prostate.

Answer b is correct. The widely accepted risk factors for prostate cancer are age, race-ethnicity, and family history of prostate cancer. The disease is rare under the age of 40, but the incidence sharply increases with each subsequent decade, most likely because the individual has had a lifetime exposure to testosterone. African American men have the highest rate of prostate cancer in the world and in the United States. Prostate cancer mortality in African Americans is more than twice that seen in Caucasian populations. Testosterone, commonly implicated in the pathogenesis of prostate cancer, is 15% higher in African American men compared with Caucasian males. Men with a brother or father with prostate cancer have twice the risk for prostate cancer compared to the rest of the population. Family clustering of prostate cancer can be explained by inheritance of a rare, autosomal, dominant allele, which accounts for 9% of all prostate cancer and 45% of disease reported in men under the age of 55.

Answer c is incorrect. Prostate cancer is related to increased exposure to testosterone over time.

Answer d is incorrect. Adenocarcinoma is the major pathologic cell type of prostate cancer. Squamous cell carcinoma is a type of lung cancer.

---

2. A prostate cancer with a Gleason score of 7 to 10 is considered:

a. Poorly differentiated
b. Differentiated
c. Moderately differentiated
d. Well differentiated

Answer a is correct. Prostate cancer can be graded systematically according to the histologic appearance of the malignant cell and then grouped into well, moderately, or poorly differentiated grades. Gland architecture is examined and then rated on a scale of 1 (well differentiated) to 5 (poorly differentiated). Two different specimens are examined, and the score for each specimen is added. Poorly differentiated tumors grow rapidly (poor prognosis), while well-differentiated tumors grow slowly (better prognosis). A Gleason score of 7 to 10 is considered poorly differentiated.

Answer b is incorrect. The term "differentiated" is not used alone in the Gleason scoring system.

Answer c is incorrect. Moderately differentiated is a Gleason score of 5 to 6.

Answer d is incorrect. Well differentiated is equal to a Gleason score of 2 to 4.

---

3. BD is a 45-year-old African American man with a family history of prostate cancer who presents to his primary care physician for his annual examination. He asks about prostate cancer screening. Which of the following is the most appropriate course of action?

a. Observation because he is not eligible for prostate cancer due to his age.
b. Perform a digital rectal examination to determine the size of the prostate.
c. Draw a PSA level to rule out benign prostatic hyperplasia.
d. Perform a digital rectal examination and draw a PSA level.

Answer a is incorrect. A baseline PSA and DRE at age 40 with annual evaluations beginning at age 50 to all men of normal risk with a 10-year or greater life expectancy is recommended. Men with an increased risk of prostate cancer, including men of African American ancestry and men with a family history of prostate cancer may begin screening earlier, at age 40 to 45. Patient is eligible for screening because he is at high risk due to his race-ethnicity and family history.

Answer b is incorrect. DRE as a single screening method, has poor compliance, and has had little effect on preventing metastatic prostate cancer. Therefore, prostate screening with a DRE alone is currently not recommended.

Answer c is incorrect. PSA may be elevated in men with acute urinary retention, acute prostatitis, and prostatic ischemia or infarction, as well as BPH. PSA elevations between 4.1 (4.1 μg/L) and 10 ng/mL (10 μg/L) cannot distinguish between BPH and prostate cancer, limiting the utility of PSA alone for the early detection of prostate cancer.

Answer d is correct. Neither DRE nor PSA is sensitive or specific enough to be used alone as a screening test. Therefore, the combination of a DRE plus PSA determination is a better method in detecting prostate cancer than DRE alone.

---

4. AJ is a 60-year-old man with a history of BPH. His most recent DRE was normal, but last PSA was 5.3 ng/mL. AJ is concerned about getting prostate cancer and wants to discuss preventative therapy. Which of the following is the most appropriate recommendation?

a. Finasteride 5 mg daily
b. Docetaxel 75 mg/m^2 + Prednisone 5 mg bid
c. Leuprolide
d. Surgery

Answer a is correct. The use of finasteride to prevent prostate cancer is currently debatable. However, in men over 50 with BPH, finasteride may provide additional benefit of prostate cancer prevention. In the 70% to 80% of men without

BPH, the benefits, side effects, and risks of finasteride should be discussed prior to initiating therapy.

Answer b is incorrect. Docetaxel and prednisone is only recommended for patients with hormone refractory metastatic prostate cancer. These agents have not been studied or used in prevention of prostate cancer.

Answer c is incorrect. LH-RH agonists such as leuprolide have not been studied in the prevention of prostate cancer.

Answer d is incorrect. Surgery is not an appropriate option for prostate cancer prevention.

---

5. SO is a 67-year-old man who was recently diagnosed with prostate cancer and is initiated on leuprolide for androgen deprivation. Which of the following agents should be added to his therapy to prevent "tumor flare"?

    a. Bicalutamide
    b. Finasteride
    c. Mitoxantrone
    d. Goserelin

Answer a is correct. The most common adverse effects reported with LH-RH agonist therapy include a disease flare-up during the first week of therapy, hot flashes, erectile impotence, decreased libido, and injection-site reactions.[8] The disease flare-up is caused by an initial induction of LH and FSH by the LH-RH agonist leading to an initial phase of increased testosterone production, and manifests clinically as either increased bone pain or increased urinary symptoms. Initiating an antiandrogen prior to the administration of the LH-RH agonist and continuing for 2 to 4 weeks is a frequently employed strategy to minimize this initial tumor flare.

Answer b is incorrect. Finasteride is a 5-alpha reductase inhibitor that is used in the prevention, not the treatment of prostate cancer.

Answer c is incorrect. Mitoxantrone is used in metastatic hormone refractory prostate cancer in patients who have failed other therapies, although the effectiveness of this agent in prostate cancer has not been determined.

Answer d is incorrect. Goserelin is a LH-RH agonist. It would not be appropriate to place the patient on two LH-RH agonists.

---

6. Which of the following side effects are associated with flutamide?

    a. Constipation
    b. Increased libido
    c. Rash
    d. Diarrhea

Answer a is incorrect. Flutamide does not cause constipation but actually causes diarrhea.

Answer b is incorrect. Flutamide is not associated with increased libido.

Answer c is incorrect. Rash is not a side effect of flutamide therapy.

Answer d is correct. Flutamide causes diarrhea. In order to minimize diarrhea, it is recommended that you initiate flutamide at 250 mg daily then titrate to 250 mg tid.

---

7. Which of the following LH-RH agonists is given subcutaneously every 12 months?

    a. Leuprolide implant (Viadur)
    b. Goserelin implant (Zoladex)
    c. Leuprolide depot (Lupron)
    d. Triptorelin depot (Trelstar Depot)

Answer a is correct. The leuprolide implant is administered subcutaneously and is a mini-osmotic pump that delivers 120 μg of leuprolide daily for 12 months. After 12 months the implant is removed, and a different implant can be placed.

Answer b is incorrect. Goserelin acetate implant contains goserelin acetate dispersed in a plastic matrix of D, L-lactic and glycolic acid copolymer and is administered subcutaneously every month or every 3 months. Hydrolysis of the copolymer material provides continuous release of goserelin over the dosing period.

Answer c is incorrect. The leuprolide depot formulation is not a mini-osmotic pump.

Answer d is incorrect. Triptorelin depot is administered intramuscularly every 28 days.

---

8. Which of the following LH-RH agonists contains coated pellets and is administered intramuscularly to allow for sustained levels throughout the dosing interval?

    a. Leuprolide implant (Viadur)
    b. Goserelin implant (Zoladex)
    c. Leuprolide depot (Lupron)
    d. Triptorelin depot (Trelstar Depot)

Answer a is incorrect. The leuprolide implant is administered subcutaneously and is a mini-osmotic pump that delivers 120 μg of leuprolide daily for 12 months. After 12 months the implant is removed, and a different implant can be placed.

Answer b is incorrect. Goserelin acetate implant contains goserelin acetate dispersed in a plastic matrix of D, L-lactic and glycolic acid copolymer and is administered subcutaneously every month or every 3 months. Hydrolysis of the copolymer material provides continuous release of goserelin over the dosing period.

Answer c is correct. The leuprolide depot formulation contains leuprolide acetate in coated pellets that is administered intramuscularly monthly, every 3 months, or every 4 months.

Answer d is incorrect. Triptorelin depot is administered intramuscularly every 28 days.

---

9. TR is a newly diagnosed prostate cancer patient being treated with androgen ablation. Which of the following are appropriate counseling points for a new patient starting on an LH-RH agonist?
   a. Patient may experience side effects such as a loss in libido, hot flushes, and impotence.
   b. Androgen deprivation therapy is associated with osteoporosis and therefore the patient should take a calcium/vitamin D supplement.
   c. Patient may experience worsening symptoms during the first week related to "tumor flare."
   d. All of the above.

Answer a is correct. TR may experience side effects such as loss in libido, hot flushes, and impotence from androgen ablation.

Answer b is correct. TR should take calcium/vitamin D supplementation because the androgen deprivation therapy is associated with osteoporosis.

Answer c is correct. TR may experience worsening of symptoms during the first week because of a tumor flare.

Answer d is correct and the best answer.

---

10. What is the mechanism of action of Degarelix?
    a. LH-RH agonist
    b. Antiandrogen
    c. Androgen synthesis inhibitors
    d. GnRH antagonist

Answer a is incorrect. Examples of LH-RH agonists are leuprolide, goserelin, and triptorelin.

Answer b is incorrect. Examples of antiandrogens include flutamide, bicalutamide, and nilutamide.

Answer c is incorrect. Examples of androgen synthesis inhibitors include aminoglutethimide and ketoconazole.

Answer d is correct. Degarelix is a GnRH antagonist.

---

11. L.B. is a 63-year-old man with hormone refractory metastatic prostate cancer. He has several other comorbid diseases including CHF, diabetes, and hypertension. Which of the following chemotherapy agents is the most appropriate for this patient?
    a. Estramustine + docetaxel
    b. Mitoxantrone + prednisone
    c. Estramustine + docetaxel + mitoxantrone + prednisone
    d. Docetaxel + prednisone

Answer a is incorrect. Although estramustine + docetaxel has survival data, it is not currently recommended first line. Additionally, estramustine would be inappropriate in this patient due to his history of cardiovascular disease.

Answer b is incorrect. Mitoxantrone + prednisone can be used in hormone refractory metastatic prostate cancer, although its benefits have yet to be determined. Therefore, it is currently not recommended first line. Additionally, mitoxantrone is associated with cardiotoxicity and may not be appropriate in a patient with CHF.

Answer c is incorrect. All four of these agents have not been studied together in combination.

Answer d is correct. Docetaxel + prednisone is the recommended chemotherapy regimen in patients with hormone refractory metastatic prostate cancer due to its overall survival benefits. Docetaxel should be administered at 75 mg/m^2 every 3 weeks combined with prednisone 5 mg tid. The most common adverse events reported with this regimen are nausea, alopecia, and bone marrow suppression. In addition, fluid retention and peripheral neuropathy, known effects of docetaxel, are observed. Docetaxel is hepatically eliminated; therefore, patients with hepatic impairment may not be eligible for treatment with docetaxel.

---

12. BB is a 69-year-old man with metastatic prostate cancer who is receiving chemotherapy and a bisphosphonate, zoledronic acid. Which of the following tests should be monitored while this patient is on zoledronic acid?
    a. LFTs
    b. Urinalysis
    c. Chem-7
    d. PFTs

Answer a is incorrect. LFTs are not necessary as zoledronic acid has renal elimination.

Answer b is incorrect. Zoledronic acid is renally eliminated, but is not associated with proteinuria.

Answer c is correct. A Chem-7 should be monitored to determine if the serum creatinine is < 3 mg/dL. If the serum creatinine is > 3 mg/dL, then zoledronic acid should be avoided.

Answer d is incorrect. PFTs are not necessary as zoledronic acid has no effect on pulmonary function.

---

13. Which of the following side effects is associated with antiandrogen use?
    a. Myelosuppression
    b. Gynecomastia
    c. Increased libido
    d. Rash

Answer a is incorrect. Antiandrogens are not associated with myelosuppression. Chemotherapy is associated with myelosuppression.

Answer b is correct. Gynecomastia is a class effect of antiandrogens.

Answer c is incorrect. Antiandrogens actually cause decreased libido.

Answer d is incorrect. Antiandrogens are not associated with a rash.

---

14. Which of the following antiandrogens is associated with alcohol intolerance?
    a. Flutamide
    b. Bicalutamide
    c. Nilutamide
    d. Leuprolide

Answer a is incorrect. Flutamide is not associated with alcohol intolerance.

Answer b is incorrect. Bicalutamide is not associated with alcohol intolerance.

Answer c is correct. Nilutamide is associated with alcohol intolerance.

Answer d is incorrect. Leuprolide is not an antiandrogen, but a LH-RH agonist.

---

15. Which of the following side effects has been associated with zoledronic acid use?
    a. Osteonecrosis of the jaw
    b. Gastroesophageal reflux disease (GERD)
    c. Diarrhea
    d. Constipation

Answer a is correct. Zoledronic acid use has been associated with osteonecrosis of the jaw.

Answer b is incorrect. IV bisphosphonates have not been associated with gastroesophageal reflux disease (GERD).

Answer c is incorrect. Zoledronic acid has not been associated with diarrhea.

Answer d is incorrect. Constipation is not a side effect of zoledronic acid.

---

16. Which of the following patients with prostate cancer can be managed with observation alone?
    a. Patient with a Gleason score of 3 and PSA of 5 ng/mL
    b. Patient with a Gleason score of 8 and PSA of 40 ng/mL
    c. Patient with a Gleason score of 2 and PSA of 15 ng/mL
    d. Patient with a Gleason score of 5 and PSA of 20 ng/mL

Answer a is correct. Asymptomatic patients with a low risk of recurrence, a Gleason score of 2 through 6, and a PSA of less than 10 ng/mL (10 μg/L) may be managed by observation, radiation (external beam or brachytherapy), or radical prostatectomy.

Answer b is incorrect. The treatment of patients at high risk of recurrence (Gleason score ranging from 8-10, or a PSA value greater than 20 ng/mL, 20 μg/L) should be treated with androgen ablation for 2 to 3 years combined with radiation therapy.

Answer c is incorrect. Individuals with moderate disease or a Gleason score of 7 or a PSA ranging from 10 to 20 ng/mL (10-20 μg/L) are considered at intermediate risk for prostate cancer recurrence.

Answer d is incorrect. Individuals with moderate disease or a Gleason score of 7 or a PSA ranging from 10 to 20 ng/mL (10-20 μg/L) are considered at intermediate risk for prostate cancer recurrence.

---

17. Which of the following statements is true?
    a. DRE is highly specific and highly sensitive for detecting prostate cancer and may be used alone for diagnosis.
    b. PSA is highly specific and highly sensitive for detecting prostate cancer and may be used alone for diagnosis.
    c. DRE and PSA are highly specific and highly sensitive for detecting prostate cancer and should be used in combination for diagnosis.
    d. Neither DRE nor PSA are highly specific or highly sensitive when used alone for detecting prostate cancer. Therefore, these agents should be used in combination for diagnosis.

Answer a is incorrect. DRE is not highly specific or highly sensitive when used alone for detection of prostate cancer.

Answer b is incorrect. PSA is not highly specific or highly sensitive when used alone for detection of prostate cancer.

Answer c is incorrect. DRE and PSA are neither highly specific nor highly sensitive for detecting prostate cancer. However, because of the lack of specificity and sensitivity when used alone, these tests *should* be used in combination for diagnosis.

Answer d is correct. Neither DRE nor PSA are highly specific or highly sensitive when used alone for detecting prostate cancer. However, because of the lack of specificity and sensitivity when used alone, these tests *should* be used in combination for diagnosis.

---

18. The use of an antiandrogen and LH-RH agonists is called:
    a. Concurrent chemoprevention
    b. Concurrent chemoradiotherapy
    c. Combined androgen blockade
    d. None of the above

Answer a is incorrect. Chemoprevention is a term that defines agents used to prevent cancer.

Answer b is incorrect. Concurrent chemoradiotherapy is the use of chemotherapy and radiation concurrently.

Answer c is correct. Combined androgen blockade is the use of an antiandrogen and LH-RH agonists concurrently.

Answer d is incorrect. Answer c is correct, therefore making answer d incorrect.

---

19. Which of the following is considered the primary site of metastases for prostate cancer?

    a. Liver
    b. Brain
    c. Lungs
    d. Bone

Answer a is incorrect. The liver is the primary site of metastases for colon cancer.

Answer b is incorrect. The brain is not the primary site of metastases for prostate cancer.

Answer c is incorrect. The lungs are not the primary site of metastases for prostate cancer.

Answer d is correct. The bone is the primary site of metastases for prostate cancer.

---

20. Which of the following is the major pathologic cell type found in 95% of prostate cancers?

    a. Adenocarcinoma
    b. Melanoma
    c. Sarcoma
    d. Carcinoma

Answer a is correct. Adenocarcinoma is the major pathologic cell type found in 95% of prostate cancers.

Answer b is incorrect. Melanoma is the major pathologic cell type in skin cancer arising from the melanocytes.

Answer c is incorrect. Sarcoma is the major pathologic cell type or cancer of the connective tissue.

Answer d is incorrect. Carcinoma is a cancer arising from epithelial cells.

CHAPTER 14 | Breast Cancer

1. Select the agent that is administered via intramuscular injection for the treatment of metastatic estrogen receptor positive breast cancer.

    a. Anastrozole
    b. Avastin
    c. Herceptin
    d. Faslodex
    e. Femara

Answer a in incorrect. Anastrozole is administered orally to patients with ER+ metastatic breast cancer.

Answer b is incorrect. Avastin is administered intravenously to patients with breast cancer characterized by an overexpression of HER-2.

Answer c is incorrect. Herceptin is administered intravenously to patients with breast cancer.

Answer d is correct. Faslodex is administered by IM injection to women with ER+ metastatic breast cancer.

---

2. Which of the following conditions would be a contraindication to administration of tamoxifen for the prevention of breast cancer in a "high-risk" premenopausal patient?

    a. History of deep venous thrombosis
    b. First-degree relative with ER negative breast cancer
    c. History of diabetes mellitus
    d. History of seizures
    e. None of the above

Answer a is correct. Tamoxifen is associated with an increased risk for developing thromboembolic events. Administration of tamoxifen to prevent breast cancer is contraindicated in patients with a history of deep venous thrombosis or pulmonary emboli.

Answer b is incorrect. The estrogen receptor status of first-degree relatives is not a contraindication to prescribing tamoxifen to reduce the risk for developing breast cancer.

Answer c is incorrect. Diabetes mellitus is not a contraindication to prescribing tamoxifen to reduce the risk for developing breast cancer.

Answer d is incorrect. A history of seizures is not a contraindication to prescribing tamoxifen to reduce the risk for developing breast cancer.

Answer e is incorrect. A history of thromboembolic events is a contraindication to prescribing tamoxifen to reduce the risk for developing cancer.

---

3. A premenopausal woman with ER negative, node positive breast cancer is starting doxorubicin and cyclophosphamide adjuvant treatment. What would you recommend to determine the severity of the most common toxicity associated with this treatment regimen?

    a. An electrocardiogram 1 week after chemotherapy.
    b. A complete blood count including platelets 1 week after administration of the chemotherapy.
    c. Serum bilirubin and aspartate transaminase 1 week after chemotherapy.
    d. Urinalysis 1 week after chemotherapy.

Answer a is incorrect. Although doxorubicin has been associated with cardiomyopathy that increases in incidence with cumulative doses exceeding 400 mg/m^2. The incidence of cardiomyopathy in patients administered cumulative doses exceeding 400 mg/m^2 is in the range of 5%. It is not the most common toxicity associated with this treatment regimen.

Answer b is correct. Myelosuppression (neutropenia, thrombocytopenia) is the most common treatment related adverse effect associated with this adjuvant treatment regimen. Nearly 100% of patients receiving this treatment regimen will experience myelosuppression.

Answer c is incorrect. Although these drugs may cause elevations of serum bilirubin and aspartate transaminase, it occurs less frequently than myelosuppression.

Answer d is incorrect. Although urinalysis could be useful in detecting hematuria caused by cyclophosphamide, this adverse effect (hemorrhagic cystitis) occurs infrequently with this adjuvant chemotherapy regimen.

---

4. Select the toxicity that has been associated with the administration of both trastuzumab and bevacizumab.
   a. Myelosuppression
   b. GI perforation
   c. Alopecia
   d. Infusion reactions

Answer a is incorrect. Trastuzumab and bevacizumab are monoclonal antibodies that are rarely associated with myelosuppression.

Answer b is incorrect. Although GI perforation is a known bevacizumab toxicity, it is not been associated with administration of trastuzumab.

Answer c is incorrect. Monoclonal antibodies are not associated with hair loss.

Answer d is correct. Trastuzumab and bevacizumab are monoclonal antibodies administered by IV infusion. Infusion reactions (the onset of chills, fever, changes in blood pressure within 1 hour of administration) have been reported to occur with both agents.

---

5. Select the appropriate premedication regimen that is recommended to be administered prior to the administration of paclitaxel?
   a. Dexamethasone, ranitidine
   b. Ranitidine and diphenhydramine
   c. Dexamethasone and diphenhydramine
   d. Dexamethasone, ranitidine, and diphenhydramine

Answers a, b, and c are incorrect.

Answer d is correct. A combination of a corticosteroid, an H1 and H2 antagonist, are recommended to be administered prior to paclitaxel infusions to decrease the incidence and severity of hypersensitivity reactions to paclitaxel.

---

6. A patient taking capecitabine for metastatic breast cancer describes to you the development of tenderness on her hands and feet that making it more difficult for her to be on her feet. Select the most appropriate recommendation for this patient.
   a. Her symptoms describe the onset of a known side effect of capecitabine. You recommend she call her physician and describe the onset of these symptoms before taking any more doses of capecitabine.
   b. Her symptoms are classic for individuals with vitamin B_6 deficiency. You recommend she schedule an appointment with her physician to discuss these symptoms.
   c. Her symptoms are commonly caused by capecitabine. You reassure her that there is nothing to worry about and recommend she avoid standing as much as possible while she completes the last week of capecitabine.
   d. Her symptoms are commonly caused by capecitabine. You recommend the symptoms are self-limiting and easily managed by spraying her hands and feet with benzocaine first aid spray four times daily.

Answer a is correct. The hand-foot syndrome is a known toxicity of capecitabine and will likely worsen if she continues taking the drug. The patient's physician should be informed and evaluate the benefits/risks of continuing therapy.

Answer b is incorrect. The symptoms are consistent with the onset of capecitabine induced hand-foot syndrome and require evaluation by the patient's physician.

Answer c is incorrect. The symptoms often become progressively worse. The patient's physician should be informed and evaluate the benefits/risks of continuing therapy.

Answer d is incorrect. The symptoms often become progressively worse. There is no clinical trial data supporting the efficacy of using a topical anesthetic to manage the symptoms while the capecitabine is continued. The patient's physician should be informed and evaluate the benefits/risks of continuing therapy.

---

7. A patient presents her prescription for capecitabine to you. Review of her medication profile documents she is also taking 5 mg of warfarin daily for atrial fibrillation and metformin for type 2 diabetes mellitus. Select the appropriate assessment of potential drug interactions for this patient.
   a. Capecitabine has been shown to increase metabolism of warfarin and results in subtherapeutic INRs. More frequent monitoring of this patient's INRs is recommended.
   b. Capecitabine has been shown to decrease metabolism of warfarin and results in elevated INRs and bleeding. More frequent monitoring of this patient's INRs is recommended.
   c. Capecitabine has been shown to decrease metabolism of metformin and results in hypoglycemia. The importance of scheduled blood glucose monitoring and possible need for holding metformin doses needs to be discussed with this patient.

   d. Capecitabine has been shown to increase metabolism of metformin and results in hyperglycemia. The importance of daily blood glucose monitoring and possible need for increasing metformin doses needs to be discussed with this patient.
   e. Metformin has been shown to decrease metabolism of capecitabine and results in the increased severity of capecitabine-induced myelosuppression. A 25% reduction in the dose of capecitabine is indicated.

Answer a is incorrect. Capecitabine has been shown to decrease metabolism of warfarin.

Answer b is correct. Case reports document significant elevation of INR values and bleeding when capecitabine was given to patients on a stable dose of warfarin. Capecitabine is responsible for elevated warfarin activity by inhibition of the CYP2C9 isoenzyme.

Answer c is incorrect. Capecitabine has been shown to alter metformin metabolism.

Answer d is incorrect. Capecitabine has been shown to alter metformin metabolism.

Answer e is incorrect. Metformin has been shown to alter capecitabine metabolism.

---

8. A patient presents a new prescription to you for tamoxifen. Her doctor said he was prescribing it as adjuvant treatment for breast cancer following her surgery last month. You review her medication profile and document that she is also taking metoprolol, hydrochlorothiazide, and Prozac. Select the appropriate assessment of potential drug interactions for this patient.
   a. There are no clinically significant drug interactions to alter her medication regimen.
   b. You explain that a number of SSRIs including Prozac have been documented to decrease the effectiveness of tamoxifen by interfering with its metabolism to an active metabolite. You will call the patient's physician to consider alternative antidepressant options.
   c. You explain that hydrochlorothiazide has been documented to decrease the effectiveness of tamoxifen by interfering with its metabolism to an active metabolite. You will call the patient's physician to consider alternative diuretic.
   d. You explain that metoprolol has been documented to decrease the effectiveness of tamoxifen by interfering with its metabolism to an active metabolite. You will call the patient's physician to consider alternative beta-blocker.

Answer a is incorrect. There is a potentially clinically significant drug interaction between tamoxifen and Prozac (fluoxetine).

Answer b is correct. SSRIs that are strong inhibitors of the cytochrome P450 system have been documented to decrease the effectiveness of tamoxifen by decreasing the metabolism of tamoxifen to its potent metabolite endoxifen. It would be appropriate to notify the patient's physician and discuss alternative antidepressant options.

Answer c is incorrect. Hydrochlorothiazide has not been shown to interfere with the activation of tamoxifen.

Answer d is incorrect. Metoprolol has not been shown to interfere with the activation of tamoxifen.

---

9. Select the statement that accurately describes breast cancer.
   a. The lifetime risk for US women developing breast cancer is 1 in 8.
   b. In the United States, the death rate from breast cancer has decreased since the widespread implementation of screening mammography guidelines.
   c. Breast cancer is the second leading cause of death from cancer in US women.
   d. Pharmacotherapy for metastatic breast cancer is palliative rather than curative.
   e. All of the above.

Answer a is correct. It accurately describes a women's lifetime risk for developing breast cancer.

Answer b is correct. It accurately describes the impact of mammography on breast cancer mortality.

Answer c is correct. It is a true statement. Breast cancer ranks behind lung cancer in cancer-related mortality.

Answer d is correct. It accurately describes the efficacy of drug therapy administered to patients with metastatic breast cancer.

Answer e is the correct and the best answer. All of the above accurately describe the current status of breast cancer.

---

10. Select the antineoplastic agent associated with an increased incidence of endometrial cancer.
    a. Letrozole
    b. Raloxifene
    c. Toremifene
    d. Fulvestrant
    e. Tamoxifen

Answer a is incorrect. Letrozole and the other aromatase inhibitors have not been proven to increase the risk for uterine cancer.

Answer b is incorrect. Raloxifene is a SERM that has less estrogenic effects on the uterus. It has not been associated with an increased risk for uterine cancer.

Answer c is incorrect. Toremifene is a SERM but has not been associated with an increased risk for uterine cancer.

Answer d is incorrect. Fulvestrant is a pure estrogen antagonist that has not been associated with an increased risk for uterine cancer.

Answer e is the correct answer. In the Breast Cancer Prevention Trial the difference in the incidence of uterine cancer was statistically significant; tamoxifen 36 cases in 6576 patients versus placebo 5 cases in 6599 patients (risk ratio 2.53 with 95% confidence interval 1.35-4.97).

---

11. Which of following conditions would be a contraindication for prescribing an aromatase inhibitor?
    a. The development of arthralgias and myalgias.
    b. A patient with a history of thromboembolic events.
    c. A premenopausal patient.
    d. A postmenopausal patient with a history of thromboembolic events.
    e. There are no contraindications for the administration of aromatase inhibitors.

Answer a is incorrect. Arthralgias and myalgias is a documented adverse effect of the aromatase inhibitors. If a patient develops these toxicities, a trial of an alternative aromatase inhibitor is indicated.

Answer b is incorrect. A patient with a history of thromboembolic events is not a contraindication for administration of aromatase inhibitors.

Answer c is correct. The administration of aromatase inhibitors to premenopausal women with breast cancer is contraindicated because they are ineffective in depleting estrogen production in women with functioning ovaries.

Answer d is incorrect. The administration of aromatase inhibitors are not contraindicated for postmenopausal patients with a history of thromboembolic events.

Answer e is incorrect. The administration of aromatase inhibitors is contraindicated in premenopausal women and in women with a known hypersensitivity to these agents or any of their excipients.

---

12. Select the brand name for letrozole.
    a. Arimidex
    b. Nolvadex
    c. Avastin
    d. Evista
    e. Femara

Answer a is incorrect. Arimidex is the trade name for anastrozole.

Answer b is incorrect. Nolvadex is the trade name for tamoxifen.

Answer c is incorrect. Avastin is the trade name for bevacizumab.

Answer d is incorrect. Evista is the trade name for raloxifene.

Answer e is correct. Femara is the trade name for letrozole.

---

13. Select the taxane effective in treating advanced breast cancer that is formulated as an albumin nanoparticle product.
    a. Abraxane
    b. Taxol
    c. Docetaxel
    d. Taxotere
    e. None of the above

Answer a is correct. Abraxane is the trade name for paclitaxel that is formulated as a nanoparticle suspension.

Answer b is incorrect. Taxol is the trade name for paclitaxel that is formulated in a Cremophor solvent.

Answer c is incorrect. Docetaxel is the generic name for Taxotere a non-nanoparticle taxane formulation.

Answer d is incorrect. Taxotere is the trade name for docetaxel a non-nanoparticle taxane formulation.

Answer e is incorrect. Abraxane is the trade name for paclitaxel that is formulated as a nanoparticle suspension.

---

14. Clinical trials that compared the efficacy of tamoxifen and AIs as adjuvant treatments for patients with breast cancer have established which of these outcomes?
    a. AIs have been better tolerated than tamoxifen.
    b. Sequential hormonal therapy (tamoxifen followed by an AI) has resulted in significantly longer progression-free survival than tamoxifen monotherapy.
    c. Tamoxifen without subsequent AI therapy resulted in superior progression-free survival.
    d. a and b.
    e. a and c are all outcomes documented in clinical trials.

Answer a is correct. Aromatase inhibitors are less likely to cause thromboembolic events and uterine cancer.

Answer b is correct. Several studies have documented improved progression-free survival rates with the sequential administration (tamoxifen followed by an AI).

Answer c is incorrect. Tamoxifen monotherapy has not resulted in superior outcomes.

Answer d is correct. Both answers a and b are correct.

Answer e is incorrect. Answer a is correct but answer c is incorrect.

---

15. A 69-year-old woman is taking anastrozole for ER+/PR+, HER-2 negative stage 4 breast cancer. Upon returning for her third refill, she tells you that she has noticed increased stiffness and joint pain in knees. She started taking ibuprofen 400 mg four times a day and at bedtime without much benefit for the past week. Your recommendation is to:
    a. Increase the ibuprofen dosage to 800 mg four times daily and at bedtime.

b. The symptoms of joint and muscle pain are likely caused by anastrozole. You offer to call her physician to discuss switching to letrozole or exemestane.
c. The symptoms are consistent with a hypersensitivity reaction to anastrozole. You recommend she take some diphenhydramine and go to the emergency room for evaluation.
d. The symptoms have not been associated with anastrozole; she is likely developing rheumatoid arthritis and should be evaluated by her physician.

Answer a is incorrect. The recommended maximum dose of ibuprofen is 3200 mg daily. Switching to an alternative AI would be the preferred option.

Answer b is correct. Aromatase inhibitors are known to cause joint and muscle pain. Switching to an alternative AI is a reasonable option as reports support other AIs may be better tolerated.

Answer c is incorrect. These symptoms are not consistent with a hypersensitivity reaction.

Answer d is incorrect. The symptoms are likely caused by anastrozole rather than symptoms consistent with the development of rheumatoid arthritis.

---

16. MK is a 63-year-old woman with newly diagnosed metastatic breast cancer is scheduled to receive her first dose of trastuzumab. She is 5 ft 6 inches tall and weighs 175 lb. You receive the following order: trastuzumab 440 mg IV infusion over 1.5 hours. Select the appropriate assessment to discuss with the prescriber.
    a. Trastuzumab causes significant nausea and vomiting warranting premedication with a serotonin antagonist antiemetic. It would be best to call the prescriber and suggest administration of an antiemetic.
    b. Trastuzumab can safely be administered as an IV bolus injection. It would be appropriate to call the prescriber and suggest the order be changed to be administered as an IV bolus injection.
    c. Trastuzumab has been shown effective as an adjuvant treatment but not treatment of metastatic disease. It would be appropriate to call the prescriber and clarify the indication for trastuzumab for this patient.
    d. The recommended initial dose of trastuzumab is 4 mg/kg (320 mg total for this patient). It would be appropriate to call the prescriber and clarify dosage for this patient.
    e. Trastuzumab ordered appropriately for this patient. No clarification is indicated.

Answer a is incorrect. Trastuzumab is not associated with nausea and vomiting that requires pretreatment antiemetic therapy.

Answer b is incorrect. Trastuzumab should not be administered as an IV bolus injection.

Answer c is incorrect. Trastuzumab has been shown effective as treatment for both micrometastatic and metastatic breast cancer characterized by overexpression of HER-2.

Answer d is correct. The standard initial dose for this patient would be 4 mg/kg or 320 mg for this patient. It would be appropriate to clarify this patient's dose.

Answer e is incorrect. Clarification of the dose ordered for this patient is warranted.

---

17. A 65-year-old patient brings in her tamoxifen prescription for a refill. Upon reviewing her medication profile you discover that she began taking tamoxifen 20 mg daily in June 2000 for the prevention of breast cancer and she has been having it refilled regularly since then. What if anything do should you discuss with the patient's physician?
    a. The recommended duration of tamoxifen when prescribed to decrease the risk of breast cancer is 10 years. There is no need to clarify this patient's tamoxifen regimen.
    b. The merits of increasing the dose to 40 mg daily based on results of a recent study documenting superior efficacy of a 40 mg daily dose.
    c. Switching this patient to an AI based on recent studies that have documented improvement in efficacy and tolerability with AIs.
    d. The merits of decreasing the dose to 10 mg daily based on results of a recent study documenting equal efficacy but superior tolerability of a 20 mg daily dose.
    e. The recommended duration of tamoxifen when prescribed to decrease the risk of breast cancer is 5 years.

Answer a is incorrect. Results from the NSABP Breast Cancer Prevention Trial established that the risks associated with of continuing tamoxifen beyond 5 years (increased incidence of uterine cancer, deep venous thrombosis) exceeded the benefits.

Answer b is incorrect. The dose of tamoxifen established as effective in the prevention of breast cancer is 20 mg daily.

Answer c is incorrect. Results from the NSABP Breast Cancer Prevention Trial established that the risks associated with continuing tamoxifen beyond 5 years (increased incidence of uterine cancer, deep venous thrombosis) exceeded the benefits.

Answer d is incorrect. The dose of tamoxifen established as effective in the prevention of breast cancer is 20 mg daily.

Answer e is correct. Results from the NSABP Breast Cancer Prevention Trial established that the risks associated with continuing tamoxifen beyond 5 years (increased incidence of uterine cancer, deep venous thrombosis) exceeded the benefits.

---

18. This patient asks you if you could recommend a dietary supplement that has been proven effective in decreasing the risk of breast cancer.

a. You explain that vitamin A 100 IU daily has been proven effective to decrease the risk of breast cancer.
b. You explain that vitamin D 200 mg daily has been proven effective to decrease the risk of breast cancer.
c. You explain that vitamin C 500 IU daily has been proven effective to decrease the risk of breast cancer.
d. You explain that there are not any dietary supplements that have been proven effective in lowering the risk of breast cancer.
e. You explain that vitamin E 100 IU daily has been proven effective to decrease the risk of breast cancer.

Answer a is incorrect. Vitamin A has not been proven effective in reducing the risk of breast cancer.

Answer b is incorrect. Vitamin D has not been proven effective in reducing the risk of breast cancer.

Answer c is incorrect. Vitamin C has not been proven effective in reducing the risk of breast cancer.

Answer d is correct. No dietary supplement has been proven effective in reducing the risk of breast cancer.

Answer e is incorrect. Vitamin E has not been proven effective in reducing the risk of breast cancer.

---

19. According to STAR trial, which of the following medications are equally effective in decreasing the risk of breast cancer in women meeting criteria for being at high risk of developing breast cancer?

a. Tamoxifen and raloxifene
b. Tamoxifen and letrozole
c. Tamoxifen and anastrozole
d. Tamoxifen and toremifene
e. Tamoxifen is the only medication proven effective in reducing the risk of breast cancer

---

Answer a is correct. The STAR trial results proved that both tamoxifen and raloxifene reduced the risk of developing breast cancer in high-risk patients by approximately 50%.

Answer b is incorrect. The STAR trial did not compare the effectiveness of tamoxifen and letrozole for breast cancer risk reduction.

Answer c is incorrect. The STAR trial did not compare the effectiveness of tamoxifen and anastrozole for breast cancer risk reduction.

Answer d is incorrect. The STAR trial did not compare the effectiveness of toremifene and tamoxifen for breast cancer risk reduction.

Answer e is incorrect. The STAR trial results proved both tamoxifen and raloxifene reduced the risk of developing breast cancer in high-risk patients by approximately 50%.

---

20. Which of the following organizations publishes on their website evidence-based clinical practice guidelines for cancers that affect over 90% of patients with cancer?

a. The American Cancer Society
b. The Eastern Cooperative Oncology Group
c. National Comprehensive Cancer Network—Clinical Practice Guidelines in Oncology
d. The National Cancer Institute
e. The American Society of Health-System Pharmacy

Answer a is incorrect. The American Cancer Society website is not a source for evidence-based clinical practice guidelines for cancers that affect over 90% of cancer patients.

Answer b is incorrect. The Eastern Cooperative Oncology Group website is not a source for evidence-based clinical practice guidelines for cancers that affect over 90% of cancer patients.

Answer c is correct. The National Comprehensive Cancer Network—Clinical Practice Guidelines are evidence-based guidelines for the treatment of cancers that affect over 90% of cancer patients. The guidelines can be accessed at the following link: http://www.nccn.org/professionals/physician_gls/f_guidelines.asp.

Answer d is incorrect. The National Cancer Institute website is not a source for evidence-based clinical practice guidelines for cancers that affect over 90% of patients with cancer.

Answer e is incorrect. American Society of Health-System Pharmacy website is not a source for evidence-based clinical practice guidelines for cancers that affect over 90% of cancer patients.

---

21. Arthralgias and myalgias are side effects that patients receiving the following antineoplastic agents are likely to experience.

a. Docetaxel, ixabepilone, letrozole, exemestane
b. Paclitaxel, ixabepilone, anastrozole
c. Anastrozole, exemestane
d. Letrozole, anastrozole, exemestane
e. All of the above

Answers a, b, c, and d are correct.

Answer e is the best answer. Arthralgias and myalgias are commonly experienced by patients taking agents belonging to the taxane, aromatase inhibitor, and epothilone classes.

---

22. Stomatitis is an adverse effect that patients administered with which of the following antineoplastic agents may experience?

a. Doxorubicin, capecitabine, tamoxifen
b. Paclitaxel, ixabepilone, anastrozole
c. Methotrexate, capecitabine, cyclophosphamide
d. Fulvestrant, paclitaxel, capecitabine
e. All of the above

Answer a is incorrect. Stomatitis is not caused by SERMs.

Answer b is incorrect. Stomatitis is not caused by AIs.

Answer c is correct. These cytotoxic chemotherapy agents can all cause stomatitis.

Answer d is incorrect. Stomatitis is not caused by fulvestrant.

Answer e is incorrect. Tamoxifen, anastrozole, fulvestrant do not cause stomatitis.

---

23. Which of the following antineoplastic agents is a vesicant?
    a. 5-Fluorouracil
    b. Fulvestrant
    c. Doxorubicin
    d. Methotrexate
    e. All of the above

Answer a is incorrect. Extravasation of 5-fluorouracil does not cause tissue necrosis.

Answer b is incorrect. Fulvestrant is not a vesicant. It is administered as an IM injection.

Answer c is correct. Extravasation of doxorubicin does cause tissue necrosis. The administration of doxorubicin and other anthracycline antitumor antibiotics should only be performed by trained personnel.

Answer d is incorrect. Extravasation of methotrexate does not cause tissue necrosis.

Answer e is incorrect. Doxorubicin is the only option that is a vesicant.

---

24. Which of the following antineoplastic agents would not be effective as adjuvant therapy for postmenopausal patients with breast cancer that is ER negative and does not overexpress HER-2?
    a. Cyclophosphamide
    b. Epirubicin
    c. Doxorubicin
    d. Letrozole
    e. All of the above antineoplastic agents have proven to be effective in such patients

---

Answer a is incorrect. Cyclophosphamide is effective in treating ER negative, HER-2 negative breast cancer.

Answer b is incorrect. Epirubicin is effective in treating ER negative, HER-2 negative breast cancer.

Answer c is incorrect. Doxorubicin is effective in treating ER negative, HER-2 negative breast cancer.

Answer d is correct. Letrozole would not be effective in treating breast cancer that is ER negative.

Answer e is incorrect. Aromatase inhibitors are only indicated for the treatment of ER positive breast cancer.

---

25. Which of the following biologic markers are used to determine appropriate pharmacotherapy for breast cancer patients?
    a. Estrogen receptor
    b. HER-2
    c. Progesterone receptor
    d. Estrogen receptor and HER-2
    e. Estrogen receptor, progesterone receptor, and HER-2

Answer a is correct. Women with breast cancer that is ER positive are likely to benefit from treatment with SERMs and aromatase inhibitors.

Answer b is correct. Women with breast cancer that overexpresses HER-2 are likely to benefit from treatment with trastuzumab.

Answer c is correct. The progesterone receptor is a biologic marker used to determine appropriate pharmacotherapy for patients with breast cancer.

Answer d is correct. Patients with breast cancer will have their cancer cells evaluated for the presence of estrogen receptors, progesterone receptors, and HER-2 overexpression to determine the appropriate therapy.

CHAPTER 15 | Colorectal Cancer

1. Which of the following statements, if any, is considered *false*?
    a. Colon and rectal cancers are usually grouped together in epidemiological studies.
    b. Colon cancer is the third leading cause of cancer incidence in men in the United States.
    c. Colon cancer is the third leading cause of cancer deaths in women in the United States.
    d. Colon cancer mortality has declined over the past few decades.
    e. None of the above is false.

Answer a is true.

Answer b is true. The three leading causes of cancer are prostate, lung, and colorectal in men.

Answer c is true. The three leading causes of cancer death are lung, breast, and colorectal in women.

Answer d is true. Colorectal cancer death rates have been decreasing for over the past 50 years.

Answer e is correct. All of the answer choices are true.

---

2. JM is a 55-year-old African American man concerned about colorectal cancer screening. He inquires about screening recommendations for someone of his age. You reply:
    a. CT/PET of chest, abdomen, and pelvis
    b. Digital rectal examination
    c. Flexible sigmoidoscopy
    d. Colonoscopy
    e. CEA blood test

Answer a is incorrect. Whole body scans have not shown to be an effective monitoring tool for colorectal or any cancer. Unnecessary imaging studies also expose the patient to unnecessary levels of radiation and put a financial burden on the health care system. In contrast, CT colonography is an accepted tool for screening, but is limited by the need for a follow up colonoscopy if any abnormalities like adenomas are discovered.

Answer b is incorrect. However, J.M. should get a digital rectal examination and PSA blood test to detect prostate cancer if he has not gotten one this year.

Answer c is incorrect. Flexible sigmoidoscopy only images the lower part of the colon and requires a follow up full colonoscopy if any abnormalities are found. However, this is a valid screening method for colorectal cancer and an option for JM if he should want it.

Answer d is correct. The advantages of colonoscopy are that the full colon is visualized and any abnormal polyps can be removed for a biopsy. The disadvantages include the invasiveness, cost, and need for sedation.

Answer e is incorrect. CEA may be elevated in other malignant and benign conditions and is not considered a valid screening method for colorectal cancer. The level may be helpful to determine extend of disease already diagnosed by other means, evaluate treatment response, and for recurrence surveillance.

3. Which of the following may decrease a person's risk of colorectal cancer?
    a. Obesity
    b. HNPCC
    c. Hormone replacement therapy (HRT)
    d. Low dietary fiber
    e. Alcoholism

Answer a is incorrect. Obesity would increase risk of colorectal cancer.

Answer b is incorrect. HNPCC would increase risk of colorectal cancer. HNPCC is an inherited disorder that leads to defects in DNA mismatch repair and predisposes a person to a number of different cancers including colorectal, endometrium, ovarian, stomach, among others.

Answer c is correct. HRT lowers risk of colorectal cancer. However, due to other risks associated with HRT, including increased risk of other types of cancers, HRT is not recommended for prophylaxis.

Answer d is incorrect. Low dietary fiber would increase risk of colorectal cancer.

Answer e is incorrect. Alcoholism would increase risk of colorectal cancer.

4. According to national guidelines, what is the recommended age to begin screening for colorectal cancer in a person with average risk?
    a. No later than 21 years old
    b. 40 years old
    c. 45 years old
    d. 50 years old
    e. 65 years old

Answer a is incorrect. Average risk women should receive Pap tests beginning 3 years after first vaginal intercourse, but no later than 21 years old.

Answer b is incorrect. Average risk women should receive annual mammograms starting at age 40.

Answer c is incorrect. High-risk men, such as African Americans, should be offered prostate cancer screening at age 45 per the American Cancer Society with careful consultation about the risks and benefits of screening. Of note, other organizations such as the National Comprehensive Cancer Network recommends a baseline evaluation and consultation begin at age 40.

Answer d is correct. The frequency of screening tests depends on the method of screening.

Answer e is incorrect.

5. Which of the following are signs or symptoms of colon cancer?
    a. Constipation
    b. Abdominal pain
    c. Weight loss
    d. Diarrhea
    e. All of the above

Answers a, b, c, and d are correct.

Answer e is correct and the best answer. Colon cancer symptoms can be nonspecific which makes screening an important method for diagnosis.

6. During a routine colonoscopy, KG was diagnosed with stage I colon cancer but is otherwise healthy. He is experiencing no symptoms and has no complications from his cancer so far. His oncologist will likely recommend which therapy?
    a. Neoadjuvant chemotherapy
    b. Surgery
    c. Radiation
    d. Adjuvant chemotherapy
    e. All of the above

Answer a is incorrect. Neoadjuvant chemotherapy would only be necessary to turn an unresectable cancer into one that can be surgically removed.

Answer b is correct. Surgical removal for cure is the primary therapy for early stage colon cancers.

Answer c is incorrect. Radiation is not commonly used for colon cancer. It is sometimes used if patients are not surgical candidates, if the tumor is very large, or as local therapy to control local recurrences. These treatment strategies are not applicable for this patient.

Answer d is incorrect. Adjuvant chemotherapy is recommended for stage III disease or stage II disease with high-risk features.

Answer e is incorrect.

---

7. Which of the following regimens is recommended first line for adjuvant treatment of stage III colon cancer?
   a. Fluorouracil plus leucovorin
   b. FOLFOX
   c. FOLFIRI
   d. IFL
   e. Fluorouracil plus radiation

Answer a is incorrect. If patients can tolerate a second chemotherapy agent, multiple clinical trials have shown a benefit of adding oxaliplatin to fluoropyrimidine based chemotherapy.

Answer b is correct. The MOSAIC trial demonstrated adding oxaliplatin to infusional fluorouracil in stage III patients. Both increased the disease-free survival and overall survival.

Answer c is incorrect. Adding irinotecan to infusional fluorouracil therapy has not demonstrated clinically significant outcomes in the adjuvant setting, but it can be considered as a first-line therapy for metastatic disease.

Answer d is incorrect. High rates of GI toxicity have made bolus fluorouracil plus irinotecan no longer recommended standard therapy for colon cancers.

Answer e is incorrect. Chemoradiation is a first-line adjuvant therapy for rectal cancers.

---

8. Which of the following statements about colorectal cancer is *false*?
   a. Surgery and other local therapies are almost never a valid option.
   b. Colon cancer tends to first spread to the liver.
   c. Survival is significantly worse than early stage disease.
   d. FOLFOX+/– bevacizumab can be used as a first-line therapy.
   e. FOLFIRI+/– bevacizumab can be used as a first-line therapy.

Answer a is false. If patient has limited metastatic disease, for example, an isolated liver metastasis, patients may still be offered local therapies including surgery. Surgery or radiation can also be palliative if patients are experiencing complications from the cancer like a malignant bowel obstruction.

Answer b is true. Lung is the second most common site of metastases.

Answer c is true. Newer therapies have extended median survival of stage IV colon cancer patients but prognosis is still poor which makes screening and early detection very important.

Answer d is true. Sequencing does not seem to be as important in metastatic disease (eg, which agents to use first) as long as a patient eventually is able to get all types of agents.

Answer e is true. Although the FDA-approved labeling for bevacizumab is for combination with IFL, FOLFIRI is generally recommended instead due to improved tolerability.

---

9. Review the following prescription for capecitabine for a female patient with colon cancer who weighs 123 lb and is 65 inches tall (BSA = 1.6 m^2):

   Capecitabine (Xenical) 500 mg tablets. Take 4 tablets po bid 30 minutes after a meal.

   Take medication for 14 days then do not take for 7 days rest period. Repeat cycle every 21 days.

   Qty: 112 tablets Refills: 2

Identify an error with the above prescription that will require clarification with the prescriber.

   a. Frequency
   b. Route
   c. Instructions in regards to food
   d. Schedule of 14 days on medicine and 7 days off medicine
   e. Drug name

Answer a is not an error. Starting doses usually range from 1000 mg/m^2/dose to 1250 mg/m^2/dose given bid.

Answer b is not an error. Be sure to recommend caution and should be handled and disposed off as hazardous materials.

Answer c is not an error. Taking capecitabine on an empty stomach may cause a higher C_{max} (maximum drug concentration) and toxicities.

Answer d is not an error. Most regimens are given 14 days on and seven days off repeated every 3 weeks. There are many exceptions, but all regimens should include built-in rest periods.

Answer e is written in error. The brand name of capecitabine is Xeloda. Xenical is orlistat, a weight loss prescription medication.

---

10. PL is a 67-year-old man with a history of diabetes mellitus (DM)and alcoholism at the clinic for his seventh cycle of oxaliplatin. He is currently taking capecitabine at home. PL's CBC (complete blood count) with differential is all within normal limits. Before preparing the oxaliplatin for infusion, which other parameters would significantly determine if he requires a dose reduction or his dose to be held?

i. Renal function estimated by creatinine clearance
ii. Liver function estimated by AST, ALT, total bilirubin
iii. Assessment of neurotoxicity side effects

a. i only
b. ii only
c. i and ii
d. i and iii
e. i, ii, and iii

Answer a is incorrect.

Answer b is incorrect. Hepatic metabolism is not a major pathway of oxaliplatin clearance and should not affect the dose. However, severe impairment should prompt you to carefully monitor capecitabine toxicities due to reduced clearance.

Answer c is incorrect.

Answer d is correct. Oxaliplatin is primarily renally excreted like other platinum chemotherapy agents. There are creatinine clearance specific recommendations in the FDA approved labeling, but caution is recommended for severe renal dysfunction. The labeling does have dose modification guidelines based on grade 2 persistent neurosensory events and recommends consideration to discontinue therapy for grade 3 events. Dose modifications are also recommended for severe GI toxicities and myelosuppression.

Answer e is incorrect.

---

11. PL is now on day 10 of his capecitabine and oxaliplatin chemotherapy (XELOX or CAPOX). He reports a dry, painful rash on the soles of his feet making it nearly impossible to ambulate and his hands are red and blistered with moist desquamation. Which of the following would you recommend?

   i. Recommend to PL's oncologist that capecitabine is the cause and to hold treatment until dermatologic toxicities resolve.
   ii. Recommend to PL's oncologist that capecitabine is the cause and to finish this current cycle and consider a dose reduction for next cycle.
   iii. Recommend to PL to liberally apply moisturizing creams, avoid constant rubbing or pressure, and/or take pyridoxine (vitamin B_6).

   a. i only
   b. ii only
   c. i and iii
   d. ii and iii
   e. None of the above

Answer a is incorrect.

Answer b is incorrect. PL's symptoms would be scored grade 3 (severe). Most capecitabine regimens and the FDA-approved labeling suggest holding therapy for grade 2 toxicities until they resolve.

Answer c is correct. Constant rubbing pressure like tight fitting shoes or clothing can increase the risk and severity of hand-foot rash. Moisturizing creams and pyridoxine may help treat and prevent this side effect and are generally recommended but evidence is lacking.

Answer d is incorrect.

Answer e is incorrect.

---

12. NK is a 47-year-old woman with stage IV colon cancer who calls your pharmacy 3 days after receiving FOLFIRI (infusional fluorouracil, leucovorin, and irinotecan). She said she picked up some over-the-counter loperamide (Imodium A-D) and is unsure how to take it. She just had a loose bowel movement, and she feels like the urgency has not gone away. What would be the best response?

   i. Loperamide 4 mg now, then 2 mg after each loose stool, not to exceed eight tablets (16 mg) per day
   ii. Loperamide 4 mg now, then 2 mg every 2 hours until diarrhea free for 12 hours
   iii. You should have taken loperamide 2 mg every 6 hours around the clock starting 1 day after irinotecan to prevent diarrhea

   a. i only
   b. ii only
   c. i and iii
   d. ii and iii
   e. None of the above

Answer a is incorrect. Irinotecan can cause severe and sometimes fatal diarrhea. Patients should not adhere to any preset limits to loperamide as long as they are still experiencing diarrhea.

Answer b is correct. If the patient is unable to keep hydrated with an electrolyte solution, have the patient contact their oncologists for an escalation to other antidiarrheals and/or IV hydration.

Answer c is incorrect.

Answer d is incorrect. Loperamide should only be taken if the patient has experienced diarrhea, and not as prophylaxis.

Answer e is incorrect.

---

13. BK is receiving FOLFOX chemotherapy. Which of the following should BK avoid most in the short term for the purpose of avoiding acute neurotoxicity exacerbations caused by oxaliplatin?

   a. Direct sunlight
   b. Cold
   c. Heat
   d. Tight fitting clothing
   e. OTC acne treatments

Answer a is incorrect. BK should still avoid direct sunlight or use protective creams because fluorouracil can cause photosensitivity.

Answer b is correct. Oxaliplatin commonly causes an acute sensory neuropathy that is precipitated or exacerbated by cold temperatures.

Answer c is incorrect. Extreme heat should be avoided with infusional fluorouracil administration to minimize complications with palmar plantar erythrodysesthesias (PPE) that can be worsened by extreme heat. PPE is more common with capecitabine or prolonged infusions of fluorouracil.

Answer d is incorrect. Tight fitting clothing can predispose that area to PPE rash.

Answer e is incorrect. OTC acne treatments potentially are used inappropriately in patients receiving EGFR1 agents such as cetuximab or panitumumab due to the rash resembling acne.

---

14. What of the following is an adverse reaction that is likely to occur with bevacizumab therapy?
    a. Hypertension
    b. Proteinuria
    c. Delayed wound healing
    d. Bleeding and thrombotic events
    e. All of the above are important adverse reactions to monitor

---

Answer a is correct. Hypertension is a frequent adverse effect and can be severe and life threatening. Monitor blood pressure regularly and initiate pharmacotherapy when indicated.

Answer b is correct. Patients have rarely progressed to nephrotic syndrome. Monitor urine protein and follow up 2+ level or greater with a 24-hour urine collection. Alternatively, some clinicians choose to monitor the urine protein/urine creatinine ratio.

Answer c is correct. The FDA-approved labeling has a black box warning to delay elective surgeries at least 28 days after bevacizumab and to hold bevacizumab at least 28 days following surgery and until the patient is fully healed. Immediately discontinue bevacizumab if a patient has any wound dehiscence.

Answer d is correct. Fatal hemorrhages have been reported with bevacizumab therapy. Thrombotic events tended to be arterial in nature (eg, CVA, MI, TIA).

Answer e is correct and the best answer.

---

15. GW is a 58-year-old man with metastatic colon cancer on irinotecan plus cetuximab therapy. When he arrives to the infusion center he is complaining of new "pimples" appearing all over his chest and face. The oncology nurse asks you to counsel him on managing this new finding. Your counselling points would include all of the following *except*:
    a. Recommend him to ask his doctor about isotretinoin, give him the FDA approved med guide, and explain about the iPLEDGE program to reduce birth defects.
    b. Recommend him to apply moisturizing lotion to the affected areas.
    c. Warn him to use sunscreen since direct sunlight can exacerbate his condition.
    d. Recommend him to ask his doctor about initiating a tetracycline like doxycycline or minocycline.
    e. Reassure him that this side effect actually may be predictive of a positive tumor response to this regimen.

Answer a is correct. This is not an appropriate counseling point. Although rash caused by EGFR agents have been described in the literature as acneiform, typical acne treatments like retinoids will have no efficacy and may even exacerbate the rash.

Answer b is incorrect. This is a valid counseling point. Moisturizing lotions and creams may be counterintuitive to patients who are not applying them to "pimples" so they will require to be educated to use these agents liberally.

Answer c is incorrect. This is a valid counseling point. Recommend sun precautions such as hats and clothing or adequate sun block.

Answer d is incorrect. This is a valid counseling point. Tetracyclines have been shown to be useful in treating EGFR rash to reduce its severity, albeit with little clinical evidence.

Answer e is incorrect. This is a valid counseling point. Although response is correlated with rash, severe rash may still require dose modifications or delays of cetuximab.

---

16. Which pair of therapies for colorectal cancer has the highest concerns for hypersensitivity reactions?
    a. Irinotecan and bevacizumab
    b. Capecitabine and oxaliplatin
    c. Panitumumab and fluorouracil
    d. Oxaliplatin and cetuximab
    e. None of the above causes hypersensitivity reactions

Answer a is incorrect. Irinotecan can cause a cholinergic syndrome acutely after administration. Bevacizumab is a humanized monoclonal antibody that has not shown particular risks for infusion or hypersensitivity reactions.

Answer b is incorrect. Capecitabine hypersensitivity reactions are rare. Oxaliplatin, like other platinum chemotherapies (cisplatin and carboplatin), should be monitored carefully for hypersensitivity reactions.

Answer c is incorrect. Panitumumab is a fully human monoclonal antibody and has shown fewer infusion or hypersensitivity reactions than cetuximab.

Answer d is correct. Both oxaliplatin and cetuximab's FDA-approved labeling contains black box warnings against hypersensitivity reactions. Monitor patients receiving these agents carefully and have reversal agents readily available (ie, antihistamines, epinephrine, corticosteroids, bronchodilators, oxygen).

Answer e is incorrect. All medications have the potential for hypersensitivity reactions. Although the risk is decreased in comparison to the chimeric monoclonal antibody cetuximab, panitumumab's FDA-approved labeling also contains a black box warning against severe infusion reactions.

---

17. UGT1A1*28 mutations have been shown to cause what change in pharmacokinetics?
    a. Decreased fluorouracil clearance
    b. Increased fluorouracil clearance
    c. Decreased irinotecan clearance
    d. Increased irinotecan clearance
    e. None of the above

Answer a is incorrect. UGT1A1*28 mediated glucuronidation is not important for fluorouracil clearance. In contrast, DPD deficiency can significantly reduce fluorouracil clearance.

Answer b is incorrect.

Answer c is correct. Patients with homozygous mutations in the UGT1A1*28 allele are recommended by the FDA-approved labeling to reduce starting doses of UGT1A1*28 by one level. Patients with heterozygous mutations have reduced clearance, but dose reductions are not empirically recommended.

Answer d is incorrect.

Answer e is incorrect.

---

18. All of the following would increase the risk of toxicity of fluorouracil *except*:
    a. DPD deficiency
    b. K-ras mutation
    c. Choose bolus administration instead of infusional administration
    d. Coadminister with leucovorin
    e. Increase the dose

Answer a is incorrect. Fluorouracil is contraindicated in patients with known DPD deficiency due to accumulation of active metabolites.

Answer b is correct. K-ras mutations are an important prognostic indicator (mutations conveys a poorer prognosis) and is predictive of nonresponse to EGFR1 agents including cetuximab and panitumumab. It has not been shown to affect fluorouracil therapy.

Answer c is incorrect. Bolus regimens such as the Mayo Clinic regimen have shown increase myelosuppression, mucositis, and diarrhea in comparison to infusional fluorouracil.

Answer d is incorrect. Leucovorin stabilizes the binding of the active metabolite of fluorouracil (FdUMP) to thymidylate synthetase, increasing the activity.

Answer e is incorrect. Fluorouracil, like most chemotherapy, shows a direct dose-response relationship.

---

19. All of the following brand names or abbreviations are correctly matched with their generic name *except*:
    a. 5-FU = fluorouracil
    b. CPT-11 = irinotecan
    c. Elitek = oxaliplatin
    d. Vectibix = panitumumab
    e. Avastin = bevacizumab

Answer a is correctly matched. 5-FU is commonly used as a shorthand abbreviation.

Answer b is correctly matched. CPT-11 is a commonly used shorthand abbreviation of irinotecan.

Answer c is incorrectly matched. Oxaliplatin's trade name is Eloxatin. Elitek is rasburicase, a drug used to prevent tumor lysis syndrome.

Answer d is correctly matched. Vectibix is the trade name for panitumumab.

Answer e is correctly matched. Avastin is the trade name for bevacizumab.

---

20. Most cancer therapies are dosed per body surface area. All of the following medications are dose in mg/m^2 *except*:
    a. Fluorouracil
    b. Oxaliplatin
    c. Irinotecan
    d. Bevacizumab
    e. Cetuximab

Answers a, b, c, and e are incorrect. These are dosed as mg/m^2.

Answer d is correct. Bevacizumab is dosed as mg/kg per the FDA-approved labeling.

CHAPTER 16 | Skin and Melanoma

1. Select the risk factor(s) associated with melanoma.
    a. Presence of multiple dysplastic nevi
    b. Presence of genetic factors
    c. Individuals with fair skin type who sunburns easily
    d. All of the above are risk factors associated with melanoma

---

Answer a is correct. Presence of multiple dysplastic nevi is a risk factor associated with melanoma.

Answer b is correct. Presences of genetic factors are risk factors associated with melanoma.

Answer c is correct. Individuals with fair skin type who sunburn easily are more likely to develop melanoma, whereas individuals with darker skin types are less likely to develop melanoma.

Answer d is incorrect and the best answer.

2. Which of the following statements is true regarding the subtypes of melanoma?
   a. Superficial spreading melanomas are the most common type of melanoma with lesions usually arising from preexisting nevus.
   b. Nodular melanomas are slow-growing lesions that develop and spread in a vertical growth phase pattern.
   c. Lentigo maligna melanomas are more commonly reported in children, with lesions less likely to metastasize.
   d. Uveal melanomas are rare lower extremity malignancies arising from pigmented epithelium of the choroids, with lesions more likely to metastasize to liver.

Answer a is correct. Superficial spreading melanoma is the most common type of melanoma, making up about 70% of all cases of melanoma, and is more common in women than men. The lesions usually arise from a *preexisting* nevus, with initial presentation appearing as flat which later develops as irregular and asymmetrical.

Answer b is incorrect. Nodular melanoma is the second most common type of melanoma, making up about 15% to 30% of all cases of melanoma, and is more common in men than women. Unlike superficial spreading melanoma, nodular melanoma has a more *aggressive and rapid growth pattern*, with lesions develop and spread in a vertical growth phase pattern. The lesions are usually dark blue-black and uniform in color, and are most commonly located on the head, neck, and trunk.

Answer c is incorrect. Lentigo maligna melanoma comprises a smaller percentage of all cases of melanoma and commonly occurs in *older age group*, typically located on the face of elderly Caucasians. Compared to the other subtypes of melanoma, lentigo maligna melanoma does not usually metastasize.

Answer d is incorrect. Uveal melanoma is an *ocular* melanoma which arises from the pigmented epithelium of the choroids. Although incidence of uveal melanoma is rare, it is the most common intraocular lesions reported in adults, with metastases most frequently occurring in the liver.

3. Which of the following is not a part of the ABCDE rule used to identify and evaluate a suspicious lesion?
   a. Asymmetry
   b. Border irregularity
   c. Color of lesions
   d. Depths of the lesions
   e. Evolving or changing characteristics of a lesion

Answer a is correct. *A* is asymmetry where one-half of the mole does not match the other half.

Answer b is correct. *B* is border irregularity where the edges of the mole are often irregular, blurred, ragged, or notched.

Answer c is correct. *C* is color where the color of the mole is not uniform, it may appear with different shades of tan or blue-black, and sometimes mixed with colors of red, purple, and white.

Answer d is incorrect. *D* is diameter where lesions are often > 6 mm in diameter, although melanoma can sometimes present with lesions of < 6 mm in diameter (ACS).

Answer e is correct. *E* is evolving or changing characteristics of a lesion.

4. Once a suspicious lesion is identified, which is the best method in confirming the diagnosis?
   a. Obtain a complete clinical examination, medical history of patient and family members.
   b. Obtain complete laboratory studies with hematology, electrolytes, liver function test, and LDH.
   c. Consider full-thickness excisional biopsy with 1 to 3 mm margin of normal-appearing skin.
   d. Consider ordering a chest x-ray and a CT scan for confirming diagnosis.

Answer a is incorrect. A complete clinical examination, medical history of patient and family members is done to identify and assess potential risk factors, but not enough to confirm the diagnosis of melanoma.

Answer b is incorrect. Laboratory studies including hematology, electrolytes, liver function test, and/or LDH are done to identify and assess the clinical status of patient, not to confirm the diagnosis of melanoma.

Answer c is correct. Biopsy of the suspicious lesions is the only way to confirm the diagnosis of melanoma. A full-thickness excisional biopsy with 1 to 3 mm margin of normal-appearing skin is the preferred method of choice as it removes the entire lesion.

Answer d is incorrect. Diagnostic tests such as chest x-ray, CT scan, MRI, PET scan, and/or bone scan are used to identify and assess for possible local regional lymph nodes involvement or metastases, and are not used to confirm the diagnosis of melanoma.

5. Select the American Cancer Society (ACS) recommendation(s) for the prevention and screening of melanoma.
   a. Wear proper protective clothing to cover as much exposed skin as possible (ie, sun glasses, hat with wide brim, long sleeve clothing, etc).
   b. Use sunscreen lotion with an SPF of at least 15 or higher.
   c. Avoid direct sun exposure between 10 AM to 4 PM when ultraviolet rays are the most intense.

d. Avoid the use of tanning beds or sunlamps to minimize exposure to ultraviolet radiation.
e. All of the above are recommendations made by ACS for the prevention and screening of melanoma.

Answer a is correct. Protect your skin from sun exposure by wearing clothing. Long-sleeved shirts, long skirts, or long pants offer the most protection. Dark colored clothing offers more protection than light colored clothing.

Answer b is correct. Use sunscreen and lip balms with at least an SPF factor of 15 or higher on areas where skin is exposed to the sun. Best to apply sunscreen about 20 to 30 minutes prior to sun exposure, and reapply at least every 2 hours or more frequently if you sweat or swim for maximum benefits.

Answer c is correct. Avoid direct sun exposure between 10 AM to 4 PM when the ultraviolet radiations are the most intense. Practice sun safety if you have to be outdoors by wearing protective clothing and use sunscreen.

Answer d is correct. Avoid the use of tanning beds or sunlamps to minimize exposure to ultraviolet radiation. There is more evidence on the potential hazards of the ultraviolet radiation they deliver and the increase risk of melanoma.

Answer e is correct and the best answer. All of the above are recommendations made by ACS for the prevention and screening of melanoma.

---

6. Select the chemotherapeutic agent regimen used for the treatment of stage IV metastatic melanoma.

a. CVD regimen
b. Dacarbazine
c. Carmustine
d. a and b
e. All of the above are chemotherapeutic agent or regimen use for the treatment of stage IV metastatic melanoma

---

Answer a is correct. The CVD regimen is a chemotherapy regimen used for the treatment of stage IV metastatic melanoma. It contains combination chemotherapy using cisplatin, vinblastine, and dacarbazine. Multiple variations of dosages and schedule exist in clinical practice.

Answer b is correct. Dacarbazine is an FDA-approved chemotherapy agent for treatment of stage IV metastatic melanoma as single agent or in combination with other chemotherapeutic agents.

Answer c is incorrect. Carmustine is part of a chemotherapeutic regimen that is used to treat stage IV melanomas, but it is not used as monotherapy.

Answer d is correct and the best answer.

Answer e is incorrect.

---

7. Which of the following oral chemotherapeutic agent has been used in the treatment of melanoma?

a. Capecitabine
b. Lapatinib
c. Erlotinib
d. Procarbazine
e. Temozolomide

Answer a is incorrect. Capecitabine (Xeloda) is FDA approved for metastatic colorectal and breast cancer, and as adjuvant for stage III colon cancer.

Answer b is incorrect. Lapatinib (Tykerb) is FDA approved for advanced or metastatic breast cancer in combination with capecitabine.

Answer c is incorrect. Erlotinib (Tarceva) is FDA approved for advanced or metastatic non–small-cell lung and pancreatic cancer.

Answer d is incorrect. Procarbazine (Matulane) is FDA approved for Hodgkin disease as part of the MOPP chemotherapy regimen which contains chemotherapy with ***M***echlorethamine, ***O***ncovin, ***P***rocarbazine, and ***P***rednisone.

Answer e is correct. Temozolomide (Temodar) is an oral chemotherapy agent which is used as an off-label, non-FDA approved indication in advanced or metastatic melanoma as single agent or in combination with other chemotherapy agent.

---

8. Select the side effect(s) associated with the use of high-dose interleukin-2 (IL-2) for the treatment of melanoma.

a. Flu-like symptoms
b. Myelosuppression
c. Constipation
d. a and b
e. All of the above

Answer a is correct. Flu-like symptoms including fever, chills, malaise, myalgias, and arthralgias were observed in all patients receiving high-dose IL-2. Consider premedication with an antipyretic (ie, acetaminophen) prior to treatment with IL-2.

Answer b is correct. Myelosuppression with neutropenia, anemia, and thrombocytopenia have all been reported, monitor patients closely for any infectious process.

Answer c is incorrect. Constipation is not commonly observed with IL-2.

Answer d is correct and the best answer. Other side effects associated with IL-2 include:

1. Vascular or capillary leak syndrome is a dose-limiting toxicity also commonly reported with IL-2. It can be observed immediately after initiation of therapy, clinical presentations may include weight gain, ascites, peripheral

edema, arrhythmias and/or tachycardia, hypotension, oliguria and renal insufficiency, pleural effusions, and pulmonary congestion.

2. Both acute and chronic neurologic or neuropsychiatric symptoms, including somnolence, delirium, and confusion have been observed and generally resolve when therapy is discontinued. **Answer e is incorrect.**

---

9. CD is a 28-year-old woman who is to start chemotherapy treatment with high-dose interferon-alfa 2b. Select the side effect(s) associated with interferon.

   a. Flu-like symptoms requiring premedication with antipyretic
   b. Fatigue
   c. Depression
   d. Somnolence and confusion
   e. All of the above

Answer a is correct. Flu-like symptoms with fever, chills headache, myalgias, and arthralgias occur in more than 80% of patients. Symptoms usually occur few hours after treatment and can last up to 24 hours and can be dose-limiting for some patients. Incidence of symptoms is lower with subsequent injections. Premedication with an antipyretic (ie, acetaminophen or indomethacin) is recommended to minimize risk and severity of fever and chills.

Answer b is correct. Fatigue (8%-96%) is a dose-limiting side effect associated with high-dose interferon-alfa 2b. Caution if used in patients (> 65 years of age) as these patients are at increased risk of developing fatigue and neurological toxicities secondary to high-dose interferon-alfa 2b.

Answer c is correct. Depression (3%-40%) is commonly associated with high-dose interferon-alfa 2b. Caution if used in patients with history of depression and/or other psychological disorders, or in patients (> 65 years of age) as these patients are at increased risk of developing neurological toxicities secondary to high-dose interferon-alfa 2b.

Answer d is correct. Somnolence and confusion are commonly associated with high-dose interferon-alfa 2b. Caution if used in patients (> 65 years of age) as these patients are at increased risk of developing neurological toxicities secondary to high-dose interferon-alfa 2b.

Answer e is correct and the best answer.

---

10. Select the medication that may be used concurrently with high-dose Aldesleukin *except*:

    a. Dexamethasone
    b. Indomethacin
    c. Losartan
    d. Granisetron

Answer a is correct. Dexamethasone is a corticosteroid. The use of corticosteroids should be avoided in patients receiving treatment with high-dose interleukin-2 (Aldesleukin). Corticosteroids decrease the antitumor effects of IL-2 due to its inhibitory effect on the immune system.

Answer b is correct. Indomethacin is a nonsteroid anti-inflammatory agent. The use of nonsteroid anti-inflammatory agents should be avoided in patients receiving treatment with high-dose interleukin-2 (Aldesleukin). NSAIDs increase the risk of capillary leak syndrome.

Answer c is correct. Losartan is an antihypertensive agent. The use of antihypertensives should be avoided in patients receiving treatment with high-dose interleukin-2 (Aldesleukin). Antihypertensives potentiate the hypotensive effects of IL-2.

Answer d is incorrect. Granisetron is a 5-HT3 receptor antagonist antiemetic agent and has no reported interaction with high-dose IL-2.

---

11. Select the side effect(s) associated with dacarbazine.

    i. Leukopenia
    ii. Increased appetite
    iii. Flu-like symptoms

    a. i
    b. i and iii
    c. ii and iii
    d. iii

Myelosuppression (eg, leukopenia and thrombocytopenia) are dose-limiting toxicities commonly associated with treatment of dacarbazine.

Increased appetite is not a side effect commonly associated with the treatment of dacarbazine. Anorexia (< 10%) has been reported with dacarbazine.

Flu-like symptoms (< 10%) including fever, chills, malaise, myalgias, and arthralgias lasting several days after therapy have been reported as side effects sometimes associated with the treatment of dacarbazine.

Other effects of dacarbazine include nausea and vomiting—dacarbazine is considered a highly emetogenic chemotherapeutic agent. Local pain and burning sensation at injection site have been reported with infusion of dacarbazine.

Answer b is correct.

---

12. CY is a 25-year-old man with stage IV metastatic melanoma receiving biochemotherapy treatment with cisplatin, vinblastine, dacarbazine, interferon-alfa 2b, and interleukin-2. His laboratory values prior to treatment are within normal limits. Select the supportive care management for CY's biochemotherapy treatment.

    i. Premedication with acetaminophen
    ii. Premedication with dolasetron and dexamethasone
    iii. Premedication with atropine 0.25 mg IV push

    a. ii only
    b. iii only
    c. ii and iii

d. i and ii
e. i and iii

Acetaminophen should be used as part of premedication for patients receiving biochemotherapy with CVD + interferon-alfa 2b + interleukin-2 to minimize risk and severity of fever and chills commonly observed with interferon-alfa 2b and interleukin-2.

Dolasetron and dexamethasone are antiemetic regimen recommended for moderate to highly emetogenic chemotherapy and should be used as part of premedication for patients receiving biochemotherapy with CVD + interferon-alfa 2b + interleukin-2 as the regimen is considered a highly emetogenic regimen with cisplatin and dacarbazine as part of the chemotherapy treatment.

Atropine is an anticholinergic agent and its use as part of premedication for patients receiving biochemotherapy with CVD + interferon-alfa 2b + interleukin-2 is not indicated.

Other supportive care treatments include: Pre- and post-hydration using 1 L of normal saline (NS) + 20 mEq KCL + 2 g magnesium sulfate infused over 3 hours before and after cisplatin (total of 2 L fluid) is an appropriate supportive care management used to minimize potential nephrotoxicity commonly associated with cisplatin, and should be used for patients receiving biochemotherapy with CVD + interferon-alfa 2b + interleukin-2.

Answer d is the correct answer.

---

13. Which of the following is the correct FDA-approved dosing of dacarbazine when used as single agent for treatment of melanoma?

a. 375 mg/m^2 IVPB on days 1 and 15 with cycle repeat every 28 days
b. 20 million IU/m^2 IVPB five times weekly for 4 weeks, then 10 million IU/m^2 subcutaneously three times weekly for 48 weeks
c. 250 mg/m^2 IVPB on days 1 to 5 with cycle repeat every 21 days
d. 600,000 IU/kg IVPB every 8 hours for a maximum of 14 doses; repeat after 9 days for a total of 28 doses per course
e. 150 mg/m^2 po daily for 5 days with cycle repeat every 28 days

---

Answers a, b, c, d are incorrect. None is correct dosing of dacarbazine when used as single agent for treatment of melanoma.

Answer c is correct. The FDA-approved dosing of dacarbazine when used as single agent for treatment of melanoma is 150 to 250 mg/m^2 IVPB on days 1 to 5 with cycle repeat every 21 days.

---

14. Which of the following is the correct FDA-approved dosing of Interferon-alfa 2b when used as single agent for treatment of melanoma?

a. 375 mg/m^2 IVPB on days 1 and 15 with cycle repeat every 28 days
b. 20 million IU/m^2 IVPB five times weekly for 4 weeks, then 10 million IU/m^2 subcutaneously three times weekly for 48 weeks
c. 250 mg/m^2 IVPB on days 1 to 5 with cycle repeat every 21 days
d. 600,000 IU/kg IVPB every 8 hours for a maximum of 14 doses; repeat after 9 days for a total of 28 doses per course
e. 150 mg/m^2 po daily for 5 days with cycle repeat every 28 days

---

Answers a, c, d, e are incorrect. None is correct dosing of interferon-alpha 2b when used as single agent for treatment of melanoma.

Answer b is correct. The FDA-approved dosing of interferon-alfa 2b when used as single agent for treatment of melanoma is 20 million IU/m^2 IVPB five times weekly for 4 weeks, then 10 million IU/m^2 subcutaneously three times weekly for 48 weeks.

---

15. Which of the following is the correct FDA-approved dosing of interleukin-2 when used as single agent for treatment of melanoma?

a. 375 mg/m^2 IVPB on days 1 and 15 with cycle repeat every 28 days
b. 20 million IU/m^2 IVPB five times weekly for 4 weeks, then 10 million IU/m^2 subcutaneously three times weekly for 48 weeks
c. 250 mg/m^2 IVPB on days 1 to 5 with cycle repeat every 21 days
d. 600,000 IU/kg IVPB every 8 hours for a maximum of 14 doses; repeat after 9 days for a total of 28 doses per course
e. 150 mg/m^2 po daily for 5 days with cycle repeat every 28 days

---

Answers a, b, c, e are incorrect. None is correct dosing of interleukin-2 when used as single agent for treatment of melanoma.

Answer d is correct. The FDA-approved dosing of interleukin-2 when used as single agent for treatment of melanoma is 600,000 IU/kg IVPB every 8 hours for a maximum of 14 doses; repeat after 9 days for a total of 28 doses per course. Retreat if needed in 7 weeks after previous course.

---

16. Select the answer that represents follow-up care recommendations for patients with melanoma.

a. Annual skin examination and surveillance by a dermatologist for all patients with melanoma regardless of stage of lesions.
b. Educate patients to perform monthly self-examination of their skin and lymph nodes.
c. Educate patients about skin cancer prevention including sun protection and proper use of sunscreen with at least SPF of 15 or higher.
d. All of the above.

Answer a is correct. Lifetime annual skin examination and surveillance by a dermatologist for all patients with melanoma regardless to stage of lesions, and including those with stage 0, in situ melanoma is recommended by the National Comprehensive Cancer Network (NCCN) clinical practice guidelines for melanoma.

Answer b is correct. The NCCN clinical practice guidelines for melanoma recommend clinicians to consider educating patients to perform monthly self-examination of their skin and lymph nodes. Any suspicious lesions should be followed up with health care professional for further work-up and evaluation.

Answer c is correct. Patients and their family should be educated on skin cancer prevention including sun protection measures and the proper use of sunscreen with at least SPF of 15 or higher.

Answer d is correct and the best answer.

---

17. Select the central nervous system side effect associated with interferon.

    i. Depression
    ii. Confusion
    iii. Somnolence
    iv. Hepatotoxicity

    a. i only
    b. iv only
    c. i, iii, and iv
    d. i, ii, and iii
    e. i and iv

Interferon is associated with a significant amount of side effects; for example, neuropsychiatric effects (depression, confusion, and somnolence) are frequently reported. The neuropsychiatric effects have led to a blackbox warning for the interferon products.

Hepatotoxicity is a side effect of interferon products, but it is not a central nervous system side effect.

Answer d is the correct answer.

---

18. Select the parameters that should be monitored with dacarbazine.

    i. Complete blood count
    ii. Liver function tests
    iii. Injection site reactions

    a. i and ii
    b. ii and iii
    c. i, ii, and iii
    d. i and iii

A complete blood count should be monitored because of myelosuppression.

Liver function tests should be monitored because of hepatotoxicity.

Injection site reactions should be monitored because of local pain, burning sensation, and irritation at the injection site (extravasation).

Answer c is the correct answer.

---

19. Select the receptor antagonists that should be administered with the alkylating agent dacarbazine.

    a. Temozolomide
    b. Interleukin-2
    c. Ondansetron
    d. Cisplatin

Answer a is incorrect. Temozolomide is an alkylating agent structurally similar to dacarbazine.

Answer b is incorrect. IL-2 is a miscellaneous antineoplastic agent/biological response modulator.

Answer c is correct. Ondansetron is a 5-HT3 receptor antagonist used for nausea and vomiting associated with the highly emetogenic dacarbazine.

Answer d is incorrect. Cisplatin is an alkylating agent/platinum analog.

---

20. Select the side effect associated with IL-2 that leads to hypotension and reduced organ perfusion.

    a. Capillary leak syndrome
    b. Myelosuppression
    c. Anemia
    d. Hepatotoxicity
    e. Delirium

Answer a is correct. IL-2 is associated with capillary leak syndrome and may lead to hypotension and reduced organ perfusion (black box warning).

Answer b is incorrect. Myelosuppression is common with IL, but does not lead to hypotension and reduced organ perfusion.

Answer c is incorrect. Anemia is associated with IL-2 therapy, but it is a type of myelosuppression. Other types of myelosuppression include leucopenia, neutropenia, and thrombocytopenia.

Answer d is incorrect. Hepatotoxicity is associated with IL-2 therapy, but it is not associated with hypotension or decrease perfusion.

Answer e is incorrect. Central nervous system (neuropsychiatric symptoms—somnolence, delirium, and confusion) side effects are associated with IL-2, but the CNS effects do not lead to hypotension or decreased perfusion.

CHAPTER 17 | Leukemia

1. AA is a 58-year-old Caucasian man who reports to his primary care physician complaining of 2-week history of fatigue and fever. A CBC with differential reveals an elevated WBC (50,000 U/L) and profound thrombocytopenia (platelets 30,000 U/L). Patient is diagnosed with acute myeloid leukemia (AML-M5). Initial induction therapy should consist of the following:

   a. Mitoxantrone
   b. Cytarabine + idarubicin
   c. Cytarabine + imatinib
   d. Asparaginase

Answer a is incorrect. Mitoxantrone is recommended in adult AML, however, is usually not given as monotherapy for induction. For patients < 60 years old, they should receive standard dose cytarabine + (daunorubicin or idarubicin) per National Comprehensive Cancer Network (NCCN) guidelines.

Answer b is correct. The most active agents in AML are anthracyclines and the antimetabolite cytarabine. Cytarabine in combination with idarubicin is often referred to as "7+3" regimen (cytarabine 100 mg/m^2 days 1-7, idarubicin 12 mg/m^2 days 1-3). Accounting for age, other comorbidities, and patient's ejection fraction, this combination should be recommended for initial induction therapy.

Answer c is incorrect. Imatinib is not recommended in AML induction. Imatinib is recommended in CML, GIST tumors, and Ph+ALL.

Answer d is incorrect. Asparaginase in not recommended in the treatment of adult AML. Asparaginase is recommended in pediatric and adult ALL regimens.

---

2. Physician asks you about tumor lysis syndrome (TLS) prevention and management for patient AA, suggestions should include:

   a. Initiating allopurinol
   b. Treating electrolyte disturbances
   c. Aggressive hydration
   d. All of the above

Answer a is correct. Allopurinol is indicated in preventing and managing TLS. Allopurinol acts as a competitive inhibitor of xanthine oxidase, thereby blocking the conversion of the purine metabolites to uric acid.

Answer b is correct. Electrolyte disturbances commonly seen in TLS include hyperuricemia, hyperkalemia, hyperphosphatemia, and hypocalcemia. Agents such as sodium polystyrene sulfonate (Kayexalate) for hyperkalemia or oral phosphate binders such as calcium acetate (PhosLo) or sevelamer (Renagel) may be warranted in some clinical situations.

Answer c is correct. Hydration enhances urine flow and promotes the excretion of uric acid and phosphate by improving intravascular volume, renal blood flow, and glomerular filtration. The use of sodium bicarbonate in IV fluids to alkalinize the urine is often performed to protect kidney function.

Answer d is correct and the best answer.

---

3. TLS is characterized by the following:

   a. Hypocalcemia, hypouricemia, hyperkalemia
   b. Hyperphosphatemia, hyperkalemia, hyperuricemia
   c. Hypercalcemia, hyperkalemia, hypomagnesium
   d. Hypokalemia, hyperphosphatemia, hypouricemia

Answer a is incorrect. Hyperuricemia is commonly seen in TLS. Uric acid levels are often > 7.5 mg/dL which may require drug therapy such as rasburicase.

Answer b is correct. Electrolyte disturbances commonly seen in TLS include hyperuricemia, hyperkalemia, hyperphosphatemia, and hypocalcemia.

Answer c is incorrect. Alterations in serum magnesium levels are not associated with TLS.

Answer d is incorrect. Serum potassium and uric acid levels are often increased in TLS.

---

4. AA achieves complete remission following induction therapy and begins high-dose cytarabine (HDAC). What toxicities should AA be counseled on?

   a. Infusion related reactions, paralytic ileus, cardiotoxicity
   b. Cerebellar toxicity, peripheral neuropathy, infusion related reactions
   c. Nausea, peripheral neuropathy, ocular toxicity
   d. Cerebellar toxicity, nausea, ocular toxicity

Answer a is incorrect. Cytarabine is not associated with infusion related reactions, paralytic ileus, or cardiotoxicity.

Answer b is incorrect. Cytarabine is not associated with peripheral neuropathy or infusion related reactions.

Answer c is incorrect. Cytarabine is not associated with peripheral neuropathy.

Answer d is correct. Cytarabine is associated with cerebellar, nausea, and ocular toxicity particularly in the high-dose (g/m^2) setting. Cerebellar toxicity is characterized by nystagmus, slurred speech, and ataxia. HDAC is listed as a moderate emetogenic risk (30%-90% frequency of emesis) agent by NCCN guidelines. Ocular toxicity manifests itself by conjunctivitis, this can be prevented with the use of prophylactic dexamethasone eye drops.

---

5. Which of the following agents is used in the treatment of relapsed AML?

   a. Rituximab (Rituxan)
   b. Mitoxantrone (Novantrone)
   c. Alemtuzumab (Campath)
   d. Imatinib (Gleevec)

Answer a is incorrect. Rituximab is indicated for CD20+ non-Hodgkin lymphoma (NHL).

Answer b is correct. For AML patients who are unable to achieve a CR, refractory/relapsed treatments are available. Cytarabine alone or in combination with fludarabine, mitoxantrone, etoposide, or clofarabine are options.

Answer c is incorrect. Alemtuzumab is a humanized MoAb that is indicated in CLL.

Answer d is incorrect. Imatinib is considered first-line treatment for chronic phase CML and continues to demonstrate durable response rates

6. A newly diagnosed patient with acute promyelocytic leukemia (APL) begins treatment with tretinoin 40 mg orally twice daily. Within 48 hours of the initiation, the patient develops fever, dyspnea, and respiratory distress. Which of the following should be immediately initiated to treat apparent differentiation syndrome (DS)?

   a. Dexamethasone
   b. Acetaminophen
   c. Diphenhydramine
   d. Epinephrine

Answer a is correct. Dexamethasone 10 mg IV every 12 hours is recommended for 3 days or until resolution of symptoms, immediately starting at onset of symptoms of DS. Steroids have shown a mortality benefit.

Answer b is incorrect. Acetaminophen is not recommended in the management of DS.

Answer c is incorrect. Diphenhydramine is not recommended in the management of DS.

Answer d is incorrect. Epinephrine is used for anaphylactic reactions, not applicable in this clinical setting.

7. SS is a 55-year-old African American woman newly diagnosed with acute lymphoblastic leukemia (ALL). Her physician has recommended she receive part A hyper-CVAD regimen (cyclophosphamide, vincristine, doxorubicin, and dexamethasone). What baseline examination should she receive prior to initiating doxorubicin on day 4?

   a. CT scan to assess distant site involvement
   b. Lumbar puncture to determine CNS disease
   c. 24-Hour urine collection to determine renal function
   d. MUGA scan to determine left ventricular ejection fraction (LVEF)

Answer a is incorrect. CT scan to assess distant site involvement is not necessary.

Answer b is incorrect. Although a lumbar puncture should be done in the initial work for ALL, it does not need to be accessed prior to initiating doxorubicin.

Answer c is incorrect. Doxorubicin is hepatically metabolized; this is not necessary prior to initiating doxorubicin.

Answer d is correct. Prior to initiating doxorubicin, an ECG and LVEF (via an ECHO or MUGA scan) to determine baseline cardiac function. The incidence of irreversible myocardial toxicity increases as the total cumulative (lifetime) dosages approach 450 to 500 mg/m^2.

8. SS is to receive CNS prophylaxis. Which of the following agents are given intrathecally (IT)?

   a. Cytarabine
   b. Methotrexate
   c. Vincristine
   d. a and b
   e. All of the above

Answer a is correct. Intrathecal cytarabine is recommended in ALL patients due to CNS involvement.

Answer b is correct. Intrathecal methotrexate is recommended in ALL patients due to CNS involvement.

Answer c is incorrect. Vincristine should never be given intrathecally; this may cause severe neurologic toxicity and/or death.

Answer d is correct and the best answer.

Answer e is incorrect because of the above mentioned information regarding vincristine.

9. You are an oncology pharmacist counseling a parent and their child undergoing treatment for pediatric ALL. Patient will be treated with a Children's Oncology Group (COG) protocol. All of the following adverse events should be discussed with them regarding asparaginase except?

   a. Hyperglycemia
   b. Risk of allergic reactions
   c. Potential for bleeding
   d. Alopecia

Answer a is incorrect. Hyperglycemia/glucose intolerance has been reported in ~10% of patients which receive asparaginase.

Answer b is incorrect. Hypersensitivity reactions are a major concern with patients which receive asparaginase. A test dose is recommended with first dose of therapy. Practitioners are instructed to have epinephrine, diphenhydramine, and hydrocortisone available at bedside due to risk.

Answer c is incorrect. Thrombosis, fatal bleeding, consumption coagulopathy, and intracranial hemorrhage have all been reported.

Answer d is correct. Asparaginase is not associated with alopecia.

10. Which of the following prophylactic agents should be recommended for a CLL patient receiving fludarabine?

    a. Enoxaparin
    b. Sulfamethoxazole/trimethoprim
    c. Pantoprazole
    d. Metronidazole

Answer a is incorrect. DVT prophylaxis is not warranted in a CLL patient receiving fludarabine unless further information was provided.

Answer b is correct. PCP prophylaxis (trimethoprim/sulfamethoxazole DS twice daily three times per week) is recommended for patients receiving fludarabine due to increased risk of opportunistic infections. Also, patients should receive antiviral and antifungal prophylaxis.

Answer c is incorrect. GI prophylaxis is not warranted in a CLL patient receiving fludarabine.

Answer d is incorrect. Although this patient is at an increased risk of infections, preemptive therapy for susceptible anaerobic bacterial and protozoal infections is not warranted.

11. Which of the following statements is false regarding the treatment of chronic lymphocytic leukemia (CLL)?

    a. Early treatment has resulted in improved overall survival.
    b. Fludarabine based therapy has benefit.
    c. Rituximab based combination regimens have demonstrated benefit.
    d. Cyclophosphamide is recommended in CLL.

Answer a is correct. Early treatment has not resulted in improved overall survival in CLL patients. Patients may defer treatment until signs and symptoms of progressive disease appear.

Answer b is incorrect. Fludarabine has shown benefit in multiple CLL regimens and is considered to be an active agent in this disease.

Answer c is incorrect. Rituximab has shown benefit in multiple CLL regimens.

Answer d is incorrect. Cyclophosphamide is used in multiple CLL regimens (in combination with fludarabine, fludarabine + rituximab, and with vincristine + prednisone).

12. Which of the following agents should be recommended in a CLL patient who is presenting with recurring infections?

    a. Annual influenza vaccine
    b. Monthly intravenous immunoglobulin
    c. Pneumococcal vaccine every 5 years
    d. All of the above

Answer a is correct. Annual influenza vaccine is recommended. In patients who have received rituximab, B-cell recovery occurs by approximately 9 months. Prior to B-cell recovery, patients generally do not respond to influenza vaccine and if given should not be considered vaccinated per NCCN guidelines.

Answer b is correct. Due to hypogammaglobinemia which occurs in most CLL patients, select patients should receive monthly IVIG infusions.

Answer c is correct. Per NCCN guidelines, patients should receive a pneumococcal vaccine every 5 years.

Answer d is correct and the best answer.

13. Which of the following is true regarding the monoclonal antibody alemtuzumab (Campath)?

    a. Humanized-targets CD33
    b. Chimeric-targets CD52
    c. Humanized-targets CD52
    d. Chimeric-targets CD20

Answer a is incorrect. A humanized MoAb that targets CD33 is gemtuzumab.

Answer b is incorrect. A chimeric MoAb that targets CD52 is not commercially available.

Answer c is correct. Alemtuzumab is a humanized MoAb that targets CD52 found on B and T lymphocytes.

Answer d is incorrect. A chimeric MoAb that targets CD20 is rituximab.

14. Which of the following should be recommended for patients receiving alemtuzumab (Campath)?

    a. Antifungal prophylaxis
    b. Herpes viral prophylaxis
    c. Pegfilgrastim (Neulasta) for neutropenia
    d. a and b
    e. a and c

Answer a is correct. Due to increased infection risk, it is recommended that patients receiving alemtuzumab receive appropriate antifungal prophylaxis.

Answer b is correct. It is recommended that patients receive herpes viral prophylaxis 2 months post completion of alemtuzumab. Recommended options include acyclovir or famciclovir.

Answer c is incorrect. Myeloid growth factors are not recommended for patients receiving alemtuzumab.

Answer d is correct. See reasons listed above.

Answer e is incorrect. See reasons listed above.

15. Common adverse events with rituximab (Rituxan) include:
    a. Infusion related reactions
    b. Tumor lysis syndrome
    c. Skin rashes
    d. Hepatitis B reactivation
    e. All of the above

Answer a is correct. Infusion related reactions are common and can be severe. Reactions include bronchospasms, hypoxia, hypotension, and in more severe cases pulmonary infiltrates. Infusion related reactions are a blackbox warning.

Answer b is correct. TLS has occurred within first 24 hours of rituximab dose. This is listed as a black box warning.

Answer c is correct. Severe skin rashes (Stevens-Johnson syndrome) have been reported 1 to 13 weeks following exposure. This is a blackbox warning.

Answer d is correct. Hepatitis B reactivation has been reported in patients treated with rituximab in combination with chemotherapy. As a result, it is recommended that hepatitis B testing be performed prior to the initiation of rituximab.

Answer e is correct and the best answer.

---

16. The Philadelphia chromosome (Ph+) results from which of the following?
    a. Translocation of chromosomes 9 and 22
    b. Translocation of chromosomes 8 and 21
    c. Inversion of chromosome 16
    d. Translocation of chromosomes 15 and 17

Answer a is correct. This is the hallmark mutation found in CML. CML results from translocation of genetic material between the long arms of chromosomes 9 and 22, which is referred to as the Philadelphia chromosome (Ph+).

Answer b is incorrect. This translocation occurs in AML and predicts a good prognosis.

Answer c is incorrect. This translocation occurs in AML and predicts a good prognosis.

Answer d is incorrect. This translocation occurs in APL.

---

17. Which of the following is a first-line treatment for chronic myelogenous leukemia?
    a. Allogeneic stem cell transplant
    b. Interferon-α + cytarabine
    c. Imatinib (Gleevec)
    d. Sunitinib (Sutent)

Answer a is incorrect. Patients will receive oral tyrosine kinase inhibitors (imatinib, dasatinib, or nilotinib) prior to stem cell transplant.

Answer b is incorrect. Imatinib was shown to provide better response rates than interferon-α + cytarabine in a clinical trial. This combination regimen is no longer recommended for first-line therapy.

Answer c is correct for the above mentioned reason. Imatinib is recommended as first-line therapy for CML at 400 mg/d in chronic phase CML.

Answer c is incorrect. Sunitinib is FDA approved for renal cell carcinoma and gastrointestinal stromal tumors (GIST).

---

18. Select the brand name for dasatinib.
    a. Tasigna
    b. Sprycel
    c. Tarceva
    d. Nexavar

Answer a is incorrect. Tasigna is the brand name for nilotinib.

Answer b is correct. Sprycel is the brand name for dasatinib.

Answer c is incorrect. Tarceva is the brand name for erlotinib.

Answer d is incorrect. Nexavar is the brand name for sorafenib.

---

19. Which of the following are adverse events associated with dasatinib?
    a. Pleural effusion
    b. Myelosuppression
    c. Alopecia
    d. a and b
    e. b and c

Answer a is correct. Fluid retention is an adverse event associated with dasatinib. Eighteen percent (all grade toxicity) of patients receiving dasatinib at 100 mg/d reported pleural effusions.

Answer b is correct. Treatment with dasatinib is associated with severe (grade 3 or 4) neutropenia, anemia, and thrombocytopenia. CBCs should be performed weekly for the first 2 months and then monthly thereafter, or as clinically indicated.

Answer d is correct and the best answer. See above mentioned reasons.

Answers c and e are incorrect. Alopecia is not a common side effect of dasatinib.

---

20. A newly diagnosed patient with CML receives a script for imatinib 400 mg orally daily. Patient is uninsured and has applied for Medicaid. They arrive at your pharmacy asking questions about this medication. What is the best course of action?

a. Instruct patient to pay with cash.
b. Refer them back to their physician for alternative agent.
c. Offer to contact pharmaceutical company for patient assistance program.
d. Instruct patient to wait on approval for Medicaid and delay therapy.

Answer a is incorrect. Oral TKI therapy is expensive and most patients will not be able to afford these without financial assistance.

Answer b is incorrect. Alternative agents such as dasatinib and nilotinib are more expensive.

Answer c is correct. The best option for this patient is to apply for an industry patient assistance program until they qualify for Medicaid.

Answer d is incorrect. Do not delay therapy. Assist patient in enrolling in patient assistance program and emphasize medication adherence.

CHAPTER 18 | Solid Organ Transplantation

1. Select the statement that most accurately describes cellular rejection after solid organ transplantation.
   a. An orchestrated immune response that involves alloantigen presentation via antigen presenting cells (APCs) that then leads to alloreactive T lymphocytes.
   b. A cytotoxic immune response mediated via preformed antibodies against antigens present on vascular endothelium.
   c. A slow process of graft fibrosis and arteriopathy, which results in graft dysfunction.
   d. A process which inhibits the entire process of immune activation, including antigen presentation by APCs, the release of cytokines such as IL-1, IL-2, IL-6 and TNF α, and subsequently lymphocyte proliferation.

Answer a is correct. This is a description of acute cellular rejection (ACR). ACR requires the production of alloreactive T cells via T-cell binding at the T-cell receptors on APCs, with subsequent cytokine release and immune activation.

Answer b is incorrect. Humoral rejection is an antibody-mediated process, which typically occurs hours to days after transplant, and can even occur intra-operatively. This type of rejection most frequently results from mismatched blood types and positive cross matches, and the incidence has decreased with the advent of screening.

Answer c is incorrect. This is a description of chronic rejection. The etiology of chronic rejection is not known and there is no treatment for this condition. However ACR has been shown to be a primary risk factor for the development of chronic rejection, thus prevention is a key modifier.

Answer d is incorrect. This is a description of the ubiquitous immunosuppressive action that steroids have on immune response.

2. You are counseling a 16-year-old patient who is waiting for a living-related renal transplantation from his brother. The patient states that he has been doing research on the Internet and has heard that acute cellular rejection (ACR) is a major complication of solid organ transplantation. He wants to know if you can inform him of his risk for this complication. You tell him the time period of greatest risk for ACR after transplant is:
   a. The first hours to days after transplantation
   b. The first several months after transplantation
   c. The risk increases with increased time from transplant
   d. The risk is the same regardless of time after transplant

Answer a is incorrect. This time period describes the time of greatest risk for antibody-mediated rejection, or humoral rejection. Humoral rejection is much less common than ACR.

Answer b is correct. The time period of greatest risk for ACR is during the first 6 months after transplantation, with risk dropping precipitously after 1 year.

Answer c is incorrect. The further out from transplant a patient is, the less likely he/she is to have an episode of ACR. However, as time passes from date of transplant, a patient is at increased risk for chronic rejection, especially if he/she has a history of multiple episodes of ACR.

Answer d is incorrect. The risk for ACR varies with time, with risk decreasing with time from transplant.

3. Select an example of the "triple drug regimen" that describes a common maintenance immunosuppression following solid organ transplantation.
   a. Cyclosporine, prednisone, and basiliximab
   b. Cyclosporine, tacrolimus, and prednisone
   c. Tacrolimus, mycophenolate mofetil, and azathioprine
   d. Prednisone, cyclosporine, and mycophenolate sodium

Answer a is incorrect. This regimen contains a calcineurin inhibitor (cyclosporine), a corticosteroid (prednisone) and an IL-2 receptor antagonist. While IL-2 receptor antagonists, such as basiliximab and daclizumab, can be used as induction agents, or to allow delayed initiation of a calcineurin inhibitor, they do not make up the maintenance regimen. This regimen should include an antiproliferative agent such as mycophenolate or azathioprine.

Answer b is incorrect. This regimen contains two calcineurin inhibitors (cyclosporine and tacrolimus) and a corticosteroid. The "triple drug regimen" is designed to optimize therapy, without excessive toxicity. A patient should never take two calcineurin inhibitors simultaneously, as their risk for serious side effects, such as nephrotoxicity, neurotoxicity, and electrolyte disturbances are greatly increased without much added benefit. The three drugs in the triple drug regimen should have different mechanisms of action, thus allowing decreased doses of each and therefore decreased incidence of dose-dependent side effects.

Answer c is incorrect. This regimen contains a calcineurin inhibitor and two antiproliferative agents (mycophenolate mofetil and azathioprine). Although mycophenolate mofetil inhibits G1-S phase and azathioprine arrests G2-M phase of cell cycle, both medications exert their effects by inhibiting lymphocyte proliferation.

Answer d is correct. This regimen contains a calcineurin inhibitor (cyclosporine), an antiproliferative agent (mycophenolate sodium), and a corticosteroid (prednisone), with three distinct mechanisms of action.

---

4. Select the drug or drug class that allowed successful solid organ transplant and ushered in the current era of large-scale transplantation and therefore is considered to be the "backbone" of the triple drug immunosuppressive regimen.
   a. Corticosteroids
   b. Azathioprine
   c. IL-2 receptor antagonists
   d. Calcineurin inhibitors

Answer a is incorrect. While corticosteroids are the oldest immunosuppressants used in solid organ transplantation, their nonspecific action resulted in significant adverse effects leading to intolerance.

Answer b is incorrect. Azathioprine, the first antiproliferative agent used in solid organ transplantation, was revolutionary, especially in combination with corticosteroids. However, toxicity due to nonspecificity limited its functionality and lead to intolerance.

Answer c is incorrect. IL-2 receptor antagonists, such as basiliximab and daclizumab, are a newer class of immunosuppressive agents used in solid organ transplantation. They are specific for the IL-2 receptor, thus suppressing T-lymphocyte-mediated immune activation. They are also very well tolerated. However, since the IL-2 receptor antagonists are large molecule monoclonal antibodies, they are only available intravenously, thereby limiting their role as maintenance immunosuppression.

Answer d is correct. The development of the calcineurin inhibitors, specifically the release of cyclosporine, ushered in the current era of transplantation. Compared to the dual drug regimen of azathioprine and corticosteroids, the cyclosporine-based regimens not only decreased the rejection rate but also increased the patient and renal allograft survival rates significantly.

---

5. A patient presents to your pharmacy with a prescription for clarithromycin. He says that his primary care physician prescribed this medication to treat community-acquired pneumonia. You review the patient's medication profile and you see that he received a renal transplant 2 years ago and his immunosuppressive regimen includes tacrolimus, mycophenolate mofetil, and prednisone. Which of the following would be most appropriate as your next course of action?
   a. Dispense clarithromycin and counsel on avoiding grape juice.
   b. Contact the prescriber about the interactions between clarithromycin and tacrolimus as clarithromycin will inhibit the metabolism of tacrolimus resulting in supratherapeutic levels and toxicity.
   c. Contact the prescriber about the interactions between clarithromycin and mycophenolate mofetil as clarithromycin will inhibit the metabolism of mycophenolate mofetil resulting in supratherapeutic levels and toxicity.
   d. Recommend an alternative as clarithromycin is not an appropriate therapy for community-acquired pneumonia in an immunosuppressed host.

Answer a is incorrect. Clarithromycin is an inhibitor of CYP 3A, and therefore will inhibit the metabolism of tacrolimus resulting in supratherapeutic concentrations and potential toxicity.

Answer b is correct. Clarithromycin is an inhibitor of CYP 3A, and therefore will inhibit the metabolism of tacrolimus resulting in supratherapeutic concentrations and potential toxicity.

Answer c is incorrect. Mycophenolate mofetil is metabolized to its active metabolite, mycophenolic acid which then undergoes enterohepatic recirculation until it is eventually cleared via hepatic glucuronidation. Clarithromycin will not significantly affect mycophenolate clearance.

Answer d is incorrect. General immunosuppressed state is not a contraindication for the use of clarithromycin, as long as the organisms isolated or suspected are susceptible to this agent.

---

6. A patient who received a lung transplant a month ago is found to have *Aspergillus* on routine bronchoscopy. The patient's transplant physician wants to begin suppressive treatment with the antifungal voriconazole and is inquiring which of the medications his patient is taking will interact with voriconazole. The patient is currently taking prednisone, cyclosporine, azathioprine, clotrimazole, rabeprazole, co-trimoxazole, valganciclovir, and inhaled amphotericin.
   a. Prednisone
   b. Azathioprine
   c. Cyclosporine
   d. Valganciclovir

Answer a is incorrect. Voriconazole is a potent inhibitor of CYP 3A and P-glycoprotein. Prednisone is not suspected to interact, as it is not involved with either of these mechanisms.

Answer b is incorrect. Voriconazole is a potent inhibitor of CYP 3A and P-glycoprotein. Azathioprine is not suspected to interact, as it is metabolized to its inactive metabolite via xanthine oxidase.

Answer c is correct. Voriconazole is a potent inhibitor of CYP 3A and P-glycoprotein. Cyclosporine is extensively metabolized via CYP 3A and also a substrate of P-glycoprotein. Voriconazole will significantly increase cyclosporine levels, and it is recommended to decrease cyclosporine dosing empirically by more than 50% to avoid toxic serum concentrations.

Answer d is incorrect. Voriconazole is a potent inhibitor of CYP 3A and P-glycoprotein. Following oral administration, valganciclovir is hydrolyzed to ganciclovir, which is then excreted renally. Therefore no interaction is suspected between these agents.

7. Which of the following best describes the mechanism of the interaction between HMG-CoA reductase inhibitors (or statins) and cyclosporine?
   a. Inhibition of CYP 3A4 resulting in increased cyclosporine concentrations in blood
   b. Inhibition of CYP 3A4 resulting in increased HMG-CoA reductase inhibitor concentrations in blood
   c. Induction of CYP 3A4 resulting in decreased cyclosporine concentrations in blood
   d. Concomitant nephrotoxicity, resulting in increased risk of renal failure

Answer a is incorrect. HMG-CoA reductase inhibitors (or statins) are substrates of CYP 3A4, but they are not potent inhibitors of the enzyme and thus increased cyclosporine concentrations are not expected. However, an interaction like this is expected with such agents as azole antifungals, macrolide antibiotics, and nondihydropyridine antihypertensive agents.

Answer b is correct. Cyclosporine can block the metabolism of HMG-CoA reductase inhibitors, resulting in increased serum concentrations of these agents and therefore increased the risk for myopathy and rhabdomyolysis.

Answer c is incorrect. HMG-CoA reductase inhibitors are substrates of CYP 3A4, but they are not inducers of this metabolic pathway and thus decreased cyclosporine concentrations are not expected. However, an interaction like this is expected with such agents as rifampin, St. John's wort, and phenytoin.

Answer d is incorrect. HMG-CoA reductase inhibitors are not nephrotoxic. This describes the pharmacodynamic interaction of cyclosporine with such agents as aminoglycosides and NSAIDs.

8. A patient approaches the counter at your pharmacy. She states that she has mild headache, and would like you to suggest an over-the-counter remedy. She is well known to you, as she received a renal transplant 3 months ago and fills her prescription for tacrolimus at your pharmacy. What would you suggest for her headache?
   a. That she proceed immediately to a local emergency room as this might be a symptom of severe tacrolimus toxicity.
   b. That she try taking OTC acetaminophen, and alert the transplant physician if the headache does not resolve.
   c. That she try taking OTC naproxen, and alert the transplant physician if the headache does not resolve.
   d. That she try taking OTC ibuprofen, and alert the transplant physician if the headache dose not resolve.

Answer a is incorrect. While neurotoxicity such as headaches and tremors are associated with supratherapeutic calcineurin-inhibitor concentrations, headache is a common side effect, especially a few hours after the dose is administered, as this is the time when drug levels in the body are highest. Because her headache is only mild, the most reasonable suggestion would be to try the OTC analgesic acetaminophen, and if the headache does not dissipate, to contact the transplant physician. If the headache was severe, immediate medical attention would be warranted.

Answer b is correct. Transplant patients who are taking calcineurin inhibitors should avoid taking nonsteroidal anti-inflammatory drugs (NSAIDs) because NSAIDs cause inhibition of renal prostaglandin production and can increase the risk for nephrotoxicity induced by calcineurin inhibitors. Therefore acetaminophen is the preferred OTC analgesic agent.

Answers c and d are incorrect. Naproxen and ibuprofen are NSAIDs, therefore they are not recommended in combination with her tacrolimus due to the pharmacodynamic interaction, which can lead to increased nephrotoxicity.

9. Which of the following represents two adverse effects specific to tacrolimus?
   a. Diarrhea and leukopenia
   b. Alopecia and hyperglycemia
   c. Hypertriglyceridemia and nephrotoxicity
   d. Hirsutism and gingival hyperplasia

Answer a is incorrect. Diarrhea and leukopenia are adverse effects specific to mycophenolate products. Diarrhea can be associated with tacrolimus, but leukopenia is not common with tacrolimus.

Answer b is correct. Alopecia and hyperglycemia are adverse effects specific to tacrolimus. Hyperglycemia is further exacerbated by the concomitant use of corticosteroids and can lead to post-transplant diabetes mellitus.

Answer c is incorrect. Both cyclosporine and tacrolimus can cause nephrotoxicity, but hypertriglyceridemia is more frequently associated with sirolimus.

Answer d is incorrect. Hirsutism and gingival hyperplasia are adverse effects specific to cyclosporine. It is important to counsel patients who are initiating cyclosporine for the importance of good oral hygiene.

---

10. Which of the following represents two adverse effects specific to corticosteroids?

    a. Diarrhea and leukopenia
    b. Alopecia and hyperglycemia
    c. Water retention and osteoporosis
    d. Hirsutism and nephrotoxicity

Answer a is incorrect. Diarrhea and leukopenia are adverse effects specific to mycophenolate products. Gastrointestinal adverse effects of corticosteroids include indigestion and ulcers, but diarrhea is not particularly associated with corticosteroids. Corticosteroids cause leukocytosis.

Answer b is incorrect. Alopecia and hyperglycemia are adverse effects specific to tacrolimus. Corticosteroids can cause hirsutism. Hyperglycemia is further exacerbated by the concomitant use of corticosteroids and can lead to post-transplant diabetes mellitus.

Answer c is correct. Water retention and osteoporosis both are adverse effects specific to corticosteroids. Water retention leads to weight gain and hypertension. It is important to ensure adequate calcium intake and screening for bone mineral density in patients taking corticosteroids chronically.

Answer d is incorrect. Hirsutism and nephrotoxicity are adverse effects specific to cyclosporine. Corticosteroids can cause hirsutism, but nephrotoxicity is not associated with corticosteroids.

---

11. Which of the following agents would be most appropriate to prevent a gout flare in a transplant patient who is currently receiving tacrolimus, azathioprine, and prednisone?

    a. Indomethacin
    b. Allopurinol
    c. Diclofenac
    d. Probenecid

Answer a is incorrect. Indomethacin is a nonsteroidal anti-inflammatory drug (NSAID). NSAIDs are not recommended in combination with calcineurin inhibitors like tacrolimus due to increased potential for nephrotoxicity via decrease in renal prostaglandin production.

Answer b is incorrect. Allopurinol inhibits xanthine oxidase and is typically the drug of choice to prevent gouty attacks. The metabolite of azathioprine (6-mercaptopurine) is inactivated via xanthine oxidase. If allopurinol is administered concomitantly with azathioprine, the other metabolic pathway that produces 6-thioguanine nucleotides can be enhanced, leading to severe pancytopenia. Allopurinol should be avoided in patients who are currently receiving azathioprine.

Answer c is incorrect. Diclofenac is a nonsteroidal anti-inflammatory drug (NSAID). NSAIDs are not recommended in combination with calcineurin inhibitors like tacrolimus due to increased potential for nephrotoxicity via decrease in renal prostaglandins.

Answer d is correct. Probenecid is indicated for the prevention of gouty attacks, and is not expected to interact with any medication in this patient's immunosuppressive regimen as it is excreted renally. However, if this patient had renal insufficiency with a CrCl < 50 mL/min, this agent should be avoided.

---

12. You are counseling a patient who is being discharged today. He received a living related renal transplant 5 days ago, and his postoperative course has been uncomplicated except for mild hypertension. When reconciling his home medications, you notice that the medical team has not restarted his home diltiazem. What course of action do you take?

    a. Notify the patient's medical team and request a discharge prescription for amlodipine.
    b. Notify the patient's medical team and instruct the patient to resume his home regimen of diltiazem after discharge.
    c. Notify the patient's medical team and request a discharge prescription for verapamil.
    d. Notify the patient's medical team and request addition of diltiazem at discharge.

Answer a is correct. Many patients will experience higher postoperative blood pressures following solid organ transplant due to high doses of steroids and calcineurin inhibitors. Patients with preexisting hypertension may have a more difficult time maintaining blood pressure control, while patients who receive renal transplants may experience resolution of their hypertension with resolution of their kidney disease. While the nondihydropyridine calcium channel blockers, such as diltiazem and verapamil may be appropriate choices for some patients prior to transplant, they may complicate management of calcineurin inhibitors postoperatively, due to their interaction-mediated via CYP 3A and P-glycoprotein. Dihydropyridine calcium channel blockers, such as nifedipine and amlodipine, have less potential for clinically significant pharmacokinetic interactions with calcineurin inhibitors.

Answers b, c, and d are incorrect. The nondihydropyridine calcium channel blockers (diltiazem and verapamil) inhibit CYP3A and P-glycoprotein, resulting in elevated concentrations and toxicity of calcineurin inhibitors. These agents can be used safely, with close monitoring of trough levels of calcineurin inhibitors, but reinitiation of these agents at discharge is not appropriate.

---

13. Which of the following statement is correct about sirolimus?
    a. Sirolimus is not metabolized via cytochrome P-450 enzymes, thus decreasing the propensity for drug interactions.
    b. Sirolimus is less nephrotoxic than calcineurin inhibitors.
    c. Sirolimus is available in many different formulations, thereby facilitating ease of dosing.
    d. Sirolimus does not require therapeutic drug monitoring.

Answer a is incorrect. CYP 3A is the major metabolic pathway for sirolimus. Like cyclosporine and tacrolimus, sirolimus is affected by inducers and inhibitors of CYP 3A.

Answer b is correct. Sirolimus has decreased risk for nephrotoxicity compared to calcineurin inhibitors, therefore it is commonly used in calcineurin inhibitor-sparing regimens to protect patients from calcineurin inhibitor-induced renal insufficiency.

Answer c is incorrect. Sirolimus is only available orally and there is no generic equivalent. Furthermore, the tablet is triangular, disallowing splitting to create unavailable tablet strengths.

Answer d is incorrect. Therapeutic drug monitoring was deemed unnecessary during clinical trials, as sirolimus was used primarily as an adjunctive agent, in the place of an antiproliferative agent. However, the risk of drug interactions and variability in pharmacokinetics warrant monitoring of sirolimus concentrations.

14. Which enzyme or protein does mycophenolic acid inhibit in order to exhibit its immunosuppressive effect?
    a. mTOR
    b. Cyclophilin
    c. FKBP-12
    d. IMPDH

Answer a is incorrect. Sirolimus is a selective immunosuppressant that exerts its effect via inhibition of the mammalian target of rapamycin (mTOR). Blockade of mTOR results in inhibition of lymphocyte proliferation via cell-cycle arrest in the G1 to S phase.

Answer b is incorrect. Cyclophilin is the binding target of cyclosporine that facilitates inhibition of calcineurin, a phosphatase enzyme that is responsible for the dephosphorylation of nuclear factor of activated T cells (NFAT), which is a required transcription factor in the process of cytokine production. This inhibition in turn suppresses T-cell activation, and thus cellular immune response.

Answer c is incorrect. FKBP-12 is the binding target of tacrolimus that facilitates inhibition of calcineurin which results in the same outcome as inhibition by cyclosporine, although the intercellular mediators are different.

Answer d is correct. Inosine monophosphate dehydrogenase (IMPDH) is an enzyme required for the de novo synthesis of purines, and is inhibited by mycophenolic acid (MPA), the active metabolite of the mycophenolate derivatives. This is the mechanism that allows these agents to selectively inhibit lymphocyte proliferation, as these cells are unable to utilize salvage pathways of purine synthesis.

15. A patient presents to the hospital with symptoms concerning for a bowel obstruction. His past medical history is significant for a liver transplant 3 months ago and he receiving Myfortic 720 mg po bid. The physician wants to convert the patient from oral Myfortic to IV due to po intolerance resulting from his bowel obstruction. Which of the following would result in comparable plasma concentrations of mycophenolic acid?
    a. Mycophenolate sodium 720 mg IV bid
    b. Mycophenolate sodium 1000 mg IV bid
    c. Mycophenolate mofetil 720 mg IV bid
    d. Mycophenolate mofetil 1000 mg IV bid

Answers a and b are incorrect. Myfortic, or mycophenolate sodium, is an enteric-coated delayed-release oral formulation and it is not available intravenously.

Answer c is incorrect. The dosing conversion between mycophenolate sodium and mycophenolate mofetil (CellCept) is not 1:1, but rather 720 mg of mycophenolate sodium is equivalent to 1000 mg of mycophenolate mofetil.

Answer d is correct. CellCept, or mycophenolate mofetil, is available in an oral and IV formulation. When converting a patient from po Myfortic (mycophenolate sodium) to IV therapy, IV mycophenolate mofetil (CellCept) can be used at a therapeutically equivalent dose. Myfortic 720 mg is equivalent to 1000 mg of CellCept.

16. Which of the following statements is *incorrect* regarding brand-name and generic tacrolimus?
    a. A sponsor of a generic tacrolimus must complete large, randomized, multiple-center studies of efficacy and safety in the patient population where the drug is intended to be used.
    b. A sponsor of a generic tacrolimus must complete bioequivalence studies.
    c. A generic tacrolimus must demonstrate a peak concentration (C_{max}) and area under the time-concentration curve (AUC) similar to the reference brand-name product.
    d. Monitoring tacrolimus trough concentrations may offer an additional degree of confidence in using generic tacrolimus products.

Answer a is incorrect. Sponsors of generic products do not need to submit clinical data to establish efficacy and safety of the active ingredients because these data were documented during the approval process for the innovator product.

Answer b is correct. Generic drug products are granted an expedited and less rigorous review process. Sponsors of generic drug products must submit clinical data demonstrating that the generic product is bioequivalent to the reference product.

Answer c is correct. The FDA defines bioequivalence as the absence of a significant difference in the rate and extent to which the active ingredient becomes available at the site of drug action. The C_{max} and AUC are assessed using a 90% confidence interval that must fall between 80% and 125%.

Answer d is correct. Therapeutic drug monitoring is a useful tool to ensure that patients maintain therapeutic drug concentrations despite generic substitution.

---

17. Which of the following is generally considered as a narrow therapeutic ratio drug?

    a. Cyclosporine
    b. Prednisone
    c. Mycophenolate mofetil
    d. Mycophenolate sodium

Answer a is correct. Cyclosporine is generally considered to have a narrow therapeutic ratio as the blood concentration ranges to effectively prevent rejection overlap with that of nephrotoxic potential, and cyclosporine-concentration monitoring is required.

The FDA does not formally designate the narrow therapeutic ratio drugs. According to 21 CFR 320.33(c), narrow therapeutic ratio is defined as follows:

1. There is less than a two-fold difference in median lethal dose (LD_{50}) and median effective dose (ED_{50}) values or there is less than a two-fold difference in the minimum toxic concentrations and minimum effective concentrations in the blood, and
2. Safe and effective use of the drug products requires careful titration and patient monitoring.

Answers b, c and d are incorrect. Prednisone and mycophenolate derivatives do not meet the FDA criteria for narrow therapeutic ratio drugs and serum concentrations are not typically monitored for these medications.

---

18. A liver transplant patient presented with elevated liver function tests and she admits to not taking her immunosuppressive regimen for the past week, as she was out of town and forgot her medications. The medical team wants to treat her for acute cellular rejection and wants you to recommend an appropriate agent. Which of the following would treat acute cellular rejection most effectively?

    a. Basiliximab
    b. Muromonab-CD3
    c. Daclizumab
    d. Rituximab

Answer a is incorrect. While the IL-2 receptor antagonists, such as basiliximab and daclizumab can be used in induction regimens, they are not indicated for the treatment of acute cellular rejection.

Answer b is correct. Muromonab-CD3 is a murine monoclonal antibody directed against CD3 antigen on the surface of T cells, which leads to T-cell inactivation. Muromonab-CD3 can be used both in induction regimens as well as treatment of acute cellular rejection.

Answer c is incorrect. While the IL-2 receptor antagonists, such as basiliximab and daclizumab can be used in induction regimens, they are not indicated for the treatment of acute cellular rejection.

Answer d is incorrect. Rituximab is a monoclonal antibody directed against CD20 on B cells. Rituximab currently has no role in the treatment of acute cellular rejection, as this type of rejection is largely mediated by T cells.

---

19. Why do patients require flow cytometry prior to administration of a second course of muromonab-CD3?

    a. To evaluate for the presence of antibodies which could make the patient more susceptible to infusion reactions
    b. To evaluate for the presence of antibodies which could result in drug inactivation
    c. To evaluate for the presence of antibodies which could result in heightened immunosuppressive effect
    d. To evaluate for the presence of antibodies indicating an episode of humoral rejection

---

Answer a is incorrect. Because muromonab-CD3 is nonhumanized murine monoclonal antibody, risk of infusion reactions is high and use of this agent requires vigorous premedication with corticosteroids, antihistamine and antipyretic agent. However, flow cytometry will not predict a patient's risk for an infusion reaction, so all patients should be universally premedicated.

Answer b is correct. Prior to a second course of muromonab-CD3 flow cytometry should be conducted to test for the presence of human anti-mouse antibodies (HAMA). If these antibodies are present and circulating, the drug will be inactivated prior to exerting its effect.

Answer c is incorrect. Flow cytometry conducted prior to muromonab-CD3 infusion is done to detect antibodies formed against the agent itself. If antibodies are present, they will bind the agent, and therefore decrease its immunosuppressive potential, not increase it.

Answer d is incorrect. Flow cytometry is conducted to determine the presence of antibody-mediated rejection or humoral rejection. However, this is unrelated to the flow cytometry that is performed prior to a second course of muromonab-CD3, which is done to detect the presence of

HAMA, which will inactivate the drug, decreasing its efficacy.

20. During interdisciplinary rounds, the medical resident states that a patient on the transplant service has a low WBC count. The patient received a combined kidney-pancreas transplant for juvenile-onset diabetes mellitus 2 months ago and presented 2 days ago with hyperglycemia and elevated amylase and lipase. Acute cellular rejection of the pancreas transplant was confirmed on a subsequent biopsy. Her rejection episode is being treated with rabbit antithymocyte globulin. Her home immunosuppressive regimen consists of tacrolimus, mycophenolate mofetil, and prednisone. She is receiving antiviral prophylaxis with valganciclovir, antibacterial prophylaxis with trimethoprim-sulfamethoxazole and antifungal prophylaxis with nystatin. Which of the following approach is most appropriate for this patient's new-onset leukopenia?
    a. Suggest the physician to hold her prednisone until her WBC count normalizes.
    b. Suggest the physician to hold her mycophenolate mofetil until her WBC count normalizes.
    c. Suggest the physician to continue her current therapy, but to closely monitor her WBC count.
    d. Suggest the physician to hold her valganciclovir until her WBC count normalizes.

Answer a is incorrect. Prednisone usually causes leukocytosis and not leukopenia.

Answer b is incorrect. While mycophenolate mofetil can cause leukopenia, the likely agent inducing this patient's leukopenia is rabbit antithymocyte globulin. It is important to review the patient's medication administration record in this case to see if her blood sample was drawn during the infusion of rabbit antithymocyte globulin, as this will produce a significant leukopenia. However, even if the blood drawn occurred after the infusion, the leukopenia is likely due to this agent, and the antiproliferative agent need not be held. This is especially true in light of her current presentation with acute cellular rejection.

Answer c is correct. This patient's leukopenia is likely caused by rabbit antithymocyte globulin infusion. WBC count along with the rest of hematology labs should be monitored closely. If there is a significant decrease in her WBC or platelet counts, a reduction of or withholding the dose of rabbit antithymocyte globulin may be warranted.

Answer d is incorrect. While valganciclovir can cause leukopenia, the likely agent inducing this patient's leukopenia is rabbit antithymocyte globulin. During an episode of rejection, patients are treated with immunosuppressive intensification, and therefore are at increased risk for reactivation of latent viral infections. Therefore, care must be taken to not inaccurately hold a patient's antiviral prophylaxis, but thoroughly investigate the cause of leukopenia and act on the most likely cause.

CHAPTER 19 | Antimicrobial Regimen Selection

1. Select the antimicrobial that may cause collateral damage by selecting for a nontargeted organism (ie, *Clostridium difficile*) leading to a colitis infection.
    a. Clindamycin
    b. Levofloxacin
    c. Ciprofloxacin
    d. b and c
    e. All of the above

Clostridium difficile, also known as *C. difficile*, is a species of gram-positive bacteria of the genus *Clostridium*. Clostridia are anaerobic, spore-forming rods (bacillus). *C. difficile* is the most serious cause of antibiotic-associated diarrhea (AAD) and can lead to pseudomembranous colitis, a severe infection of the colon, often resulting from eradication of the normal gut flora by antibiotics. The *C. difficile* bacteria, which naturally reside in the body, become overpopulated. The overpopulation is harmful because the bacterium releases toxins that can cause bloating, constipation, and diarrhea with abdominal pain, which may become severe. Discontinuation of causative antibiotic treatment is often curative. http://en.wikipedia.org/wiki/Clostridium_difficile - cite_note-Sherris-1. In more serious cases, oral administration of metronidazole or vancomycin is the treatment of choice. Relapses of *C. difficile* AAD have been reported in up to 20% of cases.

Answer a is correct. Clindamycin may cause/select for a *C. difficile* infection.

Answer b is correct. Levofloxacin may cause/select for a *C. difficile* infection.

Answer c is correct. Ciprofloxacin may cause/select for a *C. difficile* infection.

Answer e is correct and the best answer. All of the above may cause/select for a *C. difficile* infection. All antibiotics have been associated with causing/selecting for *C. difficile* infections.

2. Select the correct dose of cefepime (Maxipime) for a patient with normal renal function and empirically treated for an infection (at this time the site or source of infection have not been identified).
    a. 1 g IV every 12 hours
    b. 2 g IV every 12 hours
    c. 2 g IV every 8 hours
    d. All of the above

Answer a is correct. Cefepime 1 g every 12 hours may be utilized for patients with community-acquired pneumonia and urinary tract infections.

Answer b is correct. Cefepime 2 g every 12 hours may be utilized for patients with intra-abdominal infections, skin and skin structure infections, and urinary tract infections.

Answer c is correct. Cefepime 2 g every 8 hours may be utilized for patients with febrile neutropenia and suspected resistant pathogens (ie, *Pseudomonas aeruginosa infections*)

Answer d is correct and the best answer. All of the above doses of cefepime may be utilized, depending upon the site of infection and the potential for bacterial resistance. High doses of cefepime are often utilized empirically, especially when the site or source of infection has not been identified, as is the situation with our current case application question. Since this patient has been diagnosed with an infection and cefepime is going to be utilized, high doses would likely be the best option until the site or source has been identified. Once the site and/or source have been identified the dose or anti-infective may be required to be changed. Also, if a patient were suspected to have a multidrug resistant organism, other methods of dosing may be utilized (ie, *extended infusion* beta lactam therapy). Please note this case application question was about dosing of anti-infectives, not selection of anti-infectives, with cefepime serving as an example.

---

3. Select the antimicrobial pharmacokinetic (PK) property that impacts the dose and/or interval.

    a. Bioavailability
    b. Volume of distribution
    c. Metabolism
    d. Elimination
    e. All of the above

Answer a is correct. Bioavailability (absorption) is a key PK property in describing antimicrobial properties.

Answer b is correct. Volume of distribution (V_d) is a key PK property in describing antimicrobial properties. V_d may change during therapy and is an important factor to monitor. Patients that may have altered V_d include: ascites, edema, pregnant, burn, obese, thin, loss of extremities (ie, above the knee amputation), and dehydrated patients.

Answer c is correct. Metabolism is a key PK property in describing antimicrobial properties. Understanding drug interactions and its impact on the antimicrobial concentration are important factors in determining anti-infective dose and/or interval.

Answer d is correct. Elimination is a key PK property in describing antimicrobial properties. Understanding renal and/or hepatic function are important factors in determining anti-infective dose and/or interval. Renally eliminated anti-infectives are usually dose-based upon results from the approximation of the glomerular filtration rate (GFR) via calculation of the creatinine clearance (Cockroft-Gault or modification of diet in renal disease [MDRD] equations). Anti-infectives eliminated via the hepatic system may be dosed upon a Child-Pugh score, although recommendations for dosing anti-infectives in patients with liver dysfunction are not as formalized as guidelines for patients with renal dysfunction.

Answer e is correct and the best answer.

---

4. Select the factor that may affect the bioavailability of an oral anti-infective.

    a. A medication that is a substrate of the CYP-450 system
    b. Dosage formulation of the anti-infective
    c. A patient that has peripheral vascular disease
    d. A patient that has renal dysfunction

Answer a is incorrect. Anti-infective CYP-450 activity (substrates, inhibitors, inducers) will not affect the bioavailability. P-450 activity will affect the metabolism and elimination, but not absorption. Anti-infectives administered orally that are circulated through the liver may be affected by the first-pass effect. The first-pass effect will eliminate some of the anti-infective and would indirectly affect the amount of medication able to be absorbed. The first-pass effect is a phenomenon of drug metabolism whereby the concentration of a drug is reduced before it reaches the systemic circulation. It is the fraction of lost drug during the process of absorption which is generally related to the liver and gut wall. Notable drugs that experience a significant first-pass effect are imipramine, propranolol, and lidocaine.

Answer b is correct. The dosage formulation of the anti-infective may have significant effects on the bioavailability. A classic example is vancomycin. Vancomycin is available as oral and parenteral formulations. Oral vancomycin is not absorbed and reserved for treatment of *Clostridium difficile* infections (antibiotic-associated diarrhea). Intravenous vancomycin has a bioavailability of 100% (F=1) and is used for treatment of systemic gram-positive infections (ie, methicillin resistant *Staphylococcus aureus*). Parenteral formulations of an anti-infective may also have various degrees of bioavailability. Examples include a potential difference in bioavailability of beta lactams when administered via IV versus intramuscular routes.

Answer c is incorrect. A patient with peripheral vascular disease would not be expected to have different bioavailability. However, comorbidities (like peripheral vascular disease) may impact other PK properties of anti-infectives like distribution and elimination.

Answer d is incorrect. Renal dysfunction would not have an impact on bioavailability. Renal dysfunction would affect the elimination of the anti-infective.

---

5. Select the factor that would usually necessitate a patient to be given IV anti-infectives.

    a. Fever of 101.9°F
    b. Severe cough

the emergence of resistance, and improve outcomes. However, there are few clinical examples in the literature to support these assertions. Double antimicrobial coverage may be beneficial for selected infections associated with high bacterial loads or for initial empirical coverage of critically ill patients in whom antimicrobial-resistant organisms are suspected. Monotherapy usually is satisfactory once antimicrobial susceptibilities are known. In the case application question above, the combination of the two anti-infectives would not be ideal because they are of the same mechanism of action (beta lactams). When the clinical situation calls for combination therapy, utilization of drugs with different mechanisms of action is preferred.

Answer d is incorrect.

---

11. Central nervous system (CNS) side effects (seizures and mental status changes) are associated with beta lactam and quinolone anti-infectives. A risk factor for development of the central nervous system reactions is:

    a. Duration of therapy
    b. Infusion interval
    c. Bioavailability
    d. Renal dysfunction

Answer a is incorrect. Duration of therapy would not be a factor in CNS side effects of beta lactams or quinolones, unless the patient was accumulating (not eliminating) the anti-infective.

Answer b is incorrect. The infusion interval would not impact the central nervous system side effect.

Answer c is incorrect. Bioavailability would not impact the central nervous system side effect.

Answer d is correct. Antibiotic-associated central nervous system toxicities may be common effects for penicillin, cephalosporin, carbapenem, and quinolone anti-infectives, especially if the dose or interval is not adjusted for renal dysfunction.

---

13. Select the anti-infective that is associated with the adverse effects of nephrotoxicity and ototoxicity.

    a. Amoxicillin / Clavulanate
    b. Cefpodoxime
    c. Moxifloxacin
    d. Gentamicin

Answer a is incorrect. The penicillin beta lactam amoxicillin/clavulanate (Augmentin) is not associated with nephrotoxicity and ototoxicity.

Answer b is incorrect. The cephalosporin beta lactam cefpodoxime (Vantin) is not associated with nephrotoxicity and ototoxicity.

Answer c is incorrect. The fluoroquinolone moxifloxacin (Avelox) is not associated with nephrotoxicity and ototoxicity.

Answer d is correct. The aminoglycoside gentamicin (Garamycin) is associated with nephrotoxicity and ototoxicity.

---

13. Select the anti-infective(s) that is associated with the adverse reaction of antibiotic- associated diarrhea (*C. difficile*).

    a. Augmentin
    b. Levaquin
    c. Cleocin
    d. Vancocin
    e. a, b, and c

Answer a is correct. Amoxicillin/clavulanate (Augmentin) and other beta lactams are associated with the adverse reaction of antibiotic-associated diarrhea (*C. difficile*). Please note that anti-infectives may also cause gastrointestinal disturbances leading to diarrhea that is different than *C. difficile* infections. Augmentin has a high rate of diarrhea from gastrointestinal disturbance as well. Just because a patient develops diarrhea on anti-infectives, it does not mean it is caused by *C. difficile*.

Answer b is correct. Levofloxacin (Levaquin) and other fluoroquinolones are associated with the adverse reaction of antibiotic-associated diarrhea (*C. difficile*).

Answer c is correct. Clindamycin (Cleocin) is associated with the adverse reaction of antibiotic-associated diarrhea (*C. difficile*). Clindamycin has the highest incidence of *C. diff* infections.

Answer d is incorrect. Vancomycin (Vancocin) is not associated with the adverse reaction of antibiotic-associated diarrhea (*C. difficile*). Oral vancomycin is used to treat *C. diff* infections.

Answer e is correct and the best answer.

---

14. JG is a patient with an immediate allergic reaction to ticarcillin/clavulanate (Timentin). Select the antimicrobial that JG may take in relation to his allergy.

    a. Piperacillin/tazobactam
    b. Amoxicillin/clavulanate
    c. Ceftriaxone
    d. Aztreonam

Answer a is incorrect. JG has an immediate allergic reaction to penicillin (Timentin) and therefore cannot take penicillin or cephalosporin antimicrobials.

Answer b is incorrect. JG has an immediate allergic reaction to penicillin (Timentin) and therefore cannot take penicillin or cephalosporin antimicrobials.

Answer c is incorrect. JG has an immediate allergic reaction to penicillin (Timentin) and therefore cannot take penicillin or cephalosporin antimicrobials.

Answer d is correct. Aztreonam (Azactam) is a monobactam antimicrobial. The place in therapy for aztreonam is for patients with a hypersensitivity reaction to penicillins.

---

15. Select the host factor(s) that may impact antimicrobial therapy.
    a. Age
    b. Pregnancy
    c. Metabolic abnormalities
    d. Organ dysfunction
    e. All of the above

Answer a is correct. Age is an important factor in determining causative pathogens for certain infections (ie, meningitis) and pharmacokinetic factors (renal dysfunction).

Answer b is correct. Antimicrobial agents must be used with caution in pregnant and nursing women. Some agents are known or likely to be teratogenic (eg, metronidazole), and others pose potential threats to the fetus or infant (eg, quinolones, tetracyclines, and sulfonamides). Pharmacokinetic variables also are altered during pregnancy. Both the clearance and volume of distribution are increased during pregnancy. As a result, increased dosages and/or more frequent administration of certain drugs may be required to achieve adequate concentrations.

Answer c is correct. Inherited or acquired metabolic abnormalities influence infectious diseases therapy. Patients with peripheral vascular disease may not absorb drugs given by intramuscular injection. Other examples include: patients who are phenotypically slow acetylators of isoniazid are at greater risk for peripheral neuropathy; patients with glucose-6-phosphate dehydrogenase deficiency can develop hemolysis when exposed to sulfonamides and dapsone.

Answer d is correct. Patients with renal or hepatic dysfunction will accumulate certain drugs unless the dosage is adjusted.

Answer e is correct and the best answer.

---

16. Select the risk factor(s) for the acquisition of exogenous pathogens.
    a. Home health care utilization
    b. Pregnancy
    c. Recent antimicrobial use
    d. a and c
    e. All of the above

Answer a is correct. Home health care utilization may expose the patient to different types of bacteria and change the patient's normal flora. This change in normal flora may necessitate a change in empiric treatment of infections.

Answer b is incorrect. Pregnancy would not change the normal (endogenous) flora. Pregnancy may change pharmacokinetic parameters such as volume of distribution.

Answer c is correct. Patients with a history of recent antimicrobial use may have altered normal flora (acquisition of exogenous pathogen).

Answer d is correct and the best answer.

Answer e is incorrect.

---

17. Select the potential cause of a fever.
    a. Infection
    b. Piperacillin
    c. Trauma
    d. Cancer
    e. All of the above

Answer a is correct. Infections may cause a fever. However, patients with infections may also present with hypothermia (eg, patients with overwhelming infection, sepsis). Elderly patients may be afebrile, as well as patients with localized infection (eg, uncomplicated urinary tract infections).

Answer b is correct. Medications may cause a fever. Examples of mediations that have been associated with a drug fever are: anticonvulsants, minocycline, penicillins, cephalosporins, allopurinol, and heparin.

Answer c is correct. Trauma may cause a fever.

Answer d is correct. Malignancy may cause a fever

Answer e is correct and the best answer. All of the above are causes of fever. Other causes of fever are autoimmune diseases and hyperthyroidism.

---

18. Select the information that is revealed by a gram stain.
    a. Minimum inhibitory concentration
    b. Genre and species of the bacteria
    c. Morphologic characteristics of the bacteria
    d. All of the above

Answer a is incorrect. Minimum inhibitory concentration (MIC) is revealed by the culture and susceptibility test.

Answer b is incorrect. The genre and species of the bacteria are revealed by the culture and susceptibility test.

Answer c is correct. A gram stain is performed to identify if bacteria are present and to determine morphologic characteristics of bacteria (such as gram positive or negative; shape—cocci or bacilli).

Answer d is incorrect.

---

19. Select the pathogen(s) that is classified as an atypical organism.
    a. *Escherichia coli*
    b. *Klebsiella pneumoniae*
    c. *Mycoplasma pneumoniae*
    d. All of the above

Answer a is incorrect. *Escherichia coli* is an aerobic lactose-positive fermenting gram-negative rod. *Escherichia coli* belongs to the Enterobacteriaceae (Enteric) family.

Answer b is incorrect. *Klebsiella* species are aerobic lactose-positive fermenting gram-negative rods. *Klebsiella* species belong to the Enterobacteriaceae (Enteric) family.

Answer c is correct. *Mycoplasma pneumoniae* is an aerobic gram-negative bacteria, but it retains the gram stain poorly and thus cannot be reliably seen on routine gram stain, and therefore referred to as an atypical pathogen. Other atypical organisms are *Legionella pneumophila* and *Chlamydia pneumoniae*.

Answer d is incorrect.

20. Select the pathogen that represents an exogenous bacteria flora (ie, acquired from the hospital). Characteristics of this pathogen are nonlactose fermenting gram-negative bacilli.
    a. *Neisseria meningitidis*
    b. *Enterobacter cloacae*
    c. *Streptococcus pneumoniae*
    d. *Pseudomonas aeruginosa*

Answer a is incorrect. *Neisseria meningitidis* is a gram-negative cocci.

Answer b is incorrect. *Enterobacter cloacae* is a lactose-fermenting gram-negative bacilli.

Answer c is incorrect. *Streptococcus pneumoniae* is a gram-positive cocci (diplococcic).

Answer d is correct. *Pseudomonas aeruginosa* is a nonlactose fermenting gram-negative bacilli. Other nonlactose fermenting gram-negative bacilli include *Proteus*, *Serratia*, *Morganella*, *Stenotrophomonas*, and *Acinetobacter*.

21. Select the penicillin antimicrobial that is broad-spectrum and has coverage against nonlactose negative (oxidase-positive) gram-negative bacilli.
    a. Amoxicillin
    b. Nafcillin
    c. Cefepime
    d. Doripenem
    e. Piperacillin/tazobactam

Answer a is incorrect. Amoxicillin is a narrow-spectrum antimicrobial and it does not have activity against the nonlactose negative (oxidase-positive) gram-negative bacilli (*P. aeruginosa*)

Answer b is incorrect. Nafcillin is a narrow-spectrum gram-positive antimicrobial and it does not have activity against the nonlactose negative (oxidase-positive) gram-negative bacilli (*P. aeruginosa*) or any gram negative.

Answer c is incorrect. Cefepime is broad-spectrum and it does have coverage against nonlactose negative (oxidase-positive) gram-negative bacilli (*P. aeruginosa*), however it is a cephalosporin.

Answer d is incorrect. Doripenem is broad-spectrum and it does have coverage against nonlactose negative (oxidase-positive) gram-negative bacilli (*P. aeruginosa*); however it is a carbapenem.

Answer e is correct. Piperacillin/tazobactam is a broad-spectrum penicillin antimicrobial that has activity against the nonlactose negative (oxidase-positive) gram-negative bacilli (*P. aeruginosa*).

22. Select the pathogen(s) that is part of the normal (endogenous) flora of the large intestine.
    a. *Escherichia coli*
    b. Viridans *streptococci*
    c. *Neisseria meningitidis*
    d. All of the above

Answer a is correct. *Escherichia coli* resides within the normal flora of the large intestine. Other organisms that reside with the large intestine include: Enterobacteriaceae, *Enterococcus* species, and Anaerobes. *Escherichia coli* also resides in the small intestine.

Answer b is incorrect. Viridans *streptococci* reside within the normal flora of the mouth and are a potential cause of endocarditis.

Answer c is incorrect. *Neisseria meningitidis* reside within the normal flora of the upper respiratory tract and may cause meningitis.

Answer d is incorrect.

23. Select the best answer that represents part of the normal (endogenous) flora of the lower respiratory tract.
    a. Enterobacteriaceae
    b. *Streptococcus pneumoniae*
    c. *Enterococcus* species
    d. Normally sterile

Answer a is incorrect. Enterobacteriaceae reside as part of the normal flora in the small and large intestine.

Answer b is incorrect. *Streptococcus pneumoniae* reside as part of the normal flora in the upper respiratory tract.

Answer c is incorrect. *Enterococcus* species reside as part of the normal flora in the small and large intestine.

Answer d is correct. The lower respiratory tract is normally sterile. Other areas that are normally sterile include the cerebrospinal fluid and urine.

24. Select the drug interaction(s) with aminoglycosides.
    a. Amphotericin B
    b. Vancomycin
    c. Furosemide
    d. Cisplatin
    e. All of the above

Answer a is correct. Amphotericin B has a drug interaction with the aminoglycosides. The mechanism/effect is additive adverse effects (nephrotoxicity).

Answer b is correct. Vancomycin has a drug interaction with the aminoglycosides. The mechanism/effect is additive adverse effects (nephrotoxicity).

Answer c is correct. Furosemide has a drug interaction with the aminoglycosides. The mechanism/effect is additive adverse effects (ototoxicity).

Answer d is correct. Cisplatin has a drug interaction with the aminoglycosides. The mechanism/effect is additive adverse effects (nephrotoxicity and ototoxicity).

Answer e is correct and the best answer. Other drug interactions with the aminoglycoside antimicrobials are neuromuscular blocking agents, cyclosporine, nonsteroidal anti-inflammatory drugs, and radio contrast. The clinical management for the aminoglycoside drug interactions is to monitor aminoglycoside serum drug concentrations and renal function (except when combined with neuromuscular blocking agents, it is best to avoid utilization of aminoglycosides and neuromuscular blocking agents).

---

25. RL is a patient with a past medical history of iron deficiency anemia. He is being treated with ferrous sulfate. Select the antimicrobial(s) that would have a decreased bioavailability when combined with ferrous sulfate.
    a. Moxifloxacin
    b. Tetracycline
    c. Azithromycin
    d. a and b
    e. All of the above

Answer a is correct. Moxifloxacin (and other fluoroquinolones) have decreased absorption when combined with multivalent cations (antacids, iron, sucralfate, zinc, vitamins, dairy, and citric acid). The clinical management for this interaction is to separate administration of the two agents by at least 2 hours.

Answer b is correct. Tetracycline antimicrobials have decreased absorption when combined with iron, antacids, calcium, and sucralfate. The clinical management for this interaction is to separate administration of the two agents by at least 2 hours.

Answer c is incorrect. Azithromycin and the macrolide antimicrobials are not affected by concurrent administration of multivalent cations.

Answer d is correct and the best answer.

Answer e is incorrect.

CHAPTER 20 | Upper Respiratory Tract Infections

1. Select the upper respiratory tract infection(s) that may be caused by viruses such as respiratory syncytial virus, influenza virus, rhinovirus, and adenovirus.
    a. Otitis media
    b. Sinusitis
    c. Pharyngitis
    d. Rhinitis
    e. All of the above

Answer a is correct. Otitis media is an upper respiratory tract infection and is often caused by viruses.

Answer b is correct. Sinusitis is an upper respiratory tract infection and is often caused by viruses.

Answer c is correct. Pharyngitis is an upper respiratory tract infection and is often caused by viruses.

Answer d is correct. Rhinitis is an upper respiratory tract infection and is often caused by viruses.

Answer e is correct and the best answer. Other viral upper respiratory tract infections include laryngitis (croup) and epiglottitis. Most upper respiratory tract infections (URTIs) have a viral etiology and tend to resolve spontaneously; therefore, antibiotics would not be appropriate for the majority of URTIs. However, URTIs are responsible for the majority of antibiotics prescribed in ambulatory practice.

---

2. Select the upper respiratory tract condition that would be defined as the presence of fluid in the middle ear without symptoms of acute illness.
    a. Otitis media with effusion
    b. Sinusitis
    c. Pharyngitis
    d. All of the above

Answer a is correct. Otitis media with effusion (OME) is the presence of fluid in the middle ear without symptoms of acute illness. It is important to differentiate between OME and acute otitis media (AOM) because antibiotics are only useful for AOM. AOM is a symptomatic middle ear infection that occurs rapidly with effusion.

Answer b is incorrect. Sinusitis is an inflammation and/or infection of the paranasal sinus mucosa.

Answer c is incorrect. Pharyngitis is an acute throat infection caused by viruses or bacteria.

Answer d is incorrect.

---

3. Select the bacterial pathogen(s) that cause upper respiratory tract infections.
   a. *Streptococcus pneumoniae*
   b. *Streptococcus pyogenes*
   c. *Haemophilus influenzae*
   d. *Moraxella catarrhalis*
   e. All of the above

Note: The majority of upper respiratory tract infections are caused by viral pathogens (respiratory syncytial virus, influenza virus, rhinovirus, and adenovirus). While this question focuses on the bacterial pathogens that cause upper respiratory tract infections, most patients have viral infections and do not require antibiotic therapy.

Answer a is correct. *Streptococcus pneumoniae* is a bacterial cause of upper respiratory tract infections (URTIs). *S. pneumoniae* causes sinusitis and otitis media.

Answer b is correct. *Streptococcus pyogenes* (also known as group A *streptococci*) is a bacterial cause of pharyngitis (strep throat).

Answer c is correct. *Haemophilus influenzae* is a gram-negative bacterial cause of URTIs.

Answer d is correct. *Moraxella catarrhalis* is a gram-negative bacterial cause of URTIs.

Answer e is correct and the best answer.

---

4. Select the nonpharmacologic management option(s) for acute otitis media.
   a. Watchful waiting
   b. Tympanostomy tubes
   c. Adenoidectomy
   d. b and c
   e. All of the above

Answer a is correct. Watchful waiting approaches are being used to attenuate microbial resistance and avoid unnecessary adverse events and costs of antibiotics. Watchful waiting involves monitoring for 48 to 72 hours after diagnosing AOM to see if spontaneous resolution will occur. Observation or delayed antibiotic therapy should only be considered in healthy children without severe or recurrent disease and if proper follow-up and good communication exist between clinicians and caregivers.

Answer b is correct. Tympanostomy tubes for patients with recurrent disease or chronic OME with impaired hearing or speech.

Answer c is correct. Adenoidectomy may be necessary for children with chronic nasal obstruction.

Answer e is correct and the best answer.

---

5. Select the pharmacologic management option(s) for acute otitis media in children.
   a. Antibiotics
   b. Acetaminophen
   c. Decongestants
   d. Aspirin
   e. a and b

Answer a is correct. Antibiotics are useful in the treatment of otitis media caused by bacteria. Antibiotics should have activity against upper respiratory pathogens such as *S. pneumoniae, H. influenza*, and *M. catarrhalis*.

Answer b is correct. Acetaminophen may alleviate pain with otitis media. Pain is a central feature of AOM and may be alleviated by acetaminophen or ibuprofen. Topical anesthetic drops such as benzocaine provide relief within 30 minutes and may be preferred over systemic analgesics when fever is absent.

Answer c is incorrect. Medications such as decongestants, antihistamines, and corticosteroids have no role in the management of AOM.

Answer d is incorrect. Due to the risk of Reye syndrome ASA should be avoided.

Answer e is correct and the best answer.

---

6. Select the bacterial resistance mechanism of action that may impact empiric therapy for acute otitis media.
   a. Altered penicillin-binding proteins
   b. Beta lactamase
   c. Penicillinase
   d. b and c
   e. All of the above

Answer a is correct. Penicillin-resistant *S. pneumoniae* (PRSP) encompasses intermediate and high level resistance. Approximately 35% of respiratory pneumococcal isolates are penicillin resistant owing to *altered penicillin binding proteins*, and almost half are highly penicillin resistant. PRSP is also commonly resistant to other antibiotic classes (sulfonamides, macrolides, clindamycin).

Answer b is correct. Beta-lactamase (penicillinase) production occurs in 30% of *H. influenzae*. Although infections caused by *H. flu* is more likely to resolve without treatment compared to *S. pneumoniae*, it must be considered in cases of treatment failure.

Answer c is correct. Beta-lactamase (penicillinase) production occurs in 100% of *M. catarrhalis*. Although infections caused by *M. cat* is more likely to resolve without treatment compared to *S. pneumoniae*, it must be considered in cases of treatment failure.

Answer e is correct and the best answer.

---

7. QW is a 35-year-old man with a diagnosis of acute bacterial sinusitis. QW has a penicillin allergy (delayed reaction—rash). Select the antibiotic that may be used to treat acute bacterial sinusitis in patients with a delayed hypersensitivity reaction to penicillin.
   a. Amoxicillin
   b. Trimethoprim-sulfamethoxazole
   c. Clarithromycin
   d. b and c
   e. All of the above

Answer a is incorrect. Amoxicillin is an amino penicillin and should not be used in patients with allergic reactions to penicillin. However, in patients without penicillin allergies, amoxicillin is the first-line antimicrobial agent for treatment of acute bacterial sinusitis. The advantages of amoxicillin include proven efficacy and safety, a narrow spectrum of activity, good tolerability, and low cost.

Answer b is correct. Trimethoprim-sulfamethoxazole may be used in the treatment of acute bacterial sinusitis in patients with a penicillin allergy. *Note: S. pneumoniae* is a bacterial cause of sinusitis infections becoming increasingly resistant to trimethoprim-sulfamethoxazole.

Answer c is correct. Clarithromycin may be used in the treatment of acute bacterial sinusitis in patients with a penicillin allergy. *Note*: *S. pneumoniae* is a bacterial cause of sinusitis infections and is becoming increasingly resistant to clarithromycin. Answer d is incorrect.

Answer d is correct and the best answer. Other antibiotics that may be utilized in patients with a penicillin allergy: cephalosporins (delayed reactions only), doxycycline (patients > 8 years of age), macrolides, respiratory quinolones (not used in children).

8. UQ is a 2-year-old child who attends day care and is diagnosed with severe acute bacterial sinusitis. Because the patient is attending a day care and is 2 years of age, penicillin-resistant *S. pneumoniae* is highly suspected. Select the antibiotic regimen that would be recommended to treat this acute bacterial sinusitis infection.
   a. Amoxicillin 45 mg/kg/d in divided doses
   b. Amoxicillin 90 mg/kg/d in divided doses
   c. Trimethoprim-sulfamethoxazole (8 mg/kg trimethoprim) in divided doses
   d. Doxycycline 100 mg in divided doses

Answer a is incorrect. Conventional dose amoxicillin (40-45 mg/kg/d in divided doses) would not produce concentrations required to treat penicillin-resistant *S. pneumoniae* (PRSP). Because PRSP is caused by altered penicillin binding proteins, higher doses of amoxicillin would be required.

Answer b is correct. Even though PRSP is referred to as penicillin-resistant *S. pneumoniae*, that does not mean we cannot use penicillin or amoxicillin. High-dose amoxicillin (90 mg/kg/d in divided doses) would produce concentrations high enough to treat cases of PRSP. Since the binding site to penicillin is altered, giving higher doses of penicillin (or amoxicillin in this case) would overcome the resistance. *Note*: Alterations in binding site may be overcome by increasing the dose; however, beta-lactamase production by *H. influenzae* and *M. catarrhalis* may not be overcome by increasing the dose. If beta-lactamase producing strains of *H. influenza* and *M. catarrhalis* were causing the bacterial sinusitis, clavulanate would have to be added to amoxicillin or use an antibiotic that is stable in beta-lactamase production (eg, cephalosporins, macrolides, doxycycline, fluoroquinolones). *Note*: this patient is 2 years of age and would not be able to take doxycycline or quinolones.

Answer c is incorrect. Increasing resistance to trimethoprim-sulfamethoxazole may limit its use in treatment of bacterial sinusitis caused by drug-resistant *S. pneumoniae*. High-dose amoxicillin should be given in this situation. If the patient has a severe penicillin allergy, clindamycin may be utilized.

Answer d is incorrect. PRSP is also commonly resistant to other antibiotic classes (sulfonamides, macrolides, tetracyclines). Also this patient is not a candidate for tetracycline antibiotics because of age.

9. Select the common side effect(s) for amoxicillin and amoxicillin-clavulanate.
   a. Nausea, vomiting, and diarrhea
   b. Rash
   c. Allergic reactions
   d. All of the above

Answer a is correct. Gastrointestinal side effects such as nausea, vomiting, and diarrhea are common adverse reactions associated with amoxicillin and amoxicillin-clavulanate. Amoxicillin-clavulanate would have a higher incidence of diarrhea because of the clavulanate component. Another gastrointestinal side effect for amoxicillin and amoxicillin-clavulanate is *C. difficile* colitis.

Answer b is correct. The dermatologic side effect of rash is associated with amoxicillin and amoxicillin-clavulanate. The rash may or may not be associated with an allergic reaction.

Answer c is correct. Allergic reactions are associated with amoxicillin and amoxicillin-clavulanate. Allergic reactions may be delayed (rash) or immediate (anaphylaxis).

Answer d is correct and the best answer.

10. Select the cephalosporin that may be used in the treatment of acute otitis media that has a bitter tasting suspension and has differing bioavailability rates depending upon the oral formulation used.

a. Ceftin
b. Vantin
c. Zithromax
d. Cleocin

Answer a is correct. Cefuroxime axetil (Ceftin) is available in tablets and suspension formulations. The tablet and suspensions are not interchangeable because of differing bioavailability rates. Cefuroxime suspension is gritty and bitter tasting. Cefuroxime is also available as an injection, but the parenteral formulation is seldom used.

Answer b is incorrect. Cefpodoxime (Vantin) has a bitter tasting suspension, but the tablets and suspension have similar bioavailability rates.

Answer c is incorrect. Azithromycin (Zithromax) is available as a suspension, tablet, and injection; however, the formulations have similar bioavailability rates and the suspension is not bitter tasting.

Answer d is incorrect. Clindamycin (Cleocin) has a poor tasting oral liquid, but the capsules and liquid are interchangeable.

---

11. Select the parenteral cephalosporin that is often administered intramuscularly as a 3-day regimen for acute otitis media.

a. Clarithromycin
b. Amoxicillin-clavulanate
c. Trimethoprim-sulfamethoxazole
d. Clindamycin
e. Ceftriaxone

Answer a is incorrect. Clarithromycin is used for treatment of otitis media; however, it is a macrolide and only available orally.

Answer b is incorrect. Amoxicillin-clavulanate is used for the treatment of otitis media; however, it is a penicillin and only available orally.

Answer c is incorrect. Trimethoprim-sulfamethoxazole is used for the treatment of otitis media; however, it is a sulfonamide antibiotic. Trimethoprim-sulfamethoxazole is available in oral and parenteral formulations; however, only the oral formulation is utilized for otitis media.

Answer d is incorrect. Clindamycin is used for the treatment of otitis media (used for PRSP—it does not have coverage against gram-negative bacteria); however, it is a lincosamide antibiotic. Clindamycin is available in oral and parenteral formulations; however, only the oral formulation is utilized for otitis media.

Answer e is correct and the best answer. Ceftriaxone is a third generation cephalosporin that is available only as a parenteral formulation. Ceftriaxone is used as a 3-day regimen.

---

12. Select the macrolide antibiotic(s) that has CYP-450 3A4 drug interactions.

a. Biaxin
b. Bactrim
c. Pediazole
d. a and c
e. All of the above

Answer a is correct. Clarithromycin (Biaxin) is a macrolide antibiotic that inhibits the CYP-450 3A4 (strong) and 1A2 (weak). Clarithromycin is also a substrate of CYP-450 3A4 (major).

Answer b is incorrect. Trimethoprim-sulfamethoxazole (Septra, Bactrim) is a sulfonamide antibiotic. Trimethoprim-sulfamethoxazole does have CYP-450 drug interactions. Sulfamethoxazole inhibits CYP-450 2C9 (moderate) and is a substrate of CYP2C9 (major) and 3A4 (minor). Trimethoprim inhibits CYP-450 2C8 (moderate) and 2C9 (moderate) and is a substrate of 2C9 (major) and 3A4 (major).

Answer c is correct. Erythromycin-sulfisoxazole (Pediazole) is a combination antibiotic consisting of a macrolide (erythromycin) and sulfonamide derivative (sulfisoxazole). Erythromycin inhibits CYP-450 1A2 (weak) and 3A4 (moderate) and is a substrate of 2B6 (minor) and 3A4 (major). Sulfisoxazole inhibits CYP-450 2C9 (strong) and is a substrate of 2C9 (major).

Answer d is correct and the best answer.

Answer e is incorrect.

---

13. IO is an 11-year-old patient with a diagnosis of acute bacterial sinusitis. IO has been prescribed 10 mg/kg of trimethoprim/sulfamethoxazole. Which component(s) of the antibiotic should the dose is based upon?

a. Trimethoprim
b. Sulfamethoxazole
c. Sulfonamide
d. All of the above

Answer a is correct. Patients receiving trimethoprim-sulfamethoxazole as a mg/kg dose should have the dose based on the trimethoprim component.

Answers b, c and d are incorrect. Sulfamethoxazole is a sulfonamide and is not used in the mg/kg dosing calculation. The trimethoprim component is used for the calculation.

---

14. YQ is a 6-year-old patient with a severe case of acute bacterial sinusitis. She has a type I (immediate) allergic reaction to penicillin. Select the antibiotic that may be utilized to treat the sinus infection.

a. Doxycycline
b. Moxifloxacin
c. Clindamycin
d. Clarithromycin

Answer a is incorrect. While patients allergic to penicillins may take tetracycline antibiotics, YQ cannot because she is less than 8 years of age.

Answer b is incorrect. While patients allergic to penicillin antibiotics may take quinolones, YQ cannot because of her age.

Answer c is incorrect. While patients allergic to penicillin antibiotics may take clindamycin as clindamycin does not have coverage against gram-negative bacteria. Clindamycin would be useful if YQ had a *S. pneumoniae* infection; however, we do not know the pathogen YQ is infected with and it could be the gram-negative *H. influenzae* or *M. catarrhalis*.

Answer d is correct. Clarithromycin may be utilized in patients allergic to penicillin and is effective in treating sinus infections.

15. TM is a 7-year-old patient with a diagnosis of strep throat. Select the bacterial pathogen that causes strep throat.
    a. *Streptococcus pyogenes*
    b. Group A *Streptococcus*
    c. Flesh-eating bacteria
    d. All of the above

Answer a is correct. Strep throat is caused by *S. pyogenes*.

Answer b is correct. Strep throat is caused by Group A *Streptococcus*.

Answer c is correct. Strep throat is caused by the flesh-eating bacteria. *Note*: Flesh-eating bacteria is a reference to characteristics of the bacteria associated with skin infections. See the skin and soft tissue chapter for further information. Strep throat is caused by the same Streptococcal species that causes skin infections.

Answer d is correct and the best answer. There are several names for *S. pyogenes* and they include group A Streptococcus (GAS), strep throat, and the flesh-eating bacteria.

16. Select the antibiotic to treat strep throat in a 4-year-old child with an immediate penicillin allergy.
    a. Trimethoprim-sulfamethoxazole
    b. Amoxicillin
    c. Cephalexin
    d. Clindamycin

Answer a is incorrect. Trimethoprim-sulfamethoxazole does not have activity against GAS and therefore would not be able to be used in treatment of pharyngitis.

Answer b is incorrect. Amoxicillin is an amino penicillin and cannot be used in patients with a penicillin allergy.

Answer c is incorrect. Cephalosporins should not be used in patients with an immediate allergic reaction to penicillin. They may be used in patients with delayed allergic reactions to penicillin antibiotics.

Answer d is correct. Clarithromycin may be used to treat pharyngitis in a patient allergic to penicillin antibiotics.

17. Select the antibiotic that may cause an abnormal taste.
    a. Biaxin
    b. Zithromax
    c. Doxycycline
    d. Amoxil

Answer a is correct. Clarithromycin (Biaxin) can cause an abnormal taste.

Answers b, c, and d are incorrect.

18. Select the antibiotic used in the treatment of upper respiratory tract infections in children less than 8 years of age that can cause photosensitivity.
    a. Doxycycline
    b. Levofloxacin
    c. Moxifloxacin
    d. All of the above
    e. None of the above

Answer a is incorrect. While doxycycline and tetracycline antibiotics can cause photosensitivity, they cannot be used in children less than 8 years of age.

Answer b is incorrect. While levofloxacin and fluoroquinolone antibiotics can cause photosensitivity, they cannot be used in children.

Answer c is incorrect. While moxifloxacin and fluoroquinolone antibiotics can cause photosensitivity, they cannot be used in children.

Answer d is incorrect.

Answer e is correct.

19. Select the brand name of cefuroxime axetil.
    a. Vantin
    b. Rocephin
    c. Ceftin
    d. Augmentin

Answer a is incorrect. Vantin is the brand name for cefpodoxime.

Answer b is incorrect. Rocephin is the brand name for ceftriaxone.

Answer c is correct. Ceftin is the brand name for oral cefuroxime axetil. Zinacef is also the brand name for injectable cefuroxime.

Answer d is incorrect. Augmentin is the brand name for amoxicillin-clavulanate.

---

20. Select the viral pathogen(s) that may cause upper respiratory tract infections.
    a. *Haemophilus influenzae*
    b. Influenza
    c. Adenovirus
    d. b and c
    e. All of the above

Answer a is incorrect. *Haemophilus influenzae* is a gram-negative pathogen. *Note:* be able to differentiate between the gram-negative *H. influenzae* and the virus influenza.

Answer b is correct. Influenza is a viral cause of lower respiratory tract infections (LRTIs).

Answer c is correct. Adenovirus is a viral cause of LRTIs.

Answer d is correct and the best answer.

Answer e is incorrect.

CHAPTER 21 | Lower Respiratory Tract Infections

1. Select the infection(s) that represents lower respiratory tract infections.
   a. Pneumonia
   b. Sinusitis
   c. Bronchitis
   d. a and c
   e. All of the above

Answer a is correct. Pneumonia is an example of lower respiratory tract infections. There are different classifications/ types of pneumonia: community-acquired, aspiration, and health care-associated. Health care-associated pneumonia represents hospital-acquired, ventilator-acquired, and health care-acquired (ie, nursing home) pneumonia.

Answer b is incorrect. Sinusitis is an example of an upper respiratory tract infection. Other examples of upper respiratory tract infections include otitis media and pharyngitis.

Answer c is correct. Bronchitis is an example of lower respiratory tract infections. Bronchitis has two subsets: acute bronchitis and chronic bronchitis. Acute bronchitis is a self-limiting viral infection and chronic bronchitis is excessive sputum production hallmarked by a smokers cough. Patients with chronic bronchitis often develop exacerbations caused by infections (acute exacerbations of chronic bronchitis—AECB).

Answer d is correct and the best answer. Bronchiolitis is another example of a lower respiratory tract infections. Bronchiolitis is a viral infection in neonates.

Answer e is incorrect.

---

2. Select the cause(s) of lower respiratory tract infections.
   a. Bacteria
   b. Virus
   c. *Streptococcus pneumoniae*
   d. Respiratory syncytial virus
   e. All of the above

Answer a is correct. Bacteria are common causes of lower respiratory tract infections, especially pneumonia.

Answer b is correct. Viruses are common causes of respiratory tract infections, especially acute bronchitis, bronchiolitis, and pediatric pneumonia. Adult pneumonia is most often caused by bacteria.

Answer c is correct. *Streptococcus pneumoniae* is the most common cause of bacterial lower respiratory tract infections.

Answer d is correct. Respiratory syncytial virus (RSV) is a common cause of lower respiratory tract infections, especially bronchiolitis.

Answer e is correct and the best answer.

---

3. Select the bacterial pathogen that is a common cause of lower respiratory tract infections.
   a. *Haemophilus influenza*
   b. Influenza
   c. Parainfluenza
   d. b and c
   e. All of the above

Answer a is correct. *Haemophilus influenza* is a gram-negative coccobacilli that is a common bacterial cause of lower respiratory tract infections.

Answer b is incorrect. Influenza is a viral pathogen that is a common cause of lower respiratory tract infections. Be able to recognize and differentiate the difference between *Haemophilus influenzae* (*H. flu*) and influenza. Both are causes of lower respiratory tract infections; however, one is a bacteria and the other a virus.

Answer c is incorrect. Parainfluenza is a viral pathogen that is a common cause of lower respiratory tract infections. Be able to recognize and differentiate the difference between *Haemophilus influenzae* (*H. flu*) and parainfluenza. Both are causes of lower respiratory tract infections; however, one is a bacteria and the other a virus.

Answer d is incorrect.

Answer e is incorrect.

---

4. Select the information that is reported by a gram stain.
   a. Presence of white blood cells or epithelial cells
   b. Morphologic characteristic of bacteria
   c. Genera and species of the bacteria
   d. a and b
   e. All of the above

Answer a is correct. A gram stain should demonstrate the presence of white blood cells if a lower respiratory tract infection is present. A gram stain should be absent of epithelial cells, presence of epithelial cells reduces the reliability of the gram stain. A sputum gram stain is less reliable than a gram stain of tracheal secretions.

Answer b is correct. A gram stain will reveal if the bacteria are-gram positive or negative and the shape (cocci or bacilli).

Answer c is incorrect. The genre and the species of the bacteria are revealed by the culture and susceptibility (C&S test).

Answer d is correct and the best answer.

Answer e is incorrect.

---

5. Health care-associated pneumonia is divided up into two subsets, early and late onset. Select the factor that is the major difference in early versus late onset.
   a. Severity of illness
   b. Pneumonia severity index score
   c. Time of onset/diagnosis
   d. All of the above

Answer a is incorrect. The severity of illness of a patient does not impact the subset classification of health care-associated pneumonia. The severity of illness may be calculated/estimated by calculating the CURB-65 (*c*onfusion, *u*remia, *r*espiratory rate, low *b*lood pressure, age 65 years or greater) score. CURB-65 is for patients with *community-acquired pneumonia*; patients with a score of two or greater, more intensive treatment is usually warranted.

Answer b is incorrect. The pneumonia severity index score (PSI) is a prognostic model for patients with *community-acquired pneumonia*. The PSI predicts patient mortality and may be used to assist in identifying patients who may be appropriate for outpatient care.

Answer c is correct. Health care-associated pneumonia is divided into two subsets, early and late onset. The major difference in early and late onset is time of onset/diagnosis (<5 days vs ≥5 days since admission to hospital). Those with late onset HCAP are at risk for infection with multidrug resistant (MDR) organisms. Examples of risk factors for MDR organisms are: current hospitalization of 5 days or more, antimicrobial therapy in preceding 90 days, high frequency of antimicrobial resistance in community or hospital, immunosuppressive disease or therapy. Patients with early onset HCAP are usually infected with organisms common to community-acquired pneumonia.

Answer d is incorrect.

---

6. Prevention of pneumonia may be achieved by:
   a. Infection control/prevention measures
   b. *Streptococcus pneumoniae* vaccine
   c. Influenza vaccine
   d. All of the above

Answer a is correct. Infection control/prevention measures may prevent pneumonia cases. Examples of infection prevention measures are: respiratory hygiene measures (use of hand hygiene and masks or tissues for patients with cough), hospitalized patients should be kept in a semirecumbent position, and enteral nutrition is preferred over parenteral.

Answer b is correct. Pneumococcal polysaccharide vaccine is recommended in the following groups:

1) Polyvalent
   a. Immunocompetent individuals
      i. Routine vaccination for persons > 50 years of age
      ii. Persons > 2 years with the following chronic conditions:
         1. Cardiovascular disease
         2. Pulmonary disease
         3. Diabetes mellitus
         4. Liver disease
      iii. Persons ≥ 2 with
         1. Alcoholism
         2. Cerebrospinal fluid leaks
         3. Asplenia
      iv. Adults 19-64 years who smoke cigarettes
   b. Immunocompromised individuals
      1. Persons ≥ 2 with HIV infection, leukemia, lymphoma, Hodgkin disease, multiple myeloma, chronic renal failure, chronic immunosuppressive therapy (including corticosteroids), person who received an organ or bone marrow transplant
2) 7-Valent
   a. Infants and toddlers

Answer c is correct. Annual influenza vaccine is recommended to high-risk groups and persons not wanting to contract influenza.

Answer d is correct and the best answer. See vaccine/immunization chapter for specific information on vaccines.

---

7. Select the anti-infective that may be used to treat pediatric community-acquired pneumonia.
   a. Levofloxacin
   b. Doxycycline
   c. Ceftriaxone
   d. All of the above

Answer a is incorrect. Levofloxacin and other fluoroquinolones should not be used to treat pediatric infections. Although the systemic use of fluoroquinolones is only FDA indicated for the treatment of complicated urinary tract infections and postexposure treatment of inhalation anthrax, use of fluoroquinolones in pediatric patients is increasing. Current recommendations by the American Academy of Pediatrics note that systemic use of these agents in children should be restricted to infections caused by multidrug resistant pathogens with no safe or effective alternative.

Answer b is incorrect. Doxycycline is incorrect. Doxycycline and tetracyclines may cause tissue hyperpigmentation, enamel hypoplasia, or permanent tooth discoloration; use of tetracyclines should be avoided during tooth development (children $\leq$ 8 years of age) unless other drugs are not likely to be effective or are contraindicated.

Answer c is correct. Ceftriaxone may used to treat pediatric infections, including pneumonia. Other antimicrobials utilized in the treatment of pediatric pneumonia include outpatient—high-dose amoxicillin, amoxicillin-clavulanate, intramuscular ceftriaxone, azithromycin, and clarithromycin; inpatient—IV cefuroxime, cefotaxime, ceftriaxone, and ampicillin-sulbactam.

Answer d is incorrect.

---

8. Select the atypical pathogen(s) that is a common cause of community-acquired pneumonia (CAP).
    a. *Mycoplasma pneumoniae*
    b. *Chlamydia pneumoniae*
    c. *Moraxella catarrhalis*
    d. a and b
    e. All of the above

Answer a is correct. *Mycoplasma pneumoniae* is an aerobic gram-negative atypical pathogen. *Mycoplasma* retains the gram stain poorly and this cannot be reliably seen on routine gram stain, hence the name atypical.

Answer b is correct. *Chlamydia pneumoniae* is an aerobic gram-negative atypical pathogen. *Chlamydia pneumoniae* is one of the three distinct species within the genus *Chlamydia.* The other two species of *Chlamydia* are *C. psittaci* (the cause of psittacosis) and *C. trachomatis* (a cause of nongonococcal urethritis).

Answer c is incorrect. *Moraxella catarrhalis* (*M. cat*) is an aerobic gram-negative diplococcus which resembles *Neisseria* species in its gram stain appearance. *Moraxella catarrhalis* is a common bacterial cause of lower respiratory tract infections.

Answer d is correct and the best answer. There are three atypical pathogens – *Mycoplasma pneumoniae, Chlamydia pneumoniae*, and *Legionella pneumophila* and three classes of antimicrobials that have activity against atypical pathogens (tetracyclines, macrolides, quinolones).

Answer e is incorrect.

---

9. Select the multidrug resistant pathogen that may cause late-onset health care-associated pneumonia.
    a. *Pseudomonas aeruginosa*
    b. Extended-spectrum beta-lactamase (ESBL) *Klebsiella pneumoniae*
    c. *Acinetobacter* species
    d. Methicillin-resistant *Staphylococcus aureus* (MRSA)
    e. All of the above

Answer a is correct. *Pseudomonas aeruginosa* is an example of a multidrug resistant (MDR) organism. Very few antimicrobials have clinical activity against *Pseudomonas* species. Examples include piperacillin/tazobactam (Zosyn), cefepime (Maxipime), ceftazidime (Fortaz), Imipenem (Primaxin), meropenem (Merrem), doripenem (Doribax), the aminoglycosides (gentamicin, tobramycin, and amikacin), and the antipseudomonal quinolones (ciprofloxacin and levofloxacin).

Answer b is correct. ESBL *Klebsiella pneumoniae* is an example of a MDR organism. Treatment of ESBL enteric gram-negative often consists of carbapenems (ertapenem, imipenem, meropenem, doripenem).

Answer c is correct. Acinetobacter species is an example of a MDR organism.

Answer d is correct. MRSA is a example of a MDR organism. Antimicrobials used to treat MRSA infections include vancomycin, linezolid, tigecycline, and daptomycin. *Note*: While daptomycin is utilized to treat MRSA infections, it *cannot* be used to treat *MRSA pneumonia* (poor lung penetration).

Answer e is correct and the best answer. The bacterial causes of late-onset health care-associated pneumonia are the early-onset pathogens plus multidrug resistant pathogens (*Pseudomonas aeruginosa*, extended-spectrum beta-lactamase [ESBL] *Klebsiella pneumoniae, Acinetobacter* species, methicillin-resistant *Staphylococcus aureus*). The early onset pathogens are: *Streptococcus pneumoniae, Haemophilus influenza, Moraxella catarrhalis*, methicillin-sensitive *Staphylococcus aureus* (MSSA), and Enterics (ie, *Klebsiella pneumoniae, Escherichia coli, Enterobacter* species, *Proteus* species, *Serratia marcescens*).

---

10. Select the risk factor(s) for health care-associated pneumonia.
    a. Hospitalization for 2 days or more in the preceding 90 days
    b. Residence in nursing home or extended-care facility
    c. Home infusion therapy
    d. All of the above

Answer a is correct. Hospitalization for 2 days or more in the preceding 90 days is a risk factor for health care-associated pneumonia.

Answer b is correct. Residence in nursing home or extended-care facility is a risk factor for health care-associated pneumonia.

Answer c is correct. Home infusion therapy is a risk factor for health care-associated pneumonia.

Answer d is correct and the best answer. Other risk factors for health care-associated pneumonia are: chronic dialysis within 30 days, home wound care, and family member with multidrug resistant organisms. Health care-associated pneumonia risk factors are considered risk factors for multidrug resistant organisms.

---

11. Select the antimicrobial that is utilized for community-acquired pneumonia, inhibits protein synthesis, and is a strong inhibitor of the CYP-450 3A4 hepatic enzyme.

    a. Azithromycin
    b. Clarithromycin
    c. Amoxicillin
    d. Cefpodoxime

Answer a is incorrect. The azalide azithromycin is utilized for community-acquired pneumonia (CAP) and inhibits protein synthesis; however, it is a weak inhibitor of the CYP-450 3A4 hepatic enzyme. Drug interactions are a major difference between the macrolides (erythromycin and clarithromycin) and the azalide azithromycin.

Answer b is correct. Clarithromycin is utilized for treatment of CAP, inhibits protein synthesis, and is a strong inhibitor of the CYP-450 3A4 hepatic enzyme. Therefore drug interactions with the macrolide antimicrobial may be common. Medications that are substrates of the CYP-450 3A4 hepatic enzyme will have their metabolism/clearance decreased. Common examples of substrates of the CYP-450 3A4 hepatic enzyme are the azole antifungals, calcium channel blockers (verapamil and diltiazem), and HMG-CoA reductase inhibitors, and many others.

Answer c is incorrect. Amoxicillin may be used as part of a treatment regimen for CAP; however, amoxicillin inhibits bacterial cell wall synthesis and *does not* inhibit the CYP-450 system.

Answer d is incorrect. Cefpodoxime may be used as part of a treatment regimen for CAP; however, cefpodoxime inhibits bacterial cell wall synthesis and *does not* inhibit the CYP-450 system.

---

12. Select the antimicrobial that may be used to treat lower respiratory tract infections in pregnant patients.

    a. Clarithromycin
    b. Azithromycin
    c. Doxycycline
    d. Cefuroxime
    e. b and d

Answer a is incorrect. Clarithromycin is pregnancy category C. Although no teratogenic effects have been reported in humans, adverse fetal effects have been documented in animal studies; therefore, clarithromycin is classified as pregnancy category C. Clarithromycin should not be used in pregnant women unless there are no alternative therapies.

Answer b is correct. Azithromycin is pregnancy category B. Adverse events were not observed in animal studies; therefore, azithromycin is classified as pregnancy category B. Although no adverse reports in human or animal fetuses have been documented, information in pregnant women is limited.

Answer c is incorrect. Doxycycline is pregnancy category D. Because use during pregnancy may cause fetal harm, doxycycline is classified as pregnancy category D. Exposure to tetracyclines during the second or third trimester may cause permanent discoloration of the teeth.

Answer d is correct. Cefuroxime is pregnancy category B. Adverse events were not observed in animal studies; therefore, cefuroxime is classified as pregnancy category B. Most cell wall antimicrobials are pregnancy category B (exception imipenem). Recommendation: If you are not familiar with pregnancy category of antimicrobials, focus on the agents that you cannot use. For example, cell wall antimicrobials are often utilized; whereas, protein synthesis and DNA gyrase inhibitors are often contraindicated.

Answer e is correct and the best answer.

---

13. Select the antimicrobial that has the same oral and IV dose.

    a. Doxycycline
    b. Amoxicillin/clavulanate
    c. Piperacillin/tazobactam
    d. Ceftriaxone
    e. Ciprofloxacin

Answer a is correct. Doxycycline is available in oral and parenteral formulations. The pneumonia dose of doxycycline for oral and IV utilization is 100 mg every 12 hours.

Answer b is incorrect. Amoxicillin/clavulanate is available in an oral formulation only. Amoxicillin/clavulanate is available in immediate and extended release formulations. The immediate release dose of amoxicillin/clavulanate is 500 mg every 8 hours or 875 mg every 12 hours; the dose for the extended release preparation is 2000 mg every 12 hours.

Answer c is incorrect. Piperacillin/tazobactam is available in a parenteral formulation only. The pneumonia dose of piperacillin/tazobactam is 3.375 g every 4 to 6 hours or 4.5 g every 6 hours.

Answer d is incorrect. Ceftriaxone is available in a parenteral formulation only. The pneumonia dose of ceftriaxone is 1 g daily.

Answer e is incorrect. Ciprofloxacin is available in oral and parenteral formulations, however the dose is different based upon the formulation utilized. The oral dose for ciprofloxacin is 500 to 750 mg every 12 hours. The IV dose is 400 mg every 8 to12 hours. *Note*: Fluoroquinolones are often referred to as medications that have excellent bioavailability. The majority of fluoroquinolones have complete absorption; however, the bioavailability of ciprofloxacin is 50% to 85%, hence the difference in the oral and IV dose of ciprofloxacin. Levofloxacin is the only other fluoroquinolone that is available in oral and IV formulation. The absorption of levofloxacin is rapid and complete. The oral and IV dose of levofloxacin is the same (500-750 mg daily).

---

14. *High-dose* amoxicillin (1 g every 8 hours) and amoxicillin/clavulanate *XR* (2 g every 12 hours) are recommended in CAP treatment. The increase in dose of the two antimicrobials is recommended because of bacterial resistance. Select the pathogen that requires an increase in the dose of amoxicillin.
    a. Drug-resistant *Streptococcus pneumoniae* (DRSP)
    b. Methicillin-resistant *Staphylococcus aureus* (MRSA)
    c. Extended-spectrum beta-lactamase (ESBL) *Klebsiella pneumoniae*
    d. All of the above

Answer a is correct. Drug-resistant *S. pneumoniae* (DRSP) is caused by alterations in the binding site (penicillin-binding protein). This alteration leads to a higher minimum inhibitory concentration (MIC). An increase in the concentration required to inhibit and kill the bacteria requires an increase in the antimicrobial dose. Therefore the higher dose of amoxicillin is needed to treat DRSP.

Answer b is incorrect. Methicillin-resistant *Staphylococcus aureus* (MRSA) is not covered by amoxicillin or amoxicillin/clavulanate; therefore, increasing the dose of amoxicillin would not have an effect on MRSA.

Answer c is incorrect. *High-dose* amoxicillin and amoxicillin/clavulanate *XR* do not cover ESBL *Klebsiella pneumoniae.* While the clavulanate part of amoxicillin/clavulanate is utilized to treat (or act as a scavenger) for beta-lactamase production by enteric gram-negatives, extended spectrum beta lactamase is a similar but different type of resistance mechanism. The beta-lactamase inhibitors : clavulanate, sulbactam, and tazobactam do not have sufficient activity against ESBL producing organisms. ESBL producing organisms are often treated with carbapenems.

Answer d is incorrect.

---

15. Select the antimicrobial(s) that is associated with the side effect photosensitivity.
    a. Doxycycline
    b. Ciprofloxacin
    c. Cefepime
    d. a and b
    e. All of the above

Answer a is correct. Tetracycline antimicrobials are associated with photosensitivity.

Answer b is correct. Fluoroquinolone antimicrobials are associated with photosensitivity.

Answer c is incorrect. Cephalosporin antimicrobials are not associated with photosensitivity.

Answer d is correct and the best answer.

Answer e is incorrect.

---

16. Select the antimicrobials that are often associated with a *Clostridium difficile* infection.
    a. Ciprofloxacin
    b. Clindamycin
    c. Cefotaxime
    d. All of the above

Answer a is correct. Fluoroquinolones may cause *C. difficile* infections.

Answer b is correct. Clindamycin may cause *C. difficile* infections.

Answer c is correct. Cephalosporins may cause *C. difficile* infections.

Answer d is correct and the best answer. The majority of antimicrobials can cause *C. difficile* infections. *Clostridium difficile* infections are treated by metronidazole or oral vancomycin.

---

17. Select the side effect that a high percentage of patients with infectious mononucleosis develop when they receive penicillin antimicrobials (amoxicillin, ampicillin, or piperacillin).
    a. Bone marrow suppression (BMS)
    b. Rash
    c. *Clostridium difficile*
    d. Thrombocytopenia

Answer a is incorrect. BMS is a rare side effect of cell wall antimicrobials and patients with infectious mononucleosis would have the same incidence of BMS compared to patients without infectious mononucleosis.

Answer b is correct. Patients with infectious mononucleosis that receive penicillin antimicrobials have a high incidence of rash.

Answer c is incorrect. *Clostridium difficile* is a serious side effect of all antimicrobials; however, patients with infectious mononucleosis would have the same incidence of *C. difficile* compared to patients without infectious mononucleosis.

Answer d is incorrect. Thrombocytopenia is a rare side effect of most penicillin antimicrobials; however, patients with infectious mononucleosis would have the same incidence of thrombocytopenia compared to patients without infectious mononucleosis. *Note*: Piperacillin has the highest incidence of thrombocytopenia of the penicillin antimicrobials.

---

18. Select the antimicrobial that a patient with a delayed allergic hypersensitivity reaction to ampicillin/sulbactam may receive.

    a. Ceftriaxone
    b. Moxifloxacin
    c. Piperacillin tazobactam
    d. a and b
    e. All of the above

Answer a is correct. Ceftriaxone and cephalosporin antimicrobials may be utilized in patients with delayed hypersensitivity (rash) reactions to penicillin. There is an 8% to 10% chance of cross reaction.

Answer b is correct. Moxifloxacin and fluoroquinolone antimicrobials may be utilized in patients with *delayed* (rash) or *immediate* (anaphylaxis) hypersensitivity reactions to penicillin.

Answer c is incorrect. Piperacillin/tazobactam is a penicillin antimicrobial and cannot be used in patients with an allergic reaction to penicillin.

Answer d is correct and the best answer.

Answer e is incorrect.

---

19. Select the penicillin antimicrobial that is combined with a beta-lactamase inhibitor.

    a. Zosyn
    b. Unasyn
    c. Augmentin
    d. All of the above

Answer a is correct. Zosyn is piperacillin/tazobactam.

Answer b is correct. Unasyn is ampicillin/sulbactam.

Answer c is correct. Augmentin is amoxicillin/clavulanate.

Answer d is correct and the best answer.

---

20. The addition of the beta-lactamase inhibitor sulbactam to ampicillin is done to:

    a. Increase bacterial coverage
    b. Decrease side effects
    c. Improve bioavailability
    d. All of the above

Answer a is correct. The addition of sulbactam to ampicillin extends the coverage of ampicillin to include beta-lactamase producing enteric gram-negatives (ie, *K. pneumoniae, E. coli, Enterobacter* species, *Proteus* species, *S. marcescens*). *Note*: Please differentiate between beta-lactamase producing enterics and extended-spectrum beta-lactamase (ESBL) producing enterics. The addition of sulbactam to ampicillin, clavulanate to amoxicillin, tazobactam to piperacillin, and clavulanate to ticarcillin extends the coverage of the penicillin antimicrobial to include beta-lactamase producing enterics, *not* ESBL producing enterics.

Answer b is incorrect. The addition of sulbactam to ampicillin would not decrease side effects. Sulbactam (and other beta-lactamase inhibitors) are beta-lactam antimicrobials; and therefore are associated with side effects. The combination would potentially increase side effects (eg, the addition of clavulanate to amoxicillin increases the gastrointestinal side effects compared to amoxicillin).

Answer c is incorrect. Ampicillin/sulbactam is an IV agent and therefore has a bioavailability of 100% (F = 1).

Answer d is incorrect.

---

21. Select the salt formation of piperacillin/tazobactam.

    a. Potassium
    b. Hydrochloride
    c. Sodium
    d. All of the above

Answer a is incorrect.

Answer b is correct. Piperacillin is a sodium salt and may increase sodium levels. 4.5 g of piperacillin/tazobactam contains 11/17 mEq of sodium and 3.375 g contains 8.38 mEq of sodium.

Answers c and d are incorrect.

---

22. Select the beta-lactam antimicrobial that *does not require* dose or interval reductions in patients with renal dysfunction.

    a. Amoxicillin
    b. Azithromycin
    c. Ceftriaxone
    d. Moxifloxacin
    e. Cefepime

Answer a is incorrect. The beta-lactam amoxicillin and other *penicillin* antimicrobials used for the treatment of pneumonia are required to have dose and/or interval modifications in patients with renal dysfunction.

Answer b is incorrect. While azithromycin does not require dose or interval reductions in patients with renal dysfunction (azithromycin undergoes hepatic metabolism/elimination), it is not a beta lactam. Azithromycin is an azalide antimicrobial; however, clinicians often refer to azithromycin as a macrolide.

Answer c is correct. The beta-lactam ceftriaxone undergoes dual elimination. Even though ceftriaxone has renal elimination, it is not required to have dose/interval reductions in patients with renal dysfunction.

Answer d is incorrect. While moxifloxacin does not require dose or interval reductions in patients with renal dysfunction (moxifloxacin undergoes hepatic metabolism and renal and feces elimination), it is not a beta lactam. Moxifloxacin is a fluoroquinolone antimicrobial. All other fluoroquinolones (levofloxacin, ciprofloxacin, gemifloxacin) require dose or interval modifications in patients with renal dysfunction.

Answer e is incorrect. The fourth generation cephalosporin cefepime is a beta lactam and requires dose or interval reductions in patients with renal dysfunction.

---

23. Select the side effect(s) associated with fluoroquinolone antimicrobials.
    a. Hypoglycemia
    b. *Clostridium difficile* infection
    c. Confusion in the elderly
    d. QTc prolongation
    e. All of the above

Answer a is correct. Fluoroquinolones can cause glucose problems. Fluoroquinolones have been associated with hypo- and hyperglycemia. Gatifloxacin (Tequin) was a fluoroquinolone pulled from the market because of this effect. While fluoroquinolones may have a different incidence of causing glucose homeostasis issues, it is a class wide effect.

Answer b is correct. Fluoroquinolones can cause *C. difficile* infections.

Answer c is correct. Fluoroquinolones can cause central nervous system side effects, such as confusion.

Answer d is correct. Fluoroquinolones can prolong the QTc interval, especially when combined with Class 1a or III antiarrhythmics. The QTc prolongation caused solely by the fluoroquinolones is usually not clinically significant. Combination with other agents that prolong the QTc interval may lead to clinically significant events.

Answer e is correct and the best answer.

---

24. Aminoglycoside antimicrobials may be dosed via conventional (1-2.5 mg/kg every 8-12 hours) or extended interval (4-7 mg/kg every 24, 36, or 48 hours) methods. Select the therapeutic drug monitoring parameter(s) associated with conventional dosing of aminoglycosides.
    a. Peak (C_{max}) 8 to 10 μg/mL for serious infections
    b. Trough (C_{min}) less than 2 mg/L
    c. Random level (between 6-14 hours) of 5 mg/L
    d. a and b
    e. All of the above

Answer a is correct. Peak concentrations for conventional dosing aminoglycosides are often 8 to 10 μg/mL for serious infections. Peak concentrations may be lower for certain types of infections (eg, urinary tract infections). Serum concentration monitoring is necessary for safe and effective therapy, particularly in patients with serious infections and those with risk factors for toxicity. Peak serum concentrations should be drawn 30 minutes after the completion of a 30-minute infusion. Serum concentrations should be drawn after 3 to 5 half-lives, usually around the third dose. Desired measured serum concentrations:

1. Gentamicin and tobramycin: Peak 4 to 10 μg/mL
2. Amikacin: Peak 20 to 30 μg/mL

Answer b is correct. Trough concentrations for conventional dosing aminoglycosides should be less than 2 mg/L (2 μg/mL). Trough serum concentrations should be drawn within 30 minutes prior to the administered dose. Serum concentrations should be drawn after 3 to 5 half-lives, usually around the third dose. Desired measured serum concentrations:

1. Gentamicin and tobramycin: Trough 0.5 to 2 μg/mL
2. Amikacin: Trough < 5 μg/mL

Answer c is incorrect. A random level between 6 and 14 hours of 5 mg/L (5 μg/mL) would be for extended interval dosing of aminoglycosides.

Answer d is correct and the best answer.

Answer e is incorrect.

---

25. Select the brand name of ceftazidime.
    a. Zyvox
    b. Rocephin
    c. Avelox
    d. Fortaz
    e. Vibramycin

Answer a is incorrect. Zyvox is the brand name for linezolid.

Answer b is incorrect. Rocephin is the brand name for ceftriaxone.

Answer c is incorrect. Avelox is the brand name for moxifloxacin.

Answer d is correct. Fortaz is the brand name for ceftazidime.

Answer e is incorrect. Vibramycin is the brand name for doxycycline.

CHAPTER 22 | Skin and Soft Tissue Infections

1. Skin and soft tissue infections (SSTIs) may involve all layers of the skin, fascia, and muscle. Select the part of the skin that represents the outermost nonvascular layer.

   a. Epidermis
   b. Dermis
   c. Subcutaneous fat
   d. Fascia
   e. All of the above

Answer a is correct. The epidermis is the outermost, nonvascular layer of the skin.

Answer b is incorrect. The dermis is the layer of skin directly beneath the epidermis. It consists of connective tissue and contains blood vessels and lymphatics, sensory nerve endings, sweat and sebaceous glands, hair follicles, and smooth muscle fibers.

Answer c is incorrect. Beneath the dermis is a layer of loose connective tissue containing primarily fat cells. This *subcutaneous fat* layer is of variable thickness over the body.

Answer d is incorrect. Beneath the subcutaneous fat lies the fascia, which separates the skin from muscle.

Answer e is incorrect.

Note: SSTIs may involve any or all layers of the skin, fascia, and muscle. SSTIs can range in severity from mild, superficial, self-limiting infections to severe, deep-seated, life-threatening infections. They may also spread far from the initial site of infection and lead to severe complications, such as sepsis, glomerulonephritis, endocarditis, or osteomyelitis.

---

2. Select the most common causative organism(s) for the majority of SSTIs.

   a. *Staphylococcus aureus*
   b. *Streptococcus pyogenes*
   c. *Pseudomonas aeruginosa*
   d. a and b
   e. All of the above

Answer a is correct. *Staphylococcus aureus* is a common cause of SSTIs. Understanding treatment of *S. aureus* requires an understanding of resistance. The majority of *S. aureus* isolates produce penicillinase (beta-lactamase). Production of penicillinase requires treatment with penicillinase stable penicillins (eg, dicloxacillin, a beta-lactam / beta-lactamase inhibitor (eg, amoxicillin-clavulanate)), or medications not affected by the penicillinase (eg, a cephalosporin (eg, cephalexin), or clindamycin). The other major resistance associated with *S. aureus* is altered target site or methicillin-resistant *Staphylococcus aureus* (MRSA). MRSA may be community acquired (caMRSA) or health care acquired (haMRSA). See Table 22-5 in the SSTI chapter for antimicrobials that treat MRSA.

Answer b is correct. *Streptococcus pyogenes* is a common cause of SSTIs. Other names for *Streptococcus pyogenes* include group A streptococci (GAS), and the flesh-eating bacteria. GAS is also an example of β-hemolytic *Streptococcus*; other examples of β-hemolytic *Streptococcus* include *Streptococcus* A,B,C,D,E. Treatment for GAS is relatively easy, it may be treated with narrow-spectrum penicillin; however, GAS may produce toxins and lead to complications, even though appropriate treatment has been initiated.

Answer c is incorrect. *Pseudomonas aeruginosa* is not a common cause of SSTIs. SSTIs are mostly caused by the gram-positives *S. aureus* and *S. pyogenes*; however, the gram-negative *P. aeruginosa* may cause SSTIs in certain situations (These situations include diabetic foot infections, pressure sores, burn wounds, and immune-compromised patients).

Answer d is correct and the best answer.

Answer e is incorrect.

---

3. Select the answer that is defined as a superficial skin infection caused by β-hemolytic *Streptococcus* and *S. aureus*. Treatment consists of soaking the lesions with soap and water, use of skin emollients to dry areas, and antimicrobials. Topical mupirocin may be used alone when there are few lesions.

   a. Erysipelas
   b. Lymphangitis
   c. Impetigo
   d. Necrotizing fasciitis
   e. All of the above

Answer a is incorrect. Erysipelas is an infection of the superficial layers of the skin and cutaneous lymphatics. The intense red color and burning pain led to the common name of St. Anthony's fire. The infection is most often caused by GAS. Mild to moderate cases of erysipelas are treated with intramuscular procaine penicillin G or oral penicillin VK.

Answer b is incorrect. Lymphangitis is an inflammation of the lymphatic channel that ensues when a local skin infection is not contained, most often caused by GAS. Lymphangitis is characterized by red linear streaks that extend from the infection site toward regional lymph nodes. Because these infections are potentially serious and rapidly progressive, initial treatment should be with IV penicillin G 1 to 2 million units every 4 to 6 hours.

Answer c is correct. Impetigo is a superficial skin infection caused by β-hemolytic *Streptococcus* and *S. aureus*. The microorganisms colonize the skin and invade through abrasions, insect bites, or other small traumas. Impetigo lesions are numerous, well-localized, and erythematous. Antimicrobials with activity against group A *Streptococcus* (GAS) and the beta-lactamase producing (penicillinase) *S. aureus* are preferred, and include first-generation cephalosporins and penicillinase-stable penicillins. Topical mupirocin may be used alone when there are few lesions.

Answer d is incorrect. Necrotizing fasciitis (NF) is an uncommon, rapidly progressive, life- threatening infection of the subcutaneous tissue and fascia. After resuscitation and hemodynamic stabilization, prompt surgical intervention is key in the treatment of NF. Broad-spectrum IV antimicrobial therapy should be initiated immediately in patients with NF.

Answer e is incorrect.

---

4. Select the SSTI that may be treated with topical antimicrobials.
   a. Impetigo
   b. Cellulitis
   c. Diabetic foot ulcers
   d. a and c
   e. All of the above

Answer a is correct. Mild cases of impetigo may be treated with topical mupirocin (mild cases defined as a patient with a few lesions).

Answer b is incorrect. Cellulitis requires treatment with systemic antimicrobials.

Answer c is incorrect. Diabetic foot ulcers require treatment with systemic antimicrobials.

Answers d and e are incorrect.

---

5. CX is a 46-year-old patient diagnosed with lymphangitis. CX has a penicillin allergy, the allergy is a rash. Select the best antimicrobial to treat the lymphangitis in CX.
   a. Penicillin G (IV)
   b. Penicillin VK (oral)
   c. Clindamycin (IV)
   d. Trimethoprim-sulfamethoxazole (IV)
   e. Vancomycin (oral)

Note: Lymphangitis is an inflammation of the lymphatic channel that ensues when a local skin infection is not contained, most often caused by *GAS*. Lymphangitis is characterized by red linear streaks that extend from the infection site toward regional lymph nodes.

Answer a is incorrect. IV penicillin G cannot be used to treat CX's infection because of penicillin allergy. In patients without penicillin allergy, IV penicillin G 1 to 2 million units every 4 to 6 hours is preferred because of the seriousness of the infection and the ability to rapidly progress. Parenteral treatment should be continued for 48 to 72 hours, followed by oral penicillin VK for a total of 10 days.

Answer b is incorrect. Oral penicillin VK cannot be used to treat CX's infection because of a penicillin allergy. Penicillin is a recommended antimicrobial in lymphangitis infections, but only in patients without penicillin allergies. Oral penicillin would be used in mild cases of lymphangitis or as a step-down therapy in patients initially started on IV penicillin.

Answer c is correct. The lincosamide antimicrobial clindamycin is effective for SSTIs that are caused by *S. aureus* and GAS. Since lymphangitis is caused by GAS, clindamycin would be an effective treatment option in patients allergic to penicillin.

Answer d is incorrect. Trimethoprim-sulfamethoxazole would not be used to treat lymphangitis infections. Although active in vitro, TMP/SMX is not clinically effective for GAS. The role of TMP-SMZ is for treatment of SSTIs caused by caMRSA.

Answer e is incorrect. Vancomycin has activity against GAS; however, oral vancomycin is not absorbed and only used to treat the antibiotic side effect of *Clostridium difficile* infection (colitis infections). Intravenous vancomycin would be effective, but will still not be used over clindamycin (use the most narrow-spectrum antibiotic as possible). Vancomycin should be reserved for treatment of MRSA infection and for allergic reactions. While CX has a history of an allergic reaction to penicillin, there are still other alternatives prior to using vancomycin.

---

6. NV is diagnosed with cellulitis. Pharmacologic treatment of cellulitis is with an antibiotic that is active against penicillinase-producing strains of *S. aureus (MSSA)*. Select the penicillin that is active against penicillinase-producing strains of *S. aureus*.
   a. Cephalexin
   b. Amoxicillin
   c. Clindamycin
   d. Doxycycline
   e. Nafcillin

Answer a is incorrect. While cephalexin is stable against penicillinase-producing strains of *S. aureus*, it is a cephalosporin. *Note:* All cephalosporins are stable/active against beta-lactamase (penicillinase) production. A newer type of beta-lactamase production is called extended-spectrum beta-lactamase (ESBL); most cephalosporins are not stable/active against ESBL production. Examples of bacteria that have ESBLs are the Enterobacteriaceae (eg, *Escherichia coli)*.

Answer b is incorrect. Amoxicillin is not stable/active against penicillinase-producing strains of *S. aureus*. Amoxicillin that is combined with clavulanate (Augmentin) would be stable against penicillinase-producing strains of *S. aureus*.

Answer c is incorrect. Clindamycin is stable against penicillinase-producing strains of *S. aureus;* however, it is a lincosamide antibiotic. Clindamycin is used to treat SSTIs in patients with a penicillin allergy or caMRSA.

Answer d is incorrect. Doxycycline is stable against penicillinase-producing strains of *S. aureus;* however, it is a tetracycline antibiotic. Doxycycline is used to treat SSTIs in patients with a penicillin allergy or caMRSA.

Answer e is correct. Nafcillin is stable against penicillinase-producing strains of *S. aureus,* and is a penicillin. Nafcillin is referred to as a penicillinase-stable penicillin or an antistaphylococcal penicillin. Other antibiotics in this class are: dicloxacillin, methicillin, and oxacillin. *Note:* Methicillin is no longer used clinically, but is referred to in *S. aureus* resistance (ie, methicillin-resistant *S. aureus*).

---

7. Select the patient risk factor(s) for health care-associated MRSA (haMRSA).
   a. Prolonged hospitalization
   b. Nursing home residence
   c. Indwelling catheters
   d. Previous antimicrobial use
   e. All of the above

Answers a, b, c, and d, are correct. These are all risk factors for haMRSA

Answer e is correct and the best answer. *Note:* haMRSA is associated with well-defined risk factors (ie, prolonged hospitalization, nursing home residence, previous antimicrobial use, indwelling catheters, pressure sores, surgery, or dialysis); however, caMRSA risk factors are not well established. caMRSA is becoming a common pathogen in SSTIs.

---

8. Select the antibiotic that would have activity against caMRSA and haMRSA.
   a. Vancomycin
   b. Clindamycin
   c. Daptomycin
   d. a and c
   e. All of the above

Answer a is correct. Vancomycin would have activity against caMRSA and haMRSA.

Answer b is incorrect. Clindamycin has activity against caMRSA. Very few strains of haMRSA are susceptible to clindamycin.

Answer c is correct. Daptomycin would have activity against caMRSA and haMRSA.

Answer d is correct and the best answer. caMRSA is susceptible to more antibiotics than haMRSA. Like haMRSA, caMRSA is sensitive to vancomycin, linezolid, daptomycin, tigecycline, and quinupristin/dalfopristin, but caMRSA is also susceptible to trimethoprim-sulfamethoxazole (TMP-SMX), clindamycin, doxycycline, and minocycline.

Answer e is incorrect.

---

9. Select the antibiotic used in combination treatment of necrotizing fasciitis. This antibiotic is used to decrease bacterial toxin production, thereby limiting tissue damage.
   a. Cleocin
   b. Primaxin
   c. Augmentin
   d. Zosyn

Answer a is correct. Clindamycin (Cleocin) should be added to decrease bacterial toxin production, thereby limiting tissue damage.

Answer b is incorrect. Imipenem-cilastatin (Primaxin) may be used in the treatment of NF, but it needs to be combined with clindamycin.

Answer c is incorrect. Amoxicillin-clavulanate (Augmentin) may be used in the treatment of NF, but it needs to be combined with clindamycin.

Answer d is incorrect. Piperacillin-tazobactam (Zosyn) may be used in the treatment of NF, but it needs to be combined with clindamycin.

---

10. Select the factor(s) that are involved in diabetic foot infections.
    a. Angiopathy
    b. Neuropathy
    c. Immunopathy
    d. All of the above

Answer a is correct. Angiopathy of large and small vessels also results from high blood glucose levels and results in ischemia and skin breakdown.

Answer b is correct. Neuropathy develops when high blood glucose levels damage motor, autonomic, and sensory nerves.

Answer c is correct. Diabetic patients develop immunopathy, which predisposes them to infections. Leukocyte function and cell-mediated immunity are compromised in poorly controlled diabetics.

Answer d is correct and the best answer.

---

11. Select the factor(s) that may reduce the rate of diabetic foot infections.
    a. Periodic foot examinations
    b. Optimal glycemic control
    c. Smoking cessation
    d. All of the above

Answer a is correct. Comprehensive foot-care programs can significantly reduce the rate of diabetic foot infections. Periodic foot examinations with monofilament testing and patient education regarding proper foot care may reduce the rate of diabetic foot infections.

Answer b is correct. Optimal glycemic control may reduce the rate of diabetic foot infections.

Answer c is correct. Smoking cessation may reduce the rate of diabetic foot infections.

Answer d is correct and the best answer.

12. Select the IV antimicrobial used in the empiric treatment of cellulitis that is active/stable against the penicillinase-producing strains of *S. aureus* and group A streptococci.

 a. Dicloxacillin
 b. Cephalexin
 c. Amoxicillin-clavulanate
 d. Cefazolin

Answer a is incorrect. Dicloxacillin is active against penicillinase-producing *S. aureus* and group A streptococci and is used in the empiric treatment of cellulitis, but is only available in the oral formulation (capsule).

Answer b is incorrect. Cephalexin is active against penicillinase-producing *S. aureus* and group A streptococci and is used in the empiric treatment of cellulitis, but is only available in the oral formulation (capsule, tablet, suspension).

Answer c is incorrect. Amoxicillin-clavulanate is active against penicillinase-producing *S. aureus* and group A streptococci and is used in the empiric treatment of cellulitis, but is only available in the oral formulation (suspension, tablet, extended-release tablet).

Answer d is correct. Cefazolin is active against penicillinase-producing *S. aureus* and group A streptococci. It is used in the empiric treatment of cellulitis, and is available in a parenteral formulation (IV).

13. PU is a 58-year-old patient diagnosed with cellulitis. It was determined that the most likely pathogens causing the infection were *S. aureus* and group A streptococci. PU has a history of chronic renal insufficiency and the provider would like to use an antibiotic that does not have to be adjusted for renal dysfunction. Select the antibiotic that is *not* required to be adjusted for renal function.

 a. Nafcillin
 b. Ertapenem
 c. Ceftriaxone
 d. a and c
 e. All of the above

Answer a is correct. Nafcillin is primarily eliminated in the feces and undergoes hepatic metabolism. Adjustment of dose or interval is only required in patients with both renal and hepatic insufficiency.

Answer b is incorrect. Ertapenem dose/interval should be modified in patients with renal dysfunction.

Answer c is correct. Ceftriaxone does not require dose/interval modifications in patients with renal dysfunction.

Answer d is correct and the best answer.

Answer e is incorrect.

14. Select the beta-lactam antibiotic(s) that is (are) renally eliminated and require dose and/or interval modification in renal dysfunction.

 a. Keflex
 b. Ceftin
 c. Unasyn
 d. Zosyn
 e. All of the above

Answer a is correct. Cephalexin (Keflex) is a beta-lactam (cephalosporin) that is renally eliminated and requires dose and/or interval modification in renal dysfunction.

Answer b is correct. Cefuroxime (Ceftin) is a beta-lactam (cephalosporin) that is renally eliminated and requires dose and/or interval modification in renal dysfunction.

Answer c is correct. Ampicillin-sulbactam (Unasyn) is a beta-lactam (penicillin: beta-lactam/beta-lactamase inhibitor) that is renally eliminated and requires dose and/or interval modification in renal dysfunction.

Answer d is correct. Piperacillin-tazobactam (Zosyn) is a beta-lactam (penicillin: beta-lactam/beta-lactamase inhibitor) that is renally eliminated and requires dose and/or interval modification in renal dysfunction.

Answer e is correct and the best answer. The majority of antibiotics are renally eliminated, especially the beta-lactams. The only **beta-lactams** that *are not renally eliminated* are nafcillin, dicloxacillin, and ceftriaxone (*note*: ceftriaxone is renally eliminated, but because it has dual methods of elimination, it is not required to be adjusted for renal dysfunction). Other antibiotics used in SSTIs and other infections that *would not require* dose modifications in renal dysfunction include: clindamycin, doxycycline, macrolides, moxifloxacin, linezolid, and tigecycline.

15. TR is a 29-year-old pregnant patient with a diagnosis of cellulitis. Select the antibiotic that may be used to treat systemic infections in a pregnant patient.

 a. Imipenem-cilastatin
 b. Doxycycline
 c. Levofloxacin
 d. Cefazolin

Answer a is incorrect. Imipenem-cilastatin has a pregnancy category of C. Other carbapenems (doripenem, meropenem, ertapenem) have a pregnancy category of B.

Answer b is incorrect. Doxycycline has a pregnancy category of D.

Answer c is incorrect. Levofloxacin has a pregnancy category of C.

Answer d is correct. Cefazolin has a pregnancy category of B.

16. Select the antibiotic with the following mechanism of action: binds to components of the cell membrane and causes rapid depolarization, inhibiting intracellular synthesis of DNA, RNA, and protein.

   a. Piperacillin-tazobactam
   b. Imipenem-cilastatin
   c. Clindamycin
   d. Daptomycin
   e. Vancomycin

Answer a is incorrect. Piperacillin/tazobactam inhibits bacterial cell wall synthesis by binding to one or more of the penicillin-binding proteins. Tazobactam binds and inhibits beta-lactamases that inactivate piperacillin resulting in piperacillin having an expanded spectrum of activity.

Answer b is incorrect. Imipenem inhibits bacterial cell wall synthesis by binding to penicillin-binding proteins, which inhibits the final transpeptidation step of peptidoglycan synthesis. Cilastatin prevents renal metabolism of imipenem by inhibition of dehydropeptidase along the brush border of the renal tubules.

Answer c is incorrect. Clindamycin reversibly binds to 50s ribosomal subunits preventing peptide bond formation thus inhibiting bacterial protein synthesis.

Answer d is correct. Daptomycin binds to components of the cell membrane and causes rapid depolarization, inhibiting intracellular synthesis of DNA, RNA, and protein.

Answer e is incorrect. Vancomycin inhibits bacterial cell wall synthesis by blocking glycopeptide polymerization through binding of the D-alanyl-D-alanine portion of cell wall precursor.

Note: Most antibiotics can be classified into three groups according to their mechanism of action: (1) beta-lactams—cell wall inhibitors; (2) protein synthesis inhibitors; and (3) miscellaneous.

---

17. Select the antimicrobial that can alter glucose levels (hyper- or hypoglycemia).

   a. Levofloxacin
   b. Clindamycin
   c. Vancomycin
   d. Daptomycin

Answer a is correct. Fluoroquinolones may cause glucose homeostasis issues (hyper- or hypoglycemia). While gatifloxacin (Tequin) was pulled from the market because of this issue, it is a class wide effect.

Answer b is incorrect. Clindamycin does not have an effect on glucose levels.

Answer c is incorrect. Vancomycin does not have an effect on glucose levels.

Answer d is incorrect. Daptomycin does not have an effect on glucose levels.

---

18. Select the fluoroquinolone that inhibits the CYP-450 system.

   a. Doxycycline
   b. Levofloxacin
   c. Trimethoprim-sulfamethoxazole
   d. Nafcillin
   e. Ciprofloxacin

Answer a is incorrect. While doxycycline is an inhibitor of the CYP-450 3A4 (moderate), it is a tetracycline antimicrobial.

Answer b is incorrect. While levofloxacin is a fluoroquinolone antimicrobial, it does not affect the CYP-450 system.

Answer c is incorrect. While trimethoprim-sulfamethoxazole is an inhibitor of the CYP-450 (Sulfamethoxazole—substrate CYP 2C9 [major], 3A4 [minor], inhibits 2C9 [moderate]; Trimethoprim—substrate 2C9 [major], 3A4 [major], inhibits 2C8 [moderate], 2C9 [moderate]), it is a sulfonamide antimicrobial.

Answer d is incorrect. While nafcillin does affect the CYP-450 system (P-450 3A4 inducer), it is a penicillin antimicrobial.

Answer e is correct. Ciprofloxacin is a fluoroquinolone antimicrobial and inhibits the CYP-450 system (1A2—strong and 3A4—weak).

---

19. Fluoroquinolones may prolong the QTc interval. Select the risk factor(s) for prolonged QTc interval.

   a. Uncorrected hypokalemia
   b. Concurrent administration of medications known to prolong QTc interval
   c. Uncorrected hypomagnesemia
   d. a and c
   e. All of the above

Answer a is correct. Uncorrected hypokalemia is a risk factor for QTc prolongation.

Answer b is correct. Concurrent administration of medications known to prolong QTc interval, examples include Class 1a and Class III antiarrhythmics, erythromycin, antipsychotics, tricyclic antidepressants.

Answer c is correct. Uncorrected hypomagnesemia is a risk factor for QTc prolongation.

Answer d is correct.

Answer e is correct and the best answer.

---

20. Select the antimicrobial utilized to treat SSTIs that may cause photosensitivity.

   a. Ciprofloxacin
   b. Doxycycline

c. Levofloxacin
d. a and c
e. All of the above

Answer a is correct. Ciprofloxacin and fluoroquinolones may cause photosensitivity.

Answer b is correct. Doxycycline and tetracyclines may cause photosensitivity.

Answer c is correct. Levofloxacin and fluoroquinolones may cause photosensitivity.

Answer d is correct.

Answer e is correct and the best answer.

21. Select the parameter(s) that should be monitored with daptomycin.

a. CPK
b. Muscle weakness
c. Serum creatinine
d. All of the above

Answer a is correct. CPK values should be monitored in patients receiving daptomycin. Daptomycin is associated with myopathy; discontinue in patients with signs and symptoms of myopathy in conjunction with increase in CPK > 5 times upper limit of normal or in asymptomatic patients with CPK > 10 times upper limit of normal.

Answer b is correct. Daptomycin is associated with myopathy, discontinue in patients with signs and symptoms of myopathy in conjunction with increase in CPK or in asymptomatic patients with CPK > 10 times upper limit of normal.

Answer c is correct. Daptomycin should be used with caution in renal dysfunction (dosage adjustment is required).

Answer d is correct and the best answer.

22. BD is a 24-year-old man with no known drug allergies who was initially treated with vancomycin for his cellulitis. His abscess culture after appropriate incision/drainage revealed caMRSA. He has clinically improved enough to receive oral antibiotics. Which of the following is an appropriate step-down antibiotic for BD?

a. Cephalexin
b. Amoxicillin-clavulanate
c. Ceftriaxone
d. Trimethoprim-sulfamethoxazole

Answer a is incorrect. Cephalexin has no activity against MRSA.

Answer b is incorrect. Amoxicillin-clavulanate has no activity against MRSA. MRSA's resistance mechanism to beta-lactams is altering the penicillin-binding protein, therefore all beta-lactams are ineffective against MRSA. Clavulanate is a beta-lactamase inhibitor and would not increase amoxicillin's activity versus MRSA.

Answer c is incorrect. Ceftriaxone has no activity against MRSA.

Answer d is correct. Trimethoprim-sulfamethoxazole has excellent activity versus MRSA. It is used primarily in uncomplicated skin/skin structure infections, but is also used as step-down therapy from IV therapy in patients requiring initial hospitalization.

23. Select the antimicrobial that may cause thrombocytopenia, especially with more than 2 weeks of therapy.

a. Cleocin
b. Zyvox
c. Cubicin
d. Tygacil

Answer a is incorrect. Cleocin is not associated with thrombocytopenia.

Answer b is correct and is the best answer. Linezolid (Zyvox) is associated with bone marrow suppression, including leukopenia, anemia, and thrombocytopenia (most common). While these side effects can occur at anytime, prolonged therapy of more than 2 weeks is associated with greater risk.

Answer c is incorrect. Cubicin is not associated with thrombocytopenia.

Answer d is incorrect. Tygacil is only rarely associated with thrombocytopenia.

24. Which of the following is a reasonable duration of antimicrobial therapy for treating osteomyelitis?

a. 1 week
b. 2 weeks
c. 3 weeks
d. 6 weeks

Answers a, b, and c are incorrect. Treatment duration of osteomyelitis generally is 4 to 6 weeks. One, two, or three weeks is too short.

Answer d is correct. Six weeks is an acceptable timeframe for the treatment of osteomyelitis.

25. Which of the following carbapenem antibiotics does *not* have coverage against *P. aeruginosa*?

a. Ertapenem
b. Doripenem
c. Imipenem-cilastatin
d. Meropenem

Answer a is correct. Ertapenem is the only carbapenem that does not have coverage against *P. aeruginosa*.

Answers b, c, and d are incorrect. These have antipseudomonal activity.

CHAPTER 23 | Urinary Tract Infections

1. Select the following organism(s) that can cause a UTI.
   a. Bacteria
   b. Fungus
   c. Virus
   d. All of the above

Answer d is correct. All of the above organisms can cause a UTI. However, most UTIs are caused by bacteria.

2. GB is a 28-year-old woman with a chief complaint of dysuria. The physician orders a urinalysis and a urine culture. What is the most likely cause of the UTI?
   a. *Acinetobacter baumannii*
   b. *Escherichia coli*
   c. *Pseudomonas aeruginosa*
   d. *Staphylococcus saprophyticus*

Answer a is incorrect. *Acinetobacter baumannii* is a nosocomial organism and a cause of catheter-associated UTIs.

Answer b is correct. The majority of UTIs are caused by gram-negative bacteria, of which *E. coli* is the most common pathogen.

Answer c is incorrect. *Pseudomonas aeruginosa* is a nosocomial organism and causes <20% of UTIs.

Answer d is incorrect. *Staphylococcus saprophyticus* only causes 5% to 10% of uncomplicated UTIs. It is the most common gram-positive bacteria causing uncomplicated UTIs.

3. What is appropriate empiric therapy for GB?
   a. Cefdinir
   b. Linezolid
   c. Penicillin
   d. TMP-SMX

Answer a is incorrect. Cefdinir is an oral third-generation cephalosporin commonly used for acute otitis media in pediatrics. It is not indicated for treatment of UTIs

Answer b is incorrect. Linezolid is an antibiotic that covers gram-positive bacteria exclusively. It is primarily used to treat methicillin-resistant *Staphylococcus aureus* (MRSA) and vancomycin-resistant enterococci (VRE). Both MRSA and VRE can cause UTIs, but GB does not need to be empirically covered with linezolid.

Answer c is incorrect. *Escherichia coli* resistance rate to ampicillin is 37%. Thus, penicillin would be a poor selection.

Answer d is correct. TMP-SMX is appropriate empiric therapy for GB. If the local *E. coli* resistance rate for TMP-SMX is high, ciprofloxacin would be an appropriate choice.

4. What is the appropriate duration of therapy for GB?
   a. 1 day
   b. 3 days
   c. 7 days
   d. 14 days

Answer a is incorrect. Multiple reviews have concluded that 3 days of therapy is better than 1 day of therapy. The Infectious Disease Society of America (IDSA) recommends 3-day therapy for treatment of uncomplicated lower tract infections in women.

Answer b is correct. The Infectious Disease Society of America (IDSA) recommends 3 day therapy for treatment of uncomplicated lower tract infections in women.

Answer c is incorrect. Seven days is recommended in pregnant women or women with a history of UTIs caused by antibiotic-resistant bacteria or >7 days of symptoms.

Answer d is incorrect. Fourteen days is the recommended duration of therapy for men and pyelonephritis.

5. Approximately what percent of uncomplicated UTIs are caused by *Escherichia coli*?
   a. <10
   b. 25
   c. 50
   d. >70

Answer d is correct. *Escherichia coli* causes 70% to 95% of uncomplicated UTIs.

6. Who should be screened for asymptomatic bacteriuria?
   a. College students
   b. Men
   c. Patients with indwelling catheters
   d. Pregnant women

Answer a is incorrect. College students do not need to be screened for asymptomatic bacteriuria.

Answer b is incorrect. Men do not need to be screened for asymptomatic bacteriuria.

Answer c is incorrect. Patients with indwelling catheters do not need to be screened for asymptomatic bacteriuria. Patients with chronic catheters universally have asymptomatic bacteriuria.

Answer d is correct. The IDSA recommends pregnant women should be screened for bacteriuria by urine culture at least once during early pregnancy (12-16 weeks gestation) or

Answer c is incorrect. Although vancomycin does have extensive gram-positive coverage, it is not a first-line therapy against *L. monocytogenes.* Therefore this regimen should include ampicillin. Additionally, the addition of vancomycin is not routinely recommended for neonates.

Answer d is incorrect. Although ceftriaxone provides adequate antimicrobial coverage, it should not be used in neonates because of the possibility of kernicterus. Additionally, when ceftriaxone is used one needs to remember that it should not be used within 48 hours of IV calcium.

---

3. When the 13-day-old former 35-week gestational age baby is examined at the pediatric hospital, she is also noted to have some lesions. The team will be sending cultures of the lesions as well as HSV PCR of the CSF. Which of the following is an appropriate pharmacologic approach in this patient?
   a. Wait for the cultures and PCR results to come back, then modify therapy if needed.
   b. Change antibiotic therapy to ceftriaxone and vancomycin.
   c. Add IV acyclovir to the current antibiotic regimen.
   d. Add oral voriconazole therapy to the current antibiotic regimen.

Answer a is incorrect because therapy against possible HSV encephalitis should not be delayed because the delay could result in devastating consequences.

Answer b is incorrect because therapy against possible HSV encephalitis would be delayed which could result in devastating consequences and ceftriaxone should not be used in infants less than 1 month old.

Answer c is correct because it provides immediate therapy that provides adequate concentrations of the drug.

Answer d is incorrect because antifungal therapy is not indicated and therapy against possible HSV encephalitis would be delayed which could result in devastating consequences.

---

4. If a neonate is begun on acyclovir for herpes simplex virus associated encephalitis, which of the following should be monitored?
   a. Serum creatinine
   b. Neutrophil count
   c. Urine output
   d. All should be routinely monitored

Answer a is correct as it is a marker of renal function that should be monitored in patients on IV acyclovir. Although the number itself is not able to be used in a valid calculation in a baby of this age, monitoring of serum creatinine is still important as increase in creatinine would provide another clue to suggest toxicity if it is seen.

Answer b is correct as it is a marker of bone marrow function that should be monitored in patients on IV acyclovir.

Answer c is correct as it is a marker of renal function that should be monitored in patients on IV acyclovir.

Answer d is correct and the best answer as it describes all of the above, which should be monitored.

---

5. Which of the following explains the pharmacokinetic differences between a neonate and an adult with regards to gentamicin?
   a. Increased volume of distribution and increased clearance
   b. Increased volume of distribution and decreased clearance
   c. Decreased volume of distribution and increased clearance
   d. Decreased volume of distribution and decreased clearance

---

Answer a is incorrect because although neonates have increased volume of distribution for hydrophilic medications such as gentamicin and they have decreased renal clearance.

Answer b is correct because neonates have increased volume of distribution for hydrophilic medications such as gentamicin and they have decreased renal clearance.

Answer c is incorrect because neonates are bags of water and as such have increased volume of distribution for hydrophilic medications. Additionally, neonates also do not have fully developed renal function as their ability to clear the medications that are renally cleared is decreased.

Answer d is incorrect because neonates are bags of water and as such have increased volume of distribution for hydrophilic medications.

---

6. Which of the following patients are *not* recommended to receive a vaccine against *Streptococcus pneumoniae.*
   a. Healthy infants
   b. A 40-year-old with chronic obstructive pulmonary disease (COPD)
   c. A healthy 55-year-old
   d. A 35-year-old asplenic patient

Answer a is incorrect because the PCV7 is recommended for all infants beginning at 6 weeks old.

Answer b is incorrect because COPD is a chronic disease and as such the patient should receive PPSV23.

Answer c is correct because the person is less than 65 years old and they do not have chronic diseases or immunocompromising conditions.

Answer d is incorrect because asplenia is an immunocompromising condition and as such they should receive PPSV23.

---

7. What is the recommended route of administration for ampicillin for the treatment of bacterial meningitis?
   a. IV
   b. Oral

may be given to pregnant women and are effective in 70%-80% of patients.

Answer b is correct. Tetracyclines should be avoided during pregnancy. An agent with low adverse effect potential and which is safe for mother and child should be selected.

---

19. Patients with chronic indwelling catheters usually have asymptomatic bacteriuria. What should be done if the patient becomes symptomatic?
    a. Remove the catheter
    b. Insert new, sterile catheter
    c. Start therapy
    d. All of the above

Answer d is correct. Asymptomatic bacteriuria is universal in patients with chronic indwelling catheters (≥30 days). Antimicrobial therapy will not prevent bacteriuria or symptomatic infection, but will aid in the emergence of resistance. However, symptomatic patients must have their catheter removed, be recatheterized, and then treated to prevent the development of pyelonephritis or bacteremia.

---

20. What is the brand name for TMP-SMX?
    a. Bactrim
    b. Macrobid
    c. Septra
    d. a and c

Answer b is incorrect. Macrobid is the brand name for nitrofurantoin.

Answer d is correct. Bactrim and Septra are both brand names for TMP-SMX.

---

21. Short-course therapy (3 days) is appropriate for which patient group.
    a. Women with a history of UTIs caused by antibiotic-resistant bacteria
    b. Men
    c. Women with >7 days of symptoms
    d. Women with uncomplicated cystitis

Answer a is incorrect. Short-course therapy (3 days) is not recommended in women with a history of UTIs caused by antibiotic-resistant bacteria. These patients should receive 7 to 14 days of therapy.

Answer b is incorrect. Short-course therapy (3 days) is not recommended in men.

Answer c is incorrect. Short-course therapy (3 days) is not recommended in women with >7 days of symptoms. These patients should receive 7 to 14 days of therapy.

Answer d is correct. The Infectious Disease Society of America (IDSA) recommends 3-day therapy for treatment of uncomplicated lower tract infections in women.

---

22. TC is a 19-year-old woman diagnosed with a UTI. She is allergic to sulfa drugs. What is an appropriate empiric regimen for her?
    a. Ciprofloxacin 250 mg po bid for 3 days
    b. Trimethoprim 100 mg po bid for 3 days
    c. Both regimens are appropriate
    d. Neither regimen is appropriate

Answer c is correct. Both ciprofloxacin and trimethoprim are appropriate for TC. TC is allergic to sulfa drugs so trimethoprim is okay. Please note that trimethoprim is usually used in combination with a sulfonamide in Bactrim/Septra. Patients allergic to sulfonamides may not take Bactrim/Septra, but could take trimethoprim.

CHAPTER 24 | Central Nervous System Infections

1. A 13-day-old former 35-week gestational age baby presents to the emergency room with a temperature of 102°F. The mother reports the baby has been feeding less, is constipated, and is very irritable. Which symptom is *not* a common symptom of meningitis in a neonate?
    a. Temperature of 102°F
    b. Decreased feeding
    c. Constipation
    d. Irritable appearance

Answer a is incorrect. A fever is a common symptom of meningitis in a neonate.

Answer b is incorrect. Decreased feeding is a very common nonspecific symptom of systemic illness, including meningitis in a neonate.

Answer c is correct. Although it is possible that the patient may appear constipated due to dehydration and decreased feeding, it is not a symptom of meningitis in an infant.

Answer d is incorrect. Irritable appearance is a common symptom of meningitis in a neonate.

---

2. The emergency physician is unable to obtain CSF fluid after multiple attempts. Based on clinical findings, the team believes that the 13-day-old former 35-week gestational age baby may have meningitis. What is the best therapy to begin in this baby before sending her to a pediatric hospital?
    a. Ampicillin and gentamicin
    b. Ceftriaxone and gentamicin
    c. Vancomycin and cefotaxime
    d. Ampicillin and ceftriaxone

Answer a is correct. It is a recommended therapy in neonates that will cover the likely pathogens and is safe to use in this age group.

Answer b is incorrect. It is not correct for multiple reasons. First the coverage does not include activity against *Listeria monocytogenes*. Secondly, ceftriaxone should not be used in neonates because of the possibility of kernicterus. Finally, IV ceftriaxone should not be used within 48 hours of IV calcium and this may be needed in a very sick baby.

Answer b is incorrect. *Staphylococcus epidermis* is an infrequent cause of UTIs. Please note that *S. epidermis* is often reported as coagulase-negative Staphylococci. *Staphylococcus saprophyticus* is also a coagulase-negative staph.

Answer c is correct. *Staphylococcus saprophyticus* is the most common gram-positive bacteria causing UTIs (5%-10%).

Answer d is incorrect. *Streptococcus pneumoniae* (pneumococcus) is an infrequent cause of UTIs. Pneumococcus is a common cause of respiratory tract infections.

---

13. Which antibiotic is recommended for prophylaxis of recurrent UTIs?
    a. Amoxicillin/clavulanic acid
    b. Levofloxacin
    c. Moxifloxacin
    d. Nitrofurantoin

Answer a is incorrect. Amoxicillin/clavulanic acid is used for the treatment of UTIs.

Answer b is incorrect. Levofloxacin is used for the treatment of UTIs.

Answer c is incorrect. Moxifloxacin is metabolized in the liver via glucuronide and sulfate conjugation, and it is not indicated for the treatment of UTIs. Ciprofloxacin and levofloxacin are the two fluoroquinolones indicated for UTIs.

Answer d in correct. Nitrofurantoin and TMP-SMX are recommended for the prophylaxis of UTIs.

---

14. Select the correct statement regarding nitrofurantoin.
    a. Does not have a renal dosing adjustment
    b. Appropriate throughout pregnancy
    c. Is not indicated for the treatment of pyelonephritis
    d. Is an antifungal

Answer a is incorrect. Nitrofurantoin is contraindicated in patients with a creatinine clearance less than 60 mL/min.

Answer b is incorrect. Nitrofurantoin is contraindicated in pregnant patients at term (38-42 weeks gestation) and during labor and delivery due to the risk of hemolytic anemia via immature erythrocyte enzyme systems.

Answer c is correct. Nitrofurantoin is an antibiotic indicated specifically for uncomplicated UTIs.

Answer d is incorrect. Nitrofurantoin is an antibiotic not an antifungal.

---

15. LA is 30-year-old pregnant woman. She is 16 weeks pregnant and reports dysuria at her appointment today. Urinalysis and urine culture are conducted, and she is started on TMP-SMX 1 DS tablet po bid. What is the appropriate duration of therapy?
    a. 3 days
    b. 7 days
    c. 14 days
    d. 28 days

Answer a is incorrect. Three days of therapy at standard doses is effective treatment for uncomplicated lower UTIs in women.

Answer b is correct. Initial therapy for pregnant women should be 7 days, and a follow-up urine culture 1 to 2 weeks post therapy and then monthly until birth is recommended.

Answer c is incorrect. Fourteen days is the recommended duration of therapy for pyelonephritis.

Answer d is incorrect. Twenty-eight days is the recommended duration of therapy for prostatitis.

---

16. Three days later the clinic calls LA to tell her the culture results are back and she needs to change therapy. The culture was positive for *E. coli*, and it is resistant to TMP-SMX. What would be the new appropriate therapy for LA?
    a. Amoxicillin 500 mg po tid for 3 days
    b. Ciprofloxacin 500 mg po bid for 7 days
    c. Nitrofurantoin 100 mg po bid for 7 days
    d. TMP-SMX 2 DS tablets po bid for 7 days

Answer a is incorrect. Three days of therapy at standard doses is effective treatment for uncomplicated lower UTIs in women.

Answer b is incorrect. Pregnant women should avoid fluoroquinolones due to the risk of arthropathies and the potential to inhibit cartilage and bone development in the newborn.

Answer c is correct. Initial therapy for pregnant women should be 7 days, and a follow-up urine culture 1 to 2 weeks post therapy and then monthly until birth is recommended. Nitrofurantoin is contraindicated in pregnant patients at term (38-42 weeks gestation) and during labor and delivery. LA is only 16 weeks pregnant; so she can take nitrofurantoin.

Answer d is incorrect. The isolate is resistant to TMP-SMX. Increasing the dose will not overcome the resistance.

---

17. Does LA need a follow-up culture? If so, when?
    a. No follow-up culture is needed
    b. Yes, in 2 days
    c. Yes, a day after the therapy is complete
    d. Yes, 7 to 14 days after the therapy is complete

Answers a, b, and c are incorrect. A follow-up culture will be needed after the therapy is complete.

Answer d is correct. Pregnant women are recommended to have a follow-up urine culture 1 to 2 weeks post therapy and then monthly until birth is recommended.

---

18. Which antibiotic is not appropriate for UTI treatment in pregnant women?
    a. Amoxicillin/clavulanic acid
    b. Doxycycline
    c. Nitrofurantoin
    d. TMP-SMX

Answers a, c, and d are incorrect. Sulfonamides, amoxicillin, amoxicillin/clavulanic acid, cephalexin, and nitrofurantoin

at their first prenatal visit. All positive urine cultures, including asymptomatic bacteriuria, should be treated in pregnant women.

7. Which of the following patient groups are considered to have complicated UTIs?
   a. Children
   b. Men
   c. Pregnant women
   d. All of the above

Answer d is correct. In general, UTIs in men, pregnant women, children, and patients who are hospitalized or in health care-associated settings are considered complicated. These infections are more likely to be caused by resistant organisms.

8. NK is a 62-year-old man presenting to urgent care today with dysuria, increased urinating frequency, and flank pain. His past medical history includes hyperlipidemia and migraines. He is allergic to penicillin and sulfa drugs. What is the probable diagnosis?
   a. Benign prostatic hyperplasia (BPH)
   b. Cystitis
   c. Prostate cancer
   d. Pyelonephritis

Answer a is incorrect. BPH produces lower urinary tract symptoms, but does not cause fever or flank pain.

Answer b is incorrect. Cystitis does not cause flank pain.

Answer c is incorrect. Prostate cancer does not present with fever or flank pain.

Answer d is correct. NK has classic symptoms of pyelonephritis. Pyelonephritis is characterized as cystitis plus fever, flank pain, nausea, and vomiting.

9. What is the most appropriate therapy for NK?
   a. Amoxicillin 500 mg po tid for 7 days
   b. Ciprofloxacin 500 mg po bid for 3 days
   c. Ciprofloxacin 500 mg po bid for 14 days
   d. TMP-SMX 1 DS tablet po bid for 14 days

Answer a is incorrect. NK is allergic to penicillin so amoxicillin would be an inappropriate choice. Men are treated for 10 to 14 days. The general rule is to treat UTIs in men for 14 days.

Answer b is incorrect. Short-course therapy (3 days) is not recommended in men.

Answer c is correct. Ciprofloxacin is the appropriate therapy because NK is allergic to penicillin and sulfa drugs. Fourteen days is the appropriate duration of therapy for men with pyelonephritis.

Answer d is incorrect. NK is allergic to sulfa drugs, and TMP-SMX includes a sulfa component.

10. NK completes his therapy and feels better. Two weeks later he returns to the emergency department (ED) with general malaise, a temperature of 101.7°F, pelvic pain, dysuria, and increased urination. What is the probable diagnosis?
    a. Acute bacterial prostatitis
    b. Benign prostatic hyperplasia
    c. Cystitis
    d. Epididymitis

Answer a is correct. NK's initial therapy resolved his pyelonephritis. The prostate is a common site of bacteria persistence. Two weeks later he displays symptoms of acute bacterial prostatitis.

Answer b is incorrect. BPH does not present with these symptoms.

Answer c is incorrect. Cystitis does not typically produce a fever.

Answer d is incorrect. Epididymitis causes unilateral testicular pain and swelling.

11. NK is admitted to the hospital. Blood and urine cultures are collected. He is started on ceftriaxone 1 g IV daily. On day three, blood cultures are negative, and the urine culture is positive for *E. coli*. The isolate is resistant to amoxicillin. On day four, NK is ready for discharge. What is the most appropriate outpatient therapy for NK?
    a. Ciprofloxacin 500 mg po bid for 3 days
    b. Ciprofloxacin 500 mg po bid for 14 days
    c. Ciprofloxacin 500 mg po bid for 28 days
    d. Nitrofurantoin 100 mg po bid for 28 days

Answer a is incorrect. Short-course therapy (3 days) is not recommended in men.

Answer b is incorrect. Fourteen days is the appropriate duration of treatment for men with a UTI.

Answer c is correct. Acute bacterial prostatitis is treated for 4 weeks to reduce the risk of developing chronic prostatitis.

Answer d is incorrect. Nitrofurantoin is indicated for uncomplicated UTIs only and not for bacterial prostatitis.

12. What is the most common gram-positive cause of a UTI?
    a. *Staphylococcus aureus*
    b. *Staphylococcus epidermidis*
    c. *Staphylococcus saprophyticus*
    d. *Streptococcus pneumoniae*

Answer a is incorrect. *Staphylococcus aureus* may cause UTI; however, it is not a common cause. *S. aurues* (including MRSA) may cause catheter-associated UTIs.

Answers b, c, and d are incorrect. These have antipseudomonal activity.

CHAPTER 23 | Urinary Tract Infections

1. Select the following organism(s) that can cause a UTI.
   a. Bacteria
   b. Fungus
   c. Virus
   d. All of the above

Answer d is correct. All of the above organisms can cause a UTI. However, most UTIs are caused by bacteria.

2. GB is a 28-year-old woman with a chief complaint of dysuria. The physician orders a urinalysis and a urine culture. What is the most likely cause of the UTI?
   a. *Acinetobacter baumannii*
   b. *Escherichia coli*
   c. *Pseudomonas aeruginosa*
   d. *Staphylococcus saprophyticus*

Answer a is incorrect. *Acinetobacter baumannii* is a nosocomial organism and a cause of catheter-associated UTIs.

Answer b is correct. The majority of UTIs are caused by gram-negative bacteria, of which *E. coli* is the most common pathogen.

Answer c is incorrect. *Pseudomonas aeruginosa* is a nosocomial organism and causes <20% of UTIs.

Answer d is incorrect. *Staphylococcus saprophyticus* only causes 5% to 10% of uncomplicated UTIs. It is the most common gram-positive bacteria causing uncomplicated UTIs.

3. What is appropriate empiric therapy for GB?
   a. Cefdinir
   b. Linezolid
   c. Penicillin
   d. TMP-SMX

Answer a is incorrect. Cefdinir is an oral third-generation cephalosporin commonly used for acute otitis media in pediatrics. It is not indicated for treatment of UTIs

Answer b is incorrect. Linezolid is an antibiotic that covers gram-positive bacteria exclusively. It is primarily used to treat methicillin-resistant *Staphylococcus aureus* (MRSA) and vancomycin-resistant enterococci (VRE). Both MRSA and VRE can cause UTIs, but GB does not need to be empirically covered with linezolid.

Answer c is incorrect. *Escherichia coli* resistance rate to ampicillin is 37%. Thus, penicillin would be a poor selection.

Answer d is correct. TMP-SMX is appropriate empiric therapy for GB. If the local *E. coli* resistance rate for TMP-SMX is high, ciprofloxacin would be an appropriate choice.

4. What is the appropriate duration of therapy for GB?
   a. 1 day
   b. 3 days
   c. 7 days
   d. 14 days

Answer a is incorrect. Multiple reviews have concluded that 3 days of therapy is better than 1 day of therapy. The Infectious Disease Society of America (IDSA) recommends 3-day therapy for treatment of uncomplicated lower tract infections in women.

Answer b is correct. The Infectious Disease Society of America (IDSA) recommends 3 day therapy for treatment of uncomplicated lower tract infections in women.

Answer c is incorrect. Seven days is recommended in pregnant women or women with a history of UTIs caused by antibiotic-resistant bacteria or >7 days of symptoms.

Answer d is incorrect. Fourteen days is the recommended duration of therapy for men and pyelonephritis.

5. Approximately what percent of uncomplicated UTIs are caused by *Escherichia coli*?
   a. <10
   b. 25
   c. 50
   d. >70

Answer d is correct. *Escherichia coli* causes 70% to 95% of uncomplicated UTIs.

6. Who should be screened for asymptomatic bacteriuria?
   a. College students
   b. Men
   c. Patients with indwelling catheters
   d. Pregnant women

Answer a is incorrect. College students do not need to be screened for asymptomatic bacteriuria.

Answer b is incorrect. Men do not need to be screened for asymptomatic bacteriuria.

Answer c is incorrect. Patients with indwelling catheters do not need to be screened for asymptomatic bacteriuria. Patients with chronic catheters universally have asymptomatic bacteriuria.

Answer d is correct. The IDSA recommends pregnant women should be screened for bacteriuria by urine culture at least once during early pregnancy (12-16 weeks gestation) or

c. Levofloxacin
d. a and c
e. All of the above

Answer a is correct. Ciprofloxacin and fluoroquinolones may cause photosensitivity.

Answer b is correct. Doxycycline and tetracyclines may cause photosensitivity.

Answer c is correct. Levofloxacin and fluoroquinolones may cause photosensitivity.

Answer d is correct.

Answer e is correct and the best answer.

---

21. Select the parameter(s) that should be monitored with daptomycin.

a. CPK
b. Muscle weakness
c. Serum creatinine
d. All of the above

Answer a is correct. CPK values should be monitored in patients receiving daptomycin. Daptomycin is associated with myopathy; discontinue in patients with signs and symptoms of myopathy in conjunction with increase in CPK > 5 times upper limit of normal or in asymptomatic patients with CPK > 10 times upper limit of normal.

Answer b is correct. Daptomycin is associated with myopathy, discontinue in patients with signs and symptoms of myopathy in conjunction with increase in CPK or in asymptomatic patients with CPK > 10 times upper limit of normal.

Answer c is correct. Daptomycin should be used with caution in renal dysfunction (dosage adjustment is required).

Answer d is correct and the best answer.

---

22. BD is a 24-year-old man with no known drug allergies who was initially treated with vancomycin for his cellulitis. His abscess culture after appropriate incision/drainage revealed caMRSA. He has clinically improved enough to receive oral antibiotics. Which of the following is an appropriate step-down antibiotic for BD?

a. Cephalexin
b. Amoxicillin-clavulanate
c. Ceftriaxone
d. Trimethoprim-sulfamethoxazole

Answer a is incorrect. Cephalexin has no activity against MRSA.

Answer b is incorrect. Amoxicillin-clavulanate has no activity against MRSA. MRSA's resistance mechanism to beta-lactams is altering the penicillin-binding protein, therefore all beta-lactams are ineffective against MRSA. Clavulanate is a beta-lactamase inhibitor and would not increase amoxicillin's activity versus MRSA.

Answer c is incorrect. Ceftriaxone has no activity against MRSA.

Answer d is correct. Trimethoprim-sulfamethoxazole has excellent activity versus MRSA. It is used primarily in uncomplicated skin/skin structure infections, but is also used as step-down therapy from IV therapy in patients requiring initial hospitalization.

---

23. Select the antimicrobial that may cause thrombocytopenia, especially with more than 2 weeks of therapy.

a. Cleocin
b. Zyvox
c. Cubicin
d. Tygacil

Answer a is incorrect. Cleocin is not associated with thrombocytopenia.

Answer b is correct and is the best answer. Linezolid (Zyvox) is associated with bone marrow suppression, including leukopenia, anemia, and thrombocytopenia (most common). While these side effects can occur at anytime, prolonged therapy of more than 2 weeks is associated with greater risk.

Answer c is incorrect. Cubicin is not associated with thrombocytopenia.

Answer d is incorrect. Tygacil is only rarely associated with thrombocytopenia.

---

24. Which of the following is a reasonable duration of antimicrobial therapy for treating osteomyelitis?

a. 1 week
b. 2 weeks
c. 3 weeks
d. 6 weeks

Answers a, b, and c are incorrect. Treatment duration of osteomyelitis generally is 4 to 6 weeks. One, two, or three weeks is too short.

Answer d is correct. Six weeks is an acceptable timeframe for the treatment of osteomyelitis.

---

25. Which of the following carbapenem antibiotics does *not* have coverage against *P. aeruginosa*?

a. Ertapenem
b. Doripenem
c. Imipenem-cilastatin
d. Meropenem

Answer a is correct. Ertapenem is the only carbapenem that does not have coverage against *P. aeruginosa*.

c. Intramuscular
d. Any of the above are reasonable

Answer a is correct because IV antibiotics are recommended for therapy of patients with bacterial meningitis to ensure adequate concentrations.

Answer b is incorrect because oral administration will not likely produce high concentrations of the ampicillin.

Answer c is incorrect because it is not optimal for administration (pain) or to ensure adequate drug concentrations. This route although not optimal, can be used in urgent situations until IV access can be obtained.

Answer d is incorrect because b and c are not correct.

---

8. Which of the following is *not* common with bacterial meningitis?
   a. CSF WBC 5000 cells/ mm^3
   b. CSF WBC with 70% lymphocytes
   c. CSF glucose 23 mg/dL
   d. CSF protein of 250 mg/dL

Answer a is incorrect because CSF WBC 5000 cells/mm^3 is consistent with bacterial meningitis (>1000 cells/mm^3).

Answer b is correct because neutrophils predominance, not lymphocytic predominance is what is usually seen with bacterial meningitis. Lymphocytic predominance is more typical of viral, fungal, or tubercular meningitis.

Answer c is correct because CSF glucose concentrations of < 40 mg/dL are common in bacterial meningitis.

Answer d is correct because CSF protein concentrations of > 100 mg/dL are expected in bacterial meningitis.

---

9. Which of the following is correct regarding bacterial meningitis?
   a. A bacteria will be identified in majority of the cases.
   b. The likelihood of a bacteria being identified is unchanged if a patient receives antibiotics prior to CSF cultures.
   c. CSF cultures are not reliable for diagnosis.
   d. There is no role for blood cultures in the diagnosis of bacterial meningitis.

Answer a is correct because more than 80% of cases of bacterial meningitis in untreated patients will reveal a pathogen.

Answer b is incorrect because prior receipt of antibiotics will decrease the likelihood of obtaining a positive culture.

Answer c is incorrect because CSF cultures are reliable when they reveal a pathogen.

Answer d is incorrect because blood cultures are very useful when they are obtained prior to the administration of antibiotics. They are in fact vital in situations when the CSF cultures cannot be performed until after antibiotic administration.

---

10. For which of the following agents is nephrotoxicity *not* one of the more common side effects that are monitored?
    a. IV gentamicin
    b. IV ceftriaxone
    c. IV vancomycin
    d. IV acyclovir

Answer a is incorrect because nephrotoxicity is a common side effect of gentamicin.

Answer b is correct because nephrotoxicity is unlikely in patients receiving ceftriaxone.

Answer c is incorrect because nephrotoxicity is one of the side effects that are monitored with vancomycin.

Answer d is incorrect because acyclovir should be monitored for nephrotoxicity.

---

11. Which of the following vaccines is recommended to be given as part of routine child-care to otherwise healthy infants?
    a. MCV4
    b. MPSV4
    c. PCV13
    d. PPSV23

Answer a is incorrect because although MCV4 is recommended for infants > 6 months that are at high risk for meningococcal disease, it is not currently part of the routine care for healthy infants.

Answer b is incorrect for multiple reasons. It is not approved in children less than 2 years because pure polysaccharide vaccines are not consistently immunogenic in this age group. Additionally, no meningococcal vaccination is currently recommended as part of the routine care for healthy infants.

Answer c is correct. PCV13 is recommended for all children under the age of 5.

Answer d is incorrect because although pneumococcal vaccination is important and recommended for infants, the PPSV23 is a pure polysaccharide vaccine and as such is only approved for patients older than 2 years. Remember that pure polysaccharide vaccines are not consistently immunogenic in children less than 2 years of age.

---

12. A 7-year-old patient with no significant past medical history presents to your hospital with fever, severe headache, photophobia, and neck pain. The physician does a lumbar puncture and sends the CSF collections to the laboratory. Based upon clinical diagnosis the patient is suspected to have bacterial meningitis. Which of the following are likely pathogens associated with bacterial meningitis in this patient?
    a. *Streptococcus pneumoniae* and *H. influenzae*
    b. *Neisseria. meningitidis* and *L. monocytogenes*
    c. *Listeria monocytogenes* and group B *Streptococcus*
    d. *Streptococcus pneumoniae* and *N. meningitidis*

Answer a is incorrect because *H. influenzae* is no longer a common pathogen-causing bacterial meningitis.

Answer b is incorrect because *L. monocytogenes* is not a common pathogen-causing bacterial meningitis in this age group.

Answer c is incorrect because neither *L. monocytogenes* nor group B *Streptococcus* are common pathogens in this age group.

Answer d is correct because both *S. pneumoniae* and *N. meningitidis* are the two likely pathogens that cause bacterial meningitis in children and adults.

13. Which of the following is consistent with the recommended empiric antibiotic therapy for a 7-year-old with bacterial meningitis.

    a. Ceftriaxone
    b. Ceftriaxone and ampicillin
    c. Cefotaxime and vancomycin
    d. Ampicillin and gentamicin

Answer a is incorrect because empiric therapy should cover the possibility of ceftriaxone-resistant *S. pneumoniae.*

Answer b is incorrect for this age patient. Remember that *S. pneumoniae* and *N. meningitidis* are the likely pathogens. Although ceftriaxone is a good choice to empirically cover the *N. meningitidis* and many *S. pneumoniae,* neither ceftriaxone nor ampicillin provides coverage against multidrug resistant *S. pneumoniae.* Therefore the regimen should include vancomycin instead of ampicillin. Ampicillin should be included in regimens for the very young and old to cover for *L. monocytogenes.*

Answer c is correct because the combination covers sensitive and multidrug resistant *S. pneumoniae* as well as *N. meningitidis* well.

Answer d is incorrect for this age patient. In neonates this regimen would be reasonable because it covers the group B *Streptococcus, E. coli,* and *L .monocytogenes.* The most common pathogens in children however are *S. pneumoniae* and *N. meningitidis.* Unfortunately, neither ampicillin nor gentamicin provides adequate empiric coverage for either common pathogen, due to potential resistance. Vancomycin should be used to cover for potential multidrug resistant *S. pneumoniae* and either cefotaxime or ceftriaxone should be used to cover for penicillin-resistant *N. meningitidis* and good coverage against noncephalosporin-resistant *S. pneumoniae.*

14. If the 7-year-old is determined to have *S. pneumoniae* meningitis, what chemoprophylaxis is suggested for close contacts?

    a. Ceftriaxone
    b. Rifampin
    c. Ciprofloxacin
    d. No chemoprophylaxis is indicated

Answers a, b, and c are incorrect because no prophylaxis is recommended for *S. pneumoniae* meningitis.

Answer d is correct because no prophylaxis is recommended for *S. pneumoniae* meningitis.

15. What is the purpose of adding vancomycin to empiric therapy for bacterial meningitis in a 4-year-old patient?

    a. To provide coverage against resistant *L. monocytogenes*
    b. To provide coverage against resistant *S. pneumoniae*
    c. To provide coverage against resistant *N. meningitidis*
    d. Vancomycin is not needed in a 4-year-old with bacterial meningitis because *S. aureus* is unlikely

Answer a is incorrect as it does not provide additional coverage against *L. monocytogenes* nor is *L. monocytogenes* a common pathogen in this age group.

Answer b is correct. Vancomycin should be used to cover for possible multidrug resistant *S. pneumoniae.* To date, almost every *S. pneumoniae* isolate has been susceptible to vancomycin.

Answer c is incorrect because vancomycin does not have coverage against any gram-negative bacteria including *N. meningitidis.*

Answer d is incorrect because although vancomycin covers *S. aureus* and is often a treatment of choice against methicillin-resistant *S. aureus.* It has coverage against most gram-positive organisms and in the case of community-associated meningitis it is recommended because *S. pneumoniae* is a likely pathogen and it is possible that the *S. pneumoniae* may be resistant to the third generation cephalosporin that is also recommended for empiric therapy.

16. Which meningococcal vaccine would be suggested for outbreak control of A, C, Y, or W135?

    a. MCV4
    b. MPSV4
    c. Either MCV4 or MPSV4 can be used
    d. Neither MCV4 or MPSV4 are used for outbreak control

Answers a, b. and d are incorrect because either MCV4 or MPSV4 is suggested for outbreak control.

Answer c is correct. MCV4 or MPSV4 may be used for meningococcal outbreak control of A, C, Y, or W135.

17. Which of the following groups has dexamethasone demonstrated a mortality benefit?

    a. A 2-week-old with group B *Streptococcus* meningitis
    b. A 17-year-old with *N. meningitidis* meningitis
    c. A 35-year-old with *S. pneumoniae* meningitis

d. It has not demonstrated clear benefit for any type of bacterial meningitis

Answer a is incorrect because dexamethasone is not suggested for patients less than 6 weeks old because there are sparse data regarding dexamethasone for neonates.

Answer b is incorrect because no benefits have been shown with either *N. meningitidis* or adolescent patients.

Answer c is correct because mortality benefit from dexamethasone has only been shown with adults with pneumococcal meningitis.

Answer d is incorrect because a benefit has been shown for adults with pneumococcal meningitis.

18. A 70-year-old man presents with fever, nausea, vomiting, severe headache, and extreme photophobia. CSF results: WBC 2500 cells/mm^3, 87% neutrophils, glucose 37 mg/dL and protein 240 mg/dL. What type of CNS infection is his clinical picture most consistent with?

    a. Bacterial meningitis
    b. Aseptic meningitis
    c. Viral encephalitis
    d. Any of the above

Answer a is correct because the laboratory values are consistent with bacterial meningitis (ie, WBC > 1000 cells/mm^3, 80% to 90% neutrophils, CSF glucose < 40 mg/dL, CSF protein > 100 mg/dL).

Answer b is incorrect because the laboratory values are consistent with bacterial meningitis. An aseptic meningitis would have WBC less than 100 cells/mm^3, a predominance of either lymphocytes or monocytes, normal CSF glucose, and a CSF protein of < 100 mg/dL.

Answer c is incorrect because the CSF laboratory values are consistent with bacterial meningitis. Viral meningitis would be more likely to have lower number of WBC, a lymphocytic predominance (although increased neutrophils are possible early in the infection), normal CSF glucose (greater than 40-50 mg/dL) and CSF protein < 100 mg/dL).

Answer d is incorrect because b and c are incorrect

19. Which of the following is consistent with the recommended antibacterial therapy for a 78-year-old patient with bacterial meningitis?

    a. Vancomycin and ceftriaxone
    b. Vancomycin, ceftriaxone, and ampicillin
    c. Ampicillin and ceftriaxone
    d. Ceftriaxone

Answer a is incorrect because it is missing additional coverage against *L. monocytogenes* recommended in elderly patients

Answer b is correct because it provides adequate coverage against all three pathogens likely to cause bacterial meningitis in this age group. Remember that coverage against *L. monocytogenes* should be added to patients over the age of 50 years.

Answer c is incorrect because it does not provide coverage against ceftriaxone-resistant *S. pneumoniae.*

Answer d is incorrect because it does not provide coverage against *L. monocytogenes* or ceftriaxone-resistant *S. pneumoniae.*

20. Which of the following patients should *not* receive the varicella vaccine?

    a. A 32-year-old with AIDS
    b. A 1-year-old with primary immunodeficiency
    c. A 25-year-old pregnant woman
    d. The vaccine is contraindicated in all of these patients

Answers a, b, c, and d are correct because these are conditions that should not receive varicella vaccine

Answer d is correct and the best answer because none of these patients, based on their conditions should receive the varicella vaccine.

21. Which of the following persons should receive the MPSV4 vaccine?

    a. A 60-year-old who just had his spleen removed after a traumatic car accident
    b. A 5-year-old with sickle cell disease
    c. A 25-year-old microbiologist that works with *N. meningitidis*
    d. A 33-year-old traveling to the meningitis belt

Answer a is correct because MPSV4 is recommended for persons at risk of meningococcal disease who are older than 55 years. MCV4 is currently not licensed for this age group.

Answers b, c, and d are incorrect because MCV4 would be recommended rather than MPSV4 because of the patient's age. Remember that the MCV4 is recommended for routine vaccination of patients < 55 years old.

CHAPTER 25 | Sepsis and Septic Shock

1. Select the phrase that most accurately describes sepsis.

    a. Presence of bacteria in the bloodstream
    b. Systemic inflammatory response to a physiologic insult
    c. Persistent hypotension and altered organ function
    d. Systemic inflammatory response due to an infection

Answer a is incorrect. Bacteremia is the presence of bacteria in the bloodstream.

Answer b is incorrect. The systemic inflammatory response to a physiologic insult can occur for reasons other than infection.

Answer c is incorrect. Persistent hypotension and altered organ function can occur for a variety of reasons other than sepsis.

Answer d is correct. Sepsis is the systemic inflammatory response secondary to infection.

---

2. Select the phrase that most accurately describes severe sepsis.
   a. Bacteremia with a high colony count
   b. Bacteremia with the systemic inflammatory response syndrome (SIRS)
   c. Bacteremia with the systemic inflammatory response syndrome (SIRS) and organ dysfunction
   d. Bacteremia with the systemic inflammatory response syndrome (SIRS), organ dysfunction, and immune failure

---

Answer a is incorrect. Bacteremia describes only the presence of bacteria in the bloodstream.

Answer b is incorrect. Nonsevere sepsis is the systemic inflammatory response in response to an infection (in this case, bacteria).

Answer c is correct. Severe sepsis is defined as sepsis (SIRS secondary to infection) with organ dysfunction.

Answer d is incorrect. Immune failure is not one of the criteria measured in defining sepsis.

---

3. Which of the following organisms cause sepsis?
   a. Gram-positive bacteria
   b. Gram-negative bacteria
   c. Viruses
   d. a and b
   e. All of the above

Answers a, b, c, and d are correct. Gram-positive and gram negative bacteria, and viruses (although less common) are possible causes of sepsis.

Answer e is correct and the best answer. Sepsis can be caused by gram-positive and gram-negative bacteria and viruses. Fungi are also a possible cause of sepsis.

---

4. TK is a 32-year-old woman admitted to the intensive care unit with possible sepsis secondary to pneumonia. Her vitals signs are temperature 38.1°C, heart rate 80 beats per minute, and respiratory rate 16 breaths per minute. She also has a white blood cell count of 15,500 cells/mm^3. Based on this information, does TK have sepsis?
   a. Yes, TK has sepsis because she has an infection source but meets no SIRS criteria.
   b. Yes, TK has sepsis because she has an infection source and meets two SIRS criteria.
   c. No, TK does not have sepsis because she has an infection source but does not have any organ failures.
   d. No, TK does not have sepsis because she does not have positive cultures.

Answer a is incorrect. The patient has sepsis because she has an infection source (likely pulmonary), but meets two SIRS criteria (elevated temperature and leucocytosis).

Answer b is correct. TK has sepsis because of the infection source (pulmonary), and meeting two SIRS criteria (elevated temperature and leucocytosis).

Answer c is incorrect. TK does have sepsis. Organ failure is not a criterion in the diagnosis of sepsis.

Answer d is incorrect. The patient does have sepsis. Positive cultures are typically not available when patients initially present with sepsis. They are therefore not included in diagnostic criteria for sepsis. Instead, possible loci of infection are determined based on clinical signs/symptoms. In this case, it appears that TK has a pulmonary source for her infection.

---

5. Which of the following can help reduce or prevent the morbidity and mortality associated with sepsis?
   a. Preventing organ failures
   b. Early goal-directed resuscitation
   c. Eliminating the infection source
   d. All of the above

Answers a, b, and c are correct because they help reduce or prevent sepsis-related morbidity and mortality.

Answer d is correct and the best answer. Reducing sepsis-related morbidity and mortality requires multiple interventions including preventing organ failure, early goal-directed resuscitation, and eliminating (or treating) infections.

---

6. XJ is a 29-year-old woman who presents with severe sepsis including hypotension and decreased urine output. She has no significant past medical history. Select the appropriate initial regimen for early fluid resuscitation in XJ.
   a. 5% dextrose 500 mL
   b. 5% albumin 1000 mL
   c. 0.9% sodium chloride 1000 mL
   d. 0.45% sodium chloride 1000 mL

Answer a is incorrect. Five percent dextrose is not an appropriate resuscitation fluid because only 8% of the administered volume stays intravascular.

Answer b is incorrect. Colloids, like albumin, can be used for fluid resuscitation in sepsis, especially in patients who can not tolerate high volumes of fluid. However, only 300 to 500 mL should be used.

Answer c is correct. It is appropriate to use 0.9% sodium chloride (normal saline) 1000 mL for fluid resuscitation in sepsis because of all crystalloids, more of it stays intravascular (~250 mL/L).

Answer d is incorrect. Sodium chloride 0.45% (1/2 normal saline) is not an appropriate fluid for resuscitation, because it provides only half of the intravascular volume that normal saline provides.

---

7. A patient with hypotension secondary to sepsis has a history of congestive heart failure and fluid overload. Select the appropriate colloid therapy for this patient.
    a. 5% albumin 500 mL
    b. 5% dextrose 500 mL
    c. 0.9% sodium chloride 500 mL
    d. 0.45% sodium chloride 500 mL

Answer a is correct. Five percent albumin is a colloid resuscitation fluid used for patients at risk for fluid overload.

Answer b is incorrect. Five percent dextrose is a crystalloid fluid and is inappropriate for fluid resuscitation.

Answer c is incorrect. An appropriate resuscitation fluid is 0.9% sodium chloride. However, it is a crystalloid, rather than colloid.

Answer d is incorrect. Sodium chloride 0.45% is a crystalloid fluid and is inappropriate for fluid resuscitation.

---

8. KT is a 65-year-old man with a history of end-state renal disease on hemodialysis admitted with severe sepsis likely secondary to an infected dialysis catheter. Which of the following represents the best order of events to manage KT sepsis?
    a. Drotrecogin alfa, fluids, microbiologic cultures, antimicrobial therapy
    b. Drotrecogin alfa, antimicrobial therapy, microbiologic cultures, fluids
    c. Fluids, microbiologic cultures, antimicrobial therapy, drotrecogin alfa
    d. Fluids, antimicrobial therapy, microbiologic cultures, drotrecogin alfa

---

Answer a is incorrect. In patients with sepsis, priority is placed on fluid resuscitation and antimicrobial therapy. Drotrecogin alfa therapy should be considered after other modalities have been used.

Answer b is incorrect. Priority should be placed on fluid resuscitation and antimicrobial therapy. Drotrecogin alfa therapy should be considered after other modalities have been used.

Answer c is correct. In patients with sepsis, early goal-directed fluid resuscitation should be administered first. Microbiologic cultures should be collected prior to antimicrobial therapy. Drotrecogin alfa therapy should be considered after other therapies and in patients with APACHE II score > 25.

Answer d is incorrect. Microbiologic cultures should be obtained prior to administration of antimicrobial therapy to help ensure their accuracy.

---

9. What therapy should be administered within 1 hour of the recognition of sepsis?
    a. Broad-spectrum antimicrobial therapy
    b. Corticosteroids in patients with documented adrenal insufficiency
    c. Drotrecogin alfa therapy
    d. Vasopressor therapy

Answer a is correct Early administration of broad-spectrum antimicrobial therapy improves mortality in sepsis.

Answer b is incorrect. Optimal timing of corticosteroids in sepsis is not well-defined.

Answer c is incorrect. Drotrecogin alfa therapy should be administered within 24 hours in patients with severe sepsis and two or more major organ failures or an APACHE II score > 25.

Answer d is incorrect. There is no specific timing of vasopressor therapy in sepsis. It should be administered in patients following fluid resuscitation with persistent hypotension.

---

10. SL is a 32-year-old man with sepsis secondary to an intra-abdominal abscess. He has no significant past medical history and currently has been fluid resuscitated with a mean arterial pressure (MAP) of 70 mm Hg. What is the best treatment plan for SL?
    a. Ampicillin/sulbactam 3 g IV every 6 hours and transfer to the intensive care unit
    b. Ampicillin/sulbactam 3 g IV every 6 hours and surgical drainage of the abscess
    c. Amoxicillin/clavulanic acid 875 mg po every 12 hours and transfer to the intensive care unit
    d. Amoxicillin/clavulanic acid 875 mg po every 12 hours and surgical drainage of the abscess

---

Answer a is incorrect. IV antimicrobial therapy with ampicillin/sulbactam is appropriate because it provides coverage of enteric gram-negatives and anaerobes likely to be present in an intra-abdominal abscess. However, definitive management and treatment of abscesses must include surgical drainage.

Answer b is correct. IV antimicrobial therapy with ampicillin/sulbactam is appropriate because it provides coverage of enteric gram-negatives and anaerobes likely to be present in an intra-abdominal abscess. In addition, treatment of abscesses should include surgical drainage, as antimicrobial therapy alone is unlikely to be curative.

Answer c is incorrect. Oral antimicrobial therapy initially is inappropriate in a patient with sepsis and hypotension. In addition, abscesses require surgical drainage.

Answer d is incorrect. Although surgical drainage of the abscess is warranted, initial oral therapy is inappropriate in a patient with sepsis.

---

11. Select the most appropriate duration of antimicrobial therapy in a patient with sepsis.

    a. 1 to 3 days
    b. 3 to 5 days
    c. 7 to 10 days
    d. 24 to 28 days

Answer a is incorrect. One to three days of therapy is too short for sepsis.

Answer b is incorrect. This duration of therapy is too short for sepsis.

Answer c is correct. Although not specifically studied, guidelines recommend at least a week to 10 days of antimicrobial therapy in sepsis.

Answer d is incorrect. Sepsis is a severe life-threatening infection. However, most patients do not benefit from an extended duration of therapy.

---

12. Which of the following is an absolute contraindication to therapy with drotrecogin alfa?

    a. Elevated endogenous levels of protein C
    b. Previous therapy with drotrecogin alfa
    c. High risk of death from sepsis
    d. Increased risk of bleeding

Answer a is incorrect. Drotrecogin alfa (Xigris) is activated protein C. Administration of drotrecogin alfa will increase protein C levels in septic patients.

Answer b is incorrect. Previous therapy is not a contraindication.

Answer c is incorrect. Drotrecogin alfa is only indicated in patients with a high risk of death (eg, APACHE II score ≥ 25).

Answer d is correct. Drotrecogin alfa is contraindicated in active internal bleeding, recent hemorrhagic stroke (within 3 months), and severe head trauma (within 2 months). Drotrecogin alfa increases the risk of bleeding; careful evaluation of risks and benefits is required prior to initiation.

---

13. Select the brand name for drotrecogin alfa.

    a. Activated protein C
    b. Xigris
    c. Levophed
    d. Solu-Medrol

Answer a is incorrect. Activated protein C is another name for drotrecogin alfa, because the product is recombinant activated protein C.

Answer b is correct. Xigris is the brand name of drotrecogin alfa.

Answer c is incorrect. Levophed is the brand name for norepinephrine.

Answer d is incorrect. Solu-Medrol is the brand name for methylprednisolone.

---

14. Identify the type of patient who is the best candidate for therapy with drotrecogin alfa.

    a. Severe sepsis and a low risk of death
    b. Severe sepsis and a high risk of death
    c. a and b
    d. None of the above

Answer a is incorrect. The ADDRESS trial demonstrated that patients with sepsis and a low risk of death (defined as an APACHE II score ≤ 25 or one organ failure) did not benefit from drotrecogin alfa therapy.

Answer b is correct. The PROWESS trial, which included patients with sepsis and a high risk of death (defined as an APACHE II score > 25 or ≥ 2 organ failures) benefited from drotrecogin alfa therapy.

Answer c is incorrect. Drotrecogin alfa is only indicated in patients with high risk of death.

Answer d is incorrect. Drotrecogin alfa is indicated in patients with sepsis and a high risk of death.

---

15. Which corticosteroid should be used to treat patients with septic shock refractory to vasopressor therapy?

    a. Prednisone
    b. Hydrocortisone
    c. Methylprednisolone
    d. Dexamethasone

Answer a is incorrect. Prednisone has not been studied in patients with septic shock.

Answer b is correct. Hydrocortisone therapy has been studied and is recommended in patients with septic shock that is refractory to vasopressors.

Answer c is incorrect. Methylprednisolone has not been studied in patients with septic shock.

Answer d is incorrect. Dexamethasone was previously used in sepsis prior to the return of cortisol levels when adrenal insufficiency is suspected.

---

16. What is the brand name for hydrocortisone?

    a. Deltasone
    b. Sterapred
    c. Solu-Medrol
    d. Solu-Cortef

Answer a is incorrect. Deltasone is the brand name for dexamethasone.

Answer b is incorrect. Sterapred is the brand name for prednisone.

Answer c is incorrect. Solu-Medrol is the brand name for methylprednisolone.

Answer d is correct. Solu-Cortef is the brand name for hydrocortisone.

---

17. What is the goal blood glucose for patients with sepsis?
    a. 80 to 110 mg/dL
    b. <120 mg/dL
    c. <150 mg/dL
    d. <200 mg/dL

Answer a is incorrect. The range for normal blood glucose is 80 to 100 mg/dL .

Answer b is incorrect. Less than 120 mg/dL is not the range for blood glucose in patients with sepsis.

Answer c is correct. The target blood glucose in patients with sepsis is <150 mg/dL, a moderate goal.

Answer d is incorrect. Less than 200 mg/dL is too high a goal for a patient with sepsis.

---

18. Select the most appropriate regimen for glycemic control in a patient with sepsis.
    a. Metformin 1000 mg po bid
    b. Sitagliptin 100 mg po daily
    c. Insulin glargine 50 units qhs
    d. Insulin infusion

Answer a is incorrect. Oral antihyperglycemic therapy is inappropriate in a patient with sepsis.

Answer b is incorrect. Oral antihyperglycemic therapy is inappropriate in a patient with sepsis.

Answer c is incorrect. Insulin glargine is a long-acting insulin. Patients with sepsis need insulin therapy that can be rapidly titrated.

Answer d is correct. Insulin infusion is appropriate for a patient with sepsis because it is rapidly titrated and can accommodate the quick changes in blood glucose seen in patients with sepsis.

---

19. Which of the following nutrition regimens is (are) appropriate in a patient with severe sepsis secondary to pneumonia?
    a. Continuous tube feeding via a nasoduodenal tube
    b. Parenteral nutrition via a central IV catheter
    c. Parenteral nutrition via a peripheral IV catheter
    d. a and b
    e. b and c

Answer a is correct. Parenteral nutrition increases a patient's risk for infection and should be avoided unless a patient can not be fed via the enteral route. Continuous tube feeding into the small intestine will avoid this risk and this location in the gut will decrease the risk for aspiration.

Answer b is incorrect. Parenteral nutrition increases a patient's risk for infection and should be avoided unless a patient can not be fed via the enteral route. In a patient with pneumonia, the patient's gastrointestinal tract is unlikely to be affected and is an appropriate route for feeding.

Answer c is incorrect. Parenteral nutrition increases a patient's infection risk. In addition, parenteral nutrition is not typically given via a peripheral line.

---

20. Which of the following is a risk factor for stress-induced gastrointestinal bleeding?
    a. Mechanical ventilation
    b. Corticosteroid therapy
    c. Warfarin therapy
    d. All of the above

Answer a is correct. Mechanical ventilation induces physiologic stress and is a risk factor for stress-induced GI bleeding.

Answer b is correct. Corticosteroids provide supraphysiologic levels of the stress hormone, cortisol, and increase the risk for GI bleeding.

Answer c is correct. Warfarin therapy induces a pharmacologic coagulopathy and increases a patient's risk for GI bleeding.

Answer d is correct and the best answer. All of the above are correct.

CHAPTER 26 Human Immunodeficiency Virus and Acquired Immunodeficiency Syndrome (HIV/AIDS)

1. Select the statement that *most* accurately describes HIV.
    a. A DNA virus
    b. An RNA virus
    c. An RNA retrovirus
    d. A parasite

Answer a is incorrect. HIV is not a DNA virus, it is an RNA retrovirus.

Answer b is incorrect. HIV is an RNA virus; however, answer c is more correct describing it as an RNA retrovirus.

Answer c is correct. HIV is an RNA retrovirus, because it transcribes its RNA into DNA, while normal cell transcription occurs from DNA to RNA.

Answer d is incorrect. HIV is a virus not a parasite.

---

2. What is the primary mode of HIV acquisition globally?
   a. Contaminated blood and tissue products
   b. Casual contact with an HIV-infected person
   c. Homosexual contact
   d. Heterosexual contact

Answer a is incorrect. Contaminated blood and tissue products are associated with HIV transmission; however, they are not the primary mode globally. Sexual transmission has the highest rates of acquisition.

Answer b is incorrect. Causal contact with an HIV-infected person is not considered a significant risk factor for HIV acquisition.

Answer c is incorrect. Homosexual contact is the primary mode of HIV acquisition in the United States, but not globally.

Answer d is correct. Heterosexual contact is the primary mode of HIV acquisition globally. It is the primary mode of transmission in Sub-Saharan Africa and that region of the world has approximately 67% of the world's HIV population.

---

3. What is the primary mode of HIV acquisition in the United States?
   a. Heterosexual contact
   b. Homosexual contact
   c. Casual contact with an HIV-infected person
   d. Contaminated blood and tissue products

Answer a is incorrect. Heterosexual contact is not the primary mode of HIV acquisition in the United States, but is it the primary mode globally.

Answer b is correct. Homosexual contact, specifically men who have sex with men (MSM), is the primary mode of HIV acquisition in the United States, with 50% of cases being associated with MSM; however, high-risk heterosexual contact represents >30% of cases in the United States based on 2006 data.

Answer c is incorrect. Contaminated blood and tissue products are associated with HIV transmission; however, they are not the primary mode in the United States or globally. Sexual transmission has the highest rates of acquisition.

Answer d is incorrect. Causal contact with an HIV-infected person is not considered a significant risk factor for HIV acquisition.

---

4. When is a person living with HIV classified as having an AIDS diagnosis?
   a. Diagnosis of *Pneumocystis jiroveci* pneumonia
   b. CD4 count decreases to 350 μL
   c. HIV viral load of > 100,000 copies/mL
   d. a and b only
   e. All of the above

Answer a is correct. *Pneumocystis jiroveci* (formerly known as *Pneumocystis carinii*) pneumonia is considered an AIDS defining condition, so an HIV patient with this diagnosis would be considered to have progressed to AIDS. Other AIDS-defining conditions include esophageal candidiasis, Kaposi sarcoma, and *Mycobacterium avium* complex.

Answer b is incorrect. A CD4 count of ≤ 200 μL or development of an AIDS-defining condition indicates an AIDS diagnosis.

Answer c is incorrect. An AIDS diagnosis is independent of viral load.

Answer d is incorrect. Answer a provides a correct answer, but answer b is incorrect.

Answer e is incorrect. Only a is the appropriate answer.

---

5. LF is 31-year-old man recently diagnosed with HIV. He presents to the HIV clinic for the first time and is eager to start treatment. What is your most appropriate course of action?
   a. Immediately begin therapy with a triple drug regimen
   b. Counsel the patient regarding HIV, transmission, prevention of transmission to others, answer his questions, and schedule another follow-up visit
   c. Obtain baseline labs and schedule another follow-up visit
   d. a and b only
   e. b and c only

Answer a is incorrect. Patients diagnosed with HIV are not immediately started on drug therapy. Baseline laboratory values need to be obtained to determine if therapy is indicated and the patient's likelihood of compliance needs to be assessed.

Answer b is correct. All newly diagnosed HIV patient need extensive counseling regarding their disease, how to prevent transmission and need their questions answered. Follow-up visits are necessary to review laboratory values and also can be used to assess if patients are candidates for therapy, because if they miss follow-up appointments, they are likely not be adherent to HIV therapy (refer to Table 26-1).

Answer c is correct. Baseline laboratory values need to be obtained to determine if therapy or opportunistic infection prophylaxis indicated and get an overall picture of the patient's general health status (refer to Table 26-1).

Answer d is incorrect. Answer b is correct, but answer a is incorrect.

Answer e is correct and the best answer. Both answers b and c are correct.

---

6. Select the most common signs of symptoms of primary HIV infection in an adult patient.
    a. Mononucleosis-like illness (fever, sore-throat, fatigue, weight loss)
    b. GI upset (nausea, vomiting, diarrhea)
    c. Lymphadenopathy
    d. Night sweats
    e. All of the above

Answers a, b, c, and d are correct.

Answer e is correct and the best answer. Mononucleosis-like illness (fever, sore-throat, fatigue, weight loss), GI upset (nausea, vomiting, diarrhea), lymphadenopathy, and night sweats are all signs and symptoms of primary HIV infection in adult patients. Symptoms are typically self-limiting, resolving often without intervention. Pediatric patients that acquire infection perinatally typically do not have symptoms.

7. Which of the following statements about HIV prevention is *true*?
    a. Condoms are 100% effective in preventing HIV transmission
    b. All pregnant women should be screened for HIV
    c. Only pregnant women who engage in high-risk behaviors should be screened for HIV
    d. IV drug abusers can reuse/share syringe hubs as long as a new needle is used
    e. None of these statements is true

Answer a is incorrect. Abstinence is the only 100% effective way to prevent sexual transmission of HIV. While condoms may reduce transmission rates, they are not 100% effective.

Answer b is correct. All pregnant women should be screened for HIV, so that if they are positive they can be placed on antiretroviral therapy to decrease their viral load and subsequently dramatically decrease the chances of transmitting the infection to the infant.

Answer c is incorrect. All pregnant women should be screened for HIV, however nonpregnant persons who engage in high-risk behaviors should be routinely screened for HIV.

Answer d is incorrect. Sharing of any drug paraphernalia can cause HIV transmission, not just needles.

Answer e is incorrect. Answer b is a true statement.

8. Which of the following are targets for currently available HIV medications?
    a. Reverse transcriptase, protease, and integrase
    b. Reverse transcriptase, protease, and proviral DNA
    c. Reverse transcriptase, mRNA, protease, and integrase
    d. Reverse transcriptase, protease, mRNA, and proviral DNA

Answer a is correct. Reverse transcriptase is the target for nucleoside/nucleotide and nonnucleoside reverse-transcriptase inhibitors. Protease is the target for protease inhibitors and integrase is the target for integrase inhibitors.

Answer b is incorrect. Proviral DNA is not a target for current antiretroviral therapies.

Answer c is incorrect. mRNA is not a target for current antiretroviral therapies.

Answer d is incorrect. Proviral DNA and mRNA are not targets for current antiretroviral therapies.

9. A health care worker has a higher risk of contracting HIV from a HIV-positive patient if:
    a. The health care worker has a deep needlestick injury and the patient has an undetectable viral load
    b. The health care worker has a superficial needlestick injury and the patient has an undetectable viral load
    c. The health care worker has a deep needlestick injury and the patient has a high viral load
    d. The health care worker has a superficial needlestick injury and the patient has a high viral load

Answer a is incorrect. A deep needlestick has a higher risk of transmission than a superficial needlestick injury, but HIV patients with undetectable viral loads are less likely to transmit disease since there is not a large amount of virus per milliliter of blood.

Answer b is incorrect. A superficial needlestick has less of a risk of transmission than a deep needlestick injury, but HIV patients with undetectable viral loads are less likely to transmit disease since there is not a large amount of virus per milliliter of blood.

Answer c is correct. A deep needlestick has a higher risk of transmission than a superficial needlestick injury, but HIV patients with high viral loads are more likely to transmit disease since there is a larger amount of virus per milliliter of blood.

Answer d is incorrect. A superficial needlestick has less of a risk of transmission than a deep needlestick injury, but HIV patients with high viral loads are more likely to transmit disease since there is a larger amount of virus per milliliter of blood.

10. One of the primary goals of HIV therapy is:
    a. Complete eradication of the virus
    b. Maintain CD4 count at the level it was when treatment began
    c. Durable and maximal suppression of HIV replication
    d. None of the above

Answer a is incorrect. Currently there is no proven strategy to completely eradicate HIV. The virus is integrated into the host chromosome and it establishes persistent infection in long-lived immune system cells like memory T lymphocytes. This helps to keep the virus hidden from immune responses.

Answer b is incorrect. The goal is to increase CD4 count as much as possible since it directly correlates to immune system function.

Answer c is correct. Suppression of HIV replication is associated with decreased morbidity and mortality, so suppression and maintenance of suppression is the primary goal of HIV therapy.

Answer d is incorrect. Answer c is correct.

11. A patient presents to the hospital with a 2-week history of a mono-like illness. All of her laboratory tests are within normal limits or are negative including her ELISA. The patient reports being sexually active with multiple partners. The most appropriate course of action is:
    a. Inform her that she does not have HIV and discharge home
    b. Inform her that she does not have HIV, but counsel her on HIV and STD prevention
    c. Inform her that she will need to complete a follow-up ELISA in 1 month
    d. Inform her that she will need to complete a follow-up ELISA in 1 month, and counsel her on HIV and STD prevention

Answer a is incorrect. HIV antibody production minimally takes 3 to 4 weeks after initial exposure and sometimes up to 6 months, so this patient could have a false negative ELISA.

Answer b is incorrect. HIV antibody production minimally takes 3 to 4 weeks after initial exposure and sometimes up to 6 months, so this patient could have a false negative ELISA. However, given her high-risk behavior it is important that she be counseled about HIV and STD prevention.

Answer c is incorrect. She should have a follow-up ELISA screen in 1 month since she is considered high risk and to give her body time to develop antibodies if HIV is present. But answer d is better because this patient will require counseling on prevention as well.

Answer d is correct. The patient should have a follow-up ELISA screen in 1 month since she is considered high risk and to give her body time to develop antibodies if HIV is present and she does need counseling regarding HIV and STD prevention.

12. In a patient receiving zidovudine therapy, which of the following could you expect to be elevated on laboratory evaluation?
    a. Blood urea nitrogen (BUN)
    b. Mean corpuscular volume (MCV)
    c. Serum creatinine
    d. Potassium

Answer a is incorrect. Zidovudine has a negligible effect on blood urea nitrogen. Zidovudine therapy does not commonly result in renal dysfunction.

Answer b is correct. Mean corpuscular volume (MCV) is a marker of RBC size and utilized in the diagnosis of anemia. An elevated MCV is common with zidovudine therapy as a result of macrocytic anemia. This can be used as an indirect marker of patient's adherence to therapy.

Answer c is incorrect. Again, zidovudine therapy does not commonly result in renal dysfunction, nor does it have a direct effect on creatinine secretion or reabsorption.

Answer d is incorrect. Zidovudine does not have a direct impact on potassium concentrations.

13. A treatment experienced patient receiving atazanavir therapy should avoid the addition of which of the following medications:
    a. Omeprazole
    b. Metronidazole
    c. Pravastatin
    d. Metoprolol

Answer a is correct. Atazanavir requires an acidic environment for optimal absorption. In treatment-experienced patients, combination therapy with proton pump inhibitors is contraindicated. In treatment-naïve patients, doses of omeprazole 20 mg equivalent or less, may be used with caution. The risk versus benefit should be weighed when combining these agents.

Answer b is incorrect. There is no known or anticipated drug interaction between metronidazole and atazanavir therapy.

Answer c is incorrect. There is no known or anticipated drug interaction between pravastatin and atazanavir therapy. Pravastatin is also the lone member of the HMG-CoA reductase inhibitor class of medications that does not undergo metabolism through the CYP-450 enzyme system.

Answer d is incorrect. There is no known or anticipated drug interaction between metoprolol and atazanavir therapy.

14. Which of the following treatment regimens would be considered appropriate in a treatment-naïve patient?
    a. Maraviroc + efavirenz + nevirapine
    b. Raltegravir + abacavir + indinavir + ritonavir
    c. Tenofovir + zidovudine + abacavir
    d. Lamviudine + zidovudine + lopinavir + ritonavir

Answer a is incorrect. Two NNRTIs (efavirenz and nevirapine) should not be used in combination. There is no two NRTI backbone in this regimen.

Answer b is incorrect. There is only one NRTI (abacavir) in this treatment regimen, whereas two is optimal for a complete NRTI backbone. Although indinavir plus ritonavir could be used, indinavir is not a preferred PI.

Answer c is incorrect. The triple combination of NRTI therapy is not preferred due to high failure rates.

Answer d is correct. This regimen includes two NRTIs (lamivudine and zidovudine) plus a preferred boosted PI (lopinavir).

---

15. In a patient with a history of acute on chronic pancreatitis, which of the following medications should be avoided?
    a. Didanosine
    b. Darunavir
    c. Tenofovir
    d. Enfuvirtide

Answer a is correct. Didanosine is a known cause of drug-induced pancreatitis and should be avoided in patients with a history of pancreatitis. In cases of unavoidable use, risk versus benefit should be carefully weighed.

Answer b is incorrect. Darunavir is not associated with drug-induced pancreatitis.

Answer c is incorrect. Tenofovir is not associated with drug-induced pancreatitis. Adverse effects from tenofovir are most commonly linked to renal impairment.

Answer d is incorrect. Enfuvirtide is not associated with drug-induced pancreatitis. Adverse effects from enfuvirtide are most commonly injection site reactions.

---

16. Which of the following properties are true of efavirenz?
    a. Should be taken with a high-fat meal.
    b. Is a common cause of vivid dreams and hallucinations.
    c. Is the NNRTI of choice in pregnancy.
    d. a and b

Answer a is incorrect. Taking efavirenz with a high-fat meal will result in significant increases in peak drug concentrations (C_{max}). These increased concentrations result in significant increase in toxicity, notably CNS-related adverse events. Thus, efavirenz should be taken on an empty stomach.

Answer b is correct. CNS-related adverse events including hallucinations, vivid dreams, and occasionally altered mental status are commonly encountered with efavirenz therapy. Dosing at bedtime on an empty stomach is preferred and may help with daytime symptoms.

Answer c is incorrect. Efavirenz is pregnancy category D, specifically during the first trimester. Careful risk versus benefit should be weighed if using this drug at any point during pregnancy, or in young women intending on becoming pregnant.

Answer d is incorrect. Choice a above is incorrect.

---

17. Which of the following antiretrovirals is/are available in an injectable form?
    a. Zidovudine
    b. Etravirine
    c. Enfuvirtide
    d. Darunavir
    e. a and c

Answer a is true, but incorrect choice. Zidovudine is the only antiretroviral available in the IV form.

Answer b is incorrect. Etravirine is only available as an oral capsule.

Answer c is true, but incorrect choice. Enfuvirtide is available as a subcutaneous injection.

Answer d is incorrect. Darunavir is only available as an oral tablet.

Answer e is correct. Both a and c are correct choices. Zidovudine and enfuvirtide are the only antiretrovirals available in an injectable form.

---

18. Which of the following patients would be at highest risk for developing hepatotoxicity secondary to nevirapine therapy?
    a. 31-year-old woman with a CD4+ count equal to 91 cells/mm^3.
    b. 21-year-old man with CD4+ count equal to 270 cells/mm^3.
    c. 50-year-old man with CD4+ count equal to 260 cells/mm^3.
    d. 25-year-old woman with CD4+ count equal to 265 cells/mm^3.

Answer a is incorrect. Women with CD4+ counts >250 cells/mm^3 are at an increased risk. Her CD4 count is below this threshold.

Answer b is incorrect. Males with CD4+ counts >400 cells/mm^3 are at an increased risk. His CD4+ count is below this threshold.

Answer c is incorrect. His CD4+ count is below 400 cells/mm^3 threshold. Also, age has not been directly linked with increased risk of hepatotoxicity.

Answer d is correct. Her CD4+ count is >250 cells/mm^3 putting this patient into a high-risk category. Nevirapine therapy should be avoided in these high-risk patients.

---

19. Which of the following combinations of antiretrovirals should be avoided?
    a. Didanosine and stavudine
    b. Tenofovir and efavirenz
    c. Lamivudine and zidovudine
    d. Fosamprenavir and ritonavir

Answer a is correct. Didanosine and stavudine, both thymidine analogues, when used together potentiate adverse effects, specifically mitochondrial toxicity. This combination should be avoided.

Answer b is incorrect. Tenofovir is an NRTI and efavirenz is an NNRTI. These drugs are coformulated together with emtricitabine in Atripla. There are no contraindications to this combination.

Answer c is incorrect. Lamivudine and zidovudine are both NRTIs and are coformulated together in Combivir. There are no contraindications to this combination.

Answer d is incorrect. Fosamprenavir and ritonavir are both PIs. Ritonavir is used in combination with fosamprenavir as a boosting agent, through its inhibition of CYP 3A4 enzyme system.

20. Which of the following antiretrovirals should be used with caution in patients with documented sulfa allergy?

    a. Fosamprenavir
    b. Tipranavir
    c. Darunavir
    d. a and b
    e. All of the above

Answer a is true, but incorrect choice. Fosamprenavir has a sulfa-moiety in its chemical structure and should be used with caution in patients with a documented sulfa allergy.

Answer b is true, but incorrect choice. Tipranavir has a sulfa-moiety in its chemical structure and should be used with caution in patients with a documented sulfa allergy.

Answer c is true, but incorrect choice. Darunavir has a sulfa-moiety in its chemical structure and should be used with caution in patients with a documented sulfa allergy.

Answer d is true, but incorrect choice. All three choices above are correct.

Answer e is correct. Fosamprenavir, tipranavir, and darunavir are all PIs that should be used with caution in patients with a documented sulfa allergy. Each of these drugs is known to cause rash.

21. Dosing of Selzentry (maraviroc) should be increased to 600 mg twice daily when combined with which of the following medications?

    a. Ketoconazole
    b. Clarithromycin
    c. Rifampin
    d. Warfarin

Answer a is incorrect. Ketoconazole is a potent inhibitor of CYP 3A. When a 3A4 inhibitor is combined with maraviroc the dose should be decreased to 150 mg twice daily.

Answer b is incorrect. Clarithromycin is a potent inhibitor of CYP 3A. When a 3A4 inhibitor is combined with maraviroc, the dose should be decreased to 150 mg twice daily.

Answer c is correct. Rifampin is a potent inducer of CYP 3A and 2C. When a 3A4 inducer is combined with maraviroc, the dose should be increased to 600 mg twice daily.

Answer d is incorrect. Warfarin is a substrate of primarily CYP 3A and 2C. There would be no dose adjustment of maraviroc when the two are combined.

CHAPTER 27 | Tuberculosis

1. JK is a 32-year-old HIV-negative new patient at the clinic you work at. He receives a Mantoux skin test that returns positive 2 days later. He was born in the United States and works as a prison guard. He injects heroin on a regular basis. His chest x-ray comes back normal, he has no symptoms of tuberculosis, and his smear culture is negative. What type of drug therapy would be appropriate for this patient?

    a. Isoniazid 300 mg daily × 9 months
    b. Rifampin 100 mg daily × 4 months
    c. No drug therapy needed
    d. Isoniazid 300 mg and rifampin 600 mg × 6 months
    e. Isoniazid, rifampin, ethambutol, and pyrazinamide

Answer a is correct. The patient does not have any symptoms or indications of active TB disease; so he needs treatment for latent TB infection. This is the correct first-line regimen for treatment of latent TB infection.

Answer b is incorrect. Rifampin is a second-line treatment for latent TB infection. It can be used in patients with intolerance to isoniazid or in areas where isoniazid-resistant strains of TB are prevalent. The dose of rifampin is also too low.

Answer c is incorrect. Treating latent TB infection significantly reduces his risk of converting to active disease. He works in a high-risk setting prison where if he were to get active disease it could be spread more easily as well.

Answer d is incorrect. Latent TB infection typically only requires monotherapy.

Answer e is incorrect. Latent TB infection typically only requires monotherapy. This four drug regimen is used in treating active TB disease.

2. BCG vaccine should be routinely given to which patient in the United States?

    a. A 10-year-old child
    b. A 2-month-old infant
    c. A 65-year-old man
    d. A 6-month-old infant
    e. None of the above

Answer a is incorrect. BCG vaccination should *not* be routinely given to any specific age group in the United States.

Answer b is incorrect. BCG vaccination should *not* be routinely given to any specific age group in the United States.

Answer c is incorrect. BCG vaccination should *not* be routinely given to any specific age group in the United States.

Answer d is incorrect. BCG vaccination should *not* be routinely given to any specific age group in the United States.

Answer e is correct.

3. Which of the following is *not* a counseling point on rifampin?
   a. This medication can cause your body secretions to be an orange-red color.
   b. This medication can decrease the effectiveness of your oral contraceptives.
   c. This medication can cause you to need a decrease in your warfarin dose.
   d. This medication may cause gastrointestinal upset.
   e. This medication can cause your phenytoin concentrations to go down.

Answer a is incorrect. Rifampin does cause secretions to turn an orange-red color.

Answer b is incorrect. Rifampin induces cytochrome P-450 enzymes that can increase the metabolism of oral contraceptives making them less effective.

Answer c is correct. Rifampin induces cytochrome P-450 enzymes that increase the metabolism of warfarin. Thus you would likely need an increase in your warfarin dose.

Answer d is incorrect. Rifampin has the potential to cause gastrointestinal upset.

Answer e is incorrect. Rifampin can induce the metabolism of phenytoin which would decrease the concentration of phenytoin.

4. RS is a 25-year-old Hispanic woman who is recently diagnosed with active tuberculosis. Her physician asks what drug regimen you would recommend to treat her disease. She does not have any contraindications to any of the tuberculosis medications. You do not have susceptibility testing back yet.
   a. INH, RIF, PZA × 8 weeks, then INH, RIF ×18 weeks
   b. INH × 9 months
   c. INH, RIF × 9 months
   d. INH, RIF, EMB, FQ × 8 weeks, then INH, RIF × 18 weeks
   e. INH, RIF, EMB, PZA × 8 weeks, then INH, RIF × 18 weeks

Answer a is incorrect. Ethambutol is also part of the initial 8-week regimen in adults.

Answer b is incorrect. This is the treatment for latent TB infection. This patient has active disease.

Answer c is incorrect. There are typically two phases of treatment in active TB disease, an initial 8 weeks and then a continuation phase of approximately 18 weeks. Ethambutol and pyrazinamide are part of the initial 8-week treatment in active TB treatment in adults unless the patient is pregnant. If the patient is pregnant the pyrazinamide is not given.

Answer d is incorrect. Fluoroquinolones are not first-line agents in active TB treatment.

Answer e is correct. This is the correct first-line initial four-drug regimen and two-drug continuation phase regimen in adults. Drug susceptibility could ultimately influence your drug choices in the future.

5. Which of the following is true regarding acid-fast bacteria?
   a. They cause the majority of bacterial infectious diseases in the United States.
   b. *Mycobacterium tuberculosis* is the only type of acid-fast bacteria.
   c. Cultures of acid-fast bacteria grow faster than other bacteria.
   d. They retain their stained color even with acid-alcohol washes.

Answer a is incorrect. Acid-fast bacilli cause a small subset of bacterial illnesses in the United States.

Answer b is incorrect. There are other acid-fast bacteria. Examples include: *Mycobacterium bovis* and *Mycobacterium leprae.*

Answer c is incorrect. Mycobacterium tuberculosis is an acid-fast bacteria and it grows in culture at a slow rate.

Answer d is correct. Acid-fast bacteria keep their stain color despite acid-alcohol washes. *Mycobacterium tuberculosis* is acid fast.

6. Select the primary method for transmission of tuberculosis.
   a. Inhalation
   b. Exposure to blood and/or bodily fluids
   c. Exposure to dead birds
   d. Hospitalization

Answer a is correct. Inhalation of respiratory droplets is the primary mechanism for contracting tuberculosis infection.

Answer b is incorrect. Tuberculosis is not transmitted this way. Viral infections such as HIV and hepatitis B/C can be transmitted this way.

Answer c is incorrect. Tuberculosis is not transmitted through animals to humans.

Answer d is incorrect. Suspected tuberculosis patients in the hospital are typically in isolation. It is possible to be exposed to TB in the hospital, but it is not the primary method for contracting TB.

7. What time period is the risk highest for conversion to active disease in those patients with latent tuberculosis infection?
   a. 10 years after exposure
   b. 8 years after exposure
   c. 6 years after exposure
   d. 4 years after exposure
   e. 2 years after exposure

Answers a, b, c, and d are incorrect. Risk of converting from latent TB infection to active disease is highest in the first 2 years. Drug therapy for latent TB reduces this risk significantly.

Answer e is correct. Risk of converting from latent TB infection to active disease is highest in the first 2 years. Drug therapy for latent TB reduces this risk significantly.

---

8. Which of the following is *not* a sign/symptom of pulmonary tuberculosis?
   a. Weight loss
   b. Productive cough
   c. Headache
   d. Fever
   e. Night sweats

Answers a, b, d, and e are incorrect. These are common signs/symptoms of pulmonary TB.

Answer c is correct. Headache is not typical with TB infection.

---

9. How long after a Mantoux skin test for TB infection is placed should it be read?
   a. 12 hours
   b. 24 hours
   c. 48 hours
   d. 96 hours
   e. 120 hours

Answer a is incorrect. This time period is too soon to read a skin test.

Answer b is incorrect. This time period is too soon to read a skin test.

Answer c is correct. Mantoux skin tests should be read within 48 to 72 hours of administering them.

Answer d is incorrect. This time period is too long to read a skin test.

Answer e is incorrect. This time period is too long to read a skin test.

---

10. Which patient group should get drug-susceptibility testing?
   a. All latent tuberculosis patients
   b. Latent tuberculosis patients over age 35
   c. All active tuberculosis disease patients
   d. Active tuberculosis patients over age 35
   e. Foreign-born cases of latent and active tuberculosis

Answer a is incorrect. Latent TB patients do not need drug-susceptibility testing.

Answer b is incorrect. Latent TB patients do not need drug-susceptibility testing regardless of age.

Answer c is correct. Drug-susceptibility testing should be initially done in all patients with active disease to determine proper drug therapy to control spread of drug-resistant strains.

Answer d is incorrect. All active TB patients should receive susceptibility regardless of age.

Answer e is incorrect. A patient being born in a foreign country does not typically affect decisions to do drug-susceptibility testing.

---

11. Which medication is typically not included in the first-line regimen for children with active TB disease?
   a. Isoniazid
   b. Rifampin
   c. Pyrazinamide
   d. Ethambutol

Answers a, b, and c are incorrect. These are first-line regimens in children with active TB disease.

Answer d is correct. Ethambutol is not typically included in a child's regimen because of the potential inability to adequately assess visual acuity. Changes in visual acuity and color vision need to be assessed during ethambutol therapy due to the drug having the potential to cause retrobulbar neuritis.

---

12. The addition of which of the following drugs necessitates follow-up liver function tests in a patient being treated for latent TB infection treated with isoniazid?
   a. Naproxen
   b. Multivitamin
   c. Sertraline
   d. Acetaminophen
   e. Lisinopril

Answer a is incorrect. Naproxen does not commonly cause changes in isoniazid metabolism and is not known to commonly cause hepatotoxicity or elevate liver enzymes.

Answer b is incorrect. Multivitamins do not commonly cause changes in isoniazid metabolism and are not known to commonly cause hepatotoxicity or elevate liver enzymes.

Answer c is incorrect. Sertraline does not commonly cause changes in isoniazid metabolism and is not known to commonly cause hepatotoxicity or elevate liver enzymes.

Answer d is correct. Acetaminophen can increase the risk of isoniazid-induced hepatotoxicity. If patients are placed on scheduled acetaminophen you need to closely monitor for hepatotoxicity including liver enzymes. You may want to recommend an alternative pain regimen while on isoniazid.

Answer e is incorrect. Lisinopril does not commonly cause changes in isoniazid metabolism and is not known to commonly cause hepatotoxicity or elevate liver enzymes.

---

13. What is the preferred regimen for treating latent tuberculosis infection in adults?

    a. Isoniazid 300 mg daily × 6 months
    b. Isoniazid 300 mg daily × 9 months
    c. Rifampin 600 mg daily × 6 months
    d. Rifampin 600 mg daily × 9 months

Answer a is incorrect. Isoniazid is the preferred drug and can be used for 6 months in certain cases; however, this is not the preferred time period of treatment.

Answer b is correct. Isoniazid is the preferred drug and 9 months is the preferred time period. It is been found to be superior to 6 months.

Answer c is incorrect. Rifampin is second-line regimen in latent TB treatment if the patient is intolerant to isoniazid or if isoniazid resistance is high in the area. Rifampin is also typically given for 4 months.

Answer d is incorrect. Rifampin is second-line regimen in latent TB treatment if the patient is intolerant to isoniazid or if isoniazid resistance is high in the area. Rifampin is also typically given for 4 months.

---

14. Which of the following group or groups are at higher risk for hepatotoxicity related to their TB treatment regimens?

    a. Pregnant
    b. Postpartum
    c. Drinks 2 beers daily
    d. 65-year-olds
    e. All of the above

Answer a is incorrect. Pregnancy puts a patient at higher risk for hepatotoxicity.

Answer b is incorrect. Postpartum women are at higher risk for hepatotoxicity.

Answer c is incorrect. Regular alcohol users are at higher risk for hepatotoxicity.

Answer d is incorrect. Advanced age puts a patient at higher risk for hepatotoxicity.

Answer e is correct and the best answer. All of the above are risk factors for hepatotoxicity.

---

15. Which of the following is *not* a second-line agent for treatment of active TB disease?

    a. Streptomycin
    b. Ciprofloxacin
    c. Amoxicillin
    d. Capreomycin
    e. Ethionamide

Answers a, b, d, e are incorrect. These can be used second-line agents against drug-resistant strains of TB.

Answer b is incorrect. Ciprofloxacin can be used second-line agent against drug-resistant strains of TB.

Answer c is correct. Amoxicillin is not typically a drug used to treat TB.

---

16. The addition of pyridoxine (vitamin B6) helps protect against which isoniazid-induced toxicity?

    a. Hepatotoxicity
    b. Peripheral neuropathy
    c. Gastrointestinal upset
    d. Rash

Answer a is incorrect. There are no protective drugs to give against isoniazid hepatotoxicity.

Answer b is correct. Isoniazid promotes excretion of pyridoxine. This pyridoxine deficiency can cause neuropathy so one can supplement with pyridoxine to prevent peripheral neuropathies from isoniazid.

Answer c is incorrect. Gastrointestinal upset can be alleviated potentially by taking the isoniazid with food.

Answer d is incorrect. There are no protective drugs to give to prevent rash.

---

17. Which rifamycin has the least drug interactions?

    a. Rifampin
    b. Rifabutin
    c. Rifapentine
    d. Rocephin

Answer a is incorrect. Rifampin is the strongest cytochrome P-450 inducer and has the most drug interactions.

Answer b is correct. Rifabutin is the least potent cytochrome P-450 inducer and has the least amount of drug interactions.

Answer c is incorrect. Rifapentine has less drug interactions than rifampin; however, rifabutin is thought to have the least and recommended in most HIV-positive patients on antiretroviral regimens.

Answer d is incorrect. Rocephin is a cephalosporin antibiotic used to treat infections other than TB.

---

18. Which of the following is an appropriate test of monitoring ethambutol toxicity?
    a. Creatinine
    b. Foot examination
    c. Snellen visual chart examination
    d. Complete blood count
    e. Triglycerides

Answer a is incorrect. Ethambutol does not cause creatinine elevations or renal toxicity.

Answer b is incorrect. Ethambutol does not cause any peripheral neuropathies that can be monitored with foot examination.

Answer c is correct. Ethambutol can cause retrobulbar neuritis which causes changes in visual acuity and red-green color blindness. Visual acuity can be checked with the Snellen visual chart examination and should be done as baseline and throughout treatment.

Answer d is incorrect. Ethambutol does not require routine complete blood counts.

Answer e is incorrect. Ethambutol does not elevate triglycerides.

---

19. Which of the following is a contraindication to pyrazinamide therapy?
    a. Acute gout attacks
    b. Chronic obstructive pulmonary disease
    c. Rheumatoid arthritis
    d. Asthma

Answer a is correct. Pyrazinamide can cause hyperuricemia which puts patients at higher risk for developing acute gout attacks.

Answer b is incorrect. Pyrazinamide does not exacerbate chronic obstructive pulmonary disease or shortness of breath.

Answer c is incorrect. Pyrazinamide does not typically exacerbate rheumatoid arthritis.

Answer d is incorrect. Pyrazinamide does not exacerbate asthma or shortness of breath.

---

20. Which of the following first-line TB drugs is recommended not to be given in pregnant patients?
    a. Isoniazid
    b. Rifampin
    c. Ethambutol
    d. Pyrazinamide

Answers a, b, and c are incorrect. These can be included in TB regimens in pregnant women.

Answer d is correct. Pyrazinamide does not have adequate safety data and is currently not recommended to be included in TB regimens given to pregnant women.

CHAPTER 28 | Invasive Fungal Infections

1. Which one of the following adjunctive measures is used to lessen the occurrence of nephrotoxicity associated with amphotericin B?
    a. Test dose of amphotericin B
    b. Diphenhydramine premedication
    c. Normal saline boluses
    d. Furosemide
    e. All of the above

Answer a is incorrect. This may help to identify patients who might develop an infusion-related adverse effects (fevers, chills, rigors, or hypotension) or anaphylaxis. Most experts do not advocate this anymore due to the poor predictive value. However, during initial dosing, the drug should be administered under close monitoring.

Answer b is incorrect. This is believed to reduce the occurrence of infusion-related adverse effects (fevers, chills, and rigors). Other medications that might be used to treat/prevent the infusion-related reactions include acetaminophen, nonsteroidal anti-inflammatory medications, and hydrocortisone. If the patient continues with severe rigors on the premedication, meperidine may be used.

Answer c is correct. Although not proven via large scale controlled trials, data from animal and small human studies suggest a decrease in nephrotoxicity. Patients will often receive a 500 mL IV bolus of normal saline solution before starting the amphotericin B infusion. Saline doses are also often administered after the dose of amphotericin B.

Answer d is incorrect. Use of furosemide can often contribute to renal insufficiency in patients receiving amphotericin B.

Answer e is incorrect. All of the above options are not used to prevent nephrotoxicity.

---

2. Which of one of the following organisms is most likely to manifest a positive India ink stain on a cerebral spinal fluid sample?
    a. *Candida albicans*
    b. *Candida glabrata*
    c. *Aspergillus fumigatus*
    d. *Cryptococcus neoformans*
    e. All of the above

Answers a, b, c, and e are incorrect.

Answer d is correct. The India ink stain adheres to the capsule around *C. neoformans.*

---

3. When preparing an IV formulation of amphotericin B deoxycholate (desoxycholate), the lyophilized amphotericin B powder must first be reconstituted with sterile water. What type of IV fluid must the reconstituted amphotericin B be placed in for IV administration?
   a. 0.9% sodium chloride
   b. 5% dextrose in water
   c. Lactated Ringer's solution
   d. Any of the above solutions

Answer a is incorrect. This solution will not maintain the micellular distribution.

Answer b is correct. This solution will maintain the micellular distribution that is required for IV amphotericin B desoxycholate.

Answer c is incorrect. This solution will not maintain the micellular distribution.

Answer d is incorrect. Only 5% dextrose in water should be used.

---

4. Which of the following agents is not recommended as therapy for invasive aspergillosis?
   a. Amphotericin B
   b. Fluconazole
   c. Voriconazole
   d. Liposomal amphotericin B

Answer a is incorrect. Amphotericin B is a drug of choice for *Aspergillus* species.

Answer b is correct. Fluconazole lacks activity against molds like *Aspergillus.*

Answer c is incorrect. Voriconazole is a drug of choice for *Aspergillus* species.

Answer d is incorrect. Lipid formulations of amphotericin B are a drug of choice for *Aspergillus* species.

---

5. Which one of the following antifungal agents is most associated with causing neutropenia and bone marrow suppression?
   a. Fluconazole
   b. Amphotericin B
   c. Voriconazole
   d. Flucytosine

Answers a and c are incorrect. The azoles have not been identified as a common cause of blood dyscrasias. *Note:* Be careful about using drug information resources when looking up or studying adverse reactions. Azole antifungals have hematologic side effects listed, but they are extremely rare.

Answer b is incorrect. Amphotericin B may cause a normocytic-normochromic anemia. The drug has been rarely associated with neutropenia.

Answer d is correct. 5-Flucytosine is known to cause blood dyscrasias. Bone marrow toxicity (as well as hepatic) is dose-related; monitor levels closely and adjust dose accordingly.

---

6. Lipid-based or liposomal amphotericin B formulations have what advantage over conventional amphotericin B (desoxycholate)?
   a. Less expensive than conventional amphotericin B
   b. Decreased mortality
   c. Decreased rates of nephrotoxicity
   d. More efficacious than conventional amphotericin B

Answer a is incorrect. Liposomal formulations are considerably more expensive.

Answer b is incorrect. This has not been shown in well-designed trials.

Answer c is correct. Changes in serum creatinine are less pronounced with lipid-based formulations.

Answer d is incorrect. This has not been shown in well-designed trials.

---

7. Which antifungal preparation carries a relative contraindication against use in patients with severe renal insufficiency (due to risk of renal complications from a carrier molecule)?
   a. IV fluconazole
   b. IV voriconazole
   c. Oral itraconazole
   d. IV caspofungin
   e. Oral voriconazole

Answer a is incorrect. No carrier molecule.

Answer b is correct. IV voriconazole uses a cyclodextrin carrier molecule. Related cyclodextrins have been associated with nephrotoxicity in some animal studies.

Answer c is incorrect. Oral itraconazole solution uses a cyclodextrin carrier molecule, but it does not enter the systemic circulation. It is possible for IV itraconazole to affect the renal system and its use is limited to 2 weeks because of concerns for potential nephrotoxicity secondary to the accumulation of the cyclodextrin vehicle.

Answer d is incorrect. No carrier molecule.

Answer e is incorrect. No carrier molecule.

---

8. A patient with a histoplasmosis infection is to be discharged from the hospital and started on oral itraconazole capsules. Which one of the following statements would you tell the patient about his medication to maximize the oral absorption?
   a. Take with food and avoid concomitant use of antacids
   b. Take on an empty stomach
   c. Food will not affect the oral absorption
   d. Do not take this with cola

Answer a is correct. For optimal dissolution and absorption of itraconazole capsules an acidic pH is desired.

Answer b is incorrect. Itraconazole should be taken with food.

Answer c is incorrect. Studies have shown that food can significantly improve oral absorption.

Answer d is incorrect. Administration with cola has been one way to provide some acidic fluid to increase dissolution and absorption.

---

9. A patient is to receive home infusion therapy with liposomal amphotericin B. What laboratory values should be monitored?

   a. Serum creatinine
   b. Serum potassium
   c. Serum magnesium
   d. All of the above

Answer a is correct. Amphotericin B is nephrotoxic.

Answer b is correct. Due to nephrotoxicity the kidney loses ability to maintain potassium.

Answer c is correct. Due to nephrotoxicity the kidney loses ability to maintain magnesium.

Answer d is correct and the best answer. All of these are generally monitored.

---

10. Which of the following antifungal agents has been shown to cause visual acuity side effects?

    a. Amphotericin B
    b. Flucytosine
    c. Fluconazole
    d. Voriconazole
    e. Caspofungin

Answers a, b, c, and e are incorrect as they have not been associated with visual disturbances.

Answer d is incorrect. About 30% of patients in clinical trials reported some degree of reversible changes in visual acuity with voriconazole.

---

11. A 54-year-old man with leukemia developed neutropenia 10 days ago after a chemotherapy course. His absolute neutrophil count (ANC) is 200, and he has been febrile for 7 days despite empiric bacterial therapy with imipenem and vancomycin. He was ordered amphotericin B 5 days ago. His CrCl has diminished to < 30 mL/min. Which one of the following antifungal agents would be the best option for a febrile neutropenic patient with renal insufficiency? The provider would like a broad-spectrum antifungal that covers yeasts and molds and an agent that does not affect the kidneys as much as conventional amphotericin B.

    a. Liposomal amphotericin B
    b. Fluconazole
    c. Caspofungin
    d. Posaconazole
    e. a and c

Answer a is correct. Although liposomal amphotericin B can still contribute to continued renal failure it affects renal function less. This agent is a broad-spectrum antifungal (yeasts and molds).

Answer b is incorrect. This agent is not advised due to narrow spectrum of activity and fungistatic killing rate.

Answer c is correct. This agent would be an acceptable agent for this indication (covers yeasts and molds) and would not contribute to renal insufficiency.

Answer d is incorrect. This drug is only available in an oral formulation with poor absorption. There is limited data on using this drug in this indication.

Answer e is correct and the best answer. Both of these agents could be considered for such a patient.

---

12. A 58-year-old febrile woman in the surgical intensive care unit has one out of two blood culture bottles growing yeast. A urine sample collected 2 days ago is growing *C. glabrata*. What is the best empiric decision for this patient?

    a. Start fluconazole 400 mg daily
    b. Wait for a susceptibility report and then start with a sensitive antifungal agent
    c. The one out of two blood bottles and the urine culture do not require therapy
    d. Initiate caspofungin 70 mg × 1 dose, then 50 mg daily

Answer a is correct. This option could be used, but many *C. glabrata* strains may require higher doses of fluconazole based on in vitro susceptibilities (S-DD). Therapy or dose could be changed after susceptibilities become known.

Answer b is incorrect. Generally antifungal therapy is initiated and changed if needed based on the susceptibility results or clinical situation.

Answer c is incorrect. All positive blood cultures growing yeast should receive treatment.

Answer d is incorrect. While caspofungin would be active against *C. glabrata*, caspofungin undergoes extensive hepatic metabolism and would not be the best agent for a urinary source.

---

13. Genetic variability in Cytochrome P-450 CYP 2C19 has been linked to significant interpatient pharmacokinetic differences for which antifungal agent?

    a. Fluconazole
    b. Voriconazole
    c. Micafungin
    d. Flucytosine

Answer a is incorrect. Fluconazole is not a significant substrate for CYP 2C19.

Answer b is correct. Studies indicated that CYP 2C19 is significantly involved in the metabolism of voriconazole. This enzyme exhibits genetic polymorphism. About 3% to 5% of Caucasians and 12% to 23% of Asians are expected to be poor metabolizers.

Answer c is incorrect. Micafungin is not a CYP-450 substrate.

Answer d is incorrect. Flucytosine is not a CYP-450 substrate.

14. A 55-year-old man is to be treated for invasive aspergillosis. He weighs 100 kg. What amphotericin B formulation dose(s) would be appropriate for this patient?
    a. Amphotericin B desoxycholate 80 mg
    b. Amphotericin B desoxycholate 400 mg
    c. Liposomal Amphotericin B 400 mg
    d. a and c
    e. None of the above

Answer a is correct. The recommended dose of amphotericin B desoxycholate is 0.7 to 1 mg/kg.

Answer b is incorrect. This dose would be too high.

Answer c is correct: The recommended dose for liposomal amphotericin B is 3 to 5 mg/kg

Answer d is correct and the best answer.

Answer e is incorrect.

15. The fungal cell wall component (1, 3) β-D-glucan is not a key structure in *C. neoformans* and therefore explains the poor activity of what class of antifungal agents for *Cryptococcus*?
    a. Triazoles
    b. Amphotericin B
    c. Echinocandins
    d. 5-Flucytosine
    e. None of the above

Answer a is incorrect. Triazoles inhibit 14-α-demethylase. They are usually effective for cryptococcal infections.

Answer b is incorrect. Amphotericin B binds to ergosterol. It usually is effective for cryptococcal infections.

Answer c is correct. Echinocandins inhibit (1, 3) β-D-glucan synthase enzyme that makes (1, 3) β-D-glucan fibrils. They lack activity for cryptococcal infections.

Answer d is incorrect. 5-Flucytosine causes defective fungal protein synthesis. It can be effective for cryptococcal infections.

Answer e is incorrect.

16. What drug interaction would be exhibited by adding fluconazole to a person's medication regimen that includes warfarin (stabilized at an INR of 2.5)?
    a. Fluconazole and warfarin concentrations would both be reduced
    b. An increase in INR would be expected
    c. Warfarin Cytochrome P-450 metabolism would be induced
    d. An interaction would not be expected

Answer a is incorrect. The major interaction causes an increase in warfarin concentrations.

Answer b is correct. Fluconazole can interact with warfarin primarily through CYP 2C9 and some CYP 3A4 inhibition.

Answer c is incorrect. The interaction is through metabolic inhibition.

Answer d is incorrect. This interaction is well reported.

17. BK is a 40-year-old HIV-positive patient. He develops CSF culture-positive cryptococcal meningitis. He has no hepatic or renal insufficiency and his complete blood count is within normal limits. Select the preferred antifungal regimen for a patient with cryptococcal meningitis?
    a. Amphotericin B desoxycholate + flucytosine
    b. Amphotericin B desoxycholate
    c. Liposomal amphotericin B
    d. Fluconazole
    e. Micafungin

Answer a is correct. This is regarded as the first-line regimen. Flucytosine has excellent CSF penetration. Historically, it was used as monotherapy, but resistance quickly developed. It is now used as adjunctive therapy with amphotericin B to avoid failure due to resistance and to optimized killing due to synergistic killing of both agents.

Answer b is incorrect. This would be a second-line alternative. Amphotericin B alone may not be as good during the initial part of the treatment. Amphotericin B does not penetrate the CSF as well as flucytosine.

Answer c is incorrect. This would be a second-line alternative. Liposomal amphotericin B alone may not be as good during the initial part of the treatment. Amphotericin B does not penetrate the CSF as well as flucytosine.

Answer d is incorrect. This would be a second-line alternative. Fluconazole is not fungicidal enough to use for induction therapy. It is however used as antifungal consolidation after about 2 weeks of amphotericin B desoxycholate + flucytosine and as a chronic suppression therapy in HIV patients.

Answer e is incorrect. Echinocandins do not have significant activity against *C. neoformans*.

18. Which antifungal agent is only available as an oral formulation?
    a. Amphotericin B lipid-complex
    b. Voriconazole
    c. Posaconazole
    d. Anidulafungin
    e. None of the above

Answer a is incorrect. Available as IV only.

Answer b is incorrect. Available as oral and IV.

Answer c is correct. Available as an oral suspension only.

Answer d is incorrect. Available as IV only.

Answer e is incorrect.

19. Which antifungal agent has the greatest 24-hour urinary excretion percentage?
    a. Amphotericin B desoxycholate
    b. Fluconazole
    c. Voriconazole
    d. Caspofungin

Answer a is incorrect. Urinary elimination of amphotericin B happens over a prolonged duration in small amounts.

Answer b is correct. About 80% of a fluconazole dose is eliminated unchanged in the urine.

Answer c is incorrect. Less than 2% of a dose of voriconazole appears in the urine.

Answer d is incorrect. Less than 2% of a dose of caspofungin appears in the urine.

Note: Most antifungals undergo hepatic metabolism and small amounts of active medication undergo renal elimination. The exception is fluconazole and flucytosine.

20. At the end of a 10-week course of treatment for cryptococcal meningitis (CSF-sterilized) in an HIV-positive patient, what is generally recommended in terms of cryptococcal infection?
    a. Once weekly doses of azithromycin
    b. Four weeks of fluconazole oral therapy
    c. Indefinite low-dose suppressive fluconazole therapy
    d. No further antifungal therapy is needed

Answer a is incorrect. This is used to prevent *Mycobacterium* avium-intracellulare complex (MAC).

Answer b is correct. Longer fluconazole therapy may be needed in some cases where CSF is still positive or was slow to sterilize. Higher doses may be used.

Answer c is correct and the best answer. HIV-positive patients will receive indefinite therapy after the patient displays clinical cure and a negative CSF. Dose is 200 mg.

Answer d is incorrect. HIV-positive patients will receive indefinite therapy after the patient displays clinical cure and a negative CSF.

CHAPTER 29 | Sexually Transmitted Diseases

1. Complications of chlamydia genital infection include which of the following?
    a. Granulomatous and cardiovascular diseases
    b. Vesicular lesions on the external genitalia
    c. Pelvic inflammatory disease and infertility
    d. General paresis, dementia, and sensory ataxia

Answer a is incorrect. Granulomatous and cardiovascular diseases are manifestations of tertiary syphilis and represent some of the long-term complications of syphilis.

Answer b is incorrect. Vesicular lesions on the external genitalia are manifestations of genital herpes infection.

Answer c is correct. Without appropriate and timely treatment for chlamydia, complications such as pelvic inflammatory disease (PID), ectopic pregnancy, premature delivery, and infertility can result.

Answer d is incorrect. General paresis, dementia, and sensory ataxia are clinical manifestations of late neurosyphilis, a form of tertiary syphilis.

2. TD is 27-year-old man who presents to a local STD clinic with complaints of painful urination and urethral discharge over the past 4 days. He is sexually active, reporting three partners within the past 30 days. He has no known drug allergies. A diagnosis of chlamydia is made. Select the most appropriate therapy for TD.
    a. Doxycycline
    b. Azithromycin +cefixime
    c. Ceftizoxime
    d. Acyclovir + ofloxacin

Answer a is incorrect. Although doxycycline is a recommended agent for the treatment of chlamydia, this is not the most appropriate answer. Because coinfection with *C. trachomatis* and *N. gonorrhoeae* commonly occurs, presumptive therapy for gonorrhea should be considered when treating chlamydia.

Answer b is correct. This is the most appropriate therapy for TD, which includes treatment for chlamydia and gonorrhea. Because coinfection with *C. trachomatis* and *N. gonorrhoeae* commonly occurs, presumptive therapy for gonorrhea should be considered when treating chlamydia.

Answer c is incorrect. Ceftizoxime is not a recommended therapy for chlamydia, although it is an alternative agent for gonorrhea treatment.

Answer d is incorrect. Acyclovir is an antiviral agent and would not be effective against a chlamydia bacterial infection. Although ofloxacin is an alternative agent for chlamydia treatment, this combination is inappropriate.

---

3. Which of the following is a contraindication to doxycycline therapy?

   a. Age less than 8 years
   b. Concomitant use of QTc interval-prolonging drugs
   c. Diabetes mellitus
   d. Documented penicillin allergy

Answer a is correct. The calcium-binding effects of tetracyclines cause permanent darkening of teeth in children and effects on developing bone. For this reason, tetracyclines are contraindicated in pregnancy and children under the age of eight.

Answer b is incorrect. This statement refers to fluoroquinolone and macrolide antibiotics, both of which can prolong the QTc interval.

Answer c is incorrect. Diabetes mellitus is not a contraindication to tetracycline therapy. However, fluoroquinolones have the potential to cause dysglycemia (hypo- or hyperglycemia), and this adverse effect has been most commonly reported in patients with underlying diabetes mellitus.

Answer d is incorrect. Tetracyclines are not contraindicated in penicillin allergy. Tetracyclines represent an alternative antibiotic class option for patients with susceptible infections and penicillin allergy.

---

4. JM is a 23-year-old woman who is 28 weeks pregnant. She presents to her primary care physician (PCP) with symptoms of dysuria and unusual vaginal discharge. A diagnosis of chlamydia is made. Assuming no drug allergies, select the most appropriate therapy for JM.

   a. Doxycycline
   b. Amoxicillin
   c. Cefixime
   d. Levofloxacin

Answer a is incorrect. While tetracyclines are effective agents against chlamydia genital infection, they are contraindicated in pregnancy.

Answer b is correct. Amoxicillin is recommended for the treatment of chlamydia in pregnancy and is classified in pregnancy category B.

Answer c is incorrect. Although cephalosporins are safe to use in pregnancy (pregnancy category B), they are not recommended agents for the treatment of chlamydia.

Answer d is incorrect. Fluoroquinolones have not adequately been studied in pregnancy, and their use is generally discouraged.

---

5. Which of the following represents an adverse effect associated with fluoroquinolone use?

   a. Permanent tooth darkening
   b. Neurologic toxicity
   c. Dysglycemia
   d. Jarisch-Herxheimer reaction

Answer a is incorrect. Permanent tooth darkening is associated with tetracycline use in children younger than 8 years of age.

Answer b is incorrect. Neurologic toxicity has been reported with the use of acyclovir and valacyclovir due to drug accumulation in renal failure.

Answer c is correct. Fluoroquinolones have the potential to cause dysglycemia (hypo- or hyperglycemia), and this adverse effect has been most commonly reported in patients with underlying diabetes mellitus.

Answer d is incorrect. The Jarisch-Herxheimer reaction is an acute febrile reaction that can occur within hours of initiation of therapy for syphilis.

---

6. Which of the following is true regarding gonococcal urethritis and/or cervicitis?

   a. Women older than 25 years are at the highest risk of infection.
   b. Men are typically asymptomatic or have minor symptoms.
   c. Increased transmission of HIV infection is associated with gonococcal infection.
   d. Antibiotic susceptibility data can be obtained using nonculture diagnostic tests for gonorrhea.

Answer a is incorrect. Women *younger* than 25 years are at the highest risk of gonococcal cervicitis.

Answer b is incorrect. Women with gonorrhea are usually asymptomatic or have only minor symptoms. In men, symptoms of gonorrhea include dysuria and purulent urethral discharge. Because of the early presentation and discomfort associated with symptoms in men, treatment is often sought early enough to prevent complications.

Answer c is correct. In both men and women, gonorrhea can cause increased susceptibility to and transmission of human immunodeficiency virus (HIV) infection.

Answer d is incorrect. Nonculture diagnostic tests cannot provide antibiotic susceptibility results, which may be necessary in cases of infection that persists after treatment.

---

7. The presence of gram-negative diplococci on Gram stain is suggestive of which organism?

   a. *Treponema pallidum*
   b. *Chlamydia trachomatis*
   c. Herpes simplex virus-2
   d. *Neisseria gonorrhoeae*

Answer a is incorrect. *Treponema pallidum* is a spiral-shaped organism that is invisible on light microscopy.

Answer b is incorrect. *Chlamydia trachomatis* is an obligate intracellular pathogen.

Answer c is incorrect. Herpes is a viral organism.

Answer d is correct. *Neisseria gonorrhoeae* is a gram-negative *Diplococcus*.

8. AF is a 19-year-old college student who is considering becoming sexually active. During her annual Pap smear she asks her gynecologist for information on STD and pregnancy prevention. Which of the following statements is true regarding STD prevention?
   a. Vaccines are currently available for chlamydia, gonorrhea, and syphilis.
   b. Diaphragm use is a reliable method of STD prevention.
   c. Hormonal contraception is effective in preventing pregnancy and STDs.
   d. Condom use reduces the acquisition and transmission of STDs.

Answer a is incorrect. Vaccines *are not* currently available for chlamydia, gonorrhea, and syphilis.

Answer b is incorrect. Diaphragm use *is not* a reliable method of STD prevention.

Answer c is incorrect. Hormonal contraception *is not* an effective method of preventing STDs.

Answer d is correct. Condom use and STD/HIV counseling have been shown to be effective in reducing the acquisition and transmission of STDs.

9. Select the mechanism of action for cephalosporin antibiotics.
   a. Bind to the 30S bacterial ribosomal subunit, ultimately inhibiting bacterial protein synthesis
   b. Bind and inactivate a family of enzymes required for bacterial cell wall synthesis, causing cell death
   c. Bind and stabilize DNA complexes with topoisomerase II and topoisomerase IV enzymes, causing DNA-strand breakage and cell death
   d. Bind to the 23S component of the 50S ribosomal subunit, inhibiting RNA-dependent protein synthesis

Answer a is incorrect. Tetracyclines bind to the 30S bacterial ribosomal subunit, ultimately inhibiting bacterial protein synthesis.

Answer b is correct. Cephalosporins bind and inactivate a family of enzymes, called penicillin-binding proteins, which are required for bacterial cell wall synthesis. This action causes cell death and is bactericidal.

Answer c is incorrect. Fluoroquinolones bind and stabilize DNA complexes with topoisomerase II and topoisomerase IV enzymes, causing DNA-strand breakage and cell death.

Answer d is incorrect. Macrolides bind to the 23S component of the 50S ribosomal subunit, inhibiting RNA-dependent protein synthesis.

10. SA is a 33-year-old man with no known drug allergies who presents to the local STD clinic with complaints of extreme pain on urination and urethral discharge for two days. A diagnosis of gonococcal urethritis is made. Select the most appropriate therapy for SA.
    a. Ceftriaxone
    b. Benzathine penicillin
    c. Azithromycin
    d. Levofloxacin

Answer a is correct. Ceftriaxone is a recommended agent for the treatment of gonococcal urethritis. Currently, cephalosporins represent the only antibiotic class available in the United States that is recommended for the treatment of gonorrhea.

Answer b is incorrect. Benzathine penicillin is a recommended agent for the treatment of syphilis.

Answer c is incorrect. Azithromycin is a recommended agent for the treatment of chlamydia.

Answer d is incorrect. Levofloxacin is an alternative agent for the treatment of chlamydia. Fluoroquinolones are no longer recommended for the treatment of gonorrhea in the United States due to increasing rates of fluoroquinolone-resistant *N. gonorrhoeae*.

11. Which of the following *does not* describe a current goal of therapy for genital herpes infection?
    a. Disease eradication
    b. Viral suppression
    c. Transmission prevention
    d. Decrease recurrence frequency

Answer a is correct. Since genital herpes cannot currently be eradicated, this is not a goal of therapy.

Answer b is incorrect. Viral suppression is a goal of therapy for genital herpes.

Answer c is incorrect. Prevention of disease transmission is a goal of therapy for genital herpes.

Answer d is incorrect. Decreasing the frequency of recurrence (outbreaks) is a goal of therapy for genital herpes.

12. Which of the following is true regarding genital herpes infection?
    a. Genital herpes is an acute, self-limiting disease.
    b. Genital lesions are typically vesicular in nature and accompanied by pain, itching, and burning.
    c. The rate of recurrence increases over time in most patients.
    d. Transmission risk in a mother with recurrent disease but no visible lesions is high.

Answer a is incorrect. Genital herpes is a chronic, lifelong viral infection.

Answer b is correct. Clinical manifestations of genital herpes include the development of papular and vesicular lesions on the external genitalia which are accompanied by pain, itching, and burning. Involvement may also include perianal, buttock, and thigh areas.

Answer c is incorrect. The rate of genital herpes recurrence generally decreases over time.

Answer d is incorrect. The risk of transmission in a mother with recurrent disease but no visible lesions is thought to be low.

13. Which of the following is true regarding genital herpes infection and pregnancy?
    a. The risk of herpes transmission is lowest in mothers who have the initial outbreak at the time of delivery.
    b. Acyclovir, famciclovir, and valacyclovir are classified in pregnancy category D.
    c. Use of antiviral therapy late in pregnancy decreases herpes transmission to the neonate.
    d. Herpes disease in the neonate commonly manifests as a scalp abscess or ophthalmic infection.

Answer a is incorrect. The risk of herpes transmission is highest in mothers who have the initial outbreak at the time of delivery.

Answer b is incorrect. Acyclovir, famciclovir, and valacyclovir are classified in pregnancy category B.

Answer c is correct. Herpes transmission from an infected mother can cause symptomatic disease in the neonate. Use of antiviral therapy late in pregnancy decreases herpes recurrences near term as well as transmission to the neonate.

Answer d is incorrect. Gonococcal disease in the neonate commonly manifests as a scalp abscess or ophthalmic infection.

14. HF is a 29-year-old woman who was diagnosed with genital herpes 6 years ago. She reports approximately one to two recurrences each year since diagnosis. Recently she has experienced an increase in outbreaks, having three in a 6-month period. The decision is made to start HF on daily suppressive therapy. Select the most appropriate therapy for HF.
    a. Valacyclovir po
    b. Erythromycin ointment
    c. Tetracycline po
    d. Acyclovir ointment

Answer a is correct. Valacyclovir is a prodrug of acyclovir that has increased oral bioavailability. It is a recommended agent for daily suppressive therapy.

Answer b is incorrect. Erythromycin is an antibacterial agent and would be ineffective against the herpes virus.

Answer c is incorrect. Tetracycline is an antibacterial agent and would be ineffective against the herpes virus.

Answer d is incorrect. Use of topical antiviral therapy (eg, acyclovir ointment) is discouraged due to limited clinical benefit.

15. Which of the following is true regarding the stages of syphilis infection?
    a. The characteristic lesion of primary syphilis is a diffuse rash, usually affecting the palms and soles.
    b. Manifestations of latent syphilis include regional lymphadenopathy and meningitis.
    c. Tertiary syphilis is highly transmissible.
    d. Neurosyphilis can present at any stage of syphilis.

Answer a is incorrect. The characteristic lesion of primary syphilis is the chancre (ulcer). The chancre is usually painless and appears at the site of *T. pallidum* entrance into the body approximately 3 weeks after transmission.

Answer b is incorrect. Latent syphilis refers to patients with a positive serologic diagnosis for syphilis, but no clinical symptoms. This stage occurs after secondary syphilis symptoms have subsided and there are two possible outcomes: progression to tertiary syphilis or clinical cure.

Answer c is incorrect. Tertiary syphilis encompasses the long-term complications of syphilitic disease such as granulomatous disease (also called gummatous syphilis) and cardiovascular syphilis. Tertiary syphilis is now uncommon due to antibiotic treatment and is not transmissible.

Answer d is correct. CNS involvement can present at any stage of syphilis. Early neurosyphilis occurs within first few years of infection and usually coexists with primary or secondary syphilis. Late neurosyphilis occurs years to decades after the initial infection and represents a tertiary manifestation of syphilis.

16. Which of the following is true regarding the diagnosis of syphilis?
    a. The diagnosis of syphilis is made through direct techniques such as culture.
    b. Serologic testing is the standard method of detecting primary, secondary, latent, and tertiary syphilis in the United States.
    c. The VDRL-CSF is the standard serologic test for secondary syphilis.
    d. Nontreponemal serologic testing alone is sufficient for a definitive diagnosis of syphilis.

Answer a is false. *Treponema pallidum* cannot be cultured, so indirect diagnostic techniques must be used.

Answer b is true. Serologic testing, including treponemal and nontreponemal tests, provides a presumptive diagnosis and is the standard method of detecting primary, secondary, latent, and tertiary syphilis in the United States.

Answer c is false. The VDRL-CSF is the standard serologic test for neurosyphilis, not secondary syphilis.

Answer d is false. Nontreponemal tests, such as the venereal disease research laboratory (VDRL) and rapid plasma reagin (RPR) are used for initial syphilis screening. Nontreponemal tests should be confirmed by treponemal-specific tests (such as the *T. pallidum* particle agglutination or fluorescent treponemal antibody absorption test) due to the rate of false-positive results.

---

17. Select the brand name for benzathine penicillin.
    a. Bicillin C-R
    b. Wycillin
    c. Bicillin L-A
    d. Pen-VK

Answer a is incorrect. Bicillin C-R is the brand name for a procaine-benzathine penicillin mix.

Answer b is incorrect. Wycillin is the brand name for procaine penicillin.

Answer c is correct. Bicillin L-A is the brand name for benzathine penicillin.

Answer d is incorrect. Pen-VK is the brand name for oral penicillin V potassium.

---

19. TP is a 26-year-old woman who is 31 weeks pregnant. She visits her obstetrician-gynecologist because of a sore throat, generalized weakness, and a rash on her palms and soles for the past week. Testing is performed and a diagnosis of secondary syphilis is made. The treating physician requests pharmacist consultation because the patient is allergic to penicillin. Select the most appropriate therapy for TP.
    a. Doxycycline
    b. Cefoxitin + probenecid
    c. Levofloxacin
    d. Desensitization + benzathine penicillin G

Answer a is incorrect. While doxycycline is an appropriate choice for the treatment of secondary syphilis in the setting of penicillin allergy, tetracyclines are contraindicated in pregnancy.

Answer b is incorrect. Cefoxitin plus probenecid is not a recommended antibiotic combination for the treatment of syphilis.

Answer c is incorrect. Levofloxacin is not a recommended agent for the treatment of syphilis. Furthermore, fluoroquinolones have not adequately been studied in pregnancy and their use is generally discouraged.

Answer d is correct. Penicillin regimens, appropriate for the stage of disease, are recommended for the treatment of syphilis in pregnant women. No proven alternatives to penicillin exist for the treatment of syphilis during pregnancy. It is recommended that pregnant patients with a penicillin allergy undergo desensitization and subsequent treatment with penicillin.

---

20. The Jarisch-Herxheimer reaction is an acute febrile reaction associated with therapy for which STD?
    a. Genital herpes
    b. Gonorrhea
    c. Chlamydia
    d. Syphilis

Answer a is incorrect. The Jarisch-Herxheimer reaction is not associated with genital herpes.

Answer b is incorrect. The Jarisch-Herxheimer reaction is not associated with gonorrhea.

Answer c is incorrect. The Jarisch-Herxheimer reaction is not associated with chlamydia.

Answer d is correct. The Jarisch-Herxheimer reaction is an acute febrile reaction that may occur within hours of initiation of therapy for syphilis. It is most common in patients with early syphilis and usually subsides within a 24-hour period. Complications of the Jarisch-Herxheimer reaction include induction of early labor and fetal distress in pregnant women.

---

21. Which of the following is true regarding the treatment of STDs in special populations?
    a. The treatment of STDs in pregnancy can decrease pregnancy complications and prevent disease transmission to the child.
    b. Children diagnosed with congenital or acquired STDs should not be treated until they reach 2 years of age due to antimicrobial toxicities.
    c. In general, adolescent patients require lower doses of recommended antimicrobials for the treatment of STDs.
    d. Management of genital herpes in patients with HIV infection is the same as the management in patient who are HIV-negative.

Answer a is correct. The treatment of STDs in pregnancy can decrease pregnancy complications and prevent disease transmission to the child.

Answer b is incorrect. Children, including neonates and infants, who are diagnosed with congenital or acquired STDs should be treated according to guideline recommendations.

Answer c is incorrect. In general, pharmacologic treatment for STDs in adolescent patients is the same as in adults.

13. YQ is a 59-year-old man with a past medical history significant for chronic obstructive pulmonary disease, diabetes mellitus, hypertension, and hyperlipidemia. YQ wanted to receive influenza vaccination, but the United States has a short supply of TIV. YQ's physician recommended postexposure prophylaxis if he is exposed to influenza. If YQ is exposed to influenza, which agent should be used as postexposure prophylaxis?

    a. Amantadine
    b. Rimantadine
    c. Oseltamivir
    d. Zanamivir
    e. LAIV

Answer a is incorrect. Amantadine should not be used for postexposure prophylaxis because it does not have activity against influenza B and because of an increase in adamantanes resistance to influenza A.

Answer b is incorrect. Rimantadine should not be used for postexposure prophylaxis because it does not have activity against influenza B and because of an increase in adamantanes resistance to influenza A.

Answer c is correct. Oseltamivir may be used as postexposure prophylaxis, but only when influenza vaccines cannot be used. Since this patient cannot obtain the vaccine because of a short supply, postexposure prophylaxis with oseltamivir would be appropriate.

Answer d is incorrect. Zanamivir may cause bronchospasm in patient's chronic obstructive pulmonary disease or asthma. Therefore, this agent is not ideal for patient YQ.

Answer e is incorrect. LAIV is currently indicated for healthy patients aged 2 to 49 years. Because of YQ's age and past medical history, he is not a candidate for LAIV. Also, LAIV is not used as postexposure prophylaxis.

---

14. A patient presents to your pharmacy to ask a question about influenza symptom resolution. She was diagnosed with influenza B. She still has cough and malaise. What should you discuss with the patient?

    a. Influenza symptoms will disappear within 48 hours. If you are still having symptoms, see your provider.
    b. Influenza symptoms typically last 3 to 7 days. Cough and malaise may last up to 2 weeks. If your symptoms have increased/worsened, you may need to see your provider.
    c. Influenza does not cause a cough. Patient should be counseled to see provider.
    d. As long as a patient does not have a fever, there is no need to worry. Cough and malaise symptoms will go away.

Answer a is incorrect. Influenza symptoms may (and often do) last longer than 48 hours.

Answer b is correct. Influenza symptoms typically last 3 to 7 days, while cough and malaise may persist for longer.

Answer c is incorrect. Influenza can (and often does) cause a cough.

Answer d is incorrect. Influenza complications can lead to high morbidity and mortality. Just because a patient lacks a fever does not mean they will not develop influenza complications.

---

15. The best agent for prevention of influenza is:

    a. TIV
    b. LAIV
    c. Adamantanes
    d. a and b
    e. b and c

Answer a is correct. TIV is effective for preventing the development of influenza for patients more than 6 months of age.

Answer b is correct. LAIV is effective for preventing the development of influenza for healthy, nonpregnant patients aged 2 to 49 years.

Answer c is incorrect. Adamantanes should not be used for prevention of influenza.

Answer d is the correct and the best answer.

Answer e is incorrect. Adamantanes should not be used for prevention of influenza. LAIV may be used in healthy, nonpregnant patients aged 2 to 49 years.

---

16. Influenza vaccination emphasis should be placed upon:

    a. Patients at high risk of complications
    b. Children 6 months to 18 years
    c. People more than 50 years of age
    d. All of the above

Answer a is correct. Patients at high risk of influenza complications should be a top priority for influenza vaccination.

Answer b is correct. Children 6 months to 18 years should be a top priority for influenza vaccination.

Answer c is correct. People more than 50 years of age should be a top priority for influenza vaccination.

Answer d is the correct and the best answer.

---

17. Select the most common adverse reaction of TIV.

    a. Injection site soreness
    b. Birth defects
    c. Bronchospasm
    d. Guillain-Barre syndrome
    e. Autism

Answer a is correct. Injection site soreness is a common adverse reaction from administration of TIV since it is administered as an intramuscular injection.

Answer b is incorrect. There is no conclusive documentation that TIV causes birth defects. TIV should be administered to pregnant patients.

Answer c is incorrect. TIV does not cause bronchospasm. Zanamivir (Relenza) may cause bronchospasm and therefore

medical history that does not exclude patients from receiving LAIV is hypertension.

Answer b is correct. Development of Guillain-Barre Syndrome (GBS) within 6 weeks of receiving an influenza vaccine (this includes both LAIV and TIV) is contraindication for receiving influenza vaccine.

Answer c is correct. Influenza vaccine (TIV and LAIV) are made from eggs and should not be utilized in patients with an egg allergy.

Answer d is correct. Antiviral agents (such as amantadine) have the potential to inhibit the replication of live vaccine virus, and could interfere with the effectiveness of the vaccine. Therefore, LAIV should not be administered within 2 weeks before or 48 hours after administration of amantadine. TIV may be administered at any time relative to amantadine.

Answer e is the correct and best answer. All of the above are contraindications for LAIV.

---

9. Which of the following condition(s) would be a contraindication for receiving TIV?
   a. Diabetes mellitus
   b. Egg allergy
   c. Recently received amantadine (within 48 hours)
   d. Concerned about development of autism from thimerosal in TIV
   e. All of the above

Answer a is incorrect. Diabetic patients can and should receive influenza vaccination with TIV unless they have a contraindication.

Answer b is correct. Patients with an egg allergy should not receive TIV. Patients with an egg allergy cannot receive LAIV either.

Answer c is incorrect. TIV may be administered within 48 hours of adamantanes (rimantadine and amantadine). LAIV should not be administered within this time frame because the adamantanes could inhibit viral replication and interfere with the effectiveness of LAIV.

Answer d is incorrect. There is no association with influenza vaccines and the development of autism or from thimerosal in the vaccines. Thimerosal is used as a preservative in the influenza vaccines and the amount of thimerosal has been reduced or eliminated from the vaccine (except from multidose vials).

Answer e is incorrect for the reasons stated above.

---

10. Adamantanes have activity against which influenza types?
    a. Influenza A
    b. Influenza B
    c. Influenza C
    d. All of the above

Answer a is correct. Adamantanes (rimantadine and amantadine) have activity against influenza A, however, over the past few influenza seasons, resistance to the adamantanes has significantly increased.

Answer b is incorrect. Adamantanes do not have activity against influenza B.

Answer c is incorrect. Influenza C is not a common cause in influenza infections.

Answer d is incorrect for the reasons listed above.

---

11. Select the brand name for zanamivir.
    a. Relenza
    b. Tamiflu
    c. FluMist
    d. Flumadine
    e. Symmetrel

Answer a is correct. Relenza is the brand name for zanamivir.

Answer b is incorrect. Tamiflu is the brand name for oseltamivir.

Answer c is incorrect. FluMist is the brand name for LAIV

Answer d is incorrect. Flumadine is the brand name for TIV. TIV has several different brand names because there are different manufacturers.

Answer e is incorrect. Symmetrel is the brand name for amantadine.

---

12. Select the anti-influenza agent that is formulated as a Rotadisk inhaler.
    c. Rimantadine
    b. Amantadine
    c. Oseltamivir
    d. Zanamivir
    e. LAIV

Answer a is incorrect. Rimantadine is formulated as syrup (50 mg/5 mL) and a tablet (100 mg).

Answer b is incorrect. Amantadine is formulated as syrup (50mg/mL), tablet (100 mg), and capsule (100 mg).

Answer c is incorrect. Oseltamivir is formulated as a capsule (75 mg) and powder for oral suspension (12 mg/mL).

Answer d is correct. Zanamivir is formulated as a Rotadisk inhaler (5 mg/blister).

Answer e is incorrect. LAIV is formulated as an intranasal mist.

Answer a, b, c, and d are correct. These are classic signs and symptoms of influenza.

Answer e is the correct and best answer. All of the above are classic signs and symptoms of influenza. Sore throat and malaise are other classic symptoms. Nausea, vomiting, and otitis media are commonly reported in children.

5. BC is a 28-month-old child with no significant past medical history. BC has not had a wheezing episode in the last 12 months. Select the best statement as it relates to influenza vaccination.
   a. BC should be vaccinated with TIV.
   b. BC should be vaccinated with LAIV.
   c. BC should be vaccinated with TIV or LAIV.
   d. BC should be administered oseltamivir for prophylaxis.
   e. BC does not meet criteria for vaccination.

Answer a is correct, but not the best answer. All children greater than 6 months of age should receive vaccination. Children greater than 2 years of age without a history of asthma or wheezing episode within past 12 months may receive TIV or LAIV. Children 6 months to 2 years should only receive TIV.

Answer b is correct, but not the best answer. All children greater than 6 months of age should receive vaccination. Children more than 2 years of age without a history of asthma or wheezing episode within past 12 months may receive TIV or LAIV.

Answer c is correct. All children more than 6 months of age should receive vaccination. Children more than 2 years of age without a history of asthma or wheezing episode within past 12 months may receive TIV or LAIV.

Answer d is incorrect. Antiviral drugs used for prophylaxis should be considered adjuncts and not a replacement for annual vaccination with TIV or LAIV.

Answer e is incorrect. Children should be recommended to receive influenza vaccination.

6. Select the agent that is administered via intramuscular injection for influenza prevention or postexposure prophylaxis.
   e. TIV
   f. LAIV
   c. Zanamivir
   d. Amantadine
   e. All of the above

Answer a is correct. TIV should be administered via intramuscular injection.

Answer b is incorrect. LAIV is administered intranasally (mist).

Answer c is incorrect. Zanamivir is administered via oral inhalation.

Answer d is incorrect. Amantadine is administered orally. Also, because of increased levels of adamantane resistance, amantadine and rimantadine are not used in the United States for postexposure prophylaxis or treatment, unless combined with other antiviral agents.

Answer e is incorrect. Only TIV is administered via intramuscular injection.

7. XW is a 28-year-old pregnant patient. She is currently receiving amoxicillin for a urinary tract infection caused by *Escherichia coli*. She comes to your pharmacy wanting an influenza vaccination. She hates shots and prefers not to receive any injection. During last year's influenza season she received treatment with oseltamivir. Select the appropriate agent for influenza vaccination for XW.
   a. LAIV
   b. TIV
   g. Oseltamivir
   h. Rimantadine

Answer a is incorrect. LAIV should not be used in pregnant patients at this time. LAIV is indicated for healthy, nonpregnant patients 2 years of age to 49 years of age.

Answer b is correct. TIV may be administered to pregnant patients. Vaccination is recommended regardless of the stage of pregnancy.

Answer c is incorrect. Oseltamivir should not replace TIV or LAIV as prevention of influenza unless the patient has a contraindication to receiving either TIV or LAIV (ie, egg allergy). Also, there are insufficient human data to determine the risk to a pregnant woman or developing fetus.

Answer d is incorrect. Rimantadine should not replace TIV or LAIV as prevention of influenza. Recent evaluations have demonstrated that the adamantanes (rimantadine and amantadine) have become resistant to seasonal influenza strains and this has limited their use. Also, rimantadine has been found to be embryotoxic in high-dose rat studies.

8. Which of the following condition(s) would be a contraindication for receiving LAIV?
   a. Diabetes mellitus
   b. Development of Guillain-Barre syndrome (GBS) within 6 weeks of receiving previous influenza vaccine
   c. Egg allergy
   d. Recently received amantadine (within 48 hours)
   e. All of the above

Answer a is correct. Diabetes is currently a contraindication for receiving LAIV. Currently, LAIV is indicated for healthy patients from the age of 2 to 49 years. Patients with a significant past medical history (diabetes, chronic obstructive pulmonary disease, asthma, atrial fibrillation, coronary heart disease, etc) will not be candidates for LAIV. The only past

Answer d is incorrect. Because severe or prolonged herpes episodes may occur in immunocompromised patients, doses for patients with HIV infection are typically higher and/or treatment durations longer than in patients who are HIV negative.

CHAPTER 30 | Influenza

1. Select the statement that most accurately describes influenza.
   a. A bacterial illness caused by *Haemophilus influenzae*
   b. A viral illness caused by respiratory syncytial virus (RSV).
   c. A viral illness caused by rhinovirus.
   d. A viral illness caused by influenza A and B.
   e. A bacterial illness caused by *Streptococcus pneumoniae.*

Answer a is incorrect. Influenza is a viral illness—not a bacterial illness. It is easy to confuse influenza viral infections with *H. influenzae* bacterial infections. Even though the species name of *Haemophilus* is *influenzae*, it is a bacterial pathogen. *Haemophilus influenzae* is a common cause of respiratory tract infections.

Answer b is incorrect. Respiratory syncytial virus (RSV) is a respiratory virus that infects the lungs and breathing passages. RSV is not influenza, although RSV is a viral infection. RSV is the most common cause of bronchiolitis (inflammation of the small airways in the lung) and pneumonia in children under 1 year of age in the United States. Most healthy people recover from RSV infection in 1 to 2 weeks. However, infection can be severe in some people, such as certain infants, young children, and older adults.

Answer c is incorrect. Rhinoviruses are the most common viral infective agents in humans, and a causative agent of the common cold.

Answer d is correct. Influenza A and B are the two types of influenza viruses that cause epidemic human disease. There are two subtypes of influenza A based upon surface antigens (hemagglutinin [H] and neuraminidase [N]). Influenza B is separated into two genetic lineages (Yamagata and Victoria), but not categorized by subtypes. Since 1977, influenza A subtype H1N1, influenza A subtype H3N2, and influenza B have been circulating globally.

Answer e is incorrect. *Streptococcus pneumoniae* is a common bacterial cause of upper and lower respiratory infections. Streptococcus is treated with penicillin and cephalosporin antibiotics.

2. ZC is a 35-year-old woman. She does not have a significant past medical history and is currently taking a multivitamin and calcium supplementation. She has a 3-year-old child. Based upon the information provided, provide influenza vaccination recommendations.
   a. ZC is too young and influenza only affects the elderly and young children. Vaccination not recommended.
   b. ZC does not have comorbidities that place her at risk for influenza complications. Vaccination not recommended.
   c. ZC has a child that is at risk for influenza complications. Vaccination recommended for ZC.
   d. ZC has a child that is at risk for influenza complications. Vaccination recommended for ZC and her 3-year-old child.

Answer a is incorrect. Influenza can cause illness in any person, regardless of age. Children and elderly individuals are often at risk for influenza complications. ZC is at low risk for influenza complications because of her age and lack of comorbidities; however, influenza vaccination is recommended for providers of children because children are at high risk for influenza complications.

Answer b is incorrect. Because of ZC's age and lack of comorbidities, she is at low risk for influenza complications. However, influenza vaccination is recommended for providers of children, because children are at high risk for influenza complications.

Answer c is incorrect. Because the child is at risk for influenza and influenza complications, it is important to vaccinate the mother and child.

Answer d is correct. Both ZC and the 3-year-old child should be recommended to receive influenza vaccination, barring any contraindication. Counseling and discussion with patient would reveal if mother or child had contraindication to receiving influenza vaccination.

3. Select the primary method for transmission of seasonal influenza.
   a. Inhalation
   b. Exposure to blood and/or bodily fluids
   c. Exposure to dead birds
   d. All of the above

Answer a is correct. Inhalation of respiratory droplets is the primacy mechanism for contracting the influenza illness.

Answer b is incorrect. Influenza is not transmitted via this route. Other viral infections such as human immunodeficiency virus (HIV) may be transmitted via blood and/or bodily fluids.

Answer c is incorrect. Exposure to dead birds has been associated with the West Nile virus and bird flu. The bird flu consists of different antigens than the traditional (seasonal) flu. Bird flu is H5N1 and traditional flu is H1N1 or H3N2.

Answer d is incorrect.

4. Select the classic signs and symptoms of influenza.
   a. Rapid onset of fever
   b. Myalgia
   c. Headache
   d. Nonproductive cough
   e. All of the above

Answer b is true. Serologic testing, including treponemal and nontreponemal tests, provides a presumptive diagnosis and is the standard method of detecting primary, secondary, latent, and tertiary syphilis in the United States.

Answer c is false. The VDRL-CSF is the standard serologic test for neurosyphilis, not secondary syphilis.

Answer d is false. Nontreponemal tests, such as the venereal disease research laboratory (VDRL) and rapid plasma reagin (RPR) are used for initial syphilis screening. Nontreponemal tests should be confirmed by treponemal-specific tests (such as the *T. pallidum* particle agglutination or fluorescent treponemal antibody absorption test) due to the rate of false-positive results.

---

17. Select the brand name for benzathine penicillin.
    a. Bicillin C-R
    b. Wycillin
    c. Bicillin L-A
    d. Pen-VK

Answer a is incorrect. Bicillin C-R is the brand name for a procaine-benzathine penicillin mix.

Answer b is incorrect. Wycillin is the brand name for procaine penicillin.

Answer c is correct. Bicillin L-A is the brand name for benzathine penicillin.

Answer d is incorrect. Pen-VK is the brand name for oral penicillin V potassium.

---

19. TP is a 26-year-old woman who is 31 weeks pregnant. She visits her obstetrician-gynecologist because of a sore throat, generalized weakness, and a rash on her palms and soles for the past week. Testing is performed and a diagnosis of secondary syphilis is made. The treating physician requests pharmacist consultation because the patient is allergic to penicillin. Select the most appropriate therapy for TP.
    a. Doxycycline
    b. Cefoxitin + probenecid
    c. Levofloxacin
    d. Desensitization + benzathine penicillin G

Answer a is incorrect. While doxycycline is an appropriate choice for the treatment of secondary syphilis in the setting of penicillin allergy, tetracyclines are contraindicated in pregnancy.

Answer b is incorrect. Cefoxitin plus probenecid is not a recommended antibiotic combination for the treatment of syphilis.

Answer c is incorrect. Levofloxacin is not a recommended agent for the treatment of syphilis. Furthermore, fluoroquinolones have not adequately been studied in pregnancy and their use is generally discouraged.

Answer d is correct. Penicillin regimens, appropriate for the stage of disease, are recommended for the treatment of syphilis in pregnant women. No proven alternatives to penicillin exist for the treatment of syphilis during pregnancy. It is recommended that pregnant patients with a penicillin allergy undergo desensitization and subsequent treatment with penicillin.

---

20. The Jarisch-Herxheimer reaction is an acute febrile reaction associated with therapy for which STD?
    a. Genital herpes
    b. Gonorrhea
    c. Chlamydia
    d. Syphilis

Answer a is incorrect. The Jarisch-Herxheimer reaction is not associated with genital herpes.

Answer b is incorrect. The Jarisch-Herxheimer reaction is not associated with gonorrhea.

Answer c is incorrect. The Jarisch-Herxheimer reaction is not associated with chlamydia.

Answer d is correct. The Jarisch-Herxheimer reaction is an acute febrile reaction that may occur within hours of initiation of therapy for syphilis. It is most common in patients with early syphilis and usually subsides within a 24-hour period. Complications of the Jarisch-Herxheimer reaction include induction of early labor and fetal distress in pregnant women.

---

21. Which of the following is true regarding the treatment of STDs in special populations?
    a. The treatment of STDs in pregnancy can decrease pregnancy complications and prevent disease transmission to the child.
    b. Children diagnosed with congenital or acquired STDs should not be treated until they reach 2 years of age due to antimicrobial toxicities.
    c. In general, adolescent patients require lower doses of recommended antimicrobials for the treatment of STDs.
    d. Management of genital herpes in patients with HIV infection is the same as the management in patient who are HIV-negative.

Answer a is correct. The treatment of STDs in pregnancy can decrease pregnancy complications and prevent disease transmission to the child.

Answer b is incorrect. Children, including neonates and infants, who are diagnosed with congenital or acquired STDs should be treated according to guideline recommendations.

Answer c is incorrect. In general, pharmacologic treatment for STDs in adolescent patients is the same as in adults.

Answer a is incorrect. Genital herpes is a chronic, lifelong viral infection.

Answer b is correct. Clinical manifestations of genital herpes include the development of papular and vesicular lesions on the external genitalia which are accompanied by pain, itching, and burning. Involvement may also include perianal, buttock, and thigh areas.

Answer c is incorrect. The rate of genital herpes recurrence generally decreases over time.

Answer d is incorrect. The risk of transmission in a mother with recurrent disease but no visible lesions is thought to be low.

13. Which of the following is true regarding genital herpes infection and pregnancy?
    a. The risk of herpes transmission is lowest in mothers who have the initial outbreak at the time of delivery.
    b. Acyclovir, famciclovir, and valacyclovir are classified in pregnancy category D.
    c. Use of antiviral therapy late in pregnancy decreases herpes transmission to the neonate.
    d. Herpes disease in the neonate commonly manifests as a scalp abscess or ophthalmic infection.

Answer a is incorrect. The risk of herpes transmission is highest in mothers who have the initial outbreak at the time of delivery.

Answer b is incorrect. Acyclovir, famciclovir, and valacyclovir are classified in pregnancy category B.

Answer c is correct. Herpes transmission from an infected mother can cause symptomatic disease in the neonate. Use of antiviral therapy late in pregnancy decreases herpes recurrences near term as well as transmission to the neonate.

Answer d is incorrect. Gonococcal disease in the neonate commonly manifests as a scalp abscess or ophthalmic infection.

14. HF is a 29-year-old woman who was diagnosed with genital herpes 6 years ago. She reports approximately one to two recurrences each year since diagnosis. Recently she has experienced an increase in outbreaks, having three in a 6-month period. The decision is made to start HF on daily suppressive therapy. Select the most appropriate therapy for HF.
    a. Valacyclovir po
    b. Erythromycin ointment
    c. Tetracycline po
    d. Acyclovir ointment

Answer a is correct. Valacyclovir is a prodrug of acyclovir that has increased oral bioavailability. It is a recommended agent for daily suppressive therapy.

Answer b is incorrect. Erythromycin is an antibacterial agent and would be ineffective against the herpes virus.

Answer c is incorrect. Tetracycline is an antibacterial agent and would be ineffective against the herpes virus.

Answer d is incorrect. Use of topical antiviral therapy (eg, acyclovir ointment) is discouraged due to limited clinical benefit.

15. Which of the following is true regarding the stages of syphilis infection?
    a. The characteristic lesion of primary syphilis is a diffuse rash, usually affecting the palms and soles.
    b. Manifestations of latent syphilis include regional lymphadenopathy and meningitis.
    c. Tertiary syphilis is highly transmissible.
    d. Neurosyphilis can present at any stage of syphilis.

Answer a is incorrect. The characteristic lesion of primary syphilis is the chancre (ulcer). The chancre is usually painless and appears at the site of *T. pallidum* entrance into the body approximately 3 weeks after transmission.

Answer b is incorrect. Latent syphilis refers to patients with a positive serologic diagnosis for syphilis, but no clinical symptoms. This stage occurs after secondary syphilis symptoms have subsided and there are two possible outcomes: progression to tertiary syphilis or clinical cure.

Answer c is incorrect. Tertiary syphilis encompasses the long-term complications of syphilitic disease such as granulomatous disease (also called gummatous syphilis) and cardiovascular syphilis. Tertiary syphilis is now uncommon due to antibiotic treatment and is not transmissible.

Answer d is correct. CNS involvement can present at any stage of syphilis. Early neurosyphilis occurs within first few years of infection and usually coexists with primary or secondary syphilis. Late neurosyphilis occurs years to decades after the initial infection and represents a tertiary manifestation of syphilis.

16. Which of the following is true regarding the diagnosis of syphilis?
    a. The diagnosis of syphilis is made through direct techniques such as culture.
    b. Serologic testing is the standard method of detecting primary, secondary, latent, and tertiary syphilis in the United States.
    c. The VDRL-CSF is the standard serologic test for secondary syphilis.
    d. Nontreponemal serologic testing alone is sufficient for a definitive diagnosis of syphilis.

Answer a is false. *Treponema pallidum* cannot be cultured, so indirect diagnostic techniques must be used.

should not be used in patients with lung disease (COPD or asthma).

Answer d is incorrect. TIV has not been associated with the development of Guillain-Barre syndrome (GBS). If a patient developed GBS within 6 weeks after an influenza vaccine, they should not receive the vaccine again.

Answer e is incorrect. TIV has not been associated with the development of autism.

---

18. Select the following patient(s) that should receive influenza vaccination.
    a. Pregnant patients
    b. Children 18 to 24 months of age
    c. Diabetes
    d. A 65-year-old healthy man
    e. All of the above

Answer a is correct. Pregnant patients should receive influenza vaccination with TIV. They would not be a candidate for LAIV.

Answer b is correct. Children 18 to 24 months of age should receive influenza vaccination with TIV. They would not be a candidate for LAIV.

Answer c is correct. Diabetic patients should receive influenza vaccination with TIV. They would not be a candidate for LAIV.

Answer d is correct. Sixty five-year-old healthy men should receive influenza vaccination with TIV. They would not be a candidate for LAIV. Patients more than 49 years of age are not candidates for LAIV.

Answer e is the correct and the best answer.

---

19. LWS is a 28-year-old man returning home from a military tour of duty from overseas. LWS is an OEF (operation enduring freedom) veteran. He received LAIV 7 days ago. Today he presents with symptoms of influenza. Select the reason LWS could develop influenza symptoms, even if he received the appropriate vaccine.
    a. LAIV is a live virus and can cause influenza.
    b. LWS was not a candidate for influenza vaccination; therefore, he should not have received LAIV.
    c. LWS does not have influenza. He has the common cold.
    d. Influenza vaccines are not 100% effective.

Answer a is incorrect. While LAIV is a live virus it is a weakened virus and cannot replicate within the lungs because it is temperature sensitive. There is currently no documentation that LAIV can cause influenza.

Answer b is incorrect. LWS was a candidate for influenza vaccine. Any person wishing to not develop influenza is a candidate for influenza vaccine.

Answer c is incorrect. The symptoms of the common cold and influenza can overlap. There is not enough information given to be able to differentiate the common cold versus influenza.

Answer d is correct. Influenza vaccines are not 100% effective. Therefore, even if you received the influenza vaccine, it is possible that you could develop influenza.

---

20. Select the two surface antigens that categorize influenza A.
    a. Hemagglutinin
    b. Thimerosal
    c. Neuraminidase
    d. Guillain-Barre syndrome
    e. a and c

Answer a is correct. Hemagglutinin is a surface antigen for influenza A (ie, H3N2)

Answer b is incorrect. Thimerosal is a preservative that is used in multidose vials of TIV. Thimerosal is not in LAIV or prefilled syringes containing TIV.

Answer c is correct. Neuraminidase is a surface antigen for influenza A (ie, H1N1).

Answer d is incorrect. Guillan-Barre syndrome is a disorder where the immune system attacks the peripheral nervous system.

Answer e is the correct and the best answer.

---

21. Select the common cause of influenza.
    a. Influenza A
    b. Influenza B
    c. *Haemophilus influenzae*
    d. *Streptococcus pneumoniae*
    e. a and b

Answer a is correct. Influenza A is a common cause of influenza.

Answer b is correct. Influenza B is a common cause of influenza.

Answer c is incorrect. *Haemophilus influenzae* is an upper respiratory gram-negative bacterial pathogen. *H. flu* is a common cause of respiratory tract infections.

Answer d is incorrect. *Streptococcus pneumoniae* is a gram-positive bacterial pathogen that is a common cause of respiratory infections.

Answer e is the correct and the best answer.

---

22. TK is a 32-year-old HIV-positive patient. He does not want influenza to develop and would like to be vaccinated since he is immunocompromised. Select the appropriate vaccination for TK.
    a. LAIV
    b. Oseltamivir
    c. TIV
    d. Amantadine
    e. Immunocompromised patients should not be vaccinated

Answer a is incorrect. LAIV is indicated for healthy, nonpregnant patients aged 2 to 49 years. Since TK has HIV, he is not a candidate for LAIV.

Answer b is incorrect. Oseltamavir cannot be used as vaccine, not should prevention or postexposure use of oseltamavir replace influenza vaccine TIV or LAIV.

Answer c is correct. TIV may be used in immunocompromised patients, including HIV.

Answer d is incorrect. Amantadine is not an influenza vaccine and because of increased resistance, it is seldom used as a preventive or treatment option.

Answer e is incorrect. Immunocompromised patients should be vaccinated with TIV, unless there is a contraindication.

CHAPTER 31 | Acid–Base Disorders

Questions 1 to 3 pertain to the following case.

A 58-year-old woman is in the intensive care unit, intubated after a recent abdominal surgery. While in the operating room, she received more than 10 L of fluid and blood products, but has been aggressively diuresed since that time. In the past 3 days she has generated 8 L of urine output, her BUN and Cr have *increased* to 40 mg/dL and 1.5 mg/dL, respectively, and her blood pressure has decreased to 100/60 mm Hg. This morning, her ABG shows the following: pH 7.51, $Paco_2$ 46 mm Hg, and HCO_3 35 mEq/L.

1. Which of the primary acid–base disturbance is present in this patient?

    a. Metabolic acidosis
    b. Metabolic alkalosis
    c. Respiratory acidosis
    d. Respiratory alkalosis

Answer a and c are incorrect because the pH is alkalotic, therefore acidosis can be excluded.

Answer b is correct because the pH is elevated, indicating alkalosis, and the bicarbonate >28, indicating metabolic alkalosis.

Answer d is incorrect because the $Paco_2$ >40 mm Hg, indicating respiratory acidosis, though the pH does not correlate with this. The reason the patient has a metabolic alkalosis is secondary to over-diuresis which has lead to volume contraction.

2. Has the patient been appropriately compensated for the primary disorder?

    a. Yes, the $Paco_2$ is elevated, indicating appropriate compensation.
    b. Yes, the HCO_3 is elevated, indicating appropriate compensation.
    c. No, the HCO_3 is low, indicating the patient has not yet been compensated.
    d. No, the $Paco_2$ is low, indicating the patient has not yet been compensated.

Answer a is correct because in metabolic alkalosis, we would expect the $Paco_2$ to be elevated as compensation to hold on to acid.

Answers b and c are incorrect because the patient does not have a primary respiratory problem.

Answer d is incorrect because the patient does not have a metabolic acidosis. Therefore the best answer is a.

3. Which of the following acid–base disturbances would *most likely* be exhibited in a person with chronic obstructive pulmonary disease (COPD)?

    a. Metabolic alkalosis with respiratory acidosis compensation
    b. Respiratory alkalosis with metabolic acidosis compensation
    c. Respiratory acidosis with metabolic alkalosis compensation
    d. Metabolic acidosis with respiratory alkalosis compensation

Answer c is correct. In patients with restrictive airway diseases, such as COPD, there is an inability to properly ventilate off CO_2. This will result in a buildup of $Paco_2$ in the lungs, leading to respiratory acidosis. As a compensatory response to the chronically elevated $Paco_2$ levels, the kidneys retain bicarbonate resulting in an apparent metabolic alkalosis.

4. Which of the following acid–base disturbances would you expect to see in an acute asthma exacerbation?

    a. Respiratory acidosis
    b. Respiratory alkalosis
    c. Metabolic acidosis
    d. Metabolic alkalosis

Answer b is correct. In acute asthma exacerbations, the bronchioles have become inflamed, resulting in airflow obstruction. This obstruction causes patients with acute exacerbations to breathe more rapidly in an effort to oxygenate their tissues more. Therefore, an increased respiratory rate causes CO_2 to be "blown off," resulting in low $Paco_2$ levels—respiratory alkalosis.

5. A patient presents to the emergency department unconscious, after ingesting a bottle of lorazepam. What acid–base disturbance would you expect to see?

    a. Increased anion gap metabolic acidosis
    b. Respiratory alkalosis
    c. Metabolic alkalosis
    d. Respiratory acidosis

Answer d is correct. Benzodiazepine overdosage results in suppression of the respiratory center of the brain. This, therefore, leads to decreased exhalation of CO_2 and increased levels of $Paco_2$. Thus, the patient who overdoses on benzodiazepines will have a respiratory acidosis. Answer a could occur if the patient was given too high a dose of intravenous lorazepam, but this is not due to the benzodiazepine, but the excipient in the formulation, propylene glycol.

Questions 6 and 7 pertain to the following case.
A 62-year-old woman has been hospitalized in the ICU for several weeks. She has had a complicated hospital course with pneumonia and sepsis, requiring prolonged courses of antibiotics. Over the past few days, she began spiking fevers and is having a lot of diarrhea. Her stool was positive for *C. difficile* by polymerase chain reaction. Laboratory values include Na 142 mEq/L, Cl 110 mEq/L, HCO_3 18 mEq/L, albumin 4.5 g/dL, pH 7.32, and $Paco_2$=33 mm Hg.

6. What is the *most likely primary* acid–base disturbance?
   a. Increased anion gap metabolic acidosis
   b. Normal anion gap metabolic acidosis
   c. Metabolic alkalosis
   d. Respiratory acidosis
   e. Respiratory alkalosis

Answer b is correct. The patient is experiencing diarrhea from an infection with *C. diff.* This leads us to believe there is a metabolic process occurring. Looking at the pH, we note the patient to be acidotic. We should examine the HCO_3 next, because we believe this to be a primary metabolic disorder, based upon patient presentation, and discover it to be low (metabolic acidosis). When we discover this, it is recommended to next check the anion gap, and it is (142– 110–18) 14. The patient's expected anion gap is 14.5 (3 × albumin of 4.5), therefore the anion gap is *not* elevated, nor is there anything in the history to point toward an increased anion gap (KILU).

---

7. Has the patient been appropriately compensated for the primary disorder?
   a. No, the $Paco_2$ is elevated, indicating the patient has not yet been compensated.
   b. Yes, the HCO_3 is elevated, indicating appropriate compensation.
   c. No, the HCO_3 is low, indicating the patient has not yet been compensated.
   d. Yes, the $Paco_2$ is low, indicating appropriate compensation.

Answers a and b are incorrect because the $Paco_2$ is low and the HCO_3 is low.

Answer c is incorrect because the primary disturbance is a metabolic acidosis; therefore, compensation has to occur through the respiratory ($Paco_2$) route.

Answer d is correct. For a primary metabolic acidosis, the lungs compensate by "blowing off" excess acid ($Paco_2$). Therefore, one should expect to see such a patient exhibit an increased respiratory rate and, on blood gas, a decreased $Paco_2$. In this case the $Paco_2$ is in fact low (<40 mm Hg), therefore, answer d is the best choice.

Questions 8 and 9 pertain to the following case.

An 18-year-old man with no known medical history is brought to the emergency department (ED) in a difficult-to-arouse state. His parents report he has been complaining of a vague abdominal pain earlier in the morning, and then began vomiting and urinating frequently in the hours before admission. Urine and blood were positive for ketones. The following laboratory values were taken: Na 142 mEq/L, K 4.5 mEq/L, Cl 100 mEq/L, HCO_3 10 mEq/L, glucose 795 mg/dL, pH 7.26, and $Paco_2$ 23 mm Hg.

8. What is the *most likely primary* acid–base disturbance?
   a. Increased anion gap metabolic acidosis
   b. Normal anion gap metabolic acidosis
   c. Metabolic alkalosis
   d. Respiratory acidosis
   e. Respiratory alkalosis

Answer a is correct. The patient is vomiting, urinating frequently, and is difficult to arouse. There is now reason to suspect any pulmonary processes based upon the information given, so we must be thinking a primary metabolic disorder. Looking at the pH, we determine the patient to be acidotic. The $Paco_2$ is low, indicating a potential respiratory alkalosis, while the HCO_3 is low, indicating a metabolic acidosis. When we discover this, it is recommended to next check the anion gap, and it is (142 – 100 – 10) 32. Without an albumin, we estimate the patient's normal anion gap to be 12, thus the anion gap is elevated. This is a classic case of diabetic ketoacidosis where a patient has been exhibiting symptoms of hyperglycemia that eventually lead to his near comatose state. Because the cells are starved of energy (no glucose is being utilized due to a lack of insulin), ketone bodies (unmeasured anions) are produced from the breakdown of free fatty acids for energy. Therefore an increase in the anion gap will be exhibited in DKA.

---

9. Has the patient been appropriately compensated for the primary disorder?
   a. Yes, the $Paco_2$ is elevated, indicating appropriate compensation.
   b. Yes, the HCO_3 is elevated, indicating appropriate compensation.
   c. Yes, the $Paco_2$ is low, indicating appropriate compensation.
   d. Yes, the HCO_3 is low, indicating appropriate compensation.

Answer a is incorrect because the $PaCO_2$ is actually decreased.

Answer c is correct. In this case of metabolic acidosis, the most appropriate compensation would be for the lungs to "blow off" acid. By doing this, one would expect to see a low $Paco_2$, and therefore a respiratory alkalosis. As we can see this to be the case, the $Paco_2$ is 23 mm Hg (lower than 40 mm Hg), thus a respiratory alkalosis is taking place.

Answers b and d are incorrect as this is a primary metabolic problem, therefore, the primary disorder, not compensatory disorder, will be a problem of bicarbonate.

Questions 10 and 11 pertain to the following case.

A 27-year-old man with no medical history is admitted after being "found down" at a party after drinking a lot of alcohol over a 30-minute time period. Upon arrival to the ER, he was neurologically unresponsive and had the following laboratory values: pH 7.15, Pao_2 55, $Paco_2$ 60 mm Hg, HCO_3 25 mEq/L, Na 132 mEq/L, Cl 95 mEq/L, and albumin 4.2 g/dL. Urine drug screen is positive for benzodiazepines.

10. What is the *primary* acid–base disturbance?

   a. Increased anion gap metabolic acidosis
   b. Normal anion gap metabolic acidosis
   c. Metabolic alkalosis
   d. Respiratory acidosis
   e. Respiratory alkalosis

Answers a, b, and c are incorrect. Upon examination of the pH, we see it is low, acidotic, and the $Paco_2$ is elevated, indicating respiratory acidosis

Answer d is correct. In this case of acute intoxication of alcohol and benzodiazepines, we would expect a primary respiratory disorder, due to the combination causing respiratory depression.

---

11. Has the patient been appropriately compensated for the primary acid–base disorder?

   a. Yes, the $Paco_2$ is elevated, indicating appropriate compensation.
   b. Yes, the $Paco_2$ is low, indicating appropriate compensation.
   c. Yes, the HCO_3 is elevated, indicating appropriate compensation.
   d. Yes, the HCO_3 is low, indicating appropriate compensation.
   e. Unsure, it is too soon after the acute respiratory event to assess metabolic compensation at this time.

Answer e is correct. Because the range in normal bicarbonate is wide (22-28 mEq/L), and because it is unknown where the patient's bicarbonate level was prior to this episode, we cannot say whether or not the patient is appropriately compensated, as the bicarbonate is within the expected range. At 25, it is certainly not high, as we would expect for a chronic respiratory acidosis (Answer b), nor is it low (Answer d). Because this is a primary respiratory disorder, Answers a and b can be excluded.

Questions 12 and 13 pertain to the following case.

A 45-year-old woman with previous peptic ulcer disease was admitted with persistent vomiting. She looked dehydrated, with dry mucus membranes and skin tenting. Her blood results were Na 141 mEq/L, K 2.6 mEq/L, Cl 87 mEq/L, pH 7.51, $Paco_2$ 50 mm Hg, and HCO_3 40 mEq/L.

12. What is the primary acid–base disorder?

   a. Increased anion gap metabolic acidosis
   b. Normal anion gap metabolic acidosis
   c. Metabolic alkalosis
   d. Respiratory acidosis
   e. Respiratory alkalosis

Answers a and b are incorrect. Looking at the HCO_3, we see it is markedly elevated, indicating a metabolic alkalosis.

Answer c is correct. Given the patient's presentation of persistent vomiting, we would expect to see a primary metabolic disorder due to loss of hydrogen ions from the upper GI tract.

Answers d and e are incorrect. Further, there is no information given to suspect a respiratory disorder, so Answers d and e can be excluded. Upon examination of the pH, we see the patient is alkalotic. Looking at the $Paco_2$, we discover it is elevated, thus eliminating Answer e, completely.

---

13. Has the patient been appropriately compensated for the primary acid–base disorder?

   a. Yes, the $Paco_2$ is elevated, indicating appropriate compensation.
   b. Yes, the $Paco_2$ is low, indicating appropriate compensation.
   c. Yes, the HCO_3 is elevated, indicating appropriate compensation.
   d. Yes, the HCO_3 is low, indicating appropriate compensation.

Answer a is correct. Knowing there is a primary metabolic disorder, we can exclude Answers c and d immediately. Because the pH is elevated secondary to metabolic alkalosis, the most appropriate respiratory compensation would be for the lungs to hold on to acid ($Paco_2$) resulting in a respiratory acidosis, which is the case here with a $Paco_2$ of 50 mm Hg. Therefore the best answer is a.

Questions 14 and 15 pertain to the following case.

A 55-year-old man was admitted to the hospital with a 3-day history of persistent vomiting. The following laboratory values are taken: pH 7.40, $Paco_2$ 40 mm Hg, HCO_3 24 mEq/L, Na 149 mEq/L, Cl 100 mEq/L, BUN 110 mg/dL, and Cr 8.7 mg/dL.

14. What would you *expect* the pH, $Paco_2$, and HCO_3 to be in a patient who has persistent vomiting (↑, ↓, N)?

   a. pH ↑; $Paco_2$ ↓; HCO_3 ↑
   b. pH ↓; $Paco_2$ ↓; HCO_3 ↓
   c. pH ↑; $Paco_2$ N; HCO_3 ↑
   d. pH ↓; $Paco_2$ N; HCO_3 ↓

Answer c is correct. In a patient with persistent vomiting, one would expect to see metabolic alkalosis, with or without respiratory compensation. Therefore, the pH should be elevated, the HCO_3 should be elevated (because of a loss of hydrogen ions from the upper GI tract), and the $Paco_2$ should be normal or elevated (depending on the duration of metabolic alkalosis). Therefore, answer c is the best choice.

15. What acid–base disturbance would you expect in this patient who has uremia?
    a. Increased anion gap metabolic acidosis
    b. Normal anion gap metabolic acidosis
    c. Metabolic alkalosis
    d. Respiratory acidosis
    e. Respiratory alkalosis

Answer a is correct. Patients with renal failure and uremia will exhibit an increased anion gap metabolic acidosis (recall: KILU, where "U" stands for uremia).

16. A 55-year-old woman with a history of severe chronic obstructive pulmonary disease is admitted after several days of worsening shortness of breath. Recently, she was discharged from the hospital with a similar episode and was doing fine until 3 days before admission, when she developed a productive cough, requiring an increase in her home O_2 and more frequent metered-dose inhaler use. What would you *expect* the pH, $Paco_2$, and HCO_3 to be in this patient (↑, ↓, N)?
    a. pH ↑; $Paco_2$ ↓; HCO_3 ↑
    b. pH ↓; $Paco_2$ ↑; HCO_3 ↑
    c. pH ↑; $Paco_2$ N; HCO_3 ↑
    d. pH ↓; $Paco_2$ N; HCO_3 ↓

Answer b is correct. In a patient with chronic obstructive pulmonary disease, one would expect to see a primary respiratory process, with metabolic compensation. Because COPD is a restrictive airway disease, patients have difficulty "blowing off" $Paco_2$. Therefore, you should see an increase in $Paco_2$ which will result in a decrease in the pH (respiratory acidosis). As compensation for this chronic process, patients with COPD hold onto bicarbonate to try and normalize the pH, therefore you will see a metabolic alkalosis. Chronically, patients with COPD will have a normal pH because the increase in $Paco_2$ is compensated for by a chronic metabolic alkalosis. However, acutely, as in this case, the increase in the $Paco_2$ that occurs will result in an acute respiratory acidosis.

17. What acid–base disturbance would you expect to see in a person hiking up Mount Everest?
    a. Increased anion gap metabolic acidosis
    b. Normal anion gap metabolic acidosis
    c. Metabolic alkalosis
    d. Respiratory acidosis
    e. Respiratory alkalosis

Answer e is correct. Hiking in high altitude areas results in a state of hypoxemia. This low level of oxygen will cause a person's respiratory system to increase ventilation in an effort to oxygenate tissues. Therefore, you would expect to see a respiratory alkalosis, answer e.

Match the following diseases to the *primary* acid–base disturbance.

18. Diabetic ketoacidosis
19. Severe anemia
20. Furosemide administration
    a. Metabolic Acidosis
    b. Metabolic Alkalosis
    c. Respiratory acidosis
    d. Respiratory alkalosis

Answers a, d, and b are the correct options for questions 18, 19, and 20, respectively. Diabetic ketoacidosis results in increased levels of unmeasured anions (ketone bodies). These unmeasured anions create a metabolic acidosis (a). Severe anemia results in tissue hypoxia. Therefore, the respiratory center is stimulated to breathe faster in order to oxygenate the tissues. The end result of this hyperventilation is a decrease in the $Paco_2$, and therefore a respiratory alkalosis (d). Furosemide administration results in volume depletion, and therefore decreased blood pressure entering the kidney. The result is that the kidneys attempt to absorb more sodium in the proximal tubule, a place where it is reabsorbed with bicarbonate. The end result is an increase in the serum bicarbonate, or a metabolic alkalosis (b).

CHAPTER 32 | Enteral Nutrition

1. Which of the following routes of supplemental nutrition would be most appropriate for a patient who is malnourished secondary to facial trauma?
    a. Parenteral nutrition
    b. Nasojejunal enteral nutrition
    c. Percutaneous gastric enteral nutrition
    d. Nasoduodenal enteral nutrition

Answer a is incorrect. A patient with facial trauma, who is unable to take food orally, but an otherwise functioning gut should be fed with enteral nutrition rather than parenteral. Parenteral nutrition should be reserved for those with nonfunctioning GI tracts.

Answer b is incorrect. There is no evidence that the patient has gastric dysfunction. As with Answer a, functional gut should be used whenever possible. Also, a patient with facial trauma is not likely to tolerate a nasojejunal tube for a long period of time.

Answer c is correct. As stated above, a functional gut should be used whenever possible, percutaneous tube placement will allow longer term access than transnasal insertion, and with a nasojejunal tube, the patient is not likely to tolerate a transnasal tube well.

Answer d is incorrect. This answer is incorrect for the same reasons as Answer b.

---

2. While administering medications via nasogastric tubes:
   a. The medication must be compatible with basic fluids.
   b. Tablets must be fully crushed and mixed with 15 to 30 mL of water.
   c. The tube must be flushed with 250 mL of water before and after medication administration.
   d. Capsule beads should be crushed and mixed with 15 to 30 mL of water.

Answer a is incorrect. The tip of a nasogastric tube terminates in the gastrum of the stomach which is acidic. There is no requirement for compatibility with basic medium.

Answer b is correct. Tablets those are able to be crushed, must be ground to a very fine powder and mixed with water prior to administration

Answer c is incorrect. Nasogastric tubes should be flushed with 30 mL before and after medication administration.

Answer d is incorrect. Capsule beads should not be crushed. For those capsules that can be opened, the beads should be given intact and flushed with 30 mL water before and after administration.

---

3. When phenytoin is administered to patient receiving tube feeds:
   a. The acidic medium of the jejunum degrades the phenytoin to inactive products.
   b. The basic medium of the duodenum degrades the phenytoin to inactive products.
   c. Phenytoin must be administered very slowly with enteral nutrition.
   d. Administration with enteral nutrition products may decrease drug absorption.

Answer a is incorrect. The gastrum, not the jejunum is acidic. Additionally, phenytoin absorption is not affected by an acidic medium.

Answer b is incorrect. Phenytoin is not degraded by the relatively (compared to the stomach) basic pH of the duodenum.

Answer c is incorrect. Phenytoin should *not* be administered concurrently with enteral nutrition.

Answer d is correct. Bezoar formation and decreased bioavailability of phenytoin has been noted when it is administered concurrently with enteral nutrition.

---

4. When administering drugs via enteral feeding tube:
   a. Liquid medications are always preferable to solid dosage forms.
   b. As long as tablets are crushed very finely they will retain their pharmacokinetic properties.
   d. All drugs that a patient receives should be given simultaneously to minimize feeding interruptions.
   e. Liquid medications may interact with nutritional formula and clog the feeding tube.

Answer a is incorrect. Liquid medications are *not* always preferable. Gastrointestinal intolerance is a common adverse effect of some liquid medications, especially those that contain sorbitol, and some may be physically incompatible with enteral nutrition.

Answer b is incorrect. Many tablets cannot be crushed at all, and crushing often changes the pharmacokinetic properties of the tablet.

Answer c is incorrect. Even in patients taking medications by mouth, there may be incompatibilities. These same restrictions apply when administering medications per tube.

Answer d is correct. As stated above, some liquid medications have physical incompatibilities with enteral nutrition products which may thicken the products or form a gel.

---

5. Which of the following statements is correct?
   a. Modular formulas contain a balanced mixture of carbohydrates and lipids.
   b. Calorically dense formulas provide nutrition targeted to a specific disease state.
   c. Elemental formulas contain intact proteins and polysaccharides.
   d. Standard formulas contain intact proteins.

Answer a is incorrect. Modular formulas contain a single nutrient entity that is used to supplement traditional formulas; targeting specific patient needs.

Answer b is incorrect. Calorically dense formulas are complete nutrition sources and contain a balanced mix of nutrients.

Answer c is incorrect. Elemental formulas contain hydrolyzed proteins; peptides and amino acids which are easier to digest than intact proteins.

Answer d is correct. Standard formulas contain intact proteins, they are meant for patients who can fully digest proteins and do not require hydrolyzed proteins.

---

6. Aspiration risks during enteral nutrition feedings are increased by:
   a. Feeding in an elevated or upright position
   b. High gastric residual prior to feeding
   c. Continuous feeding regimens
   d. High-protein modular feeding

Answer a is incorrect. An elevated or upright position is preferable to a supine position if a risk of aspiration exists.

Answer b is correct. Initiating enteral feeds when the gastric residual is high increases the risk for aspiration.

Answer c is incorrect. Continuous feeding regimens are protective against aspiration.

Answer d is incorrect. High-protein modular feeding does not have an effect on aspiration risk.

7. Aspiration pneumonia:
   a. Is usually polymicrobial
   b. Is usually preceded by a bacterial infection
   c. Is a chemical pneumonia initially
   d. Is decreased by H_2 blockers

Answer a is incorrect. Aspiration pneumonia is initially a chemical pneumonia and in most cases sterile.

Answer b is incorrect. Aspiration pneumonia is caused by aspirating the stomach contents into the lung. Bacterial pneumonia is a separate phenomenon.

Answer c is correct.

Answer d is incorrect. H_2 blockers do not appear to have an effect on susceptibility to aspiration pneumonia, but by lowering the acid content of the stomach they allow bacteria to remain in the gut. So if a patient does develop aspiration pneumonia, it is more likely to be complicated by bacterial growth if the patient is taking an H_2 blocker (or PPI).

8. Which of the following factors is most important for initial selection of an enteral formulation?
   a. Formula osmolality
   b. Cost of formulation
   c. Location of tube
   d. Nutritional needs

Answer a is incorrect. Osmolality, while important because it may influence tolerability, is not usually the primary concern when making the initial product selection.

Answer b is incorrect. Again, while important, cost is not the overriding factor in product selection.

Answer c is incorrect. Tube location is dictated by patient's disease state, and while it may have some influence on the decision of which formula to select, it is not the primary consideration.

Answer d is correct. Nutritional needs of the patient should be the guiding factor in all decisions about enteral nutrition. While osmolality, cost, and tube location are certainly important, attaining optimal nutrition status is the overall goal.

9. Enteral nutrition may be contraindicated in which of the following situations?
   a. Gastrointestinal bleeding
   b. Gastric cancer
   c. Short bowel syndrome
   d. Colostomy

Answer a is correct. Enteral feeding is contraindicated in gastrointestinal bleeding as it may potentiate bleeding. In some cases, once the cause of the GI bleeding has been determined, it may be acceptable, and even preferred to restart the feeding.

Answer b is incorrect. Gastric cancer is a common reason to initiate enteral nutrition. Patients with gastric cancer often have obstruction or gastric pain associated with their disease, and enteral feeds beyond the point of blockage are beneficial.

Answer c is incorrect. As with answer b, short bowel syndrome is a common reason to initiate enteral feeding. Those with short bowel syndrome do not absorb nutrients well, so close attention to nutrient content is warranted.

Answer d is incorrect. The colon is beyond the point that most nutrients are absorbed, and as such, colostomies do not interfere with enteral feeds any more than oral feeding.

10. MJ is a hospitalized man who weighs 78 kg and has a BMI of 24 kg/m^2. What is his calculated daily fluid requirement?
    a. 2160 mL
    b. 2660 mL
    c. 3160 mL
    d. 3660 mL

Answer a is incorrect.

Answer b is correct. The average adult requires 1500 mL for the first 20 kg of body weight and 20 mL/kg of body weight over 20 kg. Therefore, the calculations for daily fluid requirement for a 78 kg adult are: 1500 mL + [(78 kg – 20 kg) × 20 mL) = 2660 mL.

Answer c is incorrect.

Answer d is incorrect.

11. Which of the following daily calorie counts would be most appropriate for MJ?
    a. 1500 kcal
    b. 2000 kcal
    c. 2500 kcal
    d. 3000 kcal

Answer a is incorrect. This regimen does not supply enough calories for a 78-kg man (19 kcal/kg/d).

Answer b is incorrect. This regimen does not supply enough calories for a 78-kg man (25 kcal/kg/d).

Answer c is correct. Adult patients on bedrest require an average of 30 to 35 kcal/kg of body weight per day. The calculations for calorie intake are from 78 kg × 30 to 78 kg × 35 kcal/day = 2340 to 2730 kcal.

Answer d is incorrect. This regimen supplies too many calories for a 78-kg man (38 kcal/kg/d).

---

12. Which of the following is a common complication of enteral nutrition therapy?
    a. Weight loss
    b. Diarrhea
    c. Weight gain
    d. Hypoglycemia

Answer a is incorrect. Weight loss is not a common complication of enteral nutrition therapy. If unintentional weight loss is thought to be caused by enteral nutrition, a reassessment of the feeding regimen needs to be performed.

Answer b is correct. Diarrhea is a common complication of enteral nutrition and may be caused by malabsorption, infection, high osmolar concentration of formula or drugs.

Answer c is incorrect. Weight gain is not a common complication of enteral nutrition and like weight loss can be managed through appropriate nutrition management.

Answer d is incorrect. Hypoglycemia is not a common complication of enteral feeding unless feedings are held in diabetic patients receiving insulin.

---

13. Fluid retention associated with enteral nutrition is a problem that is commonly encountered in all of the following disease states *except*:
    a. Heart failure
    b. Respiratory distress
    c. Renal insufficiency
    d. Hepatic failure

Answer a is incorrect. Heart failure will likely cause increased fluid retention.

Answer b is correct. Respiratory distress is not a cause of fluid retention, increased respiratory rate will actually increase fluid losses because expired air has higher water content than inspired air.

Answer c is incorrect. Renal failure is a common cause of fluid retention.

Answer d is incorrect. Those with hepatic failure often experience fluid retention.

---

14. ED is a 62-year-old woman with type 2 diabetes and end stage renal disease who requires enteral nutrition. She was recently placed on hemodialysis therapy 3 times/wk. Please select the most appropriate nutrition combination.
    a. Low protein, high carbohydrate
    b. Low protein, low carbohydrate
    c. Moderate protein, moderate carbohydrate
    d. High protein, high carbohydrate

Answer a is incorrect. Low-protein diet in hemodialysis may lead to protein malnutrition due to increased protein loss, high carbohydrate diet is likely to lead to loss of glycemic control.

Answer b is incorrect. Low-protein diet in hemodialysis may lead to protein malnutrition due to increased protein loss, low carbohydrate diet may prove beneficial for patient with diabetes.

Answer c is correct. A moderate protein diet in a hemodialysis patient decreases the risk of protein malnutrition; there is no risk of further renal deterioration. Low carbohydrate diet may prove beneficial for patient with diabetes.

Answer d is incorrect. High-protein diets have not been proved to be beneficial in preventing protein malnutrition, high-carbohydrate diet is likely to lead to loss of glycemic control.

---

15. Patients with hepatic encephalopathy may benefit from nutritional formulations containing:
    a. High branched chain amino acids (BCAA), low aromatic amino acids (AAA)
    b. Low branched chain amino acids, low aromatic amino acids
    c. High protein, low amino acids
    d. Protein and amino acid content does not affect hepatic encephalopathy

---

Answer a is correct. Patients with hepatic encephalopathy tend to have low levels of BCAA and high levels of AAA.

Answer b is incorrect. Supplementing already high AAA may worsen hepatic encephalopathy.

Answer c is incorrect. High-protein diets may worsen hepatic encephalopathy through elevated blood ammonia levels because the impaired liver cannot synthesize the excess nitrogen into urea for disposal.

Answer d is incorrect. See Answer c for explanation of protein content and hepatic encephalopathy.

---

16. TR is a 72-year-old man with diabetes and COPD. He is currently hospitalized and on a ventilator for community-acquired pneumonia. Which of the following regimens would be most appropriate dietary therapy?
    a. 50% carbohydrate, 30% fat, 20% protein
    b. 65% carbohydrate, 30% fat, 35% protein
    c. 35% carbohydrate, 25% fat, 40% protein
    d. 35% carbohydrate, 50% fat, 15% protein

Answer a is incorrect. Patients with pulmonary disease should be given a low carbohydrate diet to decrease CO_2

production as well as to decrease the risk of hyperglycemia in a diabetic patient.

Answer b is incorrect. See Answer a above.

Answer c is incorrect. The carbohydrate load is appropriate, but the caloric deficit should be replaced with fat.

Answer d is correct. The low carbohydrate diet has been supplemented by a higher fat content. This will help decrease the CO_2 load while providing adequate calories.

---

17. TR (from Question 16) has been in your facility on the ventilator for 4 days and the resident asks how the risk of aspiration can be decreased. Which of the following methods in *not* an appropriate intervention for this patient?
    a. Elevating head of the bed during and after feedings
    b. Initiating continuous feedings rather than intermittent bolus feedings
    c. Placing gastric tube and stopping proton-pump inhibitor use
    d. Placing duodenal tube placement instead of gastric tube

---

Answer a is incorrect. Elevating the head of the bed is an appropriate method to decrease the risk of aspiration.

Answer b is incorrect. Use of continuous feeds decreases the risk of aspiration compared to intermittent bolus feeds.

Answer c is correct. Gastric tube placement actually increases the risk of aspiration compared to duodenal placement; proton-pump inhibitor use is appropriate in this patient for stress ulcer prophylaxis since he has been intubated for >48 hours.

Answer d is incorrect. Duodenal tube placement decreases the risk of aspiration when compared to gastric tube placement.

---

18. Fiber in enteral formulations:
    a. Decreases tolerability in most patients
    b. May increase diarrhea
    c. May increase constipation
    d. May contribute to GI obstruction

Answer a is incorrect. Fiber increases the tolerability of enteral feedings for most patients.

Answer b is incorrect. Fiber-containing formulas are often given to decrease the incidence of diarrhea.

Answer c is incorrect. Fiber-containing formulas are often given to decrease the incidence of constipation.

Answer d is correct. Fiber-containing products may increase the risk of GI obstruction in those already at risk.

---

19. Which of the following tubes are correctly matched to their preferred use or tube type?
    a. Nasogastric tube, long-term use
    b. Orogastric tube, small bore
    c. Percutaneous gastric tube, short-term use
    d. Nasojejunal tube, large bore

Answer a is incorrect. Nasogastric tubes should not be used long term as they are not well tolerated.

Answer b is correct. Orogastric tubes should be small bore to increase patient comfort and tolerability.

Answer c is incorrect. Percutaneous placement is typically reserved for long-term feeding access.

Answer d is incorrect. Small-bore tubes are preferred for both oral and nasal tube placement to decrease the risk of physical irritation from the tube and increase tolerability.

---

20. All of the following patient groups have increased metabolic needs *except*:
    a. Type 1 diabetics
    b. Trauma patients
    c. Burn patients
    d. Critically ill patients

Answer a is correct. Patients with type 1 diabetes do not have increased metabolic/caloric needs over those of a nondiabetic patient.

Answer b is incorrect. Trauma patients do have increased metabolic needs; recovering from trauma is a catabolic process that increases baseline energy needs.

Answer c is incorrect. Burn patients are in a highly catabolic state and have greatly increased metabolic rates.

Answer d is incorrect. Critical illness induces a catabolic state and energy needs are increased over baseline.

CHAPTER 33 | Parenteral Nutrition

1. VB is a 54-year-old man who underwent small bowel resection for bowel necrosis. He is receiving PN and has required a nasogastric tube for suction. He develops metabolic alkalosis. Which one of the following is the most appropriate adjustment to VB's PN solution?
    a. Add sodium bicarbonate
    b. Decrease acetate and increase chloride
    c. Increase acetate and decrease chloride
    d. Increase sodium and chloride

Answer a is incorrect. Sodium bicarbonate is generally not added to PN solutions due to compatibility issues. When a source of base is desired to be added to a PN solution, acetate is usually utilized. Acetate is converted to bicarbonate in the liver. Adding sodium bicarbonate to a PN solution would tend to worsen a metabolic alkalosis rather than to improve this condition.

Answer b is correct. Acetate in PN solutions tends to have an alkalinizing effect (because of its conversion to bicarbonate in the liver), whereas chloride has an acidifying effect. Therefore, decreasing acetate and increasing chloride should help to improve a metabolic alkalosis.

Answer c is incorrect. As explained above for Answer b, increasing acetate and decreasing chloride in a PN solution might be helpful in correcting a metabolic acidosis, but it would be expected to worsen a metabolic alkalosis and would therefore be inappropriate for a patient with metabolic alkalosis.

Answer d is not the best answer. Although increasing chloride in the PN might be useful for a patient with metabolic alkalosis, not enough information is given to determine whether increasing sodium in the PN is appropriate for this patient. Fluid overload can be a problem in some PN patients, and excess sodium in the PN could exacerbate this problem.

---

2. Which one of the following statements is most correct regarding macrosubstrates found in PN solutions?
   a. Dextrose and amino acids can be mixed together by the manufacturer, heat sterilized, and then shipped to hospitals.
   b. Glycerin and amino acids can be mixed together by the manufacturer, heat sterilized, and then shipped to hospitals.
   c. Premixed PN solutions containing dextrose, amino acid, and fat all in a single chamber are available from various manufacturers.
   d. Combinations of dextrose and amino acid solution must be used within 24 hours of mixing, even if they are stored in the refrigerator.

Answer a is incorrect. When heated, carbonyl groups on dextrose will react with amino groups on amino acids in what is called the Maillard or browning reaction. Therefore, dextrose and amino acid combinations are not available premixed by the manufacturer.

Answer b is correct. Because glycerin does not contain a carbonyl group, the Maillard reaction does not occur when combinations of glycerin and amino acids are heat sterilized. The commercially available product called ProcalAmine contains these components in a premixed formulation.

Answer c is incorrect. So-called premixed or ready-to-use PN solutions available in the United States are supplied in two compartment bags, with each compartment containing either amino acid or dextrose. A septum between the two chambers is broken immediately before use and the two solutions are mixed together. In other parts of the world, three-chamber, premixed PN solutions are available with dextrose, amino acid, and lipid filling the three chambers.

Answer d is incorrect. Dextrose/amino acid combinations can be stored in the refrigerator for various lengths of time. Patients receiving home PN may receive several days' supply at a time that can be stored in the refrigerator until use. Although TNA are inherently less stable than dextrose/amino acid solutions, even TNA may be stable for several days in the refrigerator.

---

3. A patient is receiving ProcalAmine postoperatively at 125 mL/h. ProcalAmine contains 3% final concentration of glycerin and 3% final concentration of amino acid. How many calories and how much protein is provided per day by this solution?
   a. 747 kcal and 90 g amino acid
   b. 666 kcal and 90g amino acid
   c. 720 kcal and 60 g amino acid
   d. 747 kcal and 60 g amino acid

Answer a is correct. Calculation of kcal and amino acid is as follows:

125 mL/h × 24 h/d = 3000 mL/d

Glycerin provides 4.3 kcal/g

3 g glycerol/100 mL = x g glycerol/3000 mL; x = 90 g

90 g × 4.3 kcal/g = 387 kcal

Amino acid provides 4 kcal/g

3 g amino acid/100 mL = x g amino acid/3000 mL; x = 90 g

90 g × 4 kcal/g = 360 kcal

387 kcal + 360 kcal = 747 kcal

Answers b, c, and d are incorrect. Note that IV dextrose supplies 3.4 kcal/g and oral carbohydrate supplies 4 kcal/g. Although ProcalAmine may be appropriate as a PPN solution, the amount of kcal and protein that it provides is limited by low concentrations. When used, it is usually appropriate to piggyback lipid onto the PN line to provide more kcal.

---

4. Which one of the following amino acid profiles best describes a specialty formulation for use in patients with hepatic encephalopathy compared to standard amino acid formulations?
   a. Higher in branched chain amino acids, same level of aromatic amino acids
   b. Higher in branched chain amino acids, lower in aromatic amino acids
   c. Higher in essential amino acids, lower in nonessential amino acids
   d. Fortified with dipeptides containing glutamine

Answer a is incorrect. Products containing more branched chain amino acids but the same amount of aromatic amino acids as in standard products have been marketed as Aminosyn-HBC or FreAmine HBC for use in highly stressed patients. Branched chain amino acids are preferentially broken down during stress and are thus fortified in these products. These products are not frequently utilized, largely because of expense and stability concerns limiting their concentration and therefore the amount that can be delivered to a patient in a reasonable fluid load.

Answer b is correct. Aromatic amino acids tend to accumulate in hepatic failure, whereas branched chain amino acids in the blood are decreased. According to the false neurotransmitter theory, aromatic amino acids compete for transport across the blood–brain barrier with branched chain amino acids and are converted to false neurotransmitters such as octopamine, leading to hepatic encephalopathy. Feeding of a parenteral amino acid formula fortified with branched chain amino acids and with lesser amounts of aromatic amino acid formulas can help normalize amino acid levels in the blood. Such formulas have been shown to help patients "wake up" from hepatic encephalopathy, but data demonstrating improved outcomes in terms of mortality with use of these products are limited. They should be reserved for use in hepatic encephalopathy patients who have failed standard medical therapy.

Answer c is incorrect. Specialty products for use in renal failure contain higher amounts of essential amino acids and lower amounts of nonessential amino acids compared to standard amino acid formulations. This allows for recycling of some endogenous urea nitrogen for synthesis of nonessential amino acids. Although some data support lowering of blood urea nitrogen in patients with renal failure receiving these products, data on improved clinical outcomes are limited.

Answer d is incorrect. Amino acid products available in the United States do not contain glutamine due to stability issues. Some products available in other parts of the world do provide dipeptides containing glutamine; the dipeptides overcome the stability issues with glutamine. Glutamine is often depleted during stress and is the preferred fuel source for small intestinal cells.

---

5. HO is a 63-year-old woman with cancer cachexia. She has lost 10% of her body weight since her diagnosis with colon cancer about 6 months ago. Her cancer treatments are causing severe nausea and vomiting. The physician wants to start PN. The dietitian expresses concern regarding refeeding syndrome. Which electrolyte abnormality is the hallmark of this syndrome?

   a. Hypermagnesemia
   b. Hypercalcemia
   c. Hyponatremia
   d. Hypophosphatemia

Refeeding syndrome occurs in the setting of chronic malnutrition when a patient is refed with aggressive amounts of dextrose. Although more likely to occur with parenteral feeding, it has also been reported with enteral and oral feedings. In extreme cases, it can be associated with pulmonary and cardiac failure and central nervous system involvement and can be life threatening.

Answer a is incorrect. Hypermagnesemia, hyperkalemia, and hyperphosphatemia are uncommon in patients with normal renal function.

Answer b is incorrect. Although hypercalcemia is common in patients with cancer, it is not the hallmark of refeeding syndrome.

Answer c is incorrect. Although not the correct option, edema may accompany refeeding syndrome related to sodium retention by the kidney.

Answer d is correct. With carbohydrate refeeding, phosphorus, magnesium, and potassium, which are primarily intracellular electrolytes, are forced intracellularly by the action of insulin. This leads to lower levels of these electrolytes in the extracellular space, including the blood, where levels are routinely measured. Therefore, hypophosphatemia, hypomagnesemia, and hypokalemia are expected with refeeding. Hypophosphatemia is the hallmark electrolyte abnormality. Phosphorus is important in diaphragm function and in energy metabolism as a component of adenosine triphosphate (ATP). Thus hypophosphatemia can contribute to respiratory failure in severe refeeding syndrome.

---

6. A national shortage of IV multivitamin products leads a hospital to ration this product in patients receiving PN. Ten days after receiving PN with minimal multivitamins, TE develops congestive heart failure symptoms that are diagnosed as wet beriberi. Deficiency of which vitamin is causing TE's symptoms?

   a. Vitamin B_{12}
   b. Vitamin K
   c. Folic acid
   d. Thiamine

Nationwide shortages of IV multivitamin products have occurred intermittently during the past several decades. In settings of shortages, patients may be given oral multivitamins if they are able to absorb them. Remaining IV multivitamin product may need to be rationed; instead of daily administration, a regimen of 2 or 3 times per week may be implemented. Some of the vitamins found in the IV multivitamin products are not available as individual IV entities. On the other hand, some vitamins are available as individual entities and should be added on a daily basis in a shortage situation. Two vitamins of particular importance available as individual IV entities are thiamine and folic acid.

Answer a is incorrect. Vitamin B_{12} deficiency develops slowly. The major concern with this deficiency is anemia.

Answer b is incorrect. Vitamin K deficiency is associated with bleeding, as vitamin K is a cofactor for several clotting factors.

Answer c is incorrect. Folic acid deficiency is associated with anemia.

Answer d is correct. The classic deficiency disease of thiamine is beriberi. Wet beriberi, characterized by a congestive heart failure picture, has been described in patients receiving short-term PN without thiamine.

---

7. Which one of the following increases the solubility of calcium and phosphate in a PN solution?
   a. Increased temperature
   b. Increased pH
   c. Use of calcium chloride instead of calcium gluconate
   d. Increased amino acid concentration in the PN

Answer a is incorrect. Although solubility of many substances increases with increased temperatures, the opposite is true for calcium and phosphate.

Answer b is incorrect. Increases in pH decrease the solubility of calcium and phosphate.

Answer c is incorrect. Calcium gluconate is the preferred form of calcium for addition to PN in the United States. Calcium gluconate is more soluble than calcium chloride.

Answer d is correct. Increasing the amino acid concentration of the PN tends to decrease the pH of the solution, thus increasing the solubility of calcium and phosphate. The low amino acid concentration of neonatal PN solutions, together with high requirements for calcium and phosphate in neonates, leads to challenges relating to calcium and phosphate solubility in PN solutions for this population. Solubility of calcium and phosphate in PN solutions is important because precipitation of these substances has led to patient harm. Precipitates large enough to cause adverse events are not always visible to the human eye, although visual checking of PN solutions is still a vital part of quality assurance. Furthermore, TNA are opaque and therefore precipitates in these admixtures are typically undetectable by visual checks. Final filtering of PN solutions is vital for prevention of infusion of large particulates into the patient.

---

8. A hospital is transitioning from use of dextrose/amino acid solutions plus piggybacked lipid for PN to a system utilizing TNA. Which one of the following best describes proper use of final filters in this setting?
   a. A switch from use of 0.22 μm filters to use of 1.2 μm filters is appropriate.
   b. A switch from use of 1.2 μm filters to use of 0.22 μm filters is appropriate.
   c. No switch in filtration practices is necessary; use of 0.22 μm filters may continue.
   d. Switching from the current 0.22 μm filters to no filters is most appropriate.

Answer a is correct. It is recommended that dextrose/amino acid solutions be filtered through a 0.22 μm final filter. Such filters remove both particulates and microbes. Lipid emulsions and TNA cannot be passed through a 0.22-μm filter, because particles within these emulsions typically range up to about 0.5 μm in size and would thus be disrupted or deformed by passage through the smaller filter. Although 5-μm filters are also available, it is recommended that TNA be passed through a 1.2-μm filter. Such filters remove particulates but do not remove most microbes. Lipid emulsions administered via piggyback are not passed through a filter.

Answer b is incorrect. TNA should not be administered through a 0.22-μm filter. Although dextrose/amino acid solutions could be administered through a 1.2-μm filter, most institutions administer them through a 0.22-μm filter.

Answer c is incorrect. Again, TNA should not be administered through a 0.22-μm filter.

Answer d is incorrect. It is very important to administer TNA through a filter. Adverse outcomes have been reported when this step was omitted. Infusion of particles greater in size than about 0.5 μm can cause lung damage.

---

9. PW is a 46-year-old man receiving PN because of intolerance to enteral feeding following multiple trauma. He is receiving 150 g of protein each day. A 24-hour urine collection for urea nitrogen (UUN) yields a value of 20 g. What is the estimated nitrogen balance in gram per day for this patient?
   a. +4
   b. 0
   c. −10
   d. −120

Answer a is incorrect. It does not take into account nonurinary urea nitrogen losses. A correction factor of 4 g/d is generally allowed for such losses.

Answer b is correct. To calculate the number of grams of nitrogen from the number of grams of protein, divide by 6.25 or multiply by 0.16. Thus, the amount of nitrogen going into the patient is 150/6.25 = 24 g. Applying the correction factor given above for nonurinary urea nitrogen losses, the nitrogen balance is calculated as follows:

$$\text{Nitrogen balance} = \text{nitrogen in} - (\text{nitrogen out} + 4), \text{ or}$$
$$\text{Nitrogen balance} = 24 - (20 + 4) = 0$$

Thus the patient is estimated to be in neutral nitrogen balance. The goal is to have patients in positive nitrogen balance, therefore increasing the protein and/or kcal of the PN may be appropriate in this situation to achieve a positive balance. Achievement of a positive nitrogen balance is frequently unrealistic in patients undergoing high stress.

Answers c and d are incorrect. Negative numbers of this magnitude would not be expected even in the setting of no feeding.

---

10. SR is a 26-year-old mechanically ventilated woman receiving propofol for sedation. The drug is provided as 10 mg/mL

propofol and is being delivered at 100 mg/h. Propofol is commercially provided in a 10% lipid emulsion vehicle. How many grams per day of lipid is SR receiving via the propofol infusion?

a. 2.4
b. 4.8
c. 24
d. 48

Propofol is commonly used as a sedative in mechanically ventilated critically ill patients. The rate of administration for this use frequently provides significant lipid kcal and should be taken into account when calculating kcal and lipid administration. In patients receiving PN concomitantly, IV lipid emulsion may need to be held or the rate of administration cut while the patient is receiving propofol.

Answers a, b, and d are incorrect.

Answer c is correct. Calculation is as follows:

Propofol being infused at 100 mg/h/10 mg/mL = 10 mL/h

10 mL/h × 24 h/d = 240 mL/d

10% lipid = 10 g/100 mL

240 mL/d × 10 g/100 mL = 24 g/d

---

11. Which one of the following statements is true regarding TNA?
    a. A cracked TNA may be safely administered to a patient, but a creamed TNA is unsafe for administration.
    b. A creamed TNA may be safely administered to a patient, but a cracked TNA is unsafe for administration.
    c. Neither a creamed nor a cracked TNA may be safely administered to a patient.
    d. Both creamed and cracked TNA may be safely administered to a patient after rehomogenization.

Total nutrient admixtures are inherently less stable than dextrose/amino acid solutions. The so-called zeta potential is a negative charge on the surface of lipid globules. This zeta potential prevents clumping of lipid globules. If this negative surface charge is neutralized by cations, coalescence of lipid globules may occur. Trivalent cations are the worst culprits for neutralizing the negative surface charge, followed by divalent cations; monovalent cations have a lesser effect. Total nutrient admixture stability is decreased with decreasing pH due to increases in hydrogen ion concentration.

A creamed TNA is one in which lipid globules have separated out of the emulsion, but gentle inversion of the container results in the globules redispersing and the original homogeneous appearance of the admixture reappears. On the other hand, in a cracked TNA, lipid globules have coalesced and separated out of the emulsion, and gentle inversion cannot result in reappearance of the original homogeneous condition of the admixture.

Answer a is incorrect. A cracked TNA may not be safely administered to a patient, whereas a creamed TNA may be administered after the separated fat globules have been redispersed.

Answer b is correct. A creamed TNA may be safely administered after redispersion, whereas a cracked TNA cannot be restored to its original condition and therefore should be discarded.

Answer c is incorrect. Creamed TNA may be safely administered to patients after redispersion to their original condition.

Answer d is incorrect. Cracked TNA cannot be rehomogenized.

---

12. Which one of the following would be most likely to cause instability when added to a TNA?
    a. Famotidine
    b. Regular insulin
    c. Iron dextran
    d. Copper

Answer a is incorrect. All parenteral H_2 antagonists are stable for at least 24 hours in PN solutions. These are commonly added to PN solutions, either dextrose/amino acids or TNA, for continuous infusion in some hospitals.

Answer b is incorrect. Regular insulin is commonly added to PN solutions. Although insulin may be adsorbed to glass, tubing, and other surfaces, it does not significantly affect stability of a TNA.

Answer c is correct. As a multivalent cation, iron dextran has the capacity to neutralize the zeta potential on fat globules, thus destabilizing a TNA. If parenteral iron is required in a patient receiving a TNA, it can either be administered outside the PN, or it can be administered via a dextrose/amino acid solution on days when the lipid is omitted from the formulation.

Answer d is incorrect. Although copper is a divalent cation, it is commonly added to PN solutions in small amounts as part of a multitrace element package.

---

13. AZ is to receive cycled PN over 16 h/d at home. The PN is to be infused at half the goal rate for the first and last hours of the 16-hour cycle. If the final concentration of amino acid in the solution is 5%, what goal rate of PN (in mL/h) will supply about 80 g of protein per day?
    a. 77
    b. 87
    c. 97
    d. 107

Answers a, b, and c are incorrect.

Answer d is correct. Calculation is as follows:

5 g/100 mL = 80 g/x mL; x = 1600 mL

14 Y + 2(1/2 Y) = 1600 mL; 15 Y = 1600 mL; Y = 107 mL; ½ Y = 53.5 mL

Therefore, infuse 107 mL/h × 14 h + 53.5 mL/h × 2 h = 1605 mL/d.

14. Which of the following most closely reflects the current recommendation for the optimal goal blood glucose range for a critically ill PN patient?
    a. 70 to 100 mg/dL
    b. 80 to 110 mg/dL
    c. 110 to 150 mg/dL
    d. 180 to 240 mg/dL

Answer a is incorrect. Although previously it was recommended to try to maintain euglycemia in critically ill patients, particularly surgical patients, concerns regarding hypoglycemia and increased morbidity in groups of patients in whom intensive insulin protocols were utilized in the NICE-SUGAR Study have led authoritative bodies to recommend less intensive blood sugar control in most patients.

Answer b is incorrect for the reasons outlined for Answer a above.

Answer c is correct. The 2009 Society for Critical Care Medicine and American Society for Parenteral and Enteral Nutrition joint guidelines for nutrition support in critically ill patients call for keeping blood sugar between 110 and 150 mg/dL in most patients. The 2009 American Diabetes Association and American Association of Clinical Endocrinologists joint guidelines for control of diabetes in the hospital setting call for a goal blood glucose of 140 to 180 mg/dL in the critical care setting and 100 to 180 mg/dL for hospitalized general medical-surgical patients.

Answer d is incorrect. Maintenance of blood glucose in the 180 to 240 mg/dL range could lead to increased risk of infection and other complications in both critically ill and other hospitalized general medical-surgical patients.

15. Which one of the following statements is most correct regarding markers of nutritional status in the hospitalized patient?
    a. Albumin, because of its short half-life, is a good marker of the adequacy of a nutritional regimen when followed serially over several days.
    b. Prealbumin has a short half-life and can be useful as a marker of nutritional status.
    c. Transferrin is a very specific marker of overall nutritional status and reflects nutritional status over a period of several days.
    d. To adequately assess nutritional status, albumin, prealbumin, and transferrin should all be monitored weekly.

Answer a is incorrect. With a half-life of about 20 days, albumin is not a good marker of nutritional status over the short term. Levels of albumin can drop precipitously following injury and are thus not good nutritional markers of acute illness. On the other hand, albumin may be a good marker of long-term nutritional status.

Answer b is correct. Prealbumin, with a half-life of only a few days, is much more useful than albumin for monitoring the adequacy of a short-term nutritional intervention in a hospitalized patient. Levels of C-reactive protein (a marker of inflammation) may be concomitantly monitored and are often elevated in the setting of acute stress. Until C-reactive protein levels start dropping toward normal, reflecting resolution of an inflammatory process, the clinician should not really expect to see the prealbumin level rise.

Answer c is incorrect. Transferrin is not a very specific marker of nutritional status. It is affected by iron status as well as other nonnutritional factors.

Answer d is incorrect. Adding monitoring of transferrin levels adds little in the setting where albumin and prealbumin are being utilized as nutritional markers.

16. NJ is a 53-year-old woman who is receiving PN following a bowel resection for mesenteric ischemia. She is receiving a dextrose/amino acid solution with final concentrations of 15% dextrose and 5% amino acid. This solution is being administered at 75 mL/h continuously over 24 hours. She is also receiving 250 mL of 20% lipid each day. Renal function is normal. NJ weighs 60 kg, which is near her ideal body weight of 62 kg. Which of the following best describes the amount of kcal, protein, and dextrose that NJ is receiving?
    a. Calories are excessive, but the amounts of protein and dextrose are within recommended ranges.
    b. The amounts of dextrose and protein are lower than recommended ranges as is the amount of calories.
    c. Protein is below the recommended range, but calories and dextrose are adequate.
    d. The number of calories, as well as the amounts of protein and dextrose, are within recommended ranges.

NJ is currently receiving the following:

Dextrose/amino acid solution: 75 mL/h × 24 h/d = 1800 mL/d

Dextrose: 15 g/100 mL = x g/1800 mL; x = 270 g/d; 270 g/60 kg = 4.5 g/kg/d; 270 g × 3.4 kcal/g = 918 kcal/d

Amino acid: 5 g/100 mL = x g/1800 mL; x = 90 g; 90 g/60 kg = 1.5 g/kg/d; 90 g × 4 kcal/g = 360 kcal/d

Lipid: 250 mL/d × 2 kcal/mL = 500 kcal/d

Total kcal/d = 918 + 360 + 500 = 1778 kcal/d; 1778 kcal/60 kg = 29 kcal/kg/d

Typical recommendations for calories are to provide about 20 to 35 kcal/kg/d to patients who are not overweight or obese.

These patients typically should receive 1.2 to 2 g protein/kg/d and no more than 7 g dextrose/kg/d. Lipid is typically recommended at <2.5 g/kg/d; some authorities recommend limiting lipid to 1 or 2 g/kg/d, especially in immunocompromised patients.

Answer a is incorrect. Calories being administered are not excessive.

Answer b is incorrect. The amounts of dextrose, protein, and calories being administered are within recommended ranges and are not too low.

Answer c is incorrect. Protein being administered is within the recommended range.

Answer d is correct. At 29 kcal/kg/d, calories are being administered within the recommended range of 20 to 35 kcal/kg/d. At 1.5 g/kg/d, protein is being administered within the recommended range of 1.2 to 2 g/kg/d. At 4.5 g/kg/d, dextrose is being administered at the recommended range of <7 g/kg/d; generally at least 100 g/d of dextrose should be provided to fuel dextrose-obligate organs such as the brain.

---

17. Which one of the following vitamins commonly included in PN solutions could interfere with warfarin anticoagulation?

    a. Vitamin D
    b. Vitamin K
    c. Thiamine
    d. Vitamin B_6

Answers a, c, and d are incorrect. Vitamin D, thiamine, and vitamin B_6 do not interfere with the anticoagulant effect of warfarin.

Answer b is correct. Warfarin acts by inhibiting the synthesis of vitamin K-dependent clotting factors II, VII, IX, and X and the anticoagulant proteins C and S. Vitamin K can actually be given in the setting of overcoagulation to reverse the effects of warfarin. Although it could be argued that patients receiving oral medications such as warfarin are not good candidates for PN, the combination of oral warfarin and PN is sometimes encountered. Most of the parenteral multivitamin preparations now commercially available contain 150 μg of vitamin K to be administered as a daily dose.

---

18. Which of the following trace elements is least commonly included in PN solutions?

    a. Iodide
    b. Zinc
    c. Manganese
    d. Copper

Answer a is correct. There is no longer a parenteral trace element product available commercially that contains iodide. Even when it was available, it was not commonly utilized.

Answers b, c, and d are incorrect. Zinc, manganese, copper, and chromium are the four most common trace elements supplied in PN solutions. Selenium is also commonly included.

---

19. What is the most common cause for hospitalization in patients receiving home PN?

    a. Metabolic bone disease
    b. Catheter-related sepsis
    c. Trace element deficiency
    d. Hyperglycemia

Answer a is incorrect. Although metabolic bone disease is a common problem in long-term home PN patients, it is not the most common cause of hospitalization in this population. The etiology of metabolic bone disease in long-term PN is not well elucidated.

Answer b is correct. Catheter-related sepsis is a common adverse event in patients on home PN that often, although not always, results in hospitalization. Because placement of a central venous catheter is an invasive procedure, and suitable venous sites for placement of such catheters are limited, efforts are made if possible to salvage infected catheters rather than removing and replacing them. Treatments include infusion of systemic antibiotics and placement of antibiotic locks within the catheter. Catheter-related sepsis is most commonly caused by gram-positive bacteria but can also be caused by gram-negative bacteria and fungi. Fungal infections almost universally require catheter removal and replacement.

Answer c is incorrect. Trace element deficiencies do occur during long-term home PN, although they can be difficult to definitively diagnose. When a trace element deficiency is suspected, higher amounts of that trace element are generally provided by the PN; this does not usually require hospitalization.

Answer d is incorrect. Hyperglycemia is a potential adverse event during PN, either short term or long term. It is prudent to stabilize blood glucose prior to initial discharge from the hospital on home PN. One setting in which hyperglycemia may develop in a patient on home PN is in the setting of infection such as catheter-related sepsis. In this situation, it is typically the signs and symptoms of infection such as fever, chills, and rigors, rather than hyperglycemia that bring the patient to the hospital.

---

20. HM is a 63-year-old critically ill, morbidly obese man (BMI 42 kg/m^2) with severe acute pancreatitis in whom enteral nutrition has failed. On day 7 of hospitalization, PN is initiated. HM weighs 150 kg; ideal body weight is 82 kg. The PN regimen consists of 1800 kcal/d and 205 g protein per day. What is the most appropriate assessment of this PN regimen?

    a. Appropriate calories and protein
    b. Appropriate calories; too much protein

c. Appropriate protein; too many calories
d. Too few calories; too much protein

Answer a is correct. According to the SCCM/ASPEN nutrition support guidelines for the critically ill, when BMI is >30 kg/m^2, goal calories are 11 to 14 kcal/kg actual body weight per day or 22 to 25 kcal/kg ideal body weight per day. HM's regimen provides 12 kcal/kg actual body weight per day and 22 kcal/kg ideal body weight per day, both of which follow the recommendations. Protein should be provided at ≥2 g/kg ideal body weight per day for BMI 30 to 40 kg/m^2 and at ≥2.5 g/kg ideal body weight per day for BMI >40 kg/m^2. HM's regimen provides 2.5 g/kg ideal body weight per day.

Answer b is incorrect. HM's regimen does not contain too much protein.

Answer c is incorrect. HM's regimen does not contain too many calories.

Answer d is incorrect. HM's regimen does not contain too few calories or too much protein.

CHAPTER 34 | Electrolyte Disorders

1. A 72-year-old man is admitted for a level of low serum sodium at a routine check-up. The patient states he feels fine. Past medical history includes chronic obstructive pulmonary disease, depression, gout, and hypertension. Current medications are albuterol, allopurinol, lisinopril, and sertraline. Physical examination is unremarkable. Pertinent laboratory values include a serum sodium of 123 mEq/L, urinary sodium of 90 mEq/L, and a urine osmolarity of 585 mOsm/L. The patient is diagnosed with SIADH. The most appropriate treatment to correct this patient's sodium abnormality includes:

   a. 3% Saline infusion
   b. Demeclocycline
   c. Stopping the offending agent and fluid restriction
   d. Normal saline infusion

Answer a is incorrect. Hypertonic saline is not indicated in asymptomatic patients. It should be reserved for patients with life-threatening symptoms, such as seizures or coma.

Answer b is incorrect. Agents that interfere with ADH activity in the collecting duct are not typically used when the causative agent can be removed. The cause in this patient is most likely sertraline. Demeclocycline and vasopressin receptor agents may be useful in patients with chronic SIADH who are unresponsive to or cannot tolerate water restriction.

Answer c is correct. In addition to stopping the offending agent, fluid restriction is the mainstay of therapy for acute management of SIADH. The negative water balance can correct serum sodium.

Answer d is incorrect. Infusion of normal saline in a patient with SIADH is inappropriate. Since the patient's renal handling of sodium is intact with an increased absorption of free water, serum sodium can actually fall with a normal saline infusion.

---

2. A medication commonly associated with SIADH is:

   a. Hydrochlorothiazide
   b. Furosemide
   c. Lithium
   d. Sertraline

Answer a is incorrect. Thiazide diuretics are commonly associated with hypovolemic hyponatremia, but do not cause SIADH. Antidiuretic hormone stimulation with thiazide therapy is an appropriate response to the modest hypovolemia caused by thiazides.

Answer b is incorrect. Loop diuretics do not typically cause hyponatremia.

Answer c is incorrect. Lithium is a common cause of nephrogenic diabetes insipidus (hypernatremia). Lithium antagonizes adenyl cyclase and cAMP, and inhibits the opening of aquaporin channels in the renal tubules. This leads to a loss of free water causing hypernatremia when water losses are not replaced.

Answer d is correct. Selective serotonin reuptake inhibitors are commonly associated with SIADH.

---

3. A 68-year-old woman is brought to the hospital because of progressive drowsiness and syncope. She complains of diarrhea for the past 3 days. She is lethargic but has no focal neurologic deficits. Past medical history is significant for lung cancer, depression, hypertension, GERD, and osteoarthritis. Medications include acetaminophen, hydrochlorothiazide, fluoxetine, ranitidine, and magnesium oxide. Physical examination reveals a blood pressure of 96/56 mm Hg, pulse of 110 beats/min, dry mucous membranes, and reduced skin turgor. Laboratory value is significant for serum sodium of 125 mEq/L. The most appropriate treatment to correct this patient's sodium abnormality includes:

   a. 3% Saline infusion
   b. Demeclocycline
   c. Fluid restriction of <1000 mL/d
   d. Normal saline infusion

Answer a is incorrect. Hypertonic saline is not indicated in patients with mild symptoms. It should be reserved for patients with life-threatening symptoms, such as seizures or coma.

Answer b is incorrect. Demeclocycline is used in chronic SIADH and is not indicated for hypovolemic hyponatremia.

Answer c is incorrect. Fluid restriction is used in isovolemic hyponatremia and is not indicated for hypovolemic hyponatremia.

Answer d is correct. Patients with hypovolemic hyponatremia require volume replacement and correction of serum sodium with isotonic saline infusion. Serum sodium should not be corrected faster than 10 to 12 mEq/L in 24 hours or 18 mEq/L in 48 hours.

---

4. A 54-year-old man is admitted to the hospital from the outpatient clinic with abdominal swelling, weight gain, and abnormal laboratory values. Medical history is significant for cirrhosis and hepatitis C. Medications include furosemide and propranolol. His physical examination is significant for distended abdomen with shifting dullness. Significant laboratory values include serum sodium of 124 mEq/L, INR of 1.9, and albumin of 2.1. The most appropriate treatment to correct this patient's sodium abnormality includes:

    a. 3% Saline with IV furosemide
    b. Fluid restriction
    c. Normal saline infusion
    d. Sodium restriction and diuretics

Answer a is incorrect. Hypertonic saline fluid is not indicated in patients without severe CNS symptoms.

Answer b is incorrect. Fluid restriction can be helpful in symptomatic hypervolemic hyponatremia. This patient, however, does not have CNS symptoms.

Answer c is incorrect. Normal saline would be inappropriate in a cirrhotic patient without evidence of volume depletion.

Answer d is correct. The cornerstone of therapy for hyponatremia associated with edema is dietary sodium restriction and diuretic therapy.

---

5. An 82-year-old man was brought to the emergency department by his daughter for worsening confusion and diarrhea. The daughter reports he has had poor oral intake over the last week. Medical history is significant for hypertension, stroke, reflux, and chronic constipation. Medications include aspirin, lactulose, lisinopril, omeprazole, and simvastatin. His physical examination is significant for orthostatic hypotension, tachycardia, and dry mucous membranes. Significant laboratory values include serum sodium of 162 mEq/L, BUN of 66, and serum creatinine of 2.5. Appropriate initial treatment for this patient would include:

    a. 0.45% Saline infusion
    b. 5% Dextrose infusion
    c. Desmopressin
    d. Normal saline infusion

Answer a is incorrect. While hypotonic fluids will help correct this patient's serum sodium, patients with hemodynamic instability (orthostatic hypotension, tachycardia) should first receive normal saline until volume status is restored. Free water, from 0.45% saline or 5% dextrose, distributes throughout the ICF and ECF. Normal saline is the appropriate initial choice. Since it is confined to the ECF, it will restore intravascular volume more efficiently than hypotonic fluids.

Answer b is incorrect. See explanation for Answer a.

Answer c is incorrect. Desmopressin is indicated in patients with central diabetes insipidus.

Answer d is correct. This patient is showing signs of hemodynamic instability (orthostatic hypotension, tachycardia) and should first receive isotonic saline until volume status is restored. After volume repletion, hypotonic fluids would be appropriate to correct serum sodium.

---

6. A 39-year-old man presents to the emergency department with abnormal laboratory values from a local psychiatric hospital. He is 4 days post neurosurgical repair of intraventricular hemorrhage secondary to bilateral self-enucleation. He is currently constrained to the hospital bed and hallucinating. Medical history includes hypertension and schizophrenia. Medications include haloperidol, fluphenazine, and benztropine. Physical examination is normal. Pertinent laboratory values include sodium of 158 mEq/L and a urine osmolarity of 76 mOsm/kg. Urine output was 6500 mL over the last 24 hours. The patient is admitted for the treatment of central diabetes insipidus. The most appropriate treatment to correct this patient's sodium abnormality includes:

    a. Desmopressin
    b. Free access to water
    c. Hydrochlorothiazide
    d. Normal saline infusion

Answer a is correct. Patients with central diabetes insipidus require exogenous ADH.

Answer b is incorrect. Oral replacement of water would be difficult in a restrained, hallucinating patient. Free water should be given in the form of intravenous hypotonic fluids when oral replacement is not possible.

Answer c is incorrect. Hydrochlorothiazide can be useful in nephrogenic diabetes insipidus. This patient requires exogenous ADH replacement.

Answer d is incorrect. Normal saline is not appropriate in hypernatremic patients without signs of volume depletion.

---

7. What is the drug of choice for lithium-induced diabetes insipidus when lithium must be continued?

    a. Amiloride
    b. Desmopressin
    c. Hydrochlorothiazide
    d. Indomethacin

Answer a is correct. Amiloride closes sodium channels in the luminal membrane of the collecting tubule cells. This is the site where lithium enters cells and interferes with the actions of ADH.

Answer b is incorrect. Patient's with nephrogenic diabetes insipidus have a defect in the vasopressin-2 receptor and have an impaired response to ADH. Desmopressin is generally not effective in nephrogenic diabetes insipidus, but may provoke a partial response at high doses.

Answer c is incorrect. Hydrochlorothiazide is useful in the treatment of other forms of nephrogenic diabetes insipidus.

Answer d is incorrect. Indomethacin is useful as adjunctive therapy in the treatment of nephrogenic diabetes insipidus.

---

8. Which is *not* an expected side effect of potassium replacement?
   a. Irritation of the vein
   b. Constipation
   c. Nausea/vomiting
   d. Cardiac arrhythmias
   e. Dyspepsia

Answer a is incorrect. Intravenous administration of potassium may cause vein irritation and phlebitis. Intravenous potassium should be diluted and infused at a slower rate when given through a peripheral vein.

Answer b is correct. Constipation is not commonly associated with potassium replacement. Adverse GI effects related to potassium replacement generally involve nausea and/or vomiting, dyspepsia, and diarrhea.

Answer c is incorrect. Nausea, vomiting, abdominal pain, diarrhea, and indigestion are common side effects of potassium chloride preparations, but all potassium salt formulations have been associated with adverse GI effects. In particular, liquid forms of potassium often have a strong, bitter smell and taste which may result in nausea and vomiting. Microencapsulated formulations are less likely to cause this effect. Administering large doses of potassium replacement orally may also increase the risk of GI upset.

Answer d is incorrect. Cardiac arrhythmias may result when the rate of potassium administration is too high. ECG monitoring is recommended when the rate of potassium administration exceeds 10 mEq/h.

Answer e is incorrect. Dyspepsia is a common adverse effect of oral potassium replacement. Administering large doses of potassium orally increases the likelihood of this effect. It is also recommended to take many formulations of potassium replacement with food and/or a full glass of water to prevent GI irritation.

---

9. A 66-year-old man is seen for annual follow-up. He has a history of hypertension, type 2 diabetes, coronary artery disease, and heart failure. Current medications include spironolactone 25 mg daily, lisinopril 20 mg daily, metoprolol 100 mg twice daily, furosemide 40 mg daily, simvastatin 40 mg daily, metformin 500 mg twice daily, and aspirin 81 mg daily. Laboratory values reveal Na 141, K 5.6, BUN 11, SCr 1.1, Phos 3.5, and Mg 2.2. Patient has no complaints at this time. What is the most likely cause of this patient's hyperkalemia?
   a. Spironolactone
   b. Metoprolol
   c. Metformin
   d. Furosemide
   e. Simvastatin

Answer a is correct. Spironolactone is a potassium-sparing diuretic. The development of hyperkalemia with spironolactone and other drugs, which decrease the activity of aldosterone, is well described. Serum potassium concentration should be monitored periodically after administration or dose titration of these types of drugs.

Answer b is incorrect. β-Blockers may cause a slight rise in serum potassium levels. However, total body potassium is not affected during treatment with these drugs. Isolated case reports of hyperkalemia with β-blocking agents in patients experiencing acute acid–base disorders can be found; however, these reports are rare.

Answer c is incorrect. Metformin is not known to cause hyperkalemia.

Answer d is incorrect. Furosemide is not associated with hyperkalemia. Conversely, this and other loop and thiazide diuretics are commonly associated with the development of hypokalemia through increased renal elimination of potassium.

Answer e is incorrect. Simvastatin is not known to cause hyperkalemia.

---

10. Which hyperkalemia treatment results in a reduction in total body potassium?
    a. IV sodium bicarbonate
    b. IV Insulin and dextrose
    c. IV calcium
    d. PO sodium polystyrene sulfonate (SPS)
    e. Nebulized albuterol

Answer a is incorrect. Intravenous sodium bicarbonate lowers the serum potassium concentration by causing potassium ions to shift intracellularly. It is most effective for hyperkalemia associated with metabolic acidosis.

Answer b is incorrect. Insulin decreases the serum potassium concentration through stimulation of the Na^+-K^+-ATPase pump. This results in the intracellular shift of potassium ions from the serum. Dextrose is usually administered concurrently to prevent the development of hypoglycemia from insulin administration. Additionally, dextrose stimulates the secretion of endogenous insulin.

Answer c is incorrect. The intent of calcium administration in the treatment of hyperkalemia is not to affect the serum potassium concentration. Rather, it slows conduction and stabilizes the cardiac membrane potential to prevent development of cardiac arrhythmias, which may result from excessive serum potassium concentrations.

Answer d is correct. Sodium polystyrene sulfonate is a cation exchange resin which works by exchanging sodium for potassium as it passes through the intestine or colon. The bound potassium ions are then excreted with normal GI transit, effectively removing potassium from the body and reducing total body potassium.

Answer e is incorrect. β-agonists result in reduction in serum potassium concentration via two separate mechanisms. β-agonists, including albuterol, stimulate the Na^+-K^+-ATPase pump to move potassium intracellularly. Additionally, these agents increase the release of insulin through stimulation of pancreatic β-cells.

---

11. Which statement best describes a mechanism of potassium homeostasis?
    a. Insulin decreases the intracellular uptake of potassium.
    b. Aldosterone increases potassium excretion.
    c. Calcitonin increases the tubular reabsorption of potassium.
    d. Increasing the plasma pH decreases the uptake of potassium into the cells.
    e. β-Receptor stimulation increases movement of potassium extracellularly.

Answer a is incorrect. Insulin increases the intracellular uptake of potassium through stimulation the Na^+-K^+-ATPase pump to move potassium intracellularly.

Answer b is correct. Aldosterone promotes urinary excretion of potassium in the distal tubule and collecting duct as it increases reabsorption of sodium and water.

Answer c is incorrect. Calcitonin increases the urinary excretion of sodium, chloride, magnesium, calcium, phosphate, and potassium by limiting tubular reabsorption.

Answer d is incorrect. Increasing the plasma pH increases the uptake of potassium inside cells as extracellular potassium is exchanged for intracellular hydrogen ions. This is the therapeutic effect desired when sodium bicarbonate is administered in the treatment of hyperkalemia.

Answer e is incorrect. Stimulation of β-receptors increases the intracellular uptake of potassium through stimulation of the Na^+-K^+-ATPase pump.

---

12. A 48-year-old man presents to the ambulatory clinic with complaints of palpitations over the past few days. Current medications are ramipril 10 mg daily, aspirin 325 mg daily, and omeprazole 20 mg daily. Vitals are blood pressure 152/90 mm Hg, pulse 90, temp 98.6°F, and respiratory rate 14 breaths/min. Laboratory values reveal Na 141, K 5.9, Cl 101, HCO_3 25, BUN 12, SCr 1.1, and glucose 115. ECG showed peaked T waves. Which is the most appropriate initial management for this patient's hyperkalemia?
    a. PO sodium polystyrene sulfonate (SPS)
    b. IV calcium
    c. IV sodium bicarbonate
    d. Nebulized albuterol
    e. IV Insulin and dextrose

Answer a is incorrect. Oral SPS should be administered early in the course of therapy for this patient, but the effect will not be seen for several hours. Because the patient is symptomatic from the hyperkalemia, IV calcium should be given initially to provide cardiovascular protection.

Answer b is correct. IV calcium should be administered initially because the patient has symptomatic ECG changes. Stabilization of the cardiac membrane potential should be addressed immediately, but quickly followed with measures to alleviate the burden of the serum potassium concentration. This can be accomplished rapidly by stimulating the shift of potassium ions intracellularly. IV sodium bicarbonate, nebulized albuterol, and IV insulin and dextrose will all stimulate transcellular potassium shifting. The best choice for this patient is likely IV insulin and dextrose. Sodium bicarbonate is especially useful for patients with concomitant metabolic acidosis which this patient lacks, and high doses of albuterol may exacerbate this patient's hypertension and tachycardia. It is important to remember that the effect of transcellular shift is transient, so additional therapy which enhances the elimination of potassium from the body should be administered early in the course of therapy. SPS is commonly employed, but it will take several hours to see the therapeutic effect.

Answer c is incorrect. Because the patient is symptomatic from the hyperkalemia, IV calcium should be given initially to provide cardiovascular protection. IV sodium bicarbonate is effective in causing intracellular shifting of potassium ions and is especially useful in patients with concomitant metabolic acidosis.

Answer d is incorrect. Because the patient is symptomatic from the hyperkalemia, IV calcium should be given initially to provide cardiovascular protection. Nebulized albuterol is effective in causing intracellular shifting of potassium ions but may exacerbate concomitant hypertension and/or tachycardia.

Answer e is incorrect. Because the patient is symptomatic from the hyperkalemia, IV calcium should be given initially to provide cardiovascular protection. IV insulin and dextrose is effective in causing intracellular shifting of potassium ions and would be the preferred therapy administered, immediately following IV calcium, to decrease the burden of the serum potassium concentration for this patient.

---

13. Which is *not* an expected symptom of hypermagnesemia?
    a. Hypotension
    b. Flushing
    c. Coma

d. ECG changes
e. Diarrhea

Answer a is incorrect. Hypotension is a common symptom of hypermagnesemia. It typically appears as the magnesium concentration exceeds 3 mEq/L.

Answer b is incorrect. Flushing is a common symptom of hypermagnesemia. Flushing results from cutaneous vasodilation.

Answer c is incorrect. Coma can result from hypermagnesemia. It does not usually appear until the serum magnesium concentration is around 10 mEq/L.

Answer d is incorrect. ECG changes associated with hypermagnesemia typically begin with QT interval prolongation but can progress to heart block and asystole.

Answer e is correct. Diarrhea is not commonly associated with hypermagnesemia. Diarrhea is a common adverse effect of oral magnesium replacement for hypomagnesemia. Additionally, diarrhea is a common cause of hypomagnesemia.

---

14. Which commonly causes hypomagnesemia?

a. Amphotericin b
b. Amiloride
c. Lithium
d. Lisinopril
e. Omeprazole

Answer a is correct. Magnesium and potassium wasting are commonly associated with amphotericin b therapy and usually require replacement.

Answer b is incorrect. Hypomagnesemia is not commonly associated with amiloride treatment.

Answer c is incorrect. Hypomagnesemia is not commonly associated with lithium treatment.

Answer d is incorrect. Hypomagnesemia is not commonly associated with lisinopril treatment.

Answer e is incorrect. Hypomagnesemia is not commonly associated with omeprazole treatment.

---

15. Loop diuretics are commonly associated with all except:

a. Hypokalemia
b. Hypocalcemia
c. Hypermagnesemia
d. Hypomagnesemia

Answer a is incorrect. Hypokalemia commonly occurs with loop diuretic administration due to decreased renal reabsorption. Monitoring of potassium concentration is required.

Answer b is incorrect. Hypocalcemia is not unexpected with loop diuretic administration. Monitoring of calcium is recommended.

Answer c is correct. Loop diuretics cause renal wasting of potassium, calcium, and magnesium. This would result in hypomagnesemia as opposed to hypermagnesemia.

Answer d is incorrect. Hypomagnesemia is not unexpected with loop diuretic administration due to decreased renal reabsorption. Monitoring of magnesium is recommended.

---

16. Which statement most accurately describes hormonal regulation of calcium and phosphate homeostasis?

a. Vitamin D reduces calcium and phosphate levels.
b. Calcitonin decreases calcium levels.
c. Parathyroid hormone (PTH) decreases calcium levels and increases phosphate levels.

Answer a is incorrect. Vitamin D increases calcium and phosphate levels by increasing intestinal absorption and renal reabsorption.

Answer b is correct. Calcitonin decreases calcium mobilization from the bone and increases renal excretion of calcium.

Answer c is incorrect. PTH increases calcium levels and decreases phosphate levels.

---

17. A 55-year-old woman with a past medical history of multiple myeloma is admitted to the hospital with nausea, abdominal pain, and severe constipation. Current laboratory values are Na 140, K 4.2, Cl 103, CO_2 24, BUN 13, SCr 0.9, Glu 123, Mg 2.2, Ca 11.5, Phos 4, and albumin 1.3. She is currently receiving normal saline and furosemide 20 mg IV q4h with adequate urine output. Select the best treatment to prevent recurrence of her hypercalcemia.

a. Intranasal calcitonin
b. IV potassium phosphate
c. Sevelamer
d. IV pamidronate 90 mg

Answer a is incorrect. Intranasal calcitonin is used to acutely manage hypercalcemia in patients who would not tolerate IV fluids and furosemide. Bisphosphonate therapy is the preferred treatment for malignancy-induced hypercalcemia.

Answer b is incorrect. This patient's potassium and phosphate are within normal limits, and she does not need to receive IV replacement of phosphate or potassium.

Answer c is incorrect. Sevelamer is a phosphate binder used to manage hyperphosphatemia. Most commonly used in patients with chronic kidney disease.

Answer d is correct. Pamidronate is a bisphosphonate. These are the drugs of choice for treatment and prevention of malignancy-induced hypercalcemia. Bisphosphonates inhibit osteoclast activity and decrease bone resorption and osteolysis.

---

18. Which adverse effect may be associated with pamidronate therapy?
    a. Constipation
    b. Tachycardia
    c. Osteonecrosis of the jaw

Answer a is incorrect. Bisphosphonate therapy is used to treat malignancy-induced hypercalcemia, which may commonly be associated with constipation.

Answer b is incorrect. Bisphosphonate therapy is not commonly associated with tachycardia.

Answer c is correct. Intravenous administration of bisphosphonate therapy has been associated with acute renal failure, and esophagitis has occurred after oral administration. Recently, numerous case reports have described a new complication: osteonecrosis of the jaw.

---

19. A patient with hyperparathyroidism is admitted to the medical intensive care unit with pneumonia and respiratory distress requiring mechanical ventilation. Current laboratory values are Na 144, K 3.4, Cl 105, CO_2 24, BUN 16, SCr 0.9, Glu 130, Mg 1.9, Ca 9, Phos 0.8, and albumin 4. Select the best medication to manage this patient's phosphate disorder.
    a. IV sodium phosphate
    b. IV potassium phosphate
    c. IV calcium chloride
    d. PO Neutra-Phos

Answer a is incorrect. Patient has a normal sodium level and should not receive sodium phosphate.

Answer b is correct. This patient's phosphate is severely low and may by contributing to the respiratory distress, which warrants intravenous phosphate administration. Additionally, the patient is hypokalemic; therefore, the patient should receive intravenous potassium phosphate. The dose should be infused over 4 to 6 hours to prevent precipitate formation.

Answer c is incorrect. This patient's calcium is within normal limits and the patient is not displaying signs and symptoms of hypocalcemia.

Answer d is incorrect. This patient has severe hypophosphatemia with respiratory distress; therefore, the patient should receive intravenous phosphate replacement.

---

20. A 70-year-old man on hemodialysis with Stage 5 chronic kidney disease (CKD) presents to the nephrology clinic for routine follow-up. Past medical history includes ESRD, hypertension, and type II diabetes. Current medications include amlodipine 10 mg daily, lisinopril 20 mg daily, glipizide 10 mg daily, aspirin 325 mg daily. Current laboratory values are BUN 60, SCr 4.5, Ca 9, Phos 8, and albumin 2. Which is the best initial management of this patient's hyperphosphatemia?
    a. Calcium acetate
    b. Sevelamer
    c. Discontinuation of lisinopril
    d. Calcium carbonate

Answer a is incorrect. This patient's corrected calcium is 10.6 (corrected calcium = measured calcium + [0.8 (4 – measured albumin)]), and his calcium-phosphate product is 84.8 mg/dL. This would increase his risk of soft tissue calcifications; therefore, he should receive a noncalcium-containing phosphate binder. It will minimize phosphate absorption in the GI tract and not further increase calcium levels.

Answer b is correct. Sevelamer (Renagel) is the best initial management for this patient because his corrected calcium is 10.6 and his calcium-phosphate product is 84.8 mg/dL. This would increase his risk of soft tissue calcifications. Sevelamer is a noncalcium-, nonaluminum-containing phosphate binder that reduces phosphate absorption in the GI tract and does not further increase calcium levels.

Answer c is incorrect. Lisinopril is an ACEI that is associated with hyperkalemia, not calcium or phosphate disorders.

Answer d is incorrect. This patient's corrected calcium is 10.6 (corrected calcium = measured calcium + [0.8 (4 – measured albumin)]), and his calcium-phosphate product is 84.8 mg/dL. This would increase his risk of soft tissue calcifications; therefore, he should receive a noncalcium-containing phosphate binder. It will minimize phosphate absorption in the GI tract and not further increase calcium levels.

---

21. Patients should be counseled to take a phosphate binder:
    a. With meals to reduce phosphate absorption
    b. With meals to increase phosphate absorption
    c. With meals to reduce GI side effects
    d. Between meals to reduce food–drug interactions

Answer a is correct. Phosphate binders are to be given with meals to minimize the absorption of dietary phosphate.

Answers b, c, and d are incorrect. Phosphate binders are taken with meals to reduce not increase phosphate absorption.

---

22. Which electrolyte abnormalities commonly occur in patients with chronic kidney disease?
    i. Hyperkalemia
    ii. Hyperphosphatemia
    iii. Hypomagnesemia

    a. i only
    b. iii only
    c. i and ii
    d. ii and ii
    e. i, ii, and iii

Answer a is incorrect. Chronic kidney disease is associated with both hyperkalemia and hyperphosphatemia.

Answer b is incorrect. Chronic kidney disease is not commonly associated with hypomagnesemia. Patients with chronic kidney disease are at increased risk of developing hypermagnesemia.

Answer c is correct. Chronic kidney disease, especially Stage 5, is most commonly associated with hyperkalemia and hyperphosphatemia.

Answer d is incorrect. Chronic kidney disease is associated with hyperphosphatemia but not hypophosphatemia.

Answer e is incorrect. Chronic kidney disease is associated with both hyperkalemia and hyperphosphatemia, but not hypomagnesemia.

CHAPTER 35 | Estimating Renal Function

1. AR is a 50-year-old Caucasian woman who is 63 in tall and weighs 165 lb. Her current serum creatinine is 1.6 mg/dL. What is her ideal body weight (IBW)?

   a. 125 lb
   b. 115 lb
   c. 135 lb
   d. 165 lb

Answer b is correct.

IBW (women) = 45.5 + 2.3 (3 in over 5 ft) = 52.4 kg × 2.2 lb/1 kg = 115 lb

---

2. What is AR's creatinine clearance as estimated by the Cockcroft-Gault equation?

   a. 41 mL/min
   b. 34 mL/min
   c. 50 mL/min
   d. 58 mL/min

Answer b is correct.

CrCl = [(140 – 50) × 52.4 kg /72 × 1.6 mg/dL] × 0.85 = ~35 mL/min

---

3. What is AR's GFR as estimated by the MDRD equation?

   a. 25 mL/min
   b. 35 mL/min
   c. 45 mL/min
   d. 55 mL/min

Answer b is correct.

GFR = $186 \times 1.6^{-1.154} \times 50^{-0.203} \times 0.742$ = ~36 mL/min

---

4. TM is a 79-year-old African American man who is 71 in tall and weighs 254 lb. His current serum creatinine is 1.2 mg/dL. What is his ideal body weight (IBW)?

   a. 145 lb
   b. 156 lb
   c. 166 lb
   d. 254 lb

Answer c is correct.

IBW (man) = 50 + 2.3 (11 in over 5 ft) = 75.3 kg × 2.2 lb/1 kg = 166 lb

---

5. What is TM's creatinine clearance as estimated by the Cockcroft-Gault equation?

   a. 69 mL/min
   b. 45 mL/min
   c. 81 mL/min
   d. 53 mL/min

Answer d is correct.

CrCl = (140 – 79) × 75.3 kg /72 × 1.2 mg/dL = ~53 mL/min

---

6. What is TM's GFR as estimated by the MDRD equation?

   a. 45 mL/min
   b. 55 mL/min
   c. 65 mL/min
   d. 75 mL/min

Answer d is correct.

GFR = $186 \times 1.2^{-1.154} \times 79^{-0.203} \times 1.210$ = ~75 mL/min

---

7. AB is a 4-year-old girl who is 42 in tall and weighs 50 lb. Her current serum creatinine is 0.6 mg/dL. What is AB's estimated GFR based on the Schwartz equation?

   a. ~30 mL/min
   b. ~60 mL/min
   c. ~80 mL/min
   d. ~100 mL/min

Answer d is correct.

42 in × 2.54 cm/in × 0.55/0.6 mg/dL = ~100 mL/min

---

8. DW is a 6-month-old infant who is 25 in long and weighs 15 lb. His current serum creatinine is 0.4 mg/dL. What is DW's estimated GFR based on the Schwartz equation?

   a. 60 mL/min
   b. 70 mL/min
   c. 80 mL/min
   d. 90 mL/min

Answer b is correct.

25 in × 2.54 cm/in × 0.45/0.4 mg/dL = ~70 mL/min

9. Which of the following factors independent from GFR affect serum creatinine?
   a. Age
   b. Diet
   c. Gender
   d. Race
   e. All of the above

Answers a, b, c, and d are correct.

Answer e is correct and the best answer. Age, diet, gender, and race all can affect serum creatinine in patients.

10. Which of the following patients would be most likely to have a baseline serum creatinine of <0.8?
    a. A 24-year-old man in very good health
    b. A 35-year-old man adhering to the Atkins diet
    c. A 93-year-old woman who is wheelchair bound
    e. A bodybuilder taking creatine supplements

Answer a is incorrect. This patient is most likely to have a serum creatinine in the normal range of 0.8 to 1.2.

Answer b is incorrect. Since the Atkins diet is extremely high in protein, this patient will likely have a serum creatinine in the high end of the normal range or slightly above the normal range. Excessive protein intake can increase serum creatinine.

Answer c is correct. This patient likely has very little muscle mass, which will contribute to a below normal serum creatinine.

Answer d is incorrect. This patient will likely have a higher than normal serum creatinine due to the addition of creatine supplements to the diet.

11. Which of the following is considered the gold standard for measurement of GFR?
    a. Cockcroft-Gault equation
    b. MDRD equation
    c. 24-hour urine creatinine
    d. Inulin clearance

Answer a is incorrect. The Cockcroft-Gault equation is the most commonly used method to estimate creatinine clearance but does not *measure* GFR.

Answer b is incorrect. The MDRD equation estimates but does not measure GFR.

Answer c is incorrect. Twenty-four hour urine creatinine analysis has shown to be no more accurate than the Cockcroft-Gault and MDRD equations and does not measure GFR.

Answer d is correct. Inulin clearance method is considered the gold standard for measurement of GFR. It is rarely done in clinical practice due to cost and complexity issues.

12. Which of the following factors are important to consider when dosing a medication based on renal function?
    a. The extent to which the drug is renally eliminated
    b. The potential for drug toxicity
    c. The manufacturer-recommended dosing guidelines for the agent
    d. All of the above are important factors to consider

Answer d is correct. All of these factors are important to consider when dosing a medication based on renal function.

13. RT is a 50-year-old man who is admitted with serum creatinine of 1.1 mg/dL. Twenty-four hours later, his serum creatinine is 2.0 mg/dL. RT is on several medications that need to be dose-adjusted for renal function. What is the most appropriate course of action?
    a. Calculate RT's GFR using the MDRD equation and dose adjust based on the result.
    b. Calculate RT's CrCl using the Cockcroft-Gault equation and dose-adjust based on the result.
    c. Discontinue all of RT's medications until his renal function improves.
    d. Assess each of RT's medications and use clinical judgment to determine the best course of action, balancing the risk of treatment failure and drug toxicity.

Answer a is incorrect. The MDRD equation may overestimate GFR is this patient who is in acute renal failure. This could lead to overdosing and potential toxicities.

Answer b is incorrect. The Cockcroft-Gault equation may also overestimate renal function in a patient with acute renal failure.

Answer c is incorrect. It would be inappropriate to simply discontinue necessary medications.

Answer d is correct. Each medication should be assessed to determine the most appropriate course of action based on the patient's condition and the combined risks of drug toxicity and treatment failure.

14. TY is an 88-year-old man who weighs 70 kg and is 71 in tall. His current serum creatinine is 0.5. What is his creatinine clearance as estimated by the Cockcroft-Gault equation?
    a. 101 mL/min
    b. 51 mL/min
    c. 92 mL/min
    d. 46 mL/min

Answer b is correct. TY has a serum creatinine <1.0 mg/dL, so we should round up to 1.0 mg/dL when using the Cockcroft-Gault equation. CrCl = (140 – 88) × 70 kg/72 × 1.0 = 51 mL/min

15. FW is a 33-year-old woman with a serum creatinine of 1.3 mg/dL. She is 64 in tall and weighs 118 lb. She has no past medical history. Which of the following methods is the most appropriate way to estimate her renal function?

a. Schwartz equation.
b. MDRD equation.
c. Cockcroft-Gault equation.
d. Both b and c are appropriate.
e. All of the above are appropriate.

Answers a and e are incorrect. The Schwartz equation is used for pediatric patients.

Answer b is correct. The MDRD may be used to estimate the renal function in this patient.

Answer c is correct. The Cockcroft-Gault equation may be used to estimate the renal function in this patient.

Answer d is correct and is the best answer. Both the MDRD and Cockcroft-Gault equations would be appropriate methods to estimate this patient's renal function. However, pharmacokinetics analysis and the National Kidney Foundation endorse the Cockcroft-Gault equation for medication dosing.

---

16. QR is a 32-year-old Caucasian woman who is 67 in tall and weighs 88 lb. Her current serum creatinine is 0.8 mg/dL. What is QRs IBW?

a. 135 lb
b. 125 lb
c. 145 lb
d. 85 lb

Answer a is correct.

IBW (women) = 45.5 + 2.3 (7 in over 5 ft) = 61.6 kg × 2.2 lb/1 kg = 135 lb

---

17. What is QRs CrCl as estimated by the Cockcroft-Gault equation?

a. 98 mL/min
b. 115 mL/min
c. 64 mL/min
d. 75 mL/min

Answer c is correct. Since QRs actual body weight is less than her IBW, actual body weight should be used.

$$\text{CrCl} = [(140 - 32) \times 40 \text{ kg}/72 \times 0.8] \times 0.85 = \sim 60 \text{ to } 65 \text{ mL/min}$$

---

18. What is QRs GFR as estimated by the MDRD equation?

a. 54 mL/min
b. 66 mL/min
c. 75 mL/min
d. 88 mL/min

Answer d is correct.

$$\text{GFR} = 186 \times 0.8^{-1.154} \times 32^{-0.203} \times 0.742 = \sim 88 \text{ mL/min}$$

---

19. Select the normal serum creatinine for an adult patient.

a. 0.3 mg/dL
b. 0.7 mg/dL
c. 1.7 mg/dL
d. 2.0 mg/dL

Answer a is incorrect. The normal range for serum creatinine is from 0.6 to 1.2 mg/dL; however, this can vary between assays. A serum creatinine value of 0.3 mg/dL may indicate low muscle mass.

Answer b is correct. The normal range for serum creatinine is from 0.6 to 1.2 mg/dL; however, just because this serum creatinine value lies within a normal range does not mean that the patient has effective kidney filtration. Other factors would have to be evaluated to estimate GFR, such as age, weight, sex, race (for the MDRD), muscle mass, and urine output.

Answer c is incorrect. A serum creatinine of 1.7 mg/dL lies outside the normal range for serum creatinine.

Answer d is incorrect. A serum creatinine of 2.0 mg/dL lies outside the normal range of serum creatinine.

---

20. Select the weight that should be used to calculate the CrCl via the Cockcroft-Gault method.

a. Ideal body weight
b. Actual body weight
c. Adjusted body weight
d. All of the above

Answer a is correct. Ideal body weight should be used to calculate CrCl. However, the Cockcroft-Gault equation is a population mathematical model used to estimate kidney filtration within an individual patient. Patient extremes may introduce variability and the mathematical model will lose accuracy. For example, the Cockcroft-Gault method was not validated on using extreme patient populations; therefore, obese patients may have an inaccurate estimation of GFR compared to nonobese patients. The ideal body weight should be used in obese patients for purposes of estimating CrCl.

Answer b is incorrect. Actual body weight should not be used in calculating the CrCl *unless* the actual body weight is less than the calculated ideal body weight.

Answer c is incorrect. Adjusted body weight takes into account the patients lean body mass and a percentage of the total body weight. Adjusted body weight = ideal body weight + 0.4 (actual body weight − ideal body weight). This equation may be used for calculation of volume of distribution for certain drugs that are heavily distributed into tissues for obese patients. Adjusted body weight would not be used for estimation of GFR.

Answer d is incorrect. Only the ideal body weight should be used for calculation of CrCl, unless the actual body weight is less than the ideal body weight.

CHAPTER 36 | Acute Kidney Injury

1. HL is a 69-year-old woman who presents to the emergency room complaining of severe nausea and vomiting for 3 days. On admission her serum creatinine is 2.0 mg/dL (her baseline is 0.8 mg/dL). She has not been able to eat or drink for 3 days and has lost 2.5 kg. Her medications on admission include: hydrochlorothiazide 25 mg po every day, lisinopril 10 mg po every day. Which of the following statements is *false* regarding HL at this time?

   a. Nausea and vomiting may have caused a decrease in her effective arterial blood volume leading to pre-renal AKI.
   b. HL should not receive radio contrast media unless absolutely necessary until her kidneys recover.
   c. Hydrochlorothiazide may have caused vasoconstriction of the afferent arteriole leading to pre-renal AKI.
   d. Lisinopril should be discontinued until HL's kidney function returns near her baseline.
   e. HL's weight loss suggests fluid volume depletion.

Answer a is a true statement. Nausea and vomiting can lead to decreased fluid volume and a decrease in EABV. A decrease in EABV will result in decreased perfusion to the kidneys and may result in pre-renal AKI.

Answer b is a true statement. Radio contrast media can cause ATN, and given that this patient already has AKI, the administration of any known nephrotoxins should be avoided if possible. If the use of radio contrast media is necessary, HL should be adequately hydrated prior to the administration.

Answer c is a *false* statement, and therefore the correct answer. Hydrochlorothiazide is a thiazide-type diuretic. It acts in the distal tubule to block sodium reabsorption and thereby enhances sodium and water excretion. While this agent may have contributed to HL's AKI by this mechanism, it does not constrict the afferent arteriole.

Answer d is a true statement. Lisinopril is an angiotensin-converting enzyme inhibitor and acts to vasodilate the efferent arteriole. This action, in combination with the volume depletion HL is experiencing may have contributed to the pre-renal AKI. While ACE-I may be beneficial in slowing progression of chronic kidney disease, further decreasing the intraglomerular pressure during any type of AKI may potentiate or prolong the damage to the kidney.

Answer e is a true statement. HL's sudden weight loss is likely due to acute water loss. Volume depletion, in combination with the other risk factors likely caused HL's pre-renal AKI.

---

2. Which of the following findings are most consistent with the diagnosis of pre-renal AKI?

   a. Specific gravity 1.029, FeNa 0.72%, uOsmol 550 mOsm/kg
   b. Specific gravity 1.013, FeNa 1.72%, uOsmol 350 mOsm/L
   c. Specific gravity 1.009, FeNa 2.02%, uOsmol 213 mOsm/L
   d. Urinalysis: 1+ protein, 10 to 15 RBC, 10 to 15 WBC
   e. Urinalysis: 3+ protein, no RBC, no WBC

Answer a is correct. A high specific gravity, low FeNa, and high urine osmolality is indicative of a pre-renal AKI, a state in which the kidneys will avidly reabsorb sodium and water in an attempt to increase the perfusion to the kidneys and increase the intraglomerular pressure.

Answer b is incorrect. The specific gravity suggests normal urine density. The FeNa is within the normal range of 1% to 2%. The urine osmolality is also normal. These urine findings are not suggestive of any specific kidney damage.

Answer c is incorrect. In this situation the specific gravity is low, suggesting a diluted urine. The FeNa is possibly a little elevated, suggesting excess sodium loss. The urine osmolality is a bit low. These findings are the opposite of what might be seen in a pre-renal AKI

Answer d is incorrect. The protein and cellular matter in this urinalysis are suggestive of some type of intrinsic AKI. Typically, in pre-renal AKI there will not be any particulate matter in the urine.

Answer e is incorrect. This urinalysis shows isolated, significant, proteinuria. Proteinuria suggests a defect within the glomerulus and intrinsic damage, not pre-renal AKI.

---

3. A patient in the intensive care unit develops AKI. You review the medications the patient has been taking to evaluate for drug-induced AKI. Which of the following agents would be *most likely* to cause AIN?

   a. Labetalol
   b. Diltiazem
   c. Cefazolin
   d. Fentanyl
   e. Propofol

Answer a is incorrect. Labetolol is a nonselective beta-1 and beta-2 antagonist as well as an alpha-1 antagonist. Although it is possible to mount an allergic response to any foreign substance, this is not a common cause of AIN. This agent would more likely contribute to a pre-renal AKI through its ability to lower blood pressure and decrease renal perfusion.

Answer b is incorrect. Diltiazem is a nondihydropyridine calcium channel antagonist. Although it is possible to mount an allergic response to any foreign substance, this is not a common cause of AIN. This agent would more likely contribute to a pre-renal AKI as it can lower blood pressure and heart rate which could decrease cardiac output and therefore decrease renal perfusion.

Answer c is correct. Cefazolin is a first generation cephalosporin, structurally related to penicillin. Acute interstitial nephritis is a hypersensitivity reaction and was most commonly associated with methacillin and penicillin derivatives.

Answer d is incorrect. Fentanyl is a narcotic analgesic that acts centrally on opioid receptors. It can cause respiratory depression and hypotension. It is an unlikely cause of a hypersensitivity reaction.

Answer e is incorrect. Propofol is a sedative agent commonly use in the critical care setting. Although it is not a common cause of an allergic reaction (or AIN), it may contribute to a pre-renal AKI due to untoward decrease in blood pressure and therefore renal perfusion.

---

4. Which of the following statements is *true* regarding the use of diuretics in patients with oliguric AKI?
   a. Diuretics may increase urine output and reverse kidney damage.
   b. Diuretics should never be used in AKI as they may cause dehydration and exacerbate AKI.
   c. Diuretics can be used in very high doses as there are no toxicities to be concerned with.
   d. Thiazides and potassium-sparing diuretics are the preferred agents in AKI.
   e. Diuretics may improve urine output and help manage fluid and electrolyte abnormalities.

Answer a is incorrect. Diuretics remove fluid, predominantly from the intravascular space. For this reason, they may actually worsen AKI and must be used with extreme caution.

Answer b is incorrect. If used unwisely, diuretics may cause acute dehydration and worsen AKI. If these agents are used properly, they may aid in the management of fluid and electrolyte disorders and enhance elimination of toxins.

Answer c is incorrect. High doses of diuretics can have serious consequences such as ototoxicity. While higher doses may be necessary to overcome diuretic resistance in AKI, careful monitoring should be employed.

Answer d is incorrect. While thiazide-type diuretics may be used in combination with loop diuretics to enhance urine production, they are not generally effective in cases of decreased kidney function. Potassium-sparing diuretics are generally contraindicated, especially if the patient is anuric/oliguric as hyperkalemia may occur rapidly and is potentially life threatening.

Answer e is the correct. While studies have shown that nonoliguric patients have better outcomes than oliguric/anuric patients, there is no evidence that demonstrates that enhancing urine production through diuretic use confers these better outcomes. Diuretics may be helpful in controlling fluid overload and electrolyte abnormalities (particularly hyperkalemia).

---

5. Which of the following agents can cause constriction of the *afferent* arteriole?
   a. Nonsteroidal anti-inflammatory agents (NSAIDs)
   b. Calcineurin inhibitors
   c. Angiotensin-converting enzyme inhibitors (ACE-I)
   d. a and b only
   e. a, b, and c

Answer a is one of the correct answers. Vasodilatory prostaglandins such as PGE2 and PGI maintain the tone in the afferent arteriole. Nonsteroidal anti-inflammatory agents act by inhibiting cyclooxygenase and thereby prevent the production of prostaglandins. Thus, NSAIDs may lead to constriction of the afferent arteriole and a decrease in intraglomerular pressure.

Answer b is one of the correct answers. The calcineurin inhibitors, such as tacrolimus and cyclosporine cause vasoconstriction of the afferent arteriole and thereby decrease intraglomerular pressure.

Answer c is incorrect. Angiotensin-converting enzyme inhibitors decrease/prevent the production of angiotensin II. Angiotensin II acts to vasoconstrict the efferent arteriole and maintain tone and pressure. A decrease in angiotensin II leads to vasodialtion of the efferent arteriole and a subsequent decrease in intraglomerular pressure.

Answer d is correct and the best answer as it combines both answer a and b.

Answer e is incorrect as it includes answer c. While ACE-I can decrease the intraglomerular pressure and may contribute to a pre-renal AKI, they have a different mechanism of action.

---

6. Which of the following combinations would be most effective to enhance urine production in a patient who has oliguric ARF secondary to ATN?
   a. Furosemide and ethacrynic acid
   b. Triamterene and hydrochlorothiazide
   c. Bumetanide and spironolactone
   d. Furosemide and metolazone
   e. Spironolactone and metolazone

Answer a is incorrect. Both furosemide and ethacrynic acid are loop-type diuretics. They share the same mechanism of action, inhibiting sodium reabsorption in the loop of Henle. The use of two agents with the same mechanism of action would not be expected to produce synergistic effects.

Answer b is incorrect. Triamterene is a potassium-sparing diuretic and would be relatively contraindicated in oliguria/anuria. Hydrochlorothiazide works in the distal tubule. In oliguria, the delivery of sodium to the distal tubule is decreased and therefore the efficacy of hydrochlorothiazide would also be decreased.

Answer c is incorrect. While bumetanide is a loop-type diuretic that would be useful in oliguric ATN, spironolactone would be relatively contraindicated. Spironolactone is aldosterone antagonist and would therefore increase the elimination of sodium (and water) but enhance the reabsorption of potassium.

Answer d is correct. The combination of a loop-type (furosemide) and a thiazide diuretic (metolazone) synergistically enhances urine production. By preventing the reabsorption in the loop of Henle more sodium remains in the tubular lumen and is delivered to the distal tubule. Blocking sodium channels in the distal tubule (thiazides) promotes the excretion of the sodium and water (now from both the loop of Henle and the distal tubule).

Answer e is incorrect. As before, spironolactone use may result in hyperkalemia. Metolzaone is a thiazide diuretic and would not be as effective in oliguria.

---

7. A patient with anuric acute tubular necrosis has a serum potassium concentration of 6.5 mEq/L with associated electrocardiogram changes of peaked T waves. Which intervention should be initiated first?

    a. Regular insulin 10 U and 25 g of dextrose IV push over 2 to 5 minutes
    b. Sodium bicarbonate 50 mEq IV push over 2 to 5 minutes
    c. Calcium chloride 1 g IV push over 2 to 5 minutes
    d. Sodium polystyrene sulfonate 15 g po
    e. Furosemide 80 mg IV push over 2 to 5 minutes

Answer a is incorrect. Insulin stimulates the cellular uptake of potassium, decreasing the extracellular concentration. This is an appropriate step to manage hyperkalemia, though not the first step in this patient.

Answer b is incorrect. Administering sodium bicarbonate causes the efflux of H^+ from within in the cell in exchange for K^+. While this might be an appropriate strategy to manage hyperkalemia (especially if the patient had a metabolic acidosis), it is not the first step in this patient.

Answer c is correct. This patient has signs of cardiotoxicity secondary to hyperkalemia. The most important first step is to antagonize the effect of potassium on the myocardial cells. One gram of calcium (either chloride or gluconate) should be given immediately if any EKG abnormalities are noted.

Answer d is incorrect. Sodium polystyrene sulfonate is an appropriate adjunctive agent to promote elimination of potassium from the body in the feces. It acts to exchange sodium for potassium ions in the gastrointestinal tract. It does not work immediately and would not be the first step.

Answer e is incorrect. Furosemide, a loop-type diuretic is an important agent in managing hyperkalemia in patients that are able to urinate. Loop diuretics promote kaleresis and diuresis to enhance potassium elimination from the body. While this is an excellent tool in the management of hyperkalemia, it is not the first step in this patient.

---

8. PH is a 68-year-old man who was admitted to the hospital yesterday with an acute myocardial infarction. The cardiologists want to perform a cardiac catheterization with radio contrast dye. Which of the following regimens would be best as prophylaxis for contrast-induced nephropathy in this patient?

    a. *N*-acetylcysteine 150 mg/kg IV for 6 hours preprocedure.
    b. Sodium chloride 0.9% IV infusion 6 hours before and 6 hours after.
    c. Theophylline 200 mg po every 12 hours, two doses before, two doses after.
    d. Dopamine 0.5 μg/kg/min IV infusion 6 hours before and 6 hours after.
    e. No prophylaxis is recommended.

Answer a is incorrect. The recommended practice is to hydrate the patient prior to the administration of contrast media. While *N*-acetylcysteine is an agent that has shown some benefit and is relatively safe, it would be used in conjunction with hydration, not alone. Additionally, this dose is the loading dose for the indication of acetaminophen toxicity, not prophylaxis of ATN.

Answer b is correct. Adequate hydration is important to protect the tubules of the kidneys. The intravenous solution of choice should be a colloid/isotonic so that it remains in the intravascular space.

Answer c is incorrect. While theophylline has been studied and may be effective in reducing the incidence of contrast-induced nephropathy, the primary prevention that is recommended is intravenous hydration.

Answer d is incorrect. The use of dopamine as well as fenoldapam has been shown to be deleterious in patients with AKI and ineffective as a prophylactic agent for ATN. The use of these agents is not recommended.

Answer e is incorrect. This patient has at least two known risk factors for the development of CIN, he is older and he is male. Contraindications to intravenous hydration include heart failure and other syndromes that cause total body fluid overload. This man does not have any known contraindications.

---

9. Which of the following circumstances can lead to acute tubular necrosis?

    a. Administration of a direct nephrotoxin
    b. Prolonged hypotension
    c. Prolonged pre-renal AKI
    d. a and b only
    e. a, b, and c

Answer a is correct. One mechanism of damage leading to acute tubular necrosis is direct toxicity. Substances that can bind to tubular cells and cause cellular damage include aminoglycosides, radio contrast agents, myoglobin, and cisplatin.

Answer b is correct. There are two basic mechanisms that can cause acute tubular necrosis. Prolonged hypotension, decreases in renal perfusion, and decreases in intraglomerular pressure will lead to ischemia and necrosis in the tubular cells.

Answer c is correct. As in Answer b, any sustained episode of hypotension of hypoperfusion can lead to apoptosis of tubular cells and ATN.

Answer d is incorrect, as it does not include all of the previous answers, a, b, and c.

Answer e is correct. All of the factors mentioned, a, b, and c, may lead to ATN.

---

10. Which of the following statements is *true* regarding drug dosing in AKI?
    a. All patients should be dosed for a creatinine clearance <10 mL/min.
    b. Pharmacokinetic parameters do not usually change so dose adjustment is not needed.
    c. Although elimination may be decreased, the volume of distribution should remain unchanged in AKI.
    d. The estimation of kidney function should include urine output.
    e. All drugs should be monitored by serum levels to ensure safety and efficacy.

Answer a is incorrect. While it is difficult to quantify renal function during an episode of AKI, many patients will retain at least some kidney function. Assuming that there is no clearance, dosing conservatively may lead to subtherapeutic concentrations and inefficacy.

Answer b is incorrect. Many of the pharmacokinetic parameters (absorption, distribution, metabolism, and excretion) may be altered during AKI. While all of the changes are difficult to quantify, they must be considered and professional judgment must be exercised when determining drug doses.

Answer c is incorrect. While decreases in elimination are easier to observe, changes in protein binding are common as metabolic byproducts, drugs and drug metabolites, and other substances accumulate in the body and compete for plasma protein binding sites.

Answer d is correct. It is difficult to quantify renal function and results from current equations and formulas should be interpreted with care. The patient's renal function should be evaluated with regard to the urine output and other clinical information. All of the available information should be used to obtain a more accurate assessment of the patient's renal function and status.

Answer e is incorrect. There are numerous reasons why serum concentrations are not obtained for every drug that is used in patients with AKI. First, there are not assays for every drug that the patient may need. Second, for many drugs the relationship between efficacy and serum levels has not been determined clearly. Lastly, this would be a very expensive practice. For most agents we must rely on careful monitoring for subjective and objective signs of efficacy and toxicity to ensure optimal outcomes.

---

11. Which of the following urinalysis findings would be *most indicative* of acute glomerulonephritis (GN)?
    a. SpGr <1.003
    b. Muddy brown casts
    c. pH 8.0
    d. Eosinophils
    e. Protein

Answer a is incorrect. This specific gravity is very low, meaning that the urine is very dilute. In cases of GN, the SpGr may vary depending on the amount of protein being excreted. However, it will generally be in the middle of the range or increased due to the proteinuria.

Answer b is incorrect. Muddy brown casts are the cellular components of necrotic tubular epithelial cells. This is the hallmark finding of acute tubular necrosis (ATN).

Answer c is incorrect. The pH of the urine may have little to do with the pathophysiology of AKI. A high pH may predispose crystal formation of alkaline substances. This information would be more useful in the evaluation of post-obstructive nephropathy.

Answer d is incorrect. The presence of eosinophils in the urine is unusual and would be more indicative of a hypersensitivity reaction (acute interstitial nephritis).

Answer e is correct. Proteins are large molecule substances that should not be able to cross the barriers in the glomerulus to be excreted in the urine. The presence of proteinuria is most indicative of glomerular nephritis.

---

12. Which of the following statements is *true* regarding urine volume?
    a. Anuria is defined as <50 mL of urine per day.
    b. Oliguria is defined as <50 mL of urine per day.
    c. Polyuria is defined as <50 mL of urine per day.
    d. Anuria is defined as no urea in the urine.
    e. Polyuria is defined as >1 g of proteinuria per day.

Answer a is correct. Anuria, the absence of urine, is defined as urine output of <50 mL/d. Quantifying urine output is very important as it provides information about the GFR, the prognosis of the patient (worse outcomes) as well as anticipating needs for RRT as fluid, electrolyte, and acid–base balance will be severely compromised.

Answer b is incorrect. Oliguria, "little urine" is defined as urine output <400 mL/d. The judicious use of diuretics may enhance urine production to convert oliguria to nonoliguira (>400 mL/d). Patients who are nonoliguric have better outcomes.

Answer c is incorrect. Polyuria means a great deal of urine, generally any amount greater than normal output (~ 1.5-2 L/d). Polyuria maybe caused by aggressive diuresis or in the recovery phase of ATN as glomerulus regains the ability to filter but the tubules have not yet regained the ability to properly reabsorb water, sodium, and other solutes.

Answer d is incorrect. The suffix "uria" refers to urine. While the urine may not contain a great deal of urea, the body is still producing urea and other nitrogenous wastes.

Answer e is incorrect. Polyuria refers to the amount of urine, not protein. The presence of any protein in the urine is pathologic so the prefixes hypo or hyper would not be used. The extent or severity of protein is quantified by the milligrams (or grams) present per volume of urine per 24 hours (1 g/d, 3 g/d, etc).

---

13. Please identify the correct interpretation of the acronym "AEIOU" as it relates to the initiation of acute RRT.

    a. A, *a*cid–base imbalance; E, *E*KG changes; I, *i*nflammation; O, obtundation, U, *u*remia
    b. A, *a*cute distress; e, *e*lectrolyte disturbance; I, *i*nflammation O, *o*vert proteinuria, U, *u*remia
    c. A, *a*cid–base imbalance, E, *e*lectrolyte disturbance; I, *i*ngestion/*i*ntoxication; O, fluid *o*verload; U, *u*remia
    d. A, *a*cid–base imbalance; E, *E*KG abnormality; I, *i*ngestion/*i*ntoxication; O, *o*liguria; U, *u*remia
    e. A, *a*nuria; E, *e*lectrolyte disturbance; I, *i*ngestion/*i*ntoxication; O, fluid *o*verload; U, *u*remia

---

Answer a is incorrect. While EKG changes may occur as a result of severe kidney insufficiency, the "E" stands for *e*lectrolytes. In fact, the most common (and potentially life-threatening) electrolyte disturbance in AKI is hyperkalemia. Increased serum potassium concentrations can lead to EKG changes, specifically peaked T waves, prolonged QRS waves, and even ventricular fibrillation. Additionally, the "I" is for *i*ngestion or *i*ntoxication, not inflammation. Inflammation is a common finding in patients with AKI and other comorbidities; unfortunately, renal replacement therapy will not help it. While obtundation is a parameter that should be carefully monitored, the "O" in the acronym stands for fluid *o*verload. Obtundation assess for "U," uremic syndrome. For explanations I and O please also see Answers b and d.

Answer b is incorrect. The "A" stands for *a*cid–base disturbances. Metabolic acidosis is the most common finding in AKI. The "I" stands for *i*ngestion or *i*ntoxication. Renal replacement therapies may be able to remove toxic substances from the body. The "O" does not stand for overt proteinuria, but refers to fluid *o*verload. See Answer d.

Answer c is correct. Remembering the acronym AEIOU can aid in the clinical evaluation of patients with AKI who may require emergent dialysis and other care.

Answer d is incorrect. The "O" stands for fluid *o*verload. While many patients with AKI may be oliguric (upon presentation or afterward), fluid accumulation secondary to decreased urine production can result in life-threatening pulmonary edema. Auscultation of the lungs should be part of the physical examination to assess rales.

Answer e is incorrect. Anuria is an important finding, however, the "A" in the acronym is for *a*cid–base abnormalities. The absence of urine does not necessitate acute RRT unless the lack of urine has caused fluid *o*verload, *a*cid–base abnormalities, *e*lectrolyte abnormalities, *i*ntoxications, or *u*remia. ("AEIOU"!)

---

14. JT is a 24-year-old woman brought to the hospital by her roommate. She states that she has been having diarrhea and vomiting for 3 days. She reports a 3 kg weight loss and cannot keep down anything, even water. In the emergency department her BP is 96/46 mmHg, HR 120 beats/min, temp is 102.6°F, weight is 48 kg. On examination her mucous membranes are dry, she has no peripheral edema. She does not recall the last time that she urinated but thinks it may have been yesterday. Which of the following findings would you expect from her serum and urine laboratory analysis?

    a. SpGr 1.016, 2+ protein, light-yellow urine, many WBC and RBCs
    b. SpGr 1.035, 0 protein, hazy-red urine, granular casts, FeNa >2%
    c. SpGr 1.016, 2+ protein, light-yellow urine, many WBC and RBCs
    d. SpGr 1.005, 0 protein, hazy-red urine, granular casts, FeNa >1%
    e. SpGr 1.035, 0 protein, dark yellow urine, no casts, FeNa <1%

Answer a is incorrect. JT is volume depleted (sudden weight loss, vomiting and diarrhea, temperature, dry mucous membranes, etc). In a state of dehydration, the kidneys should retain sodium and water and excrete only a small amount of dark, concentrated urine. The SpGr = 1.016 is near normal, not suggesting a concentrated urine.

Answer b is incorrect. The FeNa >2% suggests that the tubules are not reabsorbing as much sodium as possible. In a volume-depleted state (pre-renal) the tubules should reabsorb as much water as possible and excrete as little as possible. In this situation the FeNa should be very low, <1%.

Answer c is incorrect. Dehydration causes a pre-renal AKI. There is no intrinsic damage to the nephrons, so there should not be any cellular matter or protein in the urine (a bland sediment).

Answer d is incorrect. This is a very dilute urine (SpGr 1.003). The FeNa is inconsistent with pre-renal AKI as is hazy-red appearance and presence of casts.

Answer e is the correct answer. The high SpGr, dark color, decreased FeNa (<1%), and the absence of cellular matter and protein are all consistent with a prerenal AKI secondary to circumstances such as dehydration.

15. Which of the following statements is *true* regarding the blood urea nitrogen (BUN) to serum creatinine (SCr) ratio?
    a. In situations of dehydration the BUN:SCr will be <10.
    b. In situations of dehydration the BUN:SCr will be >15.
    c. In situations of volume overload the BUN:SCr will be <10.
    d. In situations of volume overload the BUN:SCr will be >15.
    e. In situations of glomerulonephritis the BUN:SCr will be <5.

Answer a is incorrect. Dehydration will cause the proximal tubule to reabsorb more sodium and water to compensate for the decreased effective arterial blood volume. Urea (blood urea nitrogen) is passively reabsorbed in the proximal tubule and the diffusion is increased with the increase in water reabsorption. This process leads to a disproportionately higher BUN than SCr concentration in states of dehydration.

Answer b is correct. Generally, the BUN:SCr is approximately 10 to 15. In states of water conservation, the increased water reabsorption in the proximal tubule leads to increased reabsorption of urea back into systemic circulation and therefore an increase in BUN:SCr.

Answer c is incorrect. While an elevated BUN:SCr is helpful in assessing dehydration or a pre-renal AKI, a low BUN:SCr is not specific or sensitive for other disorders.

Answer d is incorrect. As noted in Answer b, an elevated BUN:SCr is indicative of a dehydrated, pre-renal AKI. It is important to remember that there are factors that may elevate the BUN that are not associated with a decline in renal function. Such factors include upper gastrointestinal bleeding or therapy with corticosteroids.

Answer e is incorrect. As with Answer c, a low BUN:SCr is not a sensitive marker for any particular type of AKI. One of the most common urinalysis findings in acute glomerulonephritis is proteinuria.

16. PL is a 38-year-old man brought to the emergency department (ED) after being found at the bottom of the stairs to his apartment. Apparently, he was intoxicated, fell down the stairs, and lay there, unconscious, for approximately 6 hours. In the ED he was diagnosed with rhabdomyolysis. Which of the following statements are *true* regarding his situation?
    a. Rhabdomyolysis may cause acute interstitial nephritis.
    b. Rhabdomyolysis may cause acute tubular necrosis.
    c. Rhabdomyolysis may cause eosinophilia and eosinophiluria.
    d. PL should undergo renal replacement therapy for his intoxication.
    e. Acute tubular necrosis is associated with a very good prognosis.

Answer a is incorrect. Acute interstitial nephritis is a hypersensitivity reaction (allergic reaction) causing inflammation and damage to the interstitium. While there may be systemic signs of allergy (urticaria, fever) the urinalysis is somewhat nonspecific. Eosinophiluria is not a sensitive or specific marker of acute interstitial nephritis. However, eosinophils and white blood cells are often present in the urine.

Answer b is the correct answer. Rhabdomyolysis is the breakdown of muscle tissue. Myoglobin is released during muscle breakdown and is directly toxic to tubular cells. Muddy brown casts are the remnants of the tubular cells that are often visualized upon urine microscopy.

Answer c is incorrect. Increased eosinophil count in the serum and the presence of eosinophils in the urine would be more indicative of either a parasitic infection or an allergic reaction, including AIN.

Answer d is incorrect. While renal replacement therapy may be useful to remove certain toxins, PL has at least 6 hours to metabolize the ethanol that he consumed. Additionally, there is no indication (AEIOU) for acute RRT.

Answer e is incorrect. Acute tubular necrosis represents intrinsic kidney disease. The time course to recovery and the extent of recovery are variable. Unlike pre-renal AKI, ATN may lead to permanent damage, loss of function, and potentially end-stage kidney disease.

17. Hyperkalemia may result from AKI and can lead to which one of the following life-threatening complications?
    a. Seizures
    b. Arrhythmias
    c. Hypertension
    d. Acidosis
    e. Encephalopathy

Answer a is incorrect. Patients with AKI may experience acid–base abnormalities or other electrolyte abnormalities that increase risk for seizures.

Answer b is correct. Hyperkalemia can lead to EKG changes such as peaked T waves, prolonged QRS waves, and eventually ventricular fibrillation.

Answer c is incorrect. Hypertension is not indicative of acute hyperkalemia, and patients with AKI may be normotensive, hypotensive, or hypertensive depending on the circumstances.

Answer d is incorrect. Metabolic acidosis can worsen hyperkalemia by causing a shift of potassium from the intracellular to extracellular space. Hyperkalemia, however, does not cause an acidosis.

Answer e is incorrect. Hyperkalemia does not directly cause encephalopathy. The accumulation of other substances (metabolic wastes and toxins) during an episode of AKI may cause changes in mental status and obtundation.

18. AB is a 60 year-old man with a history of chronic kidney disease and heart failure. His baseline SCr is 1.6 mg/dL with a corresponding CrCl of approximately 50 mL/min. Today he is brought by ambulance to the emergency room with dyspnea at rest and lower extremity edema all the way up to his thighs. His laboratory analysis shows a SCr of 3.2 mg/dL and he does not recall urinating at all in the past 24 hours. Which of the following statements is *true* regarding the estimation of AB's kidney function today?

   a. His CrCl is essentially zero as his is not making urine.
   b. His CrCl is approximately 25 mL/min.
   c. His CrCl is still approximately 50 mL/min.
   d. He has AKI and so we cannot estimate his CrCl.
   e. Wait to calculate the CrCl until after giving diuretics.

Answer a is correct. Clearance is defined as the volume of solvent cleared of solute per unit time. If the patient is not urinating, his clearance is essentially zero.

Answer b is incorrect. This answer seems appropriate given that AB's SCr doubled. Doubling of the SCr would cause the CrCl to decrease by one-half, from 50 mL/min to 25 mL/min. However, the SCr is the amount of creatinine in the serum at the time. If the patient stops urinating the GFR is zero, but the SCr will not reflect this change until more SCr is made and accumulates in the serum. The laboratory value lags behind the clinical situation.

Answer c is incorrect. AB's CrCl on presentation was approximately 50 mL/min. Now that he is not urinating and his SCr has started to increase, this value is no longer valid. This baseline value would be a good reference point and goal to achieve during his recovery from AKI.

Answer d is incorrect. While it is true that our equations to quantify kidney function are not very accurate during AKI, we must use the information and our professional judgment to recommend appropriate drug therapy for this patient.

Answer e is incorrect. While diuretics may be able to convert anuria/oliguria to nonoliguria, the patient may require other pharmacotherapy in the meantime. For instance, AB may require inotropes for his heart failure before diuresis can be attempted.

---

19. CG is a 58-year-old woman with a history of stage 4 ovarian cancer. She has metastases in her colon, abdominal cavity, liver, and bone. Recently she has undergone chemotherapy and radiation as palliative treatment. Today she is admitted due to 1-week history of fatigue, malaise, nausea, vomiting, and she notes that she has not urinated for days. Upon examination the doctor notes that her bladder is palpable and distended. Which of the following tests would be best to confirm a post-renal obstruction in this patient?

   a. MRI with contrast media
   b. CT abdomen with contrast media
   c. X-ray of the abdomen
   d. Ultrasound of the kidneys, ureters, and bladder
   e. MRI of the bladder without contrast

Answer a is incorrect. A different, less expensive, or time-consuming test would evaluate the bladder as effectively and contrast media could potentially worsen or further AKI.

Answer b is incorrect. As with answer a, a CT scan would not evaluate the presence of hydronephrosis as effectively, and contrast media is relatively contraindicated in this patient.

Answer c is incorrect. An X-ray is an effective tool in identifying bone and structural abnormalities.

Answer d is correct. An ultrasound of the kidneys, ureters, and bladder ("KUB") is a noninvasive procedure that can be done at the bedside. This study is particularly well suited to detecting hydronephrosis.

Answer e is incorrect. Again, an MRI is an expensive diagnostic test that is not always available. An ultrasound is the easiest, least invasive procedure to determine hydronephrosis.

---

20. Which of the following agents may be used to treat acute interstitial nephritis?

   a. Prednisone
   b. Furosemide
   c. Lisinopril
   d. Ibuprofen
   e. Metformin

Answer a is correct. Although the data is not strong, corticosteroids can be used to treat the immune reaction and inflammation that causes the damage to the interstitium. The decision to use steroids should be made on a case-by-case basis.

Answer b is incorrect. While furosemide can be used to enhance urine production and manage fluid balance, it does not treat the underlying pathophysiology of AIN. In fact, furosemide contains a sulfonamide moiety, and rarely has caused AIN.

Answer c is incorrect. Lisinopril has no role in the treatment of AIN. Additionally, the use of ACE-I or ARB during an episode of AKI is relatively contraindicated. By vasodilating the efferent arteriole, these agents may decrease the intraglomerular pressure, thwarting filtering.

Answer d is incorrect. While ibuprophen is an anti-inflammatory agent, the effects of inhibiting vasodilatory prostaglandins in the afferent arteriole may cause a worsening of kidney function in the setting of AKI.

Answer e is incorrect. Metformin does not treat the pathophysiologic changes of AIN. It is important to remember, however, that metformin may need to be temporarily discontinued during an episode of AKI as it can cause lactic acidosis in patients with decreased CrCl. Additionally, when AKI is suspected, all medications should be reviewed to ensure that they are appropriate and dosed properly for the patients' kidney function.

CHAPTER 37 Liver Cirrhosis and Complications

1. Which of the following drugs causes the most cases of hepatic cirrhosis in the western world?
   a. HMG-CoA reductase inhibitors (statins)
   b. Valproic acid
   c. Methotrexate
   d. Ethanol

Answer a is incorrect. Statin drugs have been related to cases of acute hepatotoxicity with a pattern of injury similar to acute hepatitis. However, with proper liver function test (LFT) monitoring, statins can be stopped if AST and ALT exceed three times the upper limit of normal and LFTs usually then return to normal. Statins are an unlikely cause of a chronic liver disease like cirrhosis.

Answer b is incorrect. Valproic acid can also cause acute hepatotoxicity but the pattern of injury is similar to acute hepatitis, not cirrhosis.

Answer c is incorrect. Methotrexate can cause a pattern of liver injury of fibrosis/cirrhosis. However, methotrexate is not the most common cause of cirrhosis in the western world.

Answer d is correct. Alcoholism and hepatitis C are the most common causes of cirrhosis in the western world. Other causes include hepatitis B, nonalcoholic steatohepatitis, primary biliary cirrhosis, primary sclerosing cholangitis, hemochromatosis, Wilson disease, and alpha-1-antitrypsin deficiency.

2. Which of the following is a sign or symptom of hepatic cirrhosis?
   a. Hypoglycemia
   b. Weight gain
   c. Ascites
   d. Pancreatitis

Answer a is incorrect. Diabetes mellitus (hyperglycemia) can result as a symptom of cirrhosis.

Answer b is incorrect. Muscle wasting, anorexia, and weight loss are likely to result in cirrhosis.

Answer c is correct. Ascites is a symptom of cirrhosis and is the most common complication related to cirrhosis.

Answer d is incorrect. Pancreatitis is not a symptom of cirrhosis, but pancreatitis can result from one of the main causes of cirrhosis: alcohol abuse.

3. Marked elevations (greater than 10 times normal) in AST and ALT are typically associated with which of the following?
   a. Cirrhosis
   b. Acute acetaminophen toxicity
   c. Chronic hepatitis C infection
   d. Chronic hepatitis B infection

Answer a is incorrect. Cirrhosis may cause elevations in AST and ALT, but typically not to the same degree as acute insults or AST and ALT may test within the normal range in patients with cirrhosis or another chronic liver disease.

Answer b is correct. Patients with marked increase in AST and ALT typically have acute liver injury, such as that which would occur after acute ingestion of toxic amounts of acetaminophen (greater than 4 g in 24 hours).

Answer c is incorrect. Chronic hepatitis C infection may cause elevations in AST and ALT, but typically not to the same degree as acute insults, or AST and ALT may test within the normal range in patients with chronic liver disease.

Answer d is incorrect. Chronic hepatitis B infection may cause elevations in AST and ALT, but typically not to the same degree as acute insults, or AST and ALT may test within the normal range in patients with chronic liver disease.

4. Which of the following is true?
   a. ALT is more specific for liver damage than AST.
   b. AST is more specific for liver damage than ALT.
   c. An elevation in alk phos is specific for liver disease.
   d. An elevation in prothrombin time is specific for liver disease.

Answer a is correct. ALT is more specific for liver damage that AST.

Answer b is incorrect. AST is less specific for liver damage than ALT. AST is present in the heart, skeletal muscle, kidneys, brain, and red blood cells. ALT only has low concentrations in skeletal muscle and kidneys.

Answer c is incorrect. An elevated alk phos may accompany liver disease or bone disease. However, alk phos is also present in the placenta, kidneys, intestines, and white blood cells. Glutamyl transpeptidase elevation, while not specific for liver disease either, is sensitive for liver disease and is often tested in order to help identify causes of alk phos elevations or other elevated levels.

Answer d is incorrect. Multiple reasons for prothrombin time elevation exist including liver disease, warfarin therapy, vitamin K deficiency, and certain clotting factor deficiencies.

5. BT is a 58-year-old man who has been diagnosed with cirrhosis for the past 2 years. BT is currently having difficulty with overactive bladder and his physician is considering starting him on darifenacin. BT presents with mild ascites and no encephalopathy. His pertinent laboratory values are as follows: total bilirubin 2.1 mg/dL (0.3-1.2), albumin 2.8 g/dL (3.2-4.6). prothrombin time 20.2 seconds (12.5-15.2). Based on the patient's Child-Pugh score (Table 37-1) and the following information from darifenacin's dosing information, what dose will you recommend for BT?

No Liver Disease	Mild Hepatic Insufficiency	Moderate Hepatic Insufficiency	Severe Hepatic Insufficiency
15 mg daily	15 mg daily	7.5 mg daily	No clinical experience

a. BT has grade A cirrhosis and should be started on 15 mg daily.
b. BT has grade A cirrhosis and should be started on 7.5 mg daily.
c. BT has grade B cirrhosis and should be started on 7.5 mg daily.
d. BT has grade C cirrhosis and should not be given darifenacin.

BT's Child-Pugh score is calculated as follows:

Bilirubin 2.1 (0.3-1.2) = 2 points

Albumin 2.8 (3.2-4.6) = 2 points

Mild ascites = 2 points

No encephalopathy = 1 point

Prothrombin time 20.2 (12.5-15.2) = 2 points

Child-Pugh score = 9 points = Grade B moderate liver dysfunction

Answer a is incorrect. BT has grade B liver disease.

Answer b is incorrect. BT has grade B liver disease.

Answer c is correct. BT has grade B liver disease and, per the darifenacin dosing. recommendation, BT should receive 7.5 mg daily as his initial dose.

Answer d is incorrect. BT has grade B liver disease.

---

6. Hepatic drug elimination is dependent upon which of the following?
    a. Blood flow, drug binding in blood, and hepatic extraction ratio
    b. Blood flow, drug binding in blood, and bioavailability
    c. Drug binding in blood, bioavailability, and hepatic extraction ratio
    d. Blood flow, drug binding in blood, hepatic intrinsic clearance

---

Answer a is incorrect. Hepatic drug elimination is dependent upon blood flow, protein binding of the drug in the blood, and hepatic intrinsic clearance. Hepatic extraction ratio is not one of the primary determinants of hepatic drug elimination.

Answer b is incorrect. Hepatic drug elimination is dependent upon blood flow, protein binding of the drug in the blood, and hepatic intrinsic clearance. Bioavailability is not one of the primary determinants of hepatic drug elimination.

Answer c is incorrect. Hepatic drug elimination is dependent upon protein binding of the drug in the blood but is not dependent upon bioavailability or hepatic extraction ratio.

Answer d is correct. Hepatic drug elimination is dependent upon blood flow, protein binding of the drug in the blood, and hepatic intrinsic clearance.

---

7. Which of the following statements is true in liver disease regarding volume of distribution and half-life of drugs normally highly protein bound to albumin in the blood?
    a. Albumin is increased in chronic liver disease leading to increased protein binding, increased volume of distribution, and potentially decreased half-life.
    b. Albumin is decreased in chronic liver disease leading to decreased protein binding, decreased volume of distribution, and potentially decreased half-life.
    c. Albumin is decreased in chronic liver disease leading to decreased protein binding, increased volume of distribution, and potentially increased half-life.
    d. No changes in albumin concentrations normally occur in chronic liver disease, and so no changes in volume of distribution or half-life normally occur.

Answer a is incorrect. Albumin is not increased in liver disease. It is potentially decreased in chronic liver disease.

Answer b is incorrect. Albumin can be decreased in chronic liver disease which may lead to decreased protein binding of drugs normally bound to albumin in the blood. This would result in increases in volume of distribution of these drugs and increases half-life.

Answer c is correct. Albumin is decreased in chronic liver disease which leads to decreased binding of drugs normally bound to albumin in the blood. This increases those drugs' volumes of distribution and potentially increases their half-lives.

Answer d is incorrect. Albumin concentrations are usually decreased in severe chronic liver disease.

---

8. Which of the following drugs would be expected to have a decreased therapeutic effect in cirrhosis due to pharmacodynamic changes associated with chronic liver
    a. Morphine
    b. Furosemide
    c. Lorazepam
    d. Zolpidem

Answer a is incorrect. Morphine (an opiate) would be expected to have an increased therapeutic effect in cirrhosis.

Answer b is correct. Certain diuretics (furosemide, triamterene, torsemide, and bumetanide) as well as β-blockers such as propranolol have been found to exert a decreased therapeutic effect due to pharmacodynamic changes that occur in cirrhosis.

Answer c is incorrect. Anxiolytics such as the benzodiazepine lorazepam would be expected to exert an increased effect in a patient with cirrhosis (and also increases the patient's risk of developing hepatic encephalopathy).

Answer d is incorrect. Zolpidem, a sedative, would be more likely to have an increased effect in a patient with cirrhosis rather than a decreased effect.

---

9. Which of the following is true about the oral bioavailability of relatively high hepatic ratio drugs in cirrhosis if portal-systemic shunting has occurred?
   a. Oral bioavailability will be increased and initial dosage should be decreased.
   b. Oral bioavailability will be decreased and initial dosage should be increased.
   c. Oral bioavailability will be increased but no dosage adjustment need be considered.
   d. Oral bioavailability will be unchanged and no initial dosage adjustment need be considered.

Answer a is correct. Oral bioavailability of a high hepatic ratio drug would be expected to be increased if portal-systemic shunting is present. Hepatic elimination of high hepatic extraction ratio drugs is dependent upon blood flow. Blood flow in portal systemic shunting is altered so that blood flows directly from the portal vein into systemic circulation bypassing the liver. If the drug is normally cleared to a large extent by first-pass effect, this could change drastically the serum concentration that would be achieved after the initial dose.

Answer b is incorrect. Oral bioavailability would be expected to be increased, not decreased.

Answer c is incorrect. Due to the possibility for significantly higher serum concentrations following initial dosing, consideration should be given to lowering the initial dose given to the patient.

Answer d is incorrect. In this situation, oral bioavailability would be expected to be increased.

---

10. Pharmacokinetic evaluation of low hepatic extraction and high plasma protein bound drugs should be based on which of the following?
    a. Unbound concentration
    b. Bound concentration
    c. Total drug concentration
    d. Hepatic blood flow

Answer a is correct. Hepatic elimination of a low hepatic extraction ratio drug is affected by protein binding and hepatic intrinsic clearance. Since this drug is said to be highly plasma protein bound, dosing should be adjusted in order to maintain a normal unbound concentration. A significant increase in unbound concentration would have the potential to significantly increase the amount of drug free to act in the body.

Answer b is incorrect. Dosing in this situation should be changed in order to maintain unbound, not bound concentration.

Answer c is incorrect. Dosing in this situation should be changed in order to maintain unbound, not total concentration.

Answer d is incorrect. Hepatic elimination of a low hepatic extraction ratio drug would not be expected to be significantly affected by changes in hepatic blood flow.

---

11. Dosage adjustment of low hepatic extraction ratio/low plasma protein bound drugs should be aimed at maintaining which of the following?
    a. Normal unbound plasma concentrations
    b. Normal bound plasma concentrations
    c. Normal total (bound plus unbound) plasma concentrations
    d. No dosage adjustments need be considered

Answer a is incorrect. Dosage adjustment for a low hepatic extraction ratio/low plasma protein bound drug should be aimed at maintaining normal total plasma concentrations. Low hepatic extraction ratio drugs are affected most by changes in protein binding and hepatic intrinsic clearance. Since this drug is not highly protein bound, a change in the amount of drug that is protein bound is unlikely to significantly change the amount of drug free to act in the body in this situation. Therefore, bound versus unbound concentration is less important. Total plasma concentration should be the target of dosage adjustments in this case.

Answer b is incorrect. Dosage adjustment for a low hepatic extraction ratio/low plasma protein bound drug should be aimed at maintaining normal total plasma concentrations.

Answer c is correct. Dosage adjustment for a low hepatic extraction ratio/low plasma protein bound drug should be aimed at maintaining normal total plasma concentrations.

Answer d is incorrect. Dosage adjustment for a low hepatic extraction ratio/low plasma protein bound drug should be aimed at maintaining normal total plasma concentrations.

---

12. Which of the following statements is true?
    a. In liver disease, phase II conjugation metabolism is affected to a greater extent than phase I oxidative reactions.
    b. In liver disease, phase I oxidative metabolism is affected to a greater extent than phase II conjugation reactions.
    c. Chronic liver disease is associated with uniform reductions in metabolism via the different cytochrome P450 pathways.
    d. Serum creatinine is an accurate reflection of renal function in chronic liver disease.

Answer a is incorrect. Phase I oxidative reactions (which typically involve the cytochrome P450 enzymatic pathways) are affected to a greater extent in cirrhosis than phase II reactions such as glucuronidation. This is because the cytochrome P450 enzymes are dependent upon oxygen to act. In cirrhosis, there is a relative lack of oxygen due to shunting, sinusoidal capillarization, and reduced liver perfusion. In severe cirrhosis, even glucuronidation may be affected, though.

Answer b is correct. Phase I oxidative reactions are affected to a greater extent in cirrhosis than phase II conjugation reactions.

Answer c is incorrect. Chronic liver disease is associated with nonuniform reductions in metabolism via the cytochrome P450 system. For example, in early-stage liver disease, drug metabolism through the cytochrome P450 2C19 enzyme can be expected to be reduced while the cytochrome P450 1A2, 2D6, and 2E1 enzyme pathways retain normal or near normal activity. As liver disease progresses, the activity levels of the different cytochrome P450 enzyme pathways change.

Answer d is incorrect. Serum creatinine is not considered a reliable predictor of renal function in chronic liver disease. This is because of the reduced muscle mass and impaired metabolism of creatine to creatinine that accompany severe liver disease.

---

13. Which of the following describes appropriate therapy for primary prevention of variceal bleeding in a patient with portal hypertension who has been found to have varices?
    a. No primary prevention therapy needed; only patients who have experienced an episode of variceal bleeding in the past should receive prophylaxis therapy.
    b. An appropriate prophylaxis therapy would be atenolol 50 mg po daily.
    c. An appropriate prophylaxis therapy would be propranolol 20 mg po daily.
    d. An appropriate prophylaxis therapy would be nadolol 40 mg po daily.

Answer a is incorrect. Patients found to have varices should receive primary prophylaxis therapy in an effort to prevent variceal hemorrhage.

Answer b is incorrect. Atenolol is a selective β_1 receptor antagonist. Nonselective β-blockers therapy is indicated in portal hypertension as prophylaxis against variceal bleeding.

Answer c is incorrect. Propranolol is an appropriate agent for the primary prophylaxis of variceal bleeding in portal hypertension, but the dosing schedule of 20 mg po daily is incorrect. An appropriate dose would be 20 mg po bid.

Answer d is correct. Nadolol 40 mg po daily is an appropriate drug and dosing schedule for primary prevention of variceal bleeding in portal hypertension. Nonselective β-blockers reduce portal pressure by reducing portal venous inflow via two mechanisms: a decrease in cardiac output through β_1 receptor antagonism and a decrease in splanchnic blood flow through β_2 receptor antagonism. Nadolol should be titrated to the maximum tolerated dose. Other goals that can be used include a reduction in the resting heart rate of 20% to 25%, an absolute heart rate of 55 to 60 beats per minute, or the development of adverse effects. Possible side effects of nonselective β-blocker therapy include fatigue, shortness of breath, inability to recognize hypoglycemia in patients with diabetes, depression, and erectile dysfunction.

---

14. RP is a 45-year-old white man with a 20-year history of heavy alcohol use, cirrhosis, and portal hypertension. He presents for emergent care after experiencing hematemesis and is diagnosed with acute esophageal variceal bleeding. Which of the following best describes appropriate therapy for RP at this time?
    a. Pantoprazole IV 40 mg daily plus norfloxacin po 400 mg bid
    b. Octreotide IV 50 μg bolus, then 50 μg/h infusion plus norfloxacin po 400 mg bid
    c. Octreotide IV 50 μg bolus, then 50 μg/h infusion plus pantoprazole IV 40 mg daily
    d. Octreotide IV 50 μg bolus then 50 μg/h infusion as monotherapy

---

Answer a is incorrect. While IV proton pump inhibitor therapy may be appropriate for a gastric bleed related to peptic ulcer disease, it is not appropriate for variceal bleeding.

Answer b is correct. Octreotide decreases splanchnic arterial blood flow as well as portal inflow and is therefore useful in the management of acute variceal hemorrhage. Octreotide has a very short half-life and therefore must be given as IV infusion. Short-term antibiotic therapy is recommended in a patient with acute variceal hemorrhage because patients with variceal hemorrhage are at risk of infection and sepsis due to multiple reasons including aspiration and translocation of the gastrointestinal bacterial flora. Norfloxacin po 400 mg bid for 7 days is appropriate. Ciprofloxacin IV can be used if oral access is impossible in the patient.

Answer c is incorrect. Octreotide is appropriate, but pantoprazole is not.

Answer d is incorrect. Antibiotic prophylaxis should be provided. Antibiotic prophylaxis in cases of acute variceal hemorrhage has been found to decrease rebleeding rates and increase rates of short-term survival.

---

15. Treatment of ascites includes po diuretic therapy with spironolactone and furosemide. What is the appropriate starting dosing ratio for these two drugs?
    a. Spironolactone 40 mg: furosemide 100 mg
    b. Spironolactone 100 mg: furosemide 40 mg
    c. Spironolactone 200 mg: furosemide 40 mg
    d. Spironolactone 40 mg: furosemide 200 mg

Answer a is incorrect. The starting ratio for spironolactone and furosemide combination therapy in the treatment of ascites is 100:40. Also with alcohol avoidance and sodium restriction, diuretic therapy is one of the mainstays of ascites management. This ratio helps to maximize fluid loss while maintaining electrolyte (particularly serum potassium) balance within normal range. Spironolactone may be increased to 400 mg po daily and furosemide may be increased to 160 mg po daily in 3 to 5 day increments as needed and as tolerated with proper electrolyte monitoring.

Answer b is correct. The starting ratio is 100:40.

Answer c is incorrect. The starting ratio is 100:40.

Answer d is incorrect. The starting ratio is 100:40.

16. Which of the following therapies is considered first line in addition to dietary protein restriction for patients with hepatic encephalopathy?

    a. Metronidazole po 250 mg bid
    b. Neomycin po 500 mg bid
    c. Lactulose po 15 to 45 mL every 8 to 12 hours
    d. Rifaximin po 400 mg tid

Answer a is incorrect. Metronidazole is an antibiotic used in hepatic encephalopathy patients to reduce the nitrogenous load from the gut by eliminating urease producing organisms from the intestinal tract. Though metronidazole can improve symptoms of hepatic encephalopathy, it is not commonly used due to a potential for neurotoxicity with the use of this agent.

Answer b is incorrect. Neomycin is a poorly absorbed aminoglycoside antibiotic used in hepatic encephalopathy patients to reduce the nitrogenous load from the gut by eliminating urease producing organisms from the intestinal tract. Though neomycin can improve symptoms of hepatic encephalopathy, it is not a first-line agent due to a potential for ototoxicity and nephrotoxicity. It is reserved for patients who have not responded to diet and lactulose therapy and when the combination may provide additive effects and improved clinical response.

Answer c is correct. Lactulose is first-line therapy to reduce the nitrogenous load from the gut in both acute and chronic cases of hepatic encephalopathy. Lactulose, a nonabsorbable disaccharide, exerts its action by increasing the osmotic pressure in the colon and producing organ acids to lower colonic pH. These actions increase peristalsis and acidify the colon which lowers ammonia levels in the blood. Typical dosing in chronic therapy is 15 to 45 mL every 8 to 12 hours. Dosing should be titrated to achieve two to three soft bowel movements per day.

Answer d is incorrect. Rifaximin is also a poorly absorbed antibiotic used in hepatic encephalopathy patients to reduce the nitrogenous load from the gut by eliminating urea producing organisms from the intestinal tract. Rifaximin is largely considered second-line therapy for patients with HE who fail therapy or have inadequate results with lactulose. Whether or not rifaximin should be considered as first-line therapy, in addition to lactulose, remains controversial. Rifaximin costs approximately 12 times more than lactulose.

17. Which of the following drugs sometimes used for hepatic encephalopathy is associated with ototoxicity?

    a. Metronidazole
    b. Neomycin
    c. Lactulose
    d. Rifaximin

Answer a is incorrect. Metronidazole is not expected to cause ototoxicity.

Answer b is correct. Patients on neomycin chronically should have annual auditory monitoring as well as regular renal function monitoring.

Answer c is incorrect. Lactulose is not expected to cause ototoxicity.

Answer d is incorrect. Rifaximin is not expected to cause ototoxicity. In fact, rifaximin likely has the least risk of side effects among the drug choices listed here.

18. Which of the following drugs increases a cirrhosis patient's risk of developing hepatic encephalopathy?

    a. Alprazolam
    b. Flumazenil
    c. Bromocriptine
    d. Zinc acetate

Answer a is correct. Drugs that agonize the GABA receptors like benzodiazepines can precipitate acute hepatic encephalopathy. Other predisposing factors include GI hemorrhage, infections, renal and electrolyte disturbances, constipation, and excessive dietary protein.

Answer b is incorrect. Actually, flumazenil can be used in patients with acute hepatic encephalopathy who are thought to have recently taken a benzodiazepine in order to reverse the effects of the benzodiazepine.

Answer c is incorrect. Bromocriptine is another choice for the treatment of acute hepatic encephalopathy in some instances. It is also used to inhibit GABA receptors.

Answer d is incorrect. Patients with hepatic encephalopathy and zinc deficiency should receive supplementation.

19. Which of the following drugs used for the management of hepatic encephalopathy has the possible side effect of neurotoxicity?

    a. Neomycin
    b. Rifaximin

Answer c is correct. Guillain-Barré syndrome is a rare side effect associated with Twinrix.

Answer d is incorrect. Red-man's syndrome is not a reported side effect of Twinrix.

---

4. Peg-interferon alpha-2a and ribavirin cotherapy is pregnancy category
   a. B
   b. C
   c. D
   d. X

Answers a, b, and c are incorrect.

Answer d is correct. Peg-interferon monotherapy is pregnancy class C but when combined with ribavirin, the cotherapy is pregnancy class X. Ribavirin is extremely teratogenic during and up to 6 months after therapy. Female partners of ribavirin treated patients are at equal risk. Women and men of childbearing age should use two forms of contraception until 6 months following discontinuation of therapy. A Ribavirin Registry tracks pregnancies that have been exposed to ribavirin.

---

5. CR is a 58-year-old man diagnosed with chronic hepatitis C (HCV) genotype 1. Today he will begin peg-interferon alpha-2b and ribavirin therapy. Which of the following counseling topics is appropriate?
   a. CR should use two forms of birth control.
   b. CR's therapy will last 24 weeks.
   c. CR likely developed HCV from a contaminated food source.
   d. CR likely acquired HCV from perinatal transmission.

Answer a is correct. Ribavirin has a black box warning about its teratogenic effects in both pregnant women taking ribavirin and in pregnant women whose partner is taking ribavirin and up to 6 months following completion of ribavirin therapy. Two forms of birth control are recommended even in patients who believe they are infertile or have low fertility. A Ribavirin Registry exists for women who became pregnant while they or their partner took ribavirin.

Answer b is incorrect. HCV genotypes 1 and 4 are treated for 48 weeks.

Answer c is incorrect. HCV is transmitted via the bloodstream.

Answer d is incorrect. There is only a 5% risk of perinatal transmission of HCV from an infected mother to her baby.

---

6. LO is a 28-year-old woman who found out her boyfriend has chronic hepatitis B (HBV). They are sexually active and plan to marry in 6 months. Which of the following is the best course of action?
   a. Administer HBIG and begin the HBV vaccine series.
   b. Administer HBIG.
   c. Begin the HBV vaccine series.
   d. Begin treating her for HBV.

Answer a is correct. The CDC recommends initiating the HBV vaccine series and giving HBIG as postexposure prophylaxis for HBV in both individuals.

Answers b and c are incorrect. Neither of these alone represents the *best* option for postexposure prophylaxis to HBV.

Answer d is incorrect. NRTIs for HBV are not useful as postexposure prophylaxis or even acute HBV. They are indicated for patients who develop chronic HBV.

---

7. Which of the following signs and symptoms may LO experience if she develops HBV?
   a. Jaundice
   b. Nausea
   c. Elevated liver enzymes
   d. She may experience no physical symptoms
   e. All of the above

Answers a, b, c, d are correct.

Answer e is correct and the best answer. Viral hepatitis may initially present with jaundice, nausea, and elevated liver enzymes. Some patients experience no physical symptoms.

---

8. MO is a 19-year-old Asian man diagnosed with chronic HBV acquired from perinatal exposure. He will begin therapy with entecavir today. Entecavir will likely
   a. Be combined with ribavirin
   b. Eradicate the HBV virus
   c. Develop resistance
   d. Cause minimal side effects

Answer a is incorrect. Ribavirin is not used in the treatment of chronic HBV. It is used to treat chronic HCV along with peg-interferon alpha-2a or 2b or interferon alfacon-1.

Answer b is incorrect. It is not possible to eradicate chronic HBV with the drugs currently on the market. The goal for therapy is to suppress the virus in order to prevent long-term complications of hepatocellular carcinoma or cirrhosis.

Answer c is incorrect. Entecavir has low viral resistance (<1% up to 4 years of use).

Answer d is correct. All of the nucleoside reverse transcriptase inhibitors are typically well tolerated with the most common adverse events being gastrointestinal in nature. This is in stark contrast to the only other drug available to treat chronic HBV (peg-interferon alpha-2a).

---

9. Which of the following medications for HCV is administered subcutaneously three times per week?
   a. Interferon alfacon-1
   b. Peg-interferon alpha-1a

c. Metronidazole
d. Cefotaxime

Answer a is incorrect. Neurotoxicity is not expected with neomycin therapy.

Answer b is incorrect. Neurotoxicity is not expected with rifaximin therapy.

Answer c is correct. Neurotoxicity can occur with metronidazole and, in fact, is more likely in a patient with liver dysfunction because of the decreased metabolism of metronidazole which can accompany declined hepatic function. Metronidazole is used infrequently for hepatic encephalopathy.

Answer d is incorrect. Cefotaxime is not a treatment for hepatic encephalopathy. Instead, it would be expected to be used in a patient with cirrhosis in the empiric treatment of spontaneous bacterial peritonitis.

---

20. PW is a 56-year-old woman with a history of cirrhosis who is admitted with severe ascites and undergoes paracentesis. PW's polymorphonuclear count is found to be 275 cells/mm^3. Which of the following antibiotics is available in IV formulation and is appropriate empiric therapy in PW at this time?

    a. Vancomycin
    b. Cephalexin
    c. Tigecycline
    d. Cefotaxime

Answer a is incorrect. Vancomycin is not the ideal antibiotic choice in this case as it would not adequately cover two of the likely pathogens often involved in spontaneous bacterial peritonitis, *Escherichia coli* and *Klebsiella pneumoniae.* Vancomycin is dosed via IV administration, however.

Answer b is incorrect. Cephalexin is not the ideal antibiotic choice in this case as it is a first-generation cephalosporin. Also, cephalexin is not available in IV formulation. A third-generation cephalosporin is preferable for empiric treatment of spontaneous bacterial peritonitis.

Answer c is incorrect. Tigecycline may be a viable option in this case as it would likely cover all three of the likely pathogens in spontaneous bacterial peritonitis, *E. coli, K. pneumoniae, and Streptococcus pneumoniae.* However, the most recent guideline statement supported by the American Association for the Study of Liver Diseases recommends the third-generation cephalosporin, cefotaxime, as empiric therapy for cases of likely spontaneous bacterial peritonitis. Tigecycline is administered via the IV route, however.

Answer d is correct. The ideal antibiotic choice in this case would be cefotaxime IV 2 g every 8 hours. Ofloxacin po 400 mg twice daily may be substituted for cefotaxime in patients without prior exposure to quinolones, vomiting, shock, grade II or higher encephalopathy, or serum creatinine greater than 3 mg/dL.

CHAPTER 38 | Hepatitis

1. Select the most common mode of transmission for the hepatitis A virus (HAV).

    a. Blood
    b. Fecal-oral route
    c. Perinatal exposure
    d. Semen

Answer a is incorrect. Intravenous drug users can acquire HAV through exposure to HAV infected blood but this is not a common mode of transmission.

Answer b is correct. The fecal-oral route is the most common mode of transmission of HAV and often occurs through contact with contaminated food, poor hygienic practices, and in poorly developed countries.

Answer c is incorrect. Perinatal transmission is not associated with HAV, but is infrequently associated with HBV and very rarely for HCV.

Answer d is incorrect. Transmission of viral hepatitis from semen is not associated with HAV, but is rarely associated with other viral hepatitis types.

---

2. Which of the following forms of viral hepatitis can be cured with drug therapy?

    a. Chronic hepatitis A
    b. Chronic hepatitis B
    c. Chronic hepatitis C
    d. Viral hepatitis can never be cured

Answer a is incorrect. Hepatitis A is an acute infection and patients eventually clear the virus. HAV does not develop into a chronic form.

Answer b is incorrect. Chronic hepatitis B cannot be cured with drug therapy. The goals are to suppress the viral load and to prevent complications (eg, cirrhosis and hepatocellular carcinoma).

Answer c is correct. Hepatitis C can be cured if a patient has no measurable HCV 6 months after completing treatment.

Answer d is incorrect. HCV can be cured.

---

3. A rare side effect associated with Twinrix (hepatitis A/B vaccine) is

    a. Stevens-Johnson syndrome
    b. Neuroleptic syndrome
    c. Guillain-Barré syndrome
    d. Red-man syndrome

Answer a is incorrect. Stevens-Johnson syndrome is not a reported side effect of Twinrix.

Answer b is incorrect. Neuroleptic syndrome is not a reported side effect of Twinrix.

Answer a is incorrect. The starting ratio for spironolactone and furosemide combination therapy in the treatment of ascites is 100:40. Also with alcohol avoidance and sodium restriction, diuretic therapy is one of the mainstays of ascites management. This ratio helps to maximize fluid loss while maintaining electrolyte (particularly serum potassium) balance within normal range. Spironolactone may be increased to 400 mg po daily and furosemide may be increased to 160 mg po daily in 3 to 5 day increments as needed and as tolerated with proper electrolyte monitoring.

Answer b is correct. The starting ratio is 100:40.

Answer c is incorrect. The starting ratio is 100:40.

Answer d is incorrect. The starting ratio is 100:40.

16. Which of the following therapies is considered first line in addition to dietary protein restriction for patients with hepatic encephalopathy?
    a. Metronidazole po 250 mg bid
    b. Neomycin po 500 mg bid
    c. Lactulose po 15 to 45 mL every 8 to 12 hours
    d. Rifaximin po 400 mg tid

Answer a is incorrect. Metronidazole is an antibiotic used in hepatic encephalopathy patients to reduce the nitrogenous load from the gut by eliminating urease producing organisms from the intestinal tract. Though metronidazole can improve symptoms of hepatic encephalopathy, it is not commonly used due to a potential for neurotoxicity with the use of this agent.

Answer b is incorrect. Neomycin is a poorly absorbed aminoglycoside antibiotic used in hepatic encephalopathy patients to reduce the nitrogenous load from the gut by eliminating urease producing organisms from the intestinal tract. Though neomycin can improve symptoms of hepatic encephalopathy, it is not a first-line agent due to a potential for ototoxicity and nephrotoxicity. It is reserved for patients who have not responded to diet and lactulose therapy and when the combination may provide additive effects and improved clinical response.

Answer c is correct. Lactulose is first-line therapy to reduce the nitrogenous load from the gut in both acute and chronic cases of hepatic encephalopathy. Lactulose, a nonabsorbable disaccharide, exerts its action by increasing the osmotic pressure in the colon and producing organ acids to lower colonic pH. These actions increase peristalsis and acidify the colon which lowers ammonia levels in the blood. Typical dosing in chronic therapy is 15 to 45 mL every 8 to 12 hours. Dosing should be titrated to achieve two to three soft bowel movements per day.

Answer d is incorrect. Rifaximin is also a poorly absorbed antibiotic used in hepatic encephalopathy patients to reduce the nitrogenous load from the gut by eliminating urea producing organisms from the intestinal tract. Rifaximin is largely considered second-line therapy for patients with HE who fail therapy or have inadequate results with lactulose. Whether or not rifaximin should be considered as first-line therapy, in addition to lactulose, remains controversial. Rifaximin costs approximately 12 times more than lactulose.

17. Which of the following drugs sometimes used for hepatic encephalopathy is associated with ototoxicity?
    a. Metronidazole
    b. Neomycin
    c. Lactulose
    d. Rifaximin

Answer a is incorrect. Metronidazole is not expected to cause ototoxicity.

Answer b is correct. Patients on neomycin chronically should have annual auditory monitoring as well as regular renal function monitoring.

Answer c is incorrect. Lactulose is not expected to cause ototoxicity.

Answer d is incorrect. Rifaximin is not expected to cause ototoxicity. In fact, rifaximin likely has the least risk of side effects among the drug choices listed here.

18. Which of the following drugs increases a cirrhosis patient's risk of developing hepatic encephalopathy?
    a. Alprazolam
    b. Flumazenil
    c. Bromocriptine
    d. Zinc acetate

Answer a is correct. Drugs that agonize the GABA receptors like benzodiazepines can precipitate acute hepatic encephalopathy. Other predisposing factors include GI hemorrhage, infections, renal and electrolyte disturbances, constipation, and excessive dietary protein.

Answer b is incorrect. Actually, flumazenil can be used in patients with acute hepatic encephalopathy who are thought to have recently taken a benzodiazepine in order to reverse the effects of the benzodiazepine.

Answer c is incorrect. Bromocriptine is another choice for the treatment of acute hepatic encephalopathy in some instances. It is also used to inhibit GABA receptors.

Answer d is incorrect. Patients with hepatic encephalopathy and zinc deficiency should receive supplementation.

19. Which of the following drugs used for the management of hepatic encephalopathy has the possible side effect of neurotoxicity?
    a. Neomycin
    b. Rifaximin

are affected to a greater extent in cirrhosis than phase II reactions such as glucuronidation. This is because the cytochrome P450 enzymes are dependent upon oxygen to act. In cirrhosis, there is a relative lack of oxygen due to shunting, sinusoidal capillarization, and reduced liver perfusion. In severe cirrhosis, even glucuronidation may be affected, though.

Answer b is correct. Phase I oxidative reactions are affected to a greater extent in cirrhosis than phase II conjugation reactions.

Answer c is incorrect. Chronic liver disease is associated with nonuniform reductions in metabolism via the cytochrome P450 system. For example, in early-stage liver disease, drug metabolism through the cytochrome P450 2C19 enzyme can be expected to be reduced while the cytochrome P450 1A2, 2D6, and 2E1 enzyme pathways retain normal or near normal activity. As liver disease progresses, the activity levels of the different cytochrome P450 enzyme pathways change.

Answer d is incorrect. Serum creatinine is not considered a reliable predictor of renal function in chronic liver disease. This is because of the reduced muscle mass and impaired metabolism of creatine to creatinine that accompany severe liver disease.

---

13. Which of the following describes appropriate therapy for primary prevention of variceal bleeding in a patient with portal hypertension who has been found to have varices?
    a. No primary prevention therapy needed; only patients who have experienced an episode of variceal bleeding in the past should receive prophylaxis therapy.
    b. An appropriate prophylaxis therapy would be atenolol 50 mg po daily.
    c. An appropriate prophylaxis therapy would be propranolol 20 mg po daily.
    d. An appropriate prophylaxis therapy would be nadolol 40 mg po daily.

Answer a is incorrect. Patients found to have varices should receive primary prophylaxis therapy in an effort to prevent variceal hemorrhage.

Answer b is incorrect. Atenolol is a selective β_1 receptor antagonist. Nonselective β-blockers therapy is indicated in portal hypertension as prophylaxis against variceal bleeding.

Answer c is incorrect. Propranolol is an appropriate agent for the primary prophylaxis of variceal bleeding in portal hypertension, but the dosing schedule of 20 mg po daily is incorrect. An appropriate dose would be 20 mg po bid.

Answer d is correct. Nadolol 40 mg po daily is an appropriate drug and dosing schedule for primary prevention of variceal bleeding in portal hypertension. Nonselective β-blockers reduce portal pressure by reducing portal venous inflow via two mechanisms: a decrease in cardiac output through β_1 receptor antagonism and a decrease in splanchnic blood flow through β_2 receptor antagonism. Nadolol should be titrated to the maximum tolerated dose. Other goals that can be used include a reduction in the resting heart rate of 20% to 25%, an absolute heart rate of 55 to 60 beats per minute, or the development of adverse effects. Possible side effects of nonselective β-blocker therapy include fatigue, shortness of breath, inability to recognize hypoglycemia in patients with diabetes, depression, and erectile dysfunction.

---

14. RP is a 45-year-old white man with a 20-year history of heavy alcohol use, cirrhosis, and portal hypertension. He presents for emergent care after experiencing hematemesis and is diagnosed with acute esophageal variceal bleeding. Which of the following best describes appropriate therapy for RP at this time?
    a. Pantoprazole IV 40 mg daily plus norfloxacin po 400 mg bid
    b. Octreotide IV 50 μg bolus, then 50 μg/h infusion plus norfloxacin po 400 mg bid
    c. Octreotide IV 50 μg bolus, then 50 μg/h infusion plus pantoprazole IV 40 mg daily
    d. Octreotide IV 50 μg bolus then 50 μg/h infusion as monotherapy

---

Answer a is incorrect. While IV proton pump inhibitor therapy may be appropriate for a gastric bleed related to peptic ulcer disease, it is not appropriate for variceal bleeding.

Answer b is correct. Octreotide decreases splanchnic arterial blood flow as well as portal inflow and is therefore useful in the management of acute variceal hemorrhage. Octreotide has a very short half-life and therefore must be given as IV infusion. Short-term antibiotic therapy is recommended in a patient with acute variceal hemorrhage because patients with variceal hemorrhage are at risk of infection and sepsis due to multiple reasons including aspiration and translocation of the gastrointestinal bacterial flora. Norfloxacin po 400 mg bid for 7 days is appropriate. Ciprofloxacin IV can be used if oral access is impossible in the patient.

Answer c is incorrect. Octreotide is appropriate, but pantoprazole is not.

Answer d is incorrect. Antibiotic prophylaxis should be provided. Antibiotic prophylaxis in cases of acute variceal hemorrhage has been found to decrease rebleeding rates and increase rates of short-term survival.

---

15. Treatment of ascites includes po diuretic therapy with spironolactone and furosemide. What is the appropriate starting dosing ratio for these two drugs?
    a. Spironolactone 40 mg: furosemide 100 mg
    b. Spironolactone 100 mg: furosemide 40 mg
    c. Spironolactone 200 mg: furosemide 40 mg
    d. Spironolactone 40 mg: furosemide 200 mg

c. Peg-interferon alpha-2b
d. Ribavirin

Answer a is correct. Interferon alfacon-1 is administered subcutaneously three times per week.

Answers b and c are incorrect. The pegylation process increases the drug's half-life and allows for the interferon to be administered weekly.

Answer d is incorrect. Ribavirin is administered orally twice a day.

10. Immune globulin (GamaSTAN) is indicated for postexposure prophylaxis of

a. Autoimmune hepatitis
b. Hepatitis A virus
c. Hepatitis B virus
d. Hepatitis C virus

Answer a is incorrect. Autoimmune hepatitis is not acquired from people or the environment but is instead an autoimmune disease.

Answer b is correct. Immune globulin (GamaSTAN) is used to provide passive immunity in susceptible individuals under the following circumstances: Hepatitis A, Measles, Varicella, Rubella, and Immunoglobulin deficiency.

Answer c is incorrect. The only immune globulin formulated for HBV exposure is the hepatitis B immune globulin (HBIG).

Answer d is incorrect. There are no products in the market that provide passive immunity to HCV.

11. Which of the following drugs has the highest incidence of hemolytic anemia?

a. Ribavirin
b. Peg-interferon alpha-2a
c. Lamivudine
d. Tenofovir

Answer a is correct. The incidence of hemolytic anemia for ribavirin is 10% to 13%. The FDA requires a black box warning regarding this risk in the package insert.

Answers b, c, and d are incorrect. While peg-interferon alpha-2a, lamivudine, and tenofovir are associated with anemia, they do not cause hemolytic anemia.

12. DP is a 42-year-old woman who has developed chronic HBV from longstanding intravenous drug use. Her physician asks you to recommend a NRTI that has both high potency and low viral resistance. The best choice is

a. Entecavir
b. Tenofovir
c. Lamivudine
d. Both a and b
e. All of the above

Answer a is incorrect. Entecavir has both a high potency and a low viral resistance but tenofovir does as well.

Answer b is incorrect. Tenofovir has both a high potency and a low viral resistance but entecavir does as well.

Answer c is incorrect. Lamivudine has moderate potency and high viral resistance.

Answer d is correct. Entecavir and tenofovir have a high potency and a low risk of viral resistance.

Answer e is incorrect. Lamivudine has moderate potency and high viral resistance.

13. Chronic HCV genotype 2 should be treated with peg-interferon and ribavirin for

a. 24 weeks
b. 48 weeks
c. 1 year
d. 5 years

Answer a is correct. Genotype 2 (and 3) only requires 24 weeks of peg-interferon and ribavirin. Patients with genotypes 2 or 3 have an 80% chance of responding to 24 weeks therapy.

Answer b is incorrect. Only genotypes 1 and 4 require 48 weeks of therapy due to the low efficacy rate (50%-60%) of peg-interferon and ribavirin in this patient population.

Answer c is incorrect. A 1 to 5 year duration of NRTI therapy for HBV is common.

Answer d is incorrect. A 1 to 5 year duration of NRTI therapy for HBV is common.

14. RM is a man who has just learned he is coinfected with HIV/HCV. When should RM's chronic HCV be treated?

a. Immediately.
b. As soon as his HIV is well controlled with medication.
c. Never. His HCV is not treatable.
d. After he develops decompensated cirrhosis.

Answer a is incorrect. RM should wait until his HIV is well controlled with medications. Treatment for both HIV and chronic HCV is difficult due to side effects, complicated regimens, and poor response to medications.

Answer b is correct. RM should wait until his HIV is well controlled with medications to increase his likelihood of response.

Answer c is incorrect. It is possible to treat his chronic HCV even though the likelihood that he will have an SVR is lower than if he had chronic HCV mono-infection.

Answer d is incorrect. Pegylated-interferon and ribavirin can only be used in compensated cirrhotic patients. It is contraindicated in patients with decompensated cirrhosis because of the risk that it may worsen the cirrhosis.

15. DA has been diagnosed with chronic HCV genotype 1. His past medical and social histories include a history of IV drug abuse, alcoholism, a wife (married 30 years) with chronic HCV, and a blood transfusion in 2002. During your patient counseling session, DA asks you how he most likely acquired HCV. You correctly tell him

a. Blood transfusion in 2002
b. Sexually transmitted from his wife
c. Intravenous drug abuse
d. Alcoholism

Answer a is incorrect. After 1992, blood banks began screening blood for HCV, his risk for acquiring HCV from his blood transfusion in 2002 is extremely low.

Answer b is incorrect. Transmission of HCV from one monogamous heterosexual partner to another is extremely low. In fact, it is not necessary for HCV patients to wear a condom to protect the partner *unless* they are on peg-interferon and ribavirin treatment, since the risk of spreading via sexual contact is very low.

Answer c is correct. Contact with blood contaminated with the HCV virus is the most common route of transmission with intravenous drug use being the number one method of transmission.

Answer d is incorrect. Chronic alcohol use and untreated chronic HCV can both lead to cirrhosis but alcoholism does increase the susceptibility of acquiring HCV.

16. BR is a 47-year-old woman coinfected with HBV and HIV. The physician wants to prescribe a nucleoside reverse transcriptase inhibitor (NRTI) monotherapy to treat BR's chronic HBV. Which of the following NRTIs should you recommend?

a. Lamivudine
b. Entecavir
c. Telbivudine
d. Tenofovir

Answers a, b, and d are incorrect because each drug is associated with the development of HIV resistance.

Answer c is correct. The only drug that does not result in HIV resistance is telbivudine. It is therefore the only NRTI that can be safely used as monotherapy in patients coinfected with HIV.

17. Which of the following drugs has been given a black box warning by the FDA for the risk of severe depression and suicidal risk?

a. Ribavirin
b. Peg-interferons
c. Nucleoside reverse transcriptase inhibitors
d. Hepatitis B immune globulin (HBIG)

Answers a, c, and d are incorrect. Ribavirin, NRTIs, and HBIG are not associated with a high incidence of severe depression and suicidal risk.

Answer b is correct. Peg-interferon as well as all forms of interferon is associated with severe depression and a risk of suicidal and homicidal thoughts. Patients should be educated and monitored for this risk.

18. Which of the following products should not be given concomitantly with live vaccines?

a. Engerix-B
b. Recombivax HB
c. Twinrix
d. GamaSTAN

Answers a, b, and c are incorrect. The HAV, HBV, and HAV/HBV combination vaccines are safe to give with both live and inactivated vaccines.

Answer d is correct. GamaSTAN is an immune globulin that stimulates the immune system. A live vaccine contains weakened live virus that can become virulent if given concomitantly with an immune globulin product.

19. When is it appropriate to treat chronic viral hepatitis with peg-interferon alpha-2a monotherapy without ribavirin?

a. When the patient has renal dysfunction (CrCl < 50 mL/min).
b. When the patient has chronic HCV genotype 1.
c. When the patient has chronic HBV.
d. Both a and c.
e. None of the above.

Answer a is correct but answer c is also correct.

Answer b is incorrect. It is never appropriate to treat HCV (any genotype) with monotherapy unless the patient is unable to tolerate ribavirin therapy.

Answer c is correct but answer a is also correct.

Answer d is correct. Ribavirin is renally cleared and is contraindicated in patients with CrCl < 50 mL/min. Ribavirin is not indicated for the treatment of HBV.

20. MM, a 21-year-old woman, has been exposed to hepatitis C. Which of the following is the most appropriate course of action?

a. Do nothing unless MM acquires hepatitis C.
b. Administer immune globulin.
c. Begin peg-interferon and ribavirin.
d. Begin lamivudine.

Answer a is correct. There is no postexposure prophylaxis available for HCV exposure (no vaccine and no immune globulin). If the patient acquires acute HCV, the goal would be symptom management. Treatment is reserved for chronic HCV therapy.

Answer b is incorrect. There is no immune globulin for postexposure prophylaxis of HCV.

Answer c is incorrect. Only chronic HCV is treated with peg-interferon and ribavirin.

Answer d is incorrect. Lamivudine is a nucleotide reverse transcriptase inhibitor indicated for the treatment of chronic HBV. It has no action against HCV.

CHAPTER 39 | Upper Gastrointestinal Disorders

1. Patients with NSAID induced ulcers are more likely to have which of the following?
   a. Superficial ulcer depth
   b. A duodenal ulcer
   c. Stress related mucosal bleeding
   d. Damage to the gastric mucosa

Answer a is incorrect. Superficial ulcer depth is more common with *H. pylori* induced ulcers.

Answer b is incorrect. Ulcers caused by *H. pylori* are more common in the duodenum than the stomach.

Answer c is incorrect. Stress related mucosal bleeding is generally associated with a major stressful event (trauma, burns, surgery, organ failure, or sepsis).

Answer d is correct. NSAID-induced ulcers typically develop in the gastric mucosa.

2. JD is a 62-year-old man with a documented NSAID-induced ulcer, who is *H. pylori* negative. He must continue the NSAID for osteoarthritis. Which is the preferred medication for treating NSAID-induced ulcer?
   a. Lansoprazole
   b. Misoprostol
   c. Ranitidine
   d. Sucralfate

Answer a is correct. A PPI is the agent of choice if the NSAID must be continued in the presence of ulcer disease. If a patient tests positive for *H. pylori*, treatment is recommended.

Answer b is incorrect. Misoprostol is indicated in the prevention of NSAID-induced gastric ulcers.

Answer c is incorrect. H2-receptor antagonists have been shown to prevent only duodenal ulcers and therefore should not be recommended for prophylaxis of gastric ulcers.

Answer d is incorrect. Sucralfate has not been shown to be effective in preventing or treating NSAID-related ulcers.

3. CT is a 40-year-old man with epigastric pain and recently diagnosed with a duodenal ulcer. A urea breath test confirmed *H. pylori*. The patient denies any allergies to medications. What is recommended as primary therapy for *H. pylori*?
   a. PPI + metronidazole + levofloxacin
   b. PPI + metronidazole + clarithromycin
   c. PPI + amoxicillin + clarithromycin
   d. PPI + metronidazole + bismuth + tetracycline

Answer a is incorrect. Levofloxacin-based triple therapy has been used outside the United States.

Answer b is incorrect. The regimen of PPI, metronidazole, and clarithromycin should be reserved for patients with a penicillin allergy or those patients unable to tolerate bismuth quadruple therapy.

Answer c is correct. The recommended primary therapy for *H. pylori* infection includes a PPI, clarithromycin, and amoxicillin (clarithromycin-based triple therapy).

Answer d is incorrect. The regimen of PPI, bismuth, metronidazole, and tetracycline (bismuth quadruple therapy) is used as salvage therapy.

4. Which of the following is a nonendoscopic test used to diagnose *H. pylori*?
   a. Urea breath test
   b. Mucosal biopsy
   c. Culture
   d. Antibody detection

Answer a is correct. Urea breath test and fecal antigen are reliable for identifying active *H. pylori* before treatment.

Answer b is incorrect. Mucosal biopsy is an endoscopic test that can be used to diagnose *H. pylori*.

Answer c is incorrect. Culture is an endoscopic test that can be used to diagnose *H. pylori*.

Answer d is incorrect. Antibody detection is a nonendoscopic test, but is unable to distinguish between active or cured infection.

5. A patient calls the pharmacy to complain about her tongue turning black after starting a new regimen for peptic ulcer disease. Which medication is causing the side effect?
   a. Amoxicillin
   b. Metronidazole
   c. Bismuth subsalicylate
   d. Clarithromycin

Answer a is incorrect. Amoxicillin may cause headache, diarrhea, or GI upset.

Answer b is incorrect. Metronidazole can cause metallic taste, dyspepsia, and disulfiram-like reaction with alcohol.

Answer c is correct. Bismuth may cause nausea and a dark tongue and/or stool.

Answer d is incorrect. Clarithromycin may cause GI upset, diarrhea, or altered taste (bitter or metallic).

---

6. If a patient was treated initially with PPI, amoxicillin, and clarithromycin, which regimen is recommended for salvage therapy?

   a. PPI + amoxicillin
   b. PPI + tetracycline + metronidazole + bismuth
   c. PPI + metronidazole + clarithromycin
   d. PPI + amoxicillin + levofloxacin

Answer a is incorrect. All regimens for the treatment of *H. pylori* should contain two antibiotics.

Answer b is correct. Bismuth quadruple therapy is commonly used as the second course or salvage therapy. Salvage therapy should avoid antibiotics that were previously used.

Answer c is incorrect. Clarithromycin was used in the initial treatment regimen.

Answer d is incorrect. Levofloxacin-based triple therapy has been used outside the United States.

---

7. What is the recommended duration of treatment for *H. pylori* using clarithromycin-based triple therapy?

   a. 5 days
   b. 7 days
   c. 10 days
   d. 14 days

Answer a is incorrect. Depending on which treatment regimen is used initially 14 days is the preferred duration.

Answer b is incorrect. Seven days of therapy is not recommended due to lower eradication rate when compared to 14 day therapy.

Answer c is incorrect. If bismuth quadruple therapy is used for initial treatment, the duration is 10 to 14 days.

Answer d is correct. In the United States, 14 days is the recommended treatment duration for clarithromycin-based triple therapy.

---

8. SL is a 62-year-old woman with rheumatoid arthritis and atrial fibrillation (AF). She controls her arthritis pain with high-dose nabumetone and takes warfarin for AF. Which medication regimen(s) is recommended for prevention of NSAID ulcer complications?

   a. Change to celecoxib plus PPI
   b. Add PPI to current NSAID
   c. Change to celecoxib
   d. b and c
   e. All of the above

Answer a is incorrect. COX-2 plus either misoprostol or PPI is recommended for patients at high risk for GI toxicity.

Answer b is correct. Patients at moderate risk (1-2 risk factors) of NSAID GI toxicity may be treated with NSAID plus either misoprostol or PPI.

Answer c is correct. Patients at moderate risk (1-2 risk factors) of NSAID GI toxicity may be treated with COX-2 inhibitor alone.

Answer d is correct and the best answer. Patients at moderate risk (1-2 risk factors) of NSAID GI toxicity may be treated with COX-2 inhibitor alone or a NSAID plus either misoprostol or PPI.

Answer e is incorrect. COX-2 plus misoprostol or PPI is recommended for patients at high risk for GI toxicity.

---

9. A patient heard on Good Morning America that indomethacin can cause ulcers. She calls the pharmacy to find out if there is a better alternative to treat her arthritis. The patient is age 58 and does not have any other significant medical problems. What recommendation would be most appropriate?

   a. Sulindac
   b. Etodolac
   c. Piroxicam
   d. Naproxen

Answer a is incorrect. Sulindac is a nonselective NSAID with higher GI toxicity.

Answer b is correct. Etodolac is a partially selective NSAID with lower GI toxicity.

Answer c is incorrect. Piroxicam is a nonselective NSAID with higher GI toxicity.

Answer d is incorrect. Naproxen is a nonselective NSAID, but may have some cardioprotective effects.

---

10. TC is a 55-year-old woman with hyperlipidemia, post-MI and HTN. Medications include atorvastatin 20 mg once daily, ASA 81 mg once daily, and metoprolol 100 mg bid. If the patient needs chronic NSAID therapy what is recommended to prevent ulcers?

    a. COX-2 inhibitor
    b. Naproxen
    c. COX-2 inhibitor plus PPI
    d. Naproxen plus PPI

Answer a is incorrect. The gastroprotective effect is lost with COX-2 inhibitors in patients taking low-dose aspirin. Also, COX-2 inhibitors should be avoided due to increase risk of cardiovascular events, and this patient has a history of cardiovascular disease.

Answer b is incorrect. Naproxen may have some cardioprotective properties, but for low- and moderate-risk patients on low-dose aspirin the addition of PPI or misoprostol is recommended.

Answer c is incorrect. The gastroprotective effect is lost with COX-2 inhibitors in patients taking low-dose aspirin despite the addition of a PPI. Also, COX-2 inhibitors should be avoided due to increase risk of cardiovascular events, and this patient has a history of cardiovascular disease.

Answer d is correct. TC is at moderate risk for NSAID-induced GI toxicity, but at high CV risk due to aspirin therapy. Naproxen is the NSAID of choice because it has been shown to be cardiovascular neutral. Guidelines recommend PPI or misoprostol because naproxen and low-dose aspirin increases the risk of GI bleeding.

---

11. Which of the following describes the clinical presentation of duodenal ulcers?
    a. Pain may be accompanied by coughing up blood.
    b. Pain is worse at night or between meals.
    c. Pain is worse with food.
    d. Pain is caused by damage from NSAIDs.

Answer a is incorrect. Coughing up blood is associated with the complications of PUD such as perforation or a GI bleed.

Answer b is correct. Pain due to a duodenal ulcer may be worse on an empty stomach.

Answer c is incorrect. Gastric ulcer pain may be worse with eating.

Answer d is incorrect. Gastric ulcers are associated with NSAID use.

---

12. Which of the following requires a negative pregnancy test prior to starting therapy?
    a. Celecoxib
    b. Misoprostol
    c. PPIs
    d. Amoxicillin

Answer a is incorrect. Does not require a pregnancy test prior to starting therapy. Celecoxib is pregnancy category C prior to 30 weeks gestation and category D at 30 or more weeks gestation.

Answer b is correct. Female patients should have a negative pregnancy test within 2 weeks prior to starting therapy. Patients should start misoprostol on the second or third day of their next normal menstrual cycle. Misoprostol is pregnancy category X.

Answer c is incorrect. Does not require a pregnancy test prior to starting therapy. PPIs are either pregnancy category B or C.

Answer d is incorrect. Does not require a pregnancy test prior to starting therapy. Amoxicillin is pregnancy category B.

---

13. A patient is admitted to the intensive care unit after a car accident. The patient has been on mechanical ventilation for 72 hours and has a head injury. Which of the following is recommended for this patient for stress ulcer prophylaxis?
    a. Ranitidine by mouth
    b. Intravenous pantoprazole
    c. Sucralfate by nasogastric tube
    d. Patient does not require stress ulcer prophylaxis

Answer a is incorrect. H2RAs and PPIs are preferred treatment options, but they are not preferred by mouth since the patient is on mechanical ventilation.

Answer b is correct. PPIs and H2RAs are preferred treatment options and IV would be the best route of delivery.

Answer c is incorrect. Sucralfate is not first line for high-risk patients on a ventilator.

Answer d is incorrect. The patient is considered at high risk for stress ulcers because mechanical ventilation has been used for more than 48 hours and head injury patients are at higher risk of SRMB.

Use the following case to answer questions 14 and 15.

AM is a 45-year-old obese woman with HTN and diabetes who presents with complaints of "severe" heartburn after meals and occasionally at night. She admits to smoking and occasional alcohol consumption. She consumes 4 to 5 caffeinated beverages daily. Medications include: hydrochlorothiazide (HCTZ) 12.5 mg daily and metformin 850 mg twice daily.

14. Which of the following factors may worsen GERD symptoms in this patient?
    a. Alcohol consumption
    b. Caffeine consumption
    c. Obesity
    d. Smoking
    e. All of the above

Answer a is correct. Alcohol consumption may worsen GERD symptoms by increasing acid secretion, reducing LES tone and esophageal motility, and slowing gastric emptying.

Answer b is correct. Caffeine is believed to reduce LES pressure causing increased GERD symptoms.

Answer c is correct. Obesity is believed to cause GERD symptoms for several reasons including increased intra-abdominal pressure and increased output of bile and pancreatic enzymes. Additionally, obese patients have a higher incidence of hiatal hernia.

Answer d is correct. Smoking has been shown to prolong acid clearance and decrease LES pressure.

Answer e is the correct and the best answer. All are factors which may worsen GERD symptoms in this patient case. Additional lifestyle modifications that may be beneficial include: avoiding foods that are acidic or directly irritating; avoiding foods that may cause reflux; avoiding eating within 3 hours of bedtime; elevating the head of the bed; eating smaller and more frequent meals; and not lying down after meals.

---

15. Which of the following represents the best initial treatment option with the highest probability of symptom control?

    a. Famotidine
    b. Metoclopramide
    c. Pantoprazole
    d. Sucralfate

Answer a is incorrect. H2RA are effective for many patients with mild to moderate GERD symptoms; however, this patient presents with severe reflux symptoms. Overall, PPIs are the most effective pharmacologic option for control of symptoms and healing of esophagitis.

Answer b is incorrect. Due to significant risk of side effects and lack of benefit in clinical trials, metoclopramide is not considered as first-line therapy. It could be used as an adjunctive medication in patients with known gastrointestinal motility disorders, but should always be used in conjunction with acid suppressive therapy.

Answer c is correct. PPIs have the highest rate of symptom control and healing rates when esophagitis is present or suspected. All PPIs are considered equally effective.

Answer d is incorrect. Sucralfate is not effective for patients with GERD and cannot be recommended.

---

16. HG is a 65-year-old woman with osteoporosis, GERD, and HTN. Medications include alendronate 70 mg weekly, calcium carbonate 600 mg + vitamin D 400 units, omeprazole 20 mg daily, and enalapril 10 mg bid. Which of the following are possible consequences of this regimen?

    a. Alendronate may worsen GERD symptoms.
    b. Enalapril may worsen GERD symptoms.
    c. Omeprazole may reduce calcium absorption.
    d. a and c.

Answer a is correct. Bisphosphonates can cause a myriad of gastrointestinal symptoms including dyspepsia, reflux, and ulcer formation. These symptoms may be worsened in patients who do not remain in an upright position for at least 30 minutes after taking bisphosphonates such as alendronate.

Answer b is incorrect. ACE-inhibitors do not cause an increase in GERD symptoms or interact with medications commonly used for treatment.

Answer c is correct. Calcium carbonate requires an acidic environment for adequate absorption. Acid suppressant therapy, particularly potent PPIs, raise the pH reducing calcium absorption. Older patients taking omeprazole had an increased risk of fracture compared to equally matched patients. Calcium citrate may be recommended in these patients as it does not require an acidic environment for adequate absorption.

Answer d is the correct and the best answer. Answers a and c represent possible consequences of this medication regimen. Bisphosphonates can cause a myriad of gastrointestinal symptoms including dyspepsia, reflux, and ulcer formation. These symptoms may be worsened in patients who do not remain in an upright position for at least 30 minutes after taking bisphosphonates such as alendronate. Calcium carbonate requires an acidic environment for adequate absorption. Acid suppressant therapy, particularly potent PPIs, raise the pH reducing calcium absorption. Older patients taking omeprazole had an increased risk of fracture compared to equally matched patients. Calcium citrate may be recommended in these patients as it does not require an acidic environment for adequate absorption.

---

17. Which of the following is a typical sign or symptom of patients with GERD?

    a. Iron deficiency anemia
    b. Dysphagia
    c. Regurgitation
    d. Weight loss

Answer a is incorrect. The presence of iron deficiency in patients with GERD is a complicating factor. This may be an indication of gastrointestinal bleeding; therefore, additional diagnostic testing (endoscopy and/or colonoscopy) would be indicated.

Answer b is incorrect. Dysphagia, or difficulty swallowing, is a concerning alarm symptom because it may indicate stricture or malignancy.

Answer c is correct. Regurgitation is a common symptom of uncomplicated GERD. Additional typical symptoms include heartburn, belching, and hypersalivation.

Answer d is incorrect. Unexplained weight loss is not a typical symptom of patients with GERD and warrants further investigation.

---

18. Which of the following acts by competitively inhibiting histamine at the H2 receptor of gastric parietal cells?

    a. Omeprazole
    b. Pantoprazole
    c. Rabeprazole
    d. Ranitidine

Answer a is incorrect. Omeprazole is a proton pump inhibitor.

Answer b is incorrect. Pantoprazole is a proton pump inhibitor.

Answer c is incorrect. Rabeprazole is a proton pump inhibitor.

Answer d is correct. Ranitidine is a H2-receptor antagonist.

19. NJ, a 50-year-old woman, presented to her physician approximately 8 weeks ago with complaints of heartburn, regurgitation, and dysphagia which resulted in an endoscopy. At that time her physician diagnosed GERD with erosive esophagitis and prescribed 2 months of lansoprazole 30 mg daily. Today at her follow-up visit, she reports improvement in her symptoms. What would you recommend as maintenance therapy for NJ?
    a. Lansoprazole 15 mg daily
    b. Lansoprazole 30 mg daily
    c. No further therapy required
    d. Either a or b

Answer a is correct. Daily maintenance with a PPI with erosive esophagitis is recommended. Many patients may tolerate dosage reduction and maintain adequate symptom control.

Answer b is correct. Daily maintenance with a PPI with erosive esophagitis is recommended. Patients may be continued on the previous dose as relapse of heartburn and other GERD symptoms is common.

Answer c is incorrect. GERD is a chronic condition requiring maintenance therapy. For most patients continuous PPI therapy is recommended to maintain the healed mucosa, and discontinuing therapy results in recurrent heartburn.

Answer d is the correct and the best answer. Chronic maintenance therapy with PPI will be required by most patients with symptoms severe enough to warrant initial therapy. Many patients may tolerate dosage reduction and maintain adequate symptom control. Other options in this patient might be a trial of H2RA or patient-directed therapy with a PPI when symptoms recur.

20. Select the brand name for pantoprazole.
    a. Axid
    b. Aciphex
    c. Prevacid
    d. Protonix
    e. Tagamet

Answer a is incorrect. Axid is the brand name for nizatidine.

Answer b is incorrect. Aciphex is the brand name for rabeprazole.

Answer c is incorrect. Prevacid is the brand name for lansoprazole

Answer d is correct. Protonix is the brand name for pantoprazole.

Answer e is incorrect. Tagamet is the brand name for cimetidine.

21. Which of the following would be appropriate health information to discuss with a patient presenting to your pharmacy with GERD symptoms?
    a. Eating smaller meals more often
    b. Elevating the head of the bed 6 to 8 in
    c. Weight reduction for patients who are overweight
    d. Smoking cessation for those who smoke
    e. All of the above

Answer a is correct. Eating smaller meals more often may be beneficial in reducing reflux symptoms.

Answer b is correct. Elevating the head of the bed may be a helpful nonpharmacologic strategy for patients who experience frequent nighttime GERD symptoms.

Answer c is correct. Patients who are overweight often have increased GERD symptoms. Losing weight has been shown to improve symptoms.

Answer d is correct. Cigarette smoking has been shown to reduce lower esophageal pressure and prolong acid clearance. The duration of smoking is also an important risk factor for GERD symptoms; smokers with more than 20-year history of tobacco use were more likely to have reflux symptoms when compared with those who smoked for less than 1 year.

Answer e is the correct and the best answer. All of these are important counseling points for patients who present with GERD symptoms.

CHAPTER 40 | Nausea and Vomiting

1. Select the correct statement. Patients more susceptible to nausea and vomiting include:
    a. Chronic alcoholics
    b. Female patients
    c. Patients older than 50 years of age
    d. Patients with a smoking history

Answer a is incorrect. Patients with a history of long-term alcohol consumption have a lower risk of nausea and vomiting.

Answer b is correct. Female patients tend to have more nausea and vomiting than male patients.

Answer c is incorrect. Patients younger than 50 years of age are more susceptible to nausea and vomiting.

Answer d is incorrect. Studies examining PONV suggest patients with a smoking history may be less likely to experience nausea and vomiting, similar to chronic alcoholics.

2. Select the correct statement. Delayed nausea and vomiting:
   a. Is easier to prevent than acute nausea and vomiting
   b. Occurs within the first day following drug administration
   c. Occurs more commonly with cisplatin and cyclophosphamide
   d. Commonly resolves within 72 hours following drug administration

---

Answer a is incorrect. Delayed nausea and vomiting is more difficult to prevent than acute nausea and vomiting. Most of the clinical studies have focused on acute nausea and vomiting, thus we have well-defined guidelines for acute CINV. Fortunately, drug therapy is improving with many of the new drugs such as aprepitant and palonosetron being helpful in the prevention of delayed nausea and vomiting.

Answer b is incorrect. Delayed nausea and vomiting is nausea and vomiting that occurs for more than 24 hours following the administration of chemotherapy.

Answer c is correct. Cisplatin and cyclophosphamide are two highly emetogenic chemotherapy agents that are associated with delayed nausea and vomiting. Studies suggest that > 90% of patients receiving cisplatin will experience delayed CINV if inadequate prophylaxis is given. When cisplatin and cyclophosphamide are given at high doses, drug therapy should include an antiemetic agent with delayed CINV coverage.

Answer d is incorrect. Delayed nausea and vomiting may persist for 7 days following chemotherapy.

---

3. Which neurotransmitter has no involvement in CINV?
   a. Dopamine
   b. Neurokinin-1
   c. Norepinephrine
   d. Serotonin

Answer a is incorrect. The neurotransmitter dopamine plays an important role in CINV. Dopamine antagonists such as promethazine are routinely prescribed in the prevention/treatment of CINV.

Answer b is incorrect. The neurotransmitter neurokinin-1 (substance P) plays an important role in CINV. Neurokinin-1 receptor antagonists such as aprepitant are prescribed in the prevention of CINV.

Answer c is correct. The neurotransmitter norepinephrine has not been shown to play a role in CINV. Thus, there are no drugs used in the treatment of CINV that inhibit norepinephrine.

Answer d is incorrect. The neurotransmitter serotonin plays an important role in CINV. Serotonin (5-HT3) antagonists such as ondansetron are routinely prescribed in the prevention of CINV.

---

4. DS is a 35-year-old woman undergoing surgery for a hysterectomy. She has a history of PONV and motion sickness. Which drug should be administered during or following surgery for the prevention of PONV?
   a. Haloperidol
   b. Ondansetron
   c. Prochlorperazine
   d. Scopolamine

Answer a is incorrect. The role of haloperidol in the prevention PONV has not been established.

Answer b is correct. Ondansetron and other serotonin (5-H3) antagonists are recommended by the anesthesia guidelines in the prevention of PONV for high-risk patients. All of the 5-HT3 antagonists have been used in PONV with most of the studies examining ondansetron. They are most effective when given during or at the end of surgery.

Answer c is incorrect. Prochlorperazine has been studied in prevention of PONV but has limited use because of its side-effect profile (sedation, dizziness, dry mouth).

Answer d is incorrect. Transdermal scopolamine has been studied in PONV but has limited use because of the 2 to 4 hour delay in onset of effect.

---

5. Select the correct dose and route of aprepitant for prevention of PONV.
   a. 40 mg orally
   b. 80 mg IV injection
   c. 115 mg IV injection
   d. 125 mg orally

Answer a is correct. The recommended dose of aprepitant for prevention of PONV is 40 mg orally administered within 3 hours prior to surgery.

Answer b is incorrect. Aprepitant 80 mg is given orally on days 2 and 3 of chemotherapy.

Answer c is incorrect. Fosaprepitant 115 mg is given intravenously on day 1 of chemotherapy.

Answer d is incorrect. Aprepitant 125 mg is given orally on day 1 of chemotherapy.

---

6. Select the serotonin (5-HT3) receptor antagonist that has a prolonged half-life and is given as a single-dose injection prior to the start of chemotherapy for the prevention of acute and delayed CINV.
   a. Aloxi
   b. Anzemet
   c. Kytril
   d. Zofran

Answer a is correct. Palonosetron (Aloxi) has a prolonged (40 hour) half-life. Aloxi is FDA approved for the prevention of acute CINV in moderately to highly emetogenic chemotherapy and in the prevention of delayed CINV in moderately emetogenic chemotherapy.

Answer b is incorrect. Dolasetron (Anzemet) has a short half-life and is not approved for prevention of delayed CINV.

Answer c is incorrect. Granisetron (Kytril) has a short half-life and is not approved for prevention of delayed CINV.

Answer d is incorrect. Ondansetron (Zofran) has a short half-life and is not approved for prevention of delayed CINV.

---

7. Which serotonin (5-HT3) receptor antagonist is available as a transdermal patch?
   a. Dolasetron
   b. Granisetron
   c. Ondansetron
   d. Palonosetron

Answer a is incorrect. Dolasetron is not available in a transdermal patch.

Answer b is correct. Sancuso is the trade name for the granisetron transdermal patch. It received FDA approval in September 2008.

Answer c is incorrect. Ondansetron is not available in a transdermal patch.

Answer d is incorrect. Palonosetron is not available in a transdermal patch.

---

8. DH is undergoing chemotherapy for breast cancer with doxorubicin and cyclophosphamide. Select which antiemetic combination will give her optimal prevention for CINV?
   a. Aprepitant, dolasetron, and prochlorperazine
   b. Aprepitant, prochlorperazine, and dexamethasone
   c. Aprepitant, haloperidol, and promethazine
   d. Aprepitant, ondansetron, and dexamethasone

Answer a is incorrect. Aprepitant is FDA approved in combination with a corticosteroid and 5-HT3 antagonist. This combination lacks the corticosteroid.

Answer b is incorrect. Aprepitant is FDA approved in combination with a corticosteroid and 5-HT3 antagonist. This combination lacks the 5-HT3 antagonist.

Answer c is incorrect. Aprepitant is FDA approved in combination with a corticosteroid and 5-HT3 antagonist. This combination lacks the corticosteroid and 5-HT3 antagonist.

Answer d is correct. Aprepitant is FDA approved in combination with a corticosteroid (dexamethasone) and 5-HT3 antagonist (ondansetron).

---

9. Select the correct statement.
   a. Dolasetron has similar efficacy to ondansetron when used at equipotent doses.
   b. Granisetron is the only 5-HT3 antagonist approved for prevention of delayed CINV with highly emetogenic chemotherapy.
   c. Palonosetron is superior to prochlorperazine for the treatment of breakthrough nausea and vomiting.
   d. The IV route of administration of ondansetron is superior to oral administration.

Answer a is correct. Studies show that when 5-HT3 antagonists are given at equipotent doses they have similar efficacy in the prevention of acute nausea and vomiting.

Answer b is incorrect. Currently, no 5-HT3 antagonist is approved for the prevention of delayed CINV with highly emetogenic chemotherapy. Palonosetron is the only 5-HT3 antagonist approved for delayed CINV in moderately emetogenic chemotherapy.

Answer c in incorrect. Dopamine antagonists such as prochlorperazine should be used in the treatment of breakthrough nausea and vomiting. Superiority of the 5-HT3 has not been shown.

Answer d is incorrect. The IV route of administration of 5-HT3 antagonists is equal to the oral route in regards to efficacy.

---

10. Select the correct dose of IV ondansetron when used in the prevention of PONV.
    a. 4 mg
    b. 12 mg
    c. 20 mg
    d. 32 mg

Answer a is correct. Ondansetron 4 to 8 mg is the preferred dose for PONV.

Answers b, c, d are incorrect. Ondansetron 4 to 8 mg is the preferred dose for PONV.

---

11. Which is the preferred antiemetic for breakthrough nausea and vomiting?
    a. Aprepitant
    b. Dronabinol
    c. Ondansetron
    d. Prochlorperazine

Answer a is incorrect. Aprepitant should not be prescribed for as needed use.

Answer b is incorrect. Dronabinol should be reserved for refractory CINV.

Answer c is incorrect. Ondansetron should not be prescribed for as needed use.

Answer d is correct. Dopamine antagonists such as prochlorperazine are effective for as needed use.

12. Significant drug interactions with aprepitant include:
    a. Dexamethasone
    b. Oral contraceptive pills (OCP)
    c. Warfarin
    d. All of the above

Answer a is incorrect. A reduced dose of dexamethasone is required when giving aprepitant.

Answer b is incorrect. Reduced efficacy of oral contraceptive pills has been shown when taken with aprepitant. Women should use backup contraceptives for 1 month after discontinuing aprepitant.

Answer c is incorrect. Aprepitant is an inducer of warfarin metabolism. Higher doses of warfarin may be required.

Answer d is correct. All of the above.

13. Which antiemetic should be diluted when given intravenously to minimize extravasation potential?
    a. Droperidol
    b. Fosaprepitant
    c. Palonosetron
    d. Promethazine

Answer a is incorrect. Extravasation is not a major concern with droperidol.

Answer b is incorrect. Extravasation is not a major concern with fosaprepitant.

Answer c is incorrect. Extravasation is not a major concern with palonosetron.

Answer d is correct. Promethazine can cause serious tissue damage when extravasation occurs. Several organizations recommend diluting promethazine prior to injection to minimize the extravasation potential.

14. Select which antiemetic has a black box warning associated with irreversible extrapyramidal side effects.
    a. Aprepitant
    b. Dexamethasone
    c. Dolasetron
    d. Metoclopramide

Answer a is incorrect. Aprepitant does not cause extrapyramidal side effects.

Answer b is incorrect. Dexamethasone does not cause extrapyramidal side effects.

Answer c is incorrect. Dolasetron does not cause extrapyramidal side effects.

Answer d is correct. Metoclopramide can cause irreversible extrapyramidal side effects.

15. Which antiemetic should be avoided in patients with the potential for a prolonged QT-interval?
    a. Aprepitant
    b. Droperidol
    c. Metoclopramide
    d. Scopolamine

Answer a is incorrect. QT-interval prolongation is not a concern with aprepitant.

Answer b is correct. QT-interval prolongation may occur with recommended doses of droperidol. Droperidol now has a black box warning alerting practitioners of the serious potential for QT-interval prolongation.

Answer c is incorrect. QT-interval prolongation is not a concern with metoclopramide.

Answer d is incorrect. QT-interval prolongation is not a concern with scopolamine.

16. Of the agents listed, select the chemotherapy agent with the highest emetic risk.
    a. Cisplatin
    b. Etoposide
    c. Paclitaxel
    d. Vincristine

Answer a is correct. Cisplatin has high emetogenic potential. More than 90% of patients experience nausea and vomiting if appropriate antiemetic prophylaxis is not given. The routine use of antiemetic is necessary when giving cisplatin.

Answer b is incorrect. Etoposide has low emetogenic potential.

Answer c is incorrect. Paclitaxel has low emetogenic potential.

Answer d is incorrect. Vincristine has minimal emetogenic potential.

17. Anticipatory nausea and vomiting may be prevented with:
    a. Dexamethasone
    b. Dronabinol
    c. Lorazepam
    d. Palonosetron

Answer a is incorrect. Dexamethasone is used for acute and delayed nausea and vomiting.

Answer b is incorrect. Dronabinol is used for breakthrough nausea and vomiting that has been refractory to other antiemetic therapies.

Answer c is correct. Lorazepam and other benzodiazepines are useful in the prevention of anticipatory nausea and vomiting.

Answer d is incorrect. Palonosetron is used for acute and delayed nausea and vomiting.

---

18. Sancuso transdermal patch delivers antiemetic activity for:
    a. 24 hours
    b. 72 hours
    c. 5 days
    d. 7 days

Answers a, b, and c are incorrect. Sancuso provides antiemetic activity over 7 days.

Answer d is correct. Sancuso provides antiemetic activity over 7 days.

---

19. Which statement is correct?
    a. Dronabinol is a Schedule II substance.
    b. Dronabinol is reserved for the treatment of CINV in patients with anorexia or HIV.
    c. Dronabinol is associated with sedation, euphoria, and dizziness.
    d. All of the above.

Answer a is incorrect. Dronabinol is a Schedule III substance per federal law.

Answer b is incorrect. Dronabinol may be used in any patient with CINV.

Answer c is correct. Dronabinol is associated with sedation, euphoria, and dizziness. Caution must be used in the elderly and when given with other sedative drugs.

Answer d is incorrect. Only Answer c is correct.

---

20. Factors that increase the risk of PONV include:
    a. Duration of surgery
    b. Type of anesthetic used
    c. Type of surgery
    d. All of the above

Answer a is incorrect. The duration of surgery may increase the risk of PONV.

Answer b is incorrect. The type of anesthetic used may increase the risk of PONV. Agents such as nitrous oxide increase the risk of PONV.

Answer c is incorrect. The type of surgery may increase the risk of PONV. Gynecological and abdominal surgeries increase the risk of PONV.

Answer d is correct. All of the above increase the risk of PONV.

CHAPTER 41 | Inflammatory Bowel Disease

1. Select the characteristic that is a feature of Crohn disease, but not of ulcerative colitis.
    a. Disease distribution limited to the colon
    b. Presence of extraintestinal manifestations
    c. Inflammation affecting only the mucosal layer
    d. Inflammation penetrating below the mucosal layer

Answer a is incorrect. Ulcerative colitis (UC) is confined to the colon, whereas Crohn disease (CD) may affect any area within the gastrointestinal (GI) tract.

Answer b is incorrect. Both UC and CD may have concomitant extraintestinal manifestations present as part of the disease.

Answer c is incorrect. Inflammation affecting only the mucosal layer of the GI tract is indicative of UC.

Answer d is correct. Crohn disease is associated with much deeper intestinal inflammation compared to UC. The inflammation often penetrates into the submucosal and muscular layers of the intestinal tract.

---

2. Which drug formulation of mesalamine is most effective as initial therapy for patients with mild to moderate ulcerative proctitis?
    a. Suppository
    b. Enema
    c. Tablet
    d. Intravenous injection

Answer a is correct. Ulcerative proctitis is a subset of UC in which inflammation is localized to the rectum. Mesalamine is a first-line agent for mild to moderate proctitis. The suppository formulation delivers mesalamine directly to the site of action and treats up to 20 cm of the rectal area, thus it is the preferred formulation for treatment of proctitis.

Answer b is incorrect. While the enema form of mesalamine would treat proctitis, it delivers the drug up to the splenic flexure. This would result in unnecessary coverage of this area of the GI tract and would be more appropriate for a patient with distal or left-sided disease.

Answer c is incorrect. While the tablet form of mesalamine would treat proctitis, it delivers the drug either throughout the small and large intestine or just throughout the colon, depending on the formulation. This would result in unnecessary coverage of this area of the GI tract and would be more appropriate for a patient with extensive disease.

Answer d is incorrect. Mesalamine is not available in the United States in an injectable formulation.

---

3. Which enzyme involved in the metabolism of azathioprine is subject to genetic polymorphism?
   a. Rasburicase
   b. Dihydrofolate reductase
   c. Thiopurine methyltransferase
   d. Hyaluronidase

Answer a is incorrect. Rasburicase is not an enzyme, but rather a drug used in the treatment of tumor lysis syndrome.

Answer b is incorrect. Dihydrofolate reductase is an enzyme that is involved in the metabolism of methotrexate and does not affect azathioprine.

Answer c is correct. Thiopurine methyltransferase is an enzyme that is partially responsible for the metabolism of azathioprine. Genetic polymorphisms of this enzyme may result in reduced enzyme activity. This may predispose patients to higher blood levels of azathioprine and increase the potential for toxicity. Patients should have their thiopurine methyltransferase activity level measured prior to initiating therapy with azathioprine.

Answer d is incorrect. Hyaluronidase is a substance which increases the permeability of connective tissue. It is often used in surgical procedures to increase drug absorption.

4. BD is a 27-year-old white man who is newly diagnosed with moderate extensive ulcerative colitis. He reports a drug allergy to sulfonamide-containing medications, which manifests as a rash. Which product would be most appropriate as initial therapy for this patient?
   a. Canasa
   b. Azulfidine
   c. Colazal
   d. Enterocort

Answer a is incorrect. Mesalamine is an appropriate agent for this patient. However, Canasa is the suppository formulation of mesalamine. This patient has extensive disease, which indicates that the majority of the colon is affected. The suppository formulation would deliver mesalamine only to the rectal area and not to the colon where it is needed.

Answer b is incorrect. Azulfidine is sulfasalazine. This would be an appropriate first-line agent for extensive UC; however, the patient has a sulfa allergy, which precludes the use of sulfasalazine.

Answer c is correct. Colazal is balsalazide, which contains mesalamine linked to an inert carrier molecule. This formulation delivers mesalamine to the colon. Since this patient has extensive disease, this would be a favorable formulation. Balsalazide also lacks a sulfa moiety and can be used safely in patients with an allergy to sulfonamide-containing drugs.

Answer d is incorrect. Enterocort is budesonide, which is a corticosteroid that is used for patients with CD who have disease located in the ileum and ascending colon.

5. Which product is available only as an intravenous solution for injection?
   a. Purinethol
   b. Colazal
   c. Flagyl
   d. Remicade

Answer a is incorrect. Mercaptopurine is available only as a tablet.

Answer b is incorrect. Balsalazide is available only as a tablet.

Answer c is incorrect. Metronidazole is available as both oral tablets and as an injection.

Answer d is correct. Infliximab is available only as an injection for intravenous use.

6. Which laboratory parameter(s) should be monitored closely in patients who are initiated on methotrexate therapy?
   a. Complete blood count
   b. Serum potassium
   c. Serum calcium
   d. Lipase

Answer a is correct. Methotrexate is a folate antagonist that can cause bone marrow suppression. A complete blood count should be routinely monitored in patients receiving methotrexate.

Answer b is incorrect. Methotrexate is not commonly associated with alterations in serum potassium concentrations except in the instance of severe nephrotoxicity caused by methotrexate.

Answer c is incorrect. Methotrexate is not commonly associated with alterations in serum calcium concentrations.

Answer d is correct. Methotrexate is not commonly associated with development of pancreatitis, which would result in alterations in lipase concentrations.

7. Which condition is considered a contraindication to receiving a TNF-α antagonist?
   a. Migraine headache
   b. Previous myocardial infarction
   c. Asthma
   d. Sepsis

Answer a is incorrect. Migraine headache is not considered a contraindication to therapy. Neurologic disorders, such as optic neuritis or demyelinating diseases, would be potential contraindications.

Answer b is incorrect. Previous myocardial infarction is not considered a contraindication to therapy; however, the presence of advanced heart failure would be a cardiac condition that is considered a contraindication.

Answer c is incorrect. Asthma or COPD are not considered contraindications to therapy.

Answer d is correct. Since TNF-α antagonists are associated with development of severe infections, patients should not have a preexisting severe infection when initiating therapy. Sepsis is a condition associated with severe infections and would be a contraindication to therapy.

8. JJ is a 37-year-old woman who has been receiving Asacol for treatment of ulcerative colitis. She is receiving maximal doses of Asacol, but continues to have daily moderate symptoms including urgency, abdominal pain, and rectal bleeding. Which therapy would be best for treatment of her symptoms at this time?

   a. Enterocort
   b. Trexall
   c. Remicade
   d. Apriso

Answer a is incorrect. Budesonide is a corticosteroid that is only indicated for patients with CD, who have involvement of the terminal ileum or ascending colon.

Answer b is incorrect. Methotrexate is used more in the setting of CD and, like azathioprine, has a delayed onset of action, taking at least 3 to 4 months to work. This patient needs more rapid control of her symptoms.

Answer c is correct. Infliximab is indicated in patients with moderate to severe symptoms who are unresponsive to other therapies, such as aminosalicylates or corticosteroids. Infliximab works faster than azathioprine and would be a better choice for this patient based on the fact that she is experiencing moderate symptoms on a daily basis.

Answer d is incorrect. Apriso is a once daily formulation of mesalamine. Since this patient is already failing maximal doses of mesalamine, switching to another mesalamine product would provide minimal benefit.

9. A 48-year-old male patient with Crohn disease is prescribed Humira for treatment of severe symptoms. Which counseling point should you provide to this patient prior to starting this therapy?

   a. Correct number of tablets to take on a daily basis
   b. Proper injection technique
   c. Monitor for development of diarrhea
   d. The next dose should be given in 8 weeks

Answer a is incorrect. Humira is an injectable product, and is not available in an oral tablet formulation.

Answer b is correct. Since Humira is administered by subcutaneous injection and is available as a single-dose syringe or a pen device, that patient should be instructed on how to use the formulation and administer the injection properly. The manufacturer medication guide has detailed instructions which can be used to educate patients on this process.

Answer c is incorrect. Humira is not commonly associated with development of diarrhea.

Answer d is incorrect. Following the initial dose, the next two doses occur at 2 week intervals, followed then by an every other week dose schedule.

10. Which medication would be most efficacious in a patient with fistulizing Crohn disease?

    a. Ciprofloxacin
    b. Mesalamine
    c. Prednisone
    d. Certolizumab

Answer a is incorrect. Antibiotics, such as ciprofloxacin, may be used as an adjunctive therapy in patients with fistulizing CD. There are other therapies that are preferred in this type of CD.

Answer b is incorrect. Mesalamine has a role as initial therapy in the management of mild to moderate CD; however, it is not effective for treating fistulizing CD.

Answer c is incorrect. Corticosteroids rapidly suppress inflammation in patients with all severities of CD; however, they are ineffective in the treatment of fistulizing CD.

Answer d is correct. Fistulizing CD has been observed to be most responsive to treatment with TNF-α antagonists, such as certolizumab. Thus, these agents are considered first-line therapies in the treatment of fistulizing CD.

11. Which drug may be most commonly associated with the development of pancreatitis as a potential adverse effect?

    a. Methotrexate
    b. Azathioprine
    c. Adalimumab
    d. Natalizumab

Answer a is incorrect. Methotrexate is associated with development of hepatic, pulmonary, renal, and bone marrow toxicity; however it is not commonly associated with development of pancreatitis.

Answer b is correct. Azathioprine is commonly associated with development of pancreatitis. This adverse effect often occurs within the first 4 to 6 weeks of therapy. Patients should be monitored for signs or symptoms that may be consistent with pancreatitis.

Answer c is incorrect. Adalimumab is associated with development of infections, heart failure, and neurologic complications among others, but is not commonly associated with development of pancreatitis.

Answer d is incorrect. Adalimumab is associated with development of infusion-related reactions, neurologic complications, and development of infection, but is not commonly associated with development of pancreatitis.

12. What is the role of oral prednisone in the treatment of inflammatory bowel disease (IBD)?

    a. Preferred treatment for maintenance of remission
    b. First line for treatment of mild disease
    c. No role in the management of IBD
    d. Short-term use in patients unresponsive to aminosalicylates

Answer a is incorrect. Corticosteroids are ineffective for the maintenance of remission in IBD and should only be used for short-term courses in patients with active disease.

Answer b is incorrect. Mild UC is typically treated with aminosalicylates as first-line therapies, while mild CD may be treated with aminosalicylates or budesonide. Prednisone would be reserved for patients with moderate to severe disease who have failed aminosalicylates.

Answer c is incorrect. Prednisone does have a role in short-term management of patients with moderate to severe symptoms or in patients who have failed aminosalicylates.

Answer d is correct. Prednisone's major role is as a short-term treatment in patients with moderate to severe symptoms or in patients who have failed aminosalicylates.

13. Which product has the ability to be administered on a once daily basis?

    a. Asacol
    b. Lialda
    c. Azulfidine
    d. Dipentum

Answer a is incorrect. Asacol is typically administered three times a day.

Answer b is correct. Lialda is a mesalamine formulation that is administered once daily.

Answer c is incorrect. Azulfidine is administered three to four times a day.

Answer d is incorrect. Dipentum is administered two times a day.

14. A patient receiving long-term therapy with metronidazole should be monitored for the development of which adverse effect?

    a. Peripheral neuropathy
    b. Hepatitis
    c. Pulmonary fibrosis
    d. Anemia

Answer a is correct. Metronidazole may cause peripheral neuropathy when administered in high doses over extended periods of time. Long-term use should be avoided if possible. Patients should be monitored for signs of peripheral neuropathy if long-term use is necessitated.

Answer b is incorrect. While metronidazole is metabolized hepatically, development of hepatitis is not commonly associated with metronidazole use.

Answer c is incorrect. Pulmonary fibrosis is associated with methotrexate use and is not commonly associated with metronidazole.

Answer d is incorrect. Metronidazole is not commonly associated with development of anemia.

15. What is the mechanism of action of natalizumab in the treatment of IBD?

    a. Antagonism of TNF-α
    b. Inhibition of arachidonic acid formation
    c. Down regulation of interleukin-1 production
    d. Inhibition of leukocyte adhesion

Answer a is incorrect. Antagonism of TNF-α is the main mechanism by which infliximab, adalimumab, and certolizumab work in IBD.

Answer b is incorrect. Inhibition of arachidonic acid formation is not a known mechanism of natalizumab.

Answer c is incorrect. Inhibition of arachidonic acid formation is not a known mechanism of natalizumab.

Answer d is correct. Natalizumab works by inhibiting leukocyte adhesion, specifically by inhibiting α-4 integrin, a glycoprotein expressed on leukocytes.

16. A patient who presents with "left-sided" ulcerative colitis has inflammation extending from the rectum to which area within the GI tract?
    a. Sigmoid colon
    b. Hepatic flexure
    c. Splenic flexure
    d. Terminal ileum

Answer a is incorrect. Inflammation extending to the sigmoid colon would be referred to as proctosigmoiditis.

Answer b is incorrect. Inflammation extending to the hepatic flexure would involve the rectum, as well as the sigmoid, descending, and transverse colon.

Answer c is correct. Inflammation extending to the splenic flexure would involve the rectum, as well as the sigmoid and descending colon. Since these landmarks are located on left side of body, this is designated "left-sided" disease.

Answer d is correct. Inflammation extending to the terminal ileum would involve the entire colon, as well as the terminal ileum.

---

17. What is the generic drug name for Enterocort?
    a. Prednisone
    b. Hydrocortisone
    c. Methylprednisolone
    d. Budesonide

Answer a is incorrect. Prednisone is available generically and is typically not referred to by brand name.

Answer b is incorrect. Hydrocortisone is a available as a suppository (Proctocort), foam (Cortifoam), tablet (Cortef, Hydrocortone), and injectable product (Solu-Cortef).

Answer c is incorrect. Methylprednisolone is available as tablets (Medrol) or injectable products (Solu-Medrol, Depo-Medrol).

Answer d is correct. Budesonide is the correct generic name for Enterocort.

---

18. Which medication requires that the prescriber registers with the manufacturer's prescribing program?
    a. Humira
    b. Cimzia
    c. Tysabri
    d. Remicade

Answer a is incorrect. The manufacturer of Humira does not require enrollment in a prescribing program if providers wish to prescribe this product.

Answer b is incorrect. The manufacturer of Cimzia does not require enrollment in a prescribing program if providers wish to prescribe this product.

Answer c is correct. The manufacturer of Tysabri does require enrollment in a prescribing program, known as the TOUCH program, if providers wish to prescribe this product. This is based on the fact that this agent is associated with serious adverse neurologic effects.

Answer d is incorrect. The manufacturer of Remicade does not require enrollment in a prescribing program if providers wish to prescribe this product.

---

19. How does sulfasalazine differ from mesalamine?
    a. Sulfasalazine is an active component of mesalamine.
    b. Sulfasalazine contains the carrier molecule sulfapyridine while mesalamine does not.
    c. Sulfasalazine can be used in patients with sulfa allergies, while mesalamine cannot.
    d. Sulfasalazine is available in enema form, while mesalamine is not.

Answer a is incorrect. Mesalamine is an active component of sulfasalazine.

Answer b is correct. Sulfasalazine is mesalamine bound to sulfapyridine via a diazo bond. Colonic bacteria degrade this bond to free mesalamine from sulfapyridine. Mesalamine can be administered by itself in various formulations designed to release at certain points within the GI tract.

Answer c is incorrect. Since mesalamine does not contain sulfapyridine, it can be used in patients who report sulfa allergies. Sulfasalazine should be avoided in sulfa-allergic patients.

Answer d is incorrect. Mesalamine is available in an enema formulation (Rowasa), while sulfasalazine is only available in tablet form.

---

20. A patient receiving Tysabri for Crohn disease develops mental status changes after 24 weeks of therapy. This may indicated development of which adverse effect?
    a. Cerebrovascular accident
    b. Progressive multifocal leukoencephalopathy
    c. Central pontine myelinolysis
    d. Multi-infarct dementia

Answer a is incorrect. Natalizumab is not commonly associated with development of cerebrovascular accident as a potential adverse neurologic effect.

Answer b is correct. Natalizumab is associated with development of progressive multifocal leukoencephalopathy as a potential adverse neurologic effect. For this reason, prescribers must enroll in the manufacturer's prescribing program in order to prescribe this agent. Patients should also be closely monitored for signs or symptoms of neurologic changes while receiving therapy.

Answer c is incorrect. Central pontine myelinolysis is an adverse neurologic event associated with nerve demyelination, often due to rapid correction of hyponatremia.

Answer d is incorrect. Multi-infarct dementia is a neurologic disorder associated with having multiple strokes over time, many of which are clinically silent. This is not a condition associated with natalizumab use.

CHAPTER 42 | Chronic Obstructive Pulmonary Disease

1. A patient presents with symptoms of shortness of breath, nonproductive cough and the following spirometry results: prebronchodilator FEV_1: 69% predicted; postbronchodilator FEV_1: 70% predicted; FEV_1/FVC ratio: 0.64. How would you interpret these findings?
   a. This patient has COPD with reversible airway obstruction
   b. This patient has COPD with irreversible airway obstruction
   c. This patient has asthma with reversible airway obstruction
   d. This patient does not have asthma since the airway obstruction is irreversible
   e. This patient does not have COPD or asthma

Answer a is incorrect. This patient does have COPD (an *irreversible* condition), and it is not reversible since the predicted FEV_1 did not change with administration of a bronchodilator.

Answer b is correct. This patient does have COPD, which is irreversible since the predicted FEV_1 did not change with administration of a bronchodilator.

Answer c is incorrect. This patient does not have asthma, since airway obstruction in this patient was irreversible (demonstrated by the lack of change in FEV_1 post-bronchodilator).

Answer d is incorrect. This patient does not have asthma, since airway obstruction is reversible.

Answer e is incorrect. This patient does have COPD, patient has a FEV_1/FVC ratio less than 0.7.

---

2. Which of the following characterized alpha 1 antitrypsin (AAT) deficiency?
   a. Onset at a late age (> 50 years)
   b. Disease caused by environmental factors
   c. Disease caused by genetic factors
   d. Prominent in African American populations
   e. Disease caused by oxidative stress

Answer a is incorrect. Alpha 1 antitrypsin deficiency presents at an *early* age (20-50 years)

Answer b is incorrect. Alpha 1 antitrypsin deficiency is caused by *genetic* factors, not environmental.

Answer c is correct. Alpha 1 antitrypsin deficiency is a *genetic* disorder.

Answer d is incorrect. Alpha 1 antitrypsin deficiency is prominent in those of Northern European descent.

Answer e is incorrect. Alpha 1 antitrypsin deficiency is a genetic disorder.

---

3. Which of the following is first-line treatment for a patient diagnosed with COPD (stage I)?
   a. Short-acting bronchodilator
   b. Long-acting anticholinergic
   c. Long-acting β-agonist
   d. Inhaled corticosteroid
   e. Oral theophylline

Answer a is correct. A short-acting bronchodilator PRN should be given to patients with mild (stage I) COPD. An example of the short-acting bronchodilator would be albuterol or levalbuterol. These β_2-agonists are similar in mechanism and dosing. The major difference is that levalbuterol has less effect on the heart rate as compared to albuterol. Along with the short-acting bronchodilator should be a spacer.

Note: All patients should utilize a spacer device or valved holding chamber when using a metered-dosed inhaler; in addition, face masks should be used in children less than 4 years of age.

Answer b is incorrect. A long-acting anticholinergic (tiotropium) can be added in moderate (stage II) COPD. Ipratropium (Atrovent) is a short-acting anticholinergic and is often used in the early stages of COPD. Ipratropium is often combined with albuterol and is coformulated with albuterol (Combivent). The major difference between ipratropium and tiotropium is the half-life. Ipratropium is taken every 6 hours and tiotropium is taken once per day. Compliance may be increased with tiotropium, but it is more expensive.

Answer c is incorrect. A long-acting β-agonist (salmeterol or formoterol) can be added in moderate (stage II) COPD.

Answer d is incorrect. Inhaled corticosteroids are recommended in severe (stage III) COPD with repeated exacerbations. In symptomatic patients with severe COPD (FEV_1 less than 50% predicted) and frequent exacerbations, regular treatment with *inhaled* corticosteroids decreases the number of exacerbations per year and improves health status; however, corticosteroids therapy does not slow the long-term decline in pulmonary function.

Answer e is incorrect. Theophylline is often the last agent prescribed in COPD patients (after the β_2-agonists, anticholinergic, and inhaled corticosteroid). Theophylline has a narrow-therapeutic index and requires close monitoring due to the pharmacokinetic considerations.

---

4. A patient with COPD complains of developing a tremor since starting one of his medications. Which medication is the most likely cause?

   a. Ipratropium
   b. Tiotropium
   c. Fluticasone
   d. Prednisone
   e. Albuterol

Answer a is incorrect. Dry mouth/hoarseness is a common side effect of inhaled anticholinergics.

Answer b is incorrect. Dry mouth/hoarseness is a common side effect of inhaled anticholinergics.

Answer c is incorrect. Oral pharyngeal candidiasis is the common side effect of inhaled corticosteroids. This is prevented by rinsing with water after use.

Answer d is incorrect. Long-term systemic corticosteroid use should be avoided due to an unfavorable risk/benefit ratio. The steroid myopathy that can result from long-term use of oral corticosteroids weakens muscles, further decreasing the respiratory drive in patients with advanced disease. Other long-term adverse effects of systemic corticosteroid therapy include osteoporosis, thinning of the skin, development of cataracts, adrenal suppression, and insufficiency.

Answer e is correct. Tremor is a common side effect of β-agonists. Other common effects include tachycardia and central nervous system stimulation/excitation.

---

5. Which of the following is the most likely side effect to be caused by inhaled corticosteroids?

   a. Oral candidiasis
   b. Glucose intolerance
   c. Tachycardia
   d. Immunosuppression
   e. Weight gain

Answer a is correct. Inhaled corticosteroids can cause candidiasis of the mouth and/or throat.

Answer b is incorrect. Long-term systemic (not inhaled) corticosteroids can cause glucose intolerance.

Answer c is incorrect. Inhaled β_2-agonists can cause tachycardia.

Answer d is incorrect. Long-term systemic (not inhaled) corticosteroids can cause immunosuppression.

Answer e is incorrect. Long-term systemic (not inhaled) corticosteroids can cause weight gain.

---

6. Which of the following are advantages of using a spacer device with a metered-dose inhaler?

   a. Decreased oropharyngeal deposition
   b. Enhanced lung delivery
   c. Less hand-lung coordination needed
   d. Reduced side effects from inhaled corticosteroids
   e. All of the above

Answers a, b, c, d are correct. Decreased oropharyngeal deposition is an advantage of using a spacer device, which means more medication may reach the lungs. Oral pharyngeal candidiasis/thrush is the reduced side effect.

Answer e is correct and the best answer. Spacer devices decrease oropharyngeal deposition, enhance lung delivery, require less hand-lung coordination, and reduce the side-effects from inhaled corticosteroids (thrush, hoarseness).

---

7. SS is a 68-year-old woman who smokes and has recently been diagnosed with mild COPD. In addition to a short-acting bronchodilator, what would you recommend for her treatment?

   i. Smoking cessation
   ii. Influenza vaccine yearly
   iii. Pneumococcal vaccine
   iv. Oxygen therapy

   a. i only
   b. i and ii
   c. i, ii and iii
   d. i and iii
   e. All of the above

Choices i, ii, and iii are recommended for all COPD patients, regardless of stage or symptoms. Choice iv, oxygen therapy, is added in stage IV (very severe) COPD. We are not given any clinical information about this patient, so modification of current COPD therapy would not be appropriate at this time (unless further patient information is given).

Answer c is correct. Choices i, ii and iii are recommended in all COPD patients.

---

8. The clinical presentation of COPD can include which of the following?

   a. Dyspnea
   b. Chronic cough
   c. Sputum production
   d. Exposure to risk factors
   e. All of the above

Answers a, b, c, and d are correct. Dyspnea and chronic cough are common in the presentation of COPD. Sputum production is common especially in COPD patients with chronic bronchitis. The most common risk factor is smoking, followed by air pollution.

Answer e is correct and the best answer. The clinical presentation of COPD includes dyspnea, chronic cough, sputum production, and exposure to risk factors.

---

9. When should a trial of inhaled corticosteroids be considered for a patient with COPD?
   a. Stage I with a short-acting β-agonist
   b. Stage II with a long-acting β-agonist
   c. Stage II with a long-acting anticholinergic
   d. Stage III with at least two other medications
   e. Stage III with repeated exacerbations

Answers a, b, c and d are incorrect. Inhaled corticosteroids are recommended for patients in stage III with repeated exacerbations.

Answer e is correct. Inhaled corticosteroids are recommended for patients in stage III with repeated exacerbations. Currently, the appropriate situations to consider corticosteroids in COPD include (1) short-term systemic use for acute exacerbations and (2) inhalation therapy for chronic stable COPD. In symptomatic patients with severe COPD (FEV_1 less than 50% predicted) and frequent exacerbations, regular treatment with *inhaled* corticosteroids decreases the number of exacerbations per year and improves health status; however, corticosteroids therapy does not slow the long-term decline in pulmonary function.

---

10. PL is a 75-year-old man who has been experiencing increased dyspnea for the last month. He was diagnosed with COPD 3 years ago and has been taking albuterol metered-dose inhaler on an as needed (prn) basis. His most recent spirometry results are: FEV_1/FVC ratio of 0.65 and FEV_1 65% of predicted. Which of the following is the best choice for changing his medication regimen?
    a. Add scheduled tiotropium and continue prn albuterol
    b. Add scheduled fluticasone and continue prn albuterol
    c. Add prn salmeterol and continue prn albuterol
    d. Add scheduled theophylline and continue prn albuterol
    e. No changes are necessary at this time.

Answer a is correct. The patient is in stage II since his FEV_1/FVC ratio is 0.7 and FEV_1 is between 50% and 80% of predicted. The guidelines recommend adding regular treatment with one or more long-acting bronchodilators.

Answer b is incorrect. Inhaled corticosteroids are only recommended in stage III with repeated exacerbations.

Answer c is incorrect. Salmeterol could be added in stage II as a long-acting bronchodilator, but it should be scheduled, not prn.

Answer d is incorrect. Theophylline can be considered in stage II as a long-acting bronchodilator, but is not the best choice due to adverse effects, drug interactions, and monitoring required.

Answer e is incorrect. The patient is symptomatic and therefore, in stage II needs additional medication.

---

11. Select the COPD medications that can be used concurrently in a maintenance regimen for a patient with stage III COPD.
    a. Levalbuterol and albuterol
    b. Albuterol and formoterol
    c. Formoterol and salmeterol
    d. Fluticasone and flunisolide
    e. Theophylline and aminophylline

Answer a is incorrect. Levalbuterol and albuterol are both short-acting $β_2$-agonists. A rule of thumb for combination therapy is to use medications with a different mechanism of action.

Answer b is correct. Albuterol is a short-acting $β_2$-agonist and formoterol is a long-acting $β_2$-agonist. Even though these medications have a similar mechanism of action ($β_2$-agonists), we can use these medications concurrently. Albuterol is coformulated with ipratropium (Combivent) and this medication may be used with a long-acting $β_2$-agonist. Long-acting $β_2$-agonists are coformulated with inhaled corticosteroids (fluticasone + salmeterol—Advair; budesonide + formoterol—Symbicort). For patients with stage III or IV COPD and frequent exacerbations, combinations like Combivent and Advair are common regimens used for COPD treatment.

Answer c is incorrect. Salmeterol and formoterol are long-acting $β_2$-agonists and because they work the same, would not be recommended for concurrent therapy. A rule of thumb for combination therapy is to use medications with a different mechanism of action.

Answer d is incorrect. Fluticasone and flunisolide are inhaled corticosteroids. Concurrent therapy with inhaled corticosteroids is not recommended (same mechanism of action). For patients with an exacerbation of COPD, acute treatment with a systemic corticosteroid (ie, prednisone) may be used for 14 days or less. In this situation, you may see an inhaled corticosteroid utilized with the systemic corticosteroid.

Answer e is incorrect. The methylxanthines, theophylline, and aminophylline would not be used concurrently. Aminophylline is a salt formulation of theophylline. Aminophylline is the methylxanthine that is used intravenously and theophylline is the methylxanthine used orally.

---

12. Select the disease state or factor that can affect the clearance of theophylline.
    a. Smoking history
    b. Hepatic cirrhosis
    c. Drug interactions (cytochrome P-450 inhibitors especially 1A2, 2E1, 3A4)
    d. a and b
    e. a, b, and c

Answer a is correct. Cigarette smokers have a theophylline clearance about 1.5 to 2 times that of nonsmokers. The effects of smoking (one pack of cigarettes per day) appear to last several months after the cigarettes have been discontinued. Therefore, patients admitted to the hospital with a recent history of smoking should be considered smokers throughout their hospitalization, even if they refrain from smoking during hospitalization.

Answer b is correct. Theophylline is eliminated hepatically. Therefore, hepatic damage will decrease theophylline clearance and leads to elevated levels.

Answer c is correct. Theophylline is a substrate of the cytochrome P-450 system (1A2—major; 2C9—minor; 2D6—minor; 2E1—major; 3A4—major). Therefore, medications that inhibit these CYP enzymes (especially the major pathways—1A2; 2E1; and 3A4) will decrease the elimination/metabolism of theophylline leading to increase in theophylline levels. Macrolide antibiotics (erythromycin and clarithromycin) decrease the clearance of theophylline by as much as 25% to 50%. Phenytoin and Phenobarbital increase the clearance of theophylline by as much as 30% to 50%. Cimetidine appears to reduce the clearance of theophylline by as much as 40%. Rifampin can increase theophylline clearance/metabolism by 20% to 25%. Unfortunately, the predictability of clearance changes secondary to the addition of these drugs is poor indicating that while some change may be expected, each patient will need to be evaluated individually. Please refer to a drug interaction reference to review the numerous agents that interact with theophylline.

Answer d is correct. Both answers a and b are correct

Answer e is correct and the best answer. All of the above are correct statements about disease states or factors that affect theophylline clearance. Other factors that may influence theophylline clearance are diet and other disease states. Congestive heart failure reduces theophylline clearance about 40%. Pulmonary edema reduces theophylline clearance (although this may be related to congestive heart failure). Premature newborns have a theophylline clearance that is very low even when adjusted for weight or body surface area (premature newborns would receive theophylline for the indication of apnea of prematurity). Diet also influences the metabolism of theophylline. Patients ingesting high-protein, low-carbohydrate diets generally metabolize theophylline more rapidly, presumably because the diet induces hepatic enzymes. Dietary intake of other methylxanthines such as caffeine can decrease the rate of theophylline metabolism to a limited extent. While the effects of diet are well documented, they usually produce minor changes in theophylline levels, except for food and once-daily sustained-release products. Food does not appreciably affect the absorption of the liquid, fast-release products, and most sustained-release products; however, food may induce a sudden release (dose-dump) of once-daily sustained-release products resulting in an increase in serum drug levels and potential toxicity.

---

13. Select the formulation of the corticosteroid that should be utilized in maintenance therapy for COPD.
    a. IV/injection (methylprednisolone)
    b. Oral (prednisone)
    c. Inhalation (fluticasone)
    d. Nasal (fluticasone)

Answer a is incorrect. IV medications are not ideal for the maintenance therapy of any disease state. Also, because of the adverse reactions of systemic therapy with corticosteroids, maintenance therapy is not recommended with systemic corticosteroids. Methylprednisolone could be utilized for exacerbations of COPD.

Answer b is incorrect. Because of the numerous adverse reactions associated with systemic oral corticosteroids (prednisone), maintenance therapy is not recommended. Prednisone could be utilized for exacerbations of COPD.

Answer c is correct. Inhalation is the preferred formulation/dosage route for maintenance therapy with COPD. This method minimizes adverse reactions.

Answer d is incorrect. Nasal preparations are used for allergic rhinitis.

---

14. Select the central nervous system side effect of aminophylline when levels exceed 20 μg/mL.
    a. Hypotension
    b. Arrhythmias
    c. Nausea and vomiting
    d. Seizures

Answer a is incorrect. Hypotension is a cardiac side effect of theophylline and usually occurs when patients have exceeded the concentration range of theophylline (>20 μg/mL).

Answer b is incorrect. Arrhythmias are cardiac side effects of theophylline and usually occur when patients have exceeded the concentration range of theophylline (>20 μg/mL).

Answer c is incorrect. Nausea and vomiting are gastrointestinal side effects of theophylline. Gastrointestinal side effects may occur when theophylline levels are within the therapeutic range (< 20 μg/mL) and they may also occur when levels are outside the therapeutic range (>20 μg/mL). Gastrointestinal side effects outside the therapeutic range are often repetitive and persistent. If a patient develops signs and symptoms of theophylline toxicity (eg, persistent, repetitive vomiting), a theophylline level should be checked and subsequent doses held until the level is confirmed and within the therapeutic range.

Answer d is correct. Seizures are the central nervous system side effect that most commonly occur when patients have supra-therapeutic theophylline levels. Other central nervous system side effects (occurring within therapeutic range) are: headache, hyperactivity (children), insomnia, and restlessness.

---

15. Albuterol is a short-acting bronchodilator recommended for treatment of COPD by treatment guidelines. Select the dose(s) of albuterol that may be utilized/preferred in the treatment of COPD.

    a. Albuterol inhalation (metered-dose inhaler—90 μg/puff)—two puffs every 6 hours
    b. Albuterol inhalation (metered-dose inhaler—90 μg/puff)—as needed "rescue" (prn)
    c. Albuterol oral—4 mg tid.
    d. a and b
    e. a, b, and c

Answer a is correct. Albuterol two puffs every 6 hours is a common dose for COPD patients prescribed albuterol on a scheduled basis. Albuterol is often utilized with ipratropium in this regard (Combivent two puffs every 6 hours). This is a major difference in COPD and asthma. Asthma patients would not use albuterol scheduled, only as a rescue, whereas COPD patients may use albuterol as rescue or scheduled.

Answer b is correct. Rescue albuterol is also common for COPD patients with acute symptoms.

Answer c is incorrect. Systemic albuterol is not preferred for COPD treatment. Inhalation treatment is the preferred method for treatment of COPD.

Answer d is correct and the best answer.

Answer e is incorrect because of answer c.

---

16. A patient is receiving 32 mg/h of aminophylline. The patient is ready to be changed to oral theophylline. What would the daily dose of theophylline be that would equal 32 mg/h of aminophylline? Aminophylline's salt factor is 0.8.

    a. 614 mg
    b. 768 mg
    c. 300 mg
    d. 900 mg

Answer a is correct. 32 mg/h of aminophylline would equal a daily theophylline dose of 614 mg. 32 mg/h × 24 h = 768 mg of aminophylline in a daily dose. Multiply by the aminophylline salt factor (0.8) to get the daily dose of theophylline equal to 614.4.

Answers b, c, and d are incorrect. 768 mg is the daily dose of aminophylline.

---

17. Select the generic name of Symbicort.

    a. Fluticasone + salmeterol
    b. Albuterol + ipratropium
    c. Budesonide + formoterol

Answer a is incorrect. The brand name of fluticasone + salmeterol is Advair.

Answer b is incorrect. The brand name of albuterol + ipratropium is Combivent.

Answer c is correct.

---

18. KT is a patient that presents to your clinic on Theo-24 (a sustained release/once a day theophylline product). She has experienced the dose-dumping effect when the agent is taken with a high-fat meal. She would like to be changed to another sustained release theophylline product that does not have the dose-dumping effect. Select the product that Theo-24 could be changed to:

    a. Theo-Dur twice daily
    b. Slo-Bid twice daily
    c. Uniphyl once daily
    d. All of the above

Answer a is correct. Theo-Dur is a sustained-release formulation that does not appear to be associated with dose-dumping. Be cautious—just because a product is labeled as sustained release that does not mean it will be dosed once a day. Sometimes, sustained- or extended-release products will be dosed twice daily.

Answer b is correct. Slo-Bid is a sustained-release formulation that does not appear to be associated with dose-dumping. Be cautious—just because a product is labeled as sustained release that does not mean it will be dosed once a day. Sometimes, sustained- or extended-release products will be dosed twice daily.

Answer c is correct. Uniphyl is a sustained-release product that is taken once daily. While no dose-dumping was observed following ingestion of Uniphyl with a high-fat meal, a change in the rate of absorption was apparent. For this reason, clinicians often use the sustained released theophylline products that are dosed twice daily more often.

Answer d is correct and the best answer. A large number of sustained-release dosage forms of theophylline have been marketed. These products are designed to release theophylline slowly so that patients who metabolize the drug rapidly (children and smokers) can maintain theophylline-plasma concentrations within the therapeutic range. Most of these drugs products are completely absorbed; however there are major differences between these products with regard to duration of absorption. Some of the dosage forms are absorbed over 3 to 4 hours, while others are absorbed over 8 to 12 hours. Nevertheless, as the duration of absorption increases, the possibility of incomplete bioavailability increases because the duration of absorption begins to exceed the gastrointestinal transit time. Therefore, when switching theophylline products/dosage forms caution must be taken and pharmacokinetic considerations taken into account.

---

19. Select the COPD bronchodilator that is a phosphodiesterase inhibitor.

    a. Albuterol
    b. Salmeterol

c. Ipratropium
d. Fluticasone
e. Theophylline

Answer a is incorrect. Albuterol increases cAMP, thereby relaxing bronchial smooth muscle.

Answer b is incorrect. Salmeterol increases cAMP, thereby relaxing bronchial smooth muscle.

Answer c is incorrect. Ipratropium blocks the action of acetylcholine at the parasympathetic sites in bronchial smooth muscle causing bronchodilation.

Answer d is incorrect. Fluticasone is not a bronchodilator.

Answer e is correct. Theophylline causes bronchodilation, diuresis, central nervous system, cardiac stimulation, and gastric acid secretion by blocking phosphodiesterase, which increases tissue concentrations of cAMP which in turn promotes catecholamine stimulation

20. Select the albuterol formulation with the fastest onset.
    a. Nebulization
    b. Inhalation
    c. Oral
    d. a and c
    e. a and b

Answer a is correct. Nebulization has an onset of 5 to 15 minutes.

Answer b is correct. Inhalation has an onset of 5 to 15 minutes.

Answer c is incorrect. Oral has an onset of 7 to 30 minutes.

Answer e is the correct and best answer. Nebulization and inhalation have the same onset when the medications are used correctly with proper inhaler technique.

CHAPTER 43 | Asthma

1. Select the statement that most accurately characterizes asthma.
    a. Airway inflammation and bronchial hyperresponsiveness
    b. Airway inflammation and esophageal hyperresponsiveness
    c. Adrenal inflammation and bronchial hyperresponsiveness
    d. Adrenal inflammation and esophageal hyperresponsiveness

Answer a is correct. The major characteristics of asthma are airway inflammation and bronchial hyperresponsiveness which cause variable degrees of airflow obstruction.

Answer b is incorrect. Esophageal hyperresponsiveness due to acid reflux may be a precipitating factor for asthma that is not well-controlled, however, is not a major characteristic.

Answer c is incorrect. Adrenal inflammation is not part of the pathological process of asthma, but suppression may occur when oral or high-dose steroids are used.

Answer d is incorrect. See answers b and c.

2. Select the mechanism(s) for development of asthma.
    a. Ectopy and exposure to environmental triggers
    b. Ectopy and activation of neutrophils
    c. Atopy and exposure to environmental triggers
    d. Atopy and activation of neutrophils

Answer a is incorrect. Ectopy does not play a roll in asthma development.

Answer b is incorrect. See answers a and d.

Answer c is correct. In the asthmatic response, a genetically predisposed or atopic individual is exposed to a specific reactive stimuli or trigger.

Answer d is incorrect. Eosinophils are the major inflammatory cell in asthma not neutrophils.

3. The late asthmatic response is caused by influx of which primary inflammatory cell?
    a. Natural killer cells
    b. Eosinophils
    c. Monocytes
    d. Immunoglobulin A

Answer a is incorrect. Natural killer cells are a type of cytotoxic lymphocyte that constitutes a major component of the innate immune system not found in the asthmatic response.

Answer b is correct. The late asthmatic response is caused by influx of inflammatory cells primarily eosinophils. Th2 lymphocytes, mast cells, macrophages, and mediators such as leukotrienes, histamine, and prostaglandin infiltrate the airway.

Answer c is incorrect. Monocytes play a major role in the immune system response to infection, but not a great role in the inflammatory response associated with asthma.

Answer d is incorrect. Immunoglobulin A plays a role in innate immunity associated with mucus membranes not in the inflammatory response associated with asthma.

4. Irreversible obstruction or airway remodeling may occur in susceptible persons with asthma due to uncontrolled inflammation within which structure?
    a. Bronchial smooth muscles
    b. Esophageal smooth muscle
    c. Pharynx
    d. Alveoli

Answer a is correct. Inflammation is postulated to cause hypertrophy and hyperplasia of the bronchial smooth muscle and mucus glands which may lead to permanent, irreversible obstruction termed airway remodeling.

Answer b is incorrect. Inflammation of esophageal muscle can play a role in uncontrolled asthma but is not the underlying reason for airway remodeling.

Answer c is incorrect. Upper respiratory inflammation can play a role in uncontrolled asthma, but is not the underlying reason for airway remodeling.

Answer d is incorrect. Alveolar inflammation plays no role in the underlying reason for airway remodeling.

5. Among children this may be the only nighttime symptom to consider a diagnostic work up for asthma.
   a. Dyspnea
   b. Cough
   c. Reflux
   d. Enuresis

Answer a is incorrect. Dyspnea is a symptom of asthma, however, has not been shown in clinical trials to correlate as a single symptom entity for asthma work up.

Answer b is correct. Although wheezing is considered one of the classic symptoms of asthma, among children nighttime cough has been shown to be a common symptom requiring further work up for asthma.

Answer c is incorrect. Reflux may play a role in asthma that does not respond to treatment ,however, not a symptom that leads to the work up for asthma.

Answer d is incorrect. There has been no correlation between asthma and enuresis.

6. What is the preferred treatment for an 18-year-old man with off and on chest tightness that occurred 4 days this past week with no nocturnal awakening, $FEV_1/FVC = 70\%$, and $FEV_1 = 75\%$.
   a. Low-dose inhaled corticosteroid
   b. Medium-dose inhaled corticosteroid
   c. High-dose inhaled corticosteroid
   d. Leukotriene modifier

Answer a is incorrect. Treatment of mild persistent asthma not moderate persistent asthma. Refer to Table 43-1.

Answer b is correct. Therapy is always recommended based on the most severe presenting sign or symptom. In the case the FEV_1 is in the moderate persistent category, preferred treatment is ICS + LABA or medium dose ICS. Refer to Table 43-1.

Answer c is incorrect. Treatment option for severe persistent asthma and not moderate persistent asthma. Refer to Table 43-1.

Answer d is incorrect. Alternative or adjunct treatment. Refer to Table 43-1.

7. You are providing follow-up education for a 3-year-old child with asthma who in the last month is scheduling their Accu-Neb 1.25 mg tid for symptoms. The child and his parents have completed the following questionnaire:

Have your child complete these questions.				
1. How is your asthma today?				
0: Very bad	1: Bad	2: Good	3: Very good	**Score: 2**
2. How much of a problem is your asthma when you run, exercise, or play sports?				
0: It is a big problem. I cannot do what I want to do.	1: It is a problem and I do not like it.	2: It is a little problem but it's okay.	3: It is not a problem.	**Score: 2**
3. Do you cough because of your asthma?				
0: Yes, all the time.	1: Yes, most of the time.	2: Yes, sometimes.	3: No, never	**Score: 2**
4. Do you wake up during the night because of your asthma?				
0: Yes, all the time.	1: Yes, most of the time.	2: Yes, sometimes.	3: No, never.	**Score: 2**

Please complete the following questions on your own.						
5. During the *last 4 weeks,* how many days did your child have any daytime asthma symptoms?						
5: Not at all	4: 1-3 days	3: 4-10 days	2: 11-18 days	1: 19-24 days	0: Everyday	**Score: 2**
6. During the *last 4 weeks,* how many days did your child wheeze during the day because of asthma?						
5: Not at all	4: 1-3 days	3: 4-10 days	2: 11-18 days	1: 19-24 days	0: Everyday	**Score: 3**
7. During the *last 4 weeks,* how many days did your child wake up during the night because of asthma?						
5: Not at all	4: 1-3 days	3: 4-10 days	2: 11-18 days	1: 19-24 days	0: Everyday	**Score: 2**

What is the best treatment option given the patients current asthma control?

a. Continue current treatment
b. Step up one step
c. Step down one step
d. Oral steroid burst

Answer a is incorrect. Symptoms present and medication used not consistent with well-controlled category. Table 43-2

Answer b is incorrect. Symptom severity and medication exceed not well- controlled category. See Table 43-2

Answer c is incorrect. Symptoms present indicate very poor control and indicate modification of current medication regiment. See Table 43-2

Answer d is correct. Control is based on daytime symptoms, nighttime awakening, SABA use, spirometry or peak flow monitoring, exacerbation frequency, any limitation on activities, and validated quality of life questionnaires. In this case the patient is used several SABA treatments a day and has an asthma control test (ACT) of ≤ 15 indicating very poor control which requires burst of oral steroids. See Table 43-2

---

8. After assessing environmental control and medication adherence What additional factor should be addressed Prior to stepping up asthma?

a. Inhaler technique
b. IgE level
c. Serum glucose
d. pH monitoring

Answer a is correct. Prior to any increase in step therapy the following three components are to be addressed: medication adherence, inhaler technique, and environmental control.

Answer b is incorrect. IgE level is assessed for omalizumab therapy ,however, is not assessed at every step increase consideration.

Answer c is incorrect. Serum glucose may be affected by overuse of β-agonist, however, is not considered in step increase therapy.

Answer d is incorrect. No merits for pH monitoring when considering step up therapy.

---

9. Independent of asthma severity all persons with asthma should have this class of medication readily available.

a. Short-acting β_2-agonist
b. Short-acting β_2-antagonist
c. Long-acting β_2-agonist
d. Long-acting β_2-antagonist

Answer a is correct. Asthma medications are classified into two broad categories of quick relief and long-term control. Independent of severity, all persons with asthma should have a quick relief medication readily available. Their mechanism of action is to stimulate β_2-receptor on bronchial smooth muscle to cause relaxation.

Answer b is incorrect. Stimulation of bronchial smooth muscle is the desired effect for symptom control not blockage.

Answer c is incorrect. Long-acting β_2-agonist in general (exception is formotorol) have too long of an onset of action to provide required quick relief.

Answer d is incorrect. Stimulation of bronchial smooth muscle is the desired effect for symptom control not blockage

---

10. Select the brand name for levalbuterol.

a. Serevent
b. Flovent
c. Xolair
d. Xopenex

Answer a is incorrect. Brand name of salmeterol.

Answer b is incorrect. Brand name of fluticasone.

Answer c is incorrect. Brand name of omalizumab.

Answer d is correct. Brand name of levalbuterol.

---

11. Which is the best medication for control of inflammation in persistent asthma?

a. Formoterol
b. Zileuton
c. Budesonide
d. Cromolyn

Answer a is incorrect. LABA do not control inflammation.

Answer b is incorrect. Inhaler corticosteroids have shown in clinical trials to be better than leukotriene modifiers at controlling inflammation.

Answer c is correct. Inhaled corticosteroids (ICS) are the best at controlling inflammation in persons with persistent asthma.

Answer d is incorrect. Cromolyn is not as potent at controlling inflammation as ICS.

---

12. Which medication would be an absolute contraindication when given alone for the treatment of persistent asthma?

a. Mometasone
b. Zafirlukast
c. Theophylline
d. Salmeterol

Answer a is incorrect. Inhaled corticosteroids are considered preferred treatment for persistent asthma either as monotherapy or in combination

Answer b is incorrect. Leukotriene modifiers may be considered as alternative monotherapy depending on patient's asthma severity.

Answer c is incorrect. Theophylline may be considered as alternative monotherapy depending on patient's asthma severity.

Answer d is correct. Increase risk of death was associated with the long-acting β_2-agonists due to small but statically significant finding from SMART trial.

13. What is the mechanism of action of montelukast?
    a. Antagonist to leukotriene receptors
    b. Agonist to leukotriene receptors
    c. Antagonist to muscarinic receptors
    d. Agonist to muscarinic receptors

Answer a is correct. Montelukast blocks the leukotriene receptor on inflammatory cell thus inhibiting the inflammatory and bronchoconstrictive properties of leukotrienes.

Answer b is incorrect. Simulation of leukotriene receptor leads to propagation of proinflammatory mediator and bronchoconstriction.

Answer c is incorrect. Montelukast is a leukotriene receptor antagonist not muscarinic

Answer d is incorrect. Montelukast is a leukotriene receptor antagonist not muscarinic

14. Select the agent that is administered as a subcutaneous injection in patients with allergic asthma not controlled with high-dose inhaled corticosteroids.
    a. Pirbuterol
    b. Omalizumab
    c. Ciclesonide
    d. Adalimumab

Answer a is incorrect. Meter-dose inhaler stimulates smooth muscle.

Answer b is correct. Omalizumab (Xolair).

Answer c is incorrect. Inhaled corticosteroid.

Answer d is incorrect. Injectable tumor necrosis factor (TNF) blocker not used in asthma management.

15. What is the preferred treatment option for a 46-year-old man with the diagnosis of asthma? Current complaints are wheezing in morning that gets better as day progresses. One episode of cough in last month required three courses of oral steroids within the last year with an FEV_1 of 55%.
    a. Medium-dose inhaled corticosteroid (ICS)
    b. Low-dose ICS and LABA
    c. Medium-dose ICS and LABA
    d. Theophylline

Answer a is incorrect. Patient is exhibiting severe persistent asthma which requires high-dose step 4 to 6 combination therapy.

Answer b is incorrect. Patient is exhibiting severe persistent asthma which requires high-dose step 4 to 6 combination therapy.

Answer c is correct. Patient is exhibiting severe persistent asthma which requires high-dose step 4 to 6 combination therapy.

Answer d is incorrect. Patient is exhibiting severe persistent asthma which requires high-dose step 4 to 6 combination therapy.

16. Select the brand name for ciclesonide.
    a. AeroBid
    b. Asmanex
    c. Azmacort
    d. Alvesco

Answer a is incorrect. AeroBid is flunisolide.

Answer b is incorrect. Asmanex is mometasone.

Answer c is incorrect. Azmacort is triamcinolone.

Answer d is correct. Alvesco is ciclesonide.

17. What is the follow-up treatment recommendation for a 16-year-old girl currently on QVAR 80 μg 2 puffs bid who is experiencing no limitation on activity and has not used her SABA in over 3 months?
    a. Step up therapy
    b. Step down therapy
    c. Continue current treatment
    d. Discontinue SABA

Answer a is incorrect. When a patient is well-controlled for at least 3 months, therapy is stepped down.

Answer b is correct. When a patient is well-controlled for at least 3 months, therapy is stepped down. Decrease to 1 puff bid.

Answer c is incorrect. Patient is well-controlled would benefit from decrease in steroid dosing.

Answer d is incorrect. All persons with asthma regardless of severity require access to SABA.

18. What is the most common adverse reaction of short-acting β-agonists?
    a. Hypernatremia
    b. Tremor
    c. Anaphylaxis
    d. Thrush

Answer a is incorrect. SABA do not cause elevated sodium but if overused and in conjunction with diuretic therapy can cause low potassium.

Answer b is correct. SABA stimulates β_2-receptors on skeletal muscle to precipitate tremor.

Answer c is incorrect. SABA are used in anaphylaxis along with epinephrine when bronchoconstriction is present.

Answer d is incorrect. Inhaled corticosteroid's side effect is thrush not SABA.

19. You are counseling the parents of a 2-year-old child who will be released from the hospital with a new prescription for a medium-dose inhaled corticosteroid. What side effect should you educate the parents about?

    a. Reduced glucose production
    b. Permanente growth suppression
    c. Intermitted expiratory wheezing
    d. Reduced growth velocity

Answer a is incorrect. Medium-does inhaled corticosteroids do not affect glucose production, however, high-does and oral corticosteroids may increase glucose levels.

Answer b is incorrect. The CAMP trials demonstrated a reduction in growth velocity by 1 cm with first year use of inhaled corticosteroids but children caught up in subsequent year to normal physiological height.

Answer c is incorrect. Inhaled corticosteroids suppress inflammation which aids in minimization of bronchoconstriction and subsequent symptoms such as wheezing.

Answer d is correct. The CAMP trials demonstrated a reduction in growth velocity by 1 cm with first year use of inhaled corticosteroids but children caught up in subsequent year to normal physiological height.

20. You are counseling a 25-year-old woman with asthma who is well-controlled with Advair 250/50 µg 1 puff bid and albuterol 2 puffs every 4 to 6 hours prn. She presents a prescription for prenatal vitamin from her initial obstetric appointment. What is the safest medication to recommend for *control* of her asthma?

    a. Albuterol 2 puffs qid
    b. Advair 250/50 1 puffs bid
    c. Alvesco 160 µg 1 puff daily
    d. Pulmicort 90 mg 1 puff bid

Answer a is incorrect. Used for quick relief of symptom not for control.

Answer b is correct. In pregnancy when a patient is well-controlled on a current regimen, continue treatment. If initiating controller therapy, budesonide is the only category B inhaled corticosteroid.

Answer c is incorrect. In pregnancy when a patient is well-controlled on a current regimen, continue treatment. If initiating controller therapy, budesonide is the only category B inhaled corticosteroid.

Answer d is incorrect. In pregnancy when a patient is well-controlled on a current regimen, continue treatment. If initiating controller therapy, budesonide is the only category B inhaled corticosteroid.

CHAPTER 44 | Cystic Fibrosis

1. JN is a 2-year-old (8 kg) with repeat visits to her physician for pneumonia. There is a positive family history for CF. What test should be ordered in this patient to diagnose CF?

    a. Chest x-ray
    b. Sputum culture
    c. Sweat test
    d. DNA test

Answers a and b are incorrect. They are tests that would be ordered to diagnose pneumonia.

Answer c is correct. With repeat pneumonias and a positive family history for CF, this patient should receive a sweat test.

Answer d is incorrect. Most patients with CF can be diagnosed with the less expensive sweat test. If the sweat test is inconclusive then DNA testing can be used for diagnosis.

2. JN is diagnosed with CF and treatment for her pneumonia needs to be initiated. Which test should be ordered to guide the antibiotic selection?

    a. Sputum culture and sensitivity
    b. Chest x-ray
    c. Chest MRI
    d. Chest CAT scan

Answer a is correct. The sputum culture and sensitivity will identify the organism(s) in the lungs and will show the organism's sensitivity to antibiotics.

Answer b is incorrect. The chest x-ray and clinical symptoms are used to diagnose pneumonia in children. This test will not help guide antibiotic selection.

Answers c and d are incorrect. These tests are used to distinguish pathologic tissue, such as a tumor, from normal tissue in the body. These tests will not help guide antibiotic selection.

3. Which organism would you empirically treat for in this patient with CF?

    a. *Burkholderia cepacia*
    b. *Pseudomonas aeruginosa*
    c. *Stenotrophomonas maltophilia*
    d. *Haemophilus influenzae*

Answers a and c are incorrect. *B. cepacia* and *S. maltophilia* are resistant organisms seen in CF patients later in life after exposure to many broad-spectrum antibiotics.

Answer b is correct. Empiric antibiotic therapy is always aimed at *P. aeruginosa* in CF patients.

Answer d is incorrect. This organism may be a co-pathogen but CF exacerbations are correlated with *P. aeruginosa* density in the airways. Antibiotic treatment should be aimed at *P. aeruginosa's* sensitivities.

4. Which combination of antibiotics would be appropriate to treat JN's pneumonia?
   a. Aminoglycoside and amoxicillin
   b. Aminoglycoside and ticarcillin
   c. Aminoglycoside and Timentin (ticarcillin plus clavulanate)
   d. Ciprofloxacin

Answer a is incorrect. Oral therapy should not be initiated in a patient with CF and pneumonia. Amoxicillin is only available in an oral dosage form.

Answer b is correct. The treatment of *P. aeruginosa* is double-antibiotic therapy with a synergistic combination of aminoglycoside and extended-spectrum penicillin.

Answer c is incorrect. A β-lactamase inhibitor would be added if resistant organisms are present.

Answer d is incorrect. Ciprofloxacin is reserved for CF patients in the outpatient setting who need oral antipseudomonal therapy.

5. High serum peaks are needed to penetrate and adequately treat gram-negative pulmonary infections. Low troughs are needed to ensure low toxicity. What are the appropriate serum levels you would aim for with JN's aminoglycoside therapy?
   a. Peak > 8 and trough > 2
   b. Peak > 8 and trough < 2
   c. Peak < 8 and trough > 2
   d. Peak < 8 and trough < 2

Answers a, c, and d are incorrect. For good lung penetration peaks need to be > 8 μg/mL. To prevent toxicity the trough needs to be < 2 μg/mL.

Answer b is correct. Ideally, the aminoglycoside peak concentration needs to be > 8 μg/mL and the trough < 2 μg/mL. The peak range is 8-10 μg/mL (some reference peak concentrations may be listed as 8-12 μg/mL).

6. What general statement can you make regarding the initial dose of antibiotics in CF patients?
   a. Higher antibiotic doses are needed in CF patients.
   b. The same doses are needed in CF patients as other patients with pneumonia.
   c. Doses vary with each patient and should be individualized.
   d. a and c.
   e. All of the above.

Answers a and c are correct. CF patients are hypermetabolizers of hepatically and renally eliminated drugs. In general, higher antibiotic doses are needed for CF patients. All patients should have doses individualized based on patient specific parameters. In the CF population, those individualized doses will be higher than those in the general population.

Answer b is incorrect. CF patients are hypermetabolizers of drugs and lower doses or usual doses would not be adequate for this population.

Answer d is the correct and the best answer.

Answer e is incorrect.

7. How long should antibiotics be continued for JN's CF exacerbation?
   a. 7 days
   b. 10 days
   c. 14 days
   d. Until her PFTs return to baseline for a 2 year old

Answers a, b, and c are incorrect. Exacerbations are treated until pulmonary functions return to baseline.

Answer d is correct. The patient with CF exacerbation is treated until they return to their baseline PFTs. If a baseline is not known the PFTs should return to normal for a 4-year-old child.

8. Give two reasons why double IV antibiotic therapy should be used to treat JN's pulmonary exacerbation.
   a. Antibiotic synergy and decreased bacterial resistance
   b. Antibiotic synergy and increased bacterial resistance
   c. Broader antibacterial coverage and antibiotic synergy
   d. Narrower antibacterial coverage and antibiotic synergy

Answer a is correct. The combination of an aminoglycoside and β-lactam antibiotic provides synergistic bacterial killing. The combination may also prevent resistance in the exposed bacteria.

Answer b is incorrect. Antibiotic synergy will be achieved with double IV antibiotic therapy (assuming we select antibiotics with a different mechanism of action, for example piperacillin and tobramycin). This double combination therapy will not increase bacterial resistance, it may prevent antibiotic resistance.

Answer c is incorrect. Two antibiotics will provide broader antibiotic coverage but this is not needed in CF patients with a definitive organism.

Answer d is incorrect. Two antibiotics will not provide narrower antibiotic coverage.

9. What other therapy should be initiated along with antibiotics for JN's pneumonia?
   a. Chest percussion and postural drainage
   b. Pancreatic enzyme replacement therapy
   c. Vitamin replacement therapy
   d. Insulin replacement therapy

Answer a is correct. Three mainstays of pulmonary treatment in CF patients are antibiotics, anti-inflammatories, and chest physiotherapy.

Answers b and c are incorrect. These are used to treat the gastrointestinal disease in CF patients.

Answer d is incorrect. This is used in late-stage CF when CFRD is present.

10. JN is ready to go home from the hospital and needs to be started on pancreatic enzyme replacement therapy. She eats three meals each day and has three snacks. She weighs 21 kg. Calculate her beginning enzyme dose per meal.

    a. 15,000 units/meal
    b. 21,000 units/meal
    c. 22,000 units/meal
    d. 23,000 units/meal

Answers a, c, and d are incorrect.

Answer b is correct. The starting dose of enzymes based on weight is 1000 units/kg/meal of the lipase component.

(1000 units/kg/meal × 21 kg = 21,000 units/meal)

11. Which product would you select for JN to receive with each meal?

    a. Pancrease MT 4 (2 with meals)
    b. Pancrease MT 10 (1 with meals)
    c. Pancrease MT 16 (1 with meals)
    d. Pancrease MT 20 (1 with meals)

Answers a, b, and c are incorrect. These products offer 4000 units, 16,000 units, and 20,000 units of lipase per capsule.

Answer d is correct. This product offers 20,000 units of lipase in each capsule. This comes closest to the calculated dose of 21,000 units of lipase per meal.

12. What is the dose of pancreatic enzyme replacement for JN to take with her three snacks each day?

    a. Pancreatic MT 4 (1 with snacks)
    b. Pancreatic MT 10 (1 with snacks)
    c. Pancreatic MT 16 (1 with snacks)
    d. Pancreatic MT 20 (1 with snacks)

Answers a, c, and d are incorrect. They offer 4000, 16,000, or 20,000 units of lipase in each capsule.

Answer b is correct. The dose of enzymes for snacks is half the dose for meals. Therefore, the dose for JN would be 10,500 units of lipase with snacks. The product that comes closest to this dose is Pancreatic MT 10.

13. How would you instruct JN's mother to administer her pancreatic enzyme replacement therapy?

    a. Administer the capsule whole with water.
    b. Administer the capsule whole with juice.
    c. Open the capsule and sprinkle over soft, nonalkaline food. Do not chew the beads.
    d. Open the capsule and sprinkle over soft, alkaline food. Do not chew the beads.

Answers a, b, and d are incorrect. This would work in an older patient but most 2 year olds will not be able to swallow a capsule. Water or juice would not breakdown the enteric coating. Alkaline food should not be taken with the pancreatic enzymes.

Answer c is correct. The beads can be sprinkled over soft food if swallowed whole and not chewed. Nonalkaline food should be used to support the enteric coating on the microspheres. Pancrelipase should be used as part of a high-calorie diet, appropriate for age and clinical status. Administer with meals or snacks and swallow whole with a generous amount of liquid. Do not crush or chew. Delayed-release capsules containing enteric-coated microspheres or microtablets may also be opened and the contents sprinkled on soft food with a low pH such as applesauce, gelatin, banana, sweet potato, baby food, or baby formula. Dairy products such as milk, custard, and ice cream may have a high pH and should be avoided.

14. How would you instruct JN's mother to monitor the effectiveness of her child's pancreatic enzyme replacement therapy?

    a. ↓ Steatorrhea, ↑ weight
    b. ↓ Steatorrhea, ↓ weight
    c. ↑ Steatorrhea, ↑ weight
    d. ↑ Steatorrhea, ↓ weight

Answer a is correct. When the pancreatic enzyme dose is correct, malabsorption will decrease and the mother will see a decrease in the fat in the stool (steatorrhea) and an increase in JN's weight.

Answer b is incorrect. The weight will increase as the malabsorption improves.

Answers c and d are incorrect. The pancreatic enzymes will improve the absorption of fat and steatorrhea will decrease.

15. What side effects would you instruct JN's mother to monitor with the pancreatic enzyme replacement therapy?

    a. Soar mouth and diaper rash
    b. Soar mouth and sunburn
    c. Diaper rash
    d. Soar mouth

Answer a is correct. If the microspheres are chewed the enzymes will breakdown the lining of the mouth. When too much enzyme is given, the excess comes through in the stool and produces a diaper rash on the skin.

Answer b is incorrect. Pancreatic enzymes do not produce sun sensitivity.

Answers c and d are incorrect. Both are side effects of enzyme therapy but answer a is more complete.

16. JN's mother has heard CF patients are deficient in vitamins. She wants to know which ones.

    a. Fat-soluble vitamins
    b. Water-soluble vitamins
    c. None
    d. All vitamins

Answer a is correct. The fat-soluble vitamins are malabsorbed in CF due to the malabsorption of fat in these patients.

Answer b is incorrect. The water-soluble vitamins are not malabsorbed. Later in life the CF patient may become deficient in all vitamins due to severe malnutrition.

Answer c is incorrect. CF patients malabsorb the fat-soluble vitamins.

Answer d is incorrect. All vitamins may be deficient when malnutrition becomes severe. The CF patient does not malabsorb all vitamins.

17. The child down the hall with CF is older and has liver failure. Her mother wants to know if there is a drug to prevent this awful disease.

 a. Pancreatic supplements
 b. Vitamin supplements
 c. Antibiotics
 d. Ursodeoxycholic acid

Answer a is incorrect. Pancreatic supplements treat the pancreatic obstruction.

Answer b is incorrect. Vitamins treat the malabsorption of fat-soluble vitamins and severe malnutrition.

Answer c is incorrect. Antibiotics treat the pulmonary infections

Answer d is correct. UDCA is a bile acid with choleretic properties. This should be used prophylactically with taurine to prevent the slowdown and blockage that occurs in the biliary tree which leads to liver failure over time.

18. When JN goes home, the doctors would like to give a medicine shown to decrease the time between pulmonary infections. What would you recommend?

 a. Inhaled tobramycin
 b. Inhaled albuterol
 c. Inhaled DNAse
 d. Inhaled hypertonic saline

Answer a is incorrect. Inhaled tobramycin has been shown to improve PFTs in CF patients.

Answer b is incorrect. Inhaled albuterol will improve gas exchange in a patient with an asthmatic component to their CF.

Answer c is correct. Inhaled DNAse has been shown to increase the time between CF exacerbations and hospitalizations.

Answer d is incorrect. Inhaled hypertonic saline has been shown to slow the progression of damage in the lungs of CF patients.

19. What other therapy can be given to JN to help prevent pulmonary infections?

 a. Influenzae vaccine
 b. Meningococcal vaccine
 c. MMR vaccine
 d. Hepatitis vaccine

Answer a is correct. The flu vaccine will prevent URIs which can progress into a lower tract infection or exacerbation in the CF patient.

Answers b, c, and d are incorrect. These vaccines do not have an effect on pulmonary infections.

20. As JN's mother leaves the hospital with JN, she wants to know the likelihood of development of CF in other children she may have. Neither of JN's parents has been diagnosed with CF.

 a. 25%
 b. 50%
 c. 75%
 d. 100%

Answer a is correct. With recessive heterozygous (homozygous) transmission, two carriers must marry. They will have normal children (25%), asymptomatic carriers (50%), and CF children (25%).

Hh (asymptomatic carrier) + Hh (asymptomatic carrier)

↓

↓

1 HH (normal child) + 2 Hh (asymptomatic carriers) + 1 hh (CF child)

25% 50% 25%

Answers b, c, and d are incorrect.

CHAPTER 45 | Gout

1. Which of the following is *not* a risk factor for increased SUA levels?

 a. Increased age
 b. Female sex
 c. Increased body weight
 d. Increased alcohol intake

Answer b is correct because men are at a higher risk factor for hyperuricemia compared to women.

Answers a, c, and d are incorrect because they are all risk factors for hyperuricemia.

2. Which of the following foods is most likely to have the highest purine content?

 a. Liver
 b. Apple

c. Popcorn
d. Potatoes

Answer a is correct because red meats, particularly organ meats, have high purine content and should be avoided in patients with gout.

Answers b, c, and d are incorrect because these foods have relatively low purine content.

3. Which of the following is *not* consistent with the typical clinical presentation of gout?
   a. Commonly affects the great toe
   b. Bilateral joint involvement
   c. Rapid onset of symptoms
   d. Self-limiting pain and erythema

Answer b is the correct answer because gout is typically a monoarthritis and is usually not characterized by bilateral joint involvement.

Answers a, c, and d are incorrect answers because patients with gout frequently present with rapid onset of self-limiting pain and erythema, commonly involving the great toe.

4. A 76-year-old woman with a 10-year history of gout presents to the clinic with recently developed painful MSU crystal deposits in her hand tissues. Which of the following terms most accurately describes this complication of gout?
   a. Atheromas
   b. Podagra
   c. Tophi
   d. Uric acid nephrolithiasis

Answer a is incorrect because an atheroma is a lipid deposit within the arterial wall and is not related to gout.

Answer b is incorrect since podagra is a term used to describe gout-related symptoms in the great toe.

Answer c is correct because tophi are painful MSU crystals which deposit in the skin and can cause tissue damage. These complications often occur in patients with long-standing hyperuricemia and chronic gout.

Answer d is incorrect because uric acid nephrolithiasis is a complication of gout characterized by MSU crystal deposits in the kidney which can contribute to renal failure.

5. A 60-year-old man presents to the pharmacy with a past medical history of hypertension and gout. After reviewing his medication profile, which of the following medications is most likely to cause elevated SUA levels?
   a. Hydrochlorothiazide
   b. Lisinopril
   c. Metoprolol
   d. Indomethacin

Answer a is correct because the antihypertensive agent hydrochlorothiazide can contribute to hyperuricemia, and if possible, it should be avoided in patients with gout.

Answers b and c are incorrect because these antihypertensive agents are not associated with elevated SUA levels and are good choices for many patients with gout.

Answer d is incorrect because this NSAID is actually used to treat pain and inflammation associated with gout, and it does not cause elevated SUA levels.

6. Which of the following is the brand name for allopurinol?
   a. Uloric
   b. Zyloprim
   c. Zebeta
   d. Benemid

Answer a is incorrect. Uloric is the brand name for febuxostat.

Answer b is correct. Zyloprim is the brand name for allopurinol.

Answer c is incorrect. Zebeta is the brand name of bisoprolol.

Answer d is incorrect. Benemid is the brand name of probenecid.

7. Which of the following is a *true* statement?
   a. Use of allopurinol increases warfarin levels and increases theophylline levels.
   b. Use of allopurinol increases warfarin levels and decreases theophylline levels.
   c. Use of allopurinol decreases warfarin levels and decreases theophylline levels.
   d. Use of allopurinol decreases warfarin levels and increases theophylline levels.

Answer a is correct. Use of allopurinol may inhibit the metabolism of warfarin and theophylline, resulting in increased levels of each drug.

Answers b, c, and d are incorrect.

8. A resident approaches you about a patient who was just admitted for an acute gout flare. He wants to start the patient on corticosteroid therapy. Which of the following would be important to communicate to the resident regarding monitoring parameters?
   a. Recommend to monitor serum creatinine for renal dysfunction.
   b. Recommend to monitor blood glucose levels.
   c. Recommend to monitor for diarrhea.
   d. Recommend to monitor for presence of skin rash.

Answer a is incorrect as corticosteroids are a gout treatment option for patients who have renal insufficiency; corticosteroids do not cause renal impairment.

Answer b is correct. It is important to monitor blood glucose levels in patients who are started on corticosteroid therapy—regardless if patients are diabetic or not, due to corticosteroid's ability to increase blood glucose levels.

Answer c is incorrect. This would be an important monitoring parameter if the patient was started on colchicine.

Answer d is incorrect. It would be important to monitor for this possible side effect if the patient was started on allopurinol once the initial episode was under control.

9. A 63-year-old man presents to your clinic complaining of excruciating pain in his left big toe. After being diagnosed with an acute gout flare, his physician wants to start him on therapy. His medical history is positive for hypertension, hyperlipidemia, peptic ulcer disease, and glaucoma. Which of the following is the most appropriate therapy for this patient?
    a. Ibuprofen
    b. Indomethacin
    c. Allopurinol
    d. Prednisone

Answers a and b are incorrect because they are both NSAIDs and should be avoided in patients with a history of peptic ulcer disease.

Answer c is incorrect because allopurinol should not be initiated as treatment for an acute gout flare as this medication may worsen the flare by rapidly decreasing uric acid and causing mobilization of uric acid stores.

Answer d is correct as this would be an option for patients who have contraindications to other acute gout therapy, such as NSAIDs with peptic ulcer disease.

10. In a patient with a creatinine clearance of less than 10 mL/min, which acute gout medication is most appropriate?
    a. Prednisone
    b. Ibuprofen
    c. Nabumetone
    d. Colchicine

Answer a is correct. Corticosteroids are the drugs of choice for acute gout in patients with renal insufficiency.

Answers b and c are incorrect because they are both NSAIDs and so should be avoided in patients with a history of renal dysfunction.

Answer d is incorrect because colchicine should also be avoided in patients with renal insufficiency due to increased risk for toxicities.

11. A patient is picking up a new prescription for colchicine. Which of the following are the appropriate counseling points to discuss with the patient?
    a. The patient should be counseled on gastrointestinal side effects of nausea, vomiting, diarrhea, and abdominal pain.
    b. The patient should be counseled on possibility of a rash.
    c. The patient should be counseled on signs and symptoms of bleeding.
    d. The patient should be counseled on close monitoring of blood glucose levels.

Answer a is correct. The major side effects which can limit the use of colchicine are gastrointestinal.

Answer b is incorrect. This would be a counseling point for allopurinol.

Answer c is incorrect. This would be a counseling point for NSAIDs.

Answer d is incorrect. This would be a counseling point for corticosteroids.

12. Which of the following statements most accurately describes how NSAIDs work in the treatment of gout?
    a. NSAIDs work by reducing phagocytosis and lactic acid production in joints, thereby reducing deposition of urate crystals.
    b. NSAIDs work by blocking the conversion of xanthine to uric acid.
    c. NSAIDs work by exerting anti-inflammatory, analgesic, and antipyretic effects by inhibiting the synthesis of prostaglandin.
    d. NSAIDs work by inhibiting proximal renal tubule reabsorption of uric acid to decrease serum levels.

Answer a is incorrect. This is the mechanism of action of colchicine.

Answer b is incorrect. This is the mechanism of action of allopurinol.

Answer c is correct.

Answer d is incorrect. This is the mechanism of action of probenecid.

13. Which of the following statements is *true* regarding febuxostat?
    a. Febuxostat is a good choice for patients with liver failure.
    b. Febuxostat is the drug of choice for acute gout.
    c. Febuxostat is an option for patients with renal insufficiency.
    d. Febuxostat has no drug interactions.

Answer a is incorrect. Febuxostat is metabolized through the liver andshould not be used in liver failure.

Answer b is incorrect. Febuxostat is used as treatment in chronic gout.

Answer c is correct.

Answer d is incorrect. Febuxostat does interact with drugs, including azathioprine, 6-mercaptopurine, and theophylline.

---

14. Intravenous colchicine is not recommended due to the possibility of which adverse effect?

    a. Leukopenia
    b. Diarrhea
    c. Hyperglycemia
    d. Abdominal pain

Answer a is correct as IV colchicine is not recommended due to the increased risk of serious adverse effects, including leukopenia, extravasation, and even death.

Answer b is incorrect as gastrointestinal effects are less commonly encountered when colchicine is given intravenously rather than orally.

Answer c is incorrect as colchicine does not affect blood glucose levels.

Answer d is incorrect as gastrointestinal effects are less commonly encountered when colchicine is given intravenously rather than orally.

---

15. Which of the following is a *true* statement regarding the use of NSAIDs in the treatment of gout?

    a. Indomethacin is the NSAID of choice for treating gout.
    b. Short-acting NSAIDs at equipotent, anti-inflammatory doses are the drugs of choice for acute gout in the absence of contraindications.
    c. Intravenous administration of NSAID is the preferred route of administration for the treatment of gout.
    d. NSAIDs are second-line treatment behind colchicine for the treatment of gout.

Answer a is incorrect as any NSAID used at anti-inflammatory doses can be efficacious for the treatment of gout.

Answer b is correct.

Answer c is incorrect as fast-acting oral administration is usually preferred.

Answer d is incorrect as colchicine is usually second-line to NSAIDs for the treatment of gout due to adverse effect profile.

---

16. A 68-year-old man presents to the clinic with a history of three acute episodes of gout in the past year. He is classified as an overproducer of uric acid. He has liver impairment but no renal insufficiency. Which of the following medications is *most* appropriate for chronic prophylaxis of gout?

    a. Allopurinol
    b. Febuxostat
    c. Probenecid
    d. Sulfinpyrazone

Answer a is correct. Allopurinol is used for chronic prophylaxis of gout in patients who are overproducers of uric acid.

Answer b is incorrect because febuxostat cannot be used in hepatic impairment.

Answers c and d are incorrect because these agents are used as underexcretors of uric acid, not overproducers.

---

17. What is the mechanism of action by which probenecid produces its effect?

    a. Inhibition of xanthine oxidase
    b. Blocks excretion of uric acid
    c. Blocks reuptake of uric acid at the proximal tubule
    d. Inhibits prostaglandin synthesis

Answer a is incorrect because it is the mechanism of action of allopurinol and febuxostat.

Answer b is incorrect because probenecid increases uric acid excretion.

Answer c is correct.

Answer d is incorrect because it is the mechanism of action of NSAIDs.

Please use the following case to answer questions 18 and 19.

A 75-year-old man is started on allopurinol for gout prevention. His baseline serum uric acid level is 11.6 mg/dL. He is overweight (BMI 30 mg/m^2) and drinks 1 to 2 cans of beer a day.

18. Which of the following statements *best* describes allopurinol and its role in gout prevention?

    a. Allopurinol is most effective when initiated within 24 to 48 hours of an acute attack.
    b. The usual starting dose is 300 mg po daily.
    c. Treatment with allopurinol should be continued for 3 to 12 months.
    d. Serous side effects include myopathy and bone marrow suppression.

Answer a is incorrect as allopurinol should not be initiated during an acute attack.

Answer b is incorrect as the usual starting dose is 50 to 100 mg daily.

Answer c is correct.

Answer d is incorrect as these side effects are reported with colchicine.

---

19. Regarding nonpharmacologic treatment of gout, which of the following measures should be avoided?

    a. Weight loss
    b. Reduction of alcohol consumption
    c. Application of cold packs
    d. Application of heat

Answers a, b, and c are all appropriate measures for non-pharmacologic treatment of gout. Heat should be avoided.

Answer d is correct.

20. The target serum uric acid level when treating gout is typically:

   a. ≤ 6 mg/dL
   b. ≤ 7 mg/dL
   c. ≤ 8 mg/dL
   d. ≤ 9 mg/dL

Answer a is correct.

Answers b, c, and d are incorrect.

CHAPTER 46 | Osteoporosis

1. Which of the following is correct?

   a. While osteoporosis is more prominent in women, osteopenia is equally common in men and women.
   b. Due to the availability of many medications, the prevalence of osteoporosis has been declining in the United States.
   c. Osteoporosis is most commonly associated with musculoskeletal pain.
   d. The most common sites for osteoporotic fractures include the spine and hip.
   e. Low bone mass is common in patients under the age of 30, but improves in time under normal physiologic conditions.

Answer a is incorrect. Osteopenia and osteoporosis are more prevalent in women, typically due to the loss of estrogen's beneficial effects following menopause. Men do develop osteopenia and osteoporosis, though much later in life when testosterone levels begin to decline or as a result of multiple risk factors.

Answer b is incorrect. Prior to the 2002 Women's Health Initiative (WHI), hormone replacement therapy (HRT) was routinely administered to postmenopausal women for numerous reasons. The WHI showed the risk of HRT on breast cancer and cardiovascular complications outweighed the beneficial effects on bone. Now, HRT is rarely used (except for the short-term treatment of hot flushes) and may increase the likelihood of developing osteoporosis. Also, the diligent use of sunscreen products has decreased the risk of certain skin cancers, but also leads to a decrease in vitamin D absorption from sunlight and subsequent low bone mass.

Answer c is incorrect. While musculoskeletal pain can occur, osteoporosis is usually asymptomatic. This is why screening for at-risk patients is critical.

Answer d is correct. In the absence of appropriate screening, many osteoporotic patients are not diagnosed until they suffer a fragility fracture. These often occur in the spine, and may present as kyphosis, lordosis, or remain asymptomatic. The hip is another common site for fragility fractures. Today, most clinical trials in osteoporosis use the fracture reduction of the vertebrae and/or hip as a clinical endpoint.

Answer e is incorrect. Around age 30 is when a person reaches peak bone mass, followed by a balance between bone formation and resorption. Then, as we age, resorption becomes favored and leads to bone mass loss.

2. SD is a 45-year-old woman. She does not have any significant past-medical history and currently smokes one-half pack a day and drinks alcohol socially. She attends a health fair and learns her T-score is −1.5. Which is the best course of action?

   a. SD has osteopenia and should be started on alendronate 70 mg po every week.
   b. SD has no physical signs or symptoms of osteoporosis and should be advised to quit smoking and to have her BMD checked again in 6 months.
   c. SD is young and should be started on teriparatide 20 μg SQ qd to rebuild her bone mass to more normal levels.
   d. SD should be started on calcium 1000 mg and vitamin D 800 IU qd.

Answer a is incorrect. While SD does have osteopenia based on the WHO guidelines, it would be prudent to do a more thorough assessment before initiating a bisphosphonate at this point. Furthermore, if a bisphosphonate is ultimately deemed appropriate, the "prevention" dose of alendronate is 5 mg po qd or 35 mg po every week.

Answer b is incorrect. Osteoporosis, as well as osteopenia, is often asymptomatic and a lack of symptoms does not justify withholding therapy. It should be recommended that SD go for a more thorough assessment and be advised to quit smoking, as this is a risk factor. However, repeating a BMD is generally not recommended more than every other year per the National Osteoporosis Foundation (NOF).

Answer c is incorrect. Teriparatide is recommended for patients with (severe) osteoporosis with high risk of fracture, not osteopenia.

Answer d is correct. SD is not currently taking calcium or vitamin D per WHO guidelines. Though this may or may not fully explain her low BMD score, it is the most logical starting point to minimize the risk of developing osteoporosis.

3. Which of the following is true?

   a. Osteoclasts are primarily responsible for the formation phase of bone remodeling and are stimulated by calcium and vitamin D.
   b. Bone remodeling is generally reserved for areas of bone that suffer acute damage.
   c. Osteoblastic function is stimulated by bisphosphonates.
   d. None of the above is true.

Answer a is incorrect. Osteoclasts are primarily responsible for bone resorption. Calcium and vitamin D supplementation help in the formation and stabilization of bone, not resorption.

Answer b is incorrect. While bone remodeling clearly occurs in bone that sustains acute damage, the entire body goes through the remodeling process throughout our lives. The bone, as it mechanically functions day-to-day, wears down and needs repair. This is not routinely an acute process, but a sustained one.

Answer c is incorrect. Bisphosphonates are in a class known as antiresorptive agents, which inhibit osteoclastic function. In fact, the use of a bisphosphonate will decrease overall bone turnover by directly inhibiting osteoclastic function, which indirectly leads to a decrease in osteoblastic function over time.

Answer d is correct. None of the statements above are correct.

---

4. Select the risk factors for osteoporosis.
   a. HRT therapy that is prescribed at a slightly higher dose than recommended by the FDA
   b. Low body mass index (BMI < 21 kg/m^2)
   c. Being African American
   d. All of the above

Answer a is incorrect. HRT therapy is not recommended for the prevention of osteoporosis due to the adverse event findings of the WHI. Nevertheless, a slightly high-dose HRT would not increase the general risk of osteoporosis.

Answer b is correct. Low weight and body mass index are risk factors for osteoporosis

Answer c is incorrect. The racial groups at higher risk for osteoporosis are Caucasian, Asian, and Latino. However, African Americans can definitely develop osteoporosis, particularly based on other common risk factors.

Answer d is incorrect. Only the low body mass index is a risk factor based on above.

---

5. JR is a 58-year-old white man who presents to the ED with a hip fracture after rolling out of his bed in his home. His vitals and laboratory values are generally unremarkable. He is 5 ft 8 in and weighs 133 lb. His medical history includes mild asthma and rheumatoid arthritis. His current medications include albuterol inhaler every 4 to 6 hours prn, prednisone 10 mg qd, and a multivitamin. After discharge from the hospital, he is sent to your clinic about 3 weeks later for further evaluation. Which of the following is the best answer?
   a. JR should have a BMD checked immediately to determine if he has osteoporosis.
   b. JR is a candidate for zoledronic acid 5 mg IV with repeat dosing every other year.
   c. JR is a candidate for raloxifene 60 mg po qd.
   d. JR is a candidate for teriparatide 20 μg SQ qd.
   e. JR should start taking calcium and vitamin D and follow-up in 6 months.

Answer a is incorrect. Whether JR should have a BMD checked immediately is a matter of clinical debate, and hence, not the best answer. It may be useful to have a BMD as a baseline to track the effects of therapy moving forward. However, JR has suffered a low-trauma hip fracture in the presence of multiple osteoporosis risk factors (low BMI, rheumatoid arthritis, and prednisone). Most clinicians, and the NOF, would diagnose JR as having osteoporosis regardless of the BMD score at this point.

Answer b is incorrect. JR may be a candidate for a bisphosphonate, including zoledronic acid. However, zoledronic acid 5 mg IV with every other year dosing is for prevention and JR is a candidate for treatment dosing.

Answer c is incorrect. Raloxifene is a selective estrogen receptor modulator (SERM) and is only indicated in women.

Answer d is correct. JR appears to have glucocorticoid-induced osteoporosis with a high risk of fracture (following his previous low-trauma fracture) and is a candidate for teriparatide.

Answer e is incorrect. JR appears to have glucocorticoid-induced osteoporosis and is a candidate for pharmacologic treatment, in addition to calcium and vitamin D. It would be unwise to not initiate treatment for another 6 months.

---

6. Select the agent that can be administered monthly for osteoporosis treatment.
   a. Risedronate
   b. Raloxifene
   c. Zoledronic acid
   d. Alendronate
   e. None of the above

Answer a is correct. Risedronate is taken orally either daily, weekly, every 2 consecutive days, or monthly. Ibandronate is also available as an oral monthly formulation.

Answer b is incorrect. Raloxifene is taken orally qd for treatment.

Answer c is incorrect. Zoledronic acid is given IV annually for treatment.

Answer d is incorrect. Alendronate is taken orally qd or every week for treatment.

Answer e is incorrect. Based on the above information answer e is incorrect.

---

7. RS is a 67-year-old Asian woman with a T-score −2.7. She is 5 ft 6 in and 127 lb. She was admitted to the hospital with leg swelling that was diagnosed as deep vein thrombosis (DVT) and was ultimately referred to your clinic upon resolution and

discharge. Her medical history includes hypertension, osteoarthritis, and diabetes. She currently takes furosemide, Accupril, celecoxib, metformin, and aspirin. Which of the following is the best answer?

a. RS should begin taking calcium 1000 mg qd and vitamin D 400 IU qd.
b. RS is a candidate for estrogen 0.625 mg po qd.
c. RS is a candidate for ibandronate 3 mg IV every 3 months.
d. RS is a candidate for raloxifene 60 mg po qd.

Answer a is incorrect. Patients at age 50+ require calcium 1200 mg qd and vitamin D 800 to 1000 IU qd.

Answer b is incorrect. Based on the WHI, it is no longer appropriate to initiate estrogen as first-line therapy for the treatment of osteoporosis. HRTs are also associated with venous thromboembolism and can lead to DVTs (particularly in this high-risk patient).

Answer c is correct. RS is a candidate for osteoporosis treatment, including ibandronate IV. She should also begin taking calcium 1200 mg qd and vitamin D 800 to 1000 IU qd.

Answer d is incorrect. The selective estrogen receptor modulators have been associated with venous thromboembolism and should be used with caution in a patient with a history of DVT.

---

8. Which of the following condition(s) would suggest caution for receiving a bisphosphonate?

a. Creatinine clearance CrCl < 30 mL/min
b. Peanut allergy
c. History of stroke
d. History of Paget disease
e. All of the above

Answer a is correct. Renal dysfunction described as a CrCl < 30mL/min is a contraindication to the oral and IV bisphosphonates.

Answer b is incorrect. There is no known association between a peanut allergy and any sensitivity to bisphosphonates.

Answer c is incorrect. There is no known association between stroke and sensitivity to bisphosphonates.

Answer d is incorrect. Paget disease, which is essentially a disorder of abnormally high, and erratic bone remodeling leading to deformities, pain and fractures, is commonly treated with bisphosphonates.

Answer e is incorrect. Based on the above information answer e is incorrect.

---

9. Which of the following is true regarding teriparatide?

a. It may be associated with hypercalcemia.
b. It is contraindicated in a patient with Paget disease.
c. It is available as a monthly IM injection.
d. It should only be used for a maximum of 3 years.
e. More than one of the above is true.

Answer a is correct. Teriparatide increases overall bone remodeling with a preference toward osteoblastic function and may cause hypercalcemia and hypercalciuria.

Answer b is correct. Paget disease is associated with high, erratic bone turnover, which could be worsened by the anabolic effects of teriparatide.

Answer c is incorrect. Teriparatide is FDA approved as a daily, SQ injection.

Answer d is incorrect. Teriparatide should only be used for a maximum of 2 years total, based on available data.

Answer e is correct for the reasons stated above (a and b are true).

---

10. Which of the following is true regarding bisphosphonates?

a. Ibandronate po should be taken with food to minimize any GI side effects.
b. Risedronate should be taken at bedtime to minimize any CNS side effects, including dizziness.
c. A patient receiving zoledronic acid should avoid drinking high-mineral water (ie, well water).
d. A patient taking alendronate should also routinely be taking calcium and vitamin D.

Answer a is incorrect. All oral bisphosphonates, including ibandronate, should be taken on an empty stomach, as food greatly diminishes absorption.

Answer b is incorrect. All oral bisphosphonates, including risedronate, should be taken first thing in the morning, with a full glass of water while the patient remains upright to avoid esophageal/GI irritation.

Answer c is incorrect. Zoledronic acid is given IV and will not be affected by water intake. Patients should avoid high-mineral water when taking oral bisphosphonates due to the decreased bioavailability

Answer d is correct. A patient taking alendronate, or any bisphosphonate, should routinely take calcium and vitamin D per WHO guidelines. One caveat for oral bisphosphonates, however, is to avoid taking supplements within 60 minutes of the BP to avoid effecting bioavailability.

---

11. Select the brand name for raloxifene.

a. Evista
b. Fosamax
c. Premarin
d. Reclast
e. Actonel

Answer a is correct. Evista is the brand name for raloxifene.

Answer b is incorrect. Fosamax is the brand name for alendronate.

Answer c is incorrect. Premarin is a brand name for estrogen. Estrogen has additional brand names and manufacturers.

Answer d is incorrect. Reclast is the brand name for zoledronic acid.

Answer e is incorrect. Actonel is the brand name for risedronate.

12. Select the osteoporosis medication that is available as a nasal spray.
    a. Ibandronate
    b. Teriparatide
    c. Calcitonin
    d. Zoledronic acid
    e. None of the above

Answer a is incorrect. Ibandronate is available in oral and IV form.

Answer b is incorrect. Teriparatide is available in SQ form.

Answer c is correct. Calcitonin is available as a nasal spray, as well as injectable (SQ or IM).

Answer d is incorrect. Zoledronic acid is available in IV form.

Answer e is incorrect. Based on the above explanation answer e is incorrect.

13. KG is a 59-year-old postmenopausal woman who is sent to you on referral. She recently had her BMD checked and had a T-score of −2.3. Her past medical history is unremarkable and she only takes a multivitamin with additional calcium and vitamin D. Her family history is remarkable for a mother who had osteoporosis and died of breast cancer and a father who has diabetes. Which of the following is the best answer?
    a. KG has osteopenia but is taking appropriate calcium and vitamin D.
    b. KG is a good candidate for risedronate 5 mg po qd.
    c. KG is a good candidate for alendronate 70 mg IV every week.
    d. KG is a good candidate for raloxifene 60 mg po qd.
    e. KG is a good candidate for calcitonin 100 IU IM qd.

Answer a is incorrect. Based on her T-score, KG is osteopenic, but may not be taking enough calcium and vitamin D. It would be prudent to consider checking a serum vitamin D, particularly in light of her family history of osteoporosis.

Answer b is incorrect. Technically, KG could be a candidate for risedronate based on her T-score and risk factors. However, daily oral bisphosphonates are rarely recommended first-line since there are weekly and monthly options (which help improve compliance). Therefore, this answer does not represent the best answer.

Answer c is incorrect. Alendronate is not available as IV.

Answer d is correct. Raloxifene is a good choice for two reasons: osteoporosis prevention (and arguably treatment based on risk factors) and prevention of breast cancer based on her potential risk. Her family history makes the SERM a logical option based on the information given.

Answer e is incorrect. Calcitonin IM is indicated for treatment of osteoporosis (she is osteopenic, but may be a candidate for treatment based on risk factors). Calcitonin IM is rarely used first-line based on cost and the availability of other agents that seem to offer greater fracture reduction.

14. MF is a 63-year-old postmenopausal woman who recently learned her T-score is −2.9 (it was −2.8 a year ago) despite being on an oral bisphosphonate, calcium, and vitamin D. She is not on any additional medications. Which of the following should her pharmacist do first?
    a. Explain to her that at 63 years and being postmenopausal, such a small change in BMD is not surprising.
    b. Suggest she talk to her doctor about taking a different bisphosphonate.
    c. Recommend to her physician that raloxifene should be added to the current regimen.
    d. Counsel the patient to see how she is taking her medications and review her refill records to see if she is filling the bisphosphonate as expected.

Answer a is incorrect. MF needs to have her T-score addressed. It is well below −2.5, appears to be worsening, and merits further investigation with her and her physician.

Answer b is incorrect. Different bisphosphonates do have different potencies, as well as different routes of administration that may need to ultimately be considered. However, the two most common reasons patients see worsening BMDs while on therapy are noncompliance with their bisphosphonate and/or inadequate calcium and vitamin D intake. These factors should be examined prior to recommending a switch.

Answer c is incorrect. Adding or changing therapy may be warranted, but not until the cause of the inadequate response is examined.

Answer d is correct. Oral bisphosphonates can be difficult to take for some patients, and are often associated with poor compliance (and poor outcomes). One of the most important roles a pharmacist has is to educate patients, in hopes of improving issues like poor compliance. The pharmacist may determine that education can solve the problem or decide that consultation with the prescribing physician is needed to redesign the therapeutic plan.

15. Which of the following is true regarding Vitamin D?
    a. Low serum vitamin D levels are common throughout the United States.
    b. For postmenopausal patients, Vitamin D 400 IU qd is typically adequate.
    c. If a patient has significantly low serum vitamin D levels, vitamin D 800 IU qd will usually correct this over time.
    d. All of the above are true.

Answer a is correct. Vitamin D deficiency is common throughout the United States. Some experts believed that it was less common in the Southeast due to the higher exposure to sunlight. However, the routine use of sunscreens (which are very effective at minimizing the risk of certain skin cancers) has made vitamin D deficiency a far more common national phenomenon.

Answer b is incorrect. 50+ year olds require vitamin D 800 to 1000 IU qd.

Answer c is incorrect. Vitamin D deficiency is often difficult to correct using typical daily doses, particularly if the level is significantly low. These patients often need an oral or IM loading dose prior to initiating qd therapy.

Answer d is incorrect. Based on the above information answer d is incorrect.

---

16. Which of the following is true?
    a. FRAX is an online tool for patients to use when learning about bisphosphonates.
    b. FRAX helps determine who might be the best candidates for osteoporosis therapy.
    c. FRAX is generally not useful for patients with a T-score > −1.4.
    d. All of the above.

Answer a is incorrect. FRAX is an online tool for physicians to help determine who is at risk for fractures. While anyone (including patients) can access the information, FRAX® does not provide information about specific therapies or therapeutic classes.

Answer b is correct. FRAX is a predictive model by the WHO that recommends considering therapy for those with a 10-year fracture probability of ≥ 3% for the hip or ≥ 20% for any major fracture.

Answer c is incorrect. BMD is not the only predictor of fracture. FRAX uses the T-score, along with 12 risk fractures to determine fracture probability.

Answer d is incorrect. Based on the above information answer d is incorrect.

---

17. Which of the following matches the medication with a commonly associated side effect.
    a. Alendronate—Nasal congestion
    b. Ibandronate—Gout
    c. Raloxifene—Hot flushes
    d. Teriparatide—Memory loss
    e. Zoledronic acid—Dry mouth

Answer a is incorrect. Alendronate is not commonly known to cause nasal congestion.

Answer b is incorrect. Ibandronate is not commonly known to cause gout.

Answer c is correct. Raloxifene has been associated with hot flushes. This is important to remember as hormone replacement therapy (HRT) is/was often used to treat these vasomotor symptoms during menopause and clinicians sometimes assume raloxifene will treat them as well.

Answer d is incorrect. Teriparatide is sometimes known to cause dizziness, but it is not commonly known to lead to memory loss.

Answer e is incorrect. Zoledronic acid is not commonly known to cause dry mouth.

---

18. SM is a 65-year-old postmenopausal woman with a T-score of −3.0. Her past medical history is notable for osteoarthritis. She currently takes naproxen, as well as calcium 1200 mg and vitamin D 1000 IU qd. Which of the following is correct?
    a. SM is on the appropriate doses of calcium and vitamin D according to WHO guidelines.
    b. SM is a candidate for risedronate 150 mg po every month, despite the fact she is on naproxen.
    c. SM should have her vitamin D level checked, despite the high dose of vitamin D she is currently taking.
    d. SM is a candidate for zoledronic acid 5 mg IV once a year, but normal renal function should be observed prior to receiving each dose.
    e. All of the above.

Answer a is correct. SM is on the appropriate doses of calcium and vitamin D according to WHO guidelines.

Answer b is correct. SM is a candidate for treatment doses of a bisphosphonate, including risedronate. The use of an NSAID, like naproxen, is not a contraindication to taking an oral bisphosphonate. However, the patient should be reminded to take the bisphosphonate separately from the NSAID and be made aware of the potential GI side effects of either medication.

Answer c is correct. Despite the fact that SM is on the recommended dose of vitamin D, she may still have low serum levels. It is important to remember that if her baseline levels were low, she may need a vitamin D loading dose to get her to goal.

Answer d is correct. SM is a candidate for treatment doses of a bisphosphonate, including zoledronic acid. Patients may only receive IV zoledronic acid if their CrCl is ≥ 35mL/min.

Answer e is the correct and the best answer.

---

19. Which of the following is true?
    a. The human skeleton is comprised of two types of bone: subcortical and trochanter.
    b. BMD is specific but not sensitive for fracture risk.
    c. A radiographic x-ray cannot determine osteoporosis.
    d. ONJ is an area of exposed bone in the maxillofacial region that does not heal within 2 weeks of its occurrence.

Answer a is incorrect. The human skeleton is comprised of 80% cortical bone and 20% trabecular. Cortical bone forms the exterior part of bone, while trabecular bone forms the porous interior and ends of long bones. The trochanter is the boney prominence at the end of the femur.

Answer b is correct. BMD is specific but not sensitive for fracture risk. While it is a necessary screening tool, over 50% of hip fractures, for example, occur in patients with a T-score > −2.5.

Answer c is incorrect. A radiographic x-ray can detect osteoporosis, though it has low sensitivity and may not be as useful at all osteoporotic sites. This is why dual X-ray absorptiometry (DX) is used.

Answer d is incorrect. Osteonecrosis of the jaw (ONJ) is defined as an area of exposed bone in the maxillofacial region that does not heal within 8 weeks. ONJ has rarely been seen in patients taking BPs, though a clear cause-and-effect relationship has not been determined.

---

20. Which of the following are risk factors for osteoporosis?
    a. History of fracture while in college playing rugby
    b. Amenorrhea starting at age 45
    c. Occasionally drinking a glass of wine with dinner
    d. b and c

Answer a is incorrect. History of fracture prior to age 50, particularly due to "high trauma," is not a risk factor for osteoporosis.

Answer b is correct. Amenorrhea, or the absence of menstruation, is a risk factor for osteoporosis, including those patients of a premenopausal age.

Answer c is incorrect. Alcoholism is a risk factor for osteoporosis and is described as consuming 2 to 3+ oz a day. The occasional glass of wine would fall below this threshold and not be considered a risk factor.

Answer d is incorrect. Based on the above information answer d is incorrect.

CHAPTER 47 | Rheumatoid Arthritis

1. Select the classic signs and symptoms of rheumatoid arthritis.
    a. Morning stiffness that lasts more than 1 hour
    b. Swelling in the small joints of the hands, wrists, and feet
    c. Positive rheumatoid factor
    d. All of the above

Answers a, b, and c are correct.

Answer d is correct and the best answer. All of the above are classic signs and symptoms of rheumatoid arthritis, though only 60% to 70% of patients will test positive for rheumatoid factor. Radiological changes such as joint erosions or decalcification are other classic symptoms.

---

2. Which of the following DMARDs would be contraindicated in a patient with a history of a sulfa allergy?
    a. Neoral
    b. Arava
    c. Rheumatrex
    d. Azulfidine
    e. Cytoxan

Answer a is incorrect. Neoral (cyclosporine) is not contraindicated in patients with a sulfa allergy.

Answer b is incorrect. Arava (leflunomide) is not contraindicated in patients with a sulfa allergy.

Answer c is incorrect. Rheumatrex (methotrexate) is not contraindicated in patients with a sulfa allergy.

Answer d is correct. Azulfidine (sulfasalazine) is contraindicated in patients with history of hypersensitivity to medications containing sulfa.

Answer e is incorrect. Cytoxan (cyclophosphamide) is not contraindicated in patients with a sulfa allergy.

---

3. JJ was diagnosed with RA with moderate disease activity and has been exhibiting symptoms for about 2 months. His physician is seeking your advice in designing an initial medication regimen for him. Which of the following medications would you include for the most appropriate recommendation?
    i. Ibuprofen
    ii. Prednisone
    iii. Leflunomide
    iv. Etanercept

    a. i only
    b. i and ii
    c. i, ii, and iii
    d. All of the above

Answer a is incorrect. NSAIDs such as ibuprofen possess analgesic and anti-inflammatory effects, which provide RA symptom relief. However, they do not affect the underlying disease process of RA, thus they should not be used as the sole treatment.

Answer b is incorrect. Corticosteroids like prednisone possess anti-inflammatory and immunosuppressive effects which improve symptoms in RA. They are recommended for "bridge therapy" to provide symptomatic relief until full onset of DMARD therapy or in short bursts for treatment of RA exacerbation. Additionally long-term, low-dose maintenance therapy may be used in patients refractive to DMARD or NSAID therapy. Long-term and high-dose corticosteroid treatment should be avoided due to risk of long-term side effects.

Answer c is correct. DMARDs reduce and prevent joint damage and preserve joint function. They should be initiated early, within the first 3 months of onset of symptoms. DMARDs take weeks to months for full onset of effect, thus NSAIDs and corticosteroids will be needed for symptom relief.

Answer d is incorrect. Biologic DMARDs should be used in patients who have moderate to severe RA and who have inadequate response to one or more DMARDs.

---

4. Corticosteroids may be used
   a. During acute RA flares
   b. During "bridge therapy" while awaiting the onset of DMARD therapy
   c. At low doses in patients who are refractive to traditional NSAID or DMARD therapy
   d. All of the above

Corticosteroid agents provide relief from inflammation but are typically used short term due to their problematic long-term adverse effects such as osteoporosis and adrenal suppression. Corticosteroids are indicated during acute flares and during "bridge therapy" while a patient awaits the onset of effect of the DMARD agent.

Long-term corticosteroid therapy may be required for patients who are refractory to NSAID or DMARD therapy, but this is not preferred and the lowest possible dose of the corticosteroid must be used. Patients must be advised to take corticosteroids with food in order to minimize the risk of gastric mucosa damage.

Answer d is the correct answer. All of the above are indications for corticosteroid use.

---

5. Which of the following nondrug therapies would be recommended for a patient with RA?
   a. Heat or cold therapy.
   b. Physical therapy.
   c. Weight reduction.
   d. All of the above.
   e. Nonpharmacologic therapy is not effective for RA.

Answer d is correct. Nonpharmacologic therapy such as heat or cold therapy, physical therapy, and weight reduction as well as education, emotional support, rest, occupational therapy, and surgery (for severe cases) can be used to improve symptoms and maintain joint function in RA.

---

6. Which of the following is the correct mechanism of action for Enbrel?
   a. Monoclonal antibody which targets the CD20 antigen on B-lymphocytes
   b. TNF-α inhibitor
   c. Immunoglobulin protein which inhibits T-lymphocytes
   d. Dihydrofolate reductase inhibitor

Answer a is incorrect. Rituximab is a monoclonal antibody that targets CD20 antigen on B-lymphocytes.

Answer b is correct. Enbrel (etanercept) is a TNF-α inhibitor.

Answer c is incorrect. Abatacept is a T-cell inhibitor.

Answer d is incorrect. Methotrexate is a dihydrofolate reductase inhibitor.

---

7. DMARDs are preferred over non-DMARD therapy because
   a. DMARD agents have fewer adverse reactions than non-DMARDs.
   b. Non-DMARD agents are less cost-effective than DMARDs.
   c. DMARD agents may reduce or prevent joint damage and preserve joint function.
   d. Non-DMARD agents require close laboratory monitoring.

Answer a is incorrect. Both DMARD and non-DMARD drug agents have associated adverse reactions and neither drug class is less likely to cause them than the other.

Answer b is incorrect. Though formulary restrictions may limit the availability of certain agents, drug costs are typically not a major factor in making therapeutic decisions.

Answer c is correct. Unlike non-DMARD agents such as NSAIDs, aspirin, and COX-2 inhibitors, DMARDs have been proven to reduce or prevent joint damage and preserve joint function and integrity.

Answer d is incorrect. Routine laboratory monitoring is recommended for patients on all types of rheumatoid arthritis medications.

---

8. Which brand/generic is correctly matched?
   a. Adalimumab/Enbrel
   b. Etanercept/Orencia
   c. Abatacept/Humira
   d. Infliximab/Remicade

Answer a is incorrect. Enbrel is the brand name of etanercept.

Answer b is incorrect. Orencia is the brand name of abatacept

Answer c is incorrect. Humira is the brand name of adalimumab.

Answer d is correct. Remicade is the brand name of infliximab.

---

9. Which of the following agents is dosed weekly?

   a. Methotrexate
   b. Leflunomide
   c. Hydroxychloroquine
   d. Sulfasalazine

Answer a is correct. Methotrexate is dosed on a weekly basis and is available orally and for intramuscular, subcutaneous, and intravenous injection. Weekly dosing of the drug appears to cause less gastrointestinal toxicity (less damage to the mucosa) and fewer side effects than daily dosing. It is important to be vigilant when reviewing methotrexate prescriptions to verify proper dosing frequency. Emphasize to your patients that this medication is taken on a weekly, not daily, basis to minimize the risk of overdose.

Answer b is incorrect. Leflunomide is dosed daily or twice daily.

Answer c is incorrect. Hydroxychloroquine is dosed daily.

Answer d is incorrect. Sulfasalazine is dosed bid or tid.

---

10. Choose the correct mechanism of action for leflunomide.

    a. Inhibits prostaglandin synthesis
    b. Interferes with the proliferation of T cells
    c. Prevents activation of inflammatory cells by binding to tumor necrosis factor
    d. Prevents tumor necrosis factor from binding to its receptor site

---

Answer a is incorrect. Nonsteroidal anti-inflammatory drugs, aspirin, selective COX-2 inhibitors, and sulfasalazine inhibit prostaglandin synthesis. Prostaglandins perform a wide range of activity, including regulation of inflammatory mediators.

Answer b is correct. Leflunomide hinders the body's immune response by interfering with the proliferation of T cells. T cells are key players in cell-mediated immunity. They are involved in the production of cytokines, recruiting other immunological cells to fight infection, and serve as memory cells to "remember" past infections.

Answer c is incorrect. Biological agents such as infliximab, etanercept, and adalimumab work by interfering with the actions of TNF-α. Infliximab, an IgG anti-TNF-α human-murine chimeric antibody, binds to TNF in order to prevent it from binding to its receptor. Etanercept also binds to TNF, thus preventing it from binding to the surfaces of inflammatory cells. Adalimumab is a recombinant human monoclonal antibody that attaches to TNF-α receptor sites, inhibiting the binding of endogenous TNF-α to those targets.

Answer d is incorrect. Biological agents such as infliximab, etanercept, and adalimumab work by interfering with the actions of TNF-α.

---

11. A serious adverse reaction of hydroxychloroquine is

    a. Bone marrow suppression
    b. Hepatic toxicity
    c. Renal impairment
    d. Retinal damage

Answer a is incorrect. Hydroxychloroquine is not associated with bone marrow suppression.

Answer b is incorrect. Hydroxychloroquine is not known to cause liver toxicity.

Answer c is incorrect. Hydroxychloroquine is not associated with kidney toxicity.

Answer d is correct. Hydroxychloroquine has been associated with various types of ocular toxicity including blurred vision, diminished visual acuity, abnormal color vision, and retinopathy. It appears that the toxicities are specific to the cornea and the macula of the eye. Retinal damage is dose-related and sometimes irreversible.

Patients taking hydroxychloroquine are recommended to have an ophthalmology examination within 1 year following initiation of the drug. High-risk patients (those who take a daily dose >6.5 mg/kg, are renally impaired, have been taking the drug for more than 10 years, or have taken a cumulative dose of 200 g) should have the examination repeated every 6 to 12 months, while low-risk patients may repeat the examination approximately every 5 years.

---

12. The adverse reaction common to all biological DMARD agents is

    a. Bone marrow suppression
    b. Heart failure exacerbation
    c. Increased susceptibility to infection
    d. Teratogenicity

Answer a is incorrect. Bone marrow suppression is not an expected side effect of biological DMARD agents.

Answer b is incorrect. Anti-TNF-α agents (infliximab, etanercept, and adalimumab) are contraindicated in patients with New York Heart Association Class III or IV heart failure, but as a class biological DMARDs have not been shown to cause or exacerbate heart failure.

Answer c is correct. All biological DMARD agents suppress the immune system by affecting various immunological components. Consequently, the body becomes more vulnerable to infection. Patients on biological DMARD therapy should be assessed regularly for any signs of infection. Localized signs may include unhealed skin wounds possibly leaking pus or other drainage, pain, swelling, or heat at the site of infection. Systemic infection symptoms include fever, chills, and other cold- or flu-like symptoms.

Answer d is incorrect. Biological agents have been assigned pregnancy category B and C by the U.S. Food and Drug Administration. Category B designation indicates that either animal reproduction studies have failed to demonstrate a risk to the fetus and there are no well-controlled studies in pregnant women or that animal studies have shown adverse effects but they have not been confirmed in controlled studies in pregnant women. Category C assignment means that animal reproduction studies have shown an adverse effect to the fetus and there are no adequate and well-controlled studies in humans, but the potential benefits may warrant use of the drug in pregnant women despite the potential risks.

---

13. All of the following biological agents work by interfering with the actions of tumor necrosis factor *except*:
    a. Adalimumab
    b. Etanercept
    c. Infliximab
    d. Rituximab

Answer a is incorrect. Adalimumab is a recombinant human monoclonal antibody that binds to TNF-α receptor sites, blocking the binding of endogenous TNF-α to those targets.

Answer b is incorrect. Etanercept competitively binds to TNF to prevent it from binding to the surfaces of inflammatory cells.

Answer c is incorrect. Infliximab is an IgG anti-TNF-α human-murine chimeric antibody that affixes to TNF, preventing it from binding to its receptor target.

Answer d is correct. Rituximab does not work by interfering with the actions of TNF-α. This drug is a monoclonal antibody that targets the CD20 antigen on B-lymphocytes.

---

14. Which of the following conditions would be a contraindication for receiving methotrexate?
    a. Slight renal impairment (ClCr = 50 mL/min)
    b. Mild thrombocytopenia (platelets = 100×10^9/L)
    c. Pregnancy
    d. Latent tuberculosis infection

Answer a is incorrect. Methotrexate should be avoided in patients with very poor renal function (ClCr <30 mL/min), but there is no limit to its use in patients with mild or moderate impairment. Patients' serum creatinine should be measured regularly to screen for renal toxicity.

Answer b is incorrect. Patients with a platelet count of less than 50×10^9/L should not use methotrexate. A complete blood count should be measured at baseline, every 2 to 4 weeks after initiation of therapy for 3 months, and then periodically thereafter to monitor for signs of thrombocytopenia and bone marrow suppression.

Answer c is correct. Methotrexate is pregnancy category X and should be avoided in women who are pregnant or may become pregnant.

Answer d is incorrect. Methotrexate should be avoided in patients with active tuberculosis, but there is not a contraindication to its use in patients latently infected. Patients with active bacterial infection, ongoing herpes zoster infection, or life-threatening fungal infection should not take methotrexate.

---

15. Which of the following is true about DMARD therapy?
    a. DMARDs reduce or prevent joint damage in RA.
    b. Onset of action is usually 1 to 2 weeks.
    c. Reserved for use in severe long-term RA.
    d. If a patient fails one DMARD, they will likely fail all DMARDs,
    e. All of the above are true.

Answer a is correct. Disease-modifying antirheumatic drugs (DMARDs) have been shown to slow or prevent disease progression.

Answer b is incorrect. DMARDs have a typical onset of 1 to 6 months.

Answer c is incorrect. It is recommended to initiate DMARDs within 3 months of the onset of symptoms. All RA patients are candidates for DMARD therapy except those with very limited disease or who have very severe disease in which little reversibility is expected.

Answer d is incorrect. If one DMARD does not provide sufficient control of RA, the dose should be increased or additional DMARDs should be added.

Answer e is incorrect.

---

16. AA is a 34-year-old woman who regularly picks up her Arava and Ortho Tri-Cyclen refills at your pharmacy. Today she arrives to pick up her Arava and states she will no longer need her Ortho Tri-Cyclen as she and her husband have decided to start trying to have a baby. Which of the following would be the most appropriate response to this information?
    a. Continue Arava at a lower dose when she becomes pregnant, as rheumatoid arthritis typically improves during pregnancy.
    b. Change Arava to methotrexate during pregnancy.
    c. Discontinue Arava 2 to 3 weeks prior to trying to get pregnant.
    d. Undergo drug-elimination with cholestyramine prior to trying to get pregnant.

Answer a is incorrect. RA symptoms may improve during pregnancy, but Arava is pregnancy category X and must be discontinued prior to conception.

Answer b is incorrect. Both methotrexate and Arava are pregnancy category X.

Answer c is incorrect. Arava must be discontinued approximately 3 months prior to conception to allow for a drug elimination and washout period.

Answer d is correct. Arava is pregnancy category X based on data suggesting increased risk for fetal death and teratogenic effects. Due to Arava's active metabolite and long half-life, patients wishing to become pregnant should undergo the drug elimination procedure with cholestyramine (8 g cholestyramine tid for 11 days; plasma levels M1 <0.02 mg/L must be verified on two separate occasions at least 14 days apart.

---

17. Folic acid supplementation is recommended for patients taking methotrexate because

    a. Folic acid can prevent renal toxicity.
    b. Folic acid can prevent gastrointestinal toxicity.
    c. Most people with rheumatoid arthritis have folic acid deficiencies.
    d. Folic acid will enhance the efficacy of methotrexate.

Answer a is incorrect. Although methotrexate may cause renal toxicity, folic acid is not indicated to reduce the nephrotoxic effects of the drug.

Answer b is correct. Folate (the naturally occurring form of folic acid, which is also known as vitamin B9) is necessary for the synthesis and maintenance of new cells. Methotrexate is a folic acid antagonist and will deplete the body's folate stores by inhibiting the enzyme dihydrofolate reductase. Since many fast-dividing cells (such as those that line the gastric mucosa) utilize folate during their replication, a deficiency of folic acid will inhibit their growth and proliferation. For this reason it is recommended that patients on methotrexate take 1 mg daily of folic acid.

Answer c is incorrect. Patients who have rheumatoid arthritis are not also likely to have a folate deficiency.

Answer d is incorrect. Folic acid will not enhance the efficacy of methotrexate.

---

18. Which of the following agents is available as an SQ injection?

    a. Abatacept
    b. Cytoxan
    c. Etanercept
    d. Remicade
    e. Rituxan

Answer a is incorrect. Abatacept is given as an IV infusion at weeks 0, 2, and 4 and then every 4 weeks thereafter.

Answer b is incorrect. Cytoxan is available orally and by IV injection.

Answer c is correct. Etanercept is given as an SQ injection and is dosed weekly or semiweekly.

Answer d is incorrect. Remicade is available as an IV infusion given at weeks 0, 2, and 6 and then every 8 weeks thereafter.

Answer e is incorrect. Rituxan is available as an injectable drug and is given by IV infusion.

---

19. Select the brand name for hydroxychloroquine.

    a. Arava
    b. Cytoxan
    c. Humira
    d. Plaquenil
    e. Rituxan

Answer a is incorrect. Arava is the brand name for leflunomide.

Answer b is incorrect. Cytoxan is the brand name for cyclophosphamide.

Answer c is incorrect. Humira is the brand name for adalimumab.

Answer d is correct. Plaquenil is the brand name for hydroxychloroquine.

Answer e is incorrect. Rituxan is the brand name for rituximab.

---

20. Which of the following is true about Rituximab?

    i. It is available for administration IV or SQ.
    ii. Premedication with corticosteroid, APAP, and antihistamine should be done prior to each dose.
    iii. Dosing may be repeated every 7 days.
    iv. Recommended infusion dose is 1000 mg.

    a. i only
    b. ii and iv
    c. i, ii, and iv
    d. All of the above

Answer a is incorrect. Rituximab is available only for IV administration.

Answer b is correct. It is necessary to premedicate with a corticosteroid, acetaminophen, and an antihistamine prior to each dose of rituximab. The usual recommended dose is 1000 mg given by IV infusion. This medication should not be given as IV push or bolus dose. Infusion should be initiated at 50 mg/h, and may be increased to a maximum rate 400 mg/h (increasing by 50 mg/h every 30 minutes) if no infusion-related reaction develops. The next infusion may be initiated at 100 mg/h, and may be increased to a maximum rate of 400 mg/h.

Answer c is incorrect. Dosing recommendations for rituximab indicated a repeat dose in 14 days for a maximum of two doses as safety data is unknown beyond two doses

Answer d is incorrect. Rituximab is not available for SQ administration and the dose is not given on a weekly basis.

CHAPTER 48 | Osteoarthritis

1. EM is a 63-year-old obese man with a history of increasing pain in his left knee. He presently cares for his 85-year-old mother who has had bilateral knee replacements secondary to osteoarthritis. During his college years, he played on the intramural football team and suffered several knee injuries. During his career as a radio announcer for sports, he maintained a sedentary lifestyle and does not presently exercise. Which of the following are risk factors for the development of osteoarthritis in EM?

   a. Age
   b. Genetics
   c. Joint injury
   d. Obesity
   e. All of the above

Answer a is correct. Osteoarthritis mainly affects adults >50 years old. This patient is over the age of 50.

Answer b is correct. Osteoarthritis can be inherited. This patient has a mother with a history of knee replacements secondary to osteoarthritis.

Answer c is correct. Acute joint injury can place a patient at risk for osteoarthritis. Tears of the meniscus as well as articular surface injury increases joint instability. This patient has a history of acute joint injury during his college years with sports participation which placed him at risk for injury.

Answer d is correct. Weight gain predisposes patients to development of osteoarthritis secondary to overload of the knee. This patient is stated as being obese.

Answer e is correct and the best answer. Since this patient does not exercise and leads a sedentary lifestyle, he may be at risk for quadriceps muscle weakness. This can be a risk factor for causing future joint damage.

2. Which of the following pathophysiological changes occur in a patient with osteoarthritis?

   a. Interarticular narrowing
   b. Bone remodeling
   c. Cytokine release
   d. Chondrocyte destruction
   e. All of the above

Answer a is correct. Interarticular narrowing may be present on radiographs. This occurs with bone remodeling, which causes thickened bone and cartilage thinning leading to joint space narrowing.

Answer b is correct. Bone remodeling occurs with subchondral sclerosis (tissue hardening), cyst formation (cavities within bone), and development of osteophytes (bony outgrowths). Despite increased bone formation, the bone formed is of poor quality and lacks strength and normal mineralization of regular bone.

Answer c is correct. Although not typically considered inflammatory in nature, osteoarthritis demonstrates the inflammatory response with cytokine release which may be a response to tissue inflammation. Interleukin-1 and tumor necrosis factor-alpha may be present within the joint.

Answer d is correct. Chondrocytes are cartilage cells and normally undergo slow turnover. Cartilage damage increases the rate of turnover, but chondrocyte formation is not able to replace tissue to normal. Further damage will occur.

Answer e is correct and the best answer. All of the above are changes that occur in osteoarthritis.

---

3. Which of the following is a sign or symptom of a patient with clinical presentation of osteoarthritis?

   a. Joint stiffness with rest
   b. Normal range of motion with joint
   c. Joint stability
   d. Joint pain with movement
   e. Frictionless joint movement

Answer a is correct. Patients will experience a stiffening of the joint at rest and improved mobility with increased movement.

Answer b is incorrect. Patients have a limited range of motion because of abnormal joint structure.

Answer c is incorrect. Patients will experience joint instability secondary to pathophysiological changes leading to abnormal anatomy.

Answer d is incorrect. Osteoarthritis patients will experience pain relief with movement of the joint. Pain worsens with rest.

Answer e is incorrect. Osteoarthritis patients experience friction with movement as bone may move against bone secondary to cartilage destruction.

---

4. Diagnosis of a patient with osteoarthritis of the hip could be made with which of the following?

   a. Pain with external rotation of the hip
   b. Age >40
   c. Osteophyte development
   d. Joint pain with osteophytes on radiograph and normal laboratory values
   e. Abnormal erythrocyte sedimentation rate

Answer a is incorrect. The American College of Rheumatology Criteria states that patients should have pain and altered movement with internal rotation of the hip in addition to other clinical criteria.

Answer b is incorrect. Age alone is not a criteria for development of osteoarthritis.

Answer c is incorrect. Clinical presentation of joint pain should accompany presence of osteophytes and/or joint space narrowing demonstrated on radiographs in addition to an erythrocyte sedimentation rate of <20 mm/h. Presence of osteophytes alone does not indicate osteoarthritis.

Answer d is correct. Diagnosis of osteoarthritis involves patient history with clinical presentation, radiographic evidence, and elimination of laboratory abnormalities. Joint pain and stiffness with tenderness confirmed by osteophytes on radiology would confirm OA. Normal laboratory values indicate patient does not have other disease.

Answer e is incorrect. While the erythrocyte sedimentation rate (ESR) is a nonspecific test, it is usually normal in patients with osteoarthritis. Elevations will occur with rheumatoid arthritis.

---

5. Preventative measures in patients without osteoarthritis but who have joint injury include:
   a. Resistance exercise
   b. Maintaining a healthy weight
   c. Surgery
   d. Joint rehabilitation
   e. All of the above

Answer a is correct. Building muscle strength with resistance exercise is a strategy for strengthening muscles, which could possibly prevent risk of osteoarthritis later in life.

Answer b is correct. Avoiding obesity can decrease risk of osteoarthritis development. Increased weight can increase load on joints and predispose them to damage.

Answer c is correct. Surgery may be needed for joint injuries to restore normal function. Surgery may assist with prevention of later life development of osteoarthritis.

Answer d is correct. Rehabilitation of the joint may involve different types of exercise and regimen of rest to improve flexibility and proprioception (unconscious movement of the body with spatial awareness).

Answer e is correct and the best answer. All of the above are measures recommended clinically to improve joint function after injury.

---

6. SL is a 62-year-old obese man with a history of degenerative joint disease in his entire left knee. Past medical history is significant for dyslipidemia treated with gemfibrozil and diabetes with NPH 10 U at bedtime and glipizide 10 mg bid. Blood sugar readings are not at goal with HgA1c of 8.5%. Current blood pressure is 130/80 mm Hg. He receives his second injection of 40 mg of Kenalog in his left knee today. Which side effect could cause a drug–disease state interaction in this patient?
   a. Skin depigmentation
   b. Adrenal insufficiency
   c. Joint infection
   d. Hyperglycemia
   e. All of the above

Answer a is incorrect. Skin depigmentation may occur with corticosteroids. However, this is not a disease drug state interaction this patient is at risk for. Increased pigmentation can be a sign associated with adrenal insufficiency.

Answer b is incorrect. Patient is not manifesting signs of hypotension, fever or symptoms of weakness, anorexia, or myalgia associated with adrenal insufficiency. Adrenal insufficiency is a life-threatening situation.

Answer c is incorrect. He does not report any joint infection with symptoms of painful joint and abnormal white blood cell count.

Answer d is correct. Patient is a diabetic. Glucocorticoid use is associated with carbohydrate intolerance and hyperglycemia. This would necessitate closer monitoring of his diabetes.

Answer e is incorrect.

---

7. What is the primary objective of medication therapy for osteoarthritis?
   a. Improve mobility
   b. Weight loss
   c. Pain relief
   d. Improve muscle and joint strength
   e. All of the above

Answer a is incorrect. Improvement of mobility without relief of pain may assist with increased movement; however, patients will not have improved quality of life. Improved mobility occurs as a result of pain relief.

Answer b is incorrect. Weight loss can improve signs and symptoms but will not provide acute pain relief. However, it is not the primary objective of medication therapy.

Answer c is correct. Pain relief is the primary objective of pharmacologic treatment.

Answer d is incorrect. Improvement of muscle and joint strength can assist with support of the joint. However, this will not improve acute pain.

Answer e is incorrect.

---

8. What is the most preventable risk factor for developing osteoarthritis?
   a. Genetics
   b. Joint trauma history
   c. Repetitive movement
   d. Obesity
   e. All of the above

Answer a is incorrect. Genetics is not modifiable.

Answer b is incorrect. History of joint trauma is not modifiable since it occurred in the past. Appropriate therapy at the time of trauma may assist to decrease development of future osteoarthritis.

Answer c is incorrect. Repetitive movement is a risk factor for development of joint damage. Certain occupations may be associated with repetitive movements. This may not be easily modified unless measures are taken to address it.

Answer d is correct. Weight loss is the most preventable risk factor for development of osteoarthritis. Decrease of load on joints can prevent damage and possible malalignment.

Answer e is incorrect.

---

9. Select the first-line pharmacologic agent for treating osteoarthritis?

    a. Acetaminophen
    b. Intra-articular corticosteroids
    c. Tramadol
    d. Ibuprofen
    e. All of the above

Answer a is correct. Acetaminophen has been shown to be the most appropriate first-line agent to relieve pain and inflammation.

Answer b is incorrect. Intra-articular corticosteroids are appropriate for exacerbations of osteoarthritis of for patients who are not candidates for NSAIDs.

Answer c is incorrect. Tramadol is used for those with contraindications to nonselective NSAIDs and COX-2 inhibitors with failure on previous drug trials.

Answer d is incorrect. Nonselective NSAIDs is second-line therapy after acetaminophen.

Answer e is incorrect.

---

10. Which of the following help to reduce NSAID-induced GI toxicity?

    a. Nonacetylated salicylates
    b. COX-2 inhibitors
    c. Addition of misoprostol
    d. Addition of PPI
    e. All of the above

Answer a is correct. Nonacetylated salicylates are associated with decrease in GI toxicity.

Answer b is correct. Celecoxib demonstrated fewer GI ulcers when compared to traditional NSAIDs.

Answer c is correct. Misoprostol is protective for ulcers and potential GI complications.

Answer d is correct. Proton pump inhibitors reduce risk for GI ulcer development.

Answer e is correct and the best answer.

---

11. Which of the following is *not* a goal of osteoarthritis treatment?

    a. Teaching patient about the disease state
    b. Curing osteoarthritis
    c. Providing pain relief
    d. Improving musculoskeletal movement
    e. Maintaining ability to perform activities of daily living

---

Answer a is incorrect. Patient education is a goal for osteoarthritis treatment.

Answer b is correct. At present, there is no cure for osteoarthritis.

Answer c is incorrect. Pain relief is the primary goal for osteoarthritis.

Answer d is incorrect. Improvement in musculoskeletal movement is a goal for osteoarthritis treatment.

Answer e is incorrect. Patients should be able to perform activities of daily living even with osteoarthritis.

---

12. Which of the following is the *correct* order in which treatment options for acute pain should be trialed?

    a. Acetaminophen → COX-2 inhibitor → nonselective NSAID → opioid → joint replacement
    b. Acetaminophen → nonselective NSAID → opioid → COX-2 inhibitor → intra-articular corticosteroid
    c. Nonselective NSAID → COX-2 inhibitor → opioid → intra-articular hyaluronic acid → joint replacement
    d. Nonselective NSAID → COX-2 inhibitor → opioid → intra-articular corticosteroid → Ultram
    e. Acetaminophen → nonselective NSAID → COX-2 inhibitor → opioid analgesic → joint replacement

---

Answer a is incorrect. Nonselective NSAIDs or nonacetylated salicylates should be tried before COX-2 inhibitors. COX-2 inhibitors should be utilized in patients with GI risk. If a COX-2 inhibitor is utilized for this reason, a nonselective NSAID would not be tried after a COX-2 inhibitor because nonselective NSAIDs cause more GI distress.

Answer b is incorrect. Opioids are the final pharmacologic option for acute pain. Intra-articular corticosteroids are used for exacerbation, not acute pain.

Answer c is incorrect. Opioids are the final pharmacologic option for acute pain. Hyaluronic acid is not used for acute pain.

Answer d is incorrect. Tramadol should be tried before prescribing an opioid. Intra-articular corticosteroids are not used for acute pain.

Answer e is correct. Acetaminophen is the first-line pharmacologic agent to treat osteoarthritis-induced acute pain. Nonselective NSAIDs or nonacetylated salicylates are the next viable option unless the patient has active or a PMH of GI bleeding. For patients with GI risk, NSAIDs + a GI protective agent or COX-2 inhibitors should be used. If all previous medications do not provide relief, tramadol can be trialed next. Opioids are last-line medications because of their addictive qualities and side effects (ie, respiratory depression).

---

13. AZ is a 72-year-old woman with a history of atrial fibrillation treated with warfarin. Her height is 5 ft 2 in, weight is 198 lb, blood pressure is 116/76 mm Hg, and SCr is 1.1. AZ is now complaining of pain and stiffness in her left knee. X-ray shows joint space narrowing and osteophytes at the joint. Which treatment should be initiated at this point?

    a. Weight reduction
    b. Tylenol
    c. Celebrex
    d. Both a and b
    e. Both a and c

Answer a is correct. Initiation of weight loss may assist with decreased load for the joint and possible symptom relief.

Answer b is correct. Acetaminophen is a first-line treatment for osteoarthritis. Acetaminophen can potentiate the anticoagulant effect of warfarin therapy, but is an appropriate choice with monitoring of the patient.

Answer c is incorrect. Celecoxib is third-line treatment for osteoarthritis and has demonstrated an increase in the anticoagulant effect of warfarin.

Answer d is correct. Both a and b are correct.

Answer e is incorrect.

---

14. BY is a 65-year-old man with confirmed osteoarthritis. He has been pain free on his current regimen of acetaminophen 1000 mg every 6 hours for 2 years. Past medical history is significant for gastrointestinal bleed 4 years ago and hypertension. He now presents to your clinic with pain in his left hip. BY's medication regimen also consists of lisinopril 40 mg daily and hydrochlorothiazide 25 mg daily. What recommendation will you present to the physician?

    a. Increase acetaminophen to 1000 mg every 4 hours, reinforce fitness program.
    b. Add pantoprazole 40 mg daily to his regimen, reinforce fitness program.
    c. Stop acetaminophen, begin ibuprofen 400 mg tid, reinforce fitness program.
    d. Stop acetaminophen, begin Anaprox 250 mg bid, Protonix 40 mg daily, reinforce fitness program.
    e. Add celecoxib 200 mg daily, reinforce fitness program.

Answer a is incorrect. The maximum dose for acetaminophen is 4000 mg daily. This answer gives a daily dose of 6000 mg daily and increases the patient's risk for developing hepatotoxicity.

Answer b is incorrect. The addition of pantoprazole would provide some GI protection, but would not provide any more pain relief.

Answer c is incorrect. BY has hypertension and is at high risk for cardiovascular disease. Though studies are not conclusive and all drugs in the nonselective NSAID class have not been studied, ibuprofen has shown some increased risk of MI, stroke, heart failure, and hypertension.

Answer d is correct. Naproxen is a member of the nonselective NSAID class. Increased cardiovascular disease may be higher in NSAIDs as a class. At this time, naproxen is the only nonselective drug studied that has a lower risk than ibuprofen or diclofenac. BY has a PMH of GI bleed, so a GI protective agent such as pantoprazole should be added to his NSAID regimen. Reinforcing muscle-strengthening and range of motion exercises should be part of every osteoarthritis treatment.

Answer e is incorrect. Studies have shown that COX-2 inhibitors have an increased risk of MI, stroke, heart failure, and HTN. Celecoxib would not be an appropriate choice as BY has hypertension and is high CV risk.

---

15. CK is a 58-year-old woman who presents to your pharmacotherapy clinic today with an INR of 4.2 (she was previously stable for 6 months). She has a PMH of diabetes, atrial fibrillation, and hypertension. The list of medications that she gives you from her pharmacy are as follows: metformin 1000 mg and glipizide 10 mg bid; warfarin 5 mg on Monday, Wednesday, and Friday and 2.5 mg on Sunday, Tuesday, Thursday, and Saturday; amlodipine 10 mg daily; potassium chloride 10 mEq daily; and hydrochlorothiazide 25 mg daily. CK has not had a warfarin dosage change in over 1 year. She tells you her right knee has been bothering her much more frequently than usual. Which of the following is the most likely reason for her INR fluctuation?

    a. CK took 5 mg warfarin tablets every day in the past week.
    b. After questioning CK about OTC use, she tells you she has been using Capsaicin-HP on her knee for the past week.
    c. After questioning CK about OTC use, she tells you she has been taking acetaminophen 650 mg every 6 hours to relieve her from knee pain for the past week.
    d. CK is not telling you about an herbal product she has begun taking.
    e. All of the above.

Answer a is incorrect. Though this is a possibility, CK has been stabilized for 6 months. She is young and has not made this mistake previously.

Answer b is incorrect. Capsaicin-HP is a topical treatment and does not affect INR.

Answer c is correct. A drug-drug interaction can occur between warfarin and acetaminophen. Acetaminophen may enhance the anticoagulant effect of warfarin. Acetaminophen is available over-the-counter. Many patients do not consider an OTC drug as part of their medication list. Patients should always be asked what OTC medications they are taking.

Answer d is incorrect. Though this is a possibility, CK has stated she is having knee pain. A proven drug interaction is seen between warfarin and acetaminophen. CK is most likely taking something for her pain, not an herbal product that is not labeled to help reduce pain.

Answer e is incorrect.

---

16. DP is a 55-year-old man who has hypertension and a positive family history of early cardiovascular disease. His medications include aspirin 81 mg daily and metoprolol 25 mg bid. DP's osteoarthritis is no longer controlled with acetaminophen 1000 mg every 6 hours. The physician wants to begin DP on a regimen including an NSAID. Which treatment do you recommend?

    a. Naproxen 250 mg bid
    b. Naproxen 500 mg tid
    c. Celebrex 200 mg daily
    d. Celebrex 800 mg daily
    e. Any of the above

Answer a is correct. NSAIDs as a class are probably not the best option for a patient with high cardiovascular (CV) risk. In this situation, the physician will prescribe an NSAID regardless, so you should provide the option that will cause the least harm. Most nonselective NSAIDs have not been studied in regards to CV risk. But of those studied, naproxen seems to have less CV risk than others.

Answer b is incorrect. The frequency of naproxen is bid, not tid.

Answer c is incorrect. COX-2 inhibitors should be avoided in patients with high CV risk. This patient does not have any absolute contraindications to nonselective NSAIDs, so this therapy should be tried before COX-2 inhibitors.

Answer d is incorrect. This is an abnormal dose for osteoarthritis treatment. In osteoarthritis, dosages should begin at 200 mg daily or 100 mg bid.

Answer e is incorrect.

---

17. The physician does not take your advice for DP in Question 16. She prescribes ibuprofen 800 mg tid. Which of the following do you need to counsel DP concerning?

    a. Do not take this medication, it might cause you harm.
    b. Take ibuprofen at least 30 minutes after aspirin or aspirin 8 hours after ibuprofen. Monitor your BP more often.
    c. Stop taking your aspirin. Do not take ibuprofen on an empty stomach.
    d. Stop taking your aspirin. Monitor your BP more often.
    e. None of the above.

Answer a is incorrect. The studies evaluating nonselective NSAIDs as a class are inconclusive. You should counsel the patient to monitor their BP more frequently, keep all appointments with their physician, and call the pharmacist or physician if any side effects are experienced.

Answer b is correct. Ibuprofen may block the antiplatelet effect of aspirin. Ibuprofen may diminish the cardioprotective effect that aspirin is providing this patient. Aspirin may decrease the effect of ibuprofen. To limit the interaction, the two drugs should be administered separately. The minimum time between these two drugs is ibuprofen at least 30 minutes after aspirin or aspirin 8 hours after ibuprofen. BP should be monitored because NSAIDs cause sodium and water retention, therefore, possibly raising BP.

Answer c is incorrect. This patient is a high-risk CV patient. Aspirin is being used for cardioprotection and should not be stopped. Ibuprofen should not be taken on an empty stomach.

Answer d is incorrect. BP should be monitored more often, but aspirin should not be discontinued without a physician's consent. The patient has a family history positive for CV disease.

Answer e is incorrect.

---

18. A 44-year-old woman with a history of GI bleed presents to your community pharmacy. She tells you her pregnancy test from last night was positive. She presents refill bottles for her prescription of ibuprofen 400 mg every 8 hours and Cytotec 200 μg bid and asks if these are okay for her to keep taking. You respond:

    a. Stop taking Cytotec. It is ok to continue ibuprofen.
    b. Stop taking ibuprofen. It is ok to continue Cytotec.
    c. Continue taking both medications. Call your physician as soon as you can.
    d. Continue taking both medications. Your pregnancy test may not be accurate.
    e. Stop taking both prescriptions. Let us call your physician together now to discuss your situation.

Answer a is incorrect. Ibuprofen has a C/D pregnancy rating. It has caused deformities and miscarriages in some cases.

Answer b is incorrect. Misoprostol has a pregnancy rating of X. It is an abortifacient.

Answer c is incorrect. Both medications should be stopped immediately if any chance of pregnancy exists. Then the physician should be called to prescribe alternative agents.

Answer d is incorrect. Pregnancy tests can have false-positives, but you should not take the risk of counseling the patient to continue an abortifacient.

Answer e is correct. The patient should stop taking the medications immediately until the physician can be reached to assess pain control and pregnancy plans.

---

19. Which of the following medications is contraindicated in patients with documented sulfa allergy?
    a. Ultram
    b. Toradol
    c. Celebrex
    d. Aspirin
    e. Hyaluronic acid

Answer a is incorrect. Tramadol may be taken in patients with a history of sulfa allergy.

Answer b is incorrect. Toradol may be taken in patients with a history of sulfa allergy.

Answer c is correct. An allergy to sulfa is a contraindication to celecoxib.

Answer d is incorrect. Aspirin is not contraindicated in patients with a sulfa allergy.

Answer e is incorrect. Hyaluronic acid is not contraindicated in patients with a sulfa allergy.

---

20. AM is a 52-year-old woman whose medications include acetaminophen 500 mg qid, gabapentin 300 mg tid, gemfibrozil 600 mg bid, and fluoxetine 20 mg daily. At the direction of her physician, AM added ibuprofen 800 mg bid and capsaicin cream 0.025% tid prn to her regimen. While putting on her contacts this morning she experienced an immediate burning pain in her eyes. She immediately takes out her contacts, flushes her eyes, and calls you, her pharmacist. Which of the following is most likely causing her eye pain?
    a. Capsaicin cream
    b. Acetaminophen
    c. Drug interaction between acetaminophen and gemfibrozil
    d. Drug interaction between acetaminophen and gabapentin
    e. None of the above

Answer a is correct. Contact with the eyes should be avoided when using capsaicin because it causes a burning sensation and irritation. AM either did not wash her hands after applying the cream or did not wash the cream completely off of her hands before touching her contacts to her eyes.

Answer b is incorrect. Eye pain is not a side effect of acetaminophen.

Answer c is incorrect. There are no drug interactions between acetaminophen and gemfibrozil.

Answer d is incorrect. There are no drug interactions between acetaminophen and gabapentin.

Answer e is incorrect.

---

21. KT is a 73-year-old woman with osteoarthritis of the hand. Her medication list includes: salsalate 500 mg bid, Lantus 10 U at bedtime, hydrochlorothiazide 25 mg daily, and ibuprofen 400 mg prn that was recently increased to 800 mg bid prn because of pain. What recommendation(s) do you give to the physician during rounds?
    a. KT should not be on more than one NSAID at a time.
    b. Ibuprofen should not be given prn for osteoarthritis.
    c. Ibuprofen should be dosed 3 to 4 times daily.
    d. Both a and b.
    e. All of the above.

Answer a is incorrect as it is not the complete answer. NSAIDs should not be used together as the anticoagulant effect is enhanced. The risk of bleeding increases.

Answer b is incorrect as it is not the complete answer. Agents being used to treat osteoarthritis should be given round the clock. A drug will never be fully effective if used prn as it will not reach steady state and produce its full effect.

Answer c is incorrect as it is not the complete answer. The duration of ibuprofen is 4 to 6 hours. Its half-life is 2 to 4 hours in adults. Dosing this drug twice daily leaves 6 or more hours at which the patient is not experiencing any pain relief from the drug.

Answer d is incorrect. This is not the best answer as it is not all inclusive.

Answer e is correct. Answers a, b, and c are correct.

---

22. GM is an 81-year-old woman with history of bilateral knee osteoarthritis for 25 years. She has contraindications to surgery and has received one injection of hyaluronic acid (Hyalgan) weekly for the last 2 weeks. She complains that she has not felt any pain relief. You explain:
    a. She will not experience pain relief at this point.
    b. She may need to complete the series of five injections before improvement.
    c. She may need concomitant administration of intra-articular glucocorticoid.
    d. She should take glucosamine and chondroitin in addition to the use of hyaluronic acid.
    e. She should stop NSAID therapy while Hyalgan is administered.

Answer a is incorrect. Patient has not received full treatment of therapy which is usually 5 weeks. Hyaluronic acid has a slow onset of action.

Answer b is correct. Patient may need to complete the full series before relief of pain.

Answer c is incorrect. Patients should receive intra-articular corticosteroids for acute exacerbations and not as treatment for chronic inflammation.

Answer d is incorrect. Use of glucosamine and chondroitin in addition to hyaluronic acid will not improve patient response.

Answer e is incorrect. Patient should continue current NSAID treatment if she is receiving it. This will continue to decrease pain and inflammation for the patient.

---

23. A 59-year-old man with history of 2 months of joint pain in his knees with movement decides to treat with glucosamine chondroitin. He reports an allergy to shellfish. He asks for your recommendation. You tell him:
   a. No significant benefit is seen with use of glucosamine chondroitin as monotherapy.
   b. Glucosamine chondroitin demonstrates benefit when used in combination with NSAIDS.
   c. Glucosamine chondroitin is contraindicated in those with shellfish allergies.
   d. Gastrointestinal symptoms of gas, bloating, and cramps may occur with use of glucosamine chondroitin.
   e. All of the above.

Answer a is correct. Use of these agents as monotherapy did not show superiority to placebo.

Answer b is correct. When used with NSAIDS, this may be of potential benefit.

Answer c is correct. Glucosamine is contraindicated with shellfish allergies.

Answer d is correct. Gastrointestinal symptoms are mild but may include gas, bloating, or cramps.

Answer e is correct and the best answer.

---

24. Corticosteroids work to provide pain relief in osteoarthritis by:
   a. Reduction of interarticular space narrowing
   b. Reduction of cytokine production
   c. Depletion of substance P
   d. Prostaglandin synthesis inhibition
   e. Inhibition of serotonin and norepinephrine

Answer a is incorrect. Corticosteroids do not work via this mechanism.

Answer b is correct. Corticosteroids are theorized to reduce antibodies, cytokines, and macrophage movement.

Answer c is incorrect. Topical agents such as capsaicin deplete and prevent CNS neurons of substance P.

Answer d is incorrect. Prostaglandin substance inhibition is associated with nonsteroidals.

Answer e is incorrect. Inhibition of serotonin and norepinephrine is the mechanism for tramadol.

---

25. Your technician brings you an IV bag to check. The label states "Cerebyx 1200 mg IV daily for pain." You check the patient's profile as your hospital does not have Cerebyx on formulary and find the patient has a history of osteoarthritis and hypertension with hospitalization for an acute gout episode. Identify the errors in this drug order.
   a. Indication
   b. Dose
   c. Route of administration
   d. Drug
   e. All of the above

Answer a is correct. Cerebyx is the brand name for fosphenytoin, which is an anticonvulsant. The drug on the label does not match the indication on the directions.

Answer b is correct. While the dose of Cerebyx is appropriate for the IV formulation, it is inappropriate for the patient who should receive a dose matched to Celebrex for osteoarthritis.

Answer c is correct. This is not the correct route of administration for the drug Celebrex. The drug is administered orally.

Answer d is correct. The drug should have been Celebrex, a COX-2 inhibitor instead of the brand name for fosphenytoin.

Answer e is correct.

CHAPTER 49 | Epilepsy

1. Select the type of epilepsy that results in a sudden interruption of activities and a blank stare.
   a. Absence seizures
   b. Tonic-clonic
   c. Myoclonic
   d. Atonic

Answer a is correct. Absence seizures or petit mal result in sudden interruption of activities and a blank stare.

Answer b is incorrect. Tonic-clonic seizures or grand mal result in alternating muscle contractions and jerking.

Answer c is incorrect. Myoclonic seizures result in brief shock-like contractions of a muscle group.

Answer d is incorrect. Atonic seizures result in sudden loss of muscle tone ("drop attacks").

---

2. Select the treatable cause of seizures.
   i. Hypoglycemia
   ii. Altered electrolytes
   iii. Infections
   iv. Cryptogenic

   a. i and ii
   b. i and iii
   c. i, ii, and iii
   d. iii and iv

Answer c is correct. Hypoglycemia, altered electrolytes, and infections are treatable causes of seizures. A seizure produced by treatable causes does not represent epilepsy. Note: medications that cause hypoglycemia and altered electrolytes could indirectly precipitate a seizure.

Cryptogenic epilepsy represents an epilepsy syndrome, which is a classification system of epilepsies based on seizure type and prognosis. Other classifications of epilepsy syndromes include idiopathic and symptomatic. Cryptogenic epilepsy is presumed to have an underlying etiology that cannot be identified. Note: The epilepsy classification system that uses terms such as absence, tonic-clonic, and myoclonic is classified upon seizure presentation.

Note: The underlying etiology of epilepsy is unknown in 80% of patients. The most common recognized causes of epilepsy are head trauma and stroke. Developmental and genetic defects represent 5% of epilepsy cases. Central nervous system tumors, infections, metabolic disturbances (hyponatremia and hypoglycemia), neurodegenerative diseases, and medications represent other causes.

---

3. Select the drug-induced cause of seizures.

   i. Bupropion
   ii. Tramadol
   iii. Amoxicillin

   a. i
   b. iii
   c. i and iii
   d. ii and iii
   e. i, ii, and iii

Answer e is correct. Bupropion, tramadol, and amoxicillin may cause seizures. The antidepressant bupropion has a dose-dependent risk of seizures and is increased in patients with a history of seizures, anorexia/bulimia, head trauma, CNS tumors, and hepatic cirrhosis. The analgesic tramadol has an increased risk of seizures in patients receiving SSRIs, tricyclic antidepressants, neuroleptics, or other drugs that lower the seizure threshold. Patients with a history of seizures or seizure risk (head trauma, metabolic disorders, CNS infection, alcohol withdrawal) are at increased risk when receiving tramadol. Excessive doses of penicillins and cephalosporins may cause seizures. When the beta-lactam antibiotics are dose-adjusted based upon renal dysfunction, the seizure risk is low.

Other medications associated with causing seizures include theophylline, antidepressants, antipsychotics, amphetamines, cocaine, imipenem, lithium, sympathomimetics, and stimulants.

---

4. Select the dose-related adverse reaction of AEDs.

   a. Neutropenia
   b. Sedation
   c. Thrombocytopenia
   d. All of the above
   e. a and c

Answer a is incorrect. Neutropenia (hematologic toxicity) is an idiosyncratic reaction and not related to dose or concentration.

Answer b is correct. Sedation is a dose-dependent adverse reaction. Other dose-dependent adverse reactions include ataxia and diplopia.

Answer c is incorrect. Thrombocytopenia (hematologic toxicity) is an idiosyncratic reaction and not related to dose or concentration. Other idiosyncratic reactions include rash and hepatotoxicity.

Answer d is incorrect.

Answer e is incorrect.

---

5. Select the patient population or condition that often leads to fast titration of AEDs.

   a. Switching AEDs
   b. Discontinuing AEDs
   c. Children
   d. Women of child-bearing potential

Answer a is incorrect. Switching AEDs requires a titration process, because abrupt discontinuation of an AED may lead to breakthrough seizures. The process requires starting the new AED at a *low dose* and titrating up to the minimal effective dose. Once the minimal effective dose is reached, the drug to be discontinued is *gradually tapered*, while the dose of the new AED continues to be increased to the target dose.

Answer b is incorrect. Epilepsy is considered a lifelong disorder; however, patients who are seizure-free may desire to discontinue their medication. Withdrawal of AEDs is done slowly with a dose tapered over at least 3 months.

Answer c is correct. Children require prompt control of seizures to avoid interference with development of the brain and cognition. AED doses are increased rapidly and frequent changes in the regimen are made to maximize control of seizures. Due to high metabolic rates in children, doses of AEDs are higher on a milligram per kilogram basis compared to adults.

Answer d is incorrect. Women of child-bearing potential or who are pregnant have recommendations for AED management because several AEDs have been implicated in minor and serious birth defects. The majority of pregnant epileptic patients receiving AEDs produce a normal infant, but special recommendations must be followed. Recommendations include: use monotherapy when possible; *use lowest dose* possible to control seizures; monitor AED serum concentrations at the start of pregnancy and monthly thereafter; give supplemental folic acid 1 to 4 mg daily to all women of child-bearing potential; administer supplemental vitamin K during the eighth month of pregnancy to women receiving enzyme-inducing AEDs.

---

6. Select the medication that exhibits dose-dependent, capacity-limited pharmacokinetics.
   i. Dilantin
   ii. Cerebyx
   iii. Keppra
   iv. Neurontin

   a. i and ii
   b. i and iii
   c. i and iv
   d. i, ii, iii, and iv

Answer a is correct. Phenytoin (Dilantin) and fosphenytoin (Cerebyx) exhibit dose-dependent, capacity-limited (Michaelis-Menten) pharmacokinetics.

---

7. Select the AED that has CYP-450 3A4 isoenzyme induction and autoinduction.
   a. Topiramate
   b. Carbamazepine
   c. Phenytoin
   d. Phenobarbital

Answer a is incorrect. Topiramate is a CYP-450 inhibitor.

Answer b is correct. Carbamazepine is a potent inducer of the cytochrome-P450 isoenzyme system leading to increased clearance of many medications and itself. Carbamazepine displays autoinduction of its own metabolism.

Answer c is incorrect. Phenytoin is an inducer of 3A4, but it is not an autoinducer.

Answer d is incorrect. Phenobarbital is an inducer of 3A4, but it is not an autoinducer.

---

8. Select the example of partial seizures.
   i. Complex
   ii. Simple
   iii. Tonic-clonic
   iv. Myoclonic

   a. i
   b. iii
   c. i and iv
   d. i and ii
   e. ii and iv

Answer d is correct. Partial seizures consist of simple, complex, and secondarily generalized seizures. Generalized seizures consist of absence, myoclonic, tonic-clonic, and atonic seizures.

---

9. Select the AED that modulates sodium channels.
   a. Clonazepam
   b. Ethosuximide
   c. Gabapentin
   d. Carbamazepine

Answer a is incorrect. Clonazepam enhances GABA activity.

Answer b is incorrect. Ethosuximide modulates calcium channels.

Answer c is incorrect. Gabapentin modulates calcium channels and enhances GABA activity.

Answer d is correct. Carbamazepine modulates sodium channels.

---

10. Select the AED which is primarily eliminated through renal route.
   a. Clonazepam
   b. Ethosuximide
   c. Gabapentin
   d. Carbamazepine

Answers a, b, and d are incorrect. They undergo hepatic metabolism and elimination.

Answer c is correct. Gabapentin undergoes renal elimination.

---

11. Select the idiosyncratic adverse reaction of carbamazepine.
   a. Aplastic anemia
   b. Hyponatremia
   c. Rash
   d. All of the above

Answers a, b, and c, are correct. Aplastic anemia, hyponatremia, and rash are idiosyncratic reactions. Because idiosyncratic reactions may be life threatening, the AED may require discontinuation. Idiosyncratic reactions are associated with an immunologic reaction; therefore cross-reactivity among AEDs is possible.

Answer d is correct and the best answer.

---

12. Select the AED that modulates sodium channels.
   i. Phenytoin
   ii. Phenobarbital
   iii. Oxcarbazepine
   iv. Lamotrigine

   a. i and ii
   b. i and iii
   c. i, ii, iii, and iv
   d. ii, iii, and iv

Answer c is correct and the best answer. Phenytoin, phenobarbital, oxcarbazepine, and lamotrigine modulate sodium channels. Other AEDs that modulate sodium channels include carbamazepine, zonisamide (Na and Ca), valproic acid, and topiramate (Na, inhibits glutamate, enhances GABA).

---

13. Select the AED that is associated with the idiosyncratic adverse effect of gingival hyperplasia.

    a. Phenobarbital
    b. Primidone
    c. Tiagabine
    d. Phenytoin

Answer a is incorrect.

Answer b is incorrect. *Note:* Primidone is rarely used; however, it is important because it is metabolized to two active metabolites, one of which is phenobarbital.

Answer c is incorrect.

Answer d is correct. Phenytoin is associated with gingival hyperplasia (gum overgrowth).

14. Select the AED that has a usual serum concentration of 50 to 100 μg/mL.

    a. Phenytoin
    b. Carbamazepine
    c. Valproic acid
    d. Oxcarbazepine

Answer a is incorrect. Phenytoin's usual total serum concentration is 10 to 20 mg/L (10-20 μg/mL).

Answer b is incorrect. Carbamazepine's usual serum concentration is 4 to 12 mg/L.

Answer c is correct. Valproic acid's usual serum concentration is 50 to 100 mg/L.

Answer d is incorrect. Oxcarbazepine does not have established serum concentrations.

15. Select the AED that has an unbound (free) concentration of 1 to 2 μg/mL.

    a. Phenytoin
    b. Carbamazepine
    c. Valproic acid
    d. Oxcarbazepine

Answer a is correct. Phenytoin is highly protein bound. The usual total (bound and unbound) concentration for phenytoin is 10 to 20 μg/mL; however, the unbound (free) concentration is 1 to 2 μg/mL. The unbound concentration is the component that produces seizure control and adverse reactions.

Answer b is incorrect. Carbamazepine is highly protein bound (75%-90%), but free carbamazepine levels are not monitored.

Answer c is incorrect. Valproic acid is highly protein bound, but free valproic acid levels are not monitored.

Answer d is incorrect. Oxcarbazepine does not have established serum concentrations.

16. Select the AED that has a primary route of elimination (substrate) of CYP-450 3A4.

    i. Carbamazepine
    ii. Zonisamide
    iii. Levetiracetam

    a. i and iii
    b. i and ii
    c. ii and iii
    d. i, ii, and iii

Answer b is correct. Carbamazepine and zonisamide have a primary route of elimination of CYP-4450 3A4. Levetiracetam is one of the few AEDs that undergo renal elimination.

17. Select the AED that is a substrate and inducer of the CYP-450 2C9.

    a. Phenytoin
    b. Phenobarbital
    c. Gabapentin
    d. All of the above
    e. A and B

Answer a is correct. Phenytoin is a substrate and inducer of the CYP-450 2C9.

Answer b is correct. Phenobarbital is a substrate and inducer of the CYP-450 2C9.

Answer c is incorrect. Gabapentin is one of the few AEDs that undergo renal elimination.

Answer d is incorrect.

Answer e is correct and the best answer.

18. Select the water-soluble prodrug of phenytoin that is rapidly converted to phenytoin in the body.

    a. Trileptal
    b. Tegretol
    c. Keppra
    d. Cerebyx
    e. Dilantin

Answer a is incorrect. Trileptal is oxcarbazepine.

Answer b is incorrect. Tegretol is carbamazepine.

Answer c is incorrect. Keppra is levetiracetam.

Answer d is correct. Cerebyx is fosphenytoin. Fosphenytoin is a prodrug of phenytoin.

Answer e is incorrect. Dilantin is phenytoin.

19. Intravenous dosing of phenytoin cannot be infused faster than 50 mg/min. Select the adverse reactions that are associated with infusions faster than 50 mg/min.

    a. Hypotension
    b. Gingival hyperplasia
    c. Anemia
    d. Rash

Answer a is correct. The dose cannot be infused faster than 50 mg/min due to the potential risks of hypotension and arrhythmias.

Answers b, c, and d are incorrect. Gingival hyperplasia, anemia, and rash are idiosyncratic reactions and not related to infusion rates or dose.

---

20. Select the AED that is available in oral and parenteral formulations.

    a. Neurontin
    b. Dilantin
    c. Keppra
    d. Trileptal

Answers a, c, and d are incorrect. They are available in oral formulations only.

Answer b is correct. Phenytoin (Dilantin) is available in oral and parenteral formulations.

CHAPTER 50 | Parkinson Disease

1. What is the primary neurotransmitter deficiency in Parkinson disease?

    a. Acetylcholine
    b. Dopamine
    c. Norepinephrine
    d. Serotonin

Answer a is incorrect. There is a relative overactivity of acetylcholine in Parkinson disease.

Answer b is correct. The deficiency is caused by a loss of nigrostriatal neurons in the substantial nigra pars compacta.

Answer c is incorrect. Adrenergic pathways may be affected by Parkinson disease, but norepinephrine is not the primary neurotransmitter deficiency.

Answer d is incorrect. Serotonergic pathways may be affected by Parkinson disease, but norepinephrine is not the primary neurotransmitter deficiency.

---

2. Which of the cardinal features of Parkinson disease is least likely to be present upon diagnosis?

    a. Bradykinesia
    b. Postural instability
    c. Rigidity
    d. Tremor

Answer a is incorrect. Bradykinesia, or slowness of movement, is frequently present at the time of diagnosis.

Answer b is correct. Postural instability is rarely present at the time of diagnosis, but frequently appears after several years.

Answer c is incorrect. Rigidity is more common upon presentation in older patients.

Answer d is incorrect. Tremor is often the first symptom noticed by patients and family members.

---

3. What is the primary goal of Parkinson disease treatment?

    a. Cessation of disease progression
    b. Facilitate an increase in the storage capacity of dopamine
    c. Maintenance of functional ability
    d. Reversal of neuronal loss

Answer a is incorrect. There are currently no therapies that stop the progression of Parkinson disease

Answer b in incorrect. As Parkinson disease progresses, additional neurons will cease to function and dopamine levels will continue to decrease. As there is no medication that stops disease progression, there is no medication that increases dopamine storage capacity.

Answer c is correct. The control of motor symptoms ultimately allows the Parkinson disease patient to continue to function and perform normal activities of daily living. As there is no medication that stops disease progression, the goal is to maintain the patient's ability to function as long as possible.

Answer d is incorrect. There are no medications capable of reversing the loss of nigrostriatal neurons.

---

4. What is the role of carbidopa in the treatment of Parkinson disease?

    a. It inhibits acetylcholine.
    b. It inhibits dopa decarboxylase.
    c. It inhibits catechol-*o*-methyltransferase.
    d. It inhibits monoamine oxidase.

Answer a is incorrect. Anticholinergics (such as benztropine) inhibit acetylcholine.

Answer b is correct. Carbidopa inhibits dopa decarboxylase to prevent the conversion of levodopa to dopamine in the periphery, allowing the drug to cross the blood–brain barrier.

Answer c is incorrect. COMT inhibitors (tolcapone and entacapone) inhibit catechol-*o*-methyltransferase.

Answer d is incorrect. MAO inhibitors (selegiline and rasagiline) inhibit monoamine oxidase.

---

5. Which of the following describes off-time associated with "on-off" phenomena?

   a. It lasts for several hours.
   b. It typically happens at the end of a dosing interval.
   c. It is associated with receptor overstimulation.
   d. It is unpredictable.

Answer a is incorrect. The duration of an episode of off-time when a patient is experiencing "on-off" phenomena is typically seconds to minutes.

Answer b is incorrect. Wearing off occurs at the end of a dosing interval.

Answer c is incorrect. Receptor overstimulation has historically been implicated in contributing to dyskinesias.

Answer d is correct. Due to the unpredictable nature of off-time associate with "on-off" phenomena, it is extremely distressing for patients, and is more difficult to treat with medication than off-time that occurs near the end of a dosing interval.

---

6. What is the maximum recommended daily dose of pramipexole?

   a. 0.375 mg
   b. 4.5 mg
   c. 24 mg
   d. 100 mg

Answer a is incorrect. A daily dose of 0.375 mg is the normal dose for initiating pramipexole use.

Answer b is correct. The maximum recommended daily dose of pramipexole is 4.5 mg.

Answer c is incorrect. The maximum daily dose of ropinirole is 24 mg.

Answer d is incorrect. Doses of bromocriptine as high as 100 mg/d have been used in some patients.

---

7. Which of the following medication has been implicated in causing impulsive behavior?

   a. Amantadine
   b. Entacapone
   c. Rasagiline
   d. Ropinirole

Answers a, b, and c are incorrect. These have not been associated with impulsive behavior.

Answer d is correct. Ropinirole is a dopamine agonist, and has been associated with impulsive behaviors including gambling, excessive shopping, and hypersexuality.

---

8. Which drug is frequently associated with insomnia due to the action of its metabolite?

   a. Amantadine
   b. Benztropine
   c. Pramipexole
   d. Selegiline

Answer a is incorrect. Although a fraction of patients taking amantadine complain of insomnia, the drug does not have a metabolite specifically associated with an increased frequency of this side effect.

Answer b is incorrect. Benztropine is not typically associated with insomnia.

Answer c is incorrect. Pramipexole has been implicated in causing insomnia, but the side-effect is not associated with its metabolite.

Answer d is correct. Selegiline has an amphetamine metabolite, and has been associated with increased incidence of insomnia. Doses should be given no later than early afternoon to help prevent this side effect.

---

9. Anticholinergics are primarily used to control which cardinal Parkinson disease symptom?

   a. Bradykinesia
   b. Postural instability
   c. Rigidity
   d. Tremor

Answers a, b, and c are incorrect. Anticholinergics are not useful for patients with significant bradykinesia and rigidity and are not help correct postural instability.

Answer d is correct. Anticholinergics help to correct the relative overactivity of acetylcholine that exists due to dopamine deficiency. It is this imbalance that is responsible for the tremor of Parkinson disease.

---

10. The use of which of the following medication requires monitoring of liver function tests?

    a. Levodopa
    b. Rasagiline
    c. Ropinirole
    d. Tolcapone

Answers a, b, and c are incorrect. Routine monitoring of liver function tests is not required with levodopa, rasagiline, and rasagiline use.

Answer d is correct. Tolcapone has been linked to liver toxicity and at least three fatalities secondary to liver failure. The drug should be reserved for patients who have failed to achieve an adequate response with other therapies. Liver function tests should be checked over 2 to 4 weeks for the first 6 months, and then periodically thereafter as deemed clinically relevant.

---

11. Which drug should be dosed simultaneously with levodopa?
    a. Amantadine
    b. Entacapone
    c. Pramipexole
    d. Rasagiline

Answer a is incorrect. Amantadine is typically dosed twice daily and may be administered to patients who are not receiving levodopa therapy.

Answer b is correct. Entacapone inhibits the action of catechol-o-methyltransferase in the periphery to avoid the breakdown of levodopa and dopamine before levodopa crosses the blood–brain barrier. It must be present with levodopa to achieve this outcome.

Answer c is incorrect. Pramipexole stimulates dopamine receptors independent of levodopa and may be used as monotherapy.

Answer d is incorrect. Rasagiline inhibits the breakdown of dopamine in the brain and may be used as monotherapy without levodopa.

12. Parkinsonian symptoms have been noted in patients exposed to which of the following medications?
    a. Haloperidol
    b. Metoclopramide
    c. Prochlorperazine
    d. All of the above

Answer a is correct. Haloperidol is a neuroleptic medication that has been associated with parkinsonism.

Answer b is correct. Metoclopramide is centrally acting and has been associated with parkinsonism.

Answer c is correct. Prochlorperazine is a phenothiazine antiemetic and has been associated with parkinsonism.

Answer d is correct. All of these medications have been associated with parkinsonism.

13. What is the mechanism of action of the ropinirole?
    a. Direct replacement of dopamine in the central nervous system
    b. Direct stimulation of postsynaptic dopamine receptors
    c. Inhibition of the enzymatic breakdown of dopamine in the central nervous system
    d. Inhibition of the enzymatic breakdown of dopamine in the periphery

Answer a is incorrect. Levodopa is converted to dopamine in the brain and serves to replace the neurotransmitter directly.

Answer b is correct. Dopamine agonists bypass the nigrostriatal neurons and provide direct receptor stimulation exerting effects like dopamine.

Answer c is incorrect. Dopamine agonists do not inhibit the enzymatic breakdown of dopamine.

Answer d is incorrect. Dopamine agonists do not inhibit the enzymatic breakdown of dopamine.

14. Which antipsychotic is preferred when treatment of psychosis is necessary in the Parkinson patient?
    a. Chlorpromazine
    b. Haloperidol
    c. Quetiapine
    d. Risperidone

Answer a is incorrect. Chlorpromazine is an antidopaminergic antipsychotic and should be avoided in patients with Parkinson disease.

Answer b is incorrect. Haloperidol is an antidopaminergic antipsychotic and should be avoided in patients with Parkinson disease.

Answer c is correct. Quetiapine is among the least likely antipsychotic agents to exacerbate the motor symptoms of Parkinson disease making it a good choice for treatment of psychosis as a comorbidity.

Answer d is incorrect. Risperidone has antidopaminergic properties, and has been shown to be more likely to exacerbate symptoms of Parkinson disease than some of the other atypical antipsychotics.

15. Which medication is available as an orally disintegrating tablet that may be taken without liquid?
    a. Carbidopa/levodopa
    b. Pramipexole
    c. Selegiline
    d. Both a and c are correct

Answer a is correct. Carbidopa/levodopa is available as an orally disintegrating tablet that may be taken without liquid.

Answer b is incorrect. There is no orally disintegrating formulation of pramipexole available.

Answer c is correct. Selegiline is available as an orally disintegrating tablet that may be taken without liquid.

Answer d is correct. Both carbidopa/levodopa and selegiline are available as tablets that may be taken without liquid.

16. Which medication can cause rebound Parkinson symptoms if stopped abruptly?
    a. Amantadine
    b. Carbidopa/levodopa
    c. Pramipexole
    d. Rasagiline

Answer a is correct. If amantadine is to be discontinued, it should be slowly tapered to avoid rebound symptoms.

Answer b is incorrect. Abrupt discontinuation of carbidopa/levodopa can lead to the development of neuroleptic malignant syndrome.

Answer c is incorrect. Abrupt discontinuation of pramipexole can lead to the development of neuroleptic malignant syndrome.

Answer d is incorrect. Rasagiline discontinuation does not require a taper.

17. GR was recently diagnosed with Parkinson disease. His family practitioner initiated therapy with carbidopa/levodopa 10/100 mg tid. He has been taking the medication with meals, but he is experiencing significant nausea. GR has noticed very little difference in his symptoms. What is the most probable reason GR is experiencing such significant nausea?
    a. Carbidopa/levodopa should be taken on an empty stomach.
    b. Carbidopa/levodopa should be taken with a meal high in protein.
    c. The levodopa component is being converted to dopamine in the periphery.
    d. Carbidopa/levodopa always causes nausea.

Answer a is incorrect. It is true that the drug should be taken on an empty stomach for optimal absorption, but administration with food often helps to relieve nausea.

Answer b is incorrect. Amino acids compete with levodopa for transport into the brain. If carbidopa/levodopa is to be taken with food, a low-protein meal is recommended.

Answer c is correct. The minimum daily dose of carbidopa necessary to prevent the peripheral conversion of levodopa to dopamine is 75 to 100 mg. The fact that GR has not noticed improvement in his symptoms supports the notion that levodopa is not crossing the blood–brain barrier to be converted to dopamine.

Answer d is incorrect. Though nausea is a frequent side-effect associated with carbidopa/levodopa, it is not inevitable.

18. Comorbid conditions frequently present in persons with Parkinson disease include which of the following?
    a. Depression
    b. Constipation
    c. Hypotension
    d. All of the above

Answer a is correct. Depression is present in over half of patients with Parkinson disease and may be part of the disease itself.

Answer b is correct. Neurological derangements in the gastrointestinal tract contribute to constipation in the Parkinson disease patient.

Answer c is correct. Hypotension in persons with Parkinson disease may be disease related or drug induced.

Answer d is correct and the best answer. All of the above are comorbidities that frequently exist with Parkinson disease.

19. Which dopamine agonist is most likely to be associated with fibrotic complications?
    a. Bromocriptine
    b. Pramipexole
    c. Ropinirole
    d. Rotigotine

Answer a is correct. Bromocriptine is an ergot derivative. It is the ergots that are most often associated with the complication of fibrosis.

Answers b, c, and d are incorrect. Nonergots are less likely to be associated with fibrotic complications..

20. Which of the following is/are true of dyskinesias in a person with Parkinson disease?
    a. They often appear when the cardinal symptoms are under good control.
    b. Intermittent dopamine receptor stimulation is believed to contribute to dyskinesia development.
    c. They are associated with extended use of levodopa.
    d. All of the above.

Answer a is correct. Dyskinesias in the Parkinson patient frequently occur when disease symptoms are well controlled and dopamine receptors are adequately stimulated. For this reason, the term "peak dose" dyskinesia is often used.

Answer b is correct. Receptor overstimulation used to be blamed for the emergence of dyskinetic movements. However, recent evidence suggests that maintaining more constant receptor stimulation is associated with a lower incidence of dyskinesia.

Answer c is correct. Dyskinesias are associated with levodopa use that has usually been continuous over several years.

Answer d is correct. All of the above are true of dyskinesias in the Parkinson patient.

CHAPTER 51 | Headache

1. Which of the following is most likely to play a role in migraine pathogenesis?
    a. Norepinephrine
    b. Serotonin
    c. Dopamine

Answer a is incorrect. There are no data that supports involvement of norepinephrine with the pathophysiology of migraine.

Answer b is correct. Serotonin is a vasoactive neurotransmitter that is released by the brainstem nuclei of the trigeminovascular system. Plasma levels of serotonin are found to be deficient during a migraine attack. Drugs that affect serotonin are often effective in treatment of migraines.

Other agents discussed as playing an active role within the trigeminovascular system are the following neuropeptides: calcitonin gene-related peptide, substance P, and neurokinin A.

Answer c is incorrect. Dopamine may also play a role in migraine headaches as dopamine receptor antagonists are effective treatments administered as monotherapy or with other antimigraine medications; however, there is a lack of clinical data to support this theory.

2. A patient presents to your community pharmacy complaining of a headache. She rates the headache as a 7 on a scale of 1 to 10, and the pulsating worsens as the headache progresses. She experiences nausea and sensitivity to light until the headache dissipates after about 12 hours. She is unable to function during the headache. Which of the following headache types is this patient likely experiencing?

   a. Migraine
   b. Tension
   c. Cluster

Answer a is correct. The International Headache Society diagnostic criteria for migraine includes:

Headache lasts for 4 to 72 hours

At least two of the following characteristics:

- Unilateral location
- Pulsating
- Moderate to severe intensity
- Aggravated by routine physical activity

At least one of the following:

- Nausea and/or vomiting
- Photophobia and phonophobia

Answer b is incorrect. Tension headache would have a gripping/tightening quality, not aggravated by activity, no nausea or vomiting, photo- and phonophobia are absent or one but not the other is present.

Answer c is incorrect. Cluster headache would last for no longer than 180 minutes and exhibits signs/symptoms of conjunctival injection, lacrimation, nasal congestion, rhinorrhea, sweating miosis, ptosis, or eyelid edema.

3. Which of the following signs/symptoms are classified as "red flags," indicating need for physician referral and diagnostic evaluation?

   a. "Worst headache of my life"
   b. Acute headache that occurs after coughing/sneezing
   c. Headache onset age ≥40 years
   d. All of the above

Answer a is correct. Headache associated with subarachnoid hemorrhage is often described by the patient as the "worst" headache.

Answer b is correct. Headache after coughing or sneezing could be benign. However, it can also be a sign of cranial mass lesion with cerebrospinal fluid path obstruction.

Answer c is correct. Headache at age ≥40 can be indicative of a new organic cause. Although it can also be benign, it requires physician evaluation.

Answer d is correct and the best answer.

4. LK suffers from chronic migraines and is currently experiencing an acute attack. Which of the following situations within the past few days could have triggered her migraine?

   a. The wine and cheese party she attended last night.
   b. She recently stopped drinking regular coffee.
   c. She started a triphasic oral contraceptive 10 days ago.
   d. All of the above.

Answer a is incorrect. Answer a lists some tyramine containing foods which are known to be triggers. Other potential food triggers include alcohol, chocolate, citrus fruits, dairy, fermented foods, and foods containing additives such as monosodium glutamate, nitrites, saccharin, sulfites, or yeast. When trying to determine a trigger of a patient's headache, it is recommended that the patient eliminate all causative agents and then gradually add back in one item at a time.

Answer b is incorrect. Answer b involves caffeine withdrawal. Caffeine intake or withdrawal can be a trigger.

Answer c is incorrect. Answer c states a change in hormone. Estrogen or oral contraceptives are known triggers of migraine.

Answer d is correct. There are numerous migraine triggers. The primary categories are behavioral, environmental, food, or medication related.

5. Which of the following would be an absolute contraindication for receiving a selective 5-HT_1 receptor agonist (triptan)?

   a. Diabetes
   b. Ischemic heart disease
   c. Anemia
   d. Controlled hypertension

Answer a is incorrect. There is no documentation of effect on blood glucose with these agents.

Answer b is correct. These medications are selective agonists for serotonin in the cranial arteries to cause vasoconstriction. Due to this constrictive nature, patients with ischemic heart disease or signs or symptoms of ischemic heart disease (including Prinzmetal angina, angina pectoris, myocardial infarction, or silent ischemia) should not take these medications.

Answer c is incorrect. There is a 1% reported incidence of hemolytic anemia as an adverse effect. A diagnosis of anemia would not be a contraindication.

Answer d is incorrect. Uncontrolled hypertension, due to the information stated above, would be a contraindication. However, a patient with controlled hypertension would not be contraindicated if using for infrequent abortive treatment.

6. Which of the following is the brand name for rizatriptan?
   a. Imitrex
   b. Maxalt
   c. Amerge
   d. Frova

Answer a is incorrect. The generic name of Imitrex is sumatriptan.

Answer b is correct.

Answer c is incorrect. The generic name for Amerge is naratriptan.

Answer d is incorrect. The generic name for Frova is frovatriptan.

7. A patient is taking Zomig ZMT. Which of the following is true regarding this medication?
   i. It is a subcutaneous injection
   ii. Liquid is not required for administration
   iii. It is an orally disintegrating tablet

   a. i and ii
   b. i and iii
   c. ii and iii
   d. i, ii, and iii

Answer c is correct. Zomig ZMT is the orally disintegrating tablet dosage form of zolmitriptan. It does not require water for administration; this may be beneficial to those patients without access to water, requiring discrete administration, or who experience nausea with their headaches, where intake of large amounts of liquid with administration may aggravate this symptom. This medication is also available as a nasal spray solution and tablet.

Answers a, b, and d are incorrect because Sumatriptan (Imitrex) is a selective serotonin agonist that is available as a subcutaneous injection. Zolmitriptan does not come in an injectable formulation.

8. A patient who currently takes oral sumatriptan often experiences headache recurrence, where the headache comes back within 24 hours after a positive response to the medication. Her physician would like a recommendation of a selective 5-HT_1 receptor agonist (triptan) with a longer half-life. Which of the following would you recommend?
   a. Frovatriptan
   b. Rizatriptan
   c. Zolmitriptan
   d. Almotriptan

Answer a is correct. Her current medication, sumatriptan (Imitrex) has an elimination half-life of 2.5 hours. Frovatriptan (Frova) has an elimination half-life of 26 hours. The longer half-life products may benefit a patient who is responsive to triptans but requires a longer-acting medication to last the duration of the headache.

Answer b is incorrect. Rizatriptan (Maxalt) has a similar elimination half-life of 2 to 3 hours.

Answer c is incorrect. Zolmitriptan (Zomig) has a similar elimination half-life of 3 hours.

Answer d is incorrect. Almotriptan (Axert) has a similar elimination half-life of 3.1 hours.

9. Which of the following are correct repeat dose instructions for the migraine medication?
   a. Zomig tablets: take one tablet now; may repeat in 2 hours
   b. Imitrex subcutaneous injection: use one injection now; may repeat in 2 hours
   c. Amerge tablets: take one tablet now; may repeat in 2 hours
   d. All of the above are correct

Answer a is correct. Zomig (zolmitriptan) tablets may be repeated in 2 hours if needed, not to exceed two doses in 24 hours.

Answer b is incorrect. Imitrex (sumatriptan) subcutaneous injection can be repeated in 1 hour if the headache has not resolved, not to exceed two injections in 24 hours.

Answer c is incorrect. Amerge (naratriptan) tablets may be repeated in 4 hours if needed, not to exceed two doses in 24 hours.

Answer d is incorrect. See rationale above.

10. Treximet is a combination headache medication made up of which of the following?
    a. Sumatriptan and naproxen
    b. Acetaminophen, aspirin, and caffeine
    c. Acetaminophen, isometheptene mucate, and dichloralphenazone
    d. Acetaminophen, butalbital, and caffeine

Answer a is correct.

Answer b is incorrect. Acetaminophen, aspirin, and caffeine are Excedrin Migraine.

Answer c is incorrect. Acetaminophen, isometheptene mucate, and dichloralphenazone are Midrin.

Answer d is incorrect. Acetaminophen, butalbital, and caffeine are Fioricet.

11. CJ is a 30-year-old patient admitted to the hospital with an unremitting migraine headache. She has tried two doses of naratriptan in the past 12 hours. She also takes lisinopril 10 mg once daily for her blood pressure and terbinafine for her onychomycosis. Her vital signs are BP 132/88 mm Hg, HR 70 bpm, Ht 5 ft 5 in, and Wt 130 lb. The physician plans to administer dihydroergotamine. Which of the following contraindications present to her receiving this treatment?
    a. Uncontrolled hypertension
    b. Elevated heart rate
    c. Terbinafine
    d. Naratriptan

Answer a is incorrect. Although uncontrolled hypertension would be a contraindication, this patient's BP is <140/90 mm Hg and would be defined as controlled.

Answer b is incorrect. Heart rate is not currently elevated for this patient at 70 bpm.

Answer c is incorrect. Ergotamine medications are contraindicated for use with potent inhibitors of CYP 3A4. Azole antifungals would be contraindicated. Terbinafine is a synthetic allylamine derivative used for treatment of onychomycosis of the toenail or fingernail. It is only a minor substrate of CYP 3A4. It has strong inhibition action on CYP 2D6 substrates.

Answer d is correct. Administration of serotonin agonists within 24 hours of ergotamine medications should be avoided due to risk of increased vasoconstriction.

12. A severe adverse effect that may result from taking ergotamine tartrate is:
    a. Purple toe syndrome
    b. Ergotism
    c. Pruritus
    d. Nausea

Answer a is incorrect. Purple toe syndrome is most commonly associated with warfarin therapy.

Answer b is correct. Ergotism is intense ischemia that results in peripheral vascular ischemia and possible gangrene.

Answer c is incorrect. Pruritus is a side effect that can result from ergotamine; however, it is not commonly severe.

Answer d is incorrect. Nausea is a side effect that can result from ergotamine; however, it is not commonly severe.

13. JB is a 55-year-old woman who has suffered from migraines for many years. Her zolmitriptan 5 mg works well to abort her headaches when they occur. Over the past few months, her headaches have increased in frequency to one every 2 weeks. She also complains of difficulty sleeping. Her vital signs today upon physical examination are Ht 5 ft 6 in, Wt 140 lb, BP 120/80 mm Hg, and HR 60 bpm. Her physician would like to start her on prophylactic drug therapy. Which of the following drug therapy options is the best option for prophylaxis for this patient?
    a. Propranolol
    b. Botulinum toxin type A
    c. Amitriptyline
    d. Phenelzine

Answer a is incorrect. The patient has a HR of 60 bpm and propranolol is a beta blocker which will slow the heart rate further.

Answer b is incorrect. Botulinum toxin type A (Botox) has an unlabeled/investigational drug use for migraine treatment and prophylaxis. Until it attains an approved indication, its efficacy is unclear.

Answer c is correct. It is always best to treat comorbid conditions whenever possible. This patient complains of difficulty sleeping and amitriptyline is a medication that has an adverse effect of drowsiness. Amitriptyline is well established in the literature for effective prophylactic therapy. It is useful in patients with comorbid depression or insomnia. Nortriptyline would be a tricyclic antidepressant that would cause less drowsiness. Caution should be used with these medications in the elderly due to the side effects.

Answer d is incorrect. Phenelzine (Nardil) is a monoamine oxidase inhibitors (MAOI). Significant lifestyle modifications regarding tyramine containing foods is necessary to avoid hypertensive crisis. This would not be an appropriate first choice for prophylactic medication for this reason.

14. Which of the following are prophylactic treatment options for migraine headache?
    i. Verapamil
    ii. Topiramate
    iii. Valproic acid

    a. i and ii
    b. i and iii
    c. ii and iii
    d. i, ii, and iii

Answer d is correct. Verapamil is a calcium channel blocker that is used for migraine prophylaxis. It would be useful for patients who cannot tolerate beta blockers or for patients with comorbid hypertension or angina.

Topiramate is an antiepileptic medication that was approved for use in migraines in 2004. It is dosed twice daily for migraine prevention. It would be useful for a patient with comorbid seizure disorder. It does have some more prominent cognitive side effects with >10% incidence, including memory difficulties, difficulty in concentrating, confusion, and speech difficulties.

Valproic acid is an antiepileptic medication also approved for migraine prophylaxis. It would be useful for those patients with comorbid seizure disorder or manic depressive illness.

15. JJ is a 49-year-old man who experiences headache cycles two times a year, usually in the spring and fall. The headaches occur for about 3 to 4 weeks. Each day during the headache series he may have up to 5 headaches. He describes the headaches as an unbearable type of pain that comes very suddenly, located in his left eye, and goes within 1to 2 hours. He experiences severe ocular and nasal symptoms, such as nasal stuffiness or rhinorrhea, ocular lacrimation, and ptosis. He tells you that in order to attempt to stop the pain, he sometimes rubs the areas of pain or even beats his head against objects. Which of the following are appropriate abortive treatment options for this patient's headache?

    a. Oxygen
    b. Imitrex (sumatriptan) tablets
    c. Amitriptyline
    d. a and c

Answer a is correct. Oxygen administered at 5 to 10 L/min by nonrebreather facemask for approximately 15 minutes is a first-line abortive treatment for cluster headache. This patient exhibits primary symptoms of cluster headache as per the International Headache Society Diagnostic Criteria for Migraine:

Headache is unilateral, orbital in location, lasting for 15 to 180 minutes

Nasal congestion, rhinorrhea, ocular lacrimation, and ptosis are present

Frequency of headaches lasts from 7 days to 1 year

Answer b is incorrect. Due to the duration of cluster headache, sumatriptan tablets will not act quick enough to have an impact before the headache dissipates.

Answer c is incorrect. Amitriptyline is a prophylactic option for migraine and tension headache. There are no data to support its use as an abortive for cluster headache.

Answer d is incorrect. See rationale above.

16. AB is a 25-year-old college student who has been having headaches 3 to 4 times a month that last for 12 to 24 hours for the past couple of months. He describes them as having a gripping quality with pressure on both sides of his head, as if someone is squeezing his head with a rubber band. He does not experience nausea or vomiting. His headaches do not stop him from going to class, but sometimes he finds himself having to turn off his radio when studying since he just can't handle any noise. Light does not bother him during his headaches.

Which of the following abortive treatment options would be appropriate recommendations for AB's headache?

    i. NSAIDS
    ii. Imitrex (sumatriptan)
    iii. Amitriptyline

    a. i only
    b. i and iii
    c. ii and iii
    d. i, ii, and iii

Answer a is correct. NSAIDs and combination analgesic products are a primary abortive treatment for patients with tension headache. The patient presents with common symptoms of tension headache based on the International Headache Society Diagnostic Criteria for Tension headache:

Headache lasts for 30 minutes to 7 days

At least two of the following characteristics:

> Pressing/tightening quality
>
> Mild intensity
>
> Bilateral location
>
> Not aggravated by routine physical activity

No nausea/vomiting

Photophobia/Phonophobia absent or one but not the other is present

Other nonpharmacologic agents effective for treatment of tension headache include stress management, relaxation therapy, biofeedback, physical therapy.

Answer b is incorrect. The triptan class of medications has no documentation of efficacy in treatment of tension headache.

Answer c is incorrect. Amitriptyline is a prophylactic treatment option for migraine and tension headache. It would not have benefit as an abortive treatment.

Answer d is incorrect.

17. DT is a 31-year-old woman who is 36 weeks pregnant. She currently has a headache with presentation most like a tension-type headache. She is requesting a recommendation for treatment. Which of the following is the best recommendation?

    a. NSAIDs
    b. Ergotamine
    c. Acetaminophen

Answer a is incorrect. NSAIDs should be avoided late in the third trimester to prevent prostaglandin alterations that could lead to premature ductus arteriosus closure.

Answer b is incorrect. Ergotamine is a pregnancy category X. It may precipitate uterine contractions and ischemia leading to hypoxemia in the fetus.

Answer c is correct. Acetaminophen is a pregnancy category B. Although it does cross the placenta, it is believed to be safe for use during pregnancy at therapeutic doses for a short period of time. The patient may also find benefit in psychophysiologic therapy, such as stress management, relaxation therapy, and biofeedback, as well as physical therapy.

18. MM presents to the emergency room (ER) with a severe migraine headache and nausea and vomiting. He has taken one dose of zolmitriptan 5 mg po within the past 6 hours, but vomited within 10 minutes. Which of the following would be the most appropriate next step for treatment?

    a. Metoclopramide 10 mg IV
    b. Biofeedback
    c. Three days of inpatient dihydroergotamine IV
    d. Acetaminophen 650 mg per rectum (PR)

Answer a is correct. A single dose of antiemetic therapy administered 15 to 30 minutes prior to taking an abortive migraine medication may assist with nausea and vomiting. Prochlorperazine and metoclopramide are commonly used. Metoclopramide may also be useful for the gastroparesis, is often associated with migraine, and improves medication absorption.

Answer b is incorrect. Biofeedback is a common nonpharmacologic treatment used for management of headache. Two types are available: electrophysiologic and thermal biofeedback. Although this may assist the patient in relaxation and minimize headache symptoms, this would not be appropriate as a primary strategy for a severe headache.

Answer c is incorrect. This patient has only had one dose of zolmitriptan and vomited after a short time. Following administration of an antiemetic agent and assuming the patient has had success in the past with serotonin receptor agonist treatment, a second dose of a triptan could be administered, either oral or subcutaneous. For intractable, severe migraine, inpatient treatment with dihydroergotamine may be an option, administered 0.5 to 1 mg every 8 hours for 3 days.

Answer d is incorrect. Acetaminophen has been found to be an ineffective sole treatment option for migraine. Treatment with acetaminophen for severe migraine is not an appropriate option.

19. A physician calls your pharmacy asking which serotonin receptor agonist migraine medications are available as a nasal spray. You respond:

    i. Sumatriptan
    ii. Rizatriptan
    iii. Zolmitriptan

    a. i and ii
    b. i and iii
    c. ii and iii
    d. i, ii, and iii

Answer b is correct. Sumatriptan is available as Imitrex nasal spray and zolmitriptan is available as Zomig nasal spray.

Answers a, c, and d are incorrect. Rizatriptan is available as Maxalt tablets and Maxalt MLT rapidly disintegrating tablets.

20. A patient is picking up a prescription for Migranal (dihydroergotamine). Which of the following is an important counseling point to provide?

    a. Remove the foil wrapper before inserting PR
    b. Once prepared, use within 8 hours
    c. Wear latex-free gloves to apply
    d. Take with a full glass of water

Answer b is correct. Migranal is a dihydroergotamine nasal spray. Once the spray applicator has been prepared, use within 8 hours and discard any remaining solution.

Answers a, c, and d are incorrect. It is not available as a suppository, topical product, or oral formulation.

21. Select the brand name for eletriptan.

    a. Maxalt
    b. Zomig
    c. Ergomar
    d. Relpax

Answer a is incorrect. Maxalt is the brand name for rizatriptan.

Answer b is incorrect. Zomig is the brand name for zolmitriptan.

Answer c is incorrect. Ergomar is the brand name for ergotamine tartrate.

Answer d is correct.

22. Which of the following herbal medications has evidence of support for the treatment of migraine?

    a. Glucosamine
    b. Black cohosh
    c. Feverfew

Answer a is incorrect. Glucosamine is commonly used for osteoarthritis, joint pain, back pain, and glaucoma.

Answer b is incorrect. Black cohosh has many uses, but it is most commonly used for symptoms of menopause, premenstrual syndrome, and dysmenorrhea. There is no claim regarding the use for treatment of migraine.

Answer c is correct. Feverfew is used for fever, headaches, prevention of migraines, and menstrual irregularities. Clinical studies have used 50 to 100 mg of feverfew extract daily for migraine prophylaxis.

23. A patient presents to pick up a new prescription for sumatriptan tablets. When verifying the prescription, the computer alerts you of a contraindication with a current prescription: Paxil 20mg. Which of the following is the reason for this contraindication?

    a. Stevens-Johnson syndrome
    b. Serotonin syndrome
    c. Neuroleptic malignant syndrome
    d. Computer error—there is no contraindication

Answer a is incorrect. There is no documentation of occurrence of these conditions with the concurrent administration of these agents.

Answer b is correct. There is a potential increased risk of serotonin syndrome with administration of sumatriptan and paroxetine (Paxil).

Answer c is incorrect. There is no documentation of occurrence of these conditions with the concurrent administration of these agents.

Answer d is incorrect. There is a potential contraindication present.

CHAPTER 52 | Pain Management

MAG is a 58-year-old woman with a chief complaint of left arm, shoulder, and axillary pain. Patient underwent a left subtotal mastectomy and chemotherapy for breast cancer 6 years ago and received radiation therapy and bone marrow transplant at that time. Patient is currently free of cancer, but complains of burning and stinging pain down her left arm and nothing has worked well for her. She is also complaining of severe constipation. Her current medications are Bupropion (Wellbutrin) 150 mg po bid, Ibuprofen 600 mg po one tablet tid, Morphine sulfate extended release (ER) 30 mg bid, Atenolol 50 mg po every morning, and Tamoxifen 10 mg po bid.

1. What is best therapeutic plan of this patient's analgesic regimen?

    a. Analgesic regimen should be discontinued, because long-acting opiate is not appropriate for this patient's pain.
    b. Increase morphine ER to 30 mg po every 4 hours since it is not providing adequate analgesia.
    c. Increase morphine ER to 60 mg po tid since it is not optimally controlling patient's pain.
    d. Add pain medication to focus on neuropathic symptoms.

Answer a is incorrect. Based upon the patient's history, her pain is most likely moderate to severe; therefore, use of opioids would be appropriate.

Answer b is incorrect. Large increases in dose or interval of opioids should be avoided to minimize risk of side effects (eg, respiratory depression).

Answer c is incorrect. The patient's pain is neuropathic, therefore, adding adjunctive therapy would be appropriate.

Answer d is correct. Adding a medication to focus on the neuropathic pain would be appropriate (eg, tricyclic antidepressant, carbamazepine, gabapentin).

2. What is the best approach for the burning pain in this patient?

    a. Add amitriptyline 50 mg po at bedtime.
    b. Add duloxetine 20 mg po at bedtime because it has less side-effects.
    c. Add nortriptyline 50 mg po at bedtime.
    d. Add gabapentin 300 mg po every bedtime, and titrate to 300 mg po tid over next 7 to 10 days for patient's neuropathic pain.

Answer a is incorrect. The TCA amitriptyline is potentially effective in neuropathic pain, however, they are associated with a significant amount of side effects and the patient is already receiving a stimulant antidepressant (bupropion).

Answer b is incorrect. Duloxetine is a serotonin-norepinephrine reuptake inhibitor (SNRI) and may be used in the treatment of neuropathic pain; however, since the patient is already receiving an antidepressant, this would not be the ideal therapy.

Answer c is incorrect. The TCS nortriptyline is potentially effective in neuropathic pain, however, they are associated with a significant amount of side effects and the patient is already receiving a stimulant antidepressant (bupropion).

Answer d is correct. Gabapentin is often used for neuropathic pain (although only indicated for postherpetic neuralgia). Pregabalin is indicated for neuropathy (diabetic) and postherpetic neuralgia.

3. Select the pain medication that has a ceiling effect (eg, higher doses do not provide better pain relief).

    a. Oxycodone
    b. Gabapentin
    c. Ibuprofen
    d. Morphine

Answer a is incorrect. Oxycodone's pain relief is dose dependent and patients will often require dosage titration for chronic use.

Answer b is incorrect. Gabapentin's pain relief is varied with dose. Patients are started on 300 mg daily and titrated up based upon response. Gabapentin is titrated up from 300 mg daily to 1800 to 3600 mg divided into three daily doses.

Answer c is correct. NSAIDs have a ceiling analgesic dose and the analgesic duration is shorter than predicted by half-life of the drug.

Answer d is incorrect. Morphine's pain relief is dose dependent and patients will often require dosage titration for chronic use.

4. NSAIDs are commonly used to treat pain. Select the potential disadvantage(s) of using NSAIDs for pain management.
   a. Gastrointestinal bleeding
   b. Antiplatelet effects
   c. Decreased renal function
   d. Fluid retention
   e. All of the above

Answer a is correct. Gastrointestinal bleeding is a major disadvantage of the NSAIDs. GI bleeding will be less with COX-2 selective NSAIDs (eg, celecoxib), but it can still occur.

Answer b is correct. All NSAIDs have antiplatelet activity.

Answer c is correct. NSAIDs are common causes of renal dysfunction and kidney function should be monitored during therapy.

Answer d is correct. Fluid retention is caused by the NSAIDs ability to retain sodium and water. Therefore, NSAIDs may adversely affect blood pressure and systolic heart failure.

Answer e is correct and the best answer.

5. Select the medication(s) that may have reduced effectiveness when used with NSAIDs.
   a. ACE inhibitors
   b. Beta-blockers
   c. Thiazide diuretics
   d. All of the above

Answers a, b, and c are correct. NSAIDs may reduce the effectiveness of these blood pressure medications because of sodium and water retention.

Answer d is correct and the best answer.

6. QP is a 44-year-old patient diagnosed with severe diabetic neuropathy. He is currently being treated with an alpha-blocker (terazosin) for an enlarged prostate. Terazosin has significantly improved the symptoms of the enlarged prostate, but the patient is having orthostatic hypotension episodes. Select the medication that would be most appropriate for QP's diabetic neuropathy.
   a. Naproxen
   b. Morphine
   c. Nortriptyline
   d. Gabapentin

Answer a is incorrect. Neuropathic pain has a poor response to NSAIDs.

Answer b is incorrect. Neuropathic pain has a poor response to opioid analgesics.

Answer c is incorrect. Neuropathic pain responds to TCAs, but TCAs have a significant amount of side effects, including orthostatic hypotension.

Answer d is correct. Gabapentin is effective in the treatment of neuropathic pain and is not associated with orthostatic hypotension.

7. Select the side effect(s) associated with tricyclic antidepressants.
   a. Gastrointestinal bleeding
   b. Heart blockade
   c. Respiratory depression
   d. Anemia

Answer a is incorrect. GI bleeding is associated with the NSAIDs.

Answer b is correct. TCAs are associated with conduction abnormalities, which may lead to heart blockade.

Answer c is incorrect. Respiratory depression is associated with opioid analgesics.

Answer d is incorrect. Anemia is associated with the anticonvulsants (ie, carbamazepine).

8. Select the medication(s) that may cause central nervous system side effects.
   a. Gabapentin
   b. Opioids
   c. TCAs
   d. All of the above

Answers a, b, and c are correct. All pain medications have activity within the CNS and therefore are associated with CNS side effects.

Answer d is correct and the best answer.

9. Select the medication that is used for trigeminal neuralgia and neuropathies and is associated with significant CYP-450 drug interactions.
   a. Valproate
   b. Gabapentin

c. Topiramate
d. Carbamazepine

Answer a is incorrect. Valproate is a substrate, inhibitor, and inducer of the CYP-450 isoenzyme system; however, it is a weak inhibitor and inducer of the CYP-450 system.

Answer b is incorrect. Gabapentin is not involved in the CYP-450 system.

Answer c is incorrect. Topiramate is an inhibitor and inducer of the CYP-450 system; however, it is a weak inhibitor and inducer.

Answer d is correct. Carbamazepine is a substrate and strong inducer of the CYP-450 system; therefore, it is associated with significant drug interactions.

---

10. Select the medication that alters function of pain-sensitive nerve endings through substance-P depletion.
    a. Capsaicin
    b. Amitriptyline
    c. Carbamazepine
    d. Topiramate

Answer a is correct. Capsaicin alters function of pain-sensitive nerve endings through substance-P depletion.

Answer b is incorrect. Amitriptyline reduces trafficking of pain signals by effects on serotonin and norepinephrine.

Answer c is incorrect. Carbamazepine prolongs the depolarization of nerves causing reduced excitability and decreased pain signals.

Answer d is incorrect. Topiramate prolongs the depolarization of nerves causing reduced excitability and decreased pain signals.

---

11. Select the side effect associated with the active metabolite of meperidine when the dose is too high or the patient has renal dysfunction.
    a. Seizures
    b. Gastrointestinal bleeding
    c. Respiratory depression
    d. a and c
    e. All of the above

Answer a is correct. Normeperidine, the active metabolite of meperidine, may cause seizures in patients that are administered high doses or patients with renal dysfunction leading to decreased clearance of normeperidine.

Answer b is incorrect. GI bleeding is associated with NSAIDs.

Answer c is correct. Respiratory depression is associated with all opioids and is dose dependent.

Answer d is correct and the best answer.

Answer e is incorrect.

---

12. Select the opioid that is available in multiple formulations, including a transdermal patch.
    a. Morphine
    b. Oxycodone
    c. Meperidine
    d. Fentanyl

Answers a, b, and c are incorrect. Opioids are available in multiple formulations including oral, solutions, extended release, rectal and parenteral formulations, but these agents are not available in a patch formulation.

Answer d is correct. Fentanyl is available as a transdermal system (patch). It is also available as injection, lozenge, powder, and tablet.

---

13. IT is a 74-year-old man with severe chronic pain. He has been previously treated with nonopioid analgesics, but is prescribed morphine today. The patient will be receiving morphine chronically. Select the medication that IT should receive in addition to morphine.
    a. Ibuprofen
    b. Gabapentin
    c. Capsaicin
    d. Bisacodyl

Answer a is incorrect. IT has been receiving nonopioid analgesics in the past and they have not been effective. We are not given enough information to know if he has taken an NSAID; however, even if he had, that does not preclude use of an NSAID with an opioid. Combination analgesic therapy with an opioid and NSAID may produce better pain relief than an opioid alone; however, it is not required to use combination analgesics to treat pain.

Answer b is incorrect. Gabapentin is used for neuropathic types of pain. We are not given enough information about the type of pain to be able to make a recommendation for gabapentin or other medications that are effective against neuropathic pain.

Answer c is incorrect. Capsaicin is used for neuropathic types of pain. We are not given enough information about the type of pain to be able to make a recommendation for capsaicin or other medications that are effective against neuropathic pain.

Answer d is correct. Patients receiving opioids, especially for chronic therapy, should receive a stimulant laxative because of the constipation. Examples of stimulant laxatives include senna, cascara, and bisacodyl.

---

14. Select the medication that can reverse respiratory depression caused by opioids.
    a. Flumazenil
    b. Naloxone
    c. Acetylcysteine
    d. All of the above

Answer a is incorrect. Flumazenil (Romazicon) is a benzodiazepine antagonist and reverses the sedative effects of benzodiazepines used in conscious sedation and general anesthesia.

Answer b is correct. Naloxone (Narcan) is an opioid antagonist that reverses respiratory depression.

Answer c is incorrect. Acetylcysteine (Mucomyst) is an antidote for acetaminophen toxicity.

Answer d is incorrect.

15. Select the dosing method that should be employed when treating acute severe pain.
    a. Intermittent
    b. Scheduled dosing
    c. Directly observed therapy
    d. b and c

Answer a is incorrect. Intermittent, or as needed (prn), is used for patients on scheduled dosing of analgesics and experiencing breakthrough pain. For example, a patient receiving oxycodone 20 mg every 12 hours and is experiencing pain relief, but it does not last the entire dosing interval, may be prescribed a short-acting opioid for breakthrough pain on an as needed basis.

Answer b is correct. Scheduled dosing or around the clock is the preferred method for controlling severe pain.

Answer c is incorrect. Directly observed therapy is utilized in patients with tuberculosis and is not related to pain management.

Answer d is incorrect.

16. Select the medication that decreases pain transmission.
    a. Naproxen
    b. Carbamazepine
    c. Oxycodone
    d. Capsaicin

Answer a is incorrect. NSAIDs decrease pain stimulus.

Answer b is correct. Carbamazepine decreases pain transmission.

Answer c is incorrect. Oxycodone alters central perception.

Answer d is incorrect. Capsaicin alters function of pain-sensitive nerve endings.

17. Select the opioid that is available in oral, parenteral, and rectal formulations.
    a. Fentanyl
    b. Hydrocodone
    c. Hydromorphone
    d. Morphine
    e. c and d

Answer a is incorrect. Fentanyl is available in the following dosage forms: injection, lozenge, powder, tablet, and transdermal patch.

Answer b is incorrect. Hydrocodone is available in the following dosage forms: capsule, elixir, solution, and tablet (above is for hydrocodone plus acetaminophen-Lortab/Vicodin).

Answer c is correct. Hydromorphone is available in the following dosage forms: capsule, injection, liquid, powder, rectal, and tablet.

Answer d is correct. Morphine is available in the following dosage forms: capsule, injection, solution, rectal, and tablet.

Answer e is the correct and the best answer.

18. Select the opioid that has the same dose when administered intramuscularly and orally.
    a. Fentanyl
    b. Oxycodone
    c. Methadone
    d. Hydrocodone

Answer a is incorrect. Equianalgesic doses for fentanyl are 150 to 200 μg IM and 400 μg orally (SL).

Answer b is incorrect. Oxycodone is not administered intramuscularly.

Answer c is correct. Equianalgesic doses for methadone are 2.5 mg IM and 2.5 mg orally.

Answer d is incorrect. Hydrocodone is not administered intramuscularly.

19. Select the nonopioid analgesic that is minimally associated with central nervous system side effects and does not slow intestinal motility.
    a. Naproxen
    b. Hydrocodone
    c. Carbamazepine
    d. Amitriptyline

Answer a is correct. Naproxen is an NSAID and NSAIDs exhibit minimal CNS side effects (especially compared to other analgesics) and is not associated with constipation.

Answer b is incorrect. Hydrocodone is an opioid and opioids are associated with central nervous system side effects and frequently cause constipation.

Answer c is incorrect. Carbamazepine has a high incidence of CNS side effects.

Answer d is incorrect. Amitriptyline is associated with CNS side effects and constipation.

20. Select the analgesic that affects pain by enhancing neurotransmitters serotonin and norepinephrine.
    a. Ibuprofen
    b. Amitriptyline

c. Carbamazepine
d. Tramadol
e. b and c

Answer a is incorrect. NSAID's analgesic properties are produced by inhibition of prostaglandins.

Answer b is correct. TCAs analgesic effects are produced by enhancing the neurotransmitters norepinephrine and serotonin.

Answer c is incorrect. Carbamazepine's analgesic effects are produced by prolonging depolarization of nerves.

Answer d is correct. Tramadol's analgesic properties are produced by binding to mu-opiate receptors causing inhibition of ascending pain pathways, altering the perception of pain. Tramadol also inhibits the reuptake of norepinephrine and serotonin.

Answer e is correct and the best answer.

CHAPTER 53 | Depression

1. The pathophysiology of major depressive disorder (MDD) is associated with:
   a. Genetic factors
   b. Stress factors
   c. Neurotransmitter factors
   d. All of the above

Answer a is correct. The occurrence of MDD exhibits a genetic pattern. First-degree relatives of MDD patients are more likely to develop MDD compared to first-degree relatives of control individuals.

Answer b is correct. Depression can occur in the absence or presence of major life stressors; however, there is an association between life stressors and depression.

Answer c is correct. Classic views for the cause of MDD focus on the neurotransmitters such as norepinephrine (NE), serotonin (5-HT), and dopamine (DA). The neurotransmitter hypothesis asserts that depression is due to a deficiency of neurotransmitters. The supporting evidence for this hypothesis is that existing antidepressants increase neurotransmitters concentrations.

Answer d is correct and the best answer.

2. Select the neurotransmitter(s) that is involved in the pathophysiology of depression.
   a. Norepinephrine
   b. Serotonin
   c. Dopamine
   d. All of the above

Answer a is correct. Norepinephrine is a neurotransmitter involved in the pathophysiology of depression. Select antidepressants inhibit the reuptake of norepinephrine (eg, tricyclic antidepressants and serotonin norepinephrine reuptake inhibitors). Antidepressants that inhibit the reuptake of NE may lead to the following effects: tremor, tachycardia, sweating, jitteriness, increased blood pressure. TCAs can also cause severe cardiovascular complications in high dose/overdose because of a change in cardiac conduction.

Answer b is correct. Serotonin is a neurotransmitter involved in the pathophysiology of depression. Select antidepressants inhibit the reuptake of serotonin (eg, selective serotonin reuptake inhibitors, serotonin norepinephrine reuptake inhibitors). Antidepressants that inhibit the reuptake of 5-HT may lead to the following effects: anxiety, insomnia, sexual dysfunction, anorexia.

Answer c is correct. Dopamine is a neurotransmitter involved in the pathophysiology of depression. Select antidepressants inhibit the reuptake of dopamine (eg, buproprion). Antidepressants that inhibit the reuptake of DA may lead to the following effects: euphoria, psychomotor activation, aggravation of psychosis.

Answer d is correct and the best answer.

3. Select the symptom(s) of major depressive disorder.
   a. Depressed mood
   b. Diminished interest in usual activities
   c. Change in appetite or weight
   d. All of the above

Answer a is correct. Depressed mood is a symptom of MDD.

Answer b is correct. Diminished interest in usual activities is a symptom of MDD.

Answer c is correct. A change in appetite or weight is a symptom of MDD.

Answer d is correct and the best answer. The diagnosis of MDD requires the presence of at least five depressive symptoms that cause clinically significant effects and the symptoms must last for a minimum of 2 weeks. Examples of the symptoms are: depressed mood, diminished interest in usual activities, change in appetite or weight, change in psychomotor activity, change in amount of sleep, loss or energy, feelings of worthlessness or guilt, diminished ability to think or concentrate, or recurrent thought of death or suicide. One of the first two symptoms (depressed mood or diminished interest in usual activities) must be present in order to diagnose MDD.

4. Select the antidepressant that inhibits the reuptake of NE and 5-HT.
   a. Tricyclics (TCAs)
   b. Serotonin norepinephrine reuptake inhibitors (SNRIs)
   c. Selective serotonin reuptake inhibitors (SSRIs)
   d. a and b
   e. All of the above

Answer a is correct. TCAs inhibit the reuptake of NE and 5-HT. All TCAs inhibit the reuptake of NE and 5-HT, but they may do so at different degrees. For example, amitriptyline inhibits the reuptake of 5-HT more than imipramine and imipramine inhibits the reuptake of NE more than amitriptyline. Therefore, TCAs have the same side effect profile based upon mechanism of action, but they may cause a particular side effect at different percentages.

Answer b is correct. SNRIs (venlafaxine and duloxetine) inhibit the reuptake of NE and 5-HT. Venlafaxine inhibits 5-HT reuptake at low doses, with additional NE reuptake inhibition at higher doses. Duloxetine inhibits 5-HT and NE across all doses.

Answer c is incorrect. SSRIs inhibit the reuptake of serotonin.

Answer d is correct and the best answer.

Answer e is incorrect.

---

5. Select the mechanism of action of trazodone that leads to the side effect of dizziness and sedation.
   a. 5-HT receptor antagonist
   b. 5-HT reuptake inhibitor
   c. $Alpha_1$ adrenergic and histaminergic antagonism
   d. All of the above

Answer a is incorrect. 5-HT receptor antagonism may lead to increased REM sleep, decreased sexual dysfunction (serotonin 2A receptor blockade), increased appetite/weight gain (serotonin 2C receptor blockade).

Answer b is incorrect. 5-HT reuptake inhibition may lead to anxiety, insomnia, sexual dysfunction, and anorexia.

Answer c is correct. $Alpha_1$ adrenergic receptor blockade and histaminergic antagonism may lead to dizziness and sedation. $Alpha_1$ adrenergic receptor blockade may lead to orthostatic hypotension, dizziness, and reflex tachycardia. Histaminergic antagonism may lead to sedation and weight gain.

Answer d is incorrect.

---

6. Select the antidepressant that has a black box warning for rare cases of liver failure.
   a. Duloxetine
   b. Bupropion
   c. Amitriptyline
   d. Nefazodone

Note: All antidepressants have the following black box warning: Antidepressants increase the risk of suicidal thinking and behavior in children, adolescents, and young adults (18-24 years of age) with major depressive disorder and other psychotic disorders.

Answers a, b, c are incorrect.

Answer d is correct. Nefazodone's use as an antidepressant has declined after reports of hepatoxicity. The FDA-approved nefazodone labeling includes a black box warning describing rare cases of liver failure. Because of the potential for hepatic injury associated with nefazodone use, treatment should not be initiated in individuals with active liver disease or with elevated baseline serum transaminases.

---

7. Select the aminoketone that is a dopamine reuptake inhibitor.
   a. Wellbutrin
   b. Elavil
   c. Prozac
   d. Cymbalta

Answer a is correct. Bupropion (Wellbutrin) is an aminoketone that inhibits the reuptake of dopamine.

Answer b is incorrect. Amitriptyline (Elavil) is a TCA that inhibits the reuptake of NE and 5-HT.

Answer c is incorrect. Fluoxetine (Prozac) is an SSRI that inhibits the reuptake of serotonin.

Answer d is incorrect. Duloxetine (Cymbalta) is an SNRI that inhibits the reuptake of serotonin and norepinehrine.

---

8. Select the answer that would represent the highest chance of developing the side effect of hypertensive crisis.
   a. Utilization of phenelzine
   b. Utilization of imipramine
   c. Utilization of phenelzine plus pseudoephedrine
   d. Utilization of imipramine plus benzodiazepine

Answer a is incorrect. Phenelzine is an MAOI and MAOIs are associated with hypertensive crisis reactions; however, the reaction is usually caused by a drug interaction of an MAOI and a sympathomimetic.

Answer b is incorrect. Imipramine is a TCA and causes cardiovascular side effects (conduction abnormalities and orthostatic hypotension).

Answer c is correct. The utilization of MAOIs and sympathomimetics leads to the pharmacodynamic interaction of hypertensive crisis.

Answer d is incorrect. The utilization of TCAs and benzodiazepines leads to the pharmacodynamic interaction of sedation (additive effect).

---

9. Select the medication that is associated with causing depression.
   a. Propranolol
   b. Clonidine
   c. Reserpine
   d. a and c
   e. All of the above

Answer a is correct. Propranolol is associated with causing depression. Propranolol blocks the action of norepinephrine, which may lead to depression. This action is associated with propranolol because propranolol is a lipophilic beta-blocker and is able to exert its mechanism of action with the central nervous system.

Answer b is correct. Clonidine is associated with causing depression. Clondine decreases sympathomimetic flow with the central nervous system. Decreasing sympathomimetic flow (decreasing the neurotransmitter norepinephinre) may lead to depression.

Answer c is correct. Reserpine is associated with causing depression. Reserpine depletes sympathomimetic amines (norepinephrine and dopamine), which may lead to depression.

Answer e is correct and the best answer. Other medications/substances associated with causing depression are: diuretics, guanethidine, hydralazine, methyldopa, oral contraceptives, steroids, isotretinoin, interferon, alcoholism, marijuana abuse and dependence, nicotine dependence, opiate abuse and dependence, and cocaine.

---

10. UW is a 49-year-old patient who suffered a myocardial infarction 5 days ago. Upon discharge, it was noted that UW appeared depressed. After a complete evaluation, UW met the criteria for diagnosis. Other past medical history includes hypertension, diabetes, and severe uncontrolled narrow angle glaucoma. Select the antidepressant that would be the most effective and safest pharmacotherapy option for UW.
    a. Elavil
    b. Effexor
    c. Zoloft
    d. a and b
    e. All of the above

Answer a is incorrect. Amitriptyline (Elavil) is a TCA antidepressant and should not be used in patients in acute recovery of myocardial infarction. TCAs have one of the most severe cardiovascular side effects of then antidepressants—conduction abnormalities.

Answer b is incorrect. Venlafaxine (Effexor) is an SNRI antidepressant and should not be used in patients with uncontrolled narrow angle glaucoma. Another venlafaxine side effect that may impact UW is the ability of venlafaxine to increase the blood pressure.

Answer c is correct. Sertraline (Zoloft) is an SSRI antidepressant and lacks significant cardiovascular side effects. SSRIs lack cardiovascular side effects because they are selective for serotonin. Inhibiting serotonin reuptake may lead to anxiety, insomnia, and sexual dysfunction.

Answers d and e are incorrect.

---

11. UW has fully recovered from his myocardial infarction and is feeling much better since initiation of his antidepressant 4 weeks ago. UW presents for a follow-up today and states that while he is happy with the results of antidepressant, he is concerned about his acquired sexual dysfunction. Select the antidepressant that would be *least* likely to cause sexual dysfunction.
    a. Wellbutrin
    b. Pamelor
    c. Prozac
    d. Cymbalta

Answer a is correct. Bupropion (Wellbutrin) is an aminoketone antidepressant that inhibits the reuptake of dopamine. This is a unique mechanism of action within the antidepressant class and is the least likely to cause sexual dysfunction.

Answer b is incorrect. Nortriptyline (Pamelor) is a TCA antidepressant that inhibits the reuptake of NE and 5-HT. 5-HT reuptake inhibition is associated with sexual dysfunction.

Answer c is incorrect. Fluoxetine (Proxac) is an SSRI antidepressant that inhibits the reuptake of 5-HT. 5-HT reuptake inhibition is associated with sexual dysfunction.

Answer d is incorrect. Duloxetine (Cymbalta) is an SSRI antidepressant that inhibits the reuptake of NE and 5-HT. 5-HT reuptake inhibition is associated with sexual dysfunction.

---

12. Select the medication property(ies) that is associated with tricyclic antidepressants.
    a. Pregnancy category B
    b. Causes orthostatic hypotension
    c. Inhibits reuptake of dopamine
    d. a and c
    e. All of the above

Answer a is incorrect. TCAs have a pregnancy category C.

Answer b is correct. TCAs may cause orthostatic hypotension; therefore patients need to be instructed about standing to quickly while receiving TCAs.

Answer c is incorrect. TCAs inhibit the reuptake of NE and 5-HT.

Answers d and e are incorrect.

13. TM is a 49-year-old patient diagnosed with major depression disorder. His past medical history is significant for alcohol-induced liver damage (patient has increased liver function tests), hypertension, and hyperlipidemia. Select the antidepressant that would be appropriate for TM.

    i. Nefazodone
    ii. Sertraline
    iii. Mirtazapine

    a. i and ii
    b. ii and iii
    c. i and iii
    d. i, ii, and iii

Nefazodone is a triazolopyridine that is associated with hepatic damage. Treatment should not be initiated in individuals with active liver disease or with elevated baseline serum transaminases.

Sertraline is an SSRI. SSRI has to undergo significant hepatic metabolism. Caution should be used with sertraline in patients with hepatic damage and a lower dose may be utilized, but the medication is not contraindicated in hepatic impairment.

Mirtazapine is a tetracyclic antidepressant. Mirtazipine undergoes significant hepatic metabolism and the clearance may be decreased by 30% in patients with hepatic damage, but the medication is not contraindicated in hepatic impairment.

Answers a, c, and d are incorrect.

Answer b is correct.

---

14. KG is a 44-year-old patient with a history of anorexia who has had several hospitalizations for anorexia because of severe weakness and electrolyte abnormalities. KG has been diagnosed with major depressive disorder. Select the antidepressant that may be utilized in KG.

    i. Wellbutrin
    ii. Paxil
    iii. Cymbalta

    a. i and ii
    b. ii and iii
    c. i and iii
    d. All of the above

Bupropion (Wellbutrin) has a dose-dependent risk of seizures and the risk is increased in patients with a history of seizures, anorexia/bulimia, head trauma, central nervous system tumor, severe hepatic cirrhosis, abrupt discontinuation of sedative-hypnotics or ethanol, medications that lower the seizure threshold (antipsychotics, theophylline, systemic steroids), stimulants, or hypoglycemic agents. Bupropion is contraindicated in patients with anorexia/bulimia because they are at increased risk for electrolyte abnormalities and therefore prone to a higher risk of seizures.

Answers a, c, and d are incorrect.

Answer b is correct.

---

15. Select the drug interaction(s) associated with TCA antidepressants.

    i. Alcohol
    ii. Antipsychotics
    iii. Meperidine

    a. i and ii
    b. ii and iii
    c. i and iii
    d. All of the above

Answers a, b, and c are correct.

Answer d is correct and the best answer. Alcohol exhibits a pharmacodynamic interaction (additive sedation) with TCAs. Antipsychotics exhibit a pharmacodynamic interaction (additive hypotension) with TCAs. Meperidine exhibits a pharmacodynamic interaction (serotonin syndrome) with TCAs.

---

16. BC is a 54-year-old patient diagnosed with major depressive disorder. BC is currently receiving the following medications: lisinopril for hyptertension and warfarin for a recent deep venous thrombosis. BC currently has an INR within range (INR = 2.5); however, the patient has had a difficult time achieving a goal INR level and has had elevated INRs in the past (most recent 14 days ago INR was 5.9). Select the antidepressant that would have the least impact on the activity of warfarin.

    a. Fluvoxamine
    b. Sertraline
    c. Fluoxetine
    d. Venlafaxine

Note: Warfarin (Coumadin) is a substrate of CYP1A2 (minor), 2C9 (major), 2C19 (minor), and 3A4 (minor). Warfarin is an inhibitor of CYP2C9 (moderate) and 2C19 (weak).

Answer a is incorrect. Fluvoxamine is a CYP450 inhibitor of 1A2 (strong), 2B6 (weak), 2C9 (weak), 2C19 (strong), 2D6 (weak), and 3A4 (weak). Since fluvoxamine is an inhibitor of 2C19, 1A2, 3A4, and 2C9 and warfarin is a substrate of the same isoenzymes, fluvoxamine could significantly increase the levels of warfarin.

Answer b is incorrect. Sertraline is a CYP450 inhibitor of 1A2 (weak), 2B6 (moderate), 2C8 (weak), 2C19 (moderate), 2D6 (moderate), and 3A4 (moderate). Since sertraline inhibits the CYP450 isoenzymes that warfarin is a substrate of, sertraline could significantly increase the levels of warfarin.

Answer c is incorrect. Fluoxetine is a CYP450 inhibitor of 1A2 (moderate), 2B6 (weak), 2C9 (weak), 2C19 (moderate), 2D6 (strong), and 3A4 (weak). Since fluoxetine inhibits the CYP450 isoenzymes that warfarin is a substrate of, fluoxetine could significantly increase the levels of warfarin.

Answer d is correct. Venlafaxine is CYP450 inhibitor of 2B6 (weak), 2D6 (weak), 3A4 (weak). Since venflaxine is a weak inhibitor of the CYP450 system and it lacks 2C inhibition, venlafaxine would be least likely to increase warfarin levels (however there would be a possibility and the INR should still be monitored).

---

17. BN is a patient with major depressive disorder currently taking a monoamine oxidase inhibitor. She has been experiencing major sinus pressure, headaches, and congestion. She approaches your pharmacy and asks if she can take a decongestant for the congestion. You inform her that she cannot take the decongestant with the MAOI because of a high incidence of what side effect.

   a. Serotonin syndrome
   b. Hypertensive crisis
   c. Orthostatic hypotension
   d. Sexual dysfunction

Answer a is incorrect. Serotonin syndrome is associated with concurrent use of MAOIs and serotonergic antidepressants, meperidine, dextromethorphan, and tramadol.

Answer b is correct. Hypertensive crisis is associated with concurrent use of MAOIs and sympathomimetics and tyramine-rich foods.

Answer c is incorrect. Orthostatic hypotension is a common side effect of antidepressants that have $alpha_1$ adrenergic receptor blockade.

Answer d is incorrect. Sexual dysfunction is a side effect of antidepressants that have activity on serotonin.

18. Select the drug interaction(s) associated with fluvoxamine.

   i. Verapamil
   ii. Carbamazepine
   iii. Lovastatin

   a. i and ii
   b. ii and iii
   c. i and iii
   d. All of the above

Note: Fluvoxamine is a CYP450 substrate of 1A2 (major) and 2D6 (major). Fluvoxamine is a CYP450 inhibitor of 1A2 (strong), 2B6 (weak), 2C9 (weak), 2C19 (strong), 2D6 (weak), and 3A4 (weak).

Verapamil is a CYP450 substrate of 1A2 (minor), 2B6 (minor), 2C9 (minor), 2C18 (minor), 2E1 (minor), and 3A4 (major). Verapamil is a CYP450 inhibitor of 1A2 (weak), 2C9 (weak), 2D6 (weak), and 3A4 (moderate). Fluvoxamine may increase levels of verapamil and slighty increase levels of fluvoxamine.

Carbamazepine is a CYP450 substrate of 2C8 (minor) and 3A4 (major). Carbamazepine is a CYP450 inducer of 1A2 (strong), 2B6 (strong), 2C8 (strong), 2C9 (strong), 2C19 (strong), 3A4 (strong). Fluvoxamine may slightly increase levels of carbamazepine, and carbamazepine will significantly decrease levels of fluvoxamine.

Lovastatin is a CYP450 substrate of 3A4 (major). Lovastatin is a CYP450 inhibitor of 2C9 (weak), 2D6 (weak), and 3A4 (weak). Fluvoxamine will slightly increase levels of lovastatin, and lovastatin will slightly increase levels of fluvoxamine.

Answers a, b, and c are correct.

Answer d is correct and the best answer.

19. Select the brand name of paroxetine.

   a. Paxil
   b. Zoloft
   c. Prozac
   d. Effexor

Answer a is correct. The brand name of paroxetine is Paxil.

Answer b is incorrect. The brand name sertraline is Zolft.

Answer c is incorrect. The brand name of fluoxetine is Prozac.

Answer d is incorrect. The brand name of venlafaxine is Effexor.

20. Select the generic name of Remeron.

   a. Duloxetine
   b. Amitriptyline
   c. Mirtazipine
   d. Trazodone

Answer a is incorrect. Duloxetine is the generic name for Cymbalta.

Answer b is incorrect. Amitriptyline is the generic name for Elavil.

Answer c is correct. Mirtazipine is the generic name of Remeron.

Answer d is incorrect. Trazodone is the generic name of Desyrel.

CHAPTER 54 | Bipolar Disorders

1. Which of the following is *not* a sign and symptom of a manic episode?

   a. Irritable mood
   b. Anhedonia
   c. Racing thoughts
   d. Psychomotor agitation
   e. Decreased need for sleep

Answer a is incorrect. Irritable mood is a symptom of mania. This may also be seen in a depressive episode, however.

Answer b is correct. Anhedonia is the inability to feel pleasure while engaging in pleasurable and enjoyable activities. This is often seen as one of the signs of major depressive disorder and not a manic episode.

Answer c is incorrect. Racing thoughts is a classic symptom of mania.

Answer d is incorrect. Psychomotor agitation is a symptom of mania. This may also be seen in a depressive episode, however.

Answer e is incorrect. Decreased need for sleep is a classic symptom of mania. Depressed patients will not report a decreased need for sleep; they wish to sleep but cannot. Manic patients in an acutely manic episode may not wish to sleep and would rather engage in goal-directed activities and stay awake.

---

2. Hypomania is characterized by:

   a. Multiple hospitalizations
   b. Psychotic episodes
   c. Impairment in social functioning
   d. Impairment in occupational functioning
   e. An inflated self-esteem

Answer a is incorrect. These patients are often able to function well; therefore they do not require hospitalization.

Answer b is incorrect. There is no psychosis (ie, auditory and visual hallucinations, delusions) involved in hypomanic states.

Answer c is incorrect. There is no impairment in social functioning.

Answer d is incorrect. There is no impairment in occupational functioning.

Answer e is correct. The symptoms of hypomania and mania are similar with respect to the target signs and symptoms. Hypomania is a less severe form of a manic episode. Inflated self-esteem can still be detected in hypomania.

---

3. Rapid cycling describes when a bipolar patient has ____ or more manic or depressive episodes within a __________ period.

   a. 2; 6-month
   b. 2; 1-year
   c. 3; 2-year
   d. 4; 1-year
   e. 4; 2-year

Answer a is incorrect. A 6-month period is not stated in the definition of rapid cycling.

Answer is b is incorrect. The correct number of episodes required in a 12-month period is four, not two.

Answer c is incorrect. A-2-year period is not stated in the definition of rapid cycling; it is 1 year.

Answer d is correct. Rapid cycling is a term to describe when a patient experiences four or more episodes of depression or mania within a 12-month period. Rapid cycling is a specified term used in the DSM-IV-TR to describe the course of recurrent episodes. This term is used to specify bipolar disorder I and II but not depressive disorders such as major depressive disorder.

Answer e is incorrect. A-2-year period is not stated in the definition of rapid cycling; it is 1 year.

---

4. In treating patients with bipolar disorder, which medications are used either as monotherapy or in combination with other agents?

   i. Lithium
   ii. Aripiprazole
   iii. Lamotrigine
   iv. Citalopram

   a. i only
   b. i and iii only
   c. i and iv only
   d. i, iii, and iv only
   e. i, ii, iii, and iv

Answer a is incorrect. Clearly, lithium is the classic mood stabilizer that is often combined with multiple agents to stabilize mood.

Answer b is incorrect. Lamotrigine is FDA approved for bipolar disorder I and is often used as an alternative to lithium for bipolar depressive episodes and may be combined with other agents.

Answer c is incorrect. Citalopram is an SSRI that may be used in conjunction with a mood stabilizer (lithium, divalproex sodium, or an atypical antipsychotic agent) for the bipolar depressive episode if lithium or lamotrigine is not used. Although citalopram should not be used as monotherapy in bipolar depression, it may be used as a combination treatment with an agent that will prevent manic episodes.

Answer d is incorrect. Combination therapies are not limited to lithium, lamotrigine and citalopram. See explanation for e below.

Answer e is correct. Aripiprazole is an atypical antipsychotic agent that is FDA-approved for the treatment of acute mania as well as maintenance treatment in bipolar disorder. All of these agents can be used either as monotherapy (lithium, lamotrigine, aripiprazole) or in combination (citalopram) for bipolar disorder, depending on the mood episode being treated.

---

5. Which of the following is a common adverse drug reaction of lithium?

   a. Alopecia
   b. Increased urination
   c. Hyperammonemia
   d. Hyperthyroidism
   e. Diplopia

Answer a is incorrect. Alopecia is associated with valproate.

Answer b is correct. Lithium causes polyuria, which is a manifestation of nephrogenic diabetes insipidus. It also causes associated polydipsia, increased thirst.

Answer c is incorrect. Hyperammonemia is associated with valproate.

Answer d is incorrect. Lithium is clearly associated with causing hypothyroidism, not hyperthyroidism; although there have been few paradoxical reports of hyperthyroidism and lithium.

Answer e is incorrect. Diplopia has been associated with carbamazepine.

---

6. What is the recommended starting dose of lithium?

   a. 300 mg tid
   b. 15 mg qhs
   c. 200 mg bid
   d. 500 mg bid
   e. 50 mg everyday

Answer a is correct. The recommended starting dose is 300 mg tid or less, depending on the patient's age and weight.

Answer b is incorrect. The recommended starting doses of 15 mg qhs is associated with olanzapine.

Answer c is incorrect. 200 mg bid is associated with carbamazepine.

Answer d is incorrect. 500 mg bid is a good starting dose for divalproex sodium.

Answer e is incorrect. 50 mg qd is a starting dose of lamotrigine if taken with carbamazepine.

---

7. The teratogenicity associated with lithium use in the first trimester of pregnancy is:

   a. Cardiovascular
   b. Renal
   c. Hepatic
   d. Neuromuscular
   e. Dermatological

Answer a is correct. Lithium is associated with causing Ebstein anomaly, a cardiac abnormality. This is a condition in which the tricuspid valve is abnormal with secondary dilation of the right ventricular outflow tract.

Answer b is incorrect. Lithium can cause renal impairment to the person using lithium, but there is no association of renal-related birth defects in the newborn.

Answer c is incorrect. Lithium is not associated with causing liver damage.

Answer d is incorrect. Carbamazepine and valproate are associated with causing spina bifida in pregnancy use.

Answer e is incorrect. Lithium can cause rash to the person taking it, but this would not be a teratogenic effect.

---

8. Which of the following is *not* something you would counsel to your lithium-user patient?

   a. "You should avoid dehydration, so maintain your water intake."
   b. "Stop your medication if you experience persistent diarrhea."
   c. "Use caution while operating machinery or driving a car."
   d. "Ask your pharmacist before starting any new pain medications."
   e. "You should reduce your sodium intake while taking lithium."

Answer a is incorrect. This should be counseled to patients. Patients should maintain consistent levels of any caffeine intake and stay hydrated to avoid changes in lithium blood concentrations.

Answer b is incorrect. This should be counseled to patients. Although diarrhea is an expected adverse reaction of lithium, persistent diarrhea may be a sign of lithium toxicity. Patients are instructed to stop the lithium and call their doctor right away. The lithium dose may be stopped for 1 day until lithium blood levels can be obtained.

Answer c is incorrect. This should be counseled to patients. Lithium can cause fatigue and sedation, therefore, as with any CNS-depressant medication, patients must be warned about lithium possibly impairing their ability to perform activities requiring mental alertness or intact physical coordination. These include operating machinery or driving a motor vehicle.

Answer d is incorrect. This should be counseled to patients. Patients taking lithium need caution about starting new pain medications such as ibuprofen or other NSAIDs that will increase the lithium blood concentration. Patients taking lithium may take sulindac (Clinoril), an NSAID that does not appear to increase lithium levels, aspirin, or acetaminophen.

Answer e is correct. This should *not* be counseled to patients. While on lithium, sodium intake should be maintained at consistent levels and not necessarily reduced. Reducing sodium intake may lead to lithium retention and higher blood concentrations which may lead to toxicity.

---

9. What is the target therapeutic concentration of a patient taking lithium for 3 years?

   a. 4 to 12 μg/mL
   b. 4 to 12 mEq/L
   c. 50 to 125 μg/mL
   d. 0.6 to 0.8 mEq/L
   e. 1 to 1.8 mEq/L

Answer a is incorrect. Levels of 4 to 12 μg/mL is associated with carbamazepine's target blood concentration in order to avoid toxicity.

Answer b is incorrect. The units are correct but the number value is incorrect. Levels >1.5 mEq/L is associated with toxicity; therefore, no patient will be maintained higher than 1.5 mEq/L.

Answer c is incorrect. Levels of 50 to 125 μg/mL is associated with valproate target concentrations.

Answer d is correct. Three years of being on lithium is considered maintenance treatment, not acute treatment. Lithium is a cation; therefore the units are in mmol/L or milliequivalents per liter (mEq/L). Levels for maintenance treatment of lithium are generally between 0.6 and 0.8 mEq/L; however, it is suggested that for bipolar depressive episode treatment, higher levels may be needed. Some sources reference 0.6 to 1.0 mEq/L as the target level range.

Answer e is incorrect. Levels >1.5 mEq/L is associated with toxicity; therefore, no patient will be maintained higher than 1.5 mEq/L.

---

10. Your 42-year-old patient is on several medications and reports the following:
 Aleve (naproxen sodium) 1 tablet twice daily for back pain when working, Motrin (ibuprofen) 400 mg 1 tablet every 8 hours as need for headache occurring three times per month, Cozaar (losartan) 50 mg 1 tablet bid, Glucophage (metformin) 850 mg 1 tablet bid. The patient smokes six to seven cigarettes per day, drinks alcohol occasionally, and has one to two cups of coffee every morning except Fridays and Saturdays.
 Which of the following factors can affect the level of lithium when he draws his blood at the next clinic visit?
 i. Aleve
 ii. Cozaar
 iii. Glucophage
 iv. Smoking
 v. Alcohol
 vi. Coffee
 a. ii and vi only
 b. ii and iii only
 c. i, ii, and vi only
 d. i and v only
 e. iv, v, and vi only

Answer a is incorrect. The choices are not limited to Cozaar and coffee (caffeine).

Answer b is incorrect. Glucophage is metformin and no drug interaction has been reported with lithium.

Answer c is correct. Aleve (Naproxen sodium) is an over-the-counter NSAID that can increase lithium blood concentrations. Motrin is also implicated in this drug interaction. NSAIDs (except sulindac) decrease the renal clearance of lithium. Cozaar (losartan) is an angiotensin-II receptor antagonist that is also associated with increasing lithium. Caffeine will increase the elimination of lithium and may decrease lithium concentrations by 20%. All three of these factors can affect the level of lithium when the patient goes in to draw his blood at the next clinic visit.

Answer d is incorrect. Alcohol does not directly affect lithium concentrations.

Answer e is incorrect. Smoking does not directly affect lithium concentrations. Lithium is not metabolized by CYP450 liver isoenzymes; therefore smoking will not affect the elimination of lithium.

---

11. The physician wants to know what extended-release preparations of lithium are available, if any. You advise that the prescription be written for:
 a. Lithium citrate
 b. Lithium carbonate tablets
 c. Lithium carbonate capsules
 d. Eskalith
 e. Lithobid

Answer a is incorrect. Lithium citrate is the oral solution dosage form containing 8 mEq of lithium per teaspoon.

Answer b is incorrect. Lithium carbonate tablets or capsules and Eskalith are all the same regular release products.

Answer c is incorrect. Lithium carbonate tablets or capsules and Eskalith are all the same regular release products.

Answer d is incorrect. If the prescription were written for Eskalith CR specifically, this is an extended-release product.

Answer e is correct. Lithobid is an extended-release, film-coated tablet.

---

12. Which of the following is *not* a required laboratory monitoring parameter for patients taking lithium?
 a. Serum creatinine
 b. Electrocardiogram
 c. Thyroid function tests
 d. Liver enzyme tests
 e. Electrolytes

Answer a is incorrect. Serum creatinine (Scr) as well as BUN are markers of kidney function. These should be monitored in all lithium patients because lithium is cleared via the kidneys. Lithium can also cause renal impairment.

Answer b is incorrect. An electrocardiogram (ECG) is recommended in patients who are already predisposed to cardiovascular disease and for those over the age of 40. Lithium can cause cardiac conduction abnormalities and worsen cardiac disease.

Answer c is incorrect. Hyperthyroidism can mimic manic states. This should be ruled out before a diagnosis of bipolar disorder is made. Moreover, lithium can cause hypothyroidism with long-term use, necessitating levothyroxine treatment.

Answer d is correct. Lithium is not metabolized by the liver; it is cleared almost exclusively by the kidneys.

Answer e is incorrect. Electrolytes should be monitored because hyponatremic (low sodium) states can increase the risk of higher blood concentrations of lithium, and therefore lithium toxicity. Hyperkalemic (high potassium) can increase the risk of lithium-induced cardiac adverse events.

13. Polycystic ovary syndrome (PCOS) has been associated with which of the following medications?

a. Aripiprazole
b. Divalproex sodium
c. Lithium
d. Lamotrigine
e. Olanzapine

Answer a is incorrect. The atypical antipsychotic, aripiprazole and others, have not been associated with PCOS.

Answer b is correct. Divalproex sodium (valproate) is associated with causing polycystic ovaries in women.

Answer c is incorrect. There is no clear relationship between lithium and PCOS.

Answer d is incorrect. There is no clear relationship between lamotrigine and PCOS.

Answer e is incorrect. The atypical antipsychotic, olanzapine and others, have not been associated with PCOS.

---

14. What is the recommended loading dose of Depakote (in kg/d) for a patient who has just been admitted into the psychiatry emergency department for an acute manic episode?

a. 5 mg
b. 10 to 15 mg
c. 20 to 30 mg
d. 40 mg
e. 50 to 55 mg

Answer a is incorrect. This is not the recommend loading dose for Depakote. It is much too low.

Answer b is incorrect. This is not the recommend loading dose for Depakote. It is too low.

Answer c is correct. The recommended loading dose of divalproex sodium (Depakote) in inpatient settings for acute mania is 20 to 30 mg/kg/d in divided oral doses. The dose is usually divided into 2 to 3 doses if the calculated loading dose exceeds 2 g/d to improve tolerability.

Answer d is incorrect. This is not the recommend loading dose for Depakote. It is too high.

Answer e is incorrect. This is not the recommend loading dose for Depakote. It is much too high.

---

15. Your bipolar patient is concerned about using certain medications for her psychiatric condition. She heard that there are some medications associated with causing a neural tube defect if taken during pregnancy. You confirm her suspicion and tell her that there are some agents associated with causing this condition in the newborn when used by the mother during pregnancy. You list the following agent(s):

i. Lithium
ii. Divalproex sodium
iii. Carbamazepine
iv. Olanzapine
v. Risperidone

a. i only
b. i and ii only
c. ii and iii only
d. ii and iv only
e. iv and v only

Answer a is incorrect. Lithium is associated mainly with causing rare instances of Ebstein anomaly.

Answer b is incorrect. Valproate is associated with spina bifida, but lithium is not.

Answer c is correct. Valproate (1%-2% risk) and carbamazepine (0.5%-1% risk) are associated with causing spina bifida, a neural tube defect, when used during pregnancy.

Answer d is incorrect. To date, the atypical antipsychotics have not been associated with causing any significantly greater structural birth defects compared to controls. Olanzapine has been reported as used during pregnancy without causing spina bifida.

Answer e is incorrect. To date, the atypical antipsychotics have not been associated with causing any significantly greater structural birth defects compared to controls. Risperidone has been reported as used during pregnancy without causing spina bifida.

---

16. It is recommended that the human leukocyte antigen type B, HLA-B*1502, allele is genotyped in Asian patients prior to taking:

a. Lithium
b. Carbamazepine
c. Lorazepam
d. Haloperidol
e. Quetiapine

Answer a is incorrect. There is no genetic marker linked with the rash induced by lithium.

Answer b is correct. Carbamazepine is associated with causing Stevens-Johnson syndrome (SJS) and toxic epidermal necrolysis (TEN), two potentially fatal dermatologic reactions. The allelic variation of the *HLA-B gene*, *HLA-B*1502*, is associated with these serious dermatologic reactions and it is recommended by the manufacturer that patient who are of ancestry in genetically at-risk populations be screened for the presence of this genetic marker. All medications can potentially cause a rash; however, there is a target genetic maker that has been linked specifically to carbamazepine. When a rash is seen with the use lamotrigine, the medication should be discontinued.

Answer c is incorrect. There is no genetic marker linked with the rash induced by lorazepam.

Answer d is incorrect. There is no genetic marker linked with the rash induced by haloperidol.

Answer e is incorrect. There is no genetic marker linked with the rash induced by quetiapine.

---

17. You discover that your bipolar patient in the hospital ward is "cheeking" his medication for the past 4 days. You decide to recommend the same medication in an orally disintegrating tablet (ODT) formulation. Which of the following medications is available in this dosage form?

    a. Carbamazepine
    b. Haloperidol
    c. Lithium
    d. Quetiapine
    e. Risperidone

Answer a is incorrect. Carbamazepine is available in an oral suspension, another viable dosage form options for "cheekers."

Answer b is incorrect. Haloperidol is available in an oral solution, which is another viable dosage form option for "cheekers."

Answer c is incorrect. Lithium is available in an oral solution, which is another viable dosage form option for "cheekers."

Answer d is incorrect. The only currently available dosage form of quetiapine is in a hard tablet formulation that must be swallowed.

Answer e is correct. Risperidone is available in Risperdal-M Tab, an orally disintegrating tablet dosage formulation. The other atypical antipsychotics available in an ODT include olanzapine (Zyprexa Zydis) and aripiprazole (Abilify Discmelt). These are good alternatives to regular tablets in instances where the patient has difficulty swallowing or is suspected of cheeking his/her medication (ie, pretending to swallow the medication when in fact the patient is holding the medication between the gums of the teeth and cheek, only to later dispose of it in order to avoid taking the medication).

---

18. Which of the following factors is *not* likely to increase the risk of lamotrigine-related rash?

    a. Coadministration with another anticonvulsant, valproate
    b. Coadministration with another anticonvulsant, carbamazepine
    c. Exceeding the recommended initial dose of lamotrigine
    d. Exceeding the recommended maximum dose of lamotrigine
    e. Exceeding the recommended dose escalation schedule of lamotrigine

---

Answer a is incorrect. This *will* increase the risk of rash. Valproate is known to increase lamotrigine almost double. Caution is advised when coadministering valproate and lamotrigine; their concomitant use is not contraindicated; rather, the dose of lamotrigine should be halved when used together.

Answer b is correct. Coadministration with carbamazepine, a drug inducer, is likely to decrease the lamotrigine levels, and not increase it. With lower lamotrigine blood levels, there is a lower risk of rash.

Answer c is incorrect. This *will* increase the risk of rash.

Answer d is incorrect. This *will* increase the risk of rash.

Answer e is incorrect. This *will* increase the risk of rash. Following the careful and slow dose escalation recommendations of lamotrigine has resulted in fewer incidences of rash.

---

19. The psychiatric treatment team decides to start Risperdal Consta on a patient who has a history of nonadherence to his mood stabilizer for bipolar disorder for the past 6 years. They ask you, the clinical pharmacist, for the recommended starting dose and directions for administration. You reply with the following:

    a. 2 mg tablet, 1 tab po bid
    b. 3 mg ODT, 1 tab on top of the tongue everyday
    c. 25 mg SQ every 2 weeks
    d. 25 mg IM every 2 weeks
    e. 50 mg IM every 2 weeks

Answer a is incorrect. This is an oral dosage formulation, not the long-acting injection formulation.

Answer b is incorrect. This is still an oral dosage formulation, not the long-acting injection formulation. ODT is the orally disintegrating tablet placed on top of the tongue with dry hands.

Answer c is incorrect. Consta is administered intramuscularly (IM), not subcutaneously (SQ).

Answer d is correct. Consta is the long-acting injection formulation of risperidone. This dosage formulation is currently FDA-approved for monotherapy or adjunctive therapy to lithium or valproate for the maintenance treatment of bipolar I disorder. The recommended starting dose is usually 25 mg. A higher dose of 37.5 mg may be started if the patient was currently stable on a higher oral dose.

Answer e is incorrect. It is not recommended to start with a high dose of 50 mg. The dose can eventually be increased to 50 mg, however, over time.

---

20. Which agent is the safest option for treating a pregnant female with acute bipolar mania?

    a. Carbamazepine
    b. Chlorpromazine
    c. Haloperidol
    d. Lithium
    e. Valproic acid

Answer a is incorrect. As one of the three classic mood stabilizers, carbamazepine is generally considered unsafe to use during pregnancy, especially during the first trimester. It is pregnancy category D, meaning that there is evidence for risk to the fetus associated with their use. However, if used, CBZ should be used with caution and careful monitoring and concomitant administration of 4 to 5 mg/d of folic acid is recommended.

Answer b is incorrect. Low-potency antipsychotics, such as chlorpromazine (Thorazine) should generally be avoided during pregnancy.

Answer c is correct. Pregnancy issues in bipolar disorder are complicated. The safest, established treatment option is a high-potency antipsychotic agent such as haloperidol.

Answer d is incorrect. As one of the three classic mood stabilizers, lithium is usually avoided during pregnancy, especially during the first trimester. During the first trimester, there is a greater risk of cardiac-related teratogenicity. Lithium is pregnancy category D, meaning that there is evidence for risk to the fetus associated with its use. However, if lithium is to be used, caution with dosing and careful monitoring is advised.

Answer e is incorrect. The three classic mood stabilizers, lithium, carbamazepine, and divalproex sodium/valproic acid, are not safe to use during pregnancy, especially during the first trimester. They are all pregnancy category D, meaning that there is evidence for risk to the fetus associated with their use. Depakote has been associated with causing spina bifida. However, if VPA is to be used, concomitant administration of 4 to 5 mg/d of folic acid is recommended.

---

21. Symbyax is a product that contains the following agents for treating bipolar depression:

    a. Lithium + divalproex sodium
    b. Risperidone + fluoxetine
    c. Olanzapine + fluoxetine
    d. Risperidone + sertraline
    e. Olanzapine + sertraline

Answer a is incorrect. There is no such combination product commercially available containing these classic moods stabilizers, although they can be used together.

Answer b is incorrect. This antipsychotic and antidepressant combination is incorrect.

Answer c is correct. Symbyax is a combination product whose only indication is bipolar depression. It contains one atypical antipsychotic, olanzapine, plus one SSRI antidepressant, fluoxetine. The active ingredients include olanzapine and fluoxetine in the following milligram ratios: 3/25, 6/25, 6/50, 12/25, and 12/50. Patients are instructed to take it at bedtime: olanzapine is sedating and fluoxetine is activating. There are no other similar combination products currently available.

Answer d is incorrect. This antipsychotic and antidepressant combination is incorrect.

Answer e is incorrect. This antipsychotic and antidepressant (sertraline) combination is incorrect.

---

22. Which antidepressant is most likely to cause a switch into mania when used in a patient with bipolar disorder?

    a. Amitriptyline
    b. Bupropion
    c. Citalopram
    d. Escitalopram
    e. Sertraline

Answer a is correct. Amitriptyline is the only agent on this list that is classified as a tricyclic antidepressant (TCA). TCAs have classically been reported to be the class of antidepressants most likely to cause a switch to mania in bipolar patients.

Answer b is incorrect. Bupropion is a dopamine and norepinephrine reuptake inhibitor that is less likely to cause a switch into mania.

Answer c is incorrect. SSRIs, as a class, have a low probability of causing treatment-emergent mania. SSRIs include citalopram (Celexa), escitalopram, fluoxetine, fluvoxamine, paroxetine, and sertraline. The SSRIs are some of the most commonly used antidepressants in treating bipolar depression and are believed to be less likely to cause drug-induced mania.

Answer d is incorrect. SSRIs, as a class, have a low probability of causing treatment-emergent mania. Escitalopram (Lexapro) is an SSRI.

Answer e is incorrect. SSRIs, as a class, have a low probability of causing treatment-emergent mania. Sertraline (Zoloft) is an SSRI.

---

23. Which of the following medication classes have *not* been used to stabilize a patient's mood in bipolar disorder?

    a. ACE-Inhibitors
    b. Anticonvulsants

c. Antidepressants
d. Antipsychotics
e. Calcium channel blockers

Answer a is correct. ACE inhibitors have no role in mood stabilization for bipolar disorders treatment.

Answer b is incorrect. Anticonvulsants such as carbamazepine, valproate, and lamotrigine are FDA approved for bipolar disorder treatment.

Answer c is incorrect. Although not FDA approved for bipolar depression (except the combination product Symbyax that contains fluoxetine), antidepressants are often used in combination therapy for bipolar depression.

Answer d is incorrect. All of the atypical antipsychotics (except clozapine) are FDA approved for various bipolar disorder mood episodes. Both oral and parenteral preparations are approved for use in bipolar disorder.

Answer e is incorrect. Although not commonly used, calcium channel blockers (ie, verapamil) have demonstrated mood stabilizing properties, especially for acute mania.

---

24. Which agent is effective for the treatment of bipolar I disorder, and may be more effective than lithium for bipolar depression?

a. Dilantin
b. Lamictal
c. Lamisil
d. Neurontin
e. Trileptal

Answer a is incorrect. Dilantin (phenytoin) is an anticonvulsant that has shown some mood-stabilizing properties, but it not widely used for bipolar disorders treatment.

Answer b is correct. Lamictal is lamotrigine, an anticonvulsant that is FDA approved for the treatment of bipolar I disorder. Where lithium may be more effective for manic episodes in bipolar disorder, there is evidence that lamotrigine may be more effective for the depressive phase.

Answer c is incorrect. Lamisil is terbinafine, an antifungal agent. Do not confuse medications that sound and look like each other.

Answer d is incorrect. Neurontin (gabapentin) is an anticonvulsant that has shown some efficacy for mood stabilization. It has not been shown to be more effective than lithium, however. It may be used as adjunctive treatment.

Answer e is incorrect. Trileptal (oxcarbazepine) is an anticonvulsant that may be used as a tertiary agent if other mood stabilizers fail to control mood. Currently, it is not FDA approved for the treatment of mood disorders. It is associated with causing hyponatremia.

CHAPTER 55 | Anxiety Disorders

1. Buspirone is most likely used in the treatment of which anxiety disorder?

a. Generalized anxiety disorder
b. Obsessive-compulsive disorder
c. Panic disorder
d. Post-traumatic stress disorder
e. Social anxiety disorder

Answer a is correct. Buspirone is only FDA indicated for use in generalized anxiety disorder. While it may be used as off-label for other anxiety disorders (Answers b, c, d, and e), Buspirone should be first or second line for generalized anxiety disorder.

---

2. Which of the following benzodiazepines has the longest duration of action at steady state?

a. Alprazolam
b. Clonazepam
c. Diazepam
d. Triazolam
e. Lorazepam

Answers a and b are incorrect. They have the shortest half-lives and do not have significant metabolites.

Answers d and e are incorrect. They have intermediate length for duration.

Answer c is correct. Diazepam has numerous metabolites which extend the half-life when administered in multiple doses.

---

3. Which of the following antidepressants is the most appropriate initial treatment for social anxiety disorder?

a. Fluvoxamine
b. Mirtazapine
c. Nefazodone
d. Trazodone
e. Venlafaxine

Answer a is incorrect. Fluvoxamine is indicated for use in obsessive-compulsive disorder.

Answers b, c, and d are incorrect. There is little evidence that they are effective as first or second line for use in social anxiety disorder.

Answer e is correct. Venlafaxine is FDA-indicated for use in social anxiety disorder and can be used in first line.

---

4. The most significant concern for patients with panic disorder starting an antidepressant is:

a. Anxiety
b. Bruxism

c. Gastrointestinal upset
d. Headache
e. Sexual dysfunction

Answer a is correct. In patients with panic disorder, initiating a new antidepressant can sometimes increase anxiety and precipitate a panic attack.

Answers b, c, d, and e are incorrect. They are not necessarily worsened significantly in patients with panic disorder compared to patients with other anxiety disorders or other mood conditions.

5. The generic name for Cymbalta is:
   a. Duloxetine
   b. Escitalopram
   c. Nefazodone
   d. Trazodone
   e. Venlafaxine

Answer a is correct. The brand names for answers b, c, d, and e are Lexapro, Serzone, Desyrel, and Effexor, respectively.

6. Which of the following medications is most effective for obsessive-compulsive disorder?
   a. Buspirone
   b. Clomipramine
   c. Clonazepam
   d. Nefazodone
   e. Venlafaxine

Answer a is incorrect. Buspirone is most effective for generalized anxiety disorder.

Answer b is correct. Clomipramine is as effective, and potentially more effective, than fluvoxamine for obsessive-compulsive disorder.

Answer c is incorrect. Clonazepam, while effective for many anxiety disorders, has been most studied for use in panic disorder.

Answer d is incorrect. Nefazodone has not been shown to be more effective than SSRIs for obsessive-compulsive disorder.

Answer e is incorrect. Venlafaxine is effective for use in generalized anxiety disorder and social anxiety disorder.

7. For the treatment of anxiety disorders, which of the following is an advantage of an SSRI compared to a tricyclic antidepressant?
   a. Safer in overdose
   b. Less likely to cause sedation
   c. Can treat comorbid depression
   d. Less likely to cause gastrointestinal upset
   e. Less likely to cause insomnia

Answer a is correct. SSRIs are not associated with significant toxicity in overdose situations.

Answer b is incorrect. SSRIs have been shown to cause weight gain similar to TCAs.

Answer c is incorrect. SSRIs and TCAs can both treat comorbid depression effectively.

Answers d and e are incorrect. One of the most common adverse effects of SSRIs is gastrointestinal upset and CNS effects (insomnia or sedation).

8. The SSRIs are effective for treating which of the following anxiety disorders?
   a. Generalized anxiety disorder
   b. Obsessive compulsive disorder
   c. Post-traumatic stress disorder
   d. Panic disorder
   e. All of the above

Answer e is correct. SSRIs are effective for treating all of the anxiety disorders.

9. Patients with significant impairment in liver function may receive which of the following benzodiazepines to minimize risk of adverse effects?
   a. Alprazolam, clonazepam, estazolam
   b. Chlordiazepoxide, clorazepate, diazepam
   c. Lorazepam, oxazepam, temazepam
   d. Lorazepam, clonazepam, triazolam
   e. Diazepam, clonazepam, lorazepam

Answers a and b are incorrect. All of the benzodiazepines listed are metabolized by oxidative metabolism and are influenced by impaired hepatic function.

Answer c is correct. Lorazepam, oxazepam, and temazepam are metabolized by glucuronidation pathway and are not affected by impaired hepatic function.

Answers d and e are incorrect because of the metabolism of clonazepam, triazolam, and diazepam.

10. The most significant dose-related adverse effect of venlafaxine is:
   a. Sedation
   b. Seizures
   c. Hypertension
   d. Hepatotoxicity
   e. Renal dysfunction

Answer a is incorrect. Sedation is not a dose-related effect of venlafaxine.

Answer b is incorrect. Seizures are not increased with venlafaxine at higher doses.

Answer c is correct. At higher doses (>150 mg/d), venlafaxine has been associated with increased blood pressure.

Answers d and e are incorrect. Liver and renal functions are not impacted in a dose-dependent manner with venlafaxine.

---

11. Valproic acid is used to treat irritability and impulse control in patients with which anxiety disorder?
    a. Panic disorder
    b. Generalized anxiety disorder
    c. Social anxiety disorder
    d. Obsessive-compulsive disorder
    e. Post-traumatic stress disorder

Answers a, b, and c are incorrect. Irritability and impulse control are generally not common features of panic disorder, generalized anxiety disorder or social anxiety disorder and valproic acid would be of little benefit in these conditions.

Answer d is incorrect. Valproic acid has not been shown to be effective in patients with obsessive-compulsive disorder.

Answer e is correct. Anticonvulsants are used frequently as adjunctive agents in post-traumatic stress disorder to treat irritability, anger, and impulse control symptoms.

---

12. Alprazolam is most likely to have a significant drug–drug interaction with which of the following medications?
    a. Citalopram
    b. Carbamazepine
    c. Paroxetine
    d. Phenytoin
    e. Warfarin

Answer a is incorrect. Citalopram does not have significant CYP3A4 enzyme- inhibitory or inducing effects.

Answer b is correct. Carbamazepine is a potent CYP3A4 inducer and can decrease the effects of alprazolam (a CYP3A4 substrate).

Answer c is incorrect. Paroxetine has potent CYP2D6-inhibitory effects, not CYP3A4.

Answer d is incorrect. Phenytoin is a potent CYP2C9/CYP2C19 inducer and does not significantly affect alprazolam metabolism.

Answer e is incorrect. Warfarin does not have significant interactions with alprazolam.

---

13. Which of the following medications has the highest risk for withdrawal symptoms?
    a. Clonazepam
    b. Diazepam
    c. Lorazepam
    d. Midazolam
    e. Triazolam

Answers a, b, c, and d are incorrect. The half-lives of citalopram, diazepam, fluoxetine, and lorazepam are adequate to prevent significant withdrawal effects when stopped abruptly.

Answer e is correct. Triazolam has a very short half-life and is associated with significant withdrawal symptoms if discontinued abruptly.

---

14. The mechanism of action of buspirone is:
    a. Selective serotonin reuptake inhibitor
    b. Serotonin and norepinephrine reuptake inhibitor
    c. Dopamine 2A partial agonist
    d. Serotonin 1A partial agonist
    e. Serotonin and dopamine antagonist

Answers a, b, c, and e are incorrect. Buspirone works primarily by acting as a serotonin 1A partial agonist.

Answer d is correct.

---

15. JK is a 38-year-old man with panic disorder who needs treatment. He has also recently completed an alcohol detoxification program. Which of the following treatment is most appropriate for JK?
    a. Alprazolam
    b. Diazepam
    c. Imipramine
    d. Phenelzine
    e. Sertraline

Answer a is incorrect. While alprazolam is effective in the treatment of panic disorder, benzodiazepines are not ideal for use in patients with a history of substance abuse.

Answer b is incorrect. Diazepam is rarely used long term for panic disorder and also it is a benzodiazepine.

Answer c is incorrect. While imipramine has been well studied for use in panic disorder, it is not the most well-tolerated medication compared to SSRIs. Also, the risk of seizures with TCAs is also of concern in a patient with a history of substance abuse.

Answer d is incorrect. Monoamine oxidase inhibitors should be considered as last line for use in panic disorder.

Answer e is correct. Sertraline is very effective in panic disorder, is very safe in patients with history of substance abuse and is well tolerated.

---

16. Which of the following nonpharmacologic treatments are effective for treating most anxiety disorders?
    a. Cognitive-behavioral therapy
    b. Dialectical behavior therapy
    c. Exposure therapy
    d. Hypnotic therapy
    e. Interpersonal therapy

Answer a is correct. Cognitive-behavioral therapy has the most evidence for its effectiveness in treating a variety of anxiety disorders compared to other types of therapy.

Answer b is incorrect. Dialectical behavior therapy has been most studied for use in borderline personality disorder.

Answer c is incorrect. Exposure therapy is most widely used for treatment of phobic disorders.

Answers d and e are incorrect. Their effectiveness in most anxiety disorders has been limited.

17. A 32-year-old pregnant woman in her first trimester presents with worsening of her OCD symptoms. Due to the potential risk of her compulsive behaviors on her fetus, she has agreed to start pharmacologic treatment. Which of the following agents should be avoided?

    a. Citalopram
    b. Fluoxetine
    c. Fluvoxamine
    d. Paroxetine
    e. Sertraline

Answers a, b, c, and e are incorrect. They can be used safely in first trimester without significant risk of causing fetal harm.

Answer d is correct. Paroxetine has been associated with cardiac malformations in the fetus when the drug is administered in the first trimester. It is labeled as a pregnancy category D while the other SSRIs are in pregnancy category C.

18. Which of the following medications has the lowest risk of causing serotonin syndrome when combined with sertraline?

    a. Clonazepam
    b. Fluoxetine
    c. Imipramine
    d. Phenelzine
    e. Venlafaxine

Answers a, c, d and e are incorrect. All of these drugs can increase the levels of serotonin and potentially increase the likelihood of serotonin syndrome when combined with an SSRI like sertraline.

Answer b is correct. Clonazepam is a benzodiazepine and does not have serotonergic properties.

19. The brand name for escitalopram is:

    a. Celexa
    b. Effexor
    c. Lexapro
    d. Paxil
    e. Zoloft

Answer c is correct. The brand name of escitalopram is Lexapro.

Answers a, b, d, and e are incorrect. The generic names for Celexa, Effexor, Paxil, and Zoloft are citalopram, venlafaxine, paroxetine, and sertraline, respectively.

20. Benzodiazepines should be avoided in pregnant women during the first trimester due to the risk of:

    a. Cleft palate
    b. Heart defects
    c. Limb abnormalities
    d. Pulmonary hypertension
    e. Renal defects

Answers b, c, d and e are incorrect.

Answer a is correct. Benzodiazepines have been associated with cleft lip or cleft palate in the fetus when administered during first trimester.

CHAPTER 56 | Schizophrenia

1. Which of the following symptoms are associated with schizophrenia?

    a. Tangentiality and disorganized speech
    b. Flat affect and alogia
    c. Impaired memory and attention
    d. All of the above

Answer a is correct. It describes positive symptoms associated with schizophrenia. Positive symptoms are symptoms which are "added" to normal functions. Positive symptoms commonly refer to hallucinations or delusions; however, there are also other positive symptoms which may be displayed by patients with schizophrenia. Disorganized speech in addition to tangential thoughts or tangential speech are other examples of positive symptoms.

Answer b is correct. It describes negative symptoms associated with schizophrenia. Negative symptoms are symptoms which are "loss" of normal functions. Alogia, which is a poverty of speech, is a negative symptom. Patients who present with a flat affect are unable to express emotion, which is also considered as a negative symptom. Avolition and anhedonia are other examples of negative symptoms.

Answer c is correct. It describes cognitive symptoms associated with schizophrenia. Impaired memory and attention are two common examples of cognitive symptoms that patients with schizophrenia may experience.

Answer d is correct and the best answer. All of the above symptoms are associated with schizophrenia.

2. Which of the following is an accepted and reliable method of diagnosing a patient with schizophrenia?
   a. Diagnosis can be confirmed by laboratory measure such as a blood test.
   b. Diagnosis can be confirmed if the patient meets the Diagnostic and Statistical Manual-IV (DSM-IV) criteria for schizophrenia.
   c. Diagnosis can be confirmed by conducting a brain imaging study on the patient.
   d. All of the above.

Answer a is incorrect. Currently there are no laboratory measures that can be used to detect or confirm schizophrenia.

Answer b is correct. Using the DSM-IV criteria for diagnosing schizophrenia is the most reliable method of diagnosing patients with schizophrenia. In order for a patient to be diagnosed with schizophrenia, the patient must meet the diagnostic criteria stated in the DSM-IV.

Answer c is incorrect. Currently brain imagining is not an accurate or accepted method for diagnosing schizophrenia.

Answer d is incorrect. Currently, the only accepted and reliable method for diagnosing schizophrenia is the diagnostic criteria provided by the DSM-IV. Brain imaging and laboratory measures may not be used for diagnostic purposes.

---

3. The best way to reduce the risk of relapse is:
   a. Acute treatment with antipsychotic therapy
   b. Acute treatment with nonpharmacologic therapy
   c. Maintenance treatment with nonpharmacologic therapy
   d. Maintenance treatment with antipsychotic therapy

Answer a is incorrect. Acute treatment with antipsychotics may temporarily treat and stabilize the patient's symptoms but in most cases it is not adequate to prevent relapse.

Answer b is incorrect. Nonpharmacologic therapy such as psychosocial support groups and programs may be useful when combined with antipsychotics; however, nonpharmacologic therapy by itself generally will not treat schizophrenia and prevent relapse. Acute treatment with nonpharmacologic therapy is not adequate to prevent relapse.

Answer c is incorrect. Nonpharmacologic therapy such as psychosocial support groups and programs may be useful when combined with antipsychotics, however, nonpharmacologic therapy by itself generally will not treat schizophrenia and prevent relapse. Maintenance treatment with nonpharmacologic therapy is not adequate to prevent relapse.

Answer d is correct. Most patients with schizophrenia require life-long antipsychotic treatment to adequately manage symptoms. Long-term treatment with an antipsychotic will treat schizophrenia and will help prevent the patient from relapsing.

---

4. Which of the following antipsychotics is most likely to improve positive symptoms, negative symptoms, and cognitive symptoms?
   a. Haloperidol
   b. Chlorpromazine
   c. Perphenazine
   d. Quetiapine

Answer a is incorrect. Haloperidol is a FGA. FGAs tend to be beneficial for the improvement of positive symptoms.

Answer b is incorrect. Chlorpromazine is a FGA. FGAs tend to be beneficial for the improvement of positive symptoms.

Answer c is incorrect. Perphenazine is a FGA. FGAs tend to be beneficial for the improvement of positive symptoms.

Answer d is correct. Quetiapine is a SGA. SGAs are helpful for improving positive symptoms; however, this class of antipsychotics will also improve negative symptoms and cognitive symptoms.

---

5. Which of the following antipsychotics exhibits a mechanism of action with greater affinity for D_2 receptors compared to serotonin receptors?
   a. Paliperidone
   b. Ziprasidone
   c. Haloperidol
   d. Olanzapine

Answer a in incorrect. Paliperidone is a SGA. SGAs have more affinity toward serotonin when compared to D_2 receptor affinity. SGAs generally exhibit moderate D_2 blockade and greater affinity toward serotonergic receptors.

Answer b is incorrect. Ziprasidone is a SGA. SGAs have more affinity toward serotonin when compared to D_2 receptor affinity. SGAs generally exhibit moderate D_2 blockade and greater affinity toward serotonergic receptors.

Answer c is correct. Haloperidol is a FGA. FGAs exhibit a mechanism of action with greater affinity toward D_2 receptor compared to serotonin affinity. FGAs generally exhibit high D_2 blockade and minimal affinity toward serotonergic receptors.

Answer d is incorrect. Olanzapine is a SGA. SGAs have more affinity toward serotonin when compared to D_2 receptor affinity. SGAs generally exhibit moderate D_2 blockade and greater affinity toward serotonergic receptors.

---

6. Which of the following is *not* a SGA?
   a. Ziprasidone
   b. Fluphenazine
   c. Paliperidone
   d. Clozapine

Answer a is incorrect. Ziprasidone is a SGA.

Answer b is correct. Fluphenazine is a FGA.

Answer c is incorrect. Paliperidone is a SGA.

Answer d is incorrect. Clozapine is a SGA.

7. MT is a 30-year-old man who is admitted to the hospital for his first psychotic episode. He is diagnosed with schizophrenia. He is not taking any medications and does not have any other medical conditions. What is the best treatment for MT?
   a. Aripiprazole
   b. Clozapine
   c. Haloperidol
   d. Chlorpromazine

Answer a is correct. SGAs are considered as first-line agents for treatment of schizophrenia. SGAs are considered as first-line agents because they are effective and there is a decreased risk of movement disorders associated with this class of antipsychotics. All SGAs, with the exception of clozapine, may be used as first-line agents. The specific SGA chosen is based on several factors such as adverse effects, patient's response, and the cost.

Answer b is incorrect. Although clozapine is a SGA, it is generally not used as a first-line agent for the treatment of schizophrenia. Clozapine is an effective SGA; however because of its adverse effect profile, it is not used as a first-line treatment. Clozapine is generally used after a patient has failed therapy on SGAs and FGAs.

Answer c is incorrect. Haloperidol is a FGA. FGAs are not considered as first-line treatment and generally are not used before trying a SGA. FGAs are an effective class of antipsychotics; however because of the risk of movement disorders associated with FGAs, this class is generally not preferred over the SGAs.

Answer d is incorrect. Chlorpromazine is a FGA. FGAs are not considered as first-line treatment and generally are not used before trying a SGA. FGAs are an effective class of antipsychotics; however because of the risk of movement disorders associated with FGAs, this class is generally not preferred over the SGAs

8. Which of the following is an adverse effect that can occur with antipsychotic use?
   a. Anticholinergic effects
   b. Orthostasis
   c. Sedation
   d. All of the above

Answer a is correct. It is an adverse effect associated with antipsychotics. Anticholinergic effects are a possibility with FGAs and SGAs.

Answer b is correct. It is an adverse effect associated with antipsychotics. Orthostasis is a possible adverse effect that may occur with FGAs and SGAs.

Answer c is correct. It is an adverse effect associated with antipsychotics. Sedation is a possible adverse effect that may occur with FGAs and SGAs.

Answer is d is correct and the best answer. All of the above are adverse effects that may occur with FGAs and SGAs. The risk of the adverse effects varies from agent to agent but in general these adverse effects may occur with the use of antipsychotics.

9. Which of the following is *not* a true statement regarding clozapine?
   a. Clozapine may cause agranulocytosis.
   b. Frequent WBC and ANC monitoring is required with clozapine.
   c. Clozapine is associated with the risk of seizures.
   d. Clozapine is not an effective agent for the treatment of schizophrenia.

Answer a is incorrect. Agranulocytosis may occur with clozapine treatment. The risk of agranulocytosis with the use of clozapine is a major concern and is one of the reasons why clozapine is not considered as first-line treatment.

Answer b is incorrect. Frequent WBC and ANC monitoring is required. Due to the risk of agranulocytosis it is important to monitor WBC and ANC values. WBC and ANC values should be obtained on weekly basis for the first 6 months of treatment. From 6 to 12 months, WBC and ANC values can be obtained every other week. Once the patient has been on clozapine treatment for 12 months, then WBC and ANC values may be obtained on a monthly basis.

Answer c is incorrect. Clozapine has been associated with decreasing seizure threshold. The risk of seizures associated with clozapine occurs in a dose-dependent manner.

Answer d is correct. This is a false statement. Clozapine is an effective treatment for schizophrenia; however, it is reserved for use after failing therapy on SGAs and FGAs. Clozapine is an effective agent however is not used in many cases due to its concerning adverse effects and precautions associated with this drug such as agranulocytosis, orthostasis, and occurrence of cardiovascular events.

10. Which of the following is a movement disorder that may occur with antipsychotic use?
    a. Akathisia
    b. Dystonia
    c. Pseudoparkinsonism
    d. Tardive dyskinesia
    e. All of the above

Answer a is correct. It is a movement disorder. Akathisia is a type of extrapyramidal symptom. Patients who experience akathisia may experience feelings of restlessness such as the inability to sit still or the need for constant movement. The onset of akathisia usually occurs within days to weeks after antipsychotic initiation.

Answer b is correct. It is a movement disorder. Dystonia is a type of extrapyramidal symptom. Dystonic reactions are described as muscle spasms. These muscle spasms or contractions usually occur in the neck, head, and trunk areas. The onset of dystonia occurs rapidly within the first few days after antipsychotic initiation.

Answer c is correct. It is a movement disorder. Pseudoparkinsonism is a type of extrapyramidal symptom. Patients experiencing this type of EPS may present with symptoms such as bradykinesia, rigidity, and tremors. The onset of pseudoparkinsonism generally occurs 1 to 2 weeks after antipsychotic initiation.

Answer d is correct. It is a movement disorder. Tardive dyskinesia is a type of extrapyramidal symptom. Patients with tardive dyskinesia experience abnormal movements which are involuntary. These movements may occur in many different areas of the body such as the facial area, extremities, or the spine. Tardive dyskinesia in many cases may be irreversible and generally develops after months or years of antipsychotic treatment.

Answer e is correct and the best answer. All of the above are movement disorders that may occur with antipsychotic treatment.

11. Which of the following adverse effects are most commonly associated with FGAs?
    a. Prolactin elevation and EPS
    b. Metabolic abnormalities and weight gain
    c. Pancreatitis and Stevens-Johnson syndrome
    d. Depression and mood swings

Answer a is correct. Prolactin elevation and EPS may occur with FGAs and is actually more likely to occur with the use of FGAs as compared to SGAs.

Answer b is incorrect. Metabolic abnormalities and weight gain are more likely to occur with SGAs. There is less risk of metabolic abnormalities and weight gain associated with FGAs.

Answer c is incorrect. Pancreatitis and Stevens-Johnson syndrome are not common adverse effects that occur with FGAs or SGAs.

Answer d is incorrect. Depression and mood swings are not common adverse effects that occur with FGAs or SGAs.

12. RT is a 35-year-old man with a recent diagnosis of schizophrenia. He is refusing to take any antipsychotics because he has read on the internet that these types of medications can cause weight gain and diabetes. After much encouragement from the psychiatrist he has agreed to try an antipsychotic. The attending psychiatrist would like to initiate RT on an antipsychotic that is least likely to cause weight gain and metabolic disturbances. Which of the following is the best option for RT?
    a. Clozapine
    b. Olanzapine
    c. Aripiprazole
    d. Any of the above agents are appropriate

Answer a is incorrect. Clozapine is not a good option because it is one of the SGAs that is associated with a greater risk of weight gain and metabolic abnormalities such as changes in glucose and lipids.

Answer b is incorrect. Olanzapine is not a good option because it is one of the SGAs that is associated with a greater risk of weight gain and metabolic abnormalities such as changes in glucose and lipids.

Answer c is correct. Aripiprazole is the best option since it is a SGA that is least associated with weight gain and metabolic abnormalities. Aripiprazole and ziprasidone are the two SGAs which are associated with the least risk of weight gain and metabolic abnormalities. Clozapine and olanzapine are most likely to cause weight gain and metabolic abnormalities. Quetiapine and risperidone may have mild to moderate effects on weight gain and metabolic abnormalities.

Answer d is incorrect. The side effect profiles of each SGA differs, therefore, the risk of weight gain and metabolic abnormalities differs among the SGAs. Some agents are more likely to cause weight gain and metabolic abnormalities while other agents have a lesser risk.

13. YM is a 55-year-old man with a 20-year history of schizophrenia. He has a significant history of stopping his medications. Which of the following is the best option for YM given his history of not adhering to his medication regimen?
    a. Haloperidol decanoate
    b. Thioridazine
    c. Ziprasidone
    d. Pimozide

Answer a is correct. Haloperidol decanoate is a long-acting injection which is administered once a month. Long-acting intramuscular injections are a good option for patients who are unable to adhere to antipsychotic treatment. This formulation allows the drug to be released slowly over a few weeks and is useful in patients who are unwilling to take medications on a daily basis. Risperidone long-acting and fluphenazine decanoate are also other long-acting injections which are available.

Answer b, c, and d are incorrect. These are not long-acting formulations.

14. Which of the following is true regarding paliperidone?
    a. Paliperidone is a FGA.
    b. Paliperidone is a metabolite of risperidone.
    c. ANC and WBC monitoring is required with paliperidone treatment.
    d. Paliperidone is considered third line treatment.

Answer a is incorrect. Paliperidone is a SGA not a FGA.

Answer b is correct. Paliperidone is the active metabolite of risperidone.

Answer c is incorrect. WBC and ANC values do not need to be monitored with paliperidone treatment. WBC and ANC values must be monitored for patients who are receiving clozapine treatment.

Answer d is incorrect. Paliperidone is not considered as third-line treatment. Paliperidone is a SGA, therefore, it is considered as first-line treatment.

---

15. Which of the following is a recommended monitoring parameter for patients receiving treatment with a SGA?
    a. Fasting glucose
    b. Blood pressure
    c. Fasting plasma lipids
    d. Weight
    e. All of the above

Answers a, b, c, and d are correct. These are recommended monitoring parameters.

Answer e is correct and the best answer. All of the above should be monitored while receiving treatment with a SGA. SGAs may cause weight gain and metabolic abnormalities, therefore, it is recommended that patients receiving treatment should be monitored. Monitoring these parameters will allow early detection of adverse effects and metabolic abnormalities that may develop.

---

16. The recommended WBC and ANC values during clozapine treatment should be
    a. WBC <3000/mm^3 and ANC <2000/mm^3
    b. WBC >2000/mm^3 and ANC >1000/mm^3
    c. WBC >3000/mm^3 and ANC >1500/mm^3
    d. WBC >3500/mm^3 and ANC >2000/mm^3

Answers a, b, and c are incorrect. The correct laboratory values are WBC >3500/mm^3 and ANC >2000/mm^3.

Answer d is correct. The patient's WBC and ANC should be in this range. Due to the risk of agranulocytosis which may occur with clozapine treatment, it is important that the WBC and ANC values do not fall below these parameters.

---

17. SW is a 45-year-old woman with a 15-year history of schizophrenia. She was started on haloperidol a few days ago. SW presents today with a stiff neck and muscle spasms. Her psychiatrist has identified this reaction as dystonia. Which of the following agents may be used to treat SW's EPS?
    a. Cyclobenzaprine
    b. Quetiapine
    c. Benztropine
    d. Clozapine

Answer a is incorrect. Cyclobenzaprine is a muscle relaxant that is not recommended for the treatment of EPS.

Answer b is incorrect. Quetiapine is a SGA.

Answer c is correct. Benztropine is an anticholinergic that can be used to treat dystonic reactions. Anticholinergics such as benztropine and diphenhydramine are usually the preferred drugs of choice for the treatment of this type of EPS.

Answer d is incorrect. Clozapine is a SGA.

---

18. MJ was recently started on fluphenazine for the treatment of schizophrenia. He has been taking the fluphenazine for 3 days now and is not feeling well on this treatment. MJ is experiencing muscle rigidity, hyperthermia, hypertension, and presents with an altered level of consciousness. Which of the following is MJ experiencing?
    a. Tardive dyskinesia
    b. Dystonia
    c. Neuroleptic malignant syndrome
    d. Serotonin syndrome
    e. Hypertensive crisis

Answer a is incorrect. Tardive dyskinesia is a type of EPS. Hyperthermia, hypertension and an altered level of consciousness do not occur with tardive dyskinesia. Tardive dyskinesia is described as abnormal involuntary movements which develop after months or years of antipsychotic treatment.

Answer b is incorrect. Dystonia is a type of EPS. Dystonic reactions are described as muscle spasms. These muscle spasms or contractions usually occur in the neck, head, and trunk areas. Dystonic reactions may occur within a few days of antipsychotic treatment; however, hyperthermia, hypertension, and an altered level of consciousness do not occur with dystonia.

Answer c is correct. Neuroleptic malignant syndrome (NMS) may occur within the first 24 to 72 hours after antipsychotic treatment. NMS may occur with FGA and SGA treatment. Common signs and symptoms associated with this syndrome include hyperthermia, hypertension, altered level of consciousness, rigidity, and increased creatine kinase.

Answer d is incorrect. Serotonin syndrome has a similar presentation as NMS, however, serotonin syndrome occurs when two or more serotonergic drugs are combined.

Answer e is incorrect. A hypertensive crisis occurs when a monoamine oxidase inhibitor (MAOI) is combined with tyramine containing foods.

---

19. Which of the following may be associated with QTc prolongation?
    a. Aripiprazole
    b. Olanzapine
    c. Ziprasidone
    d. Quetiapine

Answer a is incorrect. There is a low risk of QTc prolongation with aripiprazole.

Answer b is incorrect. There is a low risk of QTc prolongation with olanzapine.

Answer c is correct. Ziprasidone has been associated with QTc prolongation.

Answer d is incorrect. There is a low risk of QTc prolongation with quetiapine.

---

20. The blockade of which of the following receptors is responsible for inducing EPS?
    a. Serotonin
    b. Dopamine-2 ($D_{2)}$
    c. Norepinephrine
    d. All of the above

Answer a is incorrect. Serotonin blockade does not cause EPS.

Answer b is correct. D_2 blockade is responsible for causing EPS. D_2 blockade is responsible for alleviating positive symptoms; however, D_2 blockade is also responsible for inducing EPS. Both FGAs and SGAs to some extent block D_2. FGAs tend to block more D_2 which is why FGAs are more likely to cause EPS.

Answer c is incorrect. Norepinephrine blockade does not cause EPS.

Answer d is incorrect. Only D_2 blockade is responsible for inducing EPS.

---

21. RT is a 35-year-old man who is being switched to a FGA. He states that he does not like being on antipsychotics because he gets unwanted side effects such as extreme dry mouth, constipation, and urinary incontinence. Which of the following is the best option for RT?
    a. Haloperidol
    b. Chlorpromazine
    c. Loxapine
    d. Thioridazine

Answer a is correct. Haloperidol is the best option since it is a high-potency FGA. FGAs which are highly potent such as haloperidol tend to exhibit less anticholinergic effects

Answer b is incorrect. Chlorpromazine is not the best option since it is a low-potency FGA. Low-potency agents such as chlorpromazine and thioridazine tend to have more anticholinergic adverse effects.

Answer c is incorrect. Loxapine is not the best option. Loxapine is not a high- or low-potency FGA, it is a medium-potency FGA. Risk of anticholinergic side effects associated with a medium-potency FGA falls in between high- and low-potency agents.

Answer d is incorrect. Thioridazine is not the best option since it is a low-potency FGA. Low-potency agents such as chlorpromazine and thioridazine tend to have more anticholinergic side effects

---

22. TS is a 30-year-old woman with a 2-year history of schizophrenia. She has been on a few FGAs in the past which have caused her prolactin levels to rise. The psychiatrist treating TS would like to avoid any agents which are likely to elevate prolactin levels. Which of the following agents should be avoided when treating TS?
    a. Aripiprazole
    b. Risperidone
    c. Ziprasidone
    d. Quetiapine

Answer a, c, and d are incorrect. There is low risk of prolactin elevation with aripiprazole, ziprasidone, and quetiapine.

Answer b is correct. Risperidone should be avoided. Risperidone is associated with hyperprolactinemia. Risperidone along with many of the FGAs may cause prolactin elevation.

CHAPTER 57 | Post-Traumatic Stress Disorder

1. Which of the following is *not* a core symptom of PTSD?
    a. Recurrent, intrusive, distressing memories of the trauma
    b. Ability to recall an important aspect of the trauma
    c. Avoidance of conversations about the trauma
    d. Hypervigilance

Answer b is correct. Hypervigilance, recurrent memories of the trauma, avoidance of conversation, and *inability* to recall an important aspect of the trauma are all core symptoms of PTSD.

---

2. Which agent would be used as a first-line treatment for PTSD?
    a. Phenelzine
    b. Paroxetine
    c. Amitriptyline
    d. Bupropion

Answer b is correct. Paroxetine is a SSRI and is a first-line agent. Phenelzine is a MAOI and usually reserved for last-line treatment. Amitriptyline is TCA and a third-line agent. Bupropion is *not* effective in PTSD.

3. Which of the following nonpharmacologic treatment for PTSD has the most evidence supporting its use?

    a. Group counseling
    b. Stress inoculation treatment
    c. Psychoeducation
    d. Cognitive behavioral treatment

Answer d is correct. Cognitive behavioral treatment is the most studied nonpharmacologic treatment in PTSD. All others have data but they are still limited.

4. Which of the following SSRIs is/are approved by FDA for the acute treatment of PTSD?

    a. Sertraline
    b. Fluoxetine
    c. Paroxetine
    d. Both a and c

Answer d is correct. Sertraline and paroxetine are the only two agents that are FDA approved for PTSD.

5. Which of the following agents is *not* effective for the treatment of PTSD?

    a. Alprazolam
    b. Imipramine
    c. Mirtazapine
    d. Phenelzine

Answer a is correct. Alprazolam is a benzodiazepine, which has not shown efficacy in clinical trials. Imipramine and mirtazapine are considered third-line agents, which have shown some clinical efficacy. Phenelzine may be used as a last-line agent.

6. Which agent is *not* effective in patients with chronic PTSD?

    a. Risperidone
    b. Venlafaxine
    c. Bupropion
    d. Prazosin

Answer c is correct. Bupropion has not shown efficacy in clinical trials. Risperidone may be used as adjunct for those with psychotic features. Venlafaxine has shown benefits and is considered a second-line agent. Prazosin may be used as adjunctive treatment in those complaining of nightmares.

7. What is the *correct* dosing range for sertraline recommended for the treatment of PTSD?

    a. 2 to 8 mg/d
    b. 20 to 60 mg/d
    c. 50 to 200 mg/d
    d. 200 to 800 mg/d

Answer c is correct. All other doses are incorrect for sertraline in the treatment for PTSD.

8. Which of the following generic-brand name matches is *incorrect*?

    a. Sertraline—Zoloft
    b. Paroxetine—Prozac
    c. Citalopram—Celexa
    d. Imipramine—Tofranil

Answer is b. The brand name for paroxetine is Paxil, while Prozac is the brand name for fluoxetine.

9. AB is a 32-year-old woman diagnosed with chronic PTSD. She asks the pharmacist how long she needs to take the medication for the prevention of symptom recurrence. What is the goal for duration of treatment for chronic PTSD?

    a. 1 month
    b. 6 months
    c. 12 months
    d. 5 years

Answer c is correct. One month is too short, 6 months is recommended for acute PTSD. No data are available for 5 years.

10. CR is a 42-year-old man who was diagnosed with acute PTSD. He was prescribed citalopram 20 mg daily. He returns for a refill 1 month later and states, "I feel somewhat better, but still have flashbacks." How would you counsel this patient?

    a. Call the MD to change the medication to another SSRI, such as paroxetine.
    b. Call the MD to change the medication to venlafaxine.
    c. Remind the patient, it may take 8 to 12 weeks for the medication to show full benefits.
    d. Advise the patient that according to Federal laws, it is not your responsibility to counsel.

Answer c is correct. Some response may be observed in 4 weeks; however, full clinical benefits may not be demonstrated until 8 to 12 weeks.

11. MN is a 23-year-old obese woman who was diagnosed with PTSD after a car accident several years ago. Although MN has been treated with a SSRI and other agents, she still has recurrent, disturbing dreams of the event with minor daytime hallucinations. Her psychiatrist wants to prescribe an atypical antipsychotic for augmentation therapy. Which agent are you *least* likely to recommend as a clinical pharmacist?

a. Risperidone
b. Quetiapine
c. Olanzapine
d. None of the above

Answer c is correct. Olanzapine is the antipsychotic with the highest propensity to cause weight gain/metabolic changes. Therefore, olanzapine should be avoided in this obese patient.

12. Which agent has pregnancy category D?

a. Paroxetine
b. Fluoxetine
c. Citalopram
d. Sertraline

Answer a is correct. Paroxetine is category D, while all other SSRIs are of category C.

13. For which of the following medication would you counsel a patient regarding drug-food interactions, especially avoiding tyramine containing foods?

a. Prazosin
b. Phenelzine
c. Venlafaxine
d. Zoloft

Answer b is correct. Phenelzine is a MAOI which can cause hypertensive crisis when taken concomitantly with tyramine containing foods (eg, red wine, aged cheeses).

14. AS is a 49-year-old woman diagnosed with PTSD. She is taking warfarin 5 mg daily. The MD decides to initiate a SSRI. Which of the following medications would you *avoid* due to CYP-450 drug interactions?

a. Luvox
b. Sertraline
c. Celexa
d. Both b and c

Answer a is correct. Luvox is a potent CYP-450 2C19 inhibitor which may increase warfarin concentrations.

15. Which are the two most important neurotransmitters implicated in PTSD?

a. 5-HT and GABA
b. GABA and NE
c. 5-HT and NE
d. NE and DA

Answer c is correct. 5-HT and NE are the primary neurotransmitters involved in PTSD. GABA and DA may also play a minor indirect role.

16. Which medication class has a black box warning for increased risk of suicidal ideations in pediatrics?

a. Antipsychotics
b. Benzodiazepines
c. SSRIs
d. None of the above

Answer c is correct. SSRIs are the only medication class listed above which requires a black box warning.

17. Which of the following are environmental triggers which can cause PTSD?

a. War
b. Rape
c. Natural disaster
d. All of the above

Answer d is correct. All of the above scenarios can increase the likelihood of developing PTSD.

18. SB is a 23-year-old woman who has PTSD and presents to the outpatient clinic with complaints of nightmares and difficulty sleeping. She is currently on paroxetine 40 mg daily and cannot tolerate higher dosages. Which of the following medications would you consider using as adjunctive therapy?

a. Olanzapine
b. Prazosin
c. Bupropion
d. Alprazolam

Answer b is correct. Prazosin has evidence to improve nightmare complaints in PTSD. Olanzapine is used as adjunct for psychotic symptoms. Bupropion and alprazolam are not effective in PTSD.

19. SSRIs have demonstrated overall effectiveness in which of the following core symptoms?

a. Reexperiencing
b. Numbing
c. Avoidance
d. All of the above

Answer b is correct. Overall, SSRIs demonstrated effectiveness in reducing numbing symptoms.

20. Which two agents are available in extended-release formulations?

a. Citalopram—escitalopram
b. Venlafaxine—paroxetine
c. Phenelzine—sertraline
d. Fluoxetine—venlafaxine

Answer b is correct. Citalopram, escitalopram, phenelzine, sertraline, and fluoxetine do not have extended-release formulations.

CHAPTER 58 | Diabetes Mellitus

Use the following patient profile to answer questions 1 to 5

JR is a 38-year-old obese African American man with a new diagnosis of T2DM. He was classified as having prediabetes 5 years before the diagnosis and has a strong family history of diabetes. JR's blood pressure was 140/92 mm Hg. His laboratory results revealed an A1c of 8.2%, normal cholesterol panel and normal renal/hepatic function.

1. What risk factor(s) does JR display for the development of diabetes?
   a. Obesity
   b. African American
   c. Family history of diabetes
   d. Prediabetes
   e. All of the above

Answer a is correct. Obesity is a risk factor and should be used as a method to identify patients to be screened for diabetes.

Answer b is correct. Patients who are African American are one of the ethnic populations that are at high risk for developing diabetes.

Answer c is correct. Family history is a strong risk factor for developing T2DM. The true genetic link is not known at this time, however, the risk for developing diabetes goes up with the more primary relatives you have with diabetes.

Answer d is correct. Prediabetes is a risk factor for the development of diabetes. JR was classified as having prediabetes 5 years previously. See Tables 58-1 and 58-2 for screening and diagnostic criteria for prediabetes.

Answer e is correct and the best answer. See rationale above.

2. What is JR's goal blood pressure?
   a. <150/90 mm Hg
   b. <140/90 mm Hg
   c. <130/80 mm Hg
   d. <110/70 mm Hg

Answer a is incorrect. This blood pressure is not a goal for any patient population and places the patient at the risk of cardiovascular and cerebral vascular accidents.

Answer b is incorrect. This blood pressure may be the blood pressure goal for patients with uncomplicated hypertension without any other disease states.

Answer c is correct. This is the current blood pressure goal for patients with diabetes. It is recommended to attain this goal blood pressure to minimize the risk of cardiovascular events.

Answer d is incorrect. This blood pressure is not a goal for any patient population. However, as long as a patient was not symptomatic of hypotension or lack of profusion to an organ system, a patient may tolerate this blood pressure.

3. JR's blood pressure was elevated at the next visit and he was diagnosed with hypertension. Which agent would be the best to start in order to achieve blood pressure control and to prevent microvascular complications?
   a. Clonidine 0.1 mg twice daily
   b. Terazosin 10 mg at bedtime
   c. Lisinopril 5 mg daily
   d. Isosorbide mononitrate 60 mg daily

Answer a is incorrect. Clonidine does not have any data to indicate renal protective properties in patients with diabetes. Dose provided would be an appropriate starting dose.

Answer b is incorrect. Terazosin does not have data to indicate renal protective properties in patients with diabetes. Although terazosin should be dosed at night time due to possible adverse effects of nocturnal orthostatic hypotension, the starting dose of 10 mg is not recommended.

Answer c is correct. Lisinopril is in the angiotensin-converting enzyme inhibitor class which is one of the drugs of choice for renal protection in patients with diabetes. ACEi and ARB have shown a reduction in the progression to overt proteinuria. The African American population may not see the maximum effect of blood pressure lowering due to a decrease amount of renin and its activity, however, for patients with diabetes of any population it is still gold standard.

Answer d is incorrect. Isosorbide mononitrate is not used for hypertension as first-line therapy. Typically it may be added if the patient is on other oral antihypertensive agents and has ischemic heart disease, uncontrolled, unstable/stable angina or heart failure.

4. Which of the following antihyperglycemic agents would be recommended for JR to use as first-line therapy to obtain glycemic control?
   a. Pramlintide 15 μg twice daily
   b. Gemfibrozil 600 mg twice daily
   c. Metformin 500 mg daily with meals and titrate up over a few weeks
   d. Acarbose 100 mg three times daily with each meals

Answer a is incorrect. Pramlintide could be used for this patient as its weight loss abilities might help and his A1c is <9%, however, the ADA medical management of hyperglycemia guidelines does not mention this agent as a first-line agent or as monotherapy. The dose indicated above is the starting dose for patients diagnosed with T1DM.

Answer b is incorrect. Gemfibrozil is an antihyperlipidemic agent and does not provide benefits to obtain glucose control. The patient may need to be on lipid-lowering medications, however for most patients with diabetes, the first-line therapy would be a statin regardless of baseline LDL-C.

Answer c is correct. Metformin is the drug of choice recommended for most patients with diabetes in addition to lifestyle modifications. Metformin has also shown to provide positive weight loss effects in obese patients. It would be important to obtain a serum creatinine level prior to initiation of this therapy.

Answer d is incorrect. Although acarbose does have data to indicate its use in prediabetes, this agent is not recommended as first-line therapy by the ADA medical management of hyperglycemia. The starting dose provided above is not recommended due to the intolerability of gastrointestinal side effects.

---

5. What preventative measures should JR be educated on to reduce the risk of complications associated with diabetes?
   a. Perform daily foot examinations
   b. See a dentist/dental hygienist routinely throughout the year
   c. Take the yearly influenza vaccine
   d. All of the above

Answer a is correct. Patients should be encouraged to look at their feet daily to assess for signs of infection. Patients should be educated on these signs and when to follow up with a health care provider. It is recommended for patients to have a physical examination of their feet and extremities with a health care provider yearly.

Answer b is correct. It is recommended to have their teeth cleaned twice a year and a yearly dentist appointment. Patients should also be educated on signs and symptoms of gingival disease and when to follow up with a health care provider.

Answer c is correct. It is recommended that all patients with diabetes (unless they have a contraindication) should receive the influenza vaccine yearly. Patients with diabetes are not candidates to receive FluMist (intranasal) influenza vaccine due to its live-attenuated formulation.

Answer d is correct and the best answer. See rationale above.

Use the following patient profile for questions 6 to 8.

PT is a 68-year-old white woman with a BMI of 32 kg/m^2. She was recently referred to a dietitian for weight reduction and lost 40 lb over the past 8 months. She is very dedicated to getting her blood glucose under control. At this time she is not willing to go on insulin therapy. She is testing her blood sugars at home: fasting blood glucose readings are all <130 mg/dL and her 2-hour postprandials are in the range of 190 to 200 mg/dL. Her past medical history (PMH) is hypertension, hyperlipidemia, T2DM, sleep apnea, and depression; family history (FHx) is unknown (patient was adopted); and social history (SHx) is (+) tobacco use—1.5 packs per day for 52 years, (+) alcohol use—2 sifters (60 oz) of gin and tonic daily. Her medications are metformin 1000 mg twice daily, enalapril 10 mg twice daily, hydrochlorothiazide 25 mg daily, citalopram 40 mg daily, rosuvastatin 5 mg daily, and gemfibrozil 600 mg twice daily. Her laboratory results revealed normal electrolyte and cholesterol panels, normal renal and hepatic function. A1c 7.9%

6. What therapy is the best option to help lower her A1c and improve glycemic control considering her specific patient profile concerns?
   a. Nateglinide 120 mg three times daily with meals
   b. Chlorpropamide 250 mg daily
   c. Increase metformin to 2000 mg twice daily
   d. Start insulin NPH 10 units at bedtime

Answer a is correct. PT is having problems with her postprandial blood sugars which are not at goal (goal: <180 mg/dL 1-2 hours after a meal). Nateglinide will help to reduce postprandial glucose excursions. PT does not have any contraindications or drug interaction with this medication. She should be able to attain her A1c goal with starting on this therapy in addition to her metformin and weight loss.

Answer b is incorrect. PT has a history of daily alcohol use. Chlorpropamide is not recommended due to the disulfiram-like reaction and the increased risk of hypoglycemia. A second-generation agent would be a better consideration in this patient.

Answer c is incorrect. The maximum daily dose of metformin is 2550 mg; however, a plateau effect is noted at 2000 mg daily

Answer d is incorrect. Insulin is an option in this patient per the ADA medical management of hyperglycemia guidelines; however the patient indicated she is not interested in taking insulin. If a patient is not going to take the insulin it will not help to be prescribed. Further understanding of why PT is psychologically resistant to insulin injections is needed. If insulin would be started for PT, NPH may not be the recommended agent, as it is a basal insulin and her morning blood sugars are controlled. Therefore a bolus insulin might be a better recommendation.

---

7. Which of the following is/are common side effect(s) of Glucophage?
   a. Weight gain
   b. Diarrhea
   c. Lactic acidosis
   d. Pancreatitis

Answer a is incorrect. Metformin is associated with 2 to 3 kg weight loss.

Answer b is correct. Diarrhea is the most common side effect with metformin use, however can be minimized with commencement of low dose and titrating slowly.

Answer c is incorrect. Lactic acidosis is a *rare* side effect that may affect patients taking metformin. Lactic acidosis is associated in patient taking metformin who have hypoprofusion to the kidneys or increased lactic acid concentrations.

Answer d is incorrect. Pancreatitis has not been reported with metformin use. Postmarketing surveillance indicated this side effect with exenatide.

8. Which of the following treatment would be the most appropriate method to treat a severe hypoglycemic reaction that PT might have?
   a. 2 to 3 glucose tablets
   b. 1can (8 oz) of soda
   c. One-half of a banana
   d. Glucagon IM injection

Answer a is incorrect. This treatment would be appropriate for a mild hypoglycemic reaction because the patient would be awake or able to treat herself.

Answer b is incorrect. This treatment would be appropriate for a mild hypoglycemic reaction because the patient would be awake or able to treat herself. However, it would be recommended to only start off with 4 to 5 oz of soda.

Answer c is incorrect. This treatment would be appropriate for a mild hypoglycemic reaction because the patient would be awake or able to treat herself.

Answer d is correct. Since PT is having a severe hypoglycemic reaction, this means she is not able to treat herself and severe neurologic deficit is occurring. Therefore, glucagon administration is the best answer.

9. Commercially available Symlin should be administered by which route?
   a. Intravenously
   b. Intramuscularly
   c. Subcutaneously
   d. Via Insulin pump

Answers a, b, and d are incorrect. Not FDA approved for these routes of administration.

Answer c is correct. Only FDA approved route of administration.

10. Insulin detemir can be mixed with which of the following insulins?
    a. Insulin aspart
    b. Insulin regular
    c. Insulin glargine
    d. Insulin detemir cannot be mixed with any insulins

Answer a is incorrect. Insulin aspart should only be mixed with insulin NPH.

Answer b is incorrect. Insulin regular should only be mixed with insulin NPH.

Answer c is incorrect. Insulin glargine cannot be mixed with any insulins. Insulin glargine and detemir are both basal insulin, therefore another reason to never have both of these agents in a patient's regimen.

Answer d is correct. Insulin detemir is not approved to mix with any insulins, even bolus insulin.

11. How should a patient on acarbose therapy treat a hypoglycemic episode?
    a. Inject 3 units of insulin NPH at the time of episode
    b. 3 to 4 glucose tablets
    c. 1 candy bar
    d. All of the above are suitable choices

Answer a is incorrect. The patient is hypoglycemic therefore providing insulin will worsen this episode.

Answer b is correct. Due to the mechanism of action for acarbose, simple sugars are needed to treat a hypoglycemic reaction.

Answer c is incorrect. The fat and carbohydrates in the candy bar will not be absorbed in a timely manner due to the mechanism of action for acarbose.

Answer d is incorrect. See the above rationales.

12. Which drug would not be recommended for a patient with an ejection fraction of 32% and in symptomatic heart failure documented by a NYHA class III?
    a. Rosiglitazone
    b. Byetta
    c. Saxagliptin
    d. Starlix

Answer a is correct. Rosiglitazone may cause or exacerbate heart failure. This is a class effect with both rosiglitazone and pioglitazone, therefore TZD therapy is contraindicated in patients with NYHA III/IV heart failure.

Answers b, c, and d are incorrect. There is no association of exenatide, saxagliptin, and nateglinide therapy and heart failure.

13. How many minutes before a meal should a patient administer glulisine insulin?
   a. 15 minutes before the start of a meal
   b. 30 minutes before the start of a meal
   c. 60 minutes before the start of a meal
   d. Glulisine is a basal insulin and administration should be regardless of the mealtime.

Answer a is correct. Due to the rapid onset (0.25 hours), it is recommended to not take glulisine more than 15 minutes before the start of a meal.

Answer b is incorrect. If taken at 30 or more minutes before the start of a meal, hypoglycemia may occur because the onset of action occurs within 15 minutes.

Answer c is incorrect. If taken at 60 or more minutes before the start of a meal, hypoglycemia may occur because the onset of action occurs within 15 minutes.

Answer d is incorrect. Glulisine is a rapid-acting insulin and should be given to before a meal time to reduce the post-prandial glucose levels.

---

14. Which of the following is true regarding the action of insulin?
   a. Enhances ketone production
   b. Stimulates glucose uptake in the periphery
   c. It activates peroxisome-proliferator-activated receptor-γ (PPAR-γ)
   d. Increases amylin production

Answer a is incorrect. Insulin inhibits ketone production.

Answer b is correct. See Table 58-5 of this chapter for insulin action.

Answer c is incorrect. This is a mechanism of action for TZDs.

Answer d is incorrect. Insulin does not increase amylin production.

---

15. What baseline laboratory results need to be obtained prior to the prescribing of Januvia?
   a. Basic metabolic panel
   b. Prothrombin time (PT)/International normalized ratio (INR)
   c. Cholesterol panel
   d. A1c
   e. a and d

Answer a is correct. Basic metabolic panel includes a serum creatinine measurement. Januvia is renally dosed based on CrCl or gender-based SCr. levels. Therefore, this laboratory result must be obtained to determine the correct starting dose.

Answer b is incorrect. PT/INR is not needed to determine appropriateness of Januvia therapy.

Answer c is incorrect. A cholesterol is not needed to determine appropriateness of Januvia. However, a cholesterol panel is recommended to be obtained yearly in most patients with diabetes.

Answer d is incorrect. An A1c is recommended to be obtained prior to starting therapy. Januvia has the ability to lower A1c by 1.1 to 1.5%, therefore, if A1c at baseline is greater than this then the patient may not be able to achieve A1c goal.

Answer e is correct. See the rationale above.

---

16. Adjustments in antihyperglycemic drug therapy should be based on which of the following concerns?
   i. Liver function tests if the patient is on a TZD
   ii. Blood glucose levels
   iii. Gynecologic examinations
   iv. Dietary habits/physical activity
   a. i only
   b. ii only
   c. i and ii only
   d. i, ii, and iv

Answer a is correct. It is important to obtain baseline and periodic liver function tests to prevent hepatotoxicity.

Answer b is correct. Blood glucose levels are important to identify patterns to facilitate management. This will help you to determine how aggressive you treat. It is important to prevent hypoglycemic reactions.

Answer c is correct. See above rationale.

Answer d is correct and the best answer. Monitoring of laboratory results that are affected by medications, glucose levels, and dietary/physical activity all allow a patients' diabetes management to be individualized.

---

17. All of the following are true of repaglinide *except*:
   a. Dosage of repaglinide should be administered regardless of meal
   b. Normal treatment of hypoglycemia is recommended for patients on repaglinide
   c. Caution for hypoglycemic in concomitant therapy with gemfibrozil
   d. Maximum dose of repaglinide is 16 mg daily (divided with meals)

Answer a is correct. Repaglinide should be given approximately 30 minutes preprandial. However, it should only be administered if a meal is planned. If a patient does not eat, this medication should not be given.

Answer b is incorrect. Only the class of α-glucosidase inhibitors has special treatment recommendation during a hypoglycemic reaction.

Answer c is incorrect. Gemfibrozil can increase blood level of repaglinide causing hypoglycemic. This interaction does not constitute a contraindication of concomitant use, however more frequent monitoring and education to the patient is needed.

Answer d is incorrect. The maximum dosage regardless of baseline A1c is 16 mg daily divided with meals.

---

18. Glipizide has which of the following mechanisms of action?
    a. Inhibits and delays carbohydrate metabolism by inhibition of intestinal/pancreatic enzymes.
    b. Improves insulin sensitivity at adipose tissue.
    c. Causes gene transcription at adipose tissue.
    d. Stimulates pancreatic β-cells to release insulin.

Answer a is incorrect. This is the mechanism of α-glucosidase inhibitors.

Answer b is incorrect. This is a mechanism that TZDs and metformin may have.

Answer c is incorrect. Sulfonylureas are not associated with gene transcription.

Answer d is correct. Sulfonylureas stimulate β-cells within the pancreas to secrete insulin.

---

19. Exenatide is not recommended in patients with which of the following diagnoses?
    a. Vitamin B12 deficiency
    b. Gastroparesis
    c. A1c >9%
    d. a and b
    e. b and c

Answer a is incorrect. Vitamin B12 deficiency is not an issue with exenatide.

Answer b is correct. Caution should be exercised in patients with gastroparesis as exenatide is not recommended due to its MOA.

Answer c is correct. Not recommended to be used in patients with an A1c >9%, as exenatide would not be able to get them A1c goal. If A1c is >9% insulin therapy would be a better option.

Answer d is incorrect. Because answer a is considered in this option.

Answer e is correct. See above rationale.

---

20. Which drug therapy may mask the signs of hypoglycemia?
    a. Atenolol
    b. Valsartan
    c. Hydrochlorothiazide
    d. Pioglitazone

Answer a is correct. Beta blockers have been known to mask signs or symptoms of hypoglycemia. The one sign that it may not mask is diaphoresis or sweaty palms.

Answer b is incorrect. Valsartan is not associated with masked hypoglycemia.

Answer c is incorrect. Hydrochlorothiazide is not noted to mask hypoglycemia, however, transiently may worsen glucose control.

Answer d is incorrect. Pioglitazone is not associated with masked hypoglycemia.

CHAPTER 59 | Thyroid Disorders

1. Which of the following statements regarding thyroid hormones is true?
    a. The majority of T_4 is formed in peripheral tissues.
    b. T_3 has greater potency than T_4.
    c. Iodine is not involved in the formation of thyroid hormones.
    d. The concentrations of circulating hormones do not affect the secretion of TSH.

Answer a is incorrect as T_4 is formed in the thyroid gland. T_3 is mainly formed in peripheral tissues.

Answer b is correct as T_3 is much more potent due to greater affinity for binding to plasma proteins.

Answer c is incorrect as iodine is needed to form the tyrosine residues that form mono- and diiodinated residues that couple to form T_3 and T_4.

Answer d is incorrect since the concentrations of thyroid hormones circulating in the body determine if more or less hormones need to be synthesized. Lower concentrations of thyroid hormones increase the production of TSH to stimulate the production of more hormones. Higher concentrations of thyroid hormones decrease the production of TSH to slow the synthesis of thyroid hormones.

---

2. Hyperthyroidism typically presents with which laboratory result?
    a. Increased TSH, increased thyroid hormones
    b. Decreased TSH, increased thyroid hormones
    c. Increased TSH, decreased thyroid hormones
    d. Decreased TSH, decreased thyroid hormones

Answer a is incorrect since hyperthyroidism occurs when excess thyroid hormones are circulating in the body. As a result of the negative feedback system, increased concentrations of thyroid hormones will suppress the production of TSH so TSH levels will be decreased in hyperthyroidism.

Answer b is correct since hyperthyroidism increased thyroid hormones that then decrease the amount of TSH needed by the thyroid gland.

Answer c is incorrect as thyroid hormones are elevated in hyperthyroidism while TSH is suppressed. These laboratory results (increased TSH and decreased thyroid hormones) are typically found in hypothyroidism.

Answer d is incorrect because thyroid hormones will be elevated in hyperthyroidism. TSH concentrations will be decreased.

---

3. What is the most common cause of hyperthyroidism?
   a. Graves disease
   b. Hashimoto disease
   c. Silent thyroiditis
   d. Excessive ingestion of levothyroxine

Answer a is correct since Graves disease is the most common cause of hyperthyroidism, it is responsible for 50% to 80% of cases of hyperthyroidism.

Answer b is incorrect. Hashimoto disease is the most common cause of hypothyroidism.

Answer c is incorrect. Silent thyroiditis does cause hypothyroidism but is not the most common cause.

Answer d is incorrect. Excessive ingestion of levothyroxine might lead to hyperthyroidism but is not the most common cause.

---

4. MM is a 27-year-old woman who is 28 weeks pregnant who has just been diagnosed with hyperthyroidism. Which symptoms might MM be experiencing due to her diagnosis?
   a. Bradycardia and cold intolerance
   b. Tachycardia and heat intolerance
   c. Depression and cognition difficulties
   d. Weight gain and constipation

Answer a is incorrect. Bradycardia and cold intolerance are typical symptoms of hypothyroidism.

Answer b is correct. Tachycardia will occur due to increased adrenergic activity due to excess thyroid hormones. Heat intolerance and sweating are other common symptoms of hyperthyroidism due to increased metabolism.

Answer c is incorrect. Depression and cognition difficulties are typical symptoms of hypothyroidism.

Answer d is incorrect. Weight gain and constipation may occur due to her pregnancy but are more typical symptoms of hypothyroidism. Patients with hyperthyroidism may be more likely to experience frequent stools and weight loss instead.

---

5. What is the optimal treatment for MM?
   a. Surgery
   b. Radioactive iodine
   c. Methimazole
   d. Propylthiouracil

Answer a is incorrect. Surgery is usually a last-line option for the treatment of hyperthyroidism. Thyroidectomy requires precise surgical skills so that other glands around the thyroid are not damaged. Patients who fail antithyroid medications and radioactive ablation may become candidates for surgery. Surgery may also be performed if the patient has thyroid cancer.

Answer b is incorrect as radioactive iodine is contraindicated in pregnancy. It can cross the placenta and cause serious consequences in the fetus. Women should wait for 6 to 12 months after treatment with radioactive iodine before trying to get pregnant.

Answer c is incorrect. Methimazole is the preferred antithyroid medication for nonpregnant patients, but propylthiouracil is preferred in pregnancy. Methimazole may be used, but has been associated with more adverse effects in the fetus including aplasia cutis—an absence of skin in a localized area, most commonly in the scalp.

Answer d is correct. Propylthiouracil is the preferred treatment for hyperthyroidism in pregnancy due to fewer adverse effects than methimazole.

---

6. Dr. M wants to know which antithyroid medication would be preferred in a nonpregnant patient with hyperthyroidism and why. What is your response?
   a. Propylthiouracil is preferred due to fewer side effects and less frequent dosing.
   b. Methimazole is preferred due to fewer side effects and less frequent dosing.
   c. Methimazole is preferred since it blocks the peripheral conversion of T_4 to T_3.
   d. Propylthiouracil is preferred since it blocks the peripheral conversion of T_4 to T_3.

Answer a is incorrect. Propylthiouracil has a higher incidence of serious side effects such as vasculitis and hepatotoxicity. Propylthiouracil must also be dosed multiple times a day.

Answer b is correct. Methimazole does not produce side effects such as vasculitis and hepatotoxicity. Methimazole can also be dosed once daily.

Answer c is incorrect. Methimazole does not block the peripheral conversion of T_4 to T_3.

Answer d is incorrect. Propylthiouracil does block the peripheral conversion of T_4 to T_3 but this does not offer any additional benefit except in thyroid storm.

---

7. TS is a 35-year-old woman started on methimazole for treatment of hyperthyroidism. Which of the following side effects might she experience that would require discontinuation of her medication?
   a. Agranulocytosis
   b. Insomnia
   c. Gastrointestinal upset
   d. Cutaneous reaction

Answer a is correct. Agranulocytosis can occur with both methimazole and propylthiouracil. Diagnosis of agranulocytosis requires prompt treatment with broad-spectrum antibiotics and discontinuation of the antithyroid drug. Crossreactivity for agranulocytosis does occur between methimazole and propylthiouracil, so patients will need to be treated with radioactive iodine or surgery to correct the hyperthyroidism.

Answer b is incorrect. Insomnia does not require discontinuation.

Answer c is incorrect. Gastrointestinal upset does not require discontinuation.

Answer d is incorrect. Cutaneous reactions can occur with methimazole but may not warrant discontinuation of her medication.

8. LR is a 32-year-old woman who is still experiencing symptoms of hyperthyroidism despite treatment with propylthiouracil. Which medication can be added to provide additional symptomatic relief?
   a. Nifedipine
   b. Prednisone
   c. Propranolol
   d. Ibuprofen

Answer a is incorrect. Certain calcium channel blockers (nondihydropyridine calcium channel blockers like verapamil and diltiazem) may be used to decrease the heart rate in patients with hyperthyroidism. Dihydropyridine calcium channel blockers like nifedipine, amlodipine, and felodipine do not slow the heart and may actually cause a reflex tachycardia, worsening hyperthyroidism symptoms.

Answer b is incorrect. Prednisone may be used to treat patients presenting in thyroid storm but has no additional symptomatic benefit for outpatient treatment of hyperthyroidism.

Answer c is correct. Beta-adrenergic blocking agents will slow the heart rate to help correct tachycardia and may improve other symptoms of hyperthyroidism including anxiety, palpitations, and tremor. These agents are added to antithyroid medications or around treatment with radioactive iodine for symptomatic relief only.

Answer d is incorrect. Ibuprofen will not provide symptomatic relief for the typical symptoms of hyperthyroidism.

9. YD presents to the emergency room in a coma with fever and tachycardia. Based on results of his thyroid function tests, YD is diagnosed with thyroid storm. Which therapy would be preferred for treatment of YD?
   a. Radioactive iodine
   b. Propylthiouracil
   c. Methimazole
   d. Surgical thyroidectomy

Answer a is incorrect. Radioactive iodine will not immediately suppress production of thyroid hormones. Return to a euthyroid state generally takes 2 months. Due to the severe nature and high mortality associated with thyroid storm, the patient needs a more immediate reduction in thyroid hormone concentrations.

Answer b is correct. Propylthiouracil is the preferred treatment for patients presenting in thyroid storm. Not only will propylthiouracil block the formation of thyroid hormones, it also blocks the peripheral conversion of T_4 to the more potent T_3. Patients will need the multiple sites of action to help correct the symptoms of hyperthyroidism in thyroid storm.

Answer c is incorrect. Methimazole only blocks the production of thyroid hormones, but does not affect the peripheral conversion of T_4 to T_3.

Answer d is incorrect. Patients presenting in thyroid storm are not optimal candidates for surgery due to hemodynamic instability. The preferred treatment is propylthiouracil.

10. What is the most common cause of hypothyroidism in the United States?
   a. Graves disease
   b. Congenital hypothyroidism
   c. Surgical thyroidectomy
   d. Autoimmune thyroiditis

Answer a is incorrect. Graves disease is the most common cause of hyperthyroidism.

Answer b is incorrect. Congenital hypothyroidism more commonly occurs in iodine-deficient areas of the world. Most people in the United States have sufficient iodine intake.

Answer c is incorrect. Surgical thyroidectomy may cause hypothyroidism but is not the most common cause.

Answer d is correct. Autoimmune thyroiditis, or Hashimoto disease, is the most common cause of hypothyroidism.

11. GB is a 55-year-old woman recently diagnosed with hypothyroidism. Which symptoms might she be experiencing?
   a. Bradycardia and cold intolerance
   b. Anxiety and nervousness
   c. Weight loss and insomnia
   d. Frequent bowel movements and edema

Answer a is correct. The decreased concentration of thyroid hormones in the body due to hypothyroidism decreases the heart rate. Patients also present with cold intolerance due to a slower metabolism.

Answer b is incorrect. Anxiety and nervousness are common symptoms of hyperthyroidism that occur due to increased adrenergic activity.

Answer c is incorrect. Patients with hypothyroidism will typically gain weight due to a slower metabolism. Sleep disturbances are more likely to occur in hyperthyroidism, particularly insomnia. Patients with hypothyroidism may experience more fatigue.

Answer d is incorrect. Constipation is a more common problem with hypothyroidism while frequent bowel movements occur more often in hyperthyroidism. Edema does occur in hypothyroidism but usually after a long history of hypothyroidism due to low cardiac output.

12. What would thyroid function tests reveal in GB?
    a. Increased TSH, increased thyroid hormones
    b. Decreased TSH, increased thyroid hormones
    c. Increased TSH, decreased thyroid hormones
    d. Decreased TSH, decreased thyroid hormones

Answer a is incorrect. TSH concentrations will increase in hypothyroidism due to insufficient concentrations of thyroid hormones, but thyroid hormone levels will be decreased.

Answer b is incorrect. These thyroid function tests more accurately depict hyperthyroidism. TSH concentrations decrease in hyperthyroidism due to excess concentrations of thyroid hormones.

Answer c is correct. Hypothyroidism occurs when sufficient concentrations of thyroid hormones are not available in the body. As a result, TSH concentrations increase to compensate and produce more thyroid hormones.

Answer d is incorrect. Thyroid hormones levels will be decreased in hypothyroidism, but TSH concentrations should increase to stimulate production of more thyroid hormones.

13. What would be the optimal treatment for GB?
    a. Desiccated thyroid hormone
    b. Liothyronine
    c. Levothyroxine
    d. The combination of liothyronine and levothyroxine

Answer a is incorrect. Desiccated thyroid hormone was one of the first treatments available for hypothyroidism, but is rarely used due to the difficulty in standardizing concentrations and maintaining a euthyroid state for the patient. It contains a combination of T_4 and T_3 along with T_1 and T_2 derived from pigs' thyroids.

Answer b is incorrect. Liothyronine (T_3) does not replace T_4 concentrations.

Answer c is correct. Levothyroxine is the preferred thyroid replacement drug for hypothyroidism. Levothyroxine not only replaces T_4 concentrations but will also then undergo peripheral conversion in the body to replace T_3.

Answer d is incorrect. The combination of levothyroxine and liothyronine has not proven to be significantly beneficial.

14. Which of the following patient counseling tips is accurate regarding levothyroxine?
    a. Levothyroxine should be taken with food to maximize absorption.
    b. Levothyroxine should be taken on an empty stomach to maximize absorption.
    c. Levothyroxine produces immediate symptomatic relief of hypothyroidism.
    d. Levothyroxine will only be needed until symptoms of hypothyroidism resolve.

Answer a is incorrect. Food will decrease the absorption of levothyroxine.

Answer b is correct. Due to the risk for decreased absorption with food or other medications, levothyroxine should be taken on an empty stomach.

Answer c is incorrect. Due to the long half-life of levothyroxine, it may take 4 to 6 weeks to reach steady state. Symptoms will not improve immediately.

Answer d is incorrect. Levothyroxine may need to be given lifelong to maintain a euthyroid state.

15. As GB picks up her first prescription of levothyroxine, she asks you when she should have her thyroid function tests rechecked. What is your response?
    a. 1 week
    b. 1 month
    c. 3 months
    d. 6 months

Answer a is incorrect. TSH concentrations may take 4 to 6 weeks to change after levothyroxine initiation or dose changes.

Answer b is correct. The half-life of levothyroxine is 7 days. It may take 4 to 6 weeks to reach steady state. Thyroid function tests should be checked 1 to 2 months after starting levothyroxine or any dose changes.

Answer c is incorrect. Thyroid function tests should be checked sooner to appropriately titrate the levothyroxine dose.

Answer d is incorrect. Thyroid function tests should be checked 4 to 6 weeks after starting levothyroxine or any dose changes.

16. Dr. Z in your clinic asks you what are the most recent dosing recommendations for initiating levothyroxine for the treatment of hypothyroidism. What is your response?

    a. Full treatment doses of levothyroxine may be started in all patients.
    b. Levothyroxine must be started at low doses and titrated up slowly in all patients.
    c. Patients with ischemic heart disease may begin levothyroxine at full treatment doses.
    d. Full treatment doses of levothyroxine should be started only in younger healthy patients.

Answer a is incorrect. Caution should be used in patients over the age of 60 and those with ischemic heart disease as the positive chronotropic and inotropic effects of thyroid hormone may exacerbate myocardial ischemia. Levothyroxine should be started at 12.5 to 25 μg daily and titrated up slowly every 4 to 6 weeks.

Answer b is incorrect. Starting all patients at a low dose and titrating up slowly prolongs recovery time. Healthy patients and those less than 60 years old may start full treatment doses safely.

Answer c is incorrect. Full treatment doses may exacerbate myocardial ischemia in patients with ischemic heart disease. These patients should start levothyroxine at 12.5 to 25 μg daily, with a slow titration every 4 to 6 weeks.

Answer d is correct. Only healthy patients should start full treatment doses of levothyroxine at 1.6 μg/kg daily. The positive chronotropic and inotropic effects of thyroid hormone may exacerbate myocardial ischemia in patients with ischemic heart disease or those over the age of 60.

---

17. PR is a 35-year-old woman admitted for uncontrollable nausea and vomiting during the first trimester of her pregnancy. Her past medical history is significant for hypothyroidism and gastroesophageal reflux disease (GERD). How should her hypothyroidism be managed during her hospitalization?

    a. Levothyroxine should be held until PR can restart her oral medication.
    b. Levothyroxine should be given intravenously until PR can restart her oral medication.
    c. Levothyroxine should be given orally at a lower dose to reduce nausea and vomiting.
    d. Levothyroxine should be changed to liothyronine to reduce nausea and vomiting.

Answer a is correct. PR may only miss a few doses while hospitalized until she gains control of her nausea and vomiting. Due to the long half-life of levothyroxine, PR will maintain her TSH concentration for several days even without receiving her levothyroxine dose.

Answer b is incorrect. IV levothyroxine is generally reserved for treatment of myxedema coma or patients unable to take oral medications for an extended period of time. Additionally, the poor stability of reconstituted levothyroxine requires immediate administration.

Answer c is incorrect. Levothyroxine should not worsen nausea and vomiting unless she is receiving too much levothyroxine. In addition, most pregnant women require higher doses of levothyroxine.

Answer d is incorrect. Levothyroxine is the preferred thyroid replacement product for hypothyroidism and has been proven safe and effective in pregnancy. There is no medical reason to change PR to liothyronine.

---

18. FN is diagnosed with Hashimoto disease during the second trimester of her pregnancy. Which medication would be preferred for FN?

    a. Desiccated thyroid hormone
    b. Liothyronine alone
    c. Levothyroxine alone
    d. Levothyroxine in combination with liothyronine

Answer a is incorrect. Desiccated thyroid hormone is not the preferred thyroid hormone replacement product used for hypothyroidism in general due to the difficulty in standardizing concentrations. Standardization is based on the iodine content instead of the hormonal content.

Answer b is incorrect. Generally, liothyronine is not used alone for the treatment of hypothyroidism. It does not replace T_4.

Answer c is correct. Levothyroxine is the preferred thyroid replacement product. It provides T_4 that can be converted to T_3 in the peripheral tissues of the body. It has a category A pregnancy rating, so is safe and effective for use in pregnancy. The risks of not treating hypothyroidism in pregnancy are much greater than the risk of treating with levothyroxine.

Answer d is incorrect. The combination of levothyroxine and liothyronine has not proven to be beneficial.

---

19. What is the treatment of choice for amiodarone-induced hypothyroidism?

    a. Desiccated thyroid hormone
    b. Liothyronine alone
    c. Levothyroxine alone
    d. Levothyroxine in combination with liothyronine

Answer a is incorrect. Desiccated thyroid hormone is not the preferred thyroid hormone replacement product used for hypothyroidism in general due to the difficulty in standardizing concentrations. Standardization is based on the iodine content instead of the hormonal content.

Answer b is incorrect. Generally, liothyronine is not used alone for the treatment of hypothyroidism. It does not replace T_4.

Answer c is correct. Amiodarone-induced hypothyroidism responds to treatment with levothyroxine. Once amiodarone is discontinued, thyroid levels usually return to normal unless antithyroid antibodies have formed.

Answer d is incorrect. The combination of levothyroxine and liothyronine has not proven to be beneficial.

---

20. Which of the following is true?
    a. Radioactive iodine will adequately treat type 1 amiodarone-induced hyperthyroidism.
    b. Amiodarone must be discontinued to adequately treat type 1 amiodarone-induced hypothyroidism.
    c. Amiodarone must be discontinued to adequately treat type 2 amiodarone-induced hypothyroidism.
    d. Antithyroid medications may offer some benefit in type 2 amiodarone-induced hypothyroidism.

Answer a is incorrect. Type 1 amiodarone-induced hyperthyroidism does not respond to radioactive iodine due to low radioiodine uptake with this form.

Answer b is correct. Resumption of a euthyroid state requires the discontinuation of amiodarone.

Answer c is incorrect. Type 2 amiodarone-induced hyperthyroidism is inflammatory in nature that may resolve after 1 to 3 months. Discontinuation of amiodarone may not be necessary.

Answer d is incorrect. Antithyroid medications only offer some benefit in type 1 amiodarone-induced hyperthyroidism. Corticosteroids may need to treat the inflammatory process associated with type 2 amiodarone-induced hyperthyroidism.

CHAPTER 60 | Contraception

1. TK is a 23-year-old woman who comes to your pharmacy stating that she is taking the mini-pill and missed her dose yesterday. Based on this information, what is the best remedy in this situation?
    a. She should take two tablets today as soon as possible, no backup method is needed.
    b. She should start taking her tablets as scheduled and use a backup method for the next 48 hours.
    c. She should take two tablets today as soon as possible and use a backup method until she gets her period.
    d. She should start taking her tablets as scheduled and use a backup method until she gets her period.

Answer a is incorrect. Since this is a progestin-only birth control pill, its mechanism of action is very dependent on the timing of administration.

Answer b is correct. Progestin-only birth control pills need to be taken at the same time every day. Missing a dose more than 3 hours of its scheduled time is considered a missed dose and may affect the effectiveness of the medication. Therefore, a backup method is required for 48 hours.

Answer c is incorrect. She does not need to use a backup method until her next period or double up on pills.

Answer d is incorrect. She does not need to use a backup method until her next period.

---

2. AC is a 26-year-old woman who presents to the pharmacy asking to buy emergency contraceptives and says she had unprotected intercourse 3 days ago. Based on the information, select the best statement as it relates to EC.
    a. EC will not be effective for AC because it has been longer than 24 hours since she has had unprotected sex.
    b. EC will not be effective for AC because it has been longer than 48 hours since she has had unprotected sex.
    c. EC cannot be provided to AC without a prescription from her doctor.
    d. EC may still work for AC because it is still within 72 hours since she has had unprotected sex.
    e. EC may still work for AC because it is still within 120 hours since she has had unprotected sex, but she will require a prescription.

Answer a is incorrect. EC is effective for up to 120 hours after unprotected intercourse.

Answer b is incorrect. EC is effective for up to 120 hours after unprotected intercourse.

Answer c is incorrect. EC for women older than 18 years old does not require a prescription.

Answer d is correct. EC is effective for up to 120 hours after unprotected intercourse.

Answer e is incorrect. EC is effective for up to 120 hours after unprotected intercourse but a prescription is not required for women older than 18 years.

---

3. Which of the following products provides the least amount of ethinyl estradiol?
    a. Contraceptive vaginal ring
    b. Contraceptive patch
    c. Low dose combined oral contraceptive (30 μg EE)
    d. All of the above provide the same amount of ethinyl estradiol

---

Answer a is correct. The contraceptive vaginal ring provides the least amount of estradiol, 15 μg/d.

Answer b is incorrect. The contraceptive patch provides the most ethinyl estradiol of choices. It provides 60% more ethinyl estradiol than a 35 μg oral formulation.

Answer c is incorrect. The combined oral contraceptive provides 30 μg of ethinyl estradiol compared to the 15 μg provided by the contraceptive vaginal ring.

Answer d is incorrect. The formulations offer varying amounts of ethinyl estradiol.

---

4. Which of the following has an FDA indication for the treatment of acne?
   a. Depo-Provera
   b. NuvaRing
   c. Ortho-Cept
   d. Estrostep

Answer a is incorrect. Depo-Provera is not FDA approved for acne treatment.

Answer b is incorrect. NuvaRing is not FDA approved for acne treatment.

Answer c is incorrect. Ortho-Cept is not FDA approved for acne treatment.

Answer d is correct. Estrostep, Ortho Tri-Cyclen, and YAZ are FDA approved for acne treatment; although, most birth control pills will help relieve acne.

---

5. Which of the following is best to avoid in overweight/obese patients due to the side effects of weight gain?
   a. Depo-Provera
   b. NuvaRing
   c. Ortho Evra
   d. Yasmin

Answer a is correct. Depo-Provera is not the best agent to use in women who are overweight or obese since it may cause more weight gain.

Answer b is incorrect. NuvaRing has not been shown to cause a significant weight gain.

Answer c is incorrect. Ortho Evra has not been shown to cause a significant weight gain but should be avoided due to decreased effectiveness in women weighing more than 198 lb.

Answer d is incorrect. Yasmin has not been shown to cause a significant weight gain.

---

6. How often is one NuvaRing inserted vaginally?
   a. 1 week
   b. 3 weeks
   c. 2 weeks
   d. 4 weeks

Answer a is incorrect. One vaginal contraceptive ring should be inserted for 3 weeks not for 1 week.

Answer b is correct. One vaginal contraceptive ring should be inserted for 3 weeks.

Answer c is incorrect. One vaginal contraceptive ring should be inserted for 3 weeks not for 2 weeks.

Answer d is incorrect. One vaginal contraceptive ring should be inserted for 3 weeks not for 4 weeks.

---

7. BW is a 28-year-old woman who delivered a baby 1 week ago. She does not plan to breast-feed and would like to start combined oral contraceptives as soon as possible. When is the earliest she can start taking combined oral contraceptives without an increased risk of blood clots?
   a. Immediately
   b. 2 weeks postpartum
   c. 6 weeks postpartum
   d. 6 months postpartum

Answer a is incorrect. There is a higher risk of blood clots if combined oral contraceptives are taken less than 6 weeks postpartum.

Answer b is incorrect. There is a higher risk of blood clots if combined oral contraceptives are taken less than 6 weeks postpartum. If BW takes COCs 2 weeks postpartum she may have an increased risk of clotting.

Answer c is correct. There is a higher risk of blood clots if combined oral contraceptives are taken less than 6 weeks postpartum. It is recommended to begin COC/CHCs at 6 weeks if the patient is interested in hormonal contraception and not breast-feeding since COC/CHCs may affect breast milk in a woman with difficulty producing milk.

Answer d is incorrect. There is no need to wait for 6 months. The patient may start COC/CHCs as soon as 6 weeks postpartum if she chooses.

---

8. AJ is a 22-year-old woman who weighs 220 lb and would like to start hormonal contraception. Which of the following products would not be as effective in preventing pregnancy for AJ?
   a. Depo-Provera
   b. NuvaRing
   c. Ortho Evra
   d. Yasmin

Answer a is incorrect. There is no issue with effectiveness of Depo-Provera in women weighing more than 198 lb. However, it may increase weight gain.

Answer b is incorrect. At this time, there is no issue with effectiveness of NuvaRing in women weighing more than 198 lb.

Answer c is correct. Ortho Evra is not recommended in patients weighing 198 lb or more due to a higher failure rate in those women.

Answer d is incorrect. There is no issue with effectiveness of Yasmin in women weighing more than 198 lb.

---

9. Which of the following products contains drospirenone and may increase potassium levels?
   a. Alesse
   b. YAZ
   c. Cyclessa
   d. Nor-QD

Answer a is incorrect. Alesse does not contain drospirenone but contains levonorgestrel.

Answer b is correct. YAZ contains drospirenone which is a derivative of spironolactone and may increase potassium levels.

Answer c is incorrect. Cyclessa does not contain drospirenone but contains desogestrel.

Answer d is incorrect. Nor-QD does not contain drospirenone. It is a progestin-only oral contraceptive.

10. RS just started a new oral combined oral contraceptive 2 weeks ago and has had some mild nausea when she takes the pill. What is the best recommendation for RS with respect to changing products?
    a. Change the oral combined contraceptive to another agent this week
    b. Wait for 3 months to see if side effects improve, if not change products
    c. Wait for 2 months to see if side effects improve, if not change products
    d. Wait for 6 months to see if side effects improve, if not change products

Answer a is incorrect. It is recommended to try a COC for at least 3 months before changing products. One week is not enough time for RS.

Answer b is correct. It is recommended to try a COC for at least 3 months before changing products. For counseling, patients may be instructed to take COCs at bedtime to help decrease nausea.

Answer c is incorrect. It is recommended to try a COC for at least 3 months before changing products. Two months is not enough time for RS.

Answer d is incorrect. It is recommended to try a COC for at least 3 months before changing products.

11. Select the generic name for Plan B.
    a. Levonorgestrel
    b. Desogestrel
    c. Norgestimate
    d. Ethinyl estradiol
    e. Norethindrone

Answer a is correct. The generic name for Plan B is levonorgestrel. It contains two tablets of levonorgestrel 0. 75 mg.

Answer b is incorrect. Desogestrel is in other formulations such as Mircette and Desogen, but is not the generic of Plan B.

Answer c is incorrect. Norgestimate is in other formulations such as Ortho-Cyclen, but is not the generic of Plan B.

Answer d is incorrect. Ethinyl estradiol is an estrogen and Plan B contains only a progestin.

Answer e is incorrect. Norethindrone in other formulations such as Ovcon-35, but is not the generic of Plan B.

12. Select the contraceptive agent that is formulated as an injection.
    a. Desogen
    b. Mirena
    c. Estrostep
    d. Ortho Evra
    e. Depo-Provera

Answer a is incorrect. Desogen is an oral combined contraceptive.

Answer b is incorrect. Mirena is an intrauterine system that provides progestin daily.

Answer c is incorrect. Estrostep is an oral combined contraceptive.

Answer d is incorrect. Ortho Evra is a transdermal contraceptive patch.

Answer e is correct. Depo-Provera is an injectable progestin-only contraceptive available intramuscularly and subcutaneously.

13. JS is a 21-year-old man who comes to your pharmacy and states, "What can my girlfriend and I use to make sure she doesn't get pregnant and protect ourselves from, you know... diseases?" Select the best regimen to recommend from the following choices below.
    a. Water-based lubricant + male latex condom
    b. Oil-based lubricant + male latex condom
    c. Female condom + male latex condom
    d. Female condom + male lamb cecum condom
    e. Oil-based lubricant + male lamb cecum condom

Answer a is correct. Water-based lubricant is safe to use with latex condoms and do not comprise its ability to protect against STIs.

Answer b is incorrect. Oil-based lubricant is not safe to use with latex condoms since it comprises its ability to protect against STIs by breaking down the latex.

Answer c is incorrect. The female condom and male latex condom should not be used together. They may stick together, cause friction, and break.

Answer d is incorrect. The female condom and male lamb cecum condom should not be used together. They may stick together, cause friction, and break.

Answer e is incorrect. Oil-based and water-based lubricants may be used with male lamb cecum condoms, however, lamb cecum condoms themselves do not protect against all STIs.

---

14. Which of the following condoms conducts heat very well and also protects against STIs?
    a. Polyurethane
    b. Latex
    c. Lamb cecum
    d. All of the above

Answer a is correct. Polyurethane condoms conduct heat better than latex condoms. They also protect against STIs, however, they may break easier than other condoms.

Answer b is incorrect. Latex condoms are best for protecting against STIs, however, they do not conduct heat as well as lamb cecum or polyurethane condoms.

Answer c is incorrect. Lamb cecum condoms conduct heat very well, but do not protect against all STIs.

Answer d is incorrect. Not all of the answers are correct.

---

15. What is the total number of active tablets contained in the product Seasonale?
    a. 24
    b. 21
    c. 44
    d. 84
    e. 91

Answer a is incorrect. There are 24 active tablets in formulations such as YAZ and Loestrin 24.

Answer b is incorrect. There are 21 active tablets in most COC formulations, but not Seasonale.

Answer c is incorrect. There are no formulations of COCs that have 44 active tablets.

Answer d is correct. There are 84 active tablets in the product Seasonale. It is an extended cycle regimen and marketed as such.

Answer e is incorrect. There are 91 tablets in the product Seasonale, but only 84 are active with 7 placebo tablets.

---

16. CS is a 36-year-old woman who admits to smoking 1 pack of cigarettes per day. She is getting married and would like to start hormonal contraception. Which of the following products is most appropriate for CS?
    a. NuvaRing
    b. Ortho Evra
    c. Mircette
    d. Tri-Levlen
    e. Nor-QD

Answer a is incorrect. NuvaRing contains ethinyl estradiol and etonogestrel. Ethinyl estradiol is contraindicated for use in women older than 35 years and who smoke more than 15 cigarettes per day. The risk of stroke and clots rise in this population.

Answer b is incorrect. Ortho Evra contains ethinyl estradiol and norgestrelomin. Ethinyl estradiol is contraindicated for use in women older than 35 years and who smoke more than 15 cigarettes per day. The risk of stroke and clots rise in this population.

Answer c is incorrect. Mircette contains ethinyl estradiol and desogestrel. Ethinyl estradiol is contraindicated for use in women older than 35 years and who smoke more than 15 cigarettes per day. The risk of stroke and clots rise in this population.

Answer d is incorrect. Tri-Levlen contains ethinyl estradiol and desogestrel. Ethinyl estradiol is contraindicated for use in women older than 35 years and who smoke more than 15 cigarettes per day. The risk of stroke and clots rise in this population.

Answer e is correct. Nor-QD is a progestin-only oral contraceptive and is not contraindicated in women older than 35 years who smoke.

---

17. Which of the following drugs may decrease the effectiveness of Ortho-Tri Cyclen?
    a. Atorvastatin
    b. Carbamazepine
    c. Lamotrigine
    d. Acetaminophen
    e. Levothyroxine

Answer a is incorrect. Atorvastatin increases the levels of ethinyl estradiol.

Answer b is correct. Carbamazepine induces the metabolism of ethinyl estradiol and decreases its effectiveness.

Answer c is incorrect. Lamotrigine may increase the levels of ethinyl estradiol.

Answer d is incorrect. Acetaminophen does not affect the levels of ethinyl estradiol or norgestimate.

Answer e is incorrect. Levothyroxine does not affect the levels of ethinyl estradiol or norgestimate.

18. DL is a 19-year-old woman who calls you and states that she forgot to take her Desogen (EE 30 μg/0.15 mg desogestrel) tablets for the last 2 days. She says she is in her second week of the cycle. Select the following statement that is most appropriate for missed tablets.

    a. DL should take two tablets the next day and use a backup method for 7 days
    b. DL should continue taking her tablets as scheduled, one per day, no backup method is necessary
    c. DL should discard her pill pack and start a new one, use a backup method for 7 days
    d. DL should take two tablets for 2 days and use a backup method for 7 days
    e. DL should take two tablets for 2 days, no backup method is necessary

---

Answer a is incorrect. If two tablets of a COC are missed, two tablets for 2 days should be taken and a backup method should be used for 7 days and. EC may also be used if unprotected intercourse occurred within the last 5 days.

Answer b is incorrect. If two tablets of a COC are missed, a backup method should be used for 7 days and two tablets for 2 days should be taken. EC may also be used if unprotected intercourse occurred within the last 5 days.

Answer c is incorrect. DL does not need to start a new pack. She may, but it is not necessary and is not the best answer considering cost.

Answer d is correct. Since DL is taking a 30 μg EE COC, if two tablets are missed, a backup method should be used for 7 days and two tablets for 2 days should be taken. EC may also be used if unprotected intercourse occurred within the last 5 days.

Answer e is incorrect. If two tablets of a COC are missed, two tablets for 2 days should be taken and a backup method should be used for 7 days and EC may also be used if unprotected intercourse occurred within the last 5 days.

---

19. Combined hormonal contraception is contraindicated in which of the conditions?

    a. History of deep vein thrombosis
    b. Migraine with aura
    c. Active liver disease
    d. Uncontrolled hypertension
    e. All of the above

Answer e is correct and the best answer. All of the answers are correct. Ethinyl estradiol can increase the risk of blood clots. Therefore, CHCs are contraindicated in patients with a history of deep vein thrombosis. There is also a higher risk of stroke in patients who experience migraines with aura and take CHCs. Therefore, CHCs are contraindicated in patients with a history of migraines with aura. CHCs are metabolized through the liver and may also have side effects on the liver. Therefore, CHCs should not be used in patients with active liver disease. Ethinyl estradiol can increase blood pressure. Patients with uncontrolled hypertension may increase their risk of stroke if they use CHCs and have uncontrolled hypertension.

---

20. Which of the following has an FDA indication for the treatment of premenstrual dysphoric disorder (PMDD)?

    a. YAZ
    b. Ortho Tri-Cyclen
    c. Estrostep
    d. Mircette
    e. Yasmin

Answer a is correct. YAZ is FDA approved for PMDD.

Answer b is incorrect. Ortho Tri-Cyclen is not FDA approved for PMDD, but is approved for acne treatment.

Answer c is incorrect. Estrostep is not FDA approved for PMDD, but is approved for acne treatment.

Answer d is incorrect. Mircette is not FDA approved for PMDD.

Answer e is incorrect. Yasmin is not FDA approved for PMDD.

CHAPTER 61 | Smoking Cessation

1. JT is a 42-year-old black man who is interested in quitting smoking. He has smoked 1 pack per day for the last 20 years. He had one successful quit attempt in the past that lasted for approximately 16 months, but went back to smoking after starting a new job 3 years ago. Based on the various components of nicotine dependence, which reason most likely caused JT to return to smoking?

    a. Psychological dependence
    b. Physiologic dependence
    c. He did not use a pharmacologic aid to quit smoking
    d. Most persons will relapse within 24 months of a quit attempt

---

Answer a is correct. While the physical addiction to nicotine resolves in 1 to 2 weeks after stopping smoking, the person will continue to have the cravings to perform the action of smoking. Because nicotine acts on the pleasure center and reward pathway in the brain, persons tend to equate smoking with pleasure and/or calming sensations. Since the body continues to achieve or recreate these sensations, the need to smoke persists indefinitely, but at diminished levels.

Answer b is incorrect. In the early weeks of tobacco cessation, persons will seek cigarettes to avoid withdrawal symptoms and the accompanying discomfort. These symptoms last for approximately 1 to 2 weeks. Since JT was abstinent from cigarettes for 16 months, the time period for physical withdrawal symptoms had passed.

Answer c is incorrect. The maintenance of a successful quit attempt is not altered by the modality in which a patient used to quit smoking. Since JT was able to quit "cold turkey," his chances of relapsing are not increased.

Answer d is incorrect. While the risk of relapse back to smoking is continual and the number of persons who remain tobacco free dwindles with time, a person cannot consider themselves without risk of relapse after 24 months.

---

2. HN has decided that she would like to quit smoking, but is not comfortable doing it without some kind of support from a nicotine replacement agent. She decides that the gum will be her best choice because it is easily concealable among friends, family, and coworkers. She has smoked 1 to 1.5 packs per day for the last 16 years. What is the appropriate starting dose for the nicotine polacrilex gum for HN?

   a. 4-mg piece of gum; not to exceed 24 doses in 24 hours
   b. 4-mg piece of gum; not to exceed 20 doses in 24 hours
   c. 2-mg piece of gum; not to exceed 24 pieces in 24 hours
   d. 2-mg piece of gum; not to exceed 20 pieces in 24 hours

Answer a is correct. HN is smoking 20 to 30 cigarettes (average 25) throughout the day. The recommended dose for this quantity of cigarettes is 4 mg so as not to under dose the person's nicotine expectations. While the maximum number of pieces of gum is 24 pieces for a 24-hour period, the person should base their usage on symptoms and signs of adverse events/nicotine toxicity.

Answer b is incorrect. While the dose of the nicotine gum is correct, the maximum number of doses per 24 hours is not correct.

Answer c is incorrect. The 2-mg dose would most likely be too low for this patient and she would experience cravings through its use or soon after stopping use.

Answer d is incorrect. Both the dose and the maximum number of pieces per day is not correct.

---

3. How long should HN continue to use the first dose/frequency of the gum before titrating down to the next dose/frequency?

   a. 8 weeks
   b. 6 weeks
   c. 4 weeks
   d. 2 weeks

Answer a is incorrect. While patients may choose to continue the initial dose/frequency of the nicotine gum longer than the recommended 6 weeks, the goal is to have the person quit using nicotine as soon as possible. Using nicotine replacement is a safer alternative to smoking cigarettes, but the effects of nicotine on the cardiovascular, gastrointestinal, and other organ systems are still a risk versus nothing.

Answer b is correct. The recommended starting dose/frequency for the gum is 6 weeks. This initial time period allows for the patient to work through the psychological and behavioral changes necessary for a successful quit attempt, without depriving the body of the nicotine it has become accustomed to. After this initial time period, the titration periods are more rapid, attempting to alleviate the physical symptoms.

Answers c and d are incorrect. While patients may be successful using these shorter schedules, they should be reserved for the later stages of tobacco cessation. Initially, the patient needs to make the necessary behavioral changes that will minimize their exposure to smoking or situations he or she associates with smoking. By shortening the initial duration of nicotine replacement therapy, there is the risk of adding physical cravings prematurely to the process of psychological change.

---

4. AP is 29 years old and starting a new job in a dental clinic. She wishes to quit smoking before she starts her new job because the clinic does not allow employees to smoke during their shift. However, she would also like to quit to preserve her lung health. She smokes approximately 15 cigarettes daily and has her first one in the car on the way to work (about 95 minutes after waking). She wishes to use the lozenges for her quit attempt. What product would you suggest that AP use?

   a. Nicotrol 4 mg
   b. Nicotrol 2 mg
   c. Commit 4 mg
   d. Commit 2 mg

Answers a and b are incorrect. Nicotrol is not commercially available as a lozenge. It is formulated as a nasal inhaler, oral inhaler, a gum, and a patch, but not as a lozenge.

Answer c is incorrect. While the nicotine gum is dosed based on how many cigarettes per day a person smokes, the nicotine lozenge dose is based on the amount of time from waking in the morning to the person's first cigarette. If less than 30 minutes, then the dose is 4 mg. Being that AP's first cigarette of the day is approximately 95 minutes after waking, this dose would be too high.

Answer d is correct. AP's first cigarette is 95 minutes after waking in the morning, qualifying her to start with the 2 mg lozenge.

---

5. AP has chosen the lozenges because she is unable to chew gum at work. She also suffers from which condition that can be made worse using nicotine polacrilex gum?

   a. Temporomandibular joint disorder
   b. Gingival hyperplasia
   c. Oropharyngeal candidiasis
   d. Episodic epistaxis

Answer a is correct. TMJ symptoms are worsened with repetitive chewing or chewing tough foods/items. Since AP would have to chew nicotine gum aggressively in order to use the nicotine gum, it may worsen her TMJ symptoms. In a case such as this, the person may experience the same quick relief of a transbuccal medication without needing to chew and park.

Answer b is incorrect. While this condition may cause discomfort, its symptoms are not made worse with aggressive or repetitive chewing. The release and absorption of nicotine would not be affected.

Answer c is incorrect. Nicotine does not affect the immune function of the mouth and pharynx and will not increase the chances of a person developing oropharyngeal candidiasis.

Answer d is incorrect. The use of oral nicotine replacement products would not affect or be altered due to nasal irritation and nose bleedings.

---

6. JE is a 68-year-old man with 1 pack per day for the last 40 years smoking history. He has never attempted to quit smoking, but feels he must try after being hospitalized for pneumonia for 3 days. While he was in the hospital he was given a nicotine patch to wear and change daily until discharge. Upon discharge, he was not given the nicotine patch, but wants to continue using it to abstain from smoking. What dose of the patch should JE start?
   a. 21 mg/d patch
   b. 14 mg/d patch
   c. 7 mg/d patch
   d. He does not smoke enough to warrant NRT with a patch

Answer a is correct. JE smokes approximately 20 cigarettes daily. The 21-mg nicotine patch is recommended for persons who smoke >10 cigarettes per day. He should continue this dose for approximately 6 weeks before decreasing to the 14-mg patch to maximize his chance of success.

Answer b is incorrect. A person would only start on a 14-mg patch daily if he or she smoked <10 cigarettes per day *or* could not tolerate the ADRs associated with the 21-mg patch. If the person were to start on the 14-mg patch, he or she should continue on this dose for approximately 6 weeks before decreasing the dose.

Answer c is incorrect. It is not recommended to start at a 7-mg patch daily unless the person requires nicotine replacement therapy and cannot tolerate the 14-mg dose.

Answer d is incorrect.

---

7. JE has been without a cigarette for 3 days with the help of the nicotine patch. On the fourth day, JE is under a great deal of stress and needs to go outside for a cigarette. Since he is still wearing the nicotine replacement patch, what adverse event will he most likely experience?
   a. Excess fatigue
   b. Lower extremity cramping
   c. Nausea, vomiting, and headache
   d. Tinnitus

Answer a is incorrect. Most likely, JE will begin to experience symptoms consistent with anxiety and nervousness.

Answer b is incorrect. Nicotine replacement therapy while a person is smoking appears to mimic a sympathetic overload. JE's lower extremities may feel anxious or overactive, but should not exhibit symptoms of traditional cramping.

Answer c is correct. Some of the most common signs and symptoms of nicotine toxicity include nausea, vomiting, headaches, increased blood pressure, and tachycardia. Since JE is already receiving a continuous supply of nicotine via the patch, the quick release of nicotine from the cigarette will only increase his chances of these side effects.

Answer d is incorrect. Nicotine toxicity will not cause tinnitus and/or other hearing disturbances.

---

8. What would be a better choice for JE to use for breakthrough cravings while he is being treated with the nicotine patch?
   a. Nicorette gum
   b. Chantix 1 mg twice daily
   c. Zyban 150 mg twice daily
   d. He should not combine therapies for smoke tobacco cessation

---

Answer a is correct. The nicotine patch will provide a basal release of nicotine to the person over a 16- to 24-hour period. The Nicorette gum has the ability to provide the "quick fix" to help a person overcome a significant daytime craving. While the chances of developing nicotine toxicity increase when combining agents, the utility has proven to be better than any agent alone.

Answers b and c are incorrect. Each of the nonnicotine products to help persons quit smoking do not affect immediate craving issues. The varenicline will block nicotine receptor binding and gently stimulate the same receptors in an attempt to alleviate cravings all day. The bupropion will stabilize the dopaminergic response and reward pathway in the brain, but not provide instant relief.

Answer d is incorrect. Many of the best therapeutic options involve a combination of long-acting nicotine replacement product with an immediate release nicotine product.

---

9. OH is a 39-year-old woman with multiple psychiatric medical conditions. She started smoking approximately 5 years ago and has slowly increased her daily cigarette consumption to 2 packs per day. She started using Nicoderm CQ 21 mg patches, but has experienced various abnormal dreams, causing her to lose sleep over the last 3 nights. She will not continue using the patches if the dreams continue. What would be the best alternative for her?

a. Nicotrol 15 mg/d patch
b. Habitrol 21 mg/d patch
c. Habitrol 14 mg/d patch
d. Nicotine transdermal patch system 21 mg/d patch

Answer a is correct. The 15 mg patch is a 16-hour release formulation, designed to not release any further drug after 16 hours. While its efficacy has been found to be equal to the 24-hour patches, it has less of a chance to cause abnormal dreaming and insomnia.

Answers b, c, and d are incorrect. All three of these agents are 24-hour formulations and (if left on) may cause excess adverse events in the evening and sleeping hours. Patients may always remove the 24-hour path prior to bedtime.

---

10. OH decides not to use the nicotine patches and switches to the Commit nicotine lozenge. Which of the following scenarios for use is the worst with regard to altered pharmacokinetics?

a. In the morning, immediately after waking
b. In the afternoon, during her scheduled work break
c. In the evening, after her dinner and coffee
d. Before bedtime, watching the evening news

Answers a, b, and d are incorrect. Since a higher oral pH can affect the absorption of nicotine transbuccally, time of day has little to do with maximum (or minimum) absorption do to pharmacokinetics.

Answer c is correct. Products such as coffee, fruit juices, and certain foods can alter the pH of the mouth and either enhance or hinder drug absorption. An acidic product will decrease the pH of the mouth and lead to less transbuccal absorption of the nicotine product.

---

11. OH's provider also decides to use a prescription, nonnicotine, smoking cessation aid because she feels that using lozenges as needed will not be sufficient. Which of the following medications would be discouraged in the patient?

a. Varenicline
b. Bupropion
c. Nortriptyline
d. Clonidine

Answer a is correct. In 2007, the FDA issued a warning and requested a label change for varenicline that informed prescribers and customers of the agent's propensity to worsen depression and other neuropsychiatric conditions.

Answers b and c are incorrect. OH has a history significant for multiple psychiatric medical conditions. Bupropion and nortriptyline could both serve as primary or adjunct therapy for these neuropsychiatric conditions as well as help prevent cravings for nicotine.

Answer d is incorrect. While clonidine is not an ideal agent to choose, it does not have the warnings or precautions that the varenicline carries with it. The patient would need to be cautious of orthostatic hypotension, anticholinergic symptoms, or rebound cardiac symptoms (if stopped abruptly).

---

12. JM is a 44-year-old woman with a history of dysmenorrhea and tobacco abuse. She has disregarded the advice to quit smoking while she was taking oral contraceptives for the past 10 or more years. Last month, she developed a deep vein thrombosis (DVT) during a long car trip and decided that she needed to quit smoking so as not to be at risk for another one. She is given a prescription for Chantix starter pack and told to start the dose titration _______ week(s) before her quit date.

a. One
b. Two
c. Three
d. Four

Answer a is correct. Chantix should be started approximately 1 week prior to the established quit date. Over this first week, the patient will titrate the dose of Chantix from 0.5 mg daily for 3 days, then 0.5 mg twice daily for days 4 through 7, and then 1 mg twice daily for up to 12 to 24 weeks. The initial week of titration and preparation allows the patient to start their tobacco abstinence close to full dose of varenicline.

Answer b is incorrect. Bupropion typically requires persons start the agent at least 2 weeks before their quit date to ensure maximum drug concentration when refraining from smoking cigarettes.

Answers c and d are incorrect. Bupropion may be continued while a person smokes for about 8 weeks. However, because varenicline antagonizes nicotine receptors in the brain as well as slightly stimulates them, continuing to smoke for an extra 2 to 3 weeks after starting Chantix will increase the person's chance of experiencing adverse events.

---

13. The most common adverse event that JM should be warned about is

a. Insomnia
b. Headache
c. Abnormal dreaming
d. Nausea

Answer a is incorrect. 18% of persons will experience insomnia.

Answer b is incorrect. 15% of persons will experience headache.

Answer c is incorrect. 13% of persons will experience abnormal dreaming.

Answer d is correct. 30% of persons will experience nausea.

---

14. Which disease should JM be screened for before starting varenicline?
    a. Hypertension
    b. Diabetes
    c. Chronic obstructive lung disease
    d. Renal insufficiency

Answer a in incorrect. Varenicline does not have an effect on the sympathetic nervous system and only reports infrequent to rare cardiac adverse events.

Answer b is incorrect. No reports of new onset of diabetes or worsening glucose control have been associated with varenicline.

Answer c is incorrect.

Answer d is correct. Varenicline is metabolized and excreted via the kidneys. Patients with a creatinine clearance less than 30 mL/min, plasma drug concentrations were at least 2.1-fold greater than normal. These individuals should only receive up to 0.5 mg twice daily.

---

15. TY is a 37-year-old obese man with a medical history significant for hypertension and dyslipidemia. He also smokes cigarettes and has smoked 1.5 packs per day for the last 17 years. His most recent blood pressure was 158/94 mm Hg, which is consistent with his previous three readings. His physician is convinced that if TY were to lose weight and quit smoking, many of his medical issues would be easier to care for. TY requests some assistance to quit smoking. Which of the following medications would be the best choice for TY?
    a. Bupropion
    b. Nicotine polacrilex gum
    c. Nicotine patch
    d. Varenicline

Answer a is incorrect. While bupropion is an acceptable agent to choose for tobacco cessation, the patient has concurrent uncontrolled hypertension. This is not a contraindication for therapy, but was worsen his hypertension or make it more difficult to control. There are other options available that would not have this impact on his other comorbidities.

Answers b and c are incorrect. Again, since the patient has uncontrolled hypertension, choosing an agent that may worsen the condition should be avoided.

Answer d is correct. In this case, varenicline is the most appropriate choice because it would have the least negative impact on his other disease states and would increase his chances of quitting over quitting without pharmacologic assistance.

---

16. Despite the best choice for TY, he starts bupropion 150 mg twice daily. How should TY begin taking this medication?
    a. One tablet daily for 3 days and then one tablet twice daily, 1 week before his quit date
    b. One tablet daily for 3 days and then one tablet twice daily, 2 weeks before his quit date
    c. One tablet daily for 7 days and then one tablet twice daily, 1 week before his quit date
    d. One tablet daily for 7 days and then one tablet twice daily, 2 weeks before his quit date

---

Answer a is incorrect. The initial titration over 3 days is appropriate, but the medication should be started at least 2 weeks before the patient's quit date.

Answer b is correct. The patient should take bupropion 150 mg sustained release (SR) once daily for 3 days and then twice daily for the remainder of treatment. This titration will help the patient better tolerate adverse events such as insomnia, anxiety, or tremors. Also, the regimen was started 2 weeks before the quit date to allow for maximum drug concentration and steady state in the body. The agent may be used for up to 8 weeks prior to a person's quit date, but should be used for at least 2 weeks.

Answer c is incorrect. The dose titration over 7 days would be appropriate if increasing to twice daily yielded side effects, but the short pretreatment period (over 7 days) is not sufficient.

Answer d is incorrect. Starting the agent 2 weeks prior to a quit attempt is appropriate, but the initial dose titration over 7 days is not correct. The medication may be taken once daily for 7 days if the person has demonstrated adverse events to bupropion, but 3 days should be sufficient for most.

---

17. Since insomnia and anxiety are common adverse events with bupropion, which of the following recommendations will help TY the most?
    a. Do not take the second dose after 5 o'clock in the evening.
    b. If the patient develops insomnia, omit the second dose of the day.
    c. Insomnia is a temporary adverse event and will resolve approximately 7 days after increasing the dose to twice daily.
    d. The insomnia and anxiety are most likely due to nicotine withdrawal and will resolve approximately 7 to 10 days after quitting smoking.

Answer a is correct. In order for a patient to avoid such adverse events as insomnia and anxiety that interfere with restful sleep, the patient should avoid taking the second dose of the medication after 5 o'clock in the evening or 5 hours before a scheduled bedtime.

Answer b is incorrect. While the patient may omit the second dose of the day to avoid evening and night adverse events, it also jeopardizes his or her ability to be able to deal with the withdrawal symptoms or cravings that the bupropion is attempting to alleviate.

Answer c is incorrect. The insomnia is not likely a temporary effect and should be expected to continue throughout the course of therapy. If the patient is told to try and wait out the adverse event, the wakefulness and inability to sleep may lead to restarting smoking.

Answer d is incorrect. Insomnia and irritability are signs and symptoms of nicotine withdrawal, but may also be attributed to the bupropion therapy. It is not appropriate to just attribute these effects to the lack of nicotine and not appropriately address the ADR.

18. While combination therapy is ideal for patients attempting to quit smoking, which of the following combinations is *not* appropriate?
    a. Bupropion and nicotine polacrilex gum
    b. Nicotine patches and nicotine polacrilex gum
    c. Varenicline and nicotine polacrilex gum
    d. Nortriptyline and nicotine polacrilex gum

Answers a, b, and d are incorrect. These three combinations use a long-acting agent in conjunction with a short-acting agent. The first agent listed will help diminish cravings and withdrawal symptoms while the nicotine polacrilex gum will help the user overcome cravings throughout the day and night.

Answer c is correct. In this combination, the nicotine gum will be less effective at controlling cravings and more likely to cause adverse events such as nausea, vomiting, and headache. Since the varenicline can block the nicotine receptors in the brain, the effect of the gum is blunted or blocked. However, varenicline also provides slight stimulation to the nicotine receptors and the nicotine from the gum, in conjunction with the varenicline, may mimic the symptoms of nicotine toxicity.

19. LK is a 66-year-old woman with osteoporosis, chronic allergic rhinitis, and a 50-pack-year history of smoking cigarettes. At a recent trip to the dentist, she was told that due to poor oral hygiene and tooth decay, she would need to have her teeth removed and fitted for dentures. He also recommends that she quit smoking during this time period as it most likely contributed to her current predicament. Which agent listed below would be the best agent for LK to choose?
    a. Nicotine polacrilex gum
    b. Nicotine lozenge
    c. Nicotine nasal inhaler
    d. Nicotine transdermal patch

Answer a is incorrect. Since the patient is having her teeth extracted and fitted to dentures, the use of nicotine gum is not ideal. The gum may stick to the dentures and pull them out of place during the day.

Answer b is incorrect. While the lozenge offers the benefits of the gum without the need to chew, it also increases the chance of nicotine toxicity in this situation. If LK used the nicotine lozenge immediately after her procedure or during the healing process, there is a chance that she will absorb too much, too quickly, given the inflamed state of her mouth and gums.

Answer c is incorrect. Since the patient has a history of chronic allergic rhinitis, the nicotine nasal spray would not be beneficial.

Answer d is correct. Since the other 3 options for therapy were not appropriate given the woman's medical conditions and limitations, she could be tried on the nicotine patch. The first dose would be used for approximately 6 weeks and then she would begin to step down with her therapy. If she started with the 21-mg patch, then she would follow up with 2 weeks of the 14-mg patch and 2 weeks of the 7-mg patch. If she started with the 14-mg patch, she would only need to follow up with the 7-mg patch for 2 weeks.

20. AI is a 27-year-old woman with a past medical history significant for polycystic ovarian syndrome (PCOS), hypertriglyceridemia, epilepsy, hyperthyroidism, and tobacco abuse for the last 11 years. Which of her medical conditions is considered a precaution for using bupropion therapy?
    a. Polycystic ovarian syndrome
    b. Hypertriglyceridemia
    c. Epilepsy
    d. Hyperthyroidism

Answer a is incorrect. Bupropion will not have an effect on PCOS or any of its accompanying abnormalities.

Answer b is incorrect. Using bupropion has not demonstrated a change in serum triglyceride levels and would not affect this woman's free fatty acid levels.

Answer c is correct. Epilepsy or seizures is a precaution for bupropion use. The use of this medication will decrease the seizure threshold and may make it easier for a person to experience a seizure. Using the medication concurrently with other medications that have the same effect on the seizure threshold further increases the risk of seizure.

Answer d is incorrect. While bupropion may worsen some of the symptoms of hyperthyroidism, it is not a contraindication. Persons with overt hyperthyroidism exhibiting symptoms should most likely not start tobacco cessation therapy with bupropion, but may consider after surgery or medical management.

CHAPTER 62 | Glaucoma

KM is a 44-year-old African American woman with decreased peripheral vision. She was found to have a blind spot on the left side (visual field defect). She was in a motor vehicle accident because she did not see the car in the left lane. She complains of brow ache and headaches that have become worse over the past 2 weeks. Intraocular pressure measures 28 in the right eye and 26 in the left eye. She is on a fixed income and buying medications is often difficult. She works odd jobs with varying shifts. Her blood pressure was 140/95 mm Hg.

Diagnosis: Primary open angle glaucoma, hypertension, and insomnia.

Medications: Amlodipine 5 mg daily, pilocarpine 2% in both eyes qid, Tylenol PM 2 at bedtime.

Allergies: Sulfa. Hazel eyes turned brown on Xalatan and she refused treatment.

1. Which of the following are true about KM?
   a. She has at least three risk factors for glaucoma.
   b. Pilocar is first-line therapy for POAG.
   c. She could have drug-induced glaucoma.
   d. Both a and b.
   e. Both a and c.

Answer e is correct. KM risks for glaucoma include age >40 years, African American descent, elevated IOP. She is also taking the antihistamine Benadryl (Tylenol PM). This can worsen glaucoma. Pilocarpine is last-line therapy due to side effects.

2. Which of the following could affect KM's glaucoma therapy?
   a. Titration of the blood pressure medication can affect glaucoma.
   b. Adherence may be an issue.
   c. Nasolacrimal occlusion should be reviewed.
   d. Both b and c.
   e. a, b, and c.

Answer e correct. Both a, b, and c affect KM's glaucoma therapy. Changes in blood pressure affect IOP. Adherence may be an issue because of financial issues or KM's work schedule. NLO will help decrease risk of side effects and improve efficacy of the eye drops.

3. Which glaucoma medication is contraindicated for KM?
   a. Timolol
   b. Iopidine
   c. Brimonidine
   d. Dorzolamide
   e. Both a and b

Answer d is correct. Dorzolamide is a carbonic anhydrase inhibitor which contains sulfa. KM has a sulfa allergy.

4. Which medication may be causing KM to have brow aches?
   a. Amlodipine
   b. Acetaminophen
   c. Benadryl
   d. Pilocarpine
   e. Latanoprost

Answer d is correct. Older, centrally acting agents such as pilocarpine can cause brow aches.

5. Which of the following are good recommendations to improve KM's therapy?
   a. Discontinue Benadryl
   b. Switch to timolol extended release drops
   c. Titrate up to pilocarpine 4% qid
   d. Both a and b
   e. a, b, and c

Answer d is correct. Benadryl may worsen glaucoma and should be discontinued. Timolol XE could improve compliance. Pilocarpine should be used as last-line therapy.

6. Diagnosis of primary open angle glaucoma includes:
   a. Review of medications
   b. Evaluation of visual fields
   c. Tonometry
   d. Both b and c
   e. a, b, and c

Answer e is correct. All of these options are useful for the diagnosis of open angle glaucoma.

7. The most common type of glaucoma is
   a. Primary open angle
   b. Acute closed angle
   c. Drug-induced glaucoma
   d. Both a and c
   e. Both b and c

Answer a is correct. POAG is most common. Drug-induced and acute closed angle glaucoma have a low incidence.

8. Goals of treatment for glaucoma include:
   a. Decreasing intraocular pressure
   b. Increasing visual field defects
   c. Decreasing eye pain
   d. Both a and b
   e. Both a and c

Answer e is correct. Goals of treatment include decreasing intraocular pressure and eye pain. We also want to decrease visual field defects.

9. Medications reduce intraocular pressure by
   a. Increased aqueous humor outflow
   b. Increased carbonic anhydrase activity
   c. Increased aqueous humor reabsorption
   d. Both a and b
   e. Both a and c

Answer a is correct. The goal of therapy is to lower intraocular pressure by increased aqueous humor outflow, decrease carbonic anhydrase activity to decrease aqueous production, and to decrease reabsorption.

10. Aqueous humor is produced in the
    a. Ciliary body
    b. Trabecular meshwork
    c. Iris
    d. Canal of Schlemm
    e. Pituitary

Answer a is correct. Aqueous humor is produced in the ciliary body. The trabecular meshwork filters aqueous humor. The iris can block the angle between the iris and cornea to promote acute closure angle glaucoma. The canal of Schlemm and pituitary are not involved with aqueous humor production.

11. Which glaucoma medication class should be avoided in patients with a sulfa allergy?
    a. Prostaglandin analogs
    b. Beta-blockers
    c. Calcium channel blockers
    d. Carbonic anhydrase inhibitors
    e. Alpha-blockers

Answer d is correct. Carbonic anhydrase inhibitors contain a sulfa moiety.

12. 12.Which medication class is considered first-line treatment of open angle glaucoma?
    a. Beta-blockers
    b. Calcium channel blockers
    c. Carbonic anhydrase inhibitors
    d. Alpha-blockers
    e. Prostaglandin analog

Answer e is correct. Prostaglandin analogs have high efficacy rates and low risk of side effects. They are first line.

13. Which class of medications is associated with darker, thicker, and longer eye lashes?
    a. Prostaglandin analogs
    b. Carbonic anhydrase inhibitors
    c. Alpha-blockers
    d. Sympathomimetics
    e. Beta-blockers

Answer a is correct. Prostaglandin analogs can cause hyperpigmentation and hypertrichosis of the eye lashes.

14. Which of the following medications can cause drug-induced glaucoma?
    a. Corticosteroids
    b. Antihistamines
    c. Cimetidine
    d. Both a and b
    e. a, b, and c

Answer e is correct. All of these medications can worsen glaucoma. Corticosteroids and antihistamines have a high risk and cimetidine has a low risk.

15. Teaching patients about nasolacrimal occlusion helps:
    a. Improve medication effectiveness
    b. Decrease side effects
    c. Decrease systemic absorption of eye drops
    d. Both a and b
    e. a, b, and c

Answer e is correct. NLO enhances eye drop absorption to improve efficacy and decrease all side effects.

16. Pharmacist can improve outcomes in glaucoma by:
    a. Reviewing refill histories
    b. Providing medication education
    c. Teaching nasolacrimal occlusion
    d. a, b, and c
    e. Both b and c

Answer d is correct. All options are important goals for pharmacist and they all improve patient outcomes.

17. Which eye disease is characterized by elevated intraocular pressure but normal visual fields?
    a. Open angle glaucoma
    b. Closed angle glaucoma
    c. Hypotensive glaucoma
    d. Ocular hypertension
    e. Both a and c

Answer d is correct. Ocular hypertension is a risk factor for glaucoma. It is marked by increased intraocular pressure but no changes in the visual fields. Glaucoma is defined by both IOP and visual field defects.

18. Which glaucoma medication is associated with bronchospasm?
    a. Carbonic anhydrase inhibitors
    b. Epinephrine
    c. Prostaglandin analogs
    d. Mannitol
    e. Alpha-blockers

Answer b is correct. Epinephrine is a centrally acting agent that can cause bronchospasm when absorbed systemically. The other options do not cause bronchospasm.

19. Carbonic anhydrase inhibitors reduce intraocular pressure by:

    a. Miosis
    b. Decreased aqueous humor production
    c. Decreased osmolarity
    d. Increased aqueous humor outflow
    e. Opening of the Canal of Schlemm

Answer b is correct. Carbonic anhydrase inhibitors decrease aqueous humor production by inhibiting the enzyme carbonic anhydrase and blocking sodium and bicarbonate secretion.

20. The most important point of nasolacrimal occlusion includes

    a. Hand washing
    b. Separation of two doses of eye drops by 30 minutes
    c. 3 minutes time for closing the nasolacrimal duct
    d. Both b and c
    e. A, B, and C

Answer c is correct. The nasolacrimal duct should be closed for 1 to 3 minutes to increase eye drop absorption into the eye and to decrease systemic absorption and side effects.

CHAPTER 63 | Urology

1. Which of the following is the brand name for dutasteride?

    a. Hytrin
    b. Flomax
    c. Proscar
    d. Avodart
    e. Cardura

Answer a is incorrect. The chemical name for Hytrin is terazosin.

Answer b is incorrect. The chemical name for Flomax is tamsulosin.

Answer c is incorrect. The chemical name for Proscar is finasteride.

Answer d is correct.

Answer e in incorrect. The chemical name for Cardura is doxazosin.

2. An 82-year-old patient who is taking 2 mg of terazosin for BPH comes into the pharmacy complaining of dizziness and generalized muscle weakness and persistent LUTS. What would you recommend to his physician?

    a. Add finasteride 5 mg daily to his regimen.
    b. Switch his terazosin to doxazosin 4 mg.
    c. Switch his terazosin to tamsulosin 0.4 mg daily.
    d. Lower the dose of his terazosin to 1 mg.
    e. Add saw palmetto twice daily.

Answer a is incorrect. The patient is complaining of dizziness associated with his α-blocker therapy. Adding finasteride will not ameliorate this and, if a 5ARI were added, it may take several months to show benefit in symptom reduction.

Answer b is incorrect. Exchanging one long-acting, second-generation agent for another would not be ideal and this patient may continue to experience the same side effects.

Answer c is correct. Tamsulosin may afford better tolerability for this patient and would be expected to provide symptom relief relatively quickly, often within 1 week of therapy, as it does not require titration.

Answer d is incorrect. Lowering his dose of terazosin may improve tolerability; however, he is still experiencing symptoms of BPH. If his dose was lowered, he would likely continue to experience his symptoms.

Answer e is incorrect. Based on lack of clinical outcomes, phytotherapy is not recommended by the American Urological Association for treatment of BPH.

3. What pregnancy category is finasteride?

    a. A
    b. B
    c. C
    d. D
    e. X

Answer e is correct. 5-α-reductase inhibitors are associated with birth defects in men. 5ARI, including finasteride and dutasteride, should not be taken or handled by women who are pregnant or women of child-bearing age.

4. A patient reports that he has been taking his finasteride daily for the last 6 months for BPH. His last PSA was 2.6 ng/mL. Today it is 1.3 ng/mL. This can be best explained by which of the following?

    a. Finasteride stops the prostate from producing PSA.
    b. Finasteride can cause erroneous results in laboratory testing for PSA.
    c. PSA levels are often significantly decreased in patients taking 5ARI.
    d. Both a and b.
    e. All of the above.

Answer a is incorrect. The prostate still produces PSA after patients begin taking 5ARI therapy.

Answer b is incorrect. The decrease in PSA is not an anomaly associated with erroneous laboratory testing for PSA.

Answer c is correct. As finasteride decreases the size of the prostate, there is less prostate volume to produce PSA. PSA levels can be expected to decrease as much as 50% after beginning therapy with either finasteride or dutasteride.

Answers d and e are incorrect.

---

5. A patient planning on having cataract surgery next week presents with a prescription for tamsulosin. His symptoms are not particularly bothersome but he reports some urinary hesitancy and straining. You decide to:
   a. Fill the prescription and counsel the patient on risk of sexual side effects.
   b. Call his physician and ophthalmologist and get his order changed to finasteride.
   c. Call his physician and ophthalmologist to determine if treatment with tamsulosin should be deferred until after his cataract surgery.
   d. Fill the prescription and counsel on risk of dizziness and orthostatic hypotension.
   e. Call his physician and get his order changed to terazosin.

Answer a is incorrect. While tamsulosin can cause sexual side effects including ejaculatory disturbances, this is not the best answer.

Answer b is incorrect. Candidates for 5ARI include those with large prostate volume (typically >40 g). Without this information, it would be difficult to recommend finasteride for this patient.

Answer c is correct. Use of tamsulosin prior to cataract surgery is associated with surgical complications. While these can be treated, it may be prudent to determine if treatment can be deferred until after this procedure. His physician and ophthalmologist should be made aware of his intention to start this medication prior to cataract surgery.

Answer d is incorrect. As stated above, use of tamsulosin prior to cataract surgery may increase risk for surgical complications that may be prevented by deferring treatment.

Answer e is incorrect. Surgical complications have been associated with all α-blockers. At this time, informing his physician and discussing this issue with the patient is the best answer.

---

6. Which of the following is *not* an advantage of tamsulosin when compared to doxazosin?
   a. Increased efficacy in reducing LUTS.
   b. Improved tolerability especially cardiovascular side effects.
   c. Quicker onset of action in lowering symptoms.
   d. Both b and c.
   e. All of the above are advantages of tamsulosin for LUTS.

Answer a is correct. Tamsulosin is not more efficacious than other α-blockers. Most α-blockers, including doxazosin, will lower the AUA Symptom Score 4 to 6 points.

Answer b is incorrect. Tolerability is improved with use of tamsulosin as it specifically targets α_{1A}-receptors in the prostate. Discontinuation rates and cardiovascular side effects are reduced in patients taking tamsulosin versus other second-generation α-blockers (doxazosin and terazosin).

Answer c is incorrect. As tamsulosin does not require titration to reach an effective dose, its effects are seen often within the first week of therapy.

Answers d and e are incorrect.

---

7. Which of the following is mainly responsible for increased prostate growth?
   a. PSA
   b. DHT
   c. 5-α-reductase
   d. Testosterone
   e. All of the above are directly responsible for prostate growth

---

Answer a is incorrect. As PSA is *produced* by the prostate, it may be high in patients with an enlarged prostate. However, it does not directly *cause* an increase in prostate growth.

Answer b is correct. Androgens, specifically dihydrotestosterone, bind to androgen receptors and increase expression of genes that control prostate growth. For this reason, use of 5-α-reductase inhibitors (5ARI), which inhibit the conversion of testosterone to dihydrotestosterone, are therapeutic targets to prevent this process.

Answer c is incorrect. While 5-α-reductase facilitates the conversion of testosterone to DHT, it is simply the enzyme and is not directly responsible for increasing prostate growth. As stated above, by inhibiting 5-α-reductase, production of DHT is reduced and the latter is what is directly responsible for prostate growth.

Answer d is incorrect. Testosterone binds to androgen receptors; however, it freely dissociates as well. DHT is the chief androgen involved in prostate growth and the target of 5ARI therapy.

Answer e is incorrect.

---

8. Select the statement that correctly describes erectile dysfunction.
   a. Individuals with diabetes are at higher risk.
   b. It is uncommon in the United States.
   c. It generally afflicts younger men.
   d. Individuals with above normal blood pressure are protected
   e. Smokers are less likely to develop the condition.

Answer a is correct. Individuals with diabetes are three times more likely to develop ED. ED develops in diabetics because of the vascular and neurologic changes that may occur.

Answer b is incorrect. It is very common in the United States, with as many as 20 million men affected.

Answer c is incorrect. The prevalence of ED increases with increasing age. At 40 years of age, up to 5% of men are afflicted with complete to severe dysfunction. This increases to 15% to 25% in men over 65.

Answer d is incorrect. Hypertension is considered a risk factor for the development of ED.

Answer e is incorrect. Smoking increases the likelihood of ED.

---

9. Select a vascular cause of erectile dysfunction.
   a. Depression
   b. Parkinson disease
   c. Hypogonadism
   d. Anxiety
   e. Dyslipidemia

Answer a is incorrect. The vascular component is an important cause of ED. Depression may have a psychological impact that could result in ED but does not affect the vascular system.

Answer b is incorrect. Parkinson disease can lead to ED because of its effect on the nervous system. It may also present as a psychological cause.

Answer c is incorrect. Decreased levels of testosterone may contribute to ED, but hypogonadism is not a vascular cause.

Answer d is incorrect. Performance anxiety may be a cause of ED. Generalized anxiety may be a psychological cause. The vascular system is not affected in anxiety.

Answer e is correct. Dyslipidemia can result in vascular changes that can result in ED.

---

10. Select the item that should be part of an evaluation of erectile dysfunction.
    a. A sexual history from the patient and partner
    b. A medical history
    c. A physical examination
    d. A psychosocial assessment
    e. All of the above

Answer a is correct. An important part of the evaluation, the sexual history should identify the duration, frequency, quality, and duration of erections and consider the nature of the sexual relationship.

Answer b is correct. The history should particularly focus on identifying potentially modifiable risk factors such as hypertension, diabetes, and dyslipidemia.

Answer c is correct. The physical examination is necessary to identify hypogonadism or neurological conditions that could result in ED.

Answer d is correct. Psychosocial issues can be the cause or may complicate the management of ED.

Answer e is correct and the best answer. All of the above items are part of a comprehensive workup for ED.

---

11. KR is a 62-year-old Hispanic man with a history of hypertension. He complains of ED for which he seeks treatment. There is no identifiable organic cause for his ED. Select the statement that correctly describes the approach to treatment in this patient.
    a. PDE-5 inhibitors would not be the treatment of choice in this patient.
    b. PDE-5 inhibitors are less efficacious in Hispanics.
    c. The use of a PDE-5 inhibitor is not likely to be effective in this patient with hypertension.
    d. A PDE-5 inhibitor would exert its activity by enhancing the effect of nitric oxide.
    e. He should not receive a PDE-5 inhibitor because sexual intercourse would not be advisable because of his cardiac status.

Answer a is incorrect. PDE-5 inhibitors are the treatment of choice in patients with ED that do not have an identifiable cause for their ED.

Answer b is incorrect. PDE-5 inhibitors are effective in all ethnic groups.

Answer c is incorrect. PDE-5 inhibitors are effective in patients with hypertension that develop ED.

Answer d is correct. PDE-5 inhibitors exert their activity by enhancing the activity of nitric oxide.

Answer e is incorrect. There is no condition present in KR that would make sexual intercourse inadvisable.

---

12. DL is a 59-year-old Caucasian man with a history of benign prostatic hyperplasia (BPH) which is adequately managed with doxazosin. He comes to the office with concerns about ED. His workup is unremarkable and a decision is made to start treatment with a PDE-5 inhibitor. Select the statement that correctly describes treatment in this patient.
    a. DL should be advised to take the medication immediately prior to sexual intercourse.
    b. Use of a PDE-5 inhibitor could lead to postural hypotension.
    c. PDE-5 inhibitors are contraindicated in patients with BPH.
    d. The medication of choice would be sildenafil.
    e. The use of a PDE-5 inhibitor is contraindicated in a patient receiving doxazosin.

Answer a is incorrect. PDE-5 inhibitors should be taken 30 to 60 minutes before anticipated intercourse.

Answer b is correct. PDE-5 inhibitors cause some decrease in blood pressure in patients with normal blood pressure. Individuals that are also receiving α-blockers may have a more significant drop in blood pressure leading to postural hypotension or dizziness. Individuals on both medications should be cautioned about this potential drug interaction.

Answer c in incorrect. PDE-5 inhibitors are effective in patients with ED that have BPH.

Answer d is incorrect. There is no convincing evidence that one PDE-5 inhibitor is more effective than another.

Answer e is incorrect. Taking the α-blocker doxazosin with a PDE-5 inhibitor may lead to postural hypotension and dizziness, but their use together is not contraindicated.

---

13. JC is a 72-year-old African American man with erectile dysfunction and no contraindication to the use of a PDE-5 inhibitor. Which of the following medications could potentially interact and lead to increased serum concentrations of the PDE-5 inhibitor?
    a. Erythromycin
    b. Aspirin
    c. Ampicillin
    d. Haloperidol
    e. Influenza vaccine

Answer a is correct. Erythromycin inhibits the CYP 3A4 enzyme system in the liver and impairs the metabolism of PDE-5 inhibitors. The dose of the PDE-5 inhibitor should be reduced.

Answer b is incorrect. Aspirin does not interact with PDE-5 inhibitors.

Answer c is incorrect. Antibiotics are not known to interact with PDE-5 inhibitors.

Answer d is incorrect. The use of antipsychotics may result in ED by causing hyperprolactinemia, but they do not affect the serum concentration of PDE-5 inhibitors.

Answer e is incorrect. Vaccines do not interact with PDE-5 inhibitors.

---

14. Select the brand name for tadalafil.
    a. Relenza
    b. Viagra
    c. Enzyte
    d. Cialis
    e. Levitra

Answer a is incorrect. The generic name of Relenza is zanamivir.

Answer b is incorrect. The generic name of Viagra is sildenafil.

Answer c is incorrect. Enzyte is an over-the-counter product marketed for the treatment of ED.

Answer d is correct.

Answer e is incorrect. The generic name of Levitra is vardenafil.

---

15. Which statement best describes alprostadil?
    a. It should be the first agent tried for the treatment of ED.
    b. It is a nonspecific PDE-5 inhibitor.
    c. It can be administered via a medicated transurethral suppository.
    d. Priapism has not been reported with the use of alprostadil.
    e. It exerts its activity by constricting smooth muscle in the penis.

Answer a is incorrect. PDE-5 inhibitors are the first-line choice for the treatment of ED unless there is a contraindication. Alprostadil is used when they are ineffective or cannot be tolerated.

Answer b is incorrect. Alprostadil works through its activity as a prostaglandin E_1 agonist. It causes vasodilation of the penile arteries by relaxing smooth muscle. Papaverine is a nonspecific phosphodiesterase inhibitor.

Answer c is correct. A unique delivery system called Muse places the drug into the urethra where it diffuses across the urethra into the body of the penis. The drug can also be administered by intracavernosal injection.

Answer d is incorrect. Priapism and prolonged erection can occur with the use of alprostadil.

Answer e is incorrect. The mechanism of action does not include vasoconstriction.

---

16. LT, a 75-year-old woman, has severe renal impairment (CrCl <30 mL/min). All of the following are viable options for urge urinary incontinence *except*:
    a. Oxybutynin transdermal patch
    b. Tolterodine ER
    c. Solifenacin
    d. Oxybutynin IR
    e. Trospium chloride ER

Answer a is incorrect. Any delivery system of oxybutynin does not need to be renally adjusted in severe renal impairment.

Answer b is incorrect. Although it is cleared renally, the dose can be decreased and be used in patients with severe renal impairment.

Answer c is incorrect. Although it is cleared renally, the dose can be decreased and be used in patients with severe renal impairment.

Answer d is incorrect. Any delivery system of oxybutynin does not need to be renally adjusted in severe renal impairment.

Answer e is correct. The extended release trospium chloride only comes in one dose for patients with CrCl >30 mL/min. It is should not be used in severe impairment due to increased side effects.

---

17. Which subtype of muscarinic receptor is the primary target of antimuscarinics in patients with urge urinary incontinence?

    a. M_1
    b. M_2
    c. M_3
    d. M_4
    e. M_5

Answer a is incorrect. A majority of the M_1 receptors are located in the CNS.

Answer b is incorrect. Although M_2 receptors can be found in the bladder, they are not clinically significant in UI.

Answer c is correct. Antimuscarinics' therapeutic target is the M_3 receptors of the bladder.

Answer d is incorrect. M_4 receptors are not clinically significant in UI.

Answer e is incorrect. M_5 receptors are not clinically significant in UI.

---

18. TV, a 55-year-old woman, is postmenopausal. Along with urinary incontinence, this patient is also suffering from symptoms of vaginal dryness, burning, and itching. Which of the following would be the best pharmacologic option for her?

    a. Oral estrogen
    b. Duloxetine
    c. Botulinum toxin
    d. Topical estrogen
    e. None of the above

Answer a is incorrect. Studies have proven that postmenopausal women taking oral estrogen have an increased risk in UI.

Answer b is incorrect. Duloxetine is used in SUI.

Answer c is incorrect. Botulinum toxin is used for patients refractory or intolerant to antimuscarinics.

Answer d is correct. The symptoms listed above describe vaginal atrophy. Micronized 17-beta estradiol (Vagifem) is indicated for vaginal atrophy.

Answer e is incorrect.

---

19. All of the following are nonpharmacologic options for a patient with urinary incontinence *except*:

    a. Weight reduction
    b. Decrease fluid intake
    c. Increase intake of caffeine
    d. Pelvic floor exercises
    e. All of the above

Answer a is incorrect. Weight reduction is a suitable nonpharmacologic option for UI.

Answer b is incorrect. Decrease fluid intake is a suitable nonpharmacologic option for UI.

Answer c is correct. A decrease in intake of caffeine is a suitable nonpharmacologic option for UI.

Answer d is incorrect. Pelvic floor exercises are a suitable nonpharmacologic option for UI.

Answer e is incorrect.

---

20. What type of incontinence can be described as having urinary urgency, frequency, and nocturia along with leakage during exercise?

    a. Stress urinary incontinence
    b. Urge urinary incontinence
    c. Overflow incontinence
    d. Mixed incontinence
    e. None of the above

Answer a is incorrect. The above symptoms are not SUI alone.

Answer b is incorrect. The above symptoms are not UUI alone.

Answer c in incorrect. The above symptoms are not OI.

Answer d is correct. The above symptoms describe both UUI (urinary urgency, frequency, and nocturia) and SUI (leakage during exercise) and therefore are defined as mixed incontinence because it is more than one type of UI.

Answer e is incorrect.

---

21. What is the brand name for darifenacin?

    a. Detrol LA
    b. Ditropan
    c. Enablex
    d. Vesicare
    e. Sanctura XR

Answer a is incorrect. The brand name is oxybutynin.

Answer b is incorrect. The brand name is tolterodine.

Answer c is correct.

Answer d is incorrect. The brand name is solifenacin.

Answer e is incorrect. The brand name is trospium chloride.

CHAPTER 64 | Allergic Rhinitis

1. All of the following are classic symptoms of allergic rhinitis *except*

   a. Rhinorrhea
   b. Congestion
   c. Sneezing
   d. Thick nasal discharge

Answers a, b, and c are incorrect. These are classic symptoms of allergic rhinitis.

Answer d is correct. Clear and thin nasal discharge is a classic symptom of allergic rhinitis. Thick or purulent nasal discharge may be a sign of infection.

2. Which of the following is a potential adverse effect when using oral antihistamines for the management of allergic rhinitis in a 3-year-old child?

   a. HPA axis suppression
   b. Paradoxical agitation
   c. Rebound congestion
   d. Medication tolerance

Answer a is incorrect. It is a potential adverse effect related to intranasal corticosteroids.

Answer b is correct. This is a potential adverse effect of oral first-generation antihistamines unique to infants and young children.

Answer c is incorrect. Rebound congestion is an adverse effect related to overuse of topical decongestants.

Answer d is incorrect. Medication tolerance is not a concern with the use of antihistamines.

3. JB is a 45-year-old man with a history of chronic nasal stuffiness nearly daily and all year round. His only other medical condition is high blood pressure. In addition to stuffiness, he has been sneezing a lot at work (which he finds very embarrassing). Also, his allergies have caused him to cancel park outings with his family. Using the ARIA guidelines, which of the following best classifies JB's symptoms?

   a. Mild intermittent
   b. Moderate to severe intermittent
   c. Mild persistent
   d. Moderate to severe persistent

Answer a is incorrect. Since this patient's symptoms are affecting his quality of life, they are not mild. Also, since his symptoms are >4 d/wk and >4 consecutive weeks, they are persistent.

Answer b is incorrect. His symptoms are year round.

Answer c is incorrect. His symptoms affect his quality of life.

Answer d is correct. His symptoms are severe and chronic.

4. Which therapeutic option would be best for JB?

   a. Oral decongestant
   b. Nonselective antihistamine
   c. Intranasal corticosteroid
   d. Intranasal decongestant

Answer a is incorrect. This patient suffers from high blood pressure and an oral decongestant can cause it to increase even more. Also, decongestants are only useful for nasal congestion and not sneezing.

Answer b is incorrect. A nonselective antihistamine is not the best option due to its sedative and anticholinergic effects, but can be a good additional agent should your first choice be ineffective.

Answer c is correct. An intranasal corticosteroid is highly effective for congestion and sneezing.

Answer d is incorrect. Since this patient has chronic symptoms, an intranasal decongestant is not indicated. Intranasal decongestants should not be used for more than a few days at a time. Also, these agents do not reduce the frequency of sneezing.

5. If the patient in Question 3 were a 30-year-old pregnant (first trimester) woman, how would the management change?

   a. The management would be the same.
   b. Initiate nonselective antihistamine.
   c. Initiate oral decongestant.
   d. Initiate mast cell stabilizer.

Answer a is correct. An intranasal corticosteroid is highly effective since this patient has chronic symptoms. A good choice would be budesonide, which is pregnancy category B.

Answer b is incorrect. An antihistamine is not as effective for the nasal congestion.

Answer c is incorrect. This medication can worsen blood pressure and this is not safe for use in the first trimester (associated with congenital malformations). Phenylephrine and pseudoephedrine are both classified as category C drugs.

Answer d is incorrect. This option is not the most effective medication for the patient.

6. Select the brand name for montelukast.

   a. Clarinex
   b. Zaditor
   c. Xyzal
   d. Singulair

Answer a is incorrect. This is the brand name for desloratadine.

Answer b is incorrect. This is the brand name for ketotifen fumarate.

Answer c is incorrect. This is the brand name for levocetirizine.

Answer d is correct. This is the brand name for montelukast.

7. The use of pseudoephedrine is concerning in a patient with which of the following disease states?

   a. Diabetes mellitus
   b. Chronic kidney disease
   c. Hypertension
   d. All of the above

Answers a, b, and c are correct.

Answer d is correct and the best answer. Pseudoephedrine can exacerbate diabetes, cause drug-related toxicity in patients with decreased renal function, and increase blood pressure.

8. Which of the following antihistamines is available by prescription only?

   a. Diphenhydramine
   b. Ketotifen fumarate
   c. Levocetirizine
   d. Loratadine

Answers a, b, and d are incorrect. Diphenhydramine, Ketotifen, and Loratadine are available over the counter.

Answer c is correct. Levocetirizine is available by prescription only.

9. Which of the following classes of medication can be used for management of allergic rhinitis in pregnancy?

   a. Oral antihistamines
   b. Intranasal corticosteroids
   c. Oral decongestants
   d. All the above

Answers a, b, and c are correct.

Answer d is correct and the best answer. Antihistamines, intranasal corticosteroids, and decongestants can be used during pregnancy. Decongestants should not be given until after the first trimester if the benefits outweigh the risks.

10. JS is a 23-year-old man with a history of seasonal allergic rhinitis. He complains of bothersome nasal stuffiness each year during the fall when ragweed pollen is prevalent. Which of the following medications is most appropriate to provide immediate relief of his nasal congestion?

    a. Cetirizine
    b. Chlorpheniramine
    c. Fluticasone
    d. Oxymetazoline

Answer a is incorrect. Oral antihistamines are better at preventing symptoms than treating them once they occur. Oral antihistamines are less effective at treating nasal congestion than intranasal corticosteroids and decongestants.

Answer b is incorrect. As above for cetirizine, chlorpheniramine will not provide adequate relief from nasal congestion.

Answer c is incorrect. Intranasal corticosteroids will provide some relief from nasal congestion 8 to 12 hours after administration, but may take up to 2 weeks for full effects to be realized.

Answer d is correct. A topical decongestant can provide relief within minutes of application.

11. Which of the following allergen avoidance techniques would be most appropriate to help reduce allergic symptoms caused by ragweed pollen?

    a. Encase pillow and mattress in allergen-proof cover.
    b. Keep windows closed and minimize outdoor activities.
    c. Reduce indoor humidity to <50%.
    d. Wash bedding in hot water.

Answer a is incorrect. Pollen is an outdoor allergen and cannot be minimized through the use of allergen-proof covers on bedding.

Answer b is correct. This prevents pollen from entering the house and minimizes the subjects' exposure.

Answer c is incorrect. This can help with indoor mold allergies, but does not assist with outdoor allergens such as pollen.

Answer d is incorrect. This can assist patients with indoor dust mite allergies, but does not assist with outdoor allergens such as pollen.

12. Which of the following medications is beneficial in reducing symptoms of seasonal allergic rhinitis when started prior to allergen exposure?

    a. Intranasal corticosteroid
    b. Leukotriene antagonist
    c. Oral antihistamine
    d. All of the above

Answers a, b, and c are correct.

Answer d is correct and the best answer Intranasal corticosteroids, leukotriene antagonists, and antihistamines can be given prior to allergen exposure to minimize allergic rhinitis symptoms.

13. CW is an 8-year-old boy with seasonal allergic rhinitis and mild persistent asthma. Which of the following medications would be most appropriate to manage symptoms of both his asthma and allergic rhinitis?
    a. Intranasal beclomethasone
    b. Intranasal cromolyn
    c. Cetirizine
    d. Montelukast

Answer a is incorrect. Intranasal corticosteroids are, at best, marginally efficacious for asthma and should not be substituted for inhaled corticosteroids and/or other methods of asthma management.

Answer b is incorrect. Although inhaled cromolyn sodium is used as an adjunct to asthma treatment, the intranasal cromolyn sodium is not indicated for management of asthma.

Answer c is incorrect. Oral antihistamines are not recommended for the treatment of asthma.

Answer d is correct. Montelukast is effective for management of both allergic rhinitis and asthma.

14. Sedation would most likely occur with which of the following antihistamines when used at recommended dosages for adult patients?
    a. Desloratadine
    b. Diphenhydramine
    c. Fexofenadine
    d. Olopatadine

Answer a is incorrect. Desloratadine is a second-generation antihistamine and has low sedation potential.

Answer b is correct. Diphenhydramine is a first-generation antihistamine (nonselective) and can cause sedation at recommended doses. It is available in many over-the-counter sleep products.

Answer c is incorrect. Fexofenadine is a second-generation antihistamine and has low sedation potential.

Answer d is incorrect. Olopatadine is an intranasal and ocular antihistamine and has a low sedation potential.

15. Which of the following antihistamines is available in an intranasal formulation?
    a. Azelastine
    b. Ketotifen fumarate
    c. Levocetirizine
    d. Loratadine

Answer a is correct. Azelastine is available as an intranasal formulation.

Answer b is incorrect. Ketotifen is available as an ocular formulation.

Answer c is incorrect. Levocetirizine is available as an oral formulation.

Answer d is incorrect. Loratadine is available as an oral formulation.

16. Which of the following categories of allergic rhinitis medications is most likely to be associated with rhinitis medicamentosa (rebound nasal congestion) with prolonged use?
    a. Intranasal corticosteroid
    b. Intranasal decongestant
    c. Oral antihistamine
    d. Oral decongestant

Answer a is incorrect. Rebound nasal congestion is not an adverse effect related to intranasal corticosteroids. Intranasal corticosteroids are effective at managing nasal congestion associated with allergic rhinitis.

Answer b is correct. Rebound nasal congestion can occur when patients use these agents for more than 3 to 5 days. If rhinitis medicamentosa occurs, patients must be weaned from the topical decongestant. The use of intranasal corticosteroids may be beneficial to manage symptoms during the weaning process.

Answer c is incorrect. Rebound nasal congestion is not an adverse effect related to oral antihistamines.

Answer d is incorrect. Rebound nasal congestion is not an adverse effect related to oral decongestants, only topical decongestants.

17. Which of the following medications must be kept behind the pharmacy counter, since it may be used in the production of methamphetamine?
    a. Brompheniramine
    b. Chlorpheniramine
    c. Phenylephrine
    d. Pseudoephedrine

Answer a is incorrect. Brompheniramine has no sales restrictions.

Answer b is incorrect. Chlorpheniramine has no sales restrictions.

Answer c is incorrect. Phenylephrine has no sales restrictions and has replaced pseudoephedrine in many over-the-counter products.

Answer d is correct. The Combat Methamphetamine Act of 2005 prohibited over-the counter sales of pseudoephedrine. It also placed restrictions on the amounts of pseudoephedrine that could be purchased by individuals during a given month. Additional rules and restrictions apply in various states, including requiring photo identification for purchase of pseudoephedrine, maintenance of pseudoephedrine purchase logs, and, in some states, designation of pseudoephedrine as a Category V–controlled substance.

---

18. NB is a 28-year-old woman who is taking a combination of cetirizine, intranasal fluticasone, pseudoephedrine, and montelukast to manage symptoms of persistent allergic rhinitis. She complains of feeling jittery and having palpitations after taking all of her medications in the morning. Which of the following medications is most likely causing her complaints?

    a. Cetirizine
    b. Fluticasone
    c. Montelukast
    d. Pseudoephedrine

Answer a is incorrect. Oral antihistamines are infrequently associated with tachycardia or feelings of anxiety.

Answer b is incorrect. Fluticasone has minimal systemic absorption and is not associated with these adverse effects.

Answer c is incorrect. Montelukast has rarely been associated with feelings of anxiety and is not known to cause tachycardia.

Answer d is correct. Because of its sympathomimetic properties, pseudoephedrine is well known to cause anxiety, restlessness, tachycardia, and palpitations.

---

19. TR is a 6-year-old boy with persistent allergic rhinitis. He is experiencing symptoms despite the use of an oral antihistamine, and the physician would like to add an intranasal corticosteroid. Which of the following is correct regarding the use of an intranasal corticosteroid for TR?

    a. Intranasal corticosteroids should not be combined with oral antihistamines in pediatric patients.
    b. Newer intranasal corticosteroids with low systemic bioavailability are unlikely to cause growth suppression in TR.
    c. The use of intranasal corticosteroids is contraindicated in children <12 years of age.
    d. TR should obtain relief of his symptoms within minutes of using the intranasal corticosteroid.

Answer a is incorrect. Intranasal corticosteroids can be combined safely with oral antihistamines in pediatric patients.

Answer b is correct. Newer intranasal corticosteroids such as fluticasone and mometasone are less likely to cause growth suppression.

Answer c is incorrect. Intranasal corticosteroids can be used in children as young as 2 years.

Answer d is incorrect. Intranasal corticosteroids do not provide immediate relief of symptoms. Partial relief may occur in several hours, but full effects may take 2 weeks to be achieved.

---

20. KW is a 39-year-old woman who experiences daily rhinorrhea despite the use of cetirizine and intranasal flunisolide. Addition of which of the following medications would be most appropriate to target the symptoms of rhinorrhea?

    a. Azelastine
    b. Ipratropium
    c. Oxymetazoline
    d. Phenylephrine

Answer a is incorrect. Since KW is already taking an oral antihistamine, addition of a topical antihistamine does not provide additional benefit.

Answer b is correct. Intranasal ipratropium specifically targets the symptom of rhinorrhea due to its antisecretory effects. Patients with problematic rhinorrhea despite existing drug therapy may benefit from addition of an intranasal anticholinergic agent such as ipratropium.

Answer c is incorrect. Intranasal decongestants do not improve rhinorrhea, only nasal congestion.

Answer d is incorrect. Oral decongestants are best for congestion, not rhinorrhea.

CHAPTER 65 | Geriatrics

1. Factors affecting medication absorption in the older adult include

    a. Elevated gastric pH
    b. Shortened gastric emptying time
    c. Increased plasma albumin
    d. Decreased elimination

Answer a is correct. Elevation in gastric pH is part of the physiologic changes in the older adult which may affect the absorption of medications. Also, use of acid suppressing medications, such a H2 antagonists and proton pump inhibitors, may further elevate the gastric pH of any patient, not just the elderly. The absorption of azole antifungals, such as ketoconazole and itraconazole, can be significantly reduced as they require an acidic environment for maximal absorption.

Answer b is incorrect. Physiologic changes in the elderly causes lengthened, not shortened, gastric emptying.

Answer c is incorrect. Plasma albumin is often decreased in elderly patients, not increased. This decrease in plasma albumin affects distribution of medications, not absorption. For example, the distribution of phenytoin is greatly affected by reduced serum albumin levels as it is highly protein bound to albumin.

Answer d is incorrect. Elimination is often effected by the physiologic changes that occur with aging. These include reduced renal and hepatic function. However, decreased elimination would not affect absorption of medications.

---

2. Pharmacotherapy management in geriatric patients is challenging. Which of the following best describes the statement and why?
   a. Physiologic changes with aging affect how medications are metabolized
   b. Reduced renal and hepatic function affect elimination of medications
   c. Side effects can often be mistaken for a new medical condition
   d. All of the above

Answers a, b, and c are correct.

Answer d is correct and best answer. Physiologic changes that occur with aging affect absorption, distribution, metabolism, and elimination of medications. Reduced renal and hepatic function in the elderly decreases the effectiveness of drug elimination. Medication side effects are often mistaken as a new medical condition in the elderly. This can lead to a "prescribing cascade" in which additional medications are prescribed to treat the side effects of the originally prescribed medication. An example is prescribing tamsulosin for a patient who experiences urinary retention after being started on an antihistamine for allergic rhinitis. The correct approach would be to discontinue the antihistamine and switch to a nasal steroid.

---

3. What types of medications are preferred to use in the older adult?
   a. Tricyclic antidepressants.
   b. Drugs that undergo phase I metabolism.
   c. Medications that undergo phase II metabolism.
   d. Those that do not go through the CYP-450 system.

Answer a is incorrect. Tricyclic antidepressants are found on the Beers list of inappropriate medications to use in the elderly. Tricyclic antidepressants are considered potentially harmful due to their anticholinergic and sedative properties.

Answer b is incorrect. Medications that undergo phase I metabolism are converted to active metabolites. Due to the decline in renal and hepatic function in the older adult, medications with active metabolites may accumulate, causing additional adverse events. For example, the metabolite of glyburide is also an active compound. Thus, an elderly patient taking glyburide would be at increased risk of developing hypoglycemia.

Answer c is correct. Medications that undergo phase II metabolism are converted to inactive metabolites. These types of medications are preferred in the elderly as they have less potential to accumulate and cause adverse events. For example, glipizide is converted to inactive metabolites, so it would be preferred over glyburide in the elderly.

Answer d is incorrect. Although hepatic function is lessened in the older adult, limiting medications only those not metabolized through the cytochrome P450 enzyme system would be virtually impossible as approximately 90% of medications are metabolized through the CYP-450 enzyme pathways.

---

4. What is the term defined by the following: When an adverse drug event is misinterpreted as a new medical condition in which the provider prescribes an additional medication to treat the side effect of the original medication?
   a. Prescribing downfall
   b. Prescribing cascade
   c. Domino effect
   d. Provider cascade

Answers a, c, and d are incorrect. These are not terms described in the geriatrics literature.

Answer b is correct. Providers often mistake the side effect of one medication as the patient presenting with a new medical diagnosis. Providers then prescribe a new medication to treat the side effect of the first medication. This is termed prescribing cascade in geriatric literature. The ideal approach would be to discontinue the first medication and switch to another agent without the offending adverse effect.

---

5. Which of the following medications is found on the Beers list of medications to avoid in the elderly?
   a. Acetaminophen
   b. Ramipril
   c. Propoxyphene
   d. Fosinopril

Answers a, b, and d are incorrect.

Answer c is correct. Propoxyphene, which is considered ineffective for pain management, causes very similar side effects in the elderly as other narcotic analgesics. Acetaminophen, ramipril, and fosinopril are all safe medications to use in the elderly. Acetaminophen is used as first-line therapy in many older adults due to its safety and efficacy when taken in recommended doses. ACE-Inhibitors such as ramipril and fosinopril are commonly used in the geriatric patient with great benefit from their cardio and renal protective effects.

---

6. Which of the following medications are among those recommended by the Beers list of the preferred medications to use in the elderly?

   a. Propoxyphene
   b. Amitriptyline
   c. Galantamine extended-release
   d. Indomethacin

Answers a, b, and d are incorrect. These are all medications found on the Beers criteria list of medications to avoid in the elderly. Propoxyphene is considered an ineffective analgesic yet carries similar side effects as other narcotic analgesics. Tricyclic antidepressants such as amitriptyline are not recommended in the elderly due to significant anticholinergic side effects. Indomethacin is also found among those listed on the Beers list of inappropriate medications. In addition to its traditional adverse events as an NSAID, it also holds central nervous system side effects.

Answer c is correct. Galantamine extended-release may be used.

7. Which of the following are pathologic signs of Alzheimer disease?

   a. Cogwheel rigidity
   b. Neurofibrillary tangles
   c. Senile plaques
   d. Essential tremor
   e. Both b and c

Answer a is incorrect. Cogwheel rigidity is a hallmark sign of Parkinson disease and is not related to Alzheimer dementia.

Answers b and c are correct. Neurofibrillary tangles and senile plaques are two hallmark signs by which the pathology of Alzheimer disease is characterized. Cerebrocortical atrophy as well as degeneration of cholinergic neurons also occurs in the disease process.

Answer d is incorrect. Essential tremor is often diagnosed in the older adult, but is not a pathological sign of Alzheimer disease.

Answer e is correct and the best answer.

8. Which of the following is one of the 10 warning signs (ie, initial symptoms) of Alzheimer disease identified by the Alzheimer's Association?

   a. Changes in vision
   b. Difficulty hearing
   c. Difficulty with abstract thinking (ie. balancing a checkbook)
   d. Constipation

Answer a is incorrect. Although visual changes often occur in the elderly due to comorbid illnesses, it has not been identified as a sign of Alzheimer disease.

Answer b is incorrect. Difficulty hearing is very common in the older adult, but has not been associated with Alzheimer disease. It is not considered as one of the 10 warning signs of Alzheimer disease.

Answer c is correct. Difficulty with abstract thinking often occurs at the beginning stages of Alzheimer disease. Performing tasks such as balancing a checkbook can be difficult for these patients, and is often accompanied by other classic symptoms such as difficulty performing familiar tasks, getting lost, forgetting recently learned information, disorientation to place and time, changes in mood or personality, as well as a loss of interest in usual activities.

Answer d is incorrect. Although constipation is a concern in Alzheimer patients, it also occurs frequently in all elderly patients. When constipation is identified as a problem in any older adult, the patient's medications should be reviewed to rule out potential causes.

9. Which of the following scales is commonly used to assess the level of dementia in Alzheimer patients?

   a. MMSA
   b. MMSE
   c. Geriatric Depression Scale
   d. Delirium Index

Answer a is incorrect. MMSA are arbitrary letters and not a scale used to assess dementia.

Answer b is correct. A patient's score on the Mini-Mental State Examination correlates with their severity of dementia. Mild Alzheimer disease is often associated with an MMSE score of greater than or equal to 20 out of 30 possible points. Moderate dementia correlates with an MMSE score of 10 to 19 points and severe Alzheimer patients often score less than 10 points.

Answer c is incorrect. The Geriatric Depression Scale is used to assess depression in the older adult, not severity of dementia.

Answer d is incorrect. The Delirium Index is used to assess delirium not dementia. Delirium is considered an acute, reversible loss of memory; whereas, Alzheimer dementia is a chronic, irreversible illness.

10. Which of the following classes of medications are used in Alzheimer disease?

    a. Dopamine agonists
    b. Cholinesterase inhibitors
    c. NMDA-antagonist
    d. Anticholinergics
    e. b and c

Answer a is incorrect. Dopamine agonists are indicated for the treatment of Parkinson disease. The primary side effect of these agents is nausea and vomiting. They can also cause confusion and hallucinations.

Answers b and c are correct. Cholinesterase inhibitors such as donepezil and galantamine, as well as the NMDA-antagonist memantine are the only classes of medications on the market for the treatment of Alzheimer disease.

Answer d is incorrect. Anticholinergics are used for the treatment of Parkinson disease and should be avoided in patients with memory impairment. Because of their significant anticholinergic properties, these agents should be avoided in the elderly. Not only can they worsen memory but may cause other adverse effects such as blurred vision, urinary retention, and constipation.

Answer e is correct and the best answer.

---

11. Which neurotransmitter is primarily involved in the disease process of Alzheimer disease?
    a. Serotonin
    b. Acetylcholine
    c. Norepinephrine
    d. Dopamine

Answer a is incorrect. A deficit in serotonin is directly correlated to depression, not Alzheimer disease. Although depression is common among older adults, and can occur in Alzheimer patients, a deficiency in acetylcholine is considered the primary cause of the symptoms of Alzheimer dementia.

Answer b is correct. A deficiency in the neurotransmitter acetylcholine is considered the primary cause of the symptoms of Alzheimer disease.

Answer c is incorrect. Norepinephrine is an excitatory neurotransmitter. When deficient in the central nervous system, it is often correlated with depression, not Alzheimer disease.

Answer d is incorrect. Dopamine can be considered the primary neurotransmitter involved in the pathologic process of Parkinson disease, not Alzheimer dementia.

---

12. What side effect(s) do patients complain of most often with cholinesterase inhibitors?
    a. Nausea, vomiting, diarrhea
    b. Dizziness
    c. Hypotension
    d. Headache

Answer a is correct. Although dizziness, headache, and hypotension can occur with the cholinesterase inhibitors, the most commonly reported adverse events with these medications are gastrointestinal side effects. For example, nausea has been reported in up to 19% of patients, and diarrhea in up to 15% of patients taking donepezil. This class of medication works by preventing breakdown of acetylcholine. These increased levels of acetylcholine, although beneficial for memory, adversely affect the GI tract.

---

13. Select the potential cause of decreased serum creatinine in elderly patients.
    a. Increased stores of body fat
    b. Decreased renal production of creatinine
    c. Loss of muscle mass
    d. Increased body mass

Answer a is incorrect. Although body fat stores are increased in the elderly, they do not cause reduced levels of serum creatinine.

Answer b is incorrect. Creatinine is a by-product of muscle breakdown, and is not produced by the kidneys.

Answer c is correct. Loss of muscle mass is part of the aging process. As creatinine is a by-product of muscle breakdown, this decrease in muscle mass accounts for less measurable creatinine by-product.

Answer d is incorrect. Elderly patients experience a decrease in body mass, not an increase.

---

14. Which of the following best describes the place in therapy for memantine?
    a. As an adjunct therapy to Sinemet for Parkinson patients without cognitive impairment
    b. As monotherapy for Parkinson disease
    c. As an augmentation to an Alzheimer patient's Cholinesterase Inhibitor
    d. In Alzheimer patients with heart disease

Answers a and b are incorrect. Memantine is indicated for Alzheimer disease, not Parkinson disease. There are multiple agents that can be used as adjunctive therapy to Sinemet in Parkinson disease such as ropinirole and pramipexole. Memantine is an NMDA-antagonist indicated for use in moderate to severe Alzheimer disease.

Answer c is correct. Memantine is an NMDA-receptor antagonist approved for use in moderate to severe Alzheimer disease. Memantine can be used as monotherapy in patients who cannot tolerate cholinesterase inhibitors; however, clinical trials demonstrate that it is most effective when given as augmentation therapy with a cholinesterase inhibitor.

Answer d is incorrect. Although heart disease is very common among the older adult, memantine is not indicated for heart disease but for Alzheimer dementia.

---

15. Which neurotransmitter is involved in the neuronal degradation of Parkinson disease?
    a. Acetylcholine
    b. GABA
    c. COMT
    d. Dopamine

Answer a is incorrect. Acetylcholine is the neurotransmitter involved in Alzheimer disease, not Parkinson disease.

Answer b is incorrect. GABA is an inhibitory neurotransmitter and is not involved in the neuronal degradation of Parkinson disease.

Answer c is incorrect. Although COMT-inhibitors are effective as adjunct agents for the treatment of Parkinson disease, the primary neurotransmitter neuronal degradation of Parkinson disease is dopamine

Answer d is correct. Dopamine is the primary neurotransmitter involved in the neuronal degradation of Parkinson disease.

16. Which of the following is the primary goal of drug therapy in patients with Parkinson disease?
    a. Provide comfort measures only
    b. To alleviate symptoms of disease that interfere with ADLs
    c. To prevent further memory loss
    d. To reverse neuronal degradation

Answer a is incorrect. Palliative care services may be necessary for Parkinson patients at the end of life, but symptom management is the primary goal of medication therapy.

Answer b is correct. Parkinson disease medications are titrated to manage the patient's symptoms of Parkinson disease that interfere with the patient's ability to perform their own activities of daily living (ADLs). These symptoms include those such as tremor, "freezing" periods, and cogwheel rigidity.

Answer c is incorrect. Memory loss may occur in later stages of Parkinson disease, but is not a primary goal of drug therapy in these patients.

Answer d is incorrect. Unfortunately, reversal of neuronal degradation that is the underlying cause of Parkinson disease is not possible. The exact pathophysiology underlying Parkinson disease is unknown. Causative factors are hypothesized to include genetic factors, environmental causes, and oxidative stress.

17. Which medication is considered the gold standard for treating Parkinson disease?
    a. Ropinirole
    b. Pramipexole
    c. Levodopa/carbidopa
    d. Bromocriptine

Answer c is correct. Although ropinirole, pramipexole, and bromocriptine are indicated for the management of Parkinson disease, the gold standard of therapy is levodopa/carbidopa and is considered the primary treatment. Ropinirole, pramipexole, and bromocriptine can be used as monotherapy but are primarily considered adjunctive therapies.

18. Which of the following medications would be the most likely to cause a Parkinson patient's nausea and vomiting?
    a. Simvastatin
    b. Diphenhydramine
    c. Levodopa/carbidopa
    d. Furosemide

Answer c is correct. Although simvastatin, diphenhydramine, and furosemide may cause nausea and vomiting in a small percentage of patients, levodopa/carbidopa would be the most likely culprit. Because carbidopa saturates the dopa decarboxylase enzyme at doses of 70 to 100 mg per day, it is imperative that patients receive this dose of carbidopa to prevent levodopa-related side effects such as nausea and vomiting.

19. Mrs. J is a 78-year-old Parkinson patient with cognitive changes who has been experiencing worsening symptoms over the past months despite her dose of Sinemet being maximized. Which would be a reasonable recommendation to her physician?
    a. Start apomorphine orally as adjunctive therapy.
    b. Start tolcapone at the highest possible dose.
    c. Consider adding ropinirole to augment the treatment she is currently receiving.
    d. None of the above.

Answer a is incorrect. Apomorphine is an injectable dopamine agonist generally reserved for advanced Parkinson disease patients to treat periods of freezing.

Answer b is incorrect. Tolcapone is rarely used due to its hepatotoxic side effects. Starting at the highest possible dose would not be appropriate.

Answer c is correct. Adding a dopamine agonist, such as ropinirole, to her current carbidopa/levodopa regimen would be an appropriate choice. Most Parkinson disease patients require levodopa/carbidopa and/or a dopamine agonist for symptom management.

Answer d is incorrect.

20. What side effect is most likely to occur with ropinirole?
    a. Possible explosive diarrhea
    b. Liver toxicity
    c. Nausea, hallucinations, and abnormal dreams
    d. Worsening memory loss

Answer a is incorrect. While up to 5% of patients may experience diarrhea when taking ropinirole, explosive diarrhea is a notable side effect of tolcapone instead. This intolerable side effect is one reason why it is no longer prescribed for Parkinson patients.

Answer b is incorrect. A very small percentage (3%) of patients on ropinirole may experience a slight increase in liver function tests. However, hepatotoxicity has been commonly reported with tolcapone, another explanation of its infrequent use.

Answer c is correct. Nausea, hallucinations, and abnormal dreams are common side effects of ropinirole due to its dopamine agonist effects.

Answer d is incorrect. In managing Parkinson disease, worsening cognitive function would be of concern when using an anticholinergic medication in the elderly. However, worsening memory loss is not a reported side effect of dopamine agonists such as ropinirole.

CHAPTER 66 | Clinical Toxicology

1. Which of the following is an appropriate poisoning first aid measure?

   a. Cutaneous acid exposures should be neutralized with an alkaline product.
   b. Emesis should be routinely induced.
   c. Patients should be observed for abnormal symptoms for 30 minutes.
   d. Poison control should be called if the patient is having difficulty in breathing.
   e. If the poison was swallowed, any residual should be removed from the mouth.

Answer a is incorrect. Attempts to neutralize an acid with a base, or base with an acid should not be performed as additional tissue damage may result. Appropriate first aid measures following dermal exposure involve taking measures to prevent secondary exposure of responders, removal of contaminated clothing, and prolonged and thorough washing with water (with exception of select reactive and finely divided metal exposures).

Answer b is incorrect. The decision to induce emesis has significant limitations and pitfalls. Attempts to induce emesis by route other than administration of syrup of ipecac should not be performed. Use of syrup of ipecac has progressively fallen out of favor over the last 15 years. In 1997 the American Academy of Clinical Toxicology position statement on syrup of ipecac concluded it should not routinely be utilized in management of the poisoned patient, and in 2003 the American Academy of Pediatrics formally recommended syrup of ipecac should no longer routinely be stocked or used as a home treatment. In select cases induction of emesis may be deemed appropriate; however, this decision should be made only after speaking with a Poison Control Center or qualified clinician.

Answer c is incorrect. Rarely will symptoms of toxicity develop following oral exposure within the first 30 minutes as products must first be absorbed and reach excessive dose. The absence of symptoms early in the course of exposure should not be seen as a favorable prognostic value.

Answer d is incorrect. 911 or appropriate emergency response should be called for patients that are having respiratory distress, are unconscious, convulsing, or uncontrollably agitated.

Answer e is correct. Following oral exposure the oral cavity should be examined and residual particulate matter should be removed to reduce additional absorption.

---

2. RC is a 35-year-old, 170 lb man. He reports a toothache for which he has been taking four 500-mg acetaminophen tablets every 3 to 4 hours for the last 3 days without relief. Additionally, he complains of nausea and new onset of right upper quadrant pain. He denies use of any other medications or other significant past medical history, but does report consuming a 12 pack of beer daily. His last dose of acetaminophen was 2 hours prior to physical examination. Which of the following would be an appropriate measure in the evaluation/treatment of RC?

   a. Acetaminophen level should be plotted on the Rumack-Matthew nomogram to determine if antidote therapy is indicated.
   b. Antidote therapy should be initiated immediately.
   c. Acetaminophen level should be ordered to determine need for antidote therapy.
   d. Activated charcoal should be administered and acetaminophen level should be ordered to determine need for antidote therapy.

Answer a is incorrect. The Rumack-Matthew nomogram is only appropriate to determine risk of acetaminophen-induced hepatic toxicity for acute ingestions of acetaminophen. It is not appropriate to use the nomogram for chronic ingestions, ingestions of extended release acetaminophen preparations, and acute ingestions with unknown time of ingestion.

Answer b is correct. In adult patients reporting repeated supratherapeutic doses of acetaminophen with evidence of acetaminophen toxicity (nausea, vomiting, malaise, diaphoresis, abdominal pain), acetaminophen antidote should be initiated as soon as possible to prevent additional toxicity.

Answer c is incorrect. In asymptomatic patients acetaminophen levels in conjunction with other factors (AST, comorbid conditions, history) are utilized in determining relative risk and need for antidote therapy in repeated supratherapeutic cases, but in the symptomatic patient intervention to prevent ongoing toxicity should be initiated as early as possible.

Answer d is incorrect. Activated charcoal would not be expected to have a high benefit-to-risk ratio 2 hours post ingestion of 2 g of acetaminophen in a patient with complaints of nausea and effective antidote available.

---

3. How much aspirin equivalent is contained in 5 mL of the topical analgesic, oil of wintergreen (100% methyl salicylate)?

   a. 140 mg
   b. 500 mg
   c. 1400 mg
   d. 5 g
   e. 7 g

Answers a, b, c, and d are incorrect.

Answer e is correct. Methyl salicylate has an aspirin equivalent factor of 1.4, in effect it is 1.4 times more potent compared to aspirin. With the given variables, 100% methyl salicylate would equate to 100 g of methyl salicylate per 100 mL of oil of wintergreen, or stated in different units 1000 mg of methyl salicylate per 1 mL of oil of wintergreen. When this is converted to aspirin equivalents by multiplying the 1000 mg/mL by 1.4 it is determined that each 1 mL of oil of wintergreen contains 1400 mg of aspirin equivalent. Adjusting for a volume of 5 mL would give the correct answer of 7 g of aspirin equivalent per 5 mL of 100% oil of wintergreen product. This highlights the potential toxicity of methyl salicylate products as 1 mL of this product would almost meet the minimum toxic dose of 150 mg/kg for a 10 kg child, and 5 mL theoretically could prove fatal.

4. Select the agent that would be associated with the toxidrome mnemonic: mad as a hatter, blind as a bat, red as a beet, hot as a hare, dry as a bone.
   a. Methylphenidate
   b. Amitriptyline
   c. Monepezil
   d. Hydromorphone

Answer a is incorrect. Methylphenidate produces sympathomimetic excess in overdose, the symptoms of which can be extremely similar to anticholinergic syndrome clinically. The deviating clinical finding will often be the fact that adrenergic toxicity is associated with diaphoresis.

Answer b is correct. Amitriptyline has strong anticholinergic properties. The mnemonic is reflective of the altered mental status, mydriasis with loss of accommodation, flushed skin, hyperthermia, and dry skin and mucous membranes associated with anticholinergic toxicity.

Answer c is incorrect. Donepezil inhibits cholinesterases resulting in increased cholinergic tone. Symptoms of cholinergic excess are associated with the mnemonic SLUDGE (salivation, lacrimation, urination, defecation, GI distress, emesis) or DUMBBELS (diarrhea and diaphoresis, urination, miosis, bronchorrhea/bronchospasm, bradycardia, emesis, lacrimation, lethargy, salivation).

Answer d is incorrect. Opioid toxicity is associated with the "opiate triad" of CNS depression, respiratory depression, and miosis.

5. Early in the course of salicylate toxicity arterial blood gases would most likely indicate which of the following acid-base derangements?
   a. Metabolic acidosis
   b. Respiratory alkalosis
   c. Partially compensated metabolic acidosis
   d. Partially compensated respiratory acidosis

Answers a, c, and d are incorrect.

Answer b is correct. Salicylates directly stimulate the respiratory center. Early in the course of toxicity this stimulation leads to an increased respiratory rate. Hyperventilation reduces systemic CO_2 levels. The effect on pH by this reduction in "respiratory acid" is an increase in systemic pH due to a respiratory alkalosis. As the course of salicylate toxicity progresses, a mixed acid-base picture develops as the initial respiratory alkalosis continues, but a metabolic acidosis that is not purely compensatory develops. This acidosis is due to increased salicylate level concentrations which are weak acids, uncoupling of oxidative phosphorylation and resultant lactic acid production, increased free fatty acid metabolism and impaired renal function, and accumulation of other organic acids.

6. Which toxin antidote combination pairing is not correct?
   a. Butorphanol and naloxone
   b. Cyanide and hydroxocobalamin
   c. Fomepizole and isopropyl alcohol
   d. Pyridoxine and isoniazid
   e. Deferoxamine and iron

Answer a is correct. Butorphanol is a synthetic mixed agonist-antagonist opioid analgesic. Excessive dose would be expected to produce general opioid toxicity and treatment with naloxone should be considered in the management of overdose.

Answer b is correct. Cyanide is a rapid-acting toxin that inhibits mitochondrial cytochrome a3 forcing a shift to cellular anaerobic respiration lactate production, metabolic acidosis, and cellular hypoxia. Death can result in minutes. Hydroxocobalamin binds cyanide molecules by substituting a hydroxo-linked ligand to the trivalent cobalt ion to form cyanocobalamin (vitamin B_{12}) which is then eliminated in the urine.

Answer c is incorrect. Fomepizole is a competitive antagonist of alcohol dehydrogenase (ADH) most commonly used in ethylene glycol and methanol poisonings. While isopropyl alcohol is metabolized via ADH, fomepizole is not utilized for blocking metabolism as the major metabolite is acetone.

Answer d is a correct. Pyridoxine is the antidote for significant isoniazid (INH) toxicity. Significant INH poisoning is classically characterized as seizures that are refractory to standard therapy (benzodiazepines, barbiturates), coma, and metabolic acidosis. INH alters the metabolism and creates a functional depletion of pyridoxine. This state of pyridoxine deficiency impairs the synthesis and metabolism of gamma aminobutyric acid (GABA), the major inhibitory neurotransmitter in the CNS, resulting in seizure activity. Pyridoxine as an INH antidote should be administered intravenously at a dose that is equivalent to the dose of INH ingested up to a maximum of 5 g. If the dose is unknown 5 g should be given empirically. Pyridoxine doses utilized in treatment of INH toxicity may deplete hospital stock.

Answer e is correct. Deferoxamine chelates free iron following iron overdose. The chelate complex ferrioxamine is then eliminated in the urine. Urine color may be a "vin-rose" (red-brown) color following deferoxamine administration, indicating presence of ferrioxamine in the urine, but color change is not always seen. Adverse effects associated with administration of deferoxamine in acute iron poisoning include infusion rate–related hypotension, pulmonary toxicity for patients treated for longer than 24 hours, and infection.

---

7. PM is a 23-year-old woman that presents to the emergency department with a history of ingesting #60 digoxin 0.25-mg tablets 6 hours ago. The tablets came from a brand new #60 count prescription for her grandfather. On presentation she is lethargic and reported to have vomited multiple times in the last 1 to 2 hours by her family. Her electrocardiogram revealed high-degree heart block with a ventricular rate of 40 to 50 beats/min and her potassium was found to be 5.8 mEq/L and a digoxin concentration of 12 ng/mL. Her urine pregnancy test was negative and her past medical history is significant for depression. The treating physician initiated antidote therapy with digoxin immune Fab fragments in an appropriate dose for the given ingestion. Within 60 minutes the patients' clinical status improved significantly but repeat digoxin concentration 6 hours after Fab administration returned at 19 ng/mL. What is the best answer to explain the increase in digoxin concentration?
   a. Continued absorption of digoxin.
   b. The time frame of ingestion was incorrect and ingestion was closer to time of presentation.
   c. Administration of digoxin immune Fab fragment has increased serum levels of total digoxin.
   d. Endogenous digoxin-like immunoreactive substance.

Answer a is incorrect. Digoxin is associated with a biphasic distribution pattern in which it is absorbed into the plasma compartment and then slowly redistributed to the tissue. This delay in steady-state plasma concentrations results in misleadingly high plasma concentrations (two- to threefold) early after ingestion (<4-6 hours) compared to more reliable steady state levels drawn 6 or more hours after ingestion. This is the opposite of what was seen with PM and as such Answer a is not the correct answer.

Answer b is incorrect. Due to the same biphasic distribution properties discussed for Answer a, the digoxin level following acute overdose would be expected to be higher in the first 4 to 6 hours than it would be after 6 hours of ingestion. As such, if the ingestion had been closer to the time of presentation, the level would be expected to be higher than it would be 6 or more hours post ingestion when the follow up digoxin serum level was drawn.

Answer c is correct. Digoxin serum levels can be determined as both free and total digoxin. Digoxin levels reported as the more frequent total digoxin value can rise dramatically following administration of digoxin immune Fab fragments. This is due to the Fab binding of circulation plasma digoxin and establishing a concentration gradient that favors redistribution of digoxin from tissue back into the plasma. However, the digoxin will almost all be bound and not able to interact with receptors. This would explain PM's digoxin level increase following Fab administration. Total digoxin levels will remain elevated and clinically misleading until Fab fragments are eliminated from the body.

Answer d is incorrect. Endogenous digoxin-like immunoreactive substance (EDLIS) is a naturally occurring substance chemically and functionally similar to exogenous digoxin. It has been noted in neonates and patients with several other conditions including renal and hepatic dysfunction, pregnancy, congestive heart failure, type 1 diabetes mellitus, and after strenuous exercise. EDLIS can cross-react with digoxin assay if present EDLIS is not expected to increase digoxin levels by more than 2 ng/mL and clinical implications are unknown. Additionally, naturally occurring digitalis glycosides from plants and animals may cross-react with the digoxin assay if ingested.

---

8. Which of the following should caution for anaphylactoid reaction be used with digoxin immune Fab fragments administration?
   a. Papaya or papain allergy
   b. Patients treated previously with digoxin immune Fab fragments
   c. Sheep protein allergy
   d. Latex allergy
   e. All of the above

Answer a is correct. Papain is used to segment whole antibody in the production of digoxin immune Fab fragments. Caution is warranted for patients with papain, papaya extract, or the pineapple enzyme bromelain.

Answer b is correct. By design, the Fab fragment lacks the antigenic determinants of the Fc fragment and is associated with significantly reduced potential of anaphylactoid reaction compared to intact immunoglobulin. However, patient previously treated with digoxin immune Fab fragment are at increased risk of immunogenic reaction.

Answer c is correct. Patients with known sheep protein allergy are at increased risk of immunogenic reaction as the manufacturer of digoxin immune Fab fragments utilizes sheep (ovine) immunized with a digoxin derivative to form the antidigoxin antibodies.

Answer d is correct. Certain latex and dust mite allergens share antigenic structures with papain and patients with these allergies may be allergic to papain.

Answer e is correct and the best answer. All of the above are instances when precautions for emergency intervention (oxygen, H1 and H2 antagonist, corticosteroids, and airway management) should be considered prior to administration of digoxin immune Fab fragment.

---

9. The administration of which of the following agents would be indicated in the setting of tricyclic antidepressant overdose associated with seizures or QRS interval >115 ms?

   a. Sodium bicarbonate
   b. Flumazenil
   c. Physostigmine
   d. Procainamide
   e. Both a and c

Answer a is correct. Serum alkalinization with a goal of establishing a systemic pH between 7.45 and 7.55 is indicated in the setting of tricyclic antidepressant (TCAD) toxicity with evidence of widening QRS interval and/or seizure activity. Mechanisms by which sodium bicarbonate administration may provide benefit are as follows:

1. Increased systemic sodium levels may overcome blocked sodium channels and/or increased systemic pH results in increased nonionized TCAD, decreasing ligand receptor interaction between ionized TCAD and the sodium channel.
2. Wide complex dysrhythmia and hypotension can be reversed by administration of sodium bicarbonate in sufficient dose. Seizures will not respond to this sodium bicarbonate therapy, and should be treated with standard measures, but if seizures occur in the setting of TCAD overdose sodium bicarbonate therapy is warranted because they indicate significant toxicity.
3. Other potential therapies could include administration of hypertonic 3% saline to increase systemic sodium levels or hyperventilation to increase systemic pH; however, these have not been found to provide the same level benefit as treatment with sodium bicarbonate.

Answer b is incorrect. Administration of flumazenil may precipitate generalized seizures in the setting of TCAD overdose and is contraindicated.

Answer c is incorrect. Physostigmine is a cholinesterase inhibitor and can reverse some anticholinergic symptoms of TCAD poisoning. Historically, it has been utilized to treat TCAD-induced antimuscarinic symptoms. However, use has been abandoned as physostigmine is associated with increased incidence of dysrhythmia, bradycardia, asystole, and seizures.

Answer d is incorrect. Procainamide is a class IA antidysrhythmic agent and has a mechanism of action that blocks cardiac fast sodium channels. These are the same channels antagonized in TCAD poisoning leading to QRS prolongation, and utilization may worsen cardiac toxicity. As such, administration of agents with sodium channel–blocking properties (class IA and IC antidysrhythmics) is an absolute contraindication in TCAD poisoning.

Answer e is incorrect.

---

10. Which vasopressor would be the best choice for hypotension due to tricyclic antidepressant toxicity that is refractory to fluid and sodium bicarbonate support?

    a. Norepinephrine
    b. Epinephrine
    c. Dopamine
    d. Isoproterenol
    e. Dobutamine

Answer a is correct. Hypotension in the setting of tricyclic antidepressant toxicity is largely due to alpha-adrenergic blockade. For this reason, a direct acting alpha-adrenergic agonist (norepinephrine, phenylephrine) is the preferred vasopressor.

Answer b is incorrect. Epinephrine acts as an agonist at beta-1, beta-2, and alpha-1 adrenergic receptor effects. Due to this mixed agonist action, alpha-adrenergic receptor-induced vasoconstriction is often cancelled out by the beta-2 adrenergic receptor vasodilation and as such is not a preferred vasopressor.

Answer c is incorrect. Dopamine is an indirect acting agent with a mixed mechanism of action depending on the dose administered. At lower doses (1-5 ug/kg/min) dopamine acts on renal and mesenteric dopamine receptors, resulting in selective vasodilation. At intermediate doses (5-15 ug/kg/min) dopaminergic and beta-1 adrenergic receptors are stimulated, but there is minimal increase in systolic or diastolic pressures. It is not until higher doses (>15 ug/kg/min) that a direct alpha-adrenergic agonist effect resulting in more significant vasoconstriction is demonstrated from dopamine. Additionally, it is possible that blockade of endogenous norepinephrine and dopamine reuptake by TCAD mechanism of action could result in catecholamine depletion, blunting the indirect action of dopamine and further reducing potential benefit as a vasopressor. If dopamine is utilized in the setting of TCAD, induced hypotension doses should be in the higher range in attempt to counter the alpha-receptor blockade.

Answer d is incorrect. Isoproterenol is a pure beta-agonist and acts as an inotrope and chronotrope. It is not an effective vasopressor unless hypotension is primarily due to significant bradycardia.

Answer e is incorrect. Dobutamine is an inotrope and not a vasopressor. Due to significant beta-1 stimulation resulting in increased cardiac output, reflex vasodilation and hypotension occur with dobutamine administration.

---

11. Which of the following is a form of acetylcysteine that can be giving intravenously as antidote therapy in acetaminophen poisoning?
    a. Mucomyst
    b. Acetadote
    c. 10% acetylcysteine
    d. 20% acetylcysteine
    e. All of the above

Answer a is correct. Mucomyst is a brand of acetylcysteine sodium solution available in 10% and 20% solutions. While not approved by the FDA for intravenous administration and not recommended unless Acetadote is unavailable and intravenous route is deemed medically necessary, it has been utilized in patients requiring intravenous administration (irretractable vomiting, pregnancy) for treatment of acetaminophen poisoning. If Mucomyst or generic equivalent is given intravenously, it should be diluted appropriately in D5W and administered through a 0.2 micron Millipore filter.

Answer b is correct. Acetadote is a brand of acetylcysteine injection and the only FDA-approved intravenous acetylcysteine product currently available. Both Acetadote and oral acetylcysteine given intravenously are associated with a significantly higher rate of anaphylactoid reaction compared to oral administration.

Answer c is correct. Acetylcysteine sodium solution 10% is not FDA approved for intravenous administration but has been administered intravenously (see Answer a comment).

Answer d is correct. Acetylcysteine sodium solution 20% is not FDA approved for intravenous administration but has been administered intravenously (see Answer a comment).

Answer e is correct and the best answer.

---

12. Which of the following are differences between calcium gluconate and calcium chloride parenteral preparations?
    a. The mechanism of action of calcium chloride is superior in calcium channel blocker poisoning.
    b. The mechanism of action of calcium gluconate is superior in calcium channel blocker poisoning.
    c. Calcium chloride provides three times more cation compared to calcium gluconate on an equal volume basis.
    d. Calcium gluconate is more irritating when given intravenously than calcium chloride.
    e. Both c and d.

Answer a is incorrect. Administration of either of the calcium salts in appropriate dose provides the body with increased cation levels to attempt to overcome competitive blockade imposed by calcium channel blockers.

Answer b is incorrect. See explanation above.

Answer c is correct. Calcium chloride contains 13.6 mEq of calcium per gram compared to calcium gluconate which provides 4.65 mEq of calcium per gram. Both products are commercially available as 10% solutions, making calcium chloride three times more potent per equivalent volume of calcium gluconate.

Answer d is incorrect. Calcium chloride is significantly more irritating when given intravenously compared to calcium gluconate.

Answer e is incorrect.

---

13. HF presents to the emergency department and states that he took an overdose of his "heart medication." He does not remember the name of the medication but states he took a handful of tablets approximately 3 hours ago and now feels lethargic and sick in his stomach. His vitals reveal a heart rate of 45 beats/min, blood pressure of 85/40 mm Hg, respiratory rate of 12 breaths/min, and temp of 98.6°F. The ED staff contacts the patient's pharmacy and is told the patient has prescriptions for atenolol, amlodipine, and digoxin. Laboratory test is ordered and is pending. Which of the following agents should not be administered prior to return of digoxin serum concentration determination?
    a. Atropine
    b. Fluid bolus
    c. Calcium salt
    d. Glucagon
    e. All of the above

Answer a is incorrect. Atropine is a first-line agent in the treatment of bradycardia due to beta-blocker, calcium channel blocker, or digoxin toxicity.

Answer b is incorrect. Appropriate fluid bolus is a first-line therapy for hypotension due to beta-blocker or calcium channel blocker toxicity and would not be expected to adversely affect patient with concomitant digoxin.

Answer c is correct. Administration of calcium salts is appropriate in the treatment of calcium channel blocker toxicity and may be effective in beta-blocker toxicity but should not be utilized in the setting of bradycardia and hypotension where digoxin cannot be ruled out as a cause or confounding factor. Administration of calcium salts in the setting of digoxin poisoning theoretically may worsen toxicity by increasing intracellular calcium levels and could precipitate asystole.

Answer d is incorrect. Administration of glucagon is appropriate in the treatment of beta-blocker toxicity and may be effective in calcium channel blocker toxicity. Glucagon is not a therapy utilized to treat digoxin toxicity, but it would not be contraindicated to use in settings of mixed agent poisoning.

Answer e is incorrect.

---

14. RC is a 36-year-old man brought to the emergency department by his wife. She states that RC has been vomiting for the last 2 hours and acting abnormal following an argument approximately 4 hours ago. RC has a history of peptic ulcer disease for which he takes omeprazole and uses minoxidil topically. In the

ED he complains of nausea, vomiting, abdominal pain, and is diaphoretic. On physical examination the patient is awake and oriented but lethargic. His blood pressure is 135/80 mm Hg, heart rate is 111 beats/min, respiratory rate is 33 breaths/min, and a temperature is 100.1°F. HEENT was unremarkable, chest was clear to auscultation, no murmurs, rubs or gallops detected, bowels sounds were present, but abdomen was tender, stool guaiac test was negative. ECG was normal. Initial laboratory data results include: sodium of 144 mEq/L, potassium 3.8 mEq/L, bicarbonate 8 mEq/L, chloride 98 mEq/L, BUN 23 mg/dL, creatinine 0.7 mg/dL, glucose 93 mg/dL, calcium 9.6 mg/dL, and albumin 4 g/dL. Arterial blood gas values on room air were determined to be: pH 7.34, PCO_2 11 mm Hg, PO_2 93 mm Hg. What is the calculated anion gap for this patient?

a. 23
b. −49.8
c. 147
d. 38
e. 14

Answer d is correct. Conventionally, the anion gap is calculated using the formula of subtracting the sum of serum chloride and bicarbonate values from the serum sodium level (for this case [Na^+ 144 − (Cl^- 98 + $HCO3^-$ 8) = 38]). There is a degree of variance depending on method of measurement in establishing a "normal" range for anion gap with some methods setting a normal value of 12 (+/−4) and others 7 (+/−4). In patients with hypoalbuminemia, a correction factor should be accounted for in determine the anion gap as it decreases approximately 3 mEq/L per 1 g/dL decrease in the serum albumin. In the setting of a metabolic acidosis, determination of the presence of a high anion gap can aid in narrowing the differential diagnosis. The mnemonic MUDPILES (methanol, uremia, diabetic ketoacidosis, phenothiazines/paraldehyde, isoniazid/iron, lactic acidosis, ethylene glycol/ethanol, salicylates) represents frequent causes of metabolic acidosis associated with a high anion gap.

---

15. Which opioid is associated with both proconvulsant and prodysrhythmic activity in overdose?

a. Meperidine
b. Methadone
c. Hydrocodone
d. Heroin
e. Propoxyphene

Answer a is incorrect. Seizures are associated with accumulation of the meperidine metabolite normeperidine, but dysrhythmias are not a frequent adverse effect in overdose.

Answer b is incorrect. Methadone is associated with prodysrhythmic properties even in therapeutic levels as it can prolong QT/QTc interval potentially precipitating torsade de pointes, but seizures are not a frequent adverse effect.

Answer c is incorrect. Hydrocodone is not commonly associated with intrinsic proconvulsant or prodysrhythmic activity in overdose.

Answer d is incorrect. Heroin is not commonly associated with intrinsic proconvulsant or prodysrhythmic activity in overdose.

Answer e is correct. Propoxyphene is associated with seizures and QRS interval prolongation due to sodium channel–blocking properties particularly in doses >10 mg/kg.

---

16. Which of the following gastric decontamination method and toxin pairs would be appropriate?

a. Syrup of ipecac and amitriptyline; 30 minutes postexposure
b. Activated charcoal and lithium; <30 minutes postexposure
c. Multiple dose–activated charcoal and carbamazepine
d. Whole bowel irrigation and acetaminophen; 30 minutes postexposure
e. Sorbitol and atenolol; 30 minutes postexposure

Answer a is incorrect. Amitriptyline poisoning can result in rapid and severe onset of CNS depression. There is no evidence that syrup of ipecac improves clinical outcomes. Induction of emesis may delay other therapies as emesis is not guaranteed to be a single episode following administration of ipecac. Emesis is contraindicated in patients with or potential for CNS depression, caustic/corrosive substance ingestions, agents that may cause seizures, or agents with high aspiration potential.

Answer b is incorrect. Activated charcoal is a carbonaceous material with an extremely high surface area capable of binding and reducing absorption of a large number of toxins; however, it does not significantly bind lithium, iron, sodium, potassium, glycols, alcohols, hydrocarbons, and various other toxins. While position papers conclude that administration of activated charcoal should not routinely be administered to the poisoned patient, it was documented as being performed in 102,896 cases reported to poison centers in 2007. For comparison in the same report, ipecac was cited in 1740 cases, gastric lavage in 8857, multiple-dose charcoal in 3114, and whole bowel irrigation in 2708. From these numbers it is easily seen that activated charcoal is the most common method of gastric decontamination used. Benefit is most likely to be expected when administered in the first hour following overdose, but benefit cannot be excluded at times beyond 1 hour. There is no data or scientific rational to support activated charcoal dosing; common doses include 0.5 to 1 g/kg for children 0 to 12 years, 1 g/kg for all persons, 10 to 25 g for children 0 to 12 months, 25 to 50 g for children 1 to 12 years, 25 to 100 g for all person >12 years, and dosing that establishes an activated charcoal to ingested toxin ratio of 10:1. Potential concerns include nausea which could induce emesis and risk aspiration or obstruction, administration via misplaced nasogastric tube directly into the trachea, and administration to a patient with GI obstruction. Activated charcoal may impair endoscopic evaluation if necessary and this should be considered prior to administration.

Answer c is correct. There is evidence to support the use of multiple dose–activated charcoal (MDAC) therapy in the setting of life-threatening carbamazepine toxicity. Clinical studies have found that MDAC significantly increases clearance of carbamazepine as well as theophylline, quinine, dapsone, and phenobarbital. Prior to initiation, it should be verified that the patient has an intact or protected airway and no evidence of gastrointestinal obstruction.

Answer d is incorrect. Whole bowel irrigation would not be appropriate in the management of acetaminophen overdose as it is readily bound to activated charcoal and an effective antidote is available to prevent acetaminophen toxicity.

Answer e is incorrect. Cathartics as a sole agent have no role in the management of the poisoned patient and are not recommended as a method of gastric decontamination. Use in combination with activated charcoal is not endorsed by position statement, but if utilized should be restricted to a single dose due to potential fluid and electrolyte imbalance that could further complicate patient management.

---

17. Which of the following is a first-line agent in the management of beta-blocker toxicity and associated with a high incidence of nausea and vomiting?

    a. Atropine
    b. Normal saline intravenous fluid
    c. Calcium gluconate
    d. Glucagon
    e. Milrinone

Answer a is incorrect. Atropine is utilized as a first-line agent for bradycardia. In the majority of moderate to severe beta-blocker poisonings, atropine will fail to significantly increase heart rate and inotropic therapy is necessary. Effects from atropine administration would be anticholinergic in nature.

Answer b is incorrect. Administration of crystalloid fluid as either a bolus or infusion is a first-line therapy in beta-blocker toxicity but is not associated with a significant increase in nausea or vomiting. Due to the potential for cardiogenic pulmonary edema associated with beta-blocker and more commonly calcium channel blocker poisoning, close attention should be paid to the volume of crystalloid administered.

Answer c is incorrect. Calcium salt administration may improve blood pressure but not heart rate in the setting of beta-blocker poisoning and is not considered a first-line therapy.

Answer d is correct. Glucagon is the agent of choice for beta-blocker toxicity not responsive to atropine and fluid administration. Beta-adrenergic receptors and glucagon are both coupled to G proteins that on stimulation result in increased adenyl cyclase and resultant cAMP. This provides the positive inotropic and chronotropic effects of beta-1-receptor stimulation. In beta-blocker poisoning, administration of glucagon provides an effective bypass of antagonized beta-receptors. Glucagon should initially be given as a 3 to 5 mg intravenous bolus and repeated until response, upon which time a continuous infusion should be initiated at the cumulative response dose per hour. Nausea and vomiting are frequent adverse effects following administration of the higher doses utilized to treat beta-blocker toxicity and close attention should be paid to the risk of aspiration or obstruction following emesis in patients with decreased levels of consciousness. Additionally, patients should be observed for hypoglycemia or hyperglycemia and hypokalemia. Glucagon has a short duration of action compared to that of the majority of beta-antagonist. This combined with higher dose therapy may deplete entire hospital supplies following significant overdose.

Answer e is incorrect. Milrinone is a phosphodiesterase inhibitor (PDI) which decreases the breakdown of cAMP allowing for increased intracellular cAMP levels and improved myocardial function. PDI will increase cardiac output as evidence of their utility in the treatment of advanced cardiac failure, but use of PDI in the management of beta-blocker toxicity is reserved for patients failing more proven therapies. Hypotension and difficulty in titration and long half-life are properties that significantly limit PDI use.

---

18. Following acute ingestion of 10 g of acetaminophen, what is the earliest time postingestion that an acetaminophen level can be drawn and plotted on the Rumack-Matthew nomogram to appropriately determine potential hepatotoxic risk and need for antidote administration?

    a. 30 minutes postingestion
    b. 1 hour postingestion
    c. 2 hours postingestion
    d. 4 hours postingestion
    e. 8 hours postingestion

Answers a, b, and c are incorrect.

Answer d is correct. The time to peak concentration following therapeutic dose of acetaminophen can range from 10 to 90 minutes depending on formulation, presence of food, or other coingestants (anticholinergics, opiates). Following acute overdose, complete absorption and peak acetaminophen levels can take longer. In order to reasonably assure complete absorption, the Rumack-Matthew nomogram was developed and validated utilizing a 4-hour postingestion time as the earliest point to evaluate acetaminophen levels and determine potential hepatotoxicity. Levels drawn prior to 4 hours postingestion cannot be used to determine potential risk unless the level returns as "nondetectable". Levels drawn after 4 hours can be plotted on the nomogram up to 24 hours postingestion; however there is some concern that the levels closer to 24 hours may not be as accurate in determining hepatotoxic risk compared to levels closer to 4 hours postingestion.

Answer e is incorrect.

---

19. ZM is a 44-year-old, 170 lb man that was found unresponsive in the middle of a city street and brought to the emergency department by ambulance. He is noted to have a blood pressure of 115/60 mm Hg, a heart rate of 61 beats/min, a respiratory rate of 6 breaths/min, his ECG reveals a normal sinus rhythm, he is afebrile, has no apparent trauma, and is noted to have an odor of alcohol on his breath. Prescription bottles for methadone and clonazepam were found in his shirt pocket. The attending physician requests recommendations on the administration of flumazenil, naloxone, thiamine, and dextrose. Which of these agents would not be appropriate with ZM's history?

    a. Flumazenil
    b. Naloxone
    c. Thiamine
    d. Dextrose

Answer a is correct. Flumazenil is an antagonist of benzodiazepine receptors, but has limited utility as an antidote. It should not be used in the setting of an undifferentiated comatose patient. Risk of precipitating withdrawal seizures at which point benzodiazepines would be rendered of limited therapeutic benefit is one concern. Additionally, in the setting of mixed overdose presence of a benzodiazepine may be providing some therapeutic seizure protection and administration of flumazenil could unmask toxicity of other agents leading to more significant toxicity.

Answer b is incorrect. Naloxone is routinely used in the setting of undifferentiated coma. While use may precipitate withdrawal, opioid withdrawal compared to benzodiazepine, ethanol, or other withdrawal syndromes is not life threatening. In order to prevent withdrawal, dosing should be initiated at a lower dose and titrated to effect or total dose of 10 mg.

Answer c is incorrect. Thiamine along with dextrose is routinely used in the setting of undifferentiated coma. Thiamine is administered in this setting due to potential thiamine deficiency and concerns of Wernicke encephalopathy. In general, it should be given prior to administration of dextrose but dextrose should not be held if thiamine administration will cause delay. The 100 mg intravenous dose is well tolerated and potential benefit outweighs risk. Need for thiamine in children would be atypical and is not routinely performed in the setting of undifferentiated coma in this population.

Answer d is incorrect. Dextrose is routinely used in the setting of undifferentiated coma unless rapid bedside glucose determination can be made. Adults should be given 25 g (50 mL) of 50% dextrose and children 0.5 to 2 g/kg of no more than 25% dextrose intravenously.

---

20. Which of the following are correct statements with regard to the Poison Prevention Packaging Act of 1970?

    a. Child-resistant effectiveness of not <85% without demonstration and not <80% after demonstration.
    b. Senior adults must have ease in opening of not <90%.
    c. Single package forms of acetaminophen of <1 g do not require child-resistant closures.
    d. It is estimated that over 900 children's lives have been saved due to implementation of child-resistant packaging of aspirin and oral prescription medications.
    e. All of the above.

Answer a is correct. The PPPA defines a safe closure to be "child-resistant closure" (CRC) when after individual 5-minute test periods not <85% of a group of 50 to 200 children without demonstration and not <80% after demonstration fail to open the container. The children participating in the study are without physical or mental handicap and age stratification of 30% percent of the children in each group shall be of age 42 to 44 months, 40% of the children in each group shall be of age 45 to 48 months, and 30% of the children in each group shall be of age 49 to 51 months. It is important to stress to parents and grandparents that child resistant does not imply child proof and other precautions should be taken to reduce children gaining control of medication. Additionally the fact that a person may not have children in their home is not sufficient reason to utilize non-child-resistant closures as it is estimated that 23% of drugs ingested by children under age 5 belonged to someone that did not live with children. Unit dose products have a different measure of pass/fail compared to closures, but are regulated by the PPPA.

Answer b is correct. The PPPA requires that "child-resistant" closures have ease of opening for not <90% of adult seniors. The test of this standard involves 100 subjects of whom 25% of the participants shall be 50 to 54 years of age, 25% of participants shall be 55 to 59 years of age, and 50% of the participants shall be 60 to 70 years old without over physical or mental handicap. Subjects are then given 5 minutes to read the instructions provided for opening of the closure and attempt to open and empty the contents of the container and then replace the closure. If at the end of 5 minutes they fail to do so or give up, they are given two different nonresistant-closure containers and given 1 minute test periods to open each closure. If they are unable to open the container, they are removed from the subject pool. After either a subject has passed the 5-minute test he or she is given 1 minute to open and close a new but same closure product to determine a passing completion.

Answer c is correct. Several different types of products are regulated by the PPPA. These include over-the-counter and prescription medications as well as some chemical products.

Answer d is correct. Since 1972, the first year when CRC were required, poisoning-related deaths in children <5 dropped from 216 to 28 in the year 2000. The Consumer Product Safety Commission study only took into account deaths related to aspirin and oral prescription medications so it is likely that more than 900 lives have been saved.

Answer e is correct and the best answer.

CHAPTER 67 | All Hazards Preparedness

1. Preparedness is achieved and maintained by which of the following?
   a. Planning
   b. Organizing
   c. Training
   d. Exercising
   e. All of the above

Answers a, b, c, and d are correct.

Answer e is correct and the best answer. Each needs to be done in order to be prepared.

---

2. Virtually all disaster plans are based on what national system?
   a. National Planning System (NPS)
   b. National Incidence Management System (NIMS)
   c. Federal Incidence Bureau System (FIBS)
   d. Strategic National Planning System (SNPS)

Answers a, c, and d are incorrect.

Answer b is correct. Most disaster plans are based on NIMS. It provides a uniform template from a local agency all the way to a federal response.

---

3. The Strategic National Stockpile provides what during an incidence of national significance?
   a. Highly trained medical personal from around the country to disseminate supplies.
   b. Pharmaceuticals only to the state.
   c. Active military medical personnel to support the public.
   d. Pharmaceuticals and medical supplies to the state in need.

Answer a is incorrect. The state is responsible for dissemination.

Answer b is incorrect. The SNS supplies not only pharmaceuticals but also supplies and equipment.

Answer c is incorrect. Active military medical personnel are to support the armed forces. However the governor may call up his state's National Guard to assist in the disaster.

Answer d is correct.

---

4. What government official must request the SNS?
   a. President of the United States
   b. Director of Health and Human Services
   c. Governor
   d. Speaker of the House

Answers a, b, and d are incorrect.

Answer c is correct. The governor must send a request to the CDC for the SNS.

---

5. The CHEMPACK Program stores nerve agent antidotes with participating local or state entities. What are the antidotes provided by this program?
   a. Atropine and pralidoxime
   b. Atropine, pyridoxine, and diazepam
   c. Atropine, pralidoxime, and diazepam
   d. Atropine and pyridoxine

Answers a, b, and d are incorrect.

Answer c is correct. CHEMPACK allows local entities to store nerve agents on site as long as they meet the requirements of storage and planning.

---

6. Which of the following is not considered a Category A threat agent?
   a. Smallpox
   b. Novel H1N1
   c. Anthrax
   d. Arenavirus

Answer a is incorrect. Smallpox is definitely considered a Category A threat.

Answer b is correct. H1N1 (formerly known as swine flu) is not a Category A threat; although it could result in the SNS being set into motion.

Answer c is incorrect. Anthrax is definitely considered a Category A threat.

Answer d is incorrect. Arenavirus is a form of hemorrhagic fever and is definitely considered a Category A threat.

---

7. Which agent is found in the SNS and is indicated for postexposure prophylaxis to inhaled *B. anthracis*?
   a. Dapsone
   b. Difloxacin
   c. Doxycycline
   d. Dicloxacillin

Answers a, b, and d are incorrect.

Answer c is correct. Doxycycline is one of two antibiotics (ciprofloxacin is the other) that is stored by the government to combat some of the threat agents.

---

8. Antibiotic therapy for postexposure prophylaxis to inhaled *B. anthracis* should last for how many days?
   a. 30
   b. 40
   c. 60
   d. 90

Answer a is incorrect. Inadequate.

Answer b is incorrect. Inadequate.

Answer c is correct. Postexposure prophylaxis to inhaled anthrax should be done for 60 days.

Answer d is incorrect. Excessive.

---

9. An 18-year-old patient has been diagnosed with a pneumonic form of *Yersinia pestis.* What is the best course of action for the individuals exposed to the patient?

   a. Start ciprofloxacin 500 mg every 12 hours once symptoms appear.
   b. Start doxycycline 100 mg every 12 hours for 7 days in all individuals exposed during the patient's clinical course.
   c. Await the patient's culture and sensitivity results and start the most appropriate antibiotic as prophylaxis in the exposed individuals.
   d. Prophylaxis is not beneficial.

Answer a is incorrect. Ciprofloxacin is an appropriate antibiotic choice, but waiting for symptoms to appear is wrong. All patients suspected to have an exposure should be treated as soon as possible regardless of signs and symptoms.

Answer b is correct. Doxycycline 100 mg every 12 hours for 7 days in an 18-year-old is an appropriate regimen.

Answer c is incorrect. Awaiting cultures and sensitivity with an invasive organism such as *Y. pestis* is inappropriate, when an exposure is known.

Answer d is incorrect.

---

10. A pharmacist working in local retail pharmacy that is adjacent to a hospital complex receives a call during a bioterrorism drill from an emergency department physician at that health care facility. He states they have a confirmed case of pneumonic tularemia. The patient states a former coworker threatened everyone in the workplace. Upon questioning from the police it was determined the coworker had released *Francisella tularensis* into the air ducts of his former workplace approximately 3 days prior. There are six individuals in that area and he has written them each a prescription for ciprofloxacin 500 mg every 12 hours for 7 days as prophylaxis. However the air duct system is shared with a daycare and eight children have been potentially exposed. All of the children are <30 kg. The physician asks for an antibiotic recommendation. Which of the following is the best treatment recommendation for all of the children?

    a. Doxycycline 50 mg every 12 hours for 7 days
    b. Doxycycline 2.2 mg/kg every 12 hours for 7 days
    c. Ciprofloxacin 500 mg once daily for 7 days
    d. Ciprofloxacin 25 mg/kg every 12 hours for 7 days

Answer a is incorrect. The dose of doxycycline is potentially too high in some and to low in others.

Answer b is correct. Doxycycline 2.2 mg/kg every 12 hours for 7 days is an appropriate dose for the all of the children <30 kg.

Answer c is incorrect. Ciprofloxacin is an appropriate antibiotic choice, but the dose is too high for children 30 kg or less.

Answer d is incorrect. Ciprofloxacin 25 mg/kg every 12 hours is an excessive dose for children 30 kg or less.

---

11. Which of the following botulism types can potentially be treated with an antitoxin obtained from the CDC?

    a. Types A and B only
    b. Types A, B, C, D, E, and F
    c. Types A, B, and E
    d. Type B only

Answer a is incorrect. Type E is also available.

Answer b is incorrect. *Experimentally the military* has an antitoxin for all types including G.

Answer c is correct. Antitoxin for A and B is available together and E is available separately from the CDC.

Answer d is incorrect.

---

12. Twelve patients with type G botulism have been diagnosed in the United States in the past 24 hours. All had recently flown through Toronto Pearson International Airport in the last 72 hours from various destinations. All are experiencing a rapid descending paralysis. What is the most likely reason for the outbreak?

    a. Contaminated seafood at an airport vendor
    b. Deliberate release of toxin within the airport
    c. Person to person contamination
    d. Serendipity

Answer a is incorrect. Although a food vendor could be implicated, the seafood suggests type E.

Answer b is correct. Type G is unusual in humans. Multiple cases of type G infection with a single source of contact (airport) is a deliberate release until otherwise ruled out.

Answer c is incorrect. Botulism is not spread from person to person contamination.

Answer d is incorrect. A virtual statistical impossibility considering it is type G.

---

13. What is presently the best course of treatment for Ebola?

    a. Fluid replacement, ventilation, and additional supportive care as needed
    b. High dose ribavirin
    c. Cryotherapy to drop the core temperature to <95°F
    d. A cocktail of acyclovir, protease inhibitor, and interferon

Answer a is correct. Although supportive care with fluid replacement, ventilation, and additional care as needed has a high mortality rate at present, no other course of treatment appears anymore effective.

Answer b is incorrect. Ribavirin can be used for other types of hemorrhagic fever. It appears ineffective for Ebola.

Answer c is incorrect. Nothing to support dropping the core temperature at present.

Answer d is incorrect. No evidence to support this.

14. A person with smallpox is no longer considered infectious when what event occurs?

 a. Defervescence
 b. The last pustule scabs over
 c. Sloughing of the last pustule scab
 d. When the rash turns to pustules

Answer a is incorrect. An afebrile patient could be infectious.

Answer b is incorrect. Although it is probably positive in the clinical course; the patient is still considered infectious.

Answer c is correct. The sloughing of the last scab is considered the point were a patient is no longer infectious.

Answer d is incorrect. A patient at this stage is highly infectious.

15. Which of the following signs and symptoms are considered clinically significant control with atropine in a postexposure organophosphate patient?

 a. Miosis, salivation, and muscle twitching
 b. Mydriasis, dry mucous membranes, flushing and tachycardia
 c. Tachycardia, bronchorrhea, and salivation
 d. Decreased bronchial secretions and increased ease of ventilation

Answer a is incorrect. This would signal marked cholinergic syndrome.

Answer b is incorrect. This would signal anticholinergic syndrome and the patient has most likely received excessive atropine.

Answer c is incorrect. This patient has been inadequately treated and needs additional atropine based on the bronchorrhea.

Answer d is correct. A patient can still have miosis and other symptoms, but adequate atropine is based on increased ease of ventilation and decreased bronchial secretions. The patient does not have to be dry, but secretions should be greatly reduced.

16. An adult patient with sarin poisoning has been decontaminated and is now in the triage area. He has small pupils, sweating, and copious salivation and nasal secretions. He begins having a seizure almost immediately after being brought to the triage area. Which is the best course of treatment?

 a. Administer diazepam 10 mg, followed by a 2 mg bolus of atropine, and then pralidoxime 2 g in 100 cc of NS infused over 30 minutes.
 b. A 2 mg bolus of atropine and repeat as needed, then pralidoxime 2 g in 100 cc of NS infused over 30 minutes. If the seizure activity has not abated post pralidoxime then give 5 mg of diazepam.
 c. Administer 10 mg of diazepam for the seizure then no additional therapy as the other signs and symptoms are not concerning.
 d. Administer 5 g of pralidoxime via IVP since it will replenish GABA, then give atropine 2 g prn until bronchorrhea decreases.

Answer a is correct. An attempt to immediately control the seizure should be made. This patient is having significant cholinergic signs and symptoms so atropine and 2-pam should be given.

Answer b is incorrect. Delaying seizure treatment for 30 minutes is inappropriate.

Answer c is incorrect. The diazepam is correct, but withholding atropine and 2-pam is inappropriate.

Answer d is incorrect. Pyridoxine (vitamin B_6), not pralidoxime, is the GABA precursor. A benzodiazepine is needed in this patient.

17. A 3-year-old child and her 65-year-old grandmother were riding in car that was involved in a three-vehicle accident at 3 am. They have only minor injuries, but one of the other vehicles was carrying I131 for use as an imaging agent. The I131 container was not properly stored or sealed and it entered the side window of the vehicle with the child and grandmother. Many of the compounded I131 capsules were ruptured and dispersed throughout the car. They are 20 minutes post accident and no one is answering the phone at the nuclear pharmacy, there is no paperwork with the I131 product and the delivery driver is unconscious. Which is the best advice for the grandmother and child?

 a. Treat both with potassium iodide.
 b. Treat the grandmother with potassium iodide and leave the child untreated.
 c. Treat the child with potassium iodide and leave the grandmother untreated.
 d. Treat both with Prussian blue.
 e. Treat neither.

Answer a is incorrect. The grandmother is in no danger from a small I131exposure. Treating the child can be debated. See Answer c.

Answer b is incorrect.

Answer c is correct. There are too many unknowns in this case. An argument could be made to withhold potassium iodide if the dose was known. However the dose is not known and the product was inadequately stored, the child was definitely exposed and given children's sensitivity to I131 treating is the appropriate course for the child. Grandmother is older than 40 years of age. Her risk of thyroid disease secondary to the exposure is virtually nil.

Answer d is incorrect. Prussian blue is not indicated for I131.

Answer e is incorrect.

---

18. Which of these is not considered a representative of the first five groups recommended to receive the novel 2009 novel H1N1 vaccine?

   a. Healthy but pregnant 28-year-old
   b. Emergency room physician
   c. 55-year-old healthy male accountant
   d. 23-year-old female with type I diabetes
   e. 32-year-old healthy daycare worker

Answer a is incorrect. Although healthy, she is pregnant and is considered a recommended individual.

Answer b is incorrect. Emergency room physician are definitely part of the recommended group.

Answer c is correct. Greater than 24-year-old and <64-year-old with no comorbid conditions, he is not part of the first five groups.

Answer d is incorrect. She meets the criteria on two fronts. She is <24 years old and has a comorbid condition (diabetes), so she is part of the recommended group.

Answer e is incorrect. Daycare workers should receive the vaccine as part of the recommended group.

---

19. As of 2009 according the to the CDC guidelines which is considered the preferred agent for influenza in the United States regardless of *viral type*?

   a. Rimantadine
   b. Amantidine
   c. Oseltamivir
   d. Zanamivir

Answer a is incorrect.

Answer b is incorrect.

Answer c is incorrect. Although preferred for some cases, it is not preferred for all.

Answer d is correct. It is the preferred agent or copreferred agent for all types.

---

20. The first case of novel H1N1 was reported in the United States in late March-early April 2009. By the end of June reported cases topped 1 million US residents. The logical reason for rapid dissemination of the disease is mostly likely which of the following?

   a. The seasonal flu vaccine weakened the immune system.
   b. The wet spring months are better for viral survival.
   c. The population lacks immunity.
   d. Antivirals are infective.

Answers a, b, and d are incorrect.

Answer c is correct. A pandemic outbreak occurs because the population lacks immunity.

CHAPTER 68 | Ergogenic Aids and Sports Pharmacy

1. A female swimmer preparing for the US National Championships has been notified that she is required to submit a random urine sample for analysis. She calls you and asks if she can provide the sample herself or if she must consent to the collector's protocol. Your best response to this question is:

   a. Yes, you can prepare a sample and send it in to the appropriate laboratory.
   b. Yes, but your coach must witness the sample.
   c. No, according to the USOC policy, all chain-of-custody protocols must be followed.
   d. No, you must report to the nearest hospital laboratory to submit the sample.

Answer a is incorrect. The sample must be witnessed by appropriate and certified collectors according to WADA/USOC criteria.

Answer b is incorrect. The witness must be a representative of the collecting laboratory, WADA, USOC, or the appropriate organization that is sanctioning the competition.

Answer c is correct. An appropriately collected sample must be collected in the presence of official representatives; once the sample is collected, sealed, and the paperwork complete, any attempt to open, contaminate, or otherwise tamper with said sample will be obvious. The athlete should feel confident that their sample should not or cannot be tampered with. Additionally, the sponsoring or testing laboratory will report any suspicions it has about the integrity of the sample before analysis.

Answer d is incorrect. The correct sampling procedure and chain-of-custody protocol must be followed. Only WADA-certified laboratories can analyze and certify a sample if the competition falls under their purview. Other athletic organizations may credential laboratories for their analysis but it is the athlete's responsibility to ascertain which laboratories are credentialed.

---

2. JM is a competing cyclist and will likely compete on the European circuit this summer. He has an underlying asthma disorder that you help to manage. He was previously managing his asthma with formoterol/budesonide 4.5 μg/80 μg actuation inhalation aerosol: two inhalations twice daily and an occasional albuterol inhalation as needed for rescue. He has recently experienced some mild worsening. His asthma medications have changed to formoterol/budesonide 4.5 μg/160 μg actuations by aerosol (Symbicort) 2 inhalations twice daily with albuterol as a rescue inhaler. Last year he obtained a "therapeutic use exemption" (TUE). He asks you if he will require another TUE. Your best response to this question is:

   a. Yes, he will require a new TUE.
   b. No, since he has already obtained one, he need not obtain another.
   c. No, asthma medicines have been removed from the "prohibited list" for international competition.
   d. Yes, but only for the albuterol since it is short acting.

Answer a is correct. The TUE program provides athletes the opportunity to request medications for treatment and management of serious injuries or medical conditions that may require the use of prohibited substances. A TUE will be granted *only* if the substance does not pose a significant health problem, does not enhance performance (beyond bringing the individual to a state of performance equivalent to one without said injury or condition), and if there is no alternative substitute available (nonprohibited drug). Internationally competing athletes should submit to international federations and nationally competing athletes should submit to national antidoping agencies. TUEs are granted for a specific drug with a defined dosage and for a specific period of time.

Answer b is incorrect. WADA regulations specifically require a new TUE for specific drugs, dosage changes, and the TUE is only granted for a specific period of time. A new dose will require a new TUE.

Answer c is incorrect. Beta-adrenergic agonists have not been removed from the list of prohibited drugs.

Answer d is incorrect. Formoterol and corticosteroids are both on the list of prohibited drugs and require TUE.

---

3. A competitor in a cross-country ski race is consuming caffeine and pseudoephedrine prior to his competition. He is likely using this combination for what purpose?

   a. To increase his heart rate
   b. To increase his blood pressure
   c. To increase his alertness
   d. To spare his glycogen stores

Answer a is incorrect. This combination will increase his HR but that is not the ergogenic effect that he is seeking.

Answer b is incorrect. This combination may increase his BP as well but that is not the ergogenic effect that he is seeking.

Answer c is incorrect. This combination may increase his alertness but no evidence exists to support this as a performance-enhancing aspect.

Answer d is correct. Several studies have suggested that the combination of caffeine and ephedrine may increase lipolysis and spare glycogenolysis to enhance endurance. Since this is an endurance event, that is likely the outcome that he is seeking.

---

4. Androstenedione (Andro) is a dietary supplement touted to act as an anabolic agent. The purported basic science behind this theory is best described by which of the following?

   a. Androstenedione blocks the breakdown of endogenous testosterone.
   b. Androstenedione is a natural anabolic steroidal compound that acts at the androgenic receptors with a higher affinity than testosterone.
   c. Androstenedione is a precursor in the cascade of steps that produces testosterone.
   d. Androstenedione has no anabolic potential.

Answer a is incorrect. Androstenedione is a precursor in the steps forming testosterone and does not inhibit the metabolism of testosterone

Answer b is incorrect. Androstenedione is not known to act at androgenic receptors.

Answer c is correct. Androstenedione is the precursor to testosterone. In theory, providing more substrate precursor should lead to higher concentrations of end product, such as testosterone. This has been shown to be the case with doses of androstenedione >300 mg daily. For this reason, it is a prohibited substance in most athletic competition.

Answer d is incorrect. In theory, given a high-enough dose, androstenedione could increase testosterone levels and, indirectly, improve anabolism.

---

5. The most common analytical test used to assess whether exogenous testosterone or one of its derivatives has been used is which of the following?

   a. Androstenedione: testosterone ratio
   b. Testosterone: epitestosterone ratio
   c. Urine sample of 19-Nandrolone
   d. Blood specimen of 19-NA

Answer a is incorrect. No established ratio for A:T has been suggested to determine exogenous administration.

Answer b is correct. The most common test (urine) conducted examines the ratio of testosterone to epitestosterone. Normally, this occurs in a 1:1 ratio. Occasionally, some athletes will have an increased ratio of 2:1, and rarely 3:1. A threshold ratio of 4:1 currently exists with WADA; values above this ratio are consistent with exogenous administration of testosterone and its derivatives, suggesting illicit use.

Answer c is incorrect. While this is a confirmatory test, it has been associated with false positives. The most common analytical test is T:E ratio.

Answer d is incorrect. While potentially doable, the feasibility and cost of blood specimens is not warranted at this time unless in-depth confirmatory testing is warranted.

---

6. JS is college football player who is training during the off-season. He asks you about supplementing his dietary regimen with creatine monophosphate. He specifically asks if the creatine supplementation will positively affect his exercise performance. Of the following, which factor is the *least* likely to affect creatine's effect on exercise performance?

   a. Dose
   b. Trained versus untrained individuals
   c. Laboratory studies versus actual studies
   d. Concomitant medications

Answer a is incorrect. The total amount of creatine ingested per day is important to achieving increases in tissue concentrations of creatine and improving performance. Studies have supported a loading dose of 15 to 20 g/d × 5 days, and then 2 to 5 g daily; this regimen has been associated with positive performance measurements in short-burst, anaerobic activities.

Answer b is incorrect. One meta-analysis concluded that creatine supplementation benefited untrained athletes; however, trained athletes saw no outcome difference. Since well-trained athletes have higher endogenous production, tissue storage, and exercise can augment creatine uptake by exercising muscle tissue, the training-naïve individual will likely realize greater response to supplementation.

Answer c is incorrect. Many discrepancies have been found in laboratory-controlled studies compared to those conducted in "field" environments. Contradictory and equivocal results have been demonstrated in both environments and under differing circumstances. Many sprint-swimming studies have produced negative results. To properly assess the effects of creatine on performance, the duration of the activity seems to be a strong variable. The shorter the duration and more intense the exercise, the stronger the benefit on improvement.

Answer d is correct. While concerns have been raised regarding the potential renal toxicity of creatine, there are no convincing data that support this theory. There have been no drug interactions of consequence reported thus far with supplemental creatine.

---

7. BB is a 24-year-old body builder that presents to you complaining of female-like breast development that is somewhat painful. Upon questioning him, you discover that he takes 2 mg daily of stanozolol, 20 mg of methandrostenolone (Dianabol), and an injection of testosterone cypionate IM once weekly. He also takes a multitude of multivitamins and supplements and eats about 6000 kcal daily. He is 5'10" and weighs 225 lbs; his HR is 80 beats/min and BP is 162/94 mm Hg. He states that he feels he is dependent on the steroids for his muscle mass and appearance. His laboratory values include Scr 1.3 mg/dL, BUN 32 mg/dL, Na 138 mEq/L, K 4.4 mEq/L, Cl 99 MEq/L, CO_2 22 mEq/L, ALT 120 U/L, AST 80 U/L, HDL 34 mg/dL, LDL 180 mg/dL, and TC 220 mg/dL. Assuming you cannot convince BB to abate his steroid abuse, what do you think his greatest risk from long term use would be?

   a. Cardiovascular risk
   b. Hepatotoxicity
   c. Breast cancer
   d. Psychoses

Answer a is correct. Based on his HTN and dyslipidemia, he is at risk for acute and long-term CV disease. While some studies have shown a reversal of dyslipidemia upon stopping the steroids, the atheromas associated with his androgen use are increasing his risk for a cardiovascular event.

Answer b is partially correct. Transaminasemias, while worrisome, most often will revert to normal levels and while hepatotoxicity is a risk, his CV risk is larger. This is often the most difficult to convince, however, because he is at an age of perceived invincibility.

Answers c and d are partially correct. The only SE he may be concerned with are likely the ones that are readily apparent or cosmetically unacceptable and even then, desired bigger biceps may outweigh his desire for normal size testicles. His gynecomastia may present a risk for breast cancer but that has never been quantified. His dependence and addictive potential are troublesome and may lead to significant problems in the future. His will be a long-term and continuous educational process and engaging with this individual will require persistence and patience.

---

8. LL is a 34-year-old single woman who likes to compete in local cycling events. She has a history of a leg DVT 3 years ago, thought secondary to her use of oral contraceptives. She currently takes no prescription medications but does take a calcium supplement and a multivitamin. She is otherwise healthy. She is employed as an LPN at an oncology clinic where she was asked to label for destruction and shipping some outdated darbepoetin. She confides in you that she took a couple of vials because she had read somewhere that substances like this can improve cycling performance. Of the following, what do you think the best response would be?

   a. Turn her to the DEA immediately.
   b. Inform her that the increase in hematocrit will likely induce a pulmonary embolus in her given her history.
   c. Educate and encourage clean competition and to disclose what she did to her superiors.
   d. The drug was outdated, it will have no effect.

Answer a is not the best response. Darbepoetin is not a controlled substance, so the DEA is not jurisdictional. This is, however, an ethics dilemma that you may run into; clearly, education is the key and lack of education gets people into more trouble than they imagined. The education must be continuous and longitudinal to be effective.

Answer b is partially correct. Her risk for thromboembolism may increase but scare tactics seldom are effective and while VTE increases with significantly increased RBC mass, one is not assured this will be the case in this individual.

Answer c is correct. At this point, it's not your duty to turn her in because no one was personally harmed, but she should be encouraged to disclose what she did and get educated regarding the legitimate use of drugs and be encouraged to compete ethically.

Answer d is incorrect. Outdating often just signifies how far out the drug was tested for (90%) activity and potency.

9. To gain an alleged ergogenic benefit from anabolic steroids, they must be used
   a. Immediately (30 minutes) before competition.
   b. 2 weeks before competition.
   c. Cyclically in one's training regimen months before competition.
   d. They offer no ergogenic benefit.

Answers a and b are incorrect. Anabolic steroids are associated with increases in lean body mass accretion when used in conjunction with rigorous and intense training techniques that are applied for long periods (eg, 6 months) of time or when stress (eg, negative nitrogen balance from starvation, chronic wasting diseases, severe injury) becomes manifest.

Answer c is correct.

Answer d is incorrect. Although an argument can be made using the available published evidence, most experts agree that use of AAS applied to intense training over long periods of time are associated with increases in lean body mass that may afford improvement in strength and mass-dominated athletic events that could not have been achieved without these drugs.

10. Fostering an antidrug mentality in sports and athletics means focusing on
    a. The ill effects and adverse reactions of the agents involved
    b. Denying any purported benefit from the drugs
    c. An appeal to communities through "town hall" meetings
    d. Behavior, drug education, and athletes' social sphere of influence

Answers a and b are incorrect. Focusing only on the adverse reactions of the drugs or dismissing pharmacologic action that could be ergogenic in nature serves only to incent curiosity and experimentation with the athlete and instills distrust.

Answer c is incorrect. While communities represent a network of friends, families, and fans, seldom do communities as a whole offer educational programs or sponsor antidrug activities via evidence-based methods.

Answer d is correct. Modifying behavior, providing continual drug education, and impacting the athletes' social sphere of influence has been shown to have the most significant difference in curbing the use of ergogenic drug use.

11. LA is a competitive cyclist. Recently, his random urine sample revealed a testosterone: epitestosterone (T:E) ratio of 12:1. His sample from 10 days ago revealed a T:E ratio of 4:1. A reasonable explanation for the difference between these two ratios would be which of the following?
    a. T:E ratios can vary widely between stages of rest and intense exercise. One of the values was likely during a rest cycle.
    b. This may be indicative of a pathology where he cannot metabolize his testosterone.
    c. This sample likely indicates exogenous testosterone supplementation.
    d. There is likely an error in the testing process.

Answer a is incorrect. T:E ratios stay remarkably stable unless exogenous testosterone (or epitestosterone) is administered.

Answer b is incorrect. T:E ratios naturally parallel each other and the ratio stays relatively constant. There are a small number of individuals in whom their "normal" T:E ratio is >2:1 (ie, 3:1 to 4:1), but their ratio would stay constant and not vary to this degree.

Answer c is correct. A T:E ratio >6:1 is indicative of exogenous testosterone use.

Answer d is possible but not the best choice. WADA-accredited analytical laboratories follow strict procedures and protocols and the chance of the sample being erroneously handled and analyzed is very rare.

12. KM comes into your pharmacy with a prescription for propranolol 20 mg. The signatura (SIG) on the prescription reads "Take as directed." As you question KM about this, you determine the propranolol is only taken during her archery competitions. She states that the competition increases her blood pressure. The most likely conclusion you should glean from this would be which of the following?
    a. Competition does, indeed, increase the BP of many competitors and, thus, for medical and safety reasons, you should dispense the prescription.
    b. KM is using the beta-adrenergic blocking drug, propranolol, to block adrenergic response peripherally (decrease tremors) and thus using the drug unethically.

c. KM is using the beta-adrenergic blocking drug, propranolol, to block beta-2 receptors in her lung bed to control her breathing while she competes, thus using the drug unethically.
d. KM is using the drug as an ergogenic aid to boost her performance, but it is permissible under international competition rules.

Answer a may be partially correct. However, physiologic exercise–induced BP increases seldom, if ever, require treatment; rather that reflects a normal physiologic response.

Answer b is correct. Competitive sports that require fine motor control prohibit agents that improve performance by abating sympathomimetic-induced or accentuated tremors. This includes beta-blockers.

Answer c is incorrect. While beta-receptor antagonists ameliorate the beta-2 response in the lung bed, this does not improve competitive performance.

Answer d is incorrect. Beta-blocking agents are included in the WADA 2009 Prohibited List.

---

13. You have been asked to serve as a consultant on a panel analyzing competitor samples. A "sample A" specimen turns up positive for the drug probenecid. The panel asks your assessment of this drug. Of the following, which would be the best response?

a. Probenecid blocks the tubular secretion of many drugs including some AAS and their metabolites and was used to mask the sample. Sample B should be tested and the appropriate administrative authorities should be notified.
b. Probenecid can act as an anabolic agent. Sample B should be tested and the appropriate administrative authorities should be notified.
c. Probenecid can act as an oxygen enhancer. Sample B should be tested and the appropriate administrative authorities should be notified.
d. Probenecid prevents catabolic breakdown of skeletal proteins in athletes, helping them to recover from training. It is not on the 2009 Prohibited List and the sample should be disregarded.

Answer a is correct. Probenecid has higher affinity in the renal tubules and will be preferentially excreted in lieu of other drugs, thus, many unethical competitors will try to "mask" other agents (eg, AAS) by taking probenecid.

Answer b is incorrect. Probenecid has no androgenic or anabolic properties.

Answer c is incorrect. Probenecid does not enhance oxygen delivery or exchange.

Answer d is incorrect. While it is a xanthine oxidase inhibitor and can prevent increase purine concentrations, it is more effective in preventing gout exacerbations and has never been shown to enhance skeletal muscle cell recovery.

---

14. Which of the following would be considered *least* likely to be an ergogenic substance that produces an "immediate" effect?

a. Marijuana
b. Albuterol
c. Modafinil
d. Erythropoietin

Answer a is incorrect. Marijuana is a CNS depressant but has no ergogenic effect with training.

Answer b is incorrect. As a short-acting beta-adrenergic agonist, albuterol will only benefit at the time of administration and out to 3 to 4 hours.

Answer c is incorrect. Modafinil is a CNS stimulant and may provide improved alertness and lessened fatigue but only during in-competition.

Answer d is correct. Erythropoietin can enhance oxygen transfer during training periods that will carry over into competition.

---

15. A group of parents approach you because they are concerned some student-athletes may be using human growth hormone in an attempt to increase muscle mass. They inquire how to test for this agent. Of the following, what would be your best response?

a. Currently, there is no definitive test for exogenously administered recombinant HGH and surrogate markers must be utilized.
b. While there may be some lean mass accretion, there are no data to confirm an actual ergogenic benefit, so the parents should not be concerned.
c. Currently, there is no definitive test for exogenously administered recombinant HGH; monitoring for a SE profile is the best way to detect its use.
d. Set up a program and threshold levels and begin measuring serum levels of HGH.

Answer a is correct. While isomeric measurement testing is still in developmental stages and may become viable, currently, unless the serum is analyzed within 24 hours of exogenous administration, much speculation and uncertainty exists with regard to identifying illicit use of HGH, thus, surrogate markers such as insulin-like growth factor-1 are used.

Answer b is incorrect. While current evidence suggests little, if any, ergogenic effect, and many harmful effects, illicit drug use for performance-enhancing purposes should be discouraged.

Answer c is incorrect. Many SE are associated with other drugs as well (eg, fluid retention) and are long term (eg, acromegaly) and so may not be readily apparent.

Answer d is incorrect. Measuring serum levels for exogenously administered HGH has not been adequately defined.

16. Which of the following is not considered legitimate criteria for granting a therapeutic use exemption (TUE)?

a. The athlete would experience significant health problems without taking the prohibited substance or method.
b. The substance is needed to treat the side effects of previously administered ergogenic aids (eg, testosterone for gonadal atrophy from previous abuse of AAS).
c. There is no reasonable therapeutic alternative to the use of the otherwise prohibited substance or method.
d. The therapeutic use of the substance would produce no additional enhancement of a performance other than that which might be anticipated by a return to a state of normal health.

Answers a, c, and d are incorrect. Athletes, like others, may have disease states that require them to take particular medications to control their condition. If that medication happens to fall under the WADA Prohibited List, a TUE may give that athlete the authorization to take the needed medicine.

Answer b is correct. Criteria are not extended to treat maladies incited by previous illicit ergogenic use.

---

17. A 22-year-old female cross-country skier is planning on national and international competition and asks you if she can consume caffeine on daily basis without concern. Which of the following provides the best response?

a. No, caffeine exists on the WADA prohibited use.
b. Yes, caffeine is monitored on an in-competition basis only and even then, can be consumed to a certain urine threshold.
c. Yes, caffeine is monitored on an in-competition basis but must be discontinued 24 hours prior to any competition.
d. Yes, but evidence exists suggesting caffeine is deleterious to endurance performance.

Answer a is incorrect. Caffeine exists on the WADA list on an "in-competition" basis. Additionally, it can be consumed to certain urine thresholds, above which, it is considered an attempt to use it for ergogenic purposes.

Answer b is correct.

Answer c is incorrect. It can be consumed while competing but must stay under established urine thresholds.

Answer d is incorrect. Most evidence is equivocal; when combined with ephedrine, endurance improvement has been shown.

---

18. JS is a football player alleged to have taken AAS. Which of the following would *not* be considered a confirmatory test to monitor for exogenous AAS?

a. Gas chromatography
b. T:E ratio
c. Ketoconazole administration
d. Polygraph test

Answer a is incorrect. Gas chromatography and mass spectrometry are technology advancements to identify specific compounds.

Answer b is incorrect. The T:E ratio has been established as an effective method to detect exogenous testosterone.

Answer c is incorrect. Ketoconazole challenge can distinguish if exogenous testosterone has been administered by analyzing a subsequent T:E ratio.

Answer d is correct. Polygraph test has not been firmly established as a confirmatory testing methodology.

---

19. RJ, an aspiring baseball player, states that he has been taking nutraceuticals and dietary supplements so as to avoid prescription drugs that are prohibited in organized baseball. He asks you what your opinion is about this. Of the following, your best response would be:

a. This is a good plan for maintaining nutrition but avoiding prohibited substances.
b. This is a good plan for avoiding prohibited substances but will not improve his performance.
c. This is not a good plan. Many prohibited substances are components of dietary supplements and nutraceuticals.
d. This is not a good plan. Many nutraceuticals and dietary supplements can be identified in the urine.

Answers a and b are incorrect. This is an incorrect thought process. Many prohibited substances such as stimulants and anabolic steroids can be components of "dietary supplements" as this is an unregulated industry.

Answer c is correct.

Answer d is incorrect. One should never condone the practice of taking ergogenic aids.

---

20. JR is a long-distance cyclist that recently suffered a transient ischemic attack (TIA). He reported to the emergency department (ED) where he related no prescription drug use. His vitals in the ED were: BP 164/90 mm Hg, RR 20 breaths/min, HR 52 beats/min and regular, temperature 99°F. His BUN was 18 mg/dL and his Scr was 1.1 mg/dL. Of note, his hemoglobin was 19 g/dL and his hematocrit was 57.2%. He was assessed as being well hydrated but not fluid overloaded. He was no longer suffering from any neurologic deficit. He did not lose consciousness. A urine test using isoelectric focusing would likely be positive for which exogenously administered substance?

a. Testosterone
b. Recombinant human growth hormone
c. Recombinant erythropoietin
d. Recombinant human chorionic gonadotropin

Answer a is partially correct. Testosterone can stimulate endogenous erythropoiesis, but has not been associated with thromboembolic events and stroke. Advanced technological testing for testosterone involves carbon isotope ratio testing or isotope ratio mass spectrometry.

Answer b is incorrect. Because recombinant HGH does not contain glycosylation process, isoelectric focusing method developed for recombinant erythropoietin cannot be directly applied to HGH. No definitive test exists currently to detect HGH. Additionally, it has not been associated with embolic events.

Answer c is correct. Stimulating erythropoiesis increases RBC mass, which if left unabated, can increase to the point of worsened HTN, increased fluid volume, and thromboembolic events including stroke and TIA. Isoelectric focusing takes advantage of the extra sugar molecules on the recombinant product and this glycosylation allows for separation of exogenous and endogenous erythropoietin in a pH-gradient electrical field, thus, differing isoform patterns.

Answer d is incorrect. Isoelectric focusing is not the method used to test for human chorionic gonadotropin nor is it associated with stroke or TIA.

CHAPTER 69 Vaccines and Immunizations

1. Which of the following can safely be given to a 6-month-old child who had an allergic reaction to the pertussis vaccine?

   a. DTaP
   b. Tdap
   c. Td
   d. DT

Answer a is incorrect. DTaP is indicated for the prevention of diphtheria, tetanus, and pertussis in children <7 years. However, it contains the pertussis vaccine and should not be used in a patient who has had an allergic reaction to the pertussis vaccine.

Answer b is incorrect. Tdap is indicated for use as a single booster dose in adolescents and adults between the ages of 11 and 64 years. It also contains the pertussis vaccine. It should not be used in a 6-month-old who is allergic to the pertussis vaccine.

Answer c is incorrect. Even though Td does not contain the pertussis vaccine, it is indicated for use as a booster dose in adolescents and adults over the age of 7 years. It would not be appropriate to use this vaccine in a 6-month-old child.

Answer d is correct. DT is indicated for the prevention of diphtheria and tetanus in children <7 years of age. It does not contain the pertussis vaccine. It should be used in children who have previously had an allergic reaction to the pertussis vaccine.

2. KS, a 5-year-old girl, has an appointment today with her pediatrician to receive vaccines. Her vaccination record shows the following: Hep B at birth, 2 months, and 6 months; RV at 2, 4, and 6 months; DTaP at 2, 4, 6, and 15 months; Hib (ActHIB) at 2, 4, 6, and 15 months; PCV at 2, 4, 6, and 15 months; IPV at 2, 4, and 6 months; MMR at 15 months; Varicella at15 months; and Hep A at 15 months. She does not have any medical conditions and is not allergic to any medications or vaccines. What vaccines should KS receive today?

   a. DT, PPSV, IPV, MMR, MCV, and Hep A
   b. DTaP, IPV, MMR, Varicella, and Hep A
   c. Tdap, IPV, MMR, Varicella, and Hep A
   d. DTaP, PPSV, IPV, MMR, Varicella, and Hep A

Answer a is incorrect. DT is indicated for children <7 years of age who have had an allergic reaction to the pertussis vaccine. KS has no vaccine allergies so DTaP should be used. PPSV should only be administered in high-risk patients—KS does not have any conditions that would warrant administration of PPSV. It is recommended that adolescents receive the MCV at age 11 or 12 years. Children may receive it earlier if they are at high risk for meningococcal disease. Since KS is only 5 years old and does not have any risk factors for meningococcal disease, she should not receive MCV. Also, she needs to receive the second doses of MMR and Varicella.

Answer b is correct. KS has received four doses in the DTaP series already and therefore needs to receive the fifth and final DTaP dose. She has also received three doses of IPV and should receive the fourth dose today. KS received her first doses of the MMR and varicella vaccines at 15 months. She needs to receive the second dose of each today. Since KS only received one dose of the Hep A vaccine at 15 months, she needs to complete the two-dose series today. Even though it has been several years since the first dose, she does not need to start the series over again. She only needs one dose of the Hep A vaccine.

Answer c is incorrect. Tdap should only be used as a single booster dose in adolescents and adults aged 11 to 64 years. KS is too young to receive Tdap. Also, she will not need a booster until she has completed the five-dose series of DTaP.

Answer d is incorrect. PPSV should only be administered in high-risk patients—KS does not have any conditions that would warrant administration of PPSV.

3. Which of the following vaccines is given as a single dose?

   a. PCV
   b. Zoster
   c. RV
   d. Td

Answer a is incorrect. PCV requires four doses given at 2, 4, 6, and 12 to 15 months of age.

Answer b is correct. The zoster vaccine only requires one dose.

Answer c is incorrect. The RV vaccines require multiple doses. RotaTeq requires three doses at 2, 4 and 6 months. Rotarix requires two doses at 2 and 4 months of age.

Answer d is incorrect. Adults require a booster dose with Td every 10 years.

4. Which of the following pediatric vaccines is administered orally?

   a. IPV
   b. PCV
   c. RV
   d. Varicella

Answer a is incorrect. IPV can be administered IM or SC. It cannot be administered orally.

Answer b is incorrect. PCV is administered IM, not orally.

Answer c is correct. RV is the only vaccine listed that is administered orally.

Answer d is incorrect. The varicella vaccine is administered SC, not orally.

5. A 69-year-old man comes into your pharmacy after receiving a letter advertising your immunization program. He has diabetes and hypertension and smokes a pack of cigarettes a day. He does not have any medication or vaccine allergies. His vaccination record shows that he completed all of his childhood vaccinations (DTaP, Hib, PCV, IPV, and MMR) as well as the Hep B series. He had chickenpox when he was 5 years old and received his last Td booster 11 years ago. Which vaccines should this patient receive?

   a. Td, Zoster, PPSV, and Hep A
   b. Tdap, Varicella, and PPSV
   c. Tdap, Zoster, and Hep A
   d. Td, Zoster, and PPSV

Answer a is incorrect. This patient needs a tetanus-diphtheria booster because it has been over 10 years since his last one. He is also a candidate for the zoster vaccine as well as the PPSV vaccine since he is over 65 years old. He is not a candidate for Hep A vaccination because he is not a child and does not have any risk factors for Hep A infection.

Answer b is incorrect. This patient needs a tetanus-diphtheria booster; however, Tdap is only indicated in patients 11 to 64 years old. He is too old to receive Tdap. Varicella is indicated in children >12 months and adults without documented evidence of varicella immunity (eg, previous vaccination or documented case of chicken pox). Since he has had chickenpox, he is not a candidate for varicella vaccination.

Answer c is incorrect. This patient needs a tetanus-diptheriea booster; however he is too old to receive Tdap. He should receive the zoster vaccine. He does not have any risk factors for Hep A infection so he does not need the Hep A vaccine.

Answer d is correct. This patient needs a tetanus-diptheria booster and therefore should receive Td. He is a candidate for zoster and PPSV vaccines because he is over the age of 60 and 65, respectively.

6. Which of the following diphtheria and tetanus vaccines should be used in adults as a one-time booster dose?

   a. Td
   b. DT
   c. Tdap
   d. DTaP

Answer a is incorrect. Adults will require a Td booster every 10 years.

Answer b is incorrect. DT is only indicated for children <7 years of age who have a contraindication to the pertussis vaccine.

Answer c is correct. Adolescents and adults will require a booster dose of the pertussis vaccine once in their lifetime. It is recommended that one Td booster be replaced by a Tdap booster once in patients between the ages of 11 and 64 years.

Answer d is incorrect. DTaP is only indicated for children <7 years of age.

7. Which of the following adults under the age of 65 would require a pneumococcal polysaccharide vaccine (PPSV)?

   a. Pregnant women
   b. Smokers
   c. Health care workers
   d. Splenic patients

Answer a is incorrect. Pregnant women are not considered to be at high risk for pneumococcal disease.

Answer b is correct. Adults who smoke are considered to be at high risk for pneumococcal disease and therefore should receive PPSV.

Answer c is incorrect. Health care workers are not considered to be at high risk for pneumococcal disease.

Answer d is incorrect. Splenic patients are not considered to be at high risk for pneumococcal disease. However, patients with either functional or anatomic asplenia (sickle cell disease or splenectomy) should receive PPSV.

8. How should the hepatitis B vaccine (Hep B) be administered?
    a. In the deltoid muscle at a 90° angle.
    b. In the deltoid muscle at a 45° angle.
    c. In the outer aspect of the triceps at a 45° angle.
    d. In the anteriolateral thigh at a 45° angle.

Answer a is correct. The Hep B vaccine is administered intramuscularly and should be given in the deltoid muscle (for adults) and the anteriolateral thigh (for infants) at a 90° angle.

Answer b is incorrect. Injections in the deltoid muscle should be given at a 90° angle.

Answer c is incorrect. Subcutaneous injections are given in the outer aspect of the triceps at a 45° angle. The Hep B vaccine is given intramuscularly.

Answer d is incorrect. Infants can receive intramuscular injections in the anteriolateral thigh; however it should be given at a 90° angle.

---

9. EP is pregnant and in her second trimester. Which of the following vaccines can EP receive?
    a. HPV
    b. Hep B
    c. MMR
    d. DTaP

Answer a is incorrect. The HPV vaccine should not be administered to pregnant females because it is contraindicated in pregnancy.

Answer b is correct. The Hep B vaccine can be administered to a pregnant female who has not received the vaccination before.

Answer c is incorrect. The MMR vaccine is a live vaccine. Pregnant women should not receive live vaccines.

Answer d is incorrect. The DTaP vaccine is indicated for children under the age of 7. If EP needed a tetanus booster, she should receive the Td vaccine.

---

10. An 11-year-old girl fainted after receiving her 11- to 12-year-old routine vaccinations. Which of the following vaccines most likely caused her to faint?
    a. Tdap
    b. HPV
    c. MCV
    d. Hep B

Answer a is incorrect. Tdap has not been associated with syncope.

Answer b is correct. The HPV vaccine has been associated with syncope after administration. It is recommended that patients remain seated or lie down for 15 minutes after receiving the vaccine.

Answer c is incorrect. MCV has not been associated with syncope.

Answer d is incorrect. The Hep B vaccine has not been associated with syncope.

---

11. Herpes zoster vaccine should be stored at what temperature?
    a. ≤5°F
    b. 6°F to 35°F
    c. 36°F to 46°F
    d. 47°F to 77°F

Answer a is correct. The herpes zoster vaccine needs to be kept frozen. Frozen vaccines should be stored in a freezer with a temperature <5°F.

Answer b is incorrect. Storing the herpes zoster vaccine at temperatures above 5°F can lead to loss of potency.

Answer c is incorrect. Vaccines that require refrigeration should be stored at temperatures between 36°F and 46°F. The herpes zoster vaccine should be kept frozen.

Answer d is incorrect. Temperatures between 47°F and 77°F are considered room temperature. The herpes zoster vaccine should be kept frozen.

---

12. JM, a 6-month-old infant, is seeing his pediatrician today in order to receive his 6 month vaccinations. His vaccination records are as follows: Hep B at birth and 2 months; DTaP at 2 and 4 months; Hib (PedvaxHIB) at 2 and 4 months; PCV at 2 and 4 months; IPV at 2 and 4 months. JM does not have any medical conditions or allergies to medications or vaccines. Which vaccines should JM receive today?
    a. Hep B, RV, DTaP, Hib, PCV, and IPV
    b. Hep B, RV, DTaP, PCV, and IPV
    c. Hep B, DTaP, Hib, PCV, and IPV
    d. Hep B, DTaP, PCV, and IPV

Answer a is incorrect. At 6 months, JM should receive the third dose of Hep B. He should not receive the RV vaccine because he is too old. The first dose of the RV vaccine needs to be administered by the age of 14 weeks 6 days. JM should receive the third dose of DTaP at 6 months. He does not need a third dose of the Hib vaccine because PedvaxHIB is only a two-dose series and he does not need the booster dose until 12 to 15 months of age. JM should receive his third dose of PCV and IPV.

Answer b is incorrect. At 6 months, JM will need his third dose of Hep B, DTaP, PCV, and IPV. However, he should not receive the RV vaccine because he is too old. It is too late to start the series in JM.

Answer c is incorrect. At 6 months, JM will need his third dose of Hep B, DTaP, PCV, and IPV. Since he received his first two Hib vaccinations with PedvaxHIB, he does not need a third dose.

Answer d is correct. At 6 months, JM will need his third dose of Hep B, DTaP, PCV, and IPV.

13. Which of the following vaccines require a booster dose:

    a. HPV
    b. MMR
    c. MCV
    d. Hib

Answer a is incorrect. The HPV vaccine does not require a booster dose. The HPV vaccine is given as a three-dose series, all of which are required to develop immunity to HPV. A booster dose is administered after the primary series in order to boost the immunity to that particular pathogen.

Answer b is incorrect. The MMR vaccine does not require a booster dose. One dose is given at 12 to 15 months of age. A second dose is given at 4 to 6 years because a small percentage of patients do not respond to the first dose.

Answer c is incorrect. MCV is given as one dose. No additional doses are required.

Answer d is correct. The Hib vaccine should be administered in two or three doses, depending on formulation. A booster dose is recommended for children aged 12 to 15 months. Recently, Hiberix was approved for use as a booster dose in children aged 15 months to 4 years who previously did not receive a Hib booster dose due to shortages of the vaccines.

14. The Haemophilus influenzae type b (Hib) vaccine can be administered to all of the following, *except*:

    a. A 4-month-old infant
    b. A 20-year-old smoker
    c. A 58-year-old man with leukemia
    d. A 26-year-old with asplenia

Answer a in incorrect. The Hib vaccine should be administered to children at 2, 4 and 12 to 15 months. An additional dose at 6 months is required if the child is vaccinated with ActHIB.

Answer b is correct. The Hib vaccine is generally not recommended in patients over the age of 5 years. However, administering one dose to patients with sickle cell disease, leukemia, HIV infection, or who have had a splenectomy, is not contraindicated and should be considered. Smoking is not an indication to receive the Hib vaccine.

Answer c is incorrect. A patient with leukemia may benefit from receiving the Hib vaccine.

Answer d is incorrect. A patient with functional or anatomical asplenia may benefit from receiving the Hib vaccine.

15. How should the herpes zoster vaccine (Zoster) be administered?

    a. In the deltoid muscle at a 90° angle.
    b. In the deltoid muscle at a 45° angle.
    c. In the outer aspect of the triceps at a 45° angle.
    d. In the anteriolateral thigh at a 45° angle.

Answer a is incorrect. The herpes zoster vaccine should be administered subcutaneously. Intramuscular injections are given in the deltoid muscle at a 90° angle.

Answer b is incorrect. The herpes zoster vaccine should be administered subcutaneously. Subcutaneous injections are given at a 45° angle; however they are not given in the deltoid muscle.

Answer c is correct. The herpes zoster vaccine should be administered subcutaneously. Subcutaneous injections are given in the outer aspect of the triceps at a 45° angle.

Answer d is incorrect. The herpes zoster vaccine should be administered subcutaneously. Intramuscular injections are given to children in the anteriolateral thigh at a 90° angle.

16. LM is an 18-year-old woman who is leaving for her first semester of college next month. She would like to know what vaccinations she needs before going to college. Her vaccination record shows the following: DTaP at 2, 4, 6, and 15 months, and 5 years; Hib (ActHIB) at 2, 4, and 6 months; PCV at 2, 4, 6, and 15 months; IPV at 2, 4, and 6 months, and 5 years; MMR at 15 months and 5 years; Varicella at 15 months and 5 years; Hep A at 12 and 18 months; Hep B at 11 years, 11 years 2 months, and 11 years 6 months; Tdap at 15 years. LM does not have any medical conditions and is not allergic to any medications or vaccines. What vaccines should LM receive today?

    a. MCV and HPV
    b. Tdap, MCV, and HPV
    c. Tdap and MCV
    d. MPSV and HPV

Answer a is correct. LM has not received the MCV or HPV vaccines. College freshman should receive the MCV vaccine if they have not previously been vaccinated. The HPV vaccine is recommended at age 11 to 12 years; however it can be given in adult women up to the age of 26 who have not previously been vaccinated.

Answer b is incorrect. LM has completed her primary DTaP series and received a Tdap dose 3 years ago at the age of 15. She does not need another dose of Tdap. She will not need another Td booster for 7 years. LM does need the MCV and HPV vaccines.

Answer c is incorrect. LM has already received a Tdap booster and does not need another Td booster for 7 years. She does need to receive the MCV vaccine. She also needs the HPV vaccine because she has not previously received it.

Answer d is incorrect. LM does need to receive the HPV vaccine because she has not been vaccinated previously. She should also receive a meningococcal vaccine; however the conjugate vaccine (MCV) is preferred over the polysaccharide vaccine (MPSV). If the MPSV vaccine is used, she would need to be revaccinated in 5 years with the MCV vaccine, provided she remained at high risk for meningococcal disease.

---

17. TR, a 4-year-old girl, is in the doctor's office for her 4- to 6-year-old vaccinations. She has completed her Hep B, Hib, PCV, and Hep A series. She has no medical conditions and is not allergic to any medications or vaccines. Five days ago she received the live-attenuated influenza vaccine. Which vaccines should TR receive today?

    a. DTaP, IPV, MMR, and Varicella
    b. DTaP, PPSV, IPV, and MMR
    c. IPV only
    d. DTaP and IPV

Answer a is incorrect. A 4-year-old girl who has completed her Hep B, Hib, PCV, and Hep A series would need to receive DTaP, IPV, MMR, and Varicella vaccinations. TR received a live vaccine 5 days ago and cannot receive another live vaccine for 23 days. Live vaccines can be administered together on the same day or 28 days apart. MMR and Varicella are live vaccines and cannot be given in TR today.

Answer b is incorrect. PPSV should only be administered to children who have certain medical conditions (diabetes, asthma, cardiovascular disease, asplenia, or HIV infection). TR does not have any of these conditions. TR cannot receive the MMR vaccine because she received a live vaccine 5 days ago.

Answer c is incorrect. TR needs the fifth dose of DTaP as well as the fourth dose of the IPV vaccine.

Answer d is correct. TR needs the fifth dose of DTaP as well as the fourth dose of the IPV vaccine.

---

18. When should the second dose of the Hepatitis A (Hep A) vaccine be administered?

    a. 28 days after the first dose
    b. 2 months after the first dose
    c. 6 months after the first dose
    d. 30 days after the first dose

Answers a, b, and d are incorrect.

Answer c is correct. The two doses of the Hep A vaccine should be given 6 months apart.

---

19. All of the following are patients at risk for hepatitis B (Hep B) infection, *except*:

    a. A man who has sex with men
    b. A woman with diabetes
    c. An injection-drug user
    d. A wound-care nurse

Answer a is incorrect. A man who has sex with men is considered at risk for hepatitis B infection and therefore should receive the Hep B vaccine.

Answer b is correct. Diabetes alone is not considered a risk factor for hepatitis B infection. If she engaged in risky behavior, such as unprotected sex with multiple partners, use of injection drugs, health care provider, etc, she would be a candidate for Hep B vaccination.

Answer c is incorrect. An injection-drug user is at risk for hepatitis B infection.

Answer d is incorrect. A wound-care nurse comes into contact with bodily fluids and is at risk for hepatitis B infection.

---

20. Which of the following patients should receive the herpes zoster vaccine?

    a. A 58-year-old diabetic
    b. A 37-year-old without a spleen
    c. A 68-year-old with hypertension
    d. A 72-year-old allergic to neomycin

Answer a is incorrect. The herpes zoster vaccine is indicated in adults over the age of 60. A 58-year-old diabetic is too young to receive the vaccination.

Answer b is incorrect. The herpes zoster vaccine should only be administered to adults over the age of 60, regardless of medical conditions.

Answer c is correct. A 68-year-old with hypertension should receive the herpes zoster vaccine.

Answer d is incorrect. The herpes zoster vaccine is a live vaccine and should not be administered to patients who are immunocompromised, pregnant, or allergic to gelatin or neomycin. This patient is 72 years old, but is also allergic to neomycin. He or she should not receive the herpes zoster vaccine.

CHAPTER 70 | Pharmacy Math

1. Identify the Roman numeral with a value of 50.

    a. X
    b. M
    c. I
    d. L

Answer a is incorrect. X = 10.

Answer b is incorrect. M = 1000.

Answer c is incorrect. I = 1.

Answer d is correct. L = 50.

2. Identify the Arabic value of DCXXIV.

   a. 624
   b. 626
   c. 1024
   d. 1026

Answer a is correct. D = 500, C = 100, X = 10, I = −1, V = 5 (500 + 100 + 10 + 10 −1 +5 = 624).

Answer b is incorrect. The Roman numeral for 626 would be DCXXVI.

Answer c is incorrect. The Roman numeral for 1024 would be MXXIV.

Answer d is incorrect. The Roman numeral for 1026 would be MCCVI.

3. If 120 mL of a cough syrup contains 0.4 g of dextromethorphan, how many milligrams are contained in 1 teaspoonful?

   a. 0.016 mg
   b. 16 mg
   c. 160 mg
   d. 1.6 mg

Answers a. c, and d are incorrect.

Answer b is correct.

$$\frac{0.4 \text{ g}}{120 \text{ mL}} = \frac{\text{x g}}{5 \text{ mL}} \quad \text{x} = 0.016 \text{ g} = 16 \text{ mg}$$

4. Interferon injection contains 5 million U/mL. How many units are in 0.65 mL?

   a. 3,250 U
   b. 32,500 U
   c. 325,000 U
   d. 3,250,000 U

Answers a, b, and c are incorrect.

Answer d is correct.

$$\frac{5{,}000{,}000 \text{ units}}{1 \text{ mL}} = \frac{\text{x units}}{0.65 \text{ mL}} \quad \text{x} = 3{,}250{,}000 \text{ units}$$

5. An inhalant solution contains 0.025% w/v of a drug in 5 mL. Calculate the number of milligrams in this solution.

   a. 0.125 mg
   b. 1.25 mg
   c. 12.5 mg
   d. 0.0125 mg

Answers a, c, and d are incorrect.

Answer b is correct. 0.025 % w/v = 0.025 g/100 mL. Convert this percent w/v to mg/mL= 25 mg/100 mL.

$$\frac{25 \text{ mg}}{100 \text{ mL}} = \frac{\text{x g}}{5 \text{ mL}} \quad \text{x} = 1.25 \text{ mg}$$

6. How many milligrams of a drug would be contained in a 10 mL container of a 0.65% w/v solution of a drug?

   a. 0.65 mg
   b. 6.5 mg
   c. 65 mg
   d. 650 mg

Answers a, b, and d are incorrect.

Answer c is correct. 0.65% w/v = 0.65 g/100 L Converted to milligrams this equals 650 mg/100 mL.

$$\frac{650 \text{ mg}}{100 \text{ mL}} = \frac{\text{x g}}{10 \text{ mL}} \quad \text{x} = 65 \text{ mg}$$

7. How many milliequivalents of potassium are in 240 mL of a 10% solution of KCL? The gram molecular weight is 74.5 g (K^+ 39 atomic weight; Cl 35.5 atomic weight).

   a. 24 mEq
   b. 0.0745 mEq
   c. 2.4 mEq
   d. 322 mEq

Answers a, b, and c are incorrect.

Answer d is correct. The molecular weight of K is 39 and the molecular weight of Cl is 35; therefore, the molecular weight of KCL is 74.5.

- 74.5 = 1 molecular weight for KCL
- 74.5 g = 1 equivalent weight
- 74.5 mg = 1 milliequivalent weight (0.0745 g)

$$\frac{10 \text{ g}}{100 \text{ mL}} = \frac{\text{x g}}{240 \text{ mL}} \quad \text{x} = 24 \text{ g KCl}$$

$$\frac{0.0745 \text{ g}}{1 \text{ mEq}} = \frac{24 \text{ g}}{\text{x mEq}} \quad \text{x} = 322.2 \text{ mEq}$$

8. How many milliosmoles (mOsmol) of sodium chloride are there in 1 L of a 0.9% solution of normal saline solution? Molecular weight of NaCl = 58.5.

   a. 58.5 mOsmol
   b. 308 mOsmol
   c. 1 mOsmol
   d. 9000 mOsmol

Answers a, c, and d are incorrect.

Answer b is correct.

- Molecular weight of NaCl = 58.5 1 mole= 58.5 g
- 1 millimole = 58.5 mg = 2 milliosmoles, since NaCl dissociates into 2 particles
- 0.9% NaCl = 0.9 g/100 mL or 900 mg/100 mL. Since a liter of NaCl is utilized:
- $\frac{900 \text{ mg}}{100 \text{ mL}} = \frac{x \text{ mg}}{1000 \text{ mL}}$

  x = 9000 mg of NaCl in a liter (1000 mL)
- $\frac{58.5 \text{ mg}}{2 \text{ mOsmol}} = \frac{9000 \text{ mg}}{x \text{ mOsmol}} \quad x = 308 \text{ mOsmol}$

9. What is the percentage concentration (w/v) of a 250 mL solution containing 100 mEq of ammonium chloride? Molecular weight of NH_4Cl is 53.5.

   a. 53.5%
   b. 5.35%
   c. 2.14%
   d. 21.4%

Answers a, b, and d are incorrect.

Answer c is correct.

- Molecular weight of NH_4 = is 53.5
- 1 equivalent weight = 53.5 g
- 1 mEq = 53.5 mg

$$\frac{53.5 \text{ mg}}{1 \text{ mEq}} = \frac{x \text{ mg}}{100 \text{ mEq}} \quad x = 5350 \text{ mg or } 5.35 \text{ g}$$

$$\frac{5.35 \text{ g}}{250 \text{ mL}} = \frac{x}{100} \quad x = 2.14\%$$

10. How many millimoles of HCl are contained in 130 mL of a 10% solution? Molecular weight = 36.5.

   a. 361 mmol
   b. 34 mmol
   c. 36.5 mmol
   d. 13 mmol

Answer a is correct.

- Molecular weight of HCl = 36.5
- 1 mole = 36.5 g
- 1 millimole = 36.5 g/1000 = 0.0365 g = 36.5 mg

$$\frac{10 \text{ g}}{100 \text{ mL}} = \frac{x \text{ g}}{130 \text{ mL}} \quad x = 13 \text{ g HCl}$$

$$\frac{0.036 \text{ g}}{1 \text{ mmol}} = \frac{13 \text{ g HCl}}{x \text{ mmol}} \quad x = 361 \text{ mmol}$$

11. How many 60 mg tablets of codeine sulfate should be used to make this cough syrup?

   Rx: | Codeine SO_4 30 mg/teaspoon
   Cherry Syrup qs ad 150 mL

   Sig: 1 teaspoonful every 6 hours as needed for cough

   a. 7
   b. 15
   c. 20
   d. 24

Answers a, c, and d are incorrect.

Answer b is correct.

- 1 teaspoon = 5 mL

$$\frac{30 \text{ mg}}{5 \text{ mL}} = \frac{x \text{ mg}}{150 \text{ mL}} \quad x = 900 \text{ mg}$$

$$\frac{60 \text{ mg}}{1 \text{ tab}} = \frac{900 \text{ mg}}{x \text{ tab}} \quad x = 15 \text{ tablets}$$

12. How many milliliter of a 17% solution of benzalonium chloride is required to prepare 350 mL of a 1:750 w/v solution?

   a. 2.75 mL
   b. 0.275 mL
   c. 27.5 mL
   d. 275 mL

Answer a is correct.

$$\frac{1 \text{ g}}{750 \text{ mL}} = \frac{x \text{ g}}{350 \text{ mL}} \quad x = 0.47 \text{ g}$$

$$\frac{17 \text{ g}}{100 \text{ mL}} = \frac{0.47 \text{ g}}{x \text{ mL}} \quad x = 2.75 \text{ mL}$$

Answers b, c, and d are incorrect.

13. If 10 mL of a diluent is added to an injectable containing 0.5 g of a drug with a final volume of 7.3 mL, what is the final concentration of the parenteral solution in mg/mL?

   a. 6.85 mg/mL
   b. 0.069 mg/mL
   c. 685 mg/mL
   d. 68.5 mg/mL

Answers a, b, and c are incorrect.

Answer d is correct.

$$\frac{500 \text{ mg}}{7.3 \text{ mL}} = \frac{x \text{ mg}}{1 \text{ mL}} \quad x = 68.5 \text{ mg}$$

Therefore the final concentration in mg/mL is 68.5 mg/mL.

14. A medication order of a drug calls for a dose of 0.6 mg/kg to be administered to a child weighing 31 lb. The drug is to be supplied from a solution containing 0.25 g in 50 mL bottles. How many milliliters of this solution are required to fill this order.

a. 8.45 mL
b. 0.00845 mL
c. 1.69 mL
d. 0.25 mL

Answers a, b, and d are incorrect.

Answer c is correct.

$$\frac{1 \text{ kg}}{2.2 \text{ lb}} = \frac{x \text{ kg}}{31 \text{ lb}} \quad x = 14 \text{ kg}$$

$$\frac{0.6 \text{ mg}}{1 \text{ kg}} = \frac{x \text{ mg}}{14 \text{ kg}} \quad x = 8.45 \text{ mg or } 0.00845 \text{ g}$$

$$\frac{0.25 \text{ g}}{50 \text{ mL}} = \frac{0.00845 \text{ g}}{x \text{ mL}} \quad x = 1.69 \text{ mL}$$

Or, solving by dimensional analysis:
31 lb × 1 kg/2.2 lb × 0.6 mg/kg × 1 g/1000 mg × 50 mL/0.25 g = 1.69 mL.

15. A solution contains 2 mEq of KCl/mL. If a TPN order calls for the addition of 180 mg of K^+, how many milliliters of this solution should be used to provide the potassium required. Atomic weight of K = 39 and the atomic weight of Cl = 35.5.

a. 343.85 mL
b. 2.3 mL
c. 39 mL
d. 74.5 mL

Answers a, c, and d are incorrect.

Answer b is correct.

$$\frac{1 \text{ mEq KCL}}{74.5 \text{ mg KCL}} = \frac{2 \text{ mEq KCL}}{x \text{ mg KCl}} \quad x = 149 \text{ mg KCL}$$

$$\frac{39 \text{ mg K}}{74.5 \text{ mg KCl}} = \frac{x \text{ mg K}}{149 \text{ mg KCl}} \quad x = 78 \text{ mg K}$$

$$\frac{78 \text{ mg K}}{149 \text{ mg KCl}} = \frac{180 \text{ mg K}}{x \text{ mg KCl}} \quad x = 343.85 \text{ mg KCl}$$

$$\frac{149 \text{ mg KCl}}{1 \text{ mL}} = \frac{343.85 \text{ mg KCl}}{x \text{ mL}} \quad x = 2.3 \text{ mL}$$

16. A TPN solution contains 750 mL of D5W. If each gram of dextrose provides 3.4 kcal, how many kcal would the TPN solution provide?

a. 127.5 kcal
b. 37.5 kcal
c. 34 kcal
d. 75 kcal

Answer a is correct.

$$\frac{5 \text{ g dextrose}}{100 \text{ mL}} = \frac{x \text{ g}}{750 \text{ mL}} \quad x = 37.5 \text{ g}$$

$$\frac{3.4 \text{ kcal}}{1 \text{ g}} = \frac{x \text{ kcal}}{37.5} \quad x = 127.5 \text{ kcal}$$

Answers b, c, and d are incorrect.

17. Select the definition of specific gravity.

a. Ratio of the weight of a material to the weight of the same volume of standard material.
b. The mixing of solutions or solids possessing different percentage strengths.
c. The expression of two ratios which are equal.
d. Grams of ingredient in 100 g of product; assumed for mixtures of solids and semisolids.

Answer a is correct. Specific gravity is defined as ratio of the weight of a material to the weight of the same volume of standard material.

Answer b is incorrect. Alligation: The mixing of solutions or solids possessing different percentage strengths presents a calculation problem which may be solved using an arithmetic method called alligation.

Answer c is incorrect. A proportion is the expression of two ratios which are equal. It is usually written in one of two ways: two equal fractions (a/b = c/d) or using a colon (a:b = c:d).

Answer d is incorrect. Percent weight-in-weight: % (w/w) = grams of ingredient in 100 g of product; assumed for mixtures of solids and semisolids.

18. Select the apothecary measure of volume.

a. Grain
b. Scruple
c. Dram
d. Minim

Answers a, b, and c are incorrect. A grain, scruple, and dram is an apothecary measure of weight.

Answer d is correct. A minum is an apothecary measure of volume.

19. 480 minims equals:

i. 8 fluidrams
ii. 1 fl oz
iii. 1 gallon

a. i and ii
b. i and iii
c. ii and iii
d. All of the above

Answer a is correct. 480 minums = 8 fluidrams and 1 fl oz 1 gallon = 61440 minums.

20. 437.5 grains equal how many ounces?

a. 1 oz
b. 16 oz
c. 30 oz
d. 38 oz

Answer a is correct. 437.5 grains = 1 oz.

Index

Note: "*f*" *and* "*t*" indicate figures and tables, respectively.

A

C

E

F

H

I

N

O

T

U

V

W

X

Y

Z